The Penguin Dictionary of
PSYCHOLOGY

Arthur S. Reber, Rhiannon Allen & Emily S. Reber

PENGUIN BOOKS

PENGUIN BOOKS

Published by the Penguin Group
Penguin Books Ltd, 80 Strand, London WC2R 0RL, England
Penguin Group (USA) Inc., 375 Hudson Street, New York, New York 10014, USA
Penguin Group (Canada), 90 Eglinton Avenue East, Suite 700, Toronto, Ontario, Canada M4P 2Y3
(a division of Pearson Penguin Canada Inc.)
Penguin Ireland, 25 St Stephen's Green, Dublin 2, Ireland (a division of Penguin Books Ltd)
Penguin Group (Australia), 250 Camberwell Road, Camberwell, Victoria 3124, Australia
(a division of Pearson Australia Group Pty Ltd)
Penguin Books India Pvt Ltd, 11 Community Centre, Panchsheel Park, New Delhi – 110 017, India
Penguin Group (NZ), 67 Apollo Drive, Rosedale, North Shore 0632, New Zealand
(a division of Pearson New Zealand Ltd)
Penguin Books (South Africa) (Pty) Ltd, 24 Sturdee Avenue, Rosebank, Johannesburg 2196, South Africa

Penguin Books Ltd, Registered Offices: 80 Strand, London WC2R 0RL, England

www.penguin.com

First published 1985
Published simultaneously by Viking
Second Edition 1995
Third Edition 2001
Fourth Edition 2009
2

Copyright © Arthur S. Reber, 1985, 1995
Copyright © Arthur S. Reber and Emily S. Reber, 2001
Copyright © Arthur S. Reber, Rhiannon Allen and Emily S. Reber, 2009
All rights reserved

The moral right of the author has been asserted

Set in ITC Stone Sans and ITC Stone Serif
Typeset by Data Standards Ltd, Frome, Somerset
Printed in England by Clays Ltd, St Ives plc

Except in the United States of America, this book is sold subject
to the condition that it shall not, by way of trade or otherwise, be lent,
re-sold, hired out, or otherwise circulated without the publisher's
prior consent in any form of binding or cover other than that in
which it is published and without a similar condition including this
condition being imposed on the subsequent purchaser

ISBN: 978-0-141-03024-1

www.greenpenguin.co.uk

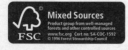

Mixed Sources
Product group from well-managed
forests and other controlled sources
www.fsc.org Cert no. SA-COC-1592
© 1996 Forest Stewardship Council
FSC

Penguin Books is committed to a sustainable future
for our business, our readers and our planet.
The book in your hands is made from paper
certified by the Forest Stewardship Council.

Contents

Preface to the First Edition

Dictionary writers incur certain obligations, the first of which is to provide the reader with a quick rundown on how the material is presented, i.e. what abbreviations are in use and what notational formats are used. This obligation is fulfilled on page xx. The second obligation is more delicate: to present the reader with a justification/ rationalization of what has been wrought. That is the first task here. This dictionary is a little different from the standard list of words and their associated meanings and it is worth initially taking up a bit of space to give the reader some background information to explain how the volume came to be written, what my aims were in compiling it and why it has its occasionally eccentric style.

I began thinking about a work such as this some twenty years ago when I was a graduate student. Students were required to write a number of essays in areas of psychology that were often quite remote from those of their particular concentration, and the first problem we had to deal with was that sudden jolt produced by the jargon of a new area. It was with interest that I discovered that when a Piagetian developmentalist used the term **accommodation** it meant something rather different from what was intended by a social psychologist studying the actions of an individual in a group or a vision scientist examining changes in the lens of the eye, that **discrimination** meant one thing to a learning theorist and another to a psychologist writing on race relations, that Jung's **self** was an entity of a rather different sort from James's. And it was with even greater interest that I began to recognize that these differences, compelling as they were, often masked subtle but critical commonalities in meaning and patterns of usage.

When stuck, as I often was, I turned to existing reference works. I found most of the dictionaries I consulted, both within psychology proper as well as the more general, comprehensive works, to be of surprisingly little help. For the most part, they gave definitions using that 'zero-redundancy' style which typifies the reference work whose editors are desperately fighting length problems. In short, if I already had a pretty good hypothesis about what a term meant the dictionary could confirm or disconfirm it, but if I went as a child to find out how the term was actually used I often ended up more frustrated than when I began.

As the years went by I began making notes on terms, notes not so much on what exactly a given technical term meant but notes that reflected more how it was actually employed, what sorts of meanings were being functionally relayed by it, what connotations were associated with it, what pragmatic force it carried and how it was used (and abused) by various authors. In my mind I always thought of my ever-growing compendium of terms as my 'lexicon' (see here page 429) although, as it now turns out, my editors would have none of this. As far back as I can recall I have never been at a meeting, conference, colloquium or even just at my desk without a pocketful of 4- × 6-inch cards upon which I jot notes should a colleague, writer or speaker present me with a new term or a novel nuance of an old one. What you hold in your hand now is the product of roughly twenty years of note-taking and a frenzied three-year period during which my collection of over 20,000 cards was collated and all earlier versions of my 'lexicon' were edited and rewritten. If you open to any random page you will see, alas, that most of the entries turned out to be rather mundane and very much like those to be found in any ordinary dictionary. After all, terms like **small group** or **T-maze** just don't have much in the way of subtlety about them. But terms like **language** and **emotion** do, and so do, surprisingly, **memory** and **self** and **unconscious**, and it is here that I do hope that my little volume can serve some useful function.

People (like my long-suffering editors) kept asking me things like, 'Who's this dictionary written for?' or 'What is the readership supposed to be here?' I honestly have never been able to supply them with a simple answer to these questions. I wrote this book for everyman, for the expert in one field who needs to know a term in a domain of our science that she or he is unfamiliar with, for the graduate student who like myself two decades back is frustrated by a new area and its terminological eccentricities, for the undergraduate student taking a first course in psychology who is told by the professor that the essence of the course is 'learning a new vocabulary', and perhaps, most significantly, for the curious layman who wants to know just what a term means. It was also written for myself, a dedicated word connoisseur who has always enjoyed thumbing through dictionaries and encyclopedias and who takes great pleasure in the playful use of the honoured tongue of English kings. All other word-lovers are free to browse.

Finally, here, a few specifics on the form of this dictionary:

1. *Scope*. The primary concern was to cover psychology and psychiatry reasonably thoroughly and to include terms from other disciplines when they shared terminological overlap with these fields. Casting this kind of net can get pretty arbitrary at times and I have to doubt that good judgement failed me on more than a few occasions. As I mention below, I would appreciate having omissions called to my attention for future editions.

2. *Alphabetization*. Unless you have written or edited a work such as this you cannot fully appreciate what a problem alphabetization can be. Where to list the terms in a reference work poses several difficulties when, as in this case, the majority of the terms are compounds made up of more than one word. For example, a term like **mixed transcortical aphasia** could legitimately be put under **mixed**, **transcortical** or **aphasia**, depending on whether one feels that the essential nature of the disorder is that it is mixed, transcortical or an aphasia. Most reference works of recent vintage have solved these problems by the simple device of adopting an 'absolute' alphabetizing rule, in which every entry is listed under the alphabetic location of the term as it is encountered. Such a dictionary would enter **mixed transcortical aphasia** under **mixed**. The obvious advantage of this technique is that terms can be located easily and unambiguously – and writers and editors do not have to suffer over where to place a given term.

However, I have eschewed this easy way out, electing instead to use the 'key'- or 'head'-word technique, whereby compound terms are listed on the basis of the most important word. In this work you will find **mixed transcortical aphasia** under **aphasia, mixed transcortical**, you will find **short-term memory** under **memory, short-term** and you will find **normal distribution** under **distribution, normal**. In a few cases this policy was carried out with a vengeance; see e.g. **reinforcement, schedules of**.

The final decision to adopt this procedure was made on the basis that I like to snoop around in dictionaries and I like all my **aphasias** together so that I can compare them; I find the grouping of several dozen kinds of **memory** deeply informative since it reveals the manner in which various theorists have been thinking about them; and I like to be able to see the relationships between the many different kinds of **distribution** that have made their way into the psychologist's lexicon. When it is appropriate terms will, of course, follow normal alphabetization rules. A term like **factitious disorder** will be found under **factitious**, since this is the operative word, and **oral eroticism** will be found under **oral**, with all the other compounds based on this keyword. In any case, all compound terms are cross-listed under each of the individual words and, where possible, under all of the various synonyms, which should minimize confusion.

3. *Names*. Since this is a dictionary and not an encyclopedia, my preference was not to include short biographies of important people. However, again since it is a dictionary, it seemed reasonable to include eponymous terms. Entries will be, therefore, found for laws, principles, syndromes and the like that are named after individuals, and occasionally extensive entries are included for those whose fame is such that an adjectivized form of their name exists. Hence, there are entries for **Freudian**, **Skinnerian**, **Pavlovian**, **Adlerian** and so forth. Moreover, since many of the terms in this volume are the direct result of neologistic exercises of individual people and often the very sense of a term cannot be dissociated from its coiner, it was often necessary to refer to the operative individual in the entry. A list of these persons, with a few simple facts about each, is printed at the end of the dictionary.

4. *Coverage*. The issue here was how completely to cover a term, how much information to provide in each definition. Most of the entries are relatively straightforward, for they present terms that are dealt with easily and coverage is short and (to that extent) sweet. However, many of the terms in psychology are not dealt with so easily: they require considerable discussion of their semantic nuances and characteristic manners of use. Perhaps not surprisingly, these typically are the most important terms in the field, the very ones that were the stimuli for this project in the first place. To deal with a term like **personality** or **mental retardation** or **perception** in half a dozen lines as some works do is to invite further confusion.

After considerable paring, I ended up with roughly 175 terms that required 'extensive' coverage ('extensive' is defined here as 200 words or more). These are terms that have (often unacknowledged) subtleties of usage or are controversial in their manner of usage or simply have meanings that are denotatively or connotatively complex. A list of them is printed on pages xxi–xxii.

5. *Style*. The writing of this book was, as much as was possible, a one-man affair. Having all the entries composed by a single author has a distinct virtue in that there

is a certain measure of consistency, a kind of continuity in style and coverage that is not going to be found in a work in which one or more editors oversee the submissions of many different writers.

Despite being basically a reference work designed to provide working definitions of the terms of a field of scholarly endeavour, this book is shot through with a singular style for which I make no apologies. Many an entry was written with the ghost of Samuel Johnson whispering in my right ear and the spectre of Ambrose Bierce hissing in my left: I am often critical of the manner in which a term has been used, I frequently object to the particular set of connotations that have come to be associated with certain key phrases and I do, on occasions, go so far as to conjecture that the very conceptual foundations of a technical term render it unworthy of being included in the psychologist's lexicon. For some samples here, see the entries on **innovative therapies**, **intelligence**, **meaning**, **parapsychology**, **psychology** and **Rorschach test**.

I am not disturbed about offending the occasional sensibility in this manner. In large measure all I have done in these cases is to review and expose the excesses of my colleagues, past and present. However, I am much concerned about offending through error, misrepresentation or misinterpretation. Since this volume ultimately needs to reflect the terms as they are actually used in our protean science, it is important that it be accurate and comprehensive. It is here that the single-author format suffers most. Although I like to think of myself as a bit of a generalist, there have been times when I have felt more than a little unhappy with my state of ignorance. The approach I took in such cases was to compose an entry based on what I knew or could discover by reading and then ask one of my wiser and more knowledgeable colleagues to critique it for me. This turns out to be an interesting technique. It does get the job done in most cases and it lets you see who your friends are – it also gave me a brand-new way to characterize a good friend: someone who is kind enough to tell you in private that if you do what you indicate you are about to do you will make a fool of yourself in public. Above I thanked those friends whose names I could recall. There must be literally hundreds of others who have been gently abused by me at a meeting or conference over the meaning of some arcane term. A general note of thanks goes out to all these nameless.

Finally here, let me put out a call for more friends. The plan is to revise this dictionary at irregular intervals and I ask readers who wish to to inform me about where I have lapsed or strayed from accuracy of meaning or pattern of usage. Simply send a note to either the publisher or, if preferred, to me directly at: Department of Psychology, Brooklyn College, The City University of New York, Brooklyn, New York, NY 11210, USA.

A. R.
Brooklyn, NY
November 21, 1984

Preface to the Second Edition

When I began working on this edition I was struck, much to my surprise, by how much the language of psychology had changed in just 10 years. While most of the classic terms are still about and still used in much the same way, there has been a subtle but most detectable drift not just in the terminology but in the very phraseology of the language of our field. Entries written back in the early 1980s that felt so modern and up to date then now often felt antiquated and stilted. I frequently found myself squirming at my own words, muttering to myself, 'No one talks that way in psychology any more.' I have tried to isolate these shifts and understand them, which has been no mean task. It is my sense that some four or five primary forces have been sculpting the language of our field in the past decade or so and contributing to these changes. Specifically:

1. *The cognitive and neuroanatomical orientations.* The increased interest in these foci have led to the outright introduction of many new terms but also have contributed to distinct shifts in the meaning and usage patterns of old ones. The majority of the revisions in this edition were stimulated by the continued increasing interest in the cognitive approach to psychological science and in the growing search for physiological and neurological explanations of behaviour. Here are a couple of examples: the old behaviourist term **connectionism**, which rated a mere three lines in the first edition, is now a major entry with a host of additional connotations reflecting its use in the cognitive sciences. A physiological staple, **hippocampus**, had to be completely rewritten and accompanied by a variety of anatomically and functionally related structures that weren't even mentioned in the first edition. And to give you a sense of the kinds of problem that can drive a lexicographer batty: the term **implicit memory**, which was (according to a recent analysis of keywords carried out by the American Psychological Society) the single most frequently cited term in psychology in the years from 1988 to 1992 was not even in the first edition! There are several hundreds of new and completely rewritten entries in the areas of cognition, neuroanatomy and physiological psychology.

2. *The extending boundaries of social psychology.* Social psychology has, in the past decade, broadened its scope considerably. Once concerned primarily with core concepts like attribution and achievement, it has become much more richly interwoven with the study of personality, developmental psychology and the cognitive sciences. These extensions have been marked both by the introduction of new terms and by the emergence of subtle shifts in meaning in old terms. These changes represent the next most important source of revisions and additions.

3. *The* DSM-IIIR *and* IV *and the* ICD-10. The first edition used the *DSM-III* and the *ICD-9* as the touchstones for psychiatric terminology; this edition has had to take into account the changes in terminology and usage mandated by the new editions. The casual reader probably doesn't understand (nor really care, I suspect), but these new editions of the *DSM* and the *ICD* made my life miserable! The problem is that I couldn't simply toss out all the old terms and meanings and slip in the new. For one, these new 'official' nosologies have not yet filtered into the literature – at least not to the point where they have displaced the older terminology. Worse, students and researchers are still working with materials that were written using the old guidelines and need to have links created between them and the new. And even worse, to be perfectly honest, much of the new officially sanctioned terminology is awkward and stilted and I suspect that, independent of insurance forms and legal documents, it is going to be resisted by many professionals. In any event, I tried to deal with these problems by keeping many (although not all) of the clinical terms from the first edition, introducing the new terms and usage patterns from the *DSM-IV* and the *ICD-10* and, where possible, identifying the common patterns of meaning and usage between the old and the new. My critics, I am sure, will let me know whether I succeeded here or not.

4. *Tests and measurements.* To be quite frank, I thought the material dealing with psychometric instruments in the first edition was weak and I wanted to make appropriate revisions for this edition. The problem, however, is that there are just too many psychometric instruments about these days. A glance at any current text in psychological assessment is enough to make a lexicographer feel weak-kneed. To include every personality test, every device designed to measure intelligence, every neurological, developmental, cognitive, vocational, educational, additudinal, sensorimotor and psychiatric instrument currently in use would double the size of this volume. There seemed only one simple way out of this conundrum: I decided to be pragmatic rather than comprehensive and to let popularity be my guide. Hence, in this edition I have entries only for some thirty or so of the most commonly used psychometric instruments. They include those most frequently used in practice and research and those that were referenced most often in the literature. As a result, many obscure and rarely used psychological tests included in the first edition have been dropped and several widely employed ones missing from that edition have been added. Admittedly my procedure here is arbitrary, but sometimes you just have to be arbitrary.

5. *Simple linguistic drift.* A subtle but real linguistic drift properly accompanies every growing scientific field as new ideas and approaches gain a foothold and old ones lose their purchase. This is as it should be: if there wasn't a need for a new edition of a dictionary every 10 years or so it would be a clear indictment of our field. But acknowledging change is not the same thing as dealing with it. The problem is that scientific fields progress in fits and starts and many hot, new topics quickly become cold and old. The nagging problem facing the lexicographer is just how many of the new terms that emerge during these local explosions of research on a new topic should be included. After all, the likely long-range prospects for most of these neologisms is pretty dim, and in any event, if I were to include them all, the

dictionary would quickly become weighty, cumbersome and too expensive. I finally decided to handle this problem in my usual egocentric fashion: I made guesses based on personal intuitions. I know this is not the optimum solution to the problem, but it was the only one I could think of – and certainly the easiest. When the third edition rolls around I will patch up errors in judgement (and, of course, replace them with new ones).

Then there is that biggie, what to do with 'old' terms, those that no longer have much lexicographic currency, especially given the pressures on length caused by all the new terms and new meanings of old ones. My decision here was to keep almost all of them, although to shorten the definitions in many cases. My reasoning took several forms. First, if things are going to keep changing so fast who knows when a term will be resuscitated (look at what happened to **connectionism**!)? Second, just because a term is not being used much these days does not mean that someone won't still need to look it up – hopefully all of us, students and professionals alike, will always maintain a healthy respect for the past. Third, it seems to me that one of the functions of a dictionary like this one is that it needs to reflect the historical elements of the field as well as its current state. Fourth, I happen to like the nuances of some of these older terms; they often provide intriguing clues about historical issues in psychology and so I have often kept a term just because I happen to like it. If you can't have fun doing lexicography you really shouldn't be doing it.

Finally, a few stylistic and editorial changes were made for this edition, as follows:

1. I eliminated cross-referenced terms where the cross-referencing seemed less than necessary. For example, in the first edition a term like **abuse, drug** was listed as a separate entry with the definition 'drug abuse'. Such entries have been dropped from this edition. Hence, to find a term, look it up under the alphabetic listing of the first word. This change does not affect the 'grouping' of definitions under a major heading. That is, all of the different specialized kinds of memory will still be found under **memory**.

I should point out that this simple stylistic shift saved dozens and dozens of pages, allowing me to introduce many new terms and expand the definitions of many others without markedly increasing the length of the book. Alas, one can only pull off a trick like this once. I have no idea what I will do for the third edition.

2. The 'minor' phobias have been dropped from the dictionary proper. Instead they have been placed in Appendix A, which begins on page 887. Part I of that appendix gives each specialized phobia and its phobic object, Part II provides the technical term for each phobic object. In the appendix you will also find a short editorial comment on phobias and terminology. Major phobias (e.g. **agoraphobia**) still have full definitions in the body of the dictionary.

3. Goaded by my friend Alan Auerbach, I had originally planned to introduce a pronunciation guide for unusual and frequently mispronounced terms. However, after much agonizing I decided against doing so. The reason is simple: dialectic variation. This book is sold in a variety of countries in which a wonderful array of standard dialects of English are spoken. It just struck me as arrogant to assume that one or another pronunciation was to be designated as the 'acceptable' one when

common sense and cross-cultural sensitivities clearly show otherwise. If you are stuck on just how to pronounce a particular word, ask someone.

Once again, let me end with a request for help for the future. I have no doubt that, despite my best efforts and those of my editors, errors both of omission and commission have crept in. As before, I would appreciate being informed (gently, of course) of any such. I can still be contacted at Department of Psychology, Brooklyn College of CUNY, Brooklyn, NY 11210, USA.

A. R.
Brooklyn, NY
February 3, 1995

Preface to the Third Edition

The most obvious change for this edition is the new co-author, Emily Reber. One advantage of taking on another Reber is that the palindromous nature of the title page remains intact.

We might as well confess right here: this is a family affair and will continue to be so for the foreseeable future. Luckily, the love of words and nuances of language seems to run in the family. Whether this is due to environment or heredity is not really an issue. It has been a delight working together to produce this latest edition of the dictionary.

As in the past, we've made significant changes across the entire breadth of psychology. And, we must admit, it is becoming increasingly difficult to do this job and continue to produce a volume that is manageable in size and cost. Psychology's range is ever increasing. The theories, findings, concepts and resulting terminology of the discipline continue to expand, seemingly with no upper bound.

Consequently, we've done something that was resisted in the previous edition: we've removed terms. We haven't liked doing this because the words that form the backbone of communication within the field have an odd way of recycling themselves. Moreover, as devoted fans of the history of our discipline, we have been loath to toss out terms that were once central, no matter how peripheralized they have become. But it has had to be done. Our apologies upfront to lovers of antiquated terminology.

The extra room created has been used up (and more) by the proliferation of new terms and concepts. The lion's share of these have come about because of the explosion of work in the cognitive neurosciences and in social psychology. Intriguingly, these areas are the same ones that stimulated growth in the previous edition. We take this as an interesting sign about how and where the field has been moving over the past twenty years. We don't know whether anyone has thought to use successive editions of a dictionary in an effort to chart the movement within a scientific field, but from our experience it would certainly seem that such a study could be carried out. In passing, we would also like to thank the American Psychiatric Association for *not* bringing out a new edition of the *Diagnostic and Statistical Manual*.

Finally, we want to thank the folks who have written over the years to offer advice and criticism. Both are accepted with equal enthusiasm. Sometimes we listened, sometimes we didn't. Such is life. Thanks go out to Elizabeth Andrews, Lisa Green, Richard Kenward, Scott Lillienfeld, Daria Michalová, Renae Montoya, Gabriel Segal and Steven Tudor, all of whom made suggestions that we took seriously.

Additionally, we'd like to thank Martin Toseland, our editor at Penguin Books, and Mark Bathurst, who, in addition to his regular duties as copy editor, took on the task of translating the work into English English. Your authors, of course, are a pair of Yanks (with Canadian links) but we have agreed to put the *u* back in *honour*.

As with earlier editions, we welcome any comments, corrections or additions that we missed. We will be glad to add your name to the growing list of friends who have let us know (for the most part rather gently) where we have strayed lexicographically.

Arthur S. Reber
Brooklyn, NY
areber@brooklyn.cuny.edu

Emily S. Reber
Newbury, NH
emily@panix.com

Preface to the Fourth Edition

The early work on the *Penguin Dictionary of Psychology* began back in the 1970s. At the time it seemed a reasonable task to undertake. Psychology was a field with sensible scope and appropriate bounds and a volume of some 16,000 or so terms pretty much covered things. Alas, the field has continued to grow and its lexicographic domain keeps expanding, seemingly without any brakes on it. Keeping up with this unrestrained expansion hasn't been easy. One obvious symptom is the increase in the number of authors in the last two editions. But, in addition to needing additional authors with backgrounds in distinct areas, we have begun to reach limits imposed by sheer physical size. Indeed, with the flood of new terminology, this edition threatened to become unwieldy and we were worried it would lose its easy portability and low cost. So, for this, the fourth edition, we have managed to overcome our resistance to cutting back on the length of entries and eliminating terms altogether. The two main victims of the blade were terms that emerged during psychology's behaviourist days and some obsolescent historical arcana whose roots go back to our beginnings in the middle and late 1800s.

This doesn't make us happy. Ideally, a volume such as this, which attempts to codify the lexical world of a scientific field, should be all-inclusive and that means keeping terms that may once have been high on the frequency-of-use charts, even if they are rarely found in the contemporary literature. Alas, idealism gave way to pragmatism.

Accordingly, in this edition there is a distinct de-emphasis of behaviourist terms and definitions. When the first edition was compiled behaviourism was in decline but was still a significant part of experimental and theoretical psychology – largely because so many trained in that tradition were still active in research, writing textbooks and editing journals. Today behaviourism is largely a historical accident and many of the definitions of those terms now seem clunky and went into too much detail. The terms are still there, we honour our history, but the entries are shorter, less developed and many of the lexicographic nuances have been dropped. In addition, the pressure to introduce new terminology from a variety of research domains has increased, forcing the elimination of many terms with primarily historic import. The obsolete terms, of course, still exist in earlier editions.

Psychology is looking more and more unwieldy, like some semantic cephalopod, sending out tentacles to an ever widening range of scientific and applied domains, drawing back concepts, terms, theories and general approaches that feed the push to understand mind and behaviour, brain and neurology, culture and society and there are hundreds, if not thousands, of new terms and novel meanings of old terms that reflect these trends. Most come from advances in related fields like social theory, economics and the neurosciences that are having an increasing impact on psychology and moulding its language and patterns of reference.

Pressure is upon us to include as much as we can, to be as faithful both to the original domains from which terms arrive and hold to our fundamental goal to present terms, not in some purist lexicographic form, but in a manner that expresses how they are used and with a sharply tuned critical eye toward misuse, misunderstanding and obfuscation. Have we succeeded? We don't know but welcome feedback.

Acknowledgements

We would like to thank the Winston Prepatory School for being so understanding of the time pressures the project has placed on Emily Reber, the Brooklyn campus of Long Island University for providing resources and leave time to Rhiannon Allen, the Brooklyn College campus of CUNY for allowing Arthur Reber to continue to use their facilities after retirement, and the Psychology Department of the University of British Columbia for providing a comfortable setting and opening its wonderful library facilities to us to complete the work.

One of the pleasures of this ongoing project has been the number and variety of comments we have received from around the world. Some make suggestions for new entries, some point out errors in existing definitions and some just write to thank us. We take all comments seriously and track down all suggestions. Several changes in this edition come from these unsolicited letters and emails, and to the list of friends whose contributions we have acknowledged in earlier editions we would like to add the following:

Hafina Allen, Mt. Sinai Hospital, NYC
Elisabeth Brauner, Brooklyn College
James Enns, University of British Columbia
Dan Gilbert, Harvard University
Alfred Kraemer
John Mace, University of New Haven, New Haven, CT
Sarvagya Narayan-Shrestha, Dharan, East Nepal
Ara Norenzayan, University of British Columbia
Mark Reber, Woods Institute, Philadelphia, PA
Jonathan Schooler, University of California, Santa Barbara
Fei Xu, University of British Columbia
Carl Zuckerman, Brooklyn College.

Arthur S. Reber
Point Roberts, WA
areber@brooklyn.cuny.edu

Rhiannon Allen
Point Roberts, WA
rhianon.allen@liu.edu

Emily S. Reber
New York, NY
emily@panix.com

Abbreviations

abbrev.	abbreviat/ed, -ion	obs.	obsolete
adj.	adjective	pl.	plural
ant.	antonym	sing.	singular
et seq.	and the following (entries)	syn.	synonym
lit.	literally	var.	variant
n.	noun	vb.	verb

Note. An asterisk (*) has been used in cross-references to indicate that the entry referred to should be looked up under the word following the asterisk. Thus, for example, the reference SPHERICAL *ABERRATION means that the reader should refer to the entry **aberration, spherical**.

List of Major Entries

The following is a list of terms which are given extensive coverage in this volume. These are terms whose definition or manner of usage is complex and/or subtle and where some degree of detail is necessary. The note 'et seq.' indicates that a term is followed by a large number of combined terms based on it.

abnormal
abstract
acquired (et seq.)
addiction
aggression (et seq.)
altered states of consciousness
Alzheimer's disease
anger
antipsychotic drugs
anxiety (et seq.)
apperception
assimilation (et seq.)
association (et seq.)
associationism
attitude
autism (et seq.)
automicity
barbiturates (et seq.)
basal ganglia
behaviour (et seq.)
behaviourism
cannabis (sativa)
category
chance
CNS depressants/stimulants
code
colour vision, theories of
concept (et seq.)
concept formation and learning
conditioning (et seq.)
connectionism
consciousness

conservation
constitutional theory
contiguity principle
correlation (et seq.)
cranial nerves
décalage
definition
degrees of freedom
delusion (et seq.)
demand characteristics
dependence (et seq.)
determinism
development (et seq.)
diagnosis
Diagnostic and Statistical Manual
discrimination
disease
dogma
dominance (et seq.)
Down syndrome
ego (et seq.)
embodied (et seq.)
emotion (et seq.)
emotion, theories of
empathy
empiricism
environment
error (et seq.)
evolutionary theory
experiment (et seq.)
factor (et seq.)
factor analysis

THE PENGUIN
DICTIONARY OF
PSYCHOLOGY

A

A 1 AMPLITUDE (2). **2** ALBEDO.

a-, an- Prefix meaning *from, away from, absent from*, etc.

ab- Prefix meaning *away from* or *opposite to*.

abasement H. Murray's term for a need to surrender one's self or will to another, to atone for real or imagined shortcomings.

abasia Inability to walk owing to impairment in motor coordination. See ASTASIA.

abdominal reflex Contraction of the abdominal muscles when the overlying skin is stroked lightly.

abducens 1 The VIth CRANIAL NERVE. It innervates the external rectus muscle in the eye, which functions to rotate the eyeball inward. Also called *abducent nerve*. **2** Pertaining to movement away from the central plane of the body. See ABDUCTION.

abducent nerve ABDUCENS (1).

abduction 1 Lateral movement of a limb away from the median plane of the body. Compare with ADDUCTION. **2** C. S. Peirce's term for the cognitive process whereby hypotheses are generated on the basis of some known facts. Abduction, in Peirce's terms, was a fundamental component of creative thought.

abductor A muscle which, upon contraction, moves a limb away from the body. Compare with ADDUCTOR.

aberration The act of wandering or straying from the normal course. The term enjoys wide currency and is used of the behaviour of an intact organism as well as for biological structures, physical systems, instruments, etc.

aberration, chromatic Unequal refraction of light of different wavelengths as it passes through a lens, producing a coloured image.

aberration, mental A nontechnical term used loosely for any mental disorder.

aberration, spherical Distortions of light waves passing through a lens produced either by the natural curvature of the lens or by irregularities in the curvature of the lens. Also called *diopteric aberration*.

ABI ACQUIRED BRAIN INJURY.

abient Characterizing movement away from something. ant., ADIENT.

ability The qualities, power, competence, faculties, proficiencies, dexterities, talents, etc. that enable one to perform a particular feat at a specified time. The essence of the term is that the person can perform this task *now*, no further training is needed. The main distinction thus is between ability and APTITUDE. Ability is an individual's potential to perform; aptitude is an individual's potential *for* performance, or the possibility of the individual being trained up to a specified level of ability. Intelligence tests, for example, are ability tests.

abiotic Not compatible with life.

ablation Removal of part of an organ. Usually refers to surgical removal. When the full organ or structure is removed, the term EXTIRPATION is generally used.

Abney's effect A perceptual phenomenon experienced when a large area is suddenly illuminated. Rather than appearing all at once, the light seems to come on first in the centre of the patch and then spread to the edges. When extinguished, the edges disappear first, the centre last.

abnormal Lit., any departure from the norm or the normal. The term is used variously to denote such things as purely quantitative deviations in statistical analyses and deviant behaviour patterns of individuals. Although this latter reference has been the dominant one in psychology for a long time, there has been some reluctance on the part of clinicians and personality theorists to use it in this fashion. The difficulty stems from the tendency to have the boundaries of 'normalness' defined by a particular theory of personality. For example, within classical *psychoanalysis* homosexuality is classified as abnormal, within a *social learning theory* analysis it is not. Note that falling back on the original 'statistical' usage will not solve the problem and will produce others: Einstein would of necessity be called abnormal. The years have layered onto this term too many value judgements and any of a number of synonyms are preferable: *maladaptive*, *maladjusted*, *deviant*, etc. Note that the tendency is to use these other terms with respect to the behaviour of the individual under consideration, and to evaluate this in terms of whether or not it is adaptive behaviour for him or her, rather than as a cold label for the behaviour itself or for any individual displaying it. None of these, however, have managed to garner much lexicographic enthusiasm.

abnormal fixation FIXATION, ABNORMAL.

abnormal psychology The branch of psychology concerned with abnormal behaviour. Because of the difficulties with the term ABNORMAL, many favour dropping this term from the psychologist's lexicon. Other terms offered as a replacement include *psychology of deviance*, *psychopathology* and *study of maladaptive behaviour*.

abortion **1** Generally, the cessation or 'arrest' of any condition. **2** More specifically and commonly, the termination of a pregnancy before the foetus becomes viable. The issue of viability is handled by some in terms of approximate length of gestation (i.e. between roughly the 20th and 25th weeks) and by others in terms of physical development (i.e. a foetus of approximately 20 cm in length and weighing roughly 500 g). Ultimately, however, viability is going to be dependent to some extent on the develop-ment of medical technology. In Great Britain, for example, 24 weeks is by law the upper limit for abortions for 'social' reasons but there is no specific limit for abortions for 'medical' reasons.

abortion, spontaneous Any expelling of a premature foetus prior to the point of viability without any specific attempt on anyone's part to produce termination of the pregnancy.

aboulia ABULIA.

abreaction A psychoanalytic term used to describe the weakening or elimination of anxiety by the 'reliving' of the original tension-evoking experience. 'Reliving' can refer to an imaginal or emotional re-experience as well as to an actual one. See also CATHARSIS.

abscissa The horizontal coordinate of a point in a plane Cartesian coordinate system. Commonly, although strictly speaking not correctly, the term is used for the x-axis. In standard notation, values of the *independent variable* are plotted on the abscissa. See also AXIS; CARTESIAN COORDINATES.

absence Momentary mental inattention, a short period during which consciousness is 'missing'. A common aspect of epilepsy; the individual typically has no memory of what transpired during the period. See AMNESIA; see also FUGUE.

absolute **1** adj. Not *relative*, not varying, characterizing a thing that has intrinsic meaning or value independent of other data, events or considerations. **2** n. CULTURAL *ABSOLUTE.

absolute, cultural A VALUE (2) that the members of a particular society or culture hold and which they believe to be universal, enduring and applicable to all societies and cultures and not merely their own.

absolute error ERROR, ABSOLUTE.

absolute limen THRESHOLD.

absolute pitch The ability to recognize the pitch of any given tone and give its name. Also called *perfect pitch*.

absolute refractory period REFRACTORY PERIOD, ABSOLUTE.

absolute scale SCALE, ABSOLUTE.

absolute sensitivity An occasional synonym for *absolute threshold*. For discussion see THRESHOLD.

absolute threshold THRESHOLD.

absolute value VALUE, ABSOLUTE.

absolute zero ZERO, ABSOLUTE.

absorption 1 In the study of sensory processes, the capture or taking in of chemical, electromagnetic or other physical stimuli by a receptor. For example, SPECTRAL ABSORPTION. **2** Preoccupation with a particular activity. The connotations here may be positive, in that one so absorbed is one whose attention is productively focused, or they may be negative in that such absorption may be viewed as a withdrawal from reality. vb., *absorb*.

absorption spectrum SPECTRAL-ABSORPTION CURVE; SPECTRAL-SENSITIVITY CURVE.

abstinence syndrome A term occasionally used for the full range of physiological disturbances caused by the sudden withdrawal of a drug on which one has developed a physical dependence. See WITHDRAWAL.

abstract 1 adj. From the Latin for *drawn away*. Most usages of the term focus on qualities of objects, events, phenomena, etc. which are considered separate or apart from the objects, events or phenomena themselves. Thus, an abstract idea is an intangible one considered apart from specific instances. For example, 'patriotism' is an abstract idea separate from particular patriotic people or events. Note that even when dealing with more concrete things an element of abstraction exists. 'Chair' can be regarded as somewhat less abstract than 'patriotism' although it still may represent an abstract class of chairs devoid of specific attributes. It is probably best to handle the term itself abstractly, relating it to a general dimension that runs from abstract to concrete. See also CONCEPT; PROTOTYPE. **2** vb. The same general notion is found here, i.e. the idea of *withdrawal*. To abstract is to extract and the cognitive processes involved are neither simple nor well understood. One may abstract a simple concept (e.g. 'red' as a property of many red things), an idealization (e.g. 'perfection' as an underlying prototype never found in reality but inducible from many nonperfect exemplars), a narrative

(e.g. a simple paraphrase capturing the main ideas of a story), and so forth. **3** n. In scientific literature, the brief summary of the main ideas of an article, usually given at the very beginning.

abstract ability A mental activity often taken as the hallmark of intellectual functioning; the ability to appreciate the ABSTRACT and/or symbolic aspects of situations.

abstract attitude A general type of cognitive functioning typified by voluntary shifting of mental set from situation to situation, moving from concrete to ABSTRACT as circumstances dictate, alternating from a focusing on a whole problem to concentrating on its parts, etc.

abstract idea (or **quality**) Any idea or quality which is *abstract* in the sense of being an element or symbol characteristic of a general conceptualization rather than of some particular or concrete instance. Presumably, all abstract ideas are inductions based upon the detection of common elements across many situations. See ABSTRACT (1); see also PROTOTYPE; SEMANTIC *MEMORY.

abstract intelligence See discussions under ABSTRACT and INTELLIGENCE.

abstraction 1 The cognitive process whereby an abstract idea or concept is isolated from a number of exemplars. **2** The result of this process; the hypothesized mental representation of an abstract concept.

abstraction theory An umbrella term for a number of theories in *cognitive psychology* that argue that memory and knowledge systems are built up by a process whereby abstract information is extracted from the numerous specific episodes or instances that one experiences. For example, if a hairy, four-legged creature should walk into the room, these theorists would argue that you know it is a dog because it fits the deep abstract representation you have of the category 'dog'. Compare with INSTANCE THEORY; PROTOTYPE.

abstract representation A mental REPRESENTATION that captures the underlying symbolic or ABSTRACT (1) character of a stimulus as distinct from specific instances. One can have a concept 'dog' that is held without any specific dog in mind.

abulia A reduction in ability to initiate actions and thoughts and a general indifference about the consequences of action. The term is properly reserved for truly pathological cases. var., *aboulia*.

abundancy motive Quite literally, the desire to attain an abundancy of things. A tendency to seek beyond simple satisfaction of needs that derive from deficiencies.

abusability The term refers to the notion that some children seem to 'invite' abuse or maltreatment from their parents. Some factors which seem to contribute are excessive crying, physical handicaps, prematurity.

abusable child ABUSABILITY.

abuse 1 n. Behaviour that is degrading, demeaning or violent toward another person. **2** n. Behaviour that is invasive of the privacy or rights of another person. **3** vb. To subject another to such behaviour. **4** vb. To misuse a drug or other substance to the point where unwanted consequences occur. These can be occupational, physical, emotional, personal, social or, of course, legal. The term, in all senses, can refer to rather different behaviours depending upon the diagnostic criteria in use and the legal system in place.

abusing parent 1 Lit., a parent guilty of CHILD ABUSE. **2** A label for a hypothetical personality type possessing a particular set of characteristics. In theory it is highly likely that a person of this type will become an abusing parent in sense 1. Research has failed to discover any clear-cut personality traits which typify abusing parents other than the fact that they were likely to have been abused themselves as children.

ABX An experimental procedure in which the subject is presented with three stimuli on each trial and must decide whether the last (X) matches the first (A) or the second (B).

academic skills disorders Any of several disorders of childhood characterized by impairment in academic function in school. Specific forms include DEVELOPMENTAL *ARITHMETIC DISORDER, DEVELOPMENTAL *EXPRESSIVE WRITING DISORDER and DEVELOPMENTAL *READING DISORDER. Also called LEARNING DISORDERS.

acalculia Lit., the inability to perform simple arithmetic operations. Generally used to refer to the loss of such ability resulting from injury and not for cases resulting from simple ignorance or lack of schooling. See and compare with DEVELOPMENTAL *ARITHMETIC DISORDER.

acatamathesia AKATAMATHESIA.

acathexis Lack of CATHEXIS, lack of emotion towards something which is (unconsciously) of considerable importance.

acathisia AKATHISIA.

acceleration Properly, the term refers not simply to increasing change in some variable, but to the *rate* of the increase in the change. Consider the following series of numbers, each of which represents, say, the speed of a car in successive seconds: (a) 0, 3, 6, 9, 12; (b) 0, 3, 7, 12, 18; (c) 0, 3, 5, 6. Here series (a) represents *zero* or *uniform* acceleration – each increase is the same as the one before; (b) displays *positive* acceleration – each increase is larger than the one before; and (c) is an example of *negative* acceleration – each increase is less than the one before. Reversing these series would produce examples of equivalent *deceleration* functions.

accent 1 Emphasis; rhythm as marked by the patterns of stress in a series of words, tones, beats, etc. See here STRESS (3). **2** An individual's speech patterns in a language which reflect habits of pronunciation acquired in speaking either another language or another dialect of that language. Compare with DIALECT.

access In addition to the standard dictionary meanings, the term is often used metaphorically to refer to retrieval of information from memory. It was borrowed from computer-sciences terminology and is used mostly, although not exclusively, in studies of human memory. It can be used for the process, as well as the actual fact, of recall.

accessible 1 Generally, available. **2** In studies of memory, retrievable, recallable. **3** In social psychology, open to personal interaction, not withdrawn.

accessory nerve SPINAL ACCESSORY NERVE.

accident An event that was unforeseen and hence unpredicted, or whose causes are at present unknown. Usually the connotation is negative. See also discussion under CHANCE for some philosophical issues which relate to the way these terms are used.

accidental error ERROR.

accident-prone A term loosely used to describe persons who display a somewhat higher than average rate of accidents. Such individuals may indeed contribute to their high accident rates by any number of conscious or unconscious reasons, or they may simply be the unlucky ones at the tail of a frequency distribution.

acclimatization Lit., adaptation or adjustment to a new climate. 'Climate' here is used loosely and can encompass simple repetition of a stimulus or the social and cultural milieu of a new country. var., *acclimation*.

accommodation **1** Generally, any movement or adjustment, either physical or psychological, which is made in preparation for incoming stimuli. This is a very rich concept and there are several specific uses, as follows: **2** In vision, adjustment of the shape of the lens of the eye to compensate for the distance of the object of focus from the retina. **3** In Piaget's theory, the modification of internal schemas to fit a changing cognizance of reality. See here the accompanying concept, ASSIMILATION (4). **4** In sociology and social psychology, a process of social adjustment designed to maintain harmony within a group, or between antagonistic groups. The adjustment may take any of several forms including compromise, conciliation, arbitration or the simple mutual acceptance of a truce. The term is used here with respect to the behaviour of single individuals as well as to that of a whole group or even a nation.

acculturation **1** With reference to children the term refers to the gradual acquisition of the behaviour patterns of the surrounding culture, in particular the subculture within which they are raised. This basic notion is also embodied in the term CULTURAL TRANSMISSION. For more on it, see also SOCIALIZATION and ENCULTURATION. **2** Somewhat more broadly, the adoption or assimilation of cultural elements from another culture.

acculturative stress Quite literally, the stress (and, by extension, the accompanying psychological difficulties) often observed in immigrants struggling to adapt to a new culture.

accuracy test Any test which emphasizes accuracy of performance independent of the time it takes to complete it. See also POWER TEST; compare with SPEED TEST.

acenaesthesia Lit., the lack of common sensation. Hence, either: **1** a general lack of well-being or **2** a lack of normal sense concerning one's body. var., *acenesthesia*.

acetophenazine One of the phenothiazine derivatives used as an antipsychotic drug.

acetylcholine (ACh) An excitatory NEUROTRANSMITTER found in a variety of locations. It is the transmitter substance liberated at the neuromuscular junctions of all skeletal muscles; it is also the neurotransmitter in the ganglia of the AUTONOMIC NERVOUS SYSTEM and functions to excite target organs of the post-ganglionic fibres of the parasympathetic division. It is found diffusely throughout the brain and concentrated specifically in neurons of the basal ganglia.

acetylcholinesterase (AChE) An enzyme produced by the post-synaptic membrane that destroys ACETYLCHOLINE by breaking it into acetate and choline, thus stopping the post-synaptic potential.

ACh ACETYLCHOLINE.

AChE ACETYLCHOLINESTERASE.

achieved role ROLE, ACHIEVED.

achievement **1** Accomplishment, the attaining of a goal. **2** The goal itself. **3** LEVEL OF ACHIEVEMENT.

achievement age AGE, ACHIEVEMENT.

achievement, level of The degree to which one has achieved on a standardized test. Used primarily in studies of education.

achievement motive **1** Generally, a personal motive manifested as a striving for success; quite literally, a motive to achieve. See NEED FOR ACHIEVEMENT. **2** In H. Murray's theory of personality, the term has a similar meaning but is conceptualized as entailing the notion of overcoming obstacles or tackling those things which are known to be difficult.

achievement test Any test designed to evaluate a person's current state of knowledge or skill. Contrast with APTITUDE TEST, which is designed to evaluate potentialities for achievement (ideally) independent of current knowledge.

achromat A person with ACHROMATOPSIA.

achromatic 1 Lit., without colour, in the sense of the dimensions of HUE and SATURATION. Hence, the term refers to visual stimuli which are describable solely in terms of BRIGHTNESS in the black–white dimension. 2 Characteristic of a lens corrected to counterbalance CHROMATIC *ABERRATION.

achromatic colour Any 'colour' lacking in HUE and SATURATION, hence describable only in terms of BRIGHTNESS, i.e. black and white.

achromatic interval 1 In vision, the interval between the absolute threshold for a monochromatic stimulus and the intensity level required for the observer to sense the hue of the given stimulus. 2 In AUDITION, the analogous interval between the absolute threshold for a pure tone and the intensity level required for the sensing of the pitch of the presented tone.

achromatism 1 Colourlessness. 2 ACHROMATOPSIA.

achromatopsia A condition wherein all visual experiences are *achromatic*, lacking in both HUE and SATURATION. Many species are naturally achromatopic; however, when the condition occurs in humans it is usually called *total colour blindness*. Such achromats are totally lacking in CONES and, as one might expect, they see everything in shades of grey, are *photophobic* (highly sensitive to bright lights) and have poor visual acuity. var., *achromatopia*. See also MONOCHROMATISM.

acid Street slang for *lysergic acid diethylamide* LSD.

acou-, acousia-, acousis- Prefixes meaning *hearing*.

acoumetre AUDIOMETER.

acoustic Pertaining to sound, especially from the point of view of the physicist. Compare with AUDITORY.

acoustic confusion Any 'confusion' (over which stimulus was presented) based upon acoustic factors. For example, hearing *bat* when the stimulus was *pat*. Compare with SEMANTIC CONFUSION.

acoustic cue Any aspect of the acoustic sig-nal in speech used to distinguish between phonetic elements. For example, VOICE ONSET TIME is an acoustic cue which distinguishes between the initial sounds in such words as 'tie' and 'die'.

acoustic filter Any device that selectively screens out ('filters') certain frequencies while permitting others to pass. See FILTER and related entries.

acoustic generalization GENERALIZATION, ACOUSTIC.

acoustic nerve VESTIBULOCOCHLEAR NERVE.

acousticoamnestic aphasia APHASIA, ACOUSTICOAMNESTIC.

acoustic pressure The average force of a sound stimulus on an area (generally measured in DYNES/cm^2). In *audition* the eardrum is the usual point of measurement.

acoustics 1 A branch of physics concerned with the study of the physical properties of sound. See PSYCHOACOUSTICS. 2 The properties of a hall or room which affect the characteristics of the sounds heard.

acoustic spectrum A term occasionally and incorrectly used when AUDITORY SPECTRUM is meant.

acoustic store A hypothesized memory system whereby auditory (and perhaps even visual) inputs are stored in a form that reflects their acoustic properties. Contrast with ARTICULATORY STORE, in which the hypothesized mechanism is based on the motor system for producing sounds. See also ICONIC, ECHOIC and SHORT-TERM *MEMORY.

acquiescence Generally, a tendency to agree with the viewpoint of others. Often used with the connotation that, if the source is an authority, the acquiescent person will tend toward agreement regardless of the nature of the content of the statement. See AUTHORITARIAN PERSONALITY.

acquired Simply, *learned*, in the sense that the behaviours, thoughts, notions, skills and propensities picked up are the results of experience and not specific genetic or inherited factors. However, it is important to keep in mind that virtually all LEARNING takes place in the context of biological propensities. It is easy for a human, by virtue of particular genetic, inherited, species-specific characteristics, to acquire the skill of roller skating; only futility would result from trying to have a fish acquire such behaviour.

acquired brain injury (ABI) Generally, any BRAIN INJURY. ABIs can result from cerebrovascular episodes such as strokes or aneurysms or physical blows to the head (see TRAUMATIC BRAIN INJURY).

acquired characteristic Quite literally, any *characteristic* which results from experience or environmental factors. The term is properly used of environmentally produced *modifications* in structural characteristics or *differences* in behavioural characteristics.

acquired characteristics, inheritance of The doctrine which states that proficiencies and attributes with survival value acquired through effort and use during the lifetime of an organism are passed on genetically to succeeding generations. When put forward by the elaborately named French naturalist Jean-Baptiste Pierre Antoine de Monet Lamarck, it was the first coherent theory of the process of evolution prior to the Darwinian theory of natural selection. Although there has been no convincing evidence to support the Lamarckian process, the concept itself seems to have some survival value. Darwin himself expressed a version of it and it has been revived in various guises by several modern biologists and psychologists, most notably Piaget. Today it is but a historic curiosity.

acquired discrimination of cues Quite literally, the process whereby two or more cues originally responded to as equivalent become functionally differentiated from each other as a result of differential reinforcement of responses made to each. Thus stated, the term is synonymous with the simple term DISCRIMINATION (1); its interest and use derives from comparison with *acquired equivalence of cues*, whereby two or more cues which are potentially discriminable are rendered functionally equivalent to each other by reinforcing responses to them equally. The point of these contrasting operations is that questions of *discrimination* or *equivalence* are not to be answered absolutely but rather functionally.

acquired drive DRIVE, ACQUIRED.

acquired dyslexia DYSLEXIA, ACQUIRED.

acquired equivalence of cues ACQUIRED DISCRIMINATION OF CUES.

acquired sociopathy A syndrome seen in some cases of frontal lobe damage, particularly the ventromedial region. Patients exhibit classic symptoms of the more common SOCIOPATHIC PERSONALITY, such as lack of planning, diminished response to punishment, lack of empathy or concern for others all in the face of unimpaired intelligence. Also called *pseudopsychopathy*.

acquisition **1** Generally, a synonym of LEARNING. **2** The process of gaining or acquiring something. This usage is very broad and the thing acquired may be a valued object, a complex skill or an ability to carry out some task. **3** In some older texts, a synonym for MATURATION. This usage is confusing and not recommended.

acquisition trial TRIAL, LEARNING.

acquisitiveness Loosely, a behavioural trait reflected by a tendency to possess or hoard things.

acro- Combining form from the Greek, meaning *extremity* or *topmost*. Used of the top of the head, hands, feet, fingers and toes, as well as to refer to heights.

acroaesthesia Hypersensitivity in one or more extremities. var., *acroesthesia*.

acroanaesthesia Loss of sensation in one or more extremities. var., *acroanesthesia*.

acromegaly Chronic disease caused by hyperfunctioning of cells in the anterior lobe of the pituitary gland resulting in an excess of growth hormone. Characteristic symptoms are elongated bones in the extremities, especially in the hands and feet and in the facial bones and the jaw.

acronym A pronounceable abbreviation of a multi-word term or phrase composed of the first letters of each word, e.g. WAT for Word Association Test, WISC for Wechsler Intelligence Scale for Children.

acroparaesthesia PARAESTHESIA (numbness, itching or tingling) in the fingers and hands. var., *acroparesthesia*.

acrotomophilia A PARAPHILIA where the individual is sexually aroused by persons who have had amputations.

act 1 n. Much has been written on this term over the decades. The only sensible meaning, in sum, is, simply, a RESPONSE or a pattern of behaviour. **2** n. Historically, ACT PSYCHOLOGY. **3** vb. To respond.

ACT An acronym for *adaptive control of thought*, an umbrella term for a family of models of human cognition developed by John R. Anderson. While there are several versions of the theory, all are based on what are known as PRODUCTION SYSTEMS, which are essentially rules for symbol manipulation. ACT has had considerable success as a theory of human reasoning and learning.

ACTH ADRENOCORTICOTROPHIC HORMONE.

acting out 1 A rather irrational, impulsive display. This meaning is usually reserved for uncontrollable outbursts in problem children. **2** The display of feeling and emotion which has previously been inhibited. Here the term is used with a neutral or even positive connotation in that such self-expression is regarded as healthy and therapeutic. **3** A coping style in which the individual deals with conflict or stress through actions rather than through reflections or feelings.

action 1 Generally, the actual performance of some function, the occurrence of a process. **2** The result of such performance or occurrence. Usage is broad: the operations may be overt and obvious, like walking or talking, when the connotation is that action is conscious and purposive; or they may be more covert and internal, like heart action, neural action potential or the action of a drug, from which this connotation is missing.

action potential The term for the whole series of changes in electrical potential which occur when an impulse is propagated by a neuron. Strictly, the term refers to the momentary difference in electrical potential between active and resting parts of an individual neuron while firing.

action readiness In the study of emotions, the tendency to shift the relationship between oneself and one's immediate environment. This definition, which may seem cryptic, is designed to capture the notion that such readinesses are culturally sensitive. In one culture a particular environmental scene might evoke an aggressive response, in another a submissive reaction and in another a diplomatic reaction.

action research As originally conceptualized by K. Lewin, research carried out with the express purpose of achieving an understanding of phenomena that leads to practical applications and solutions of real-world problems.

action-specific energy In classical ethological theory a hypothetical well of energy assumed to be associated with a particular unlearned response. Immediately after the response is made the action-specific energy is very low; it recovers over time and, according to Lorenz's analysis, should the specific SIGN-STIMULUS (or RELEASER) not occur, the energy 'spills over' and VACUUM ACTIVITY or, in some situations, DISPLACEMENT (2) occurs.

action tremor A tremor associated with cerebellar damage that emerges when intentional action is carried out. It is characterized by a staggered movement and is distinct from the tremor associated with PARKINSON'S DISEASE, which occurs during rest. Also called *intention tremor*.

activation Basically, preparing for action. The use of the term, however, is generally restricted to the activating effect of one internal organ upon another (e.g. *reticular activating system*). It is, therefore, not properly a synonym for either AROUSAL, which is more often used in a general fashion, or STIMULATION, which is used to refer to 'activation' produced by external means.

activation-synthesis model Allan Hobson's theory of dreams as cortical synthesizing of random neural activations that take place during sleep, particularly REM SLEEP.

activation theory of emotion THEORIES OF *EMOTION. This theory is more commonly referred to as the *arousal theory*.

active 1 Functioning, operational. **2** Characterizing a particular attitude or stance whereby one spontaneously initiates events and influences a situation. **3** Descriptive of a posture of control and initiative, particularly in sexual matters. See here ACTIVE AND PASSIVE for Freud's usage of the term and its opposite.

active analysis ACTIVE *THERAPY.

active and passive Classical psychoanalysis assumed the existence of a polarized dimension of activity–passivity. The former was associated with masculinity, aggression, sadism and voyeurism; the latter with femininity, submissiveness, masochism and exhibitionism. Moreover, Freud added the possibility that each of these 'natural' modes can be reversed to its opposite, so that a masochistic male is viewed as one who has 'reversed' his sadistic instincts. The whole active–passive apparatus can certainly be viewed as a respectable starting-point for a general theory, although, as many have argued, it soon leads into absurdities, as in the not uncommon syndrome of a female who is characterized as one who 'actively pursues passive aims'.

active avoidance AVOIDANCE.

active therapy THERAPY, ACTIVE.

active vocabulary VOCABULARY, ACTIVE.

activity 1 A generic term safely applicable as a synonym for action, movement, behaviour, mental process, physiological functions, etc. Because of its great generality, activity is usually bound up with a qualifying adjective, e.g. goal-directed activity, random activity, problem-solving activity **2** One of the three hypothesized universal dimensions of SEMANTIC SPACE in C. Osgood's theory of word meaning. See also SEMANTIC DIFFERENTIAL.

activity analysis 1 Generally, the objective analysis of the various activities engaged in by a person. **2** In industrial/organizational psychology, an analysis of this kind carried out with respect to the job the individual is expected to do.

activity cage Any cage designed to record general activity. Typically used with animals, the most common ones use sensitive gauges or photoelectric cells to record movements.

activity cycle Lit., a cycle or rhythm in activity. Most organisms display activity cycles which can be traced to metabolic and hormonal cycles associated with hunger, thirst, sex, diurnal rhythms, etc.

activity drive A hypothesized drive introduced in an attempt to account for the fact that virtually all organisms display a fairly constant level of activity, which takes place in the absence of any (obvious) physiologic-ally produced motivating drive state. See DRIVE.

activity inventory An objective listing ('inventory') of the various components ('activities') of a particular job; often included as part of a full *activity analysis*.

act psychology A philosophical psychological system espoused originally by Franz Brentano. His position was formulated in opposition to the so-called 'content' focus of STRUCTURALISM (1). Structuralists argued that the basic subject matter of psychology was the conscious content of mind; the acts psychologists focused on were the acts or processes of mind as the fundamental source of empirical data. As an empirical system it made few lasting contributions to psychology but it served an important historical role. It formulated the base for others such as the WÜRZBURG SCHOOL to build upon and provided many of the philosophical foundations that helped give rise to FUNCTIONALISM.

act, pure-stimulus A term introduced by the behaviourist Clark Hull to refer to any behaviour that does not explicitly lead an organism toward a goal.

actual conflict CONFLICT, ACTUAL.

actual neurosis A term originally used by Freud to refer to a neurosis which resulted from the tension of real, 'actual' frustrations or real organic dysfunctions. It was later taken up by W. Reich and assumed by him to represent the basis of all neurosis.

acuity Generally, the capacity to discriminate fine detail; keenness of perception. The term is usually used with a qualifier to denote the specific form of acuity under consideration; when found unqualified it almost always refers to VISUAL *ACUITY.

acuity, auditory 1 Sensitivity of hearing with reference to the absolute threshold for detection of sounds of various frequencies. **2** The ability to discriminate fine distinctions in sound stimuli. Meaning 2 more accurately captures the meaning of the base term ACUITY than does 1, although it is less common.

acuity grating A set of dark bars presented on a white background. By adjusting the distance between the bars until the *minimum separable* is achieved one gets an estimate of visual acuity.

acuity, sensory Generally, fineness or keenness of perception. An umbrella term which is used to cover the classic issues of sensory psychophysics; namely, detection and discrimination of stimuli. A viewer of high sensory acuity can detect stimuli of low intensity and/or short duration and discriminate small differences between stimuli. See VISUAL *ACUITY.

acuity, stereoscopic A measure of visual acuity given as the minimum difference in depth (distance from the viewer) that can be perceived using both eyes.

acuity, vernier Visual acuity in which the measure of fine detail that can be perceived is given by the minimum amount of displacement between the top and bottom halves of a line that can just be detected.

acuity, visual The capacity to see fine details of objects in the visual field. Visual acuity is typically expressed by the number of degrees of visual arc subtended by the visual object that can just be seen or by the width of the object itself. In clinical practice standard displays are used (e.g. the Snellen chart) and acuity is given as a ratio, D'/D, D' being the standard or normal viewing distance and D the distance at which the object viewed would subtend an angle of 1 minute of arc. For example, a person who, from a distance of 20 ft (6.1 m), can distinguish an object that would subtend 1 minute of arc were he or she standing 50 ft (15.2 m) away, has poor visual acuity. Visual acuity is measured in a variety of ways, the most common being *recognition* (of which the above example using the Snellen chart is one), *resolution* (see ACUITY GRATING) and *localization* (see e.g. VERNIER *ACUITY and STEREOSCOPIC *ACUITY).

acupuncture A technique for producing regional anaesthesia. Following ancient charts developed over centuries, largely by the Chinese, each region of the body is associated with a particular locale. Anaesthesia is produced by inserting a long thin needle at the critical point and often either twirling it or passing a mild electric current through it. How, why, and indeed whether acupuncture works (that is, from the mechanistic viewpoint of the Western scientist) is not known and until recently the technique received very little attention from Western researchers. The most frequently cited hypothesis is that some form of neural blocking is involved whereby neural firing patterns set up by the needles block the transmission of the pain fibres in another region of the body. See GATE-CONTROL THEORY. Some practitioners of ALTERNATIVE MEDICINE use acupuncture for various disorders such as alcoholism and drug abuse.

acute 1 Generally, highly sensitive, extremely responsive. 2 Sharp, intense. See ACUTE *PAIN. 3 With respect to diseases or to the symptoms of a disease, sudden in onset and relatively short-lived. 4 With respect to experimental work in physiology, the term characterizes preparations which are short-term or temporary. Contrast (3) and (4) with CHRONIC. A variety of diseases and syndromes often have an *acute* (3) stage which is of special significance; these are found under the alphabetical listing of the disease or syndrome itself.

acute brain disorder A cover term for any disability due to a reversible (hence, temporary) impairment of brain tissue.

acute delusional psychosis SCHIZOPHRENI-FORM DISORDER.

acute hallucinatory psychosis SCHIZO-PHRENIFORM DISORDER.

acute pain PAIN, ACUTE.

acute polymorphic psychotic disorder SCHIZOPHRENIFORM DISORDER.

acute preparation PREPARATION, ACUTE.

acute schizophrenic episode SCHIZO-PHRENIC EPISODE, ACUTE.

acute (drug) tolerance TOLERANCE, ACUTE.

AD ALZHEIMER'S DISEASE.

adaptation 1 In experimental psychology, a change in the responsiveness or sensitivity of a sensory receptor or a sense organ which is temporary in nature. Generally speaking, increases in stimulation decrease sensitivity while decreases in stimulation increase sensitivity, and the term is applicable to both processes. This meaning is captured in a number of combined phrases in which the particular stimulus dimension under consideration is specified, e.g. *chromatic* (or *spectral*) *adaptation, brightness adaptation, dark adapta-*

tion, phonetic adaptation, etc. Compare this pattern of use with HABITUATION and DESENSITIZATION. Only such phrases of which the intended meaning is not immediately apparent or important aspects need specifying are listed in this volume. **2** In social psychology and sociology, a shift in sociological or cultural disposition. Thus, one is said to 'adapt' to a new environment. **3** In evolutionary theory, any structural or behavioural change that has survival value.

adaptation, cross ADAPTATION (1) to all stimuli of a group after exposure to but one stimulus from that group. Cross adaptation is common in smell, where adapting the subject to one odour will produce a diminution in sensitivity to a large variety of other odours.

adaptation level (AL) A neutral position on a sensory continuum; specifically, the level to which the sense organ has adapted. A full theory of sensory-context effects was built up around this notion by Harry Helson. Generally the theory maintains that the neutral, adapted background provides a standard against which new stimuli are perceived. Thus, for example, originally cool water may be made to feel warm if the subject first adapts to rather cold water. Although the theory was designed with sensory processes in mind, it has been widely applied to fields far removed from simple sensory continua, particularly the study of attitudes and attitude change.

adaptation level theory ADAPTATION LEVEL.

adaptation, selective Quite literally, adaptation that is selective. Thus, if a subject is presented repeatedly with a particular stimulus, ADAPTATION (1) will occur and the subject will show a diminished sensitivity to that stimulus. If, however, the subject still displays a normal response to similar but discernibly different stimuli then one can say that selective adaptation has occurred.

adaptation syndrome GENERAL ADAPTATION SYNDROME (GAS).

adaptation time The length of time it takes for *adaptation* (1) to occur, i.e. the time from onset of stimulation to the point after which no further changes in the sensory system occur.

adaptive **1** Functioning so as to facilitate adaptation. **2** Appropriate, useful, aiding in adjustment. This term, particularly when used in the phrase *adaptive behaviour*, has become increasingly common and many use it where terms such as *sane* and *normal* were once used. That is, one who is 'sane' or 'normal' is one whose behaviour is 'adaptive'. See also MALADAPTIVE.

adaptive behaviour ADAPTIVE.

adaptive testing Assessment in which only a small subset of items of a test is administered. The testing is 'adaptive' to the individual's ability level so that only those items appropriate for the person being evaluated are used. The term is used in ability testing, not in areas like personality assessment.

ADD ATTENTION-DEFICIT HYPERACTIVITY DISORDER.

addiction **1** Any psychological or physiological overdependence of an organism on a drug. Originally the term was used only for physiological dependencies where a drug had altered the biochemistry of an individual such that continued doses (often of increasing size – see TOLERANCE) were required, as is the case with the opiates and with alcohol. However, the line between purely physiological addiction and psychological dependence is far from clear and over the years the semantic realm of the term expanded. Even in the technical literature one can find gems like 'the patient was addicted to chocolate cake'. The confusions attending such loose usage, plus the definitional problems that emerged with the attempts of different governmental bodies to circumscribe the use of various illicit drugs, led the World Health Organization to recommend that the term *dependence* be used, with proper qualifiers for cases in which drugs are involved. See DRUG *DEPENDENCE et seq. **2** Somewhat more loosely, a compelling need to carry out some behaviour. For example, individuals with various IMPULSE-CONTROL DISORDERS such as *pathological gambling* will sometimes be referred to as having an 'addiction'. This usage is not strictly correct but is quite common.

additive bilingualism BILINGUALISM, ADDITIVE.

additive mixture COLOUR MIXING.

additive scale SCALE, ADDITIVE.

additive task A type of group task in which the performance of the group as a whole is the sum of the performance of the individual group members. The classic example is a game of tug-of-war. Compare with CONJUNCTIVE TASK and DISJUNCTIVE TASK.

address The location in a computer where a particular piece of information is stored and, by extension, the place in the brain where a particular memory is located. While the term enjoyed a certain currency in theories of INFORMATION PROCESSING, few contemporary researchers believe that memory displays this kind of location-specificity.

adduction Movement of a limb or the eyes toward the median plane of the body. Compare with ABDUCTION (1).

adductor A muscle which, upon contraction, moves a limb toward the median plane of the body. Compare with ABDUCTOR.

A-delta fibres FREE NERVE ENDINGS.

adenine One of four nucleotide bases which make up both DEOXYRIBONUCLEIC ACID and RIBONUCLEIC ACID.

adenohypophysis PITUITARY GLAND.

adenosine A NEUROMODLATOR found in the brain. Released by both GLIA and neurons when they are oxygen deprived, it causes nearby blood vessels to dilate and increases the supply of nutrients.

adenosine triphosphate (ATP) A molecule involved in cellular energy metabolism. When ATP is converted into adenosine diphosphate energy is released; when converted into CYCLIC ADENOSINE MONOPHOSPHATE it serves as a messenger in the production of postsynaptic potentials. .

adenylate cyclase An enzyme that converts ADENOSINE TRIPHOSPHATE into CYCLIC ADENOSINE MONOPHOSPHATE. It operates as part of the process of mediating the intracellular effects of many neurotransmitters and peptide hormones.

adequate sample SAMPLE, ADEQUATE.

adequate stimulus STIMULUS, ADEQUATE.

ADH Abbreviation for *antidiuretic hormone.* See VASOPRESSIN.

ADHD ATTENTION-DEFICIT HYPERACTIVITY DISORDER.

ad hoc Latin, meaning *for this purpose.* Generally applied to any hypothesis or hypothetical explanation developed to explain a particular set of data that does not fit into an existing theoretical framework. An *ad hoc* hypothesis is one developed after the data have been collected.

ad hominem From the Latin for 'toward the man', a form of argument in which a position is attacked by making aspersions about an individual holding it. The technique can be effective because the negative feelings for the person generalize to the position.

adiadochokinesia DYSDIADOCHOKINESIA.

adient Characterizing movement toward something. Contrast with ABIENT.

adipocytes Lit., *fat cells.* Interest in these cells has increased recently because of the fact that obese people have more and larger adipocytes than those of normal weight.

adipose Fatty, pertaining to fat.

adipsia Lit., the absence of drinking. As a chronic syndrome it can be produced by lesions in the lateral hypothalamus.

adjective check-list Any of several self-inventory personality-assessment instruments consisting of a number of adjectives. The respondent simply checks those which are considered to be self-descriptive.

adjunctive Characterizing that which is used concurrently with another process, factor or variable. The connotation of the term varies. It may be supportive, as when *adjunctive therapies* (e.g. the use of groups) buttress other methods (e.g. ones with psychodynamic focus); it may be secondary, as when *adjunctive behaviours* emerge with other conditioned responses (see SCHEDULE-INDUCED *POLYDIPSIA*); or it may imply an interaction, as when *adjunctive drugs* enhance the therapeutic effects of other compounds. n., *adjunct.*

adjusting schedule SCHEDULES OF *REINFORCEMENT.*

adjustment 1 Generally, the relationship that any organism establishes with respect to its environment. The term usually refers to social or psychological adjustment and when used in this sense it carries clear positive connotations, e.g. *well-adjusted*. The implication is that the individual is involved in a rich, ongoing process of developing his or her potential, reacting to and in turn changing the environment in a healthy, effective manner. On the other hand, a subtle, negative connotation of the term can be found. This is reflected by the semantic overlap that it has with the term CONFORMITY, with the implication that, in adjusting, the person has given up personal initiative. **2** A state of complete equilibrium between an organism and its environment; a state wherein all needs are satisfied and all organismic functions are being carried out smoothly. **3** In statistics, any procedure for correcting, weighting or reinterpreting data so as to be able to 'adjust' for unusual or atypical conditions.

adjustment disorder A general psychiatric category used for a maladaptive reaction to a stressful situation occurring soon (the criterion usually stated is three months) after the onset of the stressor. Put simply, the individual fails to adjust properly to the new conditions of his or her life. Such 'disorders' are quite common and usually temporary; either the stressor is removed or else the person finds a new mode of adaptation to the situation.

adjustment, method of METHODS OF *SCALING.

adjustment reaction Loosely, any relatively temporary, maladaptive reaction to stressful situations or events in one's life. In some older classification systems (e.g. early versions of the DSM) the terms *transient situational personality disorder* and *transient situational disturbance* were used for these reactions and may still be found in some texts. The current *DSM* classification system groups all of them under ADJUSTMENT DISORDERS.

adjuvant Descriptive of supplementary therapeutic techniques. Psychotherapeutic drugs are often referred to as adjuvant procedures.

Adlerian Characterizing the theory and psychoanalytic practices put forward by Alfred Adler (1870–1937). Often referred to as *individual psychology*, the primary concept is that of *inferiority* and the crux of the human condition is assumed to be the struggle against feelings of inferiority, be they conscious or unconscious, physical, psychological or social.

ad lib From the Latin *ad libitum*, meaning *without restriction*. Generally used in the term 'ad lib body weight', meaning the weight approached by a fully mature organism given unlimited access to a balanced diet, i.e. one on ad lib feeding (also called *free-feeding*). Also used in a variety of contexts in which lack of restriction is the intended meaning.

adolescence The period of development marked at the beginning by the onset of puberty and at the end by the attainment of physiological or psychological maturity. It should be noted that the term is much less precise than it appears since both the onset of puberty and the attainment of maturity are effectively impossible to define or specify.

adoption The legal process of permanently placing a child in a family other than its birth family. See also CLOSED ADOPTION and OPEN ADOPTION.

ad populum From the Latin 'toward the people', a form of argument in which a position is defended on the grounds that many others hold it. The BANDWAGON EFFECT is based on this, basically fallacious, form of reasoning.

adrenal 1 Pertaining to the kidney. **2** Pertaining to the ADRENAL GLAND and/or its secretions.

adrenal gland An endocrine gland located adjacent to and covering the upper part of the surface of the kidney. The inner *adrenal medulla*, composed of modified sympathetic ganglion cells, secretes EPINEPHRINE (*adrenalin*) and small amounts of NOREPINEPHRINE (*noradrenalin*) and DOPAMINE. The outer *adrenal cortex* arises, embryonically, from the urogenital mesoderm and produces several groups of hormones: the *glucocorticoids* (CORTISOL; CORTISONE; CORTICOSTERONE), the *mineralocorticoids* (ALDOSTERONE) and various sex hormones including *androgens* (KETOSTEROID), *oestrogens* (OESTRADIOL) and PROGESTERONE. Also called *suprarenal gland*.

adrenalin EPINEPHRINE. The word *adrenalin* comes from the Latin and means *towards the kidney*, which is where the adrenal gland is located. The contemporary use of *epinephrine* as the term of choice (from the Greek, meaning *on the kidney*) was spurred by the adoption of *Adrenalin* as a proprietary name by a drug company. It should be noted, however, that the adjectival form ADRENERGIC is used uniformly. var., *adrenaline*.

adrenaline ADRENALIN.

adrenergic Characterizing neurons and neural fibres and pathways which, when stimulated, release EPINEPHRINE (*adrenalin*). It should be noted that while *epinephrine* is the preferred term for the substance itself, *adrenergic* is the preferred adjectival form. See ADRENALIN for the reasons behind this terminological peculiarity.

adreno- Combining form meaning *adrenal*.

adrenocorticotrophic hormone (ACTH) A hormone secreted by the anterior pituitary gland that functions in the growth and development of the adrenal cortex. It also plays a critical role in the continued functioning of the adrenal cortices by stimulating the production of glucocorticoids and has been implicated in suppressing the production of testosterone. vars., *adrenocorticotropic hormone, corticotrophic hormone*.

adrenogenital syndrome A congenital defect in the adrenal cortices. The abnormality begins *in utero* and requires treatment soon after birth, failing which, in severe cases, death ensues from salt loss and dehydration. Affected females typically display ambiguous external genitalia; males are superficially normal in appearance. If untreated, in addition to the salt loss and dehydration, both sexes undergo rapid premature sexual development in the first years of life.

adrenosterone A weak ANDROGEN secreted by the adrenal cortices.

adult intelligence INTELLIGENCE, ADULT.

adultomorphism Interpreting the behaviour of a child from an adult point of view; an unwarranted attribution of adult characteristics, traits or processes to a child.

Advanced Progressive Matrices Test See PROGRESSIVE MATRICES TEST.

advantage by illness A general term used for the 'beneficial' aspects that accompany some mental disorders. The gain may be *primary* (or *paranosic*), in that a symptom may function to relieve immediate anxiety (e.g. the primary gain of claustrophobia is freedom from the anxiety that comes with being in a confined space), or it may be *secondary* (or *epinosic*), in that the disability serves as a device to avoid unpleasant duties (e.g. an agoraphobic who cannot leave home cannot be expected to hold down a job). Also called *gain by illness*. See also FLIGHT INTO ILLNESS.

adventitious reinforcement Reinforcement delivered independently of any response on the part of the subject. Despite the lack of a 'true' cause-and-effect relationship between an organism's responses and the received reinforcements, adventitious reinforcement can have a powerful effect upon behaviour. See e.g. SUPERSTITIOUS BEHAVIOUR.

aerial perspective A fuzziness and/or relative blueness of distant objects caused by the atmosphere. The effect is caused by filtering out short wavelengths and loss of brightness contrast as light travels through air. It is one of the monocular cues for depth perception.

aero- Combining form meaning *air* or *gas*.

aerobic Pertaining to or characteristic of organisms (or tissues) which require, or are not destroyed by, free oxygen.

aerobic exercise Any exercise that increases oxygen uptake by the body.

aerophagia Lit., air-eating. The gulping and swallowing of air.

-aesthesia, -aesthesis, aesthesio- Combining forms from the Greek for *sensation* and used to denote *feeling, sensibility, sensitivity*, etc. var., *-esthesia*.

aesthesiometer Any device for measuring sensitivity to touch, specifically a compass-like instrument for determining the two-point threshold on the skin. var., *aesthesiometer*.

aetiology The study of the causes of disease. var., *etiology*.

affect A general term used more or less interchangeably with various others, such as *emotion, emotionality, feeling, mood,* etc. Historically, it has had various, more specialized usages. It was once applied to one of the three 'mental functions', the other two being *cognition* and *volition.* Later, Titchener used it as a label for the pleasantness–unpleasantness dimension of feeling. Contemporary usage is, however, very loose, although the *DSM-IV* recommends that, in reference to various psychological disorders, it be differentiated from MOOD, which is properly used for more pervasive and sustained emotional states. Distinguish from the verb *to affect,* and from EFFECT, in which the accent is on the final syllable. See also EMOTION.

affect, appropriateness of The extent to which an individual's emotional response to a particular situation is considered (from a 'normal' or 'acceptable' point of view) to be appropriate. Inappropriate affect is, generally speaking, the hallmark of all psychological or psychiatric disorders.

affect, displacement of The shifting (i.e. displacing) of feeling or emotion from the object or person toward which it was originally experienced on to another object or person.

affective Pertaining to or characteristic of AFFECT.

affective attack A violent, highly emotional attack on one animal by another.

affective components In social psychology, those subjective feeling or mood states that accompany an attitude. The term is often used with the connotation that these states are the result of physiological actions.

affective disorder MOOD DISORDERS.

affective fixation FIXATION, AFFECTIVE.

affective forecasting Judging the emotional impact that some upcoming event or thing will have on one. People turn out to be rather poor at this, particularly when assessing how happy some desired object or event will make them. See MISWANTING.

affective neuroscience A cover term for the interdisciplinary approach to the study of emotions and affect that focuses primarily on the underlying neurological and psychological mechanisms.

affective prosody See PROSODY.

affective psychosis Loosely, any psychosis with severe disturbances in mood or feeling. See MOOD DISORDERS.

affective syndrome, organic ORGANIC MOOD SYNDROME.

afferent The conduction of nerve impulses from the periphery (the sense organs) to or toward the central nervous system. Thus, *afferent pathways* are neural pathways that carry sensory information from the receptors to the central nervous system. Contrast with EFFERENT.

afferent code Loosely, the pattern of neural action in the *afferent* (sensory) pathways. The term *code* is used because these patterns are not simple (and only partly known). For example, increasing the intensity of a stimulus does not merely increase the number of neurons firing or the number of responses each makes, rather it results in a complex change in the overall pattern of firing at various locations in the nervous system.

affiliation The standard dictionary meaning here is appropriate for most uses in psychology: bringing into close contact or association. The connotation is always positive; affiliation is associated with co-operation, companionship, even love. Several personality theorists, particularly Henry Murray, have hypothesized the existence of a basic human NEED FOR AFFILIATION.

affordance In J. J. Gibson's theory of perception, the 'invitational' quality of a PERCEPT or an event. Thus, a part of the affordance of a hammer is its graspability, of a chair its sit-on-ability. In a sense, affordance refers to the intrinsic properties of items and events.

affricate A speech sound which, in simplest terms, is made up of a stop and a *fricative,* e.g. [j] in *jaw* or [č] in *chair.*

a fortiori Latin for *with stronger reason* or, more loosely, *from firmer ground.* Used of a conclusion or inference that follows logically from an even more compelling chain of logic than one previously accepted as logically sound.

afterdischarge Generally, any neural activity that continues after the stimulus that initiated it has been terminated.

aftereffect Generally, and quite literally, any effect of a stimulus that either exceeds in duration that of the stimulus itself or occurs after the stimulus has been removed.

afterimage A perceptual experience that occurs after the original source of stimulation has been removed. Afterimages (as the name implies) are most readily detected in the visual modality. Various forms of afterimages are known to exist, as the following entries detail.

afterimage, movement MOTION AFTER-EFFECT

afterimage, negative Generally, an *afterimage* with properties antagonistic to those of the original stimulus. Although occasionally the term *complementary* is used for such afterimages (particularly when discussing colour vision), there are doubts that they are true complements; e.g. the afterimages induced from short-wavelength stimuli (blues) are too red compared with the values obtained from colour mixing to be true complements (see the various entries on COLOUR VISION). Negative afterimages are relatively long-lasting, particularly when compared with POSITIVE *AFTERIMAGES.

afterimage, positive An *afterimage* seen immediately after the termination of a visual stimulus which has the same qualitative characteristics as the original. Positive afterimages are fleeting and are best observed when a very brief, very intense light is used and the eye has been thoroughly dark adapted. There are several different such images: HERING AFTERIMAGE, HESS IMAGE, PURKINJE AFTERIMAGE.

agamogenesis **1** Asexual reproduction. **2** Parthenogenesis.

agape love LOVE, AGAPE.

age Unless used with a qualifying term (see following entries) this word should be taken to signify the length of time since the birth of an organism, i.e. its CHRONOLOGICAL *AGE.

age, achievement A measure of achievement given as the average or 'normal' age at which a particular level of performance is reached. The term, although loosely used by many, is really only applicable when age norms have been established for the skills being assessed. Occasionally called *educational age* when school performance is under consideration.

age, anatomical Body development as assessed primarily in terms of skeletal growth and ossification. The most common index is the degree of ossification of the carpal bones in the wrist. See CARPAL *AGE.

age, basal On standardized tests, the highest age level at which *all* test items for that age are passed by an individual.

age, carpal Bone development as determined by the degree of ossification of the carpal (wrist) bones. It is the most common index for assessing ANATOMICAL *AGE.

age, chronological (CA) Simply, AGE, i.e. time since birth. Note, however, that various notational systems are used to mark CA. For children up to 3 or 4 years old CA is generally given in months; from here until adolescence the figure is usually presented in years and months, denoted, for example, as 9–6, standing for 9 years and 6 months; after adolescence the months are generally considered negligible.

age, conception Age as measured from the (estimated) time of conception. Also called *gestational age.*

age, dental An assessment of dental development based upon the number of permanent teeth which have emerged at a particular chronological age relative to the norms for that age.

age, developmental **1** Very generally, any assessment of development expressed in terms of AGE NORMS. **2** A composite assessment of development based upon a combined index of a variety of developmental indices. The term is also used by some authors to refer only to physical, sensory and motor processes and not to the cognitive and intellectual. This distinction is inappropriate and fails to reflect the degree of interaction between these several functions.

age, educational Simply, the grade-level performance of a child as assessed by standardized tests. See ACHIEVEMENT *AGE.

age-equivalent The level or stage of development of any characteristic trait, skill, etc. expressed as relative to what is typical of the average at an equivalent age. For many important developmental variables like physical growth, intelligence, reading skills, etc., age-equivalent scales have been constructed which are used to reflect the level of development of an individual child relative to the norms in the population as a whole.

age-grade scaling The standardizing of educational materials by determining the norms for a population of children who are at the appropriate grade level for their age.

ageism A PREJUDICE based on age, specifically one based on the fact that the individuals discriminated against are elderly.

age, mental (MA) The level of intellectual development as measured by an INTELLIGENCE TEST. In the normal case (i.e. the statistically average case) the MA is equal to the CHRONOLOGICAL *AGE (CA). The concept of a mental age is only meaningful when the testing procedures used are clearly specified and *age-equivalent* scales have been established; it is of little value when dealing with adults. See also INTELLIGENCE QUOTIENT.

agency The state of being an AGENT.

agency detection In evolutionary psychology, the adaptive capacity to detect an AGENT (1). In prey species it aids in detection of predators and other dangerous agents so that evasive or defensive actions can be taken; in predators it enables spotting of prey. Phylogenetically, it is assumed that this capacity evolved early and is widespread among species. It is also hypothesized to lie behind the human tendency to see faces and beings (often ones with religious significance) in clouds, ponds and burnt pieces of toast.

agenesis 1 Lack of reproductive capacity. 2 Complete or partial failure of an organ or organ part to develop properly.

age norm 1 The average score on a standardized test observed in a large, representative sample of children of a particular age. 2 The average age at which particular performances are expected to emerge. Note that the

'expectation' implied in meaning 2 is based upon the empirical scores from meaning 1.

agent 1 An individual or entity (since the term is often used of beings other than humans, see AGENCY DETECTION) that has the capacity to act, to perform, to behave. 2 By extension, an individual who can carry out such functions on behalf of another. 3 By further extension, an individual whose actions are the direct result of personal choice and FREE WILL. 4 The means through which some outcome occurs, as in *infectious agent*. 5 In linguistics, an animate noun, particularly in various theories of grammar.

age, physiological A person's age, in terms of level of physiological development. Although there are no really clear criteria for making such measurements, some rough estimates can be provided on the basis of such factors as hormonal levels, glandular secretions, musculature, neural development, etc.

agerasia Vigorous, healthy appearance in a person of advanced years.

age scale An AGE-EQUIVALENT scale.

age score A score on any standardized test expressed in terms of the age at which the average child achieves that score.

age, test A score on a test that has been standardized for various ages; one for which an AGE-EQUIVALENT scale exists.

ageusia Partial or complete loss of the sense of taste. Usually used with a qualifier to identify the locus of the dysfunction: *central ageusia* is due to a cerebral lesion; *conduction ageusia* to lesions in the afferent pathway; and *peripheral ageusia* to dysfunctions of the taste buds.

agglutination Lit., 'gluing together'. Hence: 1 In physiology a term used in a variety of contexts in which substances (microorganisms, tissues, blood corpuscles, etc.) become clumped by mutual adhesion. 2 In linguistics, a process whereby new words are formed by combining existing words.

aggression An extremely general term used for a wide variety of acts that involve attack, hostility, etc. Typically, it is used for such acts as can be assumed to be motivated by any of the following: (a) fear or frustration;

(b) a desire to produce fear or flight in others; or (c) a tendency to push forward one's own ideas or interests. While this will do as a loose but acceptable definition, it barely touches on the nuances of usage in the psychological literature. Patterns of usage typically reflect some theoretical bias on the part of the writer. For example, ethologists treat aggression as an evolutionarily determined ('instinctive') pattern of reaction to specific stimuli such as invasion of territory or attack upon offspring; those with a Freudian orientation treat it as a conscious manifestation of Thanatos (the hypothesized death instinct); Adler's followers regard it as a display of the will to power, the desire to control others; those who tie together the notions of aggression and frustration define it as any response to a frustrating situation (see FRUSTRATION–AGGRESSION HYPOTHESIS for a discussion); and social-learning theorists view aggressive acts as responses learned through observation and imitation of others and subsequent reinforcement of such behaviour. The point to be emphasized here is that different concepts of aggression play a central role in many theoretical conceptions and, as is so often the case in the social sciences, usage follows theory and no mutually accepted definition can be found. There are many combined phrases also; important ones follow.

aggression, altruistic Aggression that functions to protect others. MATERNAL *AGGRESSION is a good example. See also ALTRUISM.

aggression, angry Generally, the kind of aggression that most think of when the term *aggression* is used, i.e. aggression evoked by frustration or the thwarting of one's goals. Aggression induced by anger.

aggression, anticipatory 1 A counterattack against a predator (PREDATORY *AGGRESSION). 2 An aggressive reaction in defence of one's territory against a potential intruder. See TERRITORIALITY.

aggression, displaced Aggression directed at an organism or object that is not responsible for the factors which initially stimulated the aggressive behaviour. In many cases simple contiguity is sufficient, i.e. the organism or object attacked was simply present when the attacker became aggressive. Other causes are more complex: a person or object may be attacked some time after the initial aggression-causing incident because they are 'safe' and are not likely to counterattack. The term is often used by clinicians as evidence of the action of the defence mechanism of DISPLACEMENT.

aggression, fear-induced Quite literally, aggressive action induced by extreme fear, as when a normally meek animal cornered by a predator suddenly turns on it and attacks.

aggression, induced Aggression which has been artifically aroused. The term is used primarily with respect to an experimental procedure developed for the study of aggressive behaviour. An experimental animal is subjected to conditions of stress (usually unavoidable electric shock) in the presence of another animal or some neutral object. The stressed animal in such a situation will often aggress on the other animal or object. See here DISPLACED *AGGRESSION.

aggression, instrumental 1 Aggressive actions which result from learning experiences; aggression acquired through the action of reinforced responding. 2 An aggressive act that is a means to another end, e.g. shoving someone aside to get out of a room quickly.

aggression, interfemale Aggression between females of a species. Much less common than INTERMALE *AGGRESSION, when it does occur it too appears to be dependent on testosterone.

aggression, intermale Aggression between males of a species. It is observed in some species as the normal reaction of one adult male to any other unfamiliar adult male, in other species it is restricted to mating situations. In all cases, however, it is behaviour that is intimately linked with the hormone testosterone: immature or castrated males do not display this pattern of aggression.

aggression, maternal Any attack-like response of a female when approaches or threatening gestures are made by another towards her offspring.

aggression, predatory Aggression against a natural prey. Note that many do not consider such behaviour true aggression but rather a (necessarily violent) natural food-gathering response. As some have suggested, it is the unfortunate labelling of this behaviour as a form of aggression which has contributed to much of the misunderstanding of the term, including misestimates of how widespread it is.

aggression, prosocial Aggression that has PROSOCIAL motivations, e.g. intervening physically to prevent a rape or attacking someone about to commit a robbery.

aggression, relational The use of a social interaction or relationship to induce emotional harm, sever a relationship or gain an advantage over another person. The classic example is the mother who always asks her married son if he is hungry – implying that his wife is a poor cook. Gossip works well too.

aggression, territorial Aggression displayed specifically in protecting one's territory and defending it against intruders. Occasionally it occurs in anticipation of another violating one's territory; see ANTICIPATORY *AGGRESSION (2). See also TERRITORIALITY.

aggression, weaning A mild form of aggressive response by parents directed against offspring who show resistance to being weaned. Although this is the literal and most common meaning, the term is also used more metaphorically to cover similarly mild attacks on overly dependent offspring independently of the weaning issue.

aggressive 1 adj. of AGGRESSION. Used here with all of the various connotative and theoretically coloured meanings of that term. **2** Vigorous and enthusiastic. This usage is common in medicine, where the phrase 'aggressive treatment' means using all available means to treat a condition. One will also occasionally see similar connotative references to 'aggressive problem-solving', 'aggressively friendly people', etc. See here AGGRESSIVENESS (2).

aggressive character In K. Horney's theory, a personality type marked by a highly competitive and often hostile nature and a desire for material possessions, power and control over others.

aggressive mimicry MIMICRY.

aggressiveness 1 Originally, the displaying of aggression. The tendency to engage in hostile, aggressive acts. By extension:

2 Self-assertiveness; the tendency to work vigorously and perhaps ruthlessly toward the fulfilment of one's aims. **3** The tendency to aim for social dominance, to control the actions and beliefs of others in a group. Note that, depending upon context, the term can be made to carry either rather positive connotations or distinctly negative ones.

aging Growing old. The process of progressive change which occurs with the passage of time, independent of the vagaries of life, the assaults of disease and the random abuses of social living. Physiologically it is a progressive, irreversible process the underlying biochemical aspects of which are extremely complex and largely unknown. var., *ageing*.

agitated depression DEPRESSION, AGITATED.

agitation Restlessness.

agitolalia AGITOPHASIA.

agitophasia Extremely rapid speech with slurring and omission of words. Also called *agitolalia*.

aglossia 1 Lit., lack of a tongue. **2** By extension, complete lack of articulate speech.

agnosia Lit., not knowing. Thus, a defect in recognition. Generally, an agnosic can sense objects and forms but is unable consciously to recognize and interpret their meaning. Agnosia is the result of neurological pathology and can be manifested in almost any perceptual/cognitive system. Various special forms follow, others are listed under their appropriate alphabetic listing (e.g. *prosopagnosia*).

agnosia, apperceptive An AGNOSIA in which recognition failure is due to an impairment in visual perception. Although patients have relatively normal acuity, they fail to recognize objects normally because they have impaired object and shape recognition. Contrast with ASSOCIATIVE *AGNOSIA.

agnosia, associative A visual AGNOSIA in which recognition failure is due to factors other than the modality-specific deficits that cause APPERCEPTIVE *AGNOSIA. Patients' perceptions are normal and they can draw objects and identify them using other modalities. But visually patients' percepts are, in H. L. Teuber's telling phrase, 'stripped of their meaning'.

agnosia, auditory Inability to recognize sounds despite the patient having normal auditory function. When the problem is with the recognition of meaningful non-speech sounds, the disorder is called *auditory sound agnosia*; when it involves speech, it is called *pure word deafness*. See AUDITORY *APHASIA.

agnosia, auditory sound AUDITORY *AGNOSIA.

agnosia, finger TACTILE *AGNOSIA.

agnosia, ideational Faulty recognition or interpretation of symbols.

agnosia, landmark A form of AGNOSIA in which the patient cannot recognize stable objects in the environment such as buildings, markets and houses. They typically can describe them in detail but do not recognize them. Also called *environmental agnosia*.

agnosia, motion A form of AGNOSIA marked by an inability to interpret motion properly. Often caused by lesions in V5, patients see motion of objects as a series of static displays rather than as smooth movement.

agnosia, tactile Inability to recognize or interpret objects by touch. Also called *tactoagnosia*. A special form in which the patient cannot name or identify the fingers is called *finger agnosia*.

agnosia, visual Inability to recognize or interpret objects in the visual field. Typically, touching the object brings immediate awareness of its identity. Also known by a host of terms including *visual object agnosia, visual form agnosia* and, in older texts, *optic agnosia*.

agnosia, visuo-spatial A form of AGNOSIA in which objects in the visual field can be identified correctly but the spatial relationships between them are impaired.

agonism, drug A set of circumstances where one drug acts to enhance or facilitate the actions of another drug. An agonistic effect may be produced in any of several ways. The one drug may mimic the effects of the other, it may act to interfere with the process of deactivation of the other, it may encourage retention of the other drug by the body, etc. See and contrast with the various forms of DRUG *ANTAGONISM.

agonist 1 A muscle that contracts and operates in opposition to another, its antagonist; when bending the elbow, for example, the biceps is the agonist, the triceps the antagonist. See here ANTAGONISTIC MUSCLES. **2** Any drug that is part of a DRUG *AGONISM.

agoraphobia Generally, a fear of open spaces. Agoraphobia is the most commonly cited phobic disorder of those persons who seek psychiatric or psychological treatment. It has a variety of manifestations, the most common being a deep fear of being caught alone in some public place (indeed, this is regarded by some authorities as the defining feature of the disorder). When placed in threatening situations agoraphobics may experience panic attacks. See PANIC DISORDERS.

agrammatism The loss of grammatical speech. The patient usually has a full vocabulary but is incapable of ordering words grammatically. Usually due to a cerebral disorder, it is sometimes a symptom of certain functional disorders.

agraphia Partial or complete loss of writing ability due to cerebral pathology, an analogue of MOTOR *APHASIA. Several special forms are often noted – see below.

agraphia, deep Similar to PHONOLOGICAL *AGRAPHIA but the patient also manifests difficulties with semantics.

agraphia, lexical A rather specific form of AGRAPHIA in which the patient can spell but relies almost entirely on standard sound-to-letter patterns, resulting in misspellings of irregular words; e.g. *cough* comes out as 'cawf'. The disorder is more disruptive for patients who write in languages like English and French as opposed to more strictly phonetic ones like Spanish.

agraphia, phonological An AGRAPHIA characterized by difficulties in spelling nonwords and unfamiliar words.

agreeableness The broad personality disposition that influences how an individual values cooperation, harmony and consideration for others.

agrypnia An occasional synonym for INSOMNIA.

a-ha experience A term used to describe the feeling that accompanies the moment of insight, that instant when the various disparate aspects of a problem-solving situation suddenly fit together to yield the solution.

ahedonia ANHEDONIA.

ahistorical General term for any approach to behaviour which stresses the role of contemporary circumstances and places little or no emphasis upon earlier events and circumstances as causes of present behaviours. *Behaviourism* is an example of an approach that leans toward the ahistorical, particularly when it is applied to clinical situations. Thus the term is used as a label to distinguish such approaches from those that are strongly historical, such as the classical psychoanalytic theories. Note, however, that no coherent psychological theory can take a totally ahistorical perspective; e.g. even a 'pure' behaviour therapist usually needs some understanding of the conditions under which a particular maladaptive behaviour pattern was acquired in order to develop a useful behaviour-modification programme.

ahypnia INSOMNIA.

ahypnosia INSOMNIA.

AI ARTIFICIAL INTELLIGENCE.

AIDS dementia DEMENTIA, AIDS.

aim **1** A goal or goal state toward which behaviour is orientated. This usage generally carries the connotation of VOLITION; successful completion of a piece of work may be an aim; one may even speak of a rat's finding the food in a maze as an aim. Nonvoluntary, reflexive actions, even though they may accomplish some purpose, are not regarded as embodying aims. **2** A symbolic thought, an image or an idea that represents the end point of directed behaviour. Here, aim is a mentalistic term and, unlike meaning 1, is used to characterize the internal state of the organism and not the external environment. **3** In psychoanalytic theory, the 'end product' of behaviour. The distinction is made here between the actual person, object, event or behaviour which serves as the end product in the outside world that the individual seeks (the so-called *external aim*), and the gratifying psychic state of the organism experienced when the external aim is achieved (the *internal aim*).

aim-inhibited A psychoanalytic term characterizing an action or a relationship in which there is no conscious recognition of the underlying motive or drive. The term is most commonly used to refer to inhibitions of the erotic or sexual component in social relationships and friendships.

air sickness MOTION SICKNESS.

air swallowing AEROPHAGIA.

AJ The initials of a woman whose memory is so extraordinary that it gave rise to the term HYPERTHYMESTIC SYNDROME. AJ can recall virtually every day of her life with astonishing detail including the day of the week it fell on, the weather, what she did, what others did, the news events of the day, etc. Her memory is unique and different in important ways from another famous subject 'S', whose feats were dependent on the use of mnemonic devices.

akatamathesia **1** Generally, loss of the ability to comprehend. **2** Specifically, loss of the ability to understand spoken language. var , *acatamathesia*.

akathisia Inability or, more accurately, extreme unwillingness to sit down. The disorder is characterized by extreme restlessness and agitation, and even the thought of sitting down causes anxiety. The syndrome is associated with some antipsychotic drugs and occurs as an occasional side effect of the phenothiazine derivatives. var., *acathisia*.

akinaesthesia Partial or complete loss of kinaesthesis. See KINAESTHETICS. var., *akinesthesia*.

akinesia Partial or complete loss of motor control; a term usually used to refer to voluntary muscle movements only.

akinetic apraxia APRAXIA, AKINETIC.

akinetic mutism A motor disorder characterized by lack of movement and speech that can result from lesions to the cingulate gyrus.

akinetopsia A loss of the ability to perceive motion.

AL ADAPTATION LEVEL.

alallia Generally, loss of ability to speak. Some authors use the term only for *functional* disorders, reserving APHASIA for those with organic origins; others use it more broadly to cover various syndromes due to psychic, anatomical and/or cerebral pathologies.

alarm reaction The first stage in the GEN-ERAL ADAPTATION SYNDROME.

albedo The reflectance of any surface; specifically, the percentage of light that is reflected by a surface measured against the total light falling on that surface.

albedo perception Quite literally, perceiving the ALBEDO. That is, using the ratio of reflected light to incident light as the primary cue for perceiving the brightness of stimuli. Since the albedos of, say, a piece of chalk and a piece of coal will be the same as the incident illumination is increased or decreased, the perceived brightnesses of the two will remain constant. Hence, albedo perception is the basis of *brightness constancy*.

albinism A category of pigment disorders characterized by a less-than-normal production of melanin in the skin. Although the term is often used as though it represents a single syndrome, in reality over a dozen varieties have been identified. *Albino* is used to designate an individual with albinism.

albino ALBINISM.

alcohol abuse A general label for any pathological syndrome associated with excessive alcohol use. A variety of characteristics are found in serious cases, including a daily need for alcohol, continuing consumption in the face of physical disorders which are exacerbated by alcohol, 'blackouts' or periods of amnesia, extended alcoholic 'binges' lasting several days, repeated but unsuccessful attempts to quit drinking, and overall mental and emotional deterioration. In modern psychiatric writings the term is used in a manner roughly equivalent to meaning (1) of the more common term ALCO-HOLISM. It is classified as a *substance use disorder* – see SUBSTANCE-RELATED DISORDER – although many of the complications that occur with extended abuse of alcohol (e.g. ALCOHOL AMNESTIC DISORDER and ALCOHOL WITH-DRAWAL DELIRIUM) are regarded as ORGANIC MEN-TAL DISORDERS.

alcohol amnestic disorder Memory impairment associated with prolonged, excessive consumption of alcohol. Also

known as KORSAKOFF'S SYNDROME. See also AMNESTIC SYNDROME.

alcohol dependence Alcohol is a drug and the discussion under DRUG *DEPENDENCE applies to this term.

alcohol hallucinosis A syndrome of vivid auditory hallucinations following the sudden cessation of alcohol intake after an extended history of alcohol abuse.

alcoholic 1 adj. Pertaining to alcohol. **2** n. One who has any of a variety of disorders associated with excessive alcohol consumption. See here ALCOHOL ABUSE.

alcoholic dementia KORSAKOFF'S SYNDROME.

alcoholic jealousy An irrational, paranoid-like jealousy often observed in cases of chronic ALCOHOL ABUSE.

alcoholic psychosis A general term used to cover the serious, disabling outcome of excessive, chronic ALCOHOL ABUSE.

alcohol intolerance See ALDEHYDE DEHYDRO-GENASE.

alcohol intoxication A loose term used to cover any state marked by erratic, maladaptive behaviour and impaired judgement resulting from consumption of alcohol. The criteria determining intoxication are usually arrived at on the basis of blood-alcohol levels and/or specific sensory and motor tests. In many locales the term carries legal implications in that various behaviours such as driving a car or piloting a plane with a blood-alcohol level above some specified threshold is a crime.

alcohol intoxication, idiosyncratic ALCO-HOL INTOXICATION with its accompanying change in mood and behaviour following ingestion of an amount of alcohol too small to produce the condition in most people. Note that in the *DSM-IV* it is no longer recognized as a separate disorder. Also called *pathological intoxication*.

alcoholism 1 The personality and behavioural syndrome characteristic of a person who abuses alcohol. See ALCOHOL ABUSE. **2** The actual state or condition of one who habitually consumes excessive amounts of alcohol.

alcoholism, acute A severe case of ALCOHOL

INTOXICATION. The qualifier 'acute' denotes single, short-lived episodes as well as severity. Compare with CHRONIC *ALCOHOLISM.

alcoholism, chronic Long-term ALCOHOL ABUSE.

alcohol withdrawal An ORGANIC MENTAL DISORDER characterized by coarse tremor of the hands, eyelids and tongue, nausea, weakness, sweating, depressed mood, anxiety and irritability. It follows, usually within a few hours, cessation of alcohol intake in an individual who has been drinking for several days or longer. This disorder is often called 'uncomplicated' to distinguish it from cases in which *delirium* is one of the symptoms.

alcohol withdrawal delirium Delirium resulting from sudden cessation of alcohol intake following an extended period of ALCOHOL ABUSE. Typical symptoms are hallucinations (usually visual), rapid and irregular heartbeat, agitation, tremors, sweating and high blood pressure. See also DELIRIUM TREMENS.

aldehyde dehydrogenase An enzyme that converts acetaldehyde into acetate and assists in the metabolism of alcohol (ethanol). Those who inherit genes that code for a deficient form of the enzyme display *alcohol intolerance*, an allergic-like reaction to alcohol marked by flushing, nasal congestion and occasionally nausea. This syndrome, found most commonly in those of East Asian extraction, is associated with lower incidence of alcohol abuse.

aldosterone A hormone produced by the adrenal cortices. It helps regulate metabolism by causing the retention of sodium by the kidneys.

alethia Lit., inability to forget. Perhaps, in its own way, a more debilitating disorder than might be supposed.

alexia Lit., without words. A language-related disability characterized by partial or complete loss of the ability to identify the printed word. The disorder is often quite specific in that alexics do not have impairment of vision and can identify spoken words normally. Sometimes called *word blindness* and *visual aphasia*. Different forms of alexia have been identified and a variety of names introduced to distinguish them. Those in common use follow. A careful reading, however, suggests that many of these distinctions are less than clear and the evidence for each as a separate form of the disorder is not always compelling. Use with care.

alexia, deep A form of ALEXIA, arguably a subcategory of PHONOLOGICAL *ALEXIA, but with additional symptoms such as confusing words of similar meanings (e.g. reading 'stool' as 'chair' or 'sand' as 'beach') and having difficulty with abstract words (e.g. 'sin', 'patriotic').

alexia, phonological A form of ALEXIA characterized by difficulty in using phonological principles in reading. Patients have problems reading made-up words (e.g. 'clishy') and with unfamiliar words that do not follow normal phonological patterns (e.g. 'gnostic'). Some authorities argue that the underlying dysfunction here is the same as that seen in DEEP *ALEXIA; others are not so sure.

alexia, pure A rather crystallized form of ALEXIA, sufferers of which can still write but cannot read; indeed, they cannot even read what they themselves have just written.

alexia, surface A form of ALEXIA characterized by difficulty in reading words with irregular spellings such as 'yacht' or 'cough'. The patients try to sound them out and 'yacht' comes out as 'yah-chu-tuh'. Distinguish from PHONOLOGICAL *ALEXIA where the ability to sound things out is lost.

alexithymia A disruption in both *affective* and *cognitive* processes. It is not treated as a 'true' psychiatric syndrome but rather as a general characterization of a number of traits which are often seen together in a variety of disorders, including those with psychosomatic origins and some addictions and drug-dependency disorders. Typically the alexithymic person has relatively undifferentiated emotions and thoughts and tends to dwell excessively on the mundane.

algedonic Relating to the pleasantness–unpleasantness or the pleasure–pain dimensions of experience.

algesia Of, or referring to, pain or the pain sense, specifically the capacity for the experiencing of pain. Occasionally used to denote a heightened sensitivity to pain, although most authors prefer *hyperesthesia* for this condition. var., *algesis*. ant., *analgesia*.

algesimetre Any device for measuring sensitivity to pain. A variety of such devices exist, ranging from the pressing of finely calibrated needles on the skin to the presentation of controlled amounts of radiant energy to a small spot on the skin. In all cases, the basic data are the subject's reports of subjective experience.

algethesia The subjective experiencing of pain.

algethesis The sense of pain. However, to appreciate that there is more than a single sensory system involved in the experience of pain, see PAIN et seq.

-algia Combining form meaning *pain*.

alg(o)- Combining form meaning *pain*.

algolagnia Lit., pain-lust. Hence, the arousal of sexual feelings through pain. The term is occasionally used as a cover for both SADISM and MASOCHISM.

algophilia Lit., a liking for pain. An occasional synonym for MASOCHISM.

algorithm A method or procedure for solving a particular problem that is guaranteed to lead, eventually, to the solution. In some instances usable algorithms exist, such as those for performing long division, solving linear equations, etc. In many cases, however, they either do not exist (e.g. proving most mathematical theorems) or they are so inefficient as to be of no practical value (e.g. finding the optimum move in a chess game). Contrast with HEURISTIC, where the search for the solution is directed and not guaranteed.

ALI defence (ruling) The American Law Institute standard for the defence of legal insanity. It specifies that the individual's behaviour must be a consequence of a mental disorder that rendered the person either (a) incapable of realizing the moral status and consequences of his or her actions or (b) incapable of controlling or inhibiting his or her own actions. Cases with a diagnosed ANTISOCIAL PERSONALITY DISORDER are specifically excluded. See also INSANITY DEFENCE.

alienation 1 Most contemporary usage reflects the standard dictionary meanings: a feeling of strangeness or separation from others; a sense of a lack of warm relations with others. **2** Existentialists, however, have made the term a central construct in their psychology and appended a subtle but important meaning to the above. Rather than concentrating solely upon alienation of one human from others, they also stress the alienation of a person from him- or herself. This separation of the individual from the presumed 'real' or 'deeper' self is assumed to result from preoccupation with conformity, the wishes of others, the pressures from social institutions, and other 'outer-directed' motivations. **3** An antiquated term for any progressive psychosis.

alienation, coefficient of A measure of the degree of departure of an empirical correlation from 1.0 (or perfect correlation). The coefficient, usually denoted as k, is given by $\sqrt{(1-r^2)}$, where r is the observed correlation. As $r \to 1.0$, $k \to 0$. Hence, k can be used as a measure of prediction error of one variable in the correlation, given the known values of the other.

alien hand syndrome A neurological disorder, usually associated with medial frontal lobe lesions, in which the patient's hand is sensed as either acting under its own volition or is perceived as being 'foreign' or 'alien'.

alienist An obsolete term once common in forensic work for a physician (usually but not necessarily a psychiatrist), who can testify in court on the competence (or lack thereof) of persons who are parties to a legal case.

alien limb syndrome A neurological condition, seen most often in cases of NEGLECT, in which the patient fails to recognize, and may even deny the existence of, one of his or her own limbs. Distinguish from PHANTOM LIMB.

aliment A PIAGETIAN term used to refer to a new object which a child incorporates into its existing schema. The root of the word is Latin and the literal meaning is 'nourishment' or 'food'. Piaget's use is metaphorical but intuitively appropriate.

alimentary canal (or tract) The system of organs comprising a tubular passage from mouth to anus that serves digestive functions. It includes the mouth, pharynx, oesophagus, stomach, small and large intestines, and the rectum.

all- Prefix meaning different, other or alternative.

allachaesthesia ALLAESTHESIA (1).

allaesthesia 1 Generally, sensing the location of a touch stimulus at a point other than where the stimulus was actually applied. Also called *allachaesthesia* and *allochaesthesia*. **2** Specifically, such a sensation referred from one limb to the other. Also called *allochiria* and *allocheiria*. var., *allesthesia*.

Allais's paradox Named after its original descriptor, Maurice Allais, it is one of several economic problems where people display risk-averse behaviour and make choices not predicted by classical economic theory. See PROSPECT THEORY for more detail.

allele (*al-leel*) One of the two (or more) different forms of a given gene. The term *allelemorph* is often used to mean the same thing, and alleles are said to be in an *allelemorphic relationship* with each other.

allelotropia In vision, the apparent shifting in lateral position of an element in the visual field when a similar element is presented to a disparate position in the other eye. Also called *displacement*.

alliaesthesia Shifts in the pleasantness or unpleasantness of a stimulus depending on internal stimuli. var., *alliesthesia*.

allo- Prefix denoting: **1** *Outside of* or *away from*, often with the connotation of 'away from one's self'. **2** In linguistics, one member of a group of forms all of which taken together constitute a linguistic unit. See here ALLOMORPH, ALLOPHONE.

allocator In a GAME, the individual who makes the initial offer.

allocentric Outside the self. Occasionally used of the senses of vision and audition.

allocentrism An approach to social situations and personal relationships characterized by thought and action that emphasizes the larger interests of one's groups. Contrast with IDIOCENTRISM and see COLLECTIVISM.

allochaesthesia ALLAESTHESIA (1).

allocheiria ALLAESTHESIA (2).

allochiria ALLAESTHESIA (2).

allochthonous Characteristic of or referring to events originating from outside the organism or the self. Compare with AUTOCHTHONOUS.

alloeroticism The focusing of sexuality toward others, the opposite of *autoeroticism*. var., *alloerotism*.

alloerotism ALLOEROTICISM.

allokinesis Movement on the opposite side of the body to that intended.

allomorph One of two or more linguistic forms that have the same meaning but differ in their form. For example, the prefixes *in-*, *il-*, *im-* and *ir-* are all allomorphic variations of a single morpheme meaning 'not', as in *invalid*, *illiterate*, *improper* and *irrespective*.

allomorphic 1 Generally, characteristic of or pertaining to the changing of the outward or superficial form of something while leaving the basic underlying character unchanged. **2** Specifically, characteristic of an ALLOMORPH.

allophone One of two or more elementary sounds in a particular language that differ in acoustic or articulatory properties but without conveying any difference in meaning. For example, the [p] in *pin* is accompanied by a distinct puff of air while the [p] in *spin* is not. Nevertheless, speakers of English treat them as the same sound: the acoustic difference does not signal a semantic distinction. These two 'p's' are said to be allophonic variations of the single PHONEME /p/.

alloplasty 1 Generally, a process of adaptation whereby modifications in the outside world are made. Alloplastic changes are changes in the external environment. **2** In psychoanalysis, the process of adjusting to the outside world in which the libido turns from self toward environmental objects and persons. Contrast with AUTOPLASTY.

allopsychic Descriptive of psychic processes in which the primary reference point is in the external world; e.g. *projection* is considered to be an allopsychic process. Contrast with AUTOPSYCHIC.

all-or-none law 1 In neurophysiology, the principle that any neuron propagates its characteristic neural impulse at full strength or not at all. See also RATE LAW. **2** In learning, the principle that associations either are formed completely on a single trial or are not formed at all. Contrast this usage with the notion expressed by the term CONTINUITY THEORY. See also ALL-OR-NONE *LEARNING.

all-or-none learning LEARNING, ALL-OR-NONE.

allospecific In ethology, an organism from a species distinct form the organism under consideration. Compare with CONSPECIFIC.

allostasis Literally, outside of a static condition. Used in the neuroclinical literature to refer to situations where stress factors (often called *allostatic load*) increase and disturb the body's natural balance. Factors may be internal (medical conditions) or external (social isolation, a high stress environment), although the two sources invariably interact.

allostatic load ALLOSTASIS.

allotriophagy Lit., strange eating. See e.g. PICA.

allotropic Lit., other-directed. Characterizing persons who are not self-centred, who are concerned with the well-being of others.

all-trans retinal RHODOPSIN.

alogia 1 An occasional synonym for APHASIA. **2** A condition marked by speech that is dramatically reduced in amount or content (or both). Here the patient is not really aphasic but appears instead to be suffering from a thought disorder.

alopecia Baldness.

alpha (α) adrenoreceptors Receptors that bind epinephrine and norepinephrine, with a higher affinity for the latter. Found on many cell types, when activated they increase heart rate, cause pupil dilation, mobilize the body and divert blood to skeletal muscle. See also BETA ADRENORECEPTORS.

alpha (α) blocker A class of drugs that block the uptake of norepinephrine and epinephrine at ALPHA ADRENORECEPTORS. They are used primarily as vasodilators.

alphabet Most simplistically, the sequence of symbols (A, B, C,...) used to express a language in written form. But buried beneath this simple notion, as the study of reading is beginning to make clear, is a sublime richness and depth. Alphabets are, historically, the most recent of all writing systems (see ORTHOGRAPHY). Unlike others such as SEMASIO-

GRAPHIES and LOGOGRAPHIES, they operate by representing the sound patterns of spoken language in visual form and thereby achieve maximum flexibility. Unlike SYLLABARIES, however, which also represent sounds, alphabets code the underlying abstract phonemic elements of a language. Interestingly, the alphabet was invented but once, in ancient Greece, as a derivation from the Phoenician syllabary, and *all* existing alphabetic writing systems share this single common ancestor. For more on this matter and contemporary terminology see READING.

alpha blocking See ALPHA SUPPRESSION.

alpha error ERROR (TYPE I and TYPE II).

alpha female ALPHA MALE.

alpha level SIGNIFICANCE LEVEL.

alpha male In ethology, a term used to designate the male at the top of a DOMINANCE HIERARCHY of a troop. Note that in several species an alpha female functions as the dominant female of the hierarchy.

alpha motion MOTION, ALPHA.

alpha response In classical eyelid conditioning, a rapid, low-amplitude response that is assumed to be an unconditioned response that develops as a result of sensitization during training. Contrast with BETA RESPONSE.

alpha rhythm (or wave) The pattern of electrical activity of the brain characteristic of a normal awake but relaxed person. The typical alpha wave is between, roughly, 8 and 12 Hz.

alpha suppression A change in the alpha rhythm of an ELECTROENCEPHALOGRAM resulting from any shift away from normal waking relaxation. Alpha rhythms may be 'suppressed' (or blocked) by the person orienting toward a stimulus such as a sound or light, by a state of apprehension or anxiety, or by a mental activity such as performing multiplication covertly.

alprazolam One of the BENZODIAZEPINES used as an ANTIANXIETY DRUG. It is one of the most rapidly acting drugs in this group, reaching peak effect within 20 to 30 minutes. Trade name Xanax.

alt Abbreviation for *alternative, alternate* or *alternating*.

altered state of consciousness Roughly, any psychological state in which emotions, perceptions, sense of self and sense of the reality around one are modified in some way so that one's CONSCIOUSNESS is experienced as distinct from a normal, waking state. A very tricky term indeed. It is used by some in a straightforward manner to refer to states induced by modifications in biological and neurological functioning such as those due to psychotropic drugs or other conditions like oxygen deprivation. Others use it for states of adjusted awareness that result from such activities as meditation, hypnosis or sensory deprivation. Still others use it for religious and mystical experiences that have elements of boundlessness or a feeling of oneness with the universe. Those who lean toward the latter two patterns of use often refer to these as 'higher' states of consciousness, with the connotation that they bring one closer to a state of transcendence or enlightenment. Those who take the more hard-nosed scientific stance reflective of the first pattern of use eschew such subjectivity and approach altered psychological states as topics for empirical and theoretical exploration. We recommend keeping in mind that the fact that all states of consciousness have a neurochemical base does not detract from the compelling, personal meaning the altered forms have for those who experience them.

alter ego A nontechnical term for a person so close to oneself that he or she seems to be a 'second self'.

alternate forms COMPARABLE *FORMS.

alternate forms reliability RELIABILITY, ALTERNATE FORMS.

alternating personality MULTIPLE PERSONALITY.

alternating perspective The shift in PERSPECTIVE that occurs when one fixates on a particular stimulus for a period of time. See the example of the Necker cube under REVERSIBLE *FIGURE to experience the effect. See BISTABLE PERCEPT.

alternating vision VISION, ALTERNATING.

alternation hypothesis In EYEWITNESS TESTIMONY, the hypothesis that misleading or false information, often introduced by questions asked of the witness after the event, contaminate the individual's memory and diminish accuracy of recall.

alternative hypothesis NULL *HYPOTHESIS.

alternative medicine An umbrella term for a variety of 'marginal' forms of the practice of medicine. Included are such nontraditional methods as acupuncture, massage therapies, homeopathy and the like.

alternative schedule SCHEDULES OF *REINFORCEMENT.

alternative therapies See INNOVATIVE THERAPIES.

altitudinal neglect See NEGLECT.

altricial Pertaining to species helpless at birth and dependent on parental care for survival. ant., PRECOCIAL.

altruism 1 The elevation of the welfare, happiness, interests or even the survival of others above one's own. **2** Behaving so as to increase the safety, interests or life of others while simultaneously jeopardizing one's own. Meaning 1 is the more general and more common: it denotes a principle as well as a practice. It is also the meaning favoured in contemporary ethology and evolutionary psychology, although here the term is restricted to circumstances in which the behaviour benefits neither the individual nor his or her own direct offspring. Meaning 2 introduces an interesting subtlety in that many species engage in what seem to be altruistic behaviours, although, from the ethological point of view, they are not. For example, in *kin-selection altruism* one acts in a manner that jeopardizes one's safety but protects or promotes that of one's own kin, hence the behaviour is arguably in one's own interests in that it increases the likelihood of the survival of one's own genes (see SELFISH GENE). Similarly, in *reciprocal altruism* the actions are often based on the notion that today's giver of supportive acts will be tomorrow's receiver. Distinguish from HELPING BEHAVIOUR, in which there is no risk involved.

altruism, reciprocal R. Trivers's term for what is best summed up by the golden rule 'Do unto others as you would have them do unto you.' The term is used primarily in EVO-LUTIONARY PSYCHOLOGY and SOCIOBIOLOGY, where a genetic basis for the behaviour is the focus of research. See also ALTRUISM.

altruistic aggression AGGRESSION, ALTRUISTIC.

altruistic suicide SUICIDE, ALTRUISTIC.

alveolar A speech sound produced by placing the tip or blade of the tongue against the ALVEOLAR RIDGE, e.g. /t/ in *tap*, /n/ in *nap*.

alveolar ridge The hard ridge of the upper gums just behind the upper teeth.

Alzheimer's disease (AD) A progressive form of dementia characterized by the gradual deterioration of intellectual abilities such as memory, judgement, the capacity for abstract thought, and other higher-level cortical functions as well as by changes in personality and behaviour. It is of insidious onset, most commonly after age 65; cases of early onset (before age 50) are rare. When it occurs after age 65 it is often referred to as *senile dementia of the Alzheimer's type (SDAT)*. In the early stages memory impairments and subtle personality changes may be the only symptoms; with progression to later stages the various cognitive and behavioural changes become apparent; in the terminal stages the patient becomes totally mute and inattentive and unable to care for him or herself. Although the atrophy of the brain and accompanying AMYLOID PLAQUES that characterize the disease can sometimes be detected by a CAT-scan (see COMPUTER AXIAL TOMOGRAPHY) or MRI (MAGNETIC RESONANCE IMAGING), it is generally diagnosed by exclusion; that is, after all other possible causes for the mental deterioration have been excluded. Recent evidence suggests that the disorder has a genetic basis, particularly in cases of early onset; the term *familial AD* is used when this is the suspected form.

amacrine cells Cells in the retina that link ganglion cells with the bipolar cells.

amaurosis Generally, complete loss of vision occurring with no evidence of any pathological condition in the eye itself. Various forms are noted and usually qualified so that the cause is apparent, e.g. *diabetic amaurosis*, *lead amaurosis*.

amaurosis, fugax A form of monocular amaurosis caused by a *transient ischemic attack*. It is usually described as a kind of grey opaque film coming down over the affected eye.

amaurotic (familial) idiocy A general term for a group of related, genetically transmitted diseases all of which are marked by retardation and vision deficits and produced by faulty metabolism.

amaurotic (familial) idiocy, infantile TAY-SACH'S DISEASE.

ambi- Prefix meaning *both*, usually with the connotation of equality of the two things under consideration, e.g. *ambidextrous*.

ambidextrous 1 Lit., equally skilled in the use of both hands. **2** More loosely, having no hand preference.

ambiguity Having two or more meanings or interpretations; a characteristic of a stimulus, statement or situation that permits more than one reading. In a very real sense all things are ambiguous to some extent. Typically, however, context, one's previous learning, and general perceptual and cognitive factors constrain the situation so that one interpretation overwhelms the others that could possibly be made. Most of the interest in psychology has concerned stimulus situations in which the constraints are loose enough for the potential multiple meanings to emerge, e.g. *projective tests*, *ambiguous figures*.

ambiguity, tolerance of A dimension representing the degree to which one is able to tolerate lack of clarity in a situation or in a stimulus. To some extent no one is fond of being continuously confronted with ambiguous situations. However, this term is typically used to denote an underlying personality dimension when the primary interest is in the pole of 'intolerance', characterized by those persons who have a great deal of difficulty in tolerating even mildly ambiguous circumstances. Such individuals tend to react with anxiety and withdrawal from uncertain situations and such a pattern of behaviour has been hypothesized to be an aspect of the *authoritarian personality*.

ambiguous figure FIGURE, AMBIGUOUS.

ambisexual Characterizing that which displays no sex or gender dominance. The term is used most often to designate traits or characteristics which are found equally in both sexes. See here SEX DIFFERENCES. Distinguish from ASEXUAL; also BISEXUAL (especially meaning 4).

ambivalence 1 Having simultaneous, contrasting or mixed feelings about some person, object or idea. **2** A tendency to 'flip-flop' one's feelings or attitudes about a person, object or idea. This sense presupposes meaning 1. **3** A state in which one is pulled in two mutually exclusive directions or towards two opposite goals. This meaning derived originally from K. Lewin's work in *field theory* and shows up most clearly in the research on behavioural reactions to various forms of CONFLICT.

ambivalent/resistant   **attachment** ATTACHMENT STYLES.

ambivert One who achieves a balance between INTROVERSION and EXTRAVERSION; such a person is said to tend toward *ambiversion*.

ambly- A combining form from the Greek meaning *dull*. Used generally to denote deficiency or dysfunction.

amblyacousia A general term for any hearing deficit.

amblyaphia A diminished sense of touch.

amblygeustia Dulled or deficient sense of taste.

amblyopia A nonorganic, permanent loss of vision, particularly spatial vision. It is typically caused by disorders that affect the degree of coordination between the two eyes such as different refractive errors in the two eyes, misalignment of the eyes, different degrees of *astigmatism*, or *strabismus*. In layman's terms, *lazy eye*.

ambulatory 1 Able to walk. **2** Not requiring confinement. These two uses do not necessarily entail each other and are used distinctly.

ameliorate To improve. Used particularly with respect to improvement in diseases, dysfunctions or other conditions.

amenorrhoea   Absence of menstrual period. Compare with DYSMENORRHOEA var., *amenorrhea*.

amentia Generally, any serious mental deficiency. The term is rarely used today.

American College Testing Program (ACT) A test of academic potential in wide use in the United States. It is designed to aid in the evaluation of applicants to colleges and universities and is the primary competitor of the Scholastic Aptitude Test (SAT), the most widely used of such tests in North America. ACT consists of four subtests in English, mathematics, natural sciences and social sciences, the scores of which are combined to give a composite score. The tests are primarily achievement-oriented and were designed to evaluate how well students can apply already developed skills and acquired knowledge.

American Sign Language (ASL) The system of gestures, hand signals and finger spelling used by the deaf in North America (and other English-speaking locales). Also called *Ameslan*.

Ameslan A contraction of **American Sign Language**.

Ames room A specially constructed room designed by the artist/psychologist Adelbert Ames which provides a striking demonstration of the cues for depth perception. The room is of distorted construction: three of the walls are actually trapezoidal and the ceiling slants markedly. However, because of the use of the cues of shading, linear perspective and interposition, the room appears normal to an outside observer. Looking into the room produces many illusions: objects and persons appear distorted, particularly in their apparent size, round objects seem to roll uphill, etc. See also TRANSACTIONAL THEORY (OF PERCEPTION), the point of view that Ames argued for.

ametropia General term for any refractive deficit in the eye, e.g. *hyperopia, myopia, astigmatism*.

amimia Partial or complete loss of the ability to express oneself with gestures or signs.

amine Any of a large group of organic compounds of nitrogen. The ones of primary interest in psychology are the BIOGENIC AMINES.

amine transmitters BIOGENIC AMINES.

amino acid Any of a large group of organic compounds marked by the presence of both an *amino group* and a *carboxyl group*. They are linked by peptide bonds to form proteins. Over 20 different amino acids are known to be necessary as sources of energy for proper metabolism and growth, and several either are precursors of neurotransmitters or function as transmitter substances themselves. See here GAMMA-AMINOBUTYRIC ACID (GABA), GLUTAMIC ACID, GLYCINE.

amitriptyline An ANTIDEPRESSANT DRUG that is an effective serotonin agonist. It is a TRICYCLIC COMPOUND and, like other drugs in this group, has significant side effects. Its current use is largely limited to pain management and the treatment of migraines.

Ammon's horn HIPPOCAMPUS.

amnesia Any partial or complete loss of memory sufficiently serious to cause difficulty in functioning. A host of AMNESTIC DISORDERS are recognized based on the origins of the disorder (e.g. POST-ENCEPHALIC *AMNESIA), its known or suspected causes (e.g. TEMPORAL LOBE *AMNESIA), its temporal features (e.g. ANTEROGRADE *AMNESIA) and whether the condition is the result of normal developmental changes (INFANTILE *AMNESIA), neurological factors (TRANSIENT GLOBAL *AMNESIA) or those with a more psychological cause (DISSOCIATIVE *AMNESIA).

amnesia, anterograde Loss of memory of events and experiences occurring subsequent to the amnesia-causing trauma. In a case of complete anterograde amnesia the patient is incapable of forming new memories, although recall of material learned prior to onset is largely unaffected. Most cases are the result of damage in the medial temporal lobes, most often in the HIPPOCAMPAL FORMATION. Compare with RETROGRADE *AMNESIA. Note also that the memory loss is only for explicit or consciously held memories. IMPLICIT *MEMORY and IMPLICIT *LEARNING functions are preserved.

amnesiac One suffering from AMNESIA. The shortened form *amnesic* is also found.

amnesia, dissociative An inability to recall important personal information resulting from a traumatic or stressful experience; despite appearing as a disorder of memory, it is regarded as a DISSOCIATIVE DISORDER.

amnesia, episodic A 'hole' in one's memory; loss of information about isolated events or episodes. Also called *lacunar amnesia* or *catathymic amnesia*.

amnesia, functional Any amnesia that occurs in the absence of any known neurological damage; a psychogenic amnesia. Some functional amnesias are nonpathological, such as the inability to remember one's dreams or INFANTILE *AMNESIA. Others are signs of psychopathological disorders such as FUGUE states.

amnesia, global Complete AMNESIA evidencing both *retrograde* and *anterograde* forms.

amnesia, infantile The term refers to the perfectly normal and universal loss of memory of events and experiences that occurred early in life, generally before the age of 2 or 3. Several theories have been put forward to explain this most intriguing finding. Psychoanalysts argue that it is due to REPRESSION; cognitivists maintain that the shift in encoding of memories that occurs with the emergence of language renders these early memories irretrievable; neuropsychologists point to the strong possibility that the neural mechanisms required for long-term memory may be functionally immature during the early years. If this last explanation turns out to be correct, the others will be redundant.

amnesia, organic A general label for any AMNESIA caused by physiological dysfunctions.

amnesia, post-encephalic Any AMNESIA that results from a viral infection, particularly one that affects the temporal lobes and the underlying *limbic system*. The most commonly implicated is the herpes simplex virus, which has an affinity for this area of the brain.

amnesia, post-traumatic Generally, any loss of memory following a traumatic experience. Note that *traumatic* here may be used to describe either a physical injury or a disturbing psychological experience. Hence, it is used to refer both to organic amnesias and to psychoneurotic amnesias, although the preferred and more commonly intended meaning is the organic.

amnesia, retrograde Loss of memory of

events and experiences occurring in a (usually fairly short, circumscribed) period of time prior to the amnesia-causing trauma. Since retrograde amnesia often involves the inability to recall material once known, most memory researchers consider it to be a failure of the ability to retrieve or recall the information rather than a true loss of that information.

amnesia, source An inability to recall the source of information. The individual knows that he or she knows something but simply cannot recall accurately where or how the knowledge was acquired. A classic case is reading a book and then some time later being unable to recall whether one read the book or saw the movie (or both). While source amnesia occurs as a neurological abnormaltity, in moderate form it is normal and ubiquitous. See SOURCE *MEMORY.

amnesia, substance-induced Any AMNESIA resulting from the use of a drug or other compound. The most common culprit is alcohol (ALCOHOL AMNESTIC DISORDER, KORSAKOFF'S SYNDROME), although a host of other drugs can cause memory disturbances including ANXIOLYTICS and SEDATIVES. Also called *substance-induced persistent amnestic disorder*.

amnesia, temporal lobe An AMNESIA resulting from damage to neurological structures in the temporal lobes, specifically the *hippocampus*, the *amygdala* and related structures. It is marked by serious deficits in LONG-TERM *MEMORY while often leaving SHORT-TERM *MEMORY and IMPLICIT *MEMORY intact.

amnesia, transient global (TGA) A relatively short-lived, although virtually complete *amnesic* episode. Most TGAs last only a few minutes (or hours at the most), during which the individual has virtually no memory. The syndrome is similar to amnesias of the Korsakoff type (see KORSAKOFF'S SYNDROME) in that long-established memories are intact, only the recently learned being forgotten. TGAs, which are rare, are seen with some head injuries, restricted blood supply to the brain and, occasionally, severe migraines.

amnesic (amnestic) Terms used to indicate pertinence to AMNESIA; the adjectival forms of amnesia. Also occasionally used of one suffering from amnesia, although *amnesiac* is preferred.

amnesic aphasia APHASIA, ANOMIC.

amnesic apraxia APRAXIA, AMNESIC.

amnestic disorder In many newer texts, including the latest edition of the DSM, this term replaces the more general term AMNESIA, a change that doesn't particularly increase clarity.

amnestic syndrome Generally, severe impairment of memory, usually affecting both the ability to learn new material (see here SHORT-TERM *MEMORY) as well as the ability to recall that which was learned in the past (see LONG-TERM *MEMORY). The term denotes a psychiatric/neurological diagnostic category for cases in which the impairment results from organic dysfunctions. The most common cause is thiamine deficiency, particularly that associated with chronic alcohol abuse.

amniocentesis A procedure in which a thin needle guided by ultrasound is inserted through the abdomen or via the vagina into the uterus of a pregnant woman. The fluid and cells withdrawn can then be analysed for possible defects in the foetus. Many hereditary biochemical disorders can be identified by examining the extracted amniotic fluid. The sex of the unborn child can, of course, also be determined.

amok An acute, murderous frenzy. It is often considered a CULTURE-SPECIFIC SYNDROME particular to certain Malaysian groups; the term itself is borrowed from one of the Malaysian languages. However, the behaviour seems to be rather more widespread than early classifiers suspected, although there is a suggestion that cultural values may make it more or less likely to occur – a truism which can be made for any culturally bounded behaviour. var., *amuck*.

amorphagnosia A form of AGNOSIA in which the patient cannot identify objects using proprioceptive cues.

amoxapine An ANTIDEPRESSANT DRUG in the TRICYCLIC COMPOUND group. Like others with similar make-up, it is an effective serotonin agonist but its potentially serious side effects limit its use.

AMPA Short for amino-3-hydroxy-5-methylisoxazole-4- propionic acid. See AMPA RECEPTOR.

AMPA receptor The most common of the ionotropic GLUTAMATE RECEPTORS, it controls a sodium channel in neurons so that when a glutamate attaches it produces an excitatory postsynaptic potential.

amphetamines A class of drugs including benzedrine, dexedrine and methedrine that act as central-nervous-system stimulants. Amphetamines suppress appetite, increase heart rate and blood pressure and, in larger doses, produce a feeling of euphoria and power. Therapeutically, they are used to alleviate depression, control appetite, relieve NARCOLEPSY and by the military to increase alertness and diminish the need for sleep. METHYPHENIDATE, a drug with similar action is used widely (and controversially) in children with ATTENTION-DEFICIT HYPERACTIVITY DISORDER. The amphetamines are widely abused and a host of derivatives are found on the street. Long-term use produces the classic pattern of DRUG *TOLERANCE, DRUG *DEPENDENCE, an accompanying set of WITHDRAWAL SYMPTOMS and with extended use a model PARANOIA.

amphi- Prefix meaning *on both sides, at both ends* or *around*.

amphigenous inversion BISEXUALITY (2 and 3).

ampho- Prefix meaning *both*.

amplitude **1** Generally, intensity, value, amount or extent of some thing. **2** More specifically, the maximum displacement of a periodic wave. This meaning is often expressed as *maximum amplitude* (symbol: A) to distinguish it from: **3** The average displacement of a wave, which is occasionally called *affective amplitude*. When the physical stimulus is highly controlled, as with a pure tone, then meanings 2 and 3 are equivalent.

amuck AMOK.

amusia Lit., loss of musical ability. Generally used for partial or complete inability to comprehend (*sensory amusia*) and/or produce (*motor* or *expressive amusia*) music as a result of organic damage. Also called *avocalia*, although some reserve this term to refer to the loss of the ability to sing.

amygdala An almond-shaped neural structure composed of several nuclei and comprising part of the temporal lobe. It is classified as part of the LIMBIC SYSTEM and is intimately connected with the *hypothalamus, hippocampus, cingulate gyrus* and *septum*. It plays a significant role in emotional behaviour and motivation, particularly aggressive behaviours, and, as part of the temporal lobe, apparently serves memory functions as well. Also (and more properly) called the *amygdaloid complex*.

amygdalotomy A form of psychosurgery in which amygdaloid fibres are severed. It has been used in cases of extreme uncontrollable violence. See PSYCHOSURGERY for discussion of this and other procedures.

amyloid plaques Abnormal protein coatings on nerve cells in the brain. They are found in the brains of patients with ALZHEIMER'S DISEASE and in individuals with DOWN SYNDROME. Also called *senile plaques*.

ana- Prefix meaning *away from, back*, or *up, upper*.

anabolic Generally, promoting a build-up or restoration of a structure or body. Anabolic agents such as testosterone or similar steroids stimulate anabolism.

anabolic steroids STEROIDS.

anabolism **1** Generally, the building up of a body structure. **2** The restorative phase of METABOLISM. Contrast with CATABOLISM.

anaclisis Generally, reclining or leaning. Typically used to refer to an emotional dependency upon another. adj., *anaclitic*.

anaclitic depression R. Spitz's term used to characterize the severe and progressive depression found in infants who had lost their mothers and not obtained a suitable substitute. Although the original usage of the term was linked closely to mothering in humans, recent research has shown that the syndrome is a general phenomenon and occurs in other species, particularly other primates, when there is a dramatic lack of normal 'creature comfort' during early childhood. The connotations of the term have broadened to reflect these findings. See REACTIVE ATTACHMENT DISORDER.

anaclitic identification A general tendency to identify with a parent who is supportive and nurturing.

anaclitic object choice A psychoanalytic term for the adult selection of a loved one who closely resembles, or is modelled on, one's own mother (or other adult upon whom one depended as a child).

anacusia Total deafness. vars., *anacousia, anacusis.*

anaerobic Pertaining to or characteristic of organisms (or tissues) which require, or are not destroyed by, an absence of free oxygen.

anaerobic exercise Exercise that is not dependent upon the use of breathed oxygen. Compare with AEROBIC EXERCISE.

anaesthesia Generally, any partial or complete loss of sensitivity. Thus, an *anaesthetic* is any chemical that induces anaesthesia, generally by raising the threshold required for the neurons to respond. See also ANALGESIA. var., *anesthesia.*

anaesthesia, glove A FUNCTIONAL DISORDER involving loss of sensitivity in the hand and wrist. Since there is no combination of neural fibres which serve this area and no other, with these symptoms we have prima facie evidence of a PSYCHOGENIC DISORDER. Similar syndromes affecting the lower extremities are known as *shoe* (or *foot*) *anaesthesia* and *stocking anaesthesia.*

anaesthesia sexualis Lack of sexual responsiveness.

anaglyph A picture printed in two complementary colours slightly offset from each other. When viewed through lenses of corresponding colours (one colour to each eye) the effect is one of stereoscopic depth. This process is used in the production of 3-D movies.

anaglyptoscope Device which shifts the angle of lighting on a test object, resulting in a reversal of areas of shadow and light. It is used to demonstrate the role of shadows in the perception of depth. var., *anaglyphoscope.*

anagogic From the Greek, meaning *leading up*, and hence pertaining to the spiritual or the ideal. Used by Jung to refer to the idealistic or moralistic aspects of unconscious thought.

anagram Any of several word problems based upon the rearranging of letters in words. There are many variations on the basic theme with the following three most often used in psychological experi-

ments: (a) the simple, *single solution* anagram, the subject being given a set of scrambled letters and required to find the word they spell (e.g. HIRAC – CHAIR); (b) the *word* anagram, the subject beginning with one word and rearranging the letters to find another word (e.g. SHORE – HORSE); (c) the *multiple solution* anagram, the subject being required to find as many different words as possible using any or all of the letters in the word supplied (e.g. there are several dozen words which can be formed using the letters in TEACHER).

anal Referring to the ANUS.

anal character An adult who compulsively displays characteristics which, according to psychoanalytic theory, are referable to the ANAL STAGE. The *anal expulsive* character typically is said to be compulsively pliant, untidy, generous, etc.; the *anal retentive* to be obstinate, orderly, miserly, etc. Generally, the theory proposes that the anal character, whether it occurs in either of these two extreme forms or, more commonly, in a form which combines these traits, is an infantile FIXATION on the anal region and the anal functions.

analepsis From the Greek, meaning *taking up*; hence, restoration of health, recovery.

anal eroticism Sensual or sexual pleasure derived from the anus either by direct stimulation or by the sequences of behaviours associated with defecation. var., *anal erotism.*

anal expulsive (stage) Some psychoanalytic theorists hypothesize two distinct aspects to the ANAL STAGE, one characterized by anal expulsiveness, in which pleasure is derived from the passing of faeces, and the other characterized by anal retentiveness, in which pleasure is associated with the withholding of faeces. See ANAL CHARACTER for the personality types assumed by psychoanalytic theory to result from fixation at the anal stage.

analgesia Insensitivity to pain. Hence, any substance that serves to relieve pain is an *analgesic*. The term is also applied to procedures which do not directly involve the introduction of a substance, e.g. *hypnotic analgesia* (see HYPNOSIS for discussion).

analgesia, belief-induced Reduction in experience of pain owing to strongly held beliefs. Seen in special instances such as intense religious ceremonies and, more often, in the use of a PLACEBO.

analgesia, situation-produced Reduction of pain due to the presence of another stimulus, such as pinching a cat's neck while giving it a normally painful injection, or providing music to patients undergoing dental surgery.

analgesia, stress-induced Analgesia produced by high levels of stress, particularly those related to issues of survival. Bullet wounds in battle are often not experienced as painful until later. The secretion of ENDOR-PHINS is responsible for much of this effect.

anal impotence A psychoanalytic term for the inability to pass faeces in the presence of other persons.

anal intercourse Sexual intercourse with the penis inserted in the anus. The term is applied to hetero- and homosexual relations.

anality That part of libidinous energy associated with the anal region.

analog ANALOGUE.

analogical reasoning Reasoning whereby decisions about objects, events or concepts depend upon perceived similarities in the relationships between pairs. See ANALOGY for further discussion.

analogies test A test in which a relationship between two terms is given and the subject is required to complete an analogous relationship. Questions typically take the form: *A* is to *B* as *C* is to...; e.g. *fence* is to *field* as *frame* is to...?

analogue 1 Generally, a correspondence or a resemblance. A thing or event is said to be an analogue of another if there is a coherent correspondence between their parts, functions, roles, etc. See ANALOGY. **2** Specifically, in biology, an organ or part similar in function to another but different in structure and origin; e.g. the wing of a bat is in an analogous relation to the wings of birds. Compare with structures which are HOMOLOGOUS. var., *analog*.

analogy Generally, likeness, similarity, correspondence. Specific usages include: **1** A description, argument or explanation based on systematic comparison of one thing with

another, already known thing. Analogical reasoning so carried through is a useful *heuristic* for revealing correspondences between things, but as a *logical* argument it fails to satisfy the principles necessary for proving the validity of a proposition. **2** In biology, a correspondence in function between two organs or parts. See ANALOGUE (2).

anal retentive ANAL EXPULSIVE.

anal sadistic Any sadistic pleasure hypothesized to originate in the ANAL STAGE. It is argued by many psychoanalysts that such behaviour derives from harsh punishment during toilet training. Some theorists have even hypothesized the existence of a separate ANAL SADISTIC STAGE in development.

anal sadistic stage (or **level** or **phase**) A stage in psychosexual development assumed by some psychoanalysts to be part of the ANAL STAGE but distinguishable as a distinct component by a focus upon *anal eroticism* and sadistic impulses toward the parents, who are the agents of toilet training.

anal stage (or **level** or **phase**) In psychoanalytic theory, the stage of psychosexual development marked by preoccupation with the anus and its functions. From the libidinal point of view, the stage is marked by the deriving of sensuous pleasure from anal stimulation and defecation; from the ego perspective the stage is characterized by the beginning of socialization, as indicated by control over the sphincter muscles. Note that two opposing tendencies are assumed to be operating here: ANAL RETENTIVE and ANAL EXPULSIVE.

anal triad In psychoanalytic theory, a hypothesized syndrome in which the three traits characteristic of the retentive variety of the *anal character* (compulsive orderliness, stinginess and obstinacy) are displayed.

analysand One undergoing analysis. According to most historians of the psychoanalytic movement this term was introduced because the medical students taking a psychoanalytic internship, who routinely underwent analysis as part of their training, objected to being called *patients*!

analysis 1 Generally, the process of separating a 'thing' into its component parts or elementary qualities. The term is ubiquitous in all scientific disciplines, hence the 'thing' may be a mechanical device, a physical entity, a chemical or biological substance, a percept, an image, idea or emotion, etc. Because of its wide application the term is usually qualified so that the form of, or the theoretical motivation for, the analysis is specified. Some of these qualified terms follow below, others are found under the appropriate alphabetical listing. **2** The particular set of techniques and procedures used in the practice of PSYCHOANALYSIS. This meaning is actually consonant with meaning 1; it is given separate listing merely because it occurs so frequently without qualification in the literature that it is sometimes taken as the dominant sense of the term. **3** The outcome of either of the above two processes. The connotation here is that of *reductionism*; it is a process designed to reveal fundamental components or root causes. Contrast with SYNTHESIS. adjs., *analytic, analytical*.

analysis by synthesis A phrase referring to a broad class of pattern-recognition schemes or, more accurately, a class of information-processing theories which seek to explain such elementary phenomena as the simple fact that yo· ca· un·er·ta·d t·e m·an·ng ·f t·is ·en·en·e c cn ·ho·gh ·ve·y t·ir· le·te· is ·is·in·fr·m t·e l·st ·ar·. Analysis-by-synthesis models operate on the assumption that humans possess a vast network of memories, strategies and schemata which enable them to evaluate inputs, anticipate incoming stimuli, form guesses based on context, exclude irrelevant kangaroo material, fill in missing features, etc. In short, 'synthesize' in order to 'analyse' the input. Such models have been used in studies of sensory psychology, psycholinguistics, thinking, reading, and cognition in general.

analysis, didactic The psychoanalysis that one who is training to become a psychoanalyst undergoes as part of the educational process.

analysis, lay Psychoanalysis carried out by a LAY ANALYST.

analysis of covariance (ANCOVA) An extension of the ANALYSIS OF VARIANCE used when one or more of the variables of interest is uncontrolled in the experimental design. The procedure allows for 'statistical control' of the uncontrolled variations so that normal analysis techniques may be carried out without distorting the results.

analysis of variance 1 A statistical method for making simultaneous comparisons between two or more means. An ANOVA yields a series of values (*F* values) which can be statistically tested to determine whether a significant relation exists between the experimental variables. See also F-TEST. **2** Any statistical technique in which variation in scores is analysed. This usage is less frequent. The two meanings are almost always distinguished by use of capitalization or the acronym ANOVA to denote the first meaning.

analyst 1 Generally, a practitioner of ANALYSIS (2), i.e. a PSYCHOANALYST. **2** A follower of Jung's principles of ANALYTIC PSYCHOLOGY.

analytic (or analytical) ANALYSIS.

analytical intelligence See INTELLIGENCE, ANALYTICAL and TRIARCHIC THEORY OF INTELLIGENCE.

analytic language Any language which tends to express grammatical relationships by the use of auxiliary words rather than inflections. Syntactic components are generally carried by word-order rules in such languages (of which English is an example). Compare with SYNTHETIC LANGUAGE.

analytic psychology 1 Generally, the form of psychoanalysis put forward by Carl Jung. **2** Occasionally, a label used for any approach to psychology that emphasizes the breaking down of phenomena into their component parts. var., *analytical psychology*.

anamnesis From the Greek, meaning *recall* or *recollection*. **1** In general, recall or the ability to recall past events. **2** In medicine, the personal case history of a disorder as provided by the patient. Originally the term referred specifically to a patient's statements concerning a particular disability and his or her considerations about important antecedents deemed relevant to it. Many others, particularly psychiatrists, use the term to encompass any and all aspects of a patient's medical history, including information other than that provided by the patient, such as biographical data, reports from family, etc. Compare with CATAMNESIS.

anandamide Probably the most important

of the cannabinoids (see CANNABIS), its name derives from the Sanskrit word for 'bliss'. For what it's worth, at least three anandamide-like chemicals are found in chocolate.

anandria Absence of normal male characteristics.

anankastia A general label for the condition in which an individual feels as though he or she is being forced to behave, think or feel in ways that go against his or her personal will. The notion of 'force' here is broad, the term being used to cover a variety of conditions involving phobias, compulsions and obsessions. var., *anancastia*.

anankastic personality COMPULSIVE PERSONALITY DISORDER and OBSESSIVE-COMPULSIVE DISORDER.

anaphia Loss of or diminution in the sense of touch.

anaphora A reference to something previously mentioned. An anaphoric word or anaphoric reference relates to another, antecedent, word or proposition. In 'Max is a millionaire, I want to be one too' *millionaire* is the antecedent, *one* is the anaphoric word. How children learn anaphoric reference patterns is a topic of some interest in developmental psycholinguistics.

anaphrodisia A condition in which the desire for sex is diminished or absent.

anaphylaxis A state of hypersensitivity to a particular substance. Seen as a reaction to various drugs (e.g. penicillin) or other foreign substances (e.g. the toxin in a bee or wasp sting). The term is restricted to states of hypersensitivity which result from previous administration or injection of the substance. The primary symptoms are wheezing, extreme difficulty in breathing, chest constriction and occasionally convulsions. Serious cases of anaphylatic shock can be fatal if untreated.

anaphylaxis, psychological An extension of the meaning of *anaphylaxis* to cover psychological hypersensitivity resulting from a previous traumatic experience such that later presentation of the original circumstances causes deep psychological distress.

anarthria Partial or complete loss of articulate speech. Usually the term is used for disorders of articulation resulting from central-nervous-system lesions. Occasionally it may be used for syndromes resulting from peripheral motor or muscular defects, although the preferred term for these is DYSARTHRIA.

anastasis A return to health.

anastomosis A general anatomical/neurological term for any direct communication or joining between two anatomical structures, organs, neural processes, tissues, etc.

anatomical age AGE, ANATOMICAL.

anchor (or **anchorage**) **1** A reference point or standard against which judgements take place; see e.g. ANCHOR POINT. **2** A foundation upon which a thing is built or to which it is attached.

anchoring A COGNITIVE *HEURISTIC in which decisions are made based on an initial 'anchor'. For example, in a classic study, one group of people was asked whether the chance of nuclear war was greater or less than 1% and estimated it to be about 10%, while another group was asked if it was greater or less than 90% and estimated it to be over 20%.

anchoring of ego The process of reaching the satisfying state of security and comfortableness with one's personal and physical surroundings.

anchor point(s) Reference point(s) or standard(s) used to provide an observer with subjective criteria against which future judgements can be made. Used in *category estimation* scaling, where the extremes of the stimulus dimension are given to the subject as anchor points, and in preference rankings, where the neutral point anchors the scale ranging from least preferred to most preferred.

ANCOVA ANALYSIS OF COVARIANCE.

-andro(s)- Combining forms from the Greek meaning *man*, *male* or *masculine*.

androgen Any of the male sex hormones responsible for the development of male sex characteristics. Androgens are secreted primarily by the testes and the adrenal cortices in the male and in small amounts by the ovaries in the female. See e.g. ANDROSTENEDIONE, TESTOSTERONE.

androgen-insensitivity syndrome A congenital condition in which normal responsiveness to androgens during gestation is lacking. Affected individuals, although they possess the Y male-sex chromosome, are externally female since the developing foetus does respond to the small amounts of oestrogen normally produced in males. They are infertile and do not menstruate. Also called *testicular-feminizing syndrome*.

androgenization Lit., the process of becoming a male. The term specifically refers to the complex processes in the developing embryo initiated by exposure to androgens and resulting in the development of male sex organs.

androgyny From Greek *andros* (= man) and *gyne* (= female), the condition in which some male and some female characteristics are present in the same individual. The term is used with respect to both biological/physical and psychological/behavioural characteristics. In general, distinguish from HERMAPHRODITE since, except in rare cases, a person displaying androgyny shows sexual differentiation and can be labelled as biologically male or female. Some authors restrict the use of the term to biological males who display physical or behavioural female characteristics, while reserving *gynandry* for biological females with male characteristics. Compare with EFFEMINATE and distinguish from BISEXUAL.

androgyny scale BEM SEX ROLE INVENTORY.

android Resembling a male.

andromania An occasional synonym for NYMPHOMANIA.

androphile 1 One who exhibits an extreme affection for males. **2** Preferring man. This latter usage is generally restricted to various parasites.

androstenedione A natural androgen found in both males and females produced mainly by the adrenal cortices and, to a lesser degree, by the gonads. Relatively weak as an androgen itself, it is the direct precursor of testosterone, the most powerful of the androgens.

anecdotal evidence Evidence which is casually observed and related like a narrative. Although generally regarded as scientifically unacceptable (how can one replicate an anecdote or verify it conclusively?), such evidence can often form the basis for further systematic experimentation.

anechoic Lit., free from echo. Anechoic chambers constructed with sound-absorbing walls have been very useful in many experiments on AUDITION.

anemotropism An orienting response (see TROPISM) to air currents.

anencephalus A congenital deformity in which the brain fails to develop.

anepia Inability to speak.

anergasia Generally, loss of function. Used of such dysfunctions as result from central-nervous-system lesions.

anergia Sluggishness, lack of energy.

anesthesia Common variant spelling of ANAESTHESIA.

angel dust PHENCYCLIDINE THIOPHENE.

Angelman syndrome A genetic disorder characterized by MICROCEPHALY, ATAXIA with stiff, jerky gait and movement problems, absent speech and learning disabilities. Children with the disorder were once called 'happy puppets' because of their pleasant disposition, prosocial behaviour and frequent bouts of excessive but usually inappropriate laughter.

anger Very generally, a fairly strong emotional reaction which accompanies a variety of situations such as being physically restrained, being interfered with, having one's possessions removed, observing or hearing of actions or events that one regards as morally repugnant, being attacked or threatened, etc. Anger is often defined (or, better, *identified*) by a collection of physical reactions, including particular facial grimaces and body positions characteristic of action in the autonomic nervous system, particularly the sympathetic division. In many species anger produces overt (or implicit) attack. As with many emotions anger is extremely difficult to define objectively. The problem is that it is a rather fuzzy concept and hedges into other emotional reactions of similar kind such as ANIMUS, RAGE, HOSTILITY, HATRED. See these, and other related entries, for discussions of the distinctions typically drawn.

angina 1 Generally, a feeling of suffocation, of being choked. **2** A disease of the pharynx characterized by attacks of choking. **3** *Angina pectoris*, a disease of the heart caused by insufficient blood supply; primary symptoms are intermittent attacks of severe chest pain with a sense of suffocating pressure.

anginophobia 1 Generally, a pathological fear of suffocation. **2** More specifically, an intense, compelling fear of an attack of *angina pectoris* (see ANGINA (3)). Many angina sufferers carry this additional psychic burden.

angio- Combining form meaning *vessel*. Used commonly in reference to blood vessels but also to that contained within a vessel such as a seed.

angiotensin RENIN.

angiotensinogen RENIN.

angry aggression AGGRESSION, ANGRY.

Angst German for *anxiety, anguish* or *psychic pain*. **1** In the existential school, this mental turmoil is regarded as *the* fundamental reality of beings who come to realize the indeterminacy of things and who must confront life as a forum within which personal choice is essential and the responsibility for decisions made must be borne. **2** For its use in psychoanalysis, see the discussion under PAIN (2).

ångström unit The internationally accepted unit of measurement of wavelength given as one ten-millionth of a millimetre (or one ten-thousandth of a micron).

angular gyrus A gyrus (cerebral convolution) of the posterior portion of the parietal lobe. The left angular gyrus has been implicated in language functions, particularly reading.

anhedonia Condition marked by a general lack of interest in living, in the pleasures of life; a loss in the ability to enjoy things. It is regarded as a defining feature of DEPRESSION. var., *ahedonia*. adj., *anhedonic*.

anhedonia, social Disinterest in social activities and contact.

anhypnia INSOMNIA.

anhypnosis INSOMNIA.

aniconia A lack of mental imagery. It has been suggested that the early behaviourist J. B. Watson was aniconic, a condition which may have contributed to his lack of sympathy for those who made imagery so important in their theories.

anima 1 Originally, the soul. **2** In the early writings of Carl Jung, one's inner being, that aspect of one's psyche in intimate association with one's unconscious. Compare here with his use of the term PERSONA. **3** In Jung's later writings, the feminine archetype, which he differentiated from ANIMUS, the masculine archetype. In arguing for the essential bisexuality of all persons, Jung hypothesized that both components were present in both sexes.

animal magnetism Mesmer's term for the universal force through which hypnotic effects were hypothesized to be mediated. Alas for Mesmer, animals are not involved, nor is magnetism. See HYPNOSIS.

animal psychology A loose term for either of the following: **1** The study of psychological processes from a phylogenetic point of view, in which comparisons between the behaviour of various species are the primary focus. See here COMPARATIVE PSYCHOLOGY. **2** Any psychological investigation which uses animals as subjects.

animal type phobia SIMPLE *PHOBIA.

animatism The belief that a kind of impersonal supernatural force exists in all things, animate or inanimate. Some anthropologists argue that it is a cultural precursor to ANIMISM.

animism 1 Loosely, the belief that all things, animate or inanimate, living or not living, possess a soul or other form of spiritual essence that transcends the physical forms. The term is used with several, more specific connotations in various areas, as follows: **2** In anthropology, it is often argued that animism, as derived from the more primitive beliefs of ANIMATISM, represents the earliest form of religion. As a religious belief system, animism actually has a sophisticated panoply of spirits with specific powers and roles to play in the nature of things and persons. **3** In developmental psychology, the term refers to early patterns of thought and speech in young children in which feelings, desires and beliefs are invested in the nonhuman and the nonliving. See ANTHROPOMORPHISM. **4** In various philosophical and psychological perspectives something akin to these notions is also found. A number of gentle euphemisms have been coined to denote these ideas since the above meanings have tarnished the term to the extent that there is a distinct reluctance to use it to represent anything that one would want others to take seriously. See here PANPSYCHISM, TELEOLOGY and VITALISM.

animistic thinking Piaget's term for a form of thinking found in children in the PRE-OPERATORY STAGE where they endow inanimate objects with lifelike characteristics. See ANIMISM (3).

animosity Intense and enduring hostility with the implication that the feelings are open and active.

animunculus Lit., the animal in the head. Hence, the sketched representations of the body of an animal as projected on the somatosensory cortex. The animal equivalent of the HOMUNCULUS (2).

animus 1 An intense and enduring dislike. See here ANGER, HOSTILITY and related entries. **2** In Jung's later writings, the unconscious masculine archetype. See ANIMA (3).

anion A negatively charged ion. See CATION

aniseikonia Dissimilarity in the size and shape of the two retinal images. var., *anisoiconia*.

anis(o)- Combining form denoting *unequal*, *dissimilar* or *nonsymmetrical*.

anisocoria A condition in which the diameters of the pupils are of unequal size.

anisoiconia ANISEIKONIA.

anisometropia Unequal refractive power in the two eyes.

anisopia A general term for any inequality of vision in the two eyes.

anisotropia Lit., unequal in or when turning. Hence: **1** Of a lens, the property of being differentially refractive when oriented in different directions. **2** In perception, the change in the apparent length of a line or rod when it

is turned through space; see e.g. FORESHORTENING.

ankle clonus A repetitive contraction–relaxation of the ankle muscles. It is a common symptom of neurological diseases of the central nervous system.

ankylo- Combining form meaning *stiffly bent* or *crooked*, or characterizing a fusing of parts.

ankyloglossia A condition in which the membrane attached to the underside of the tongue is abnormally short and inflexible. Hence, tongue-tied.

ankylosis Generally, any abnormal fusing of the cartilage and bones of a joint resulting in stiffness and immobility.

Anlage German for *laying on*. Hence: **1** A primordial cluster of cells which forms the foundation for the development of an organ or part. **2** By extension, a predisposing factor or condition which functions as the basis for the development of a mental process.

Anna O., the case of One of the first and most famous case studies in psychoanalysis. The patient known as Anna O. (subsequently revealed to have been Bertha Pappenheim, who later in her life became a well-known and much respected humanitarian and social-relief worker) was originally diagnosed as a hysteric with functional limb paralysis and a tendency toward a multiple personality. She was treated by Josef Breuer and is frequently cited as the first demonstrated success of psychoanalytic therapy. The term 'talking cure' was actually coined by Anna to describe the cathartic outcome of working through her problems verbally.

annihilation anxiety Profound and disturbing anxiety that has loss of self and loss of identity at its core.

anniversary reaction A strong emotional reaction occurring at the same time of the year as an original event. Most commonly seen as a depressed state on the anniversary of some earlier tragedy such as the death of a loved one.

annoyer E. L. Thorndike's term for any stimulus possessing noxious or unpleasant properties. Defined operationally, an annoyer is any stimulus which an organism will learn to escape or avoid. Contrast with SATISFIER.

annulment A psychoanalytic term for the process through which painful, anxiety-provoking ideas and images are neutralized or 'annulled'. The standard theory maintains that annulment operates through the use of day-dreams, fantasies and the like. Compare with REPRESSION, wherein the assumption is that painful ideas are removed from awareness entirely.

annulus Any ring-shaped structure. The term is used broadly to describe stimuli with circular shapes, ring-like anatomical structures, etc. var., *anulus*.

anodyne Any pain-relieving agent, an analgesic.

anoesia Lacking the ability to comprehend or understand; idiocy. var., *anoia*.

anoetic From the Greek, meaning *unable to think*. Hence: **1** Not relevant to cognition. Affects or emotions are sometimes called anoetic functions. **2** Not relevant to or on the borderline of consciousness. Passive, implicit processing of information is occasionally referred to as anoetic processing.

anoetic memory See MEMORY, NOETIC.

anoia ANOESIA.

anomalous contour SUBJECTIVE *CONTOUR.

anomalous dichromatism (or **dichromacy**) DICHROMACY, ANOMALOUS.

anomalous sentence Any sentence that is syntactically correct but makes no (obvious) semantic sense. Perhaps the most famous is Chomsky's example, 'Colourless green ideas sleep furiously.'

anomalous stimulus STIMULUS, INADEQUATE.

anomalous trichromatism (or **trichromacy**) TRICHROMACY, ANOMALOUS.

anomaly Generally, any marked deviation from the norm or the expected. The usual connotation is the literal 'a-norm'; that is, characterizing something distinguishable from social or statistical norms without any implication of pathology or perversion. See discussion under NORMAL.

anomia **1** Partial or complete loss of the ability to recall names. The term is used in this manner only for aphasic and amnestic syndromes and not for the common condition endured by so many. Occasionally, milder forms are called *dysnomia*. **2** Occasionally ANOMIE (2), but this usage is not recommended.

anomic aphasia APHASIA, ANOMIC.

anomic suicide SUICIDE, ANOMIC.

anomie (or **anomy**) **1** In a society or group, a condition in which there is a breakdown of social structure, a general lack of social values and a dissolution of cultural norms. The term connotes confusion, disorganization and a collective insecurity, and anomie may occur in a variety of circumstances, such as in the aftermath of a catastrophe like an earthquake, during a war, or, less obviously, when large numbers of persons from rural backgrounds emigrate to urban centres where their original social values are rendered irrelevant yet assimilation is resisted by the urban society. **2** A condition in which the members of a superficially well-organized society feel isolated and disconnected, resulting from an excessively specialized social structure which limits closeness and intimacy. This meaning is used to characterize the psychological state of many who live in highly developed, technological, urban societies. To prevent confusion, some writers use *anomie* for meaning 1 and *anomy* or *anomia* for 2. *Anomy* is a useful term here, *anomia* is not since it already has a very different meaning.

anomy See discussion under ANOMIE.

anonymity The meaning in psychology is basically that of standard usage: any condition in which one's identity is unknown to others. The interest in the concept in the social sciences derives from considerable evidence that under such conditions people tend to behave in more immoral, unethical, and even lethal, ways than they ordinarily would. Compare with DEINDIVIDUATION.

anoopsia ANOPSIA (1).

anopia **1** A general term for defective vision. **2** Lack of one or both eyes. **3** ANOPSIA. **4** HEMIANOPIA.

anopsia **1** A tendency for one or both eyes to turn upward. var., *anoopsia*. **2** Failure of normal use of vision, resulting from strabismus, cataract or serious refractive errors.

anorchism Congenital lack of one or both testes.

anorectant An APPETITE SUPPRESSANT.

anorectic Lacking in appetite. var., *anorectous*.

anorexia Lit., lacking in appetite. The term is most commonly used with respect to eating (see ANOREXIA NERVOSA), although 'appetite' is occasionally extended to cover other desires such as sex (see SEXUAL *ANOREXIA).

anorexia nervosa An EATING DISORDER characterized by intense fear of becoming obese, dramatic weight loss, obsessive concern with one's weight, disturbances of body image such that the patient 'feels fat' when of normal weight or even when emaciated, and, in females, *amenorrhoea*. The classic *anorexic* is young (rarely over 30), female (roughly 95% of all cases) and from a middle- or upper-class family. Anorexics are frequently described as 'model children'. The disorder is rather resistant to treatment and can have an unremitting course leading to death, although in the large majority of cases there is spontaneous full recovery. The shortened term *anorexia*, use of which is widespread, is actually somewhat misleading in that the real loss of appetite does not occur until late in the course of the disorder – at the outset the patient is typically hungry like anyone on a sharply reduced food-intake regimen.

anorexia, sexual A lack of appetite for sex, a loss of sexual desire.

anorgasmia A total inability to achieve orgasm.

anorthopia 1 Visual defect in which straight lines are not perceived as straight, the perception of symmetry and parallel stimuli being distorted. 2 STRABISMUS.

anorthoscopic Lit., abnormally viewed. Characterizing perception under unusual or highly artificial conditions.

anosmia General term for any deficiency in the sense of smell.

anosodiaphoria A lack of concern for a serious neurological condition. Unlike *anosognosia*, the patient is aware of the condition but just doesn't care.

anosognosia 1 An unwillingness or failure to recognize and deal with a deficiency or disease. 2 A neurological disorder marked by an inability to recognize that one has a disorder. Fascinatingly, in what is known as Anton's syndrome, a brain-injured patient may be completely blind as a result of the injury but have no conscious sense of his or her own blindness, or a hemiplegic patient may be completely unaware of his or her inability to use one arm and hand.

A not B error An error of persistence first reported by Piaget. An infant watches an object hidden under one of two covers (A) and is then allowed to retrieve it. The sequence of hiding and retrieving is repeated several times. Then the child watches as the object is hidden under the other cover (B). Infants younger than 8–10 months tend to erroneously search under A. At this age the infant's mental representation of the object appears to be linked with the earlier bodily actions.

A not B paradigm (or **task**) The experimental procedure in which the A NOT B ERROR is often observed.

ANOVA ANALYSIS OF VARIANCE.

anovulatory Lit., without ovulation. The necessarily infertile menstrual cycle that occurs when there is a failure of the ovary to release an egg.

anoxia A marked deficiency in the supply of oxygen to the body tissues. Typically, the tissues of interest are cerebral and anoxic episodes, whether caused by strokes, aneurisms, heart attacks, or physical trauma, can produce a host of cognitive and memorial deficits depending on the sites affected and how widespread the damage is.

ANS (or **ans**) AUTONOMIC NERVOUS SYSTEM.

ant- Prefix meaning *against, opposed to, counter to*. var., *anti-*.

Antabuse Brand name for DISULFIRAM.

antagonism Generally, a state of affairs between two processes, stimuli, structures or organisms such that their effects are in opposition to each other.

antagonism, drug Generally, a state of affairs resulting from an interaction between two drugs such that their joint effect is less than that of either drug taken alone. *Pharmacological antagonism* results when one drug (the *antagonist*) prevents another drug (the *agonist*) from combining with its receptors. *Physiological antagonism* (or *functional antagonism*) occurs when two drugs have their effects upon different receptor sites but yield counterbalancing physiological effects. *Biochemical antagonism* takes place when one drug has an indirect inhibiting effect upon another; e.g. it may produce more rapid excretion of the first drug from the body. *Chemical antagonism* is the result of two drugs simply neutralizing each other and yielding an inactive substance.

antagonist Generally, an opponent. Anything which operates in opposite fashion with respect to another thing (its AGONIST).

antagonistic Generally, having the property of counteracting, neutralizing or inhibiting the effects of something else. For the various special usages see the following entries and ANTAGONISM et seq. Compare with SYNERGIC, SYNERGISTIC.

antagonistic colour COMPLEMENTARY *COLOUR. See also THEORIES OF *COLOUR VISION for more detail.

antagonistic muscles Pairs of muscles that work in opposition: one muscle contracts a limb, the other extends it. When one muscle is flexed the other is relaxed; they never flex simultaneously. This coordinated functioning is termed *reciprocal*. See also EXTENSOR, FLEXOR.

ante- Prefix meaning *before*, either in time or in space.

antecedent 1 Generally, something which precedes a phenomenon in a manner which 'invites' the inference of causality. **2** In logic, the conditional or hypothetical proposition, the so-called 'if' clause. See CONSEQUENT.

antedating goal response, fractional FRACTIONAL ANTEDATING GOAL RESPONSE.

antedating response Generally, any anticipatory response; a response that occurs earlier in a sequence of responses than was originally learned.

anterior 1 In the temporal sense, to precede. **2** In the spatial sense, to be in front of. Contrast with POSTERIOR. Note that in anatomical terminology for upright species like *Homo sapiens*, *anterior* is frequently found as a synonym for *ventral*, and *posterior* becomes a synonym for *dorsal*. Many brain structures have distinct anterior (and posterior) regions. Rather than list them all here, see the base term for information about location and function. **3** In phonetics, a distinctive feature for distinguishing the sounds of a language. Anterior sounds are produced toward the front of the mouth (e.g. *z* in 'zoo'), *nonanterior* sounds are further back (e.g. *sh* in 'shoe').

anterior cingulate cortex The frontal part of the CINGULATE CORTEX, thought to mediate a variety of functions including memory consolidation and emotion regulation.

anterior commissure A band of myelinated fibres that connects the olfactory structures and the lateral regions of the temporal lobes in the two hemispheres of the brain.

anterior nuclei (of the thalamus) Collectively, the anterodorsal, anteromedial and anteroventral nuclei in the *thalamus*. Part of the LIMBIC SYSTEM, these nuclei receive input from the *hippocampus* and the mammillary bodies of the *hypothalamus* and project their axons to the *cingulate gyrus*.

anterior prefrontal cortex The most anterior (forward) part of the PREFRONTAL CORTEX. Also called the *frontopolar cortex*, it is primarily involved in EXECUTIVE FUNCTIONS including balancing two or more plans of action and enabling choices based on long-term memories and estimates about potential rewards associated with each possibility.

anterior root SPINAL ROOT.

anterior thalamic nuclei ANTERIOR NUCLEI (OF THE THALAMUS).

antero- Combining form denoting *front*, *before*, *prior to*.

anterograde Extending forward in space or progressing forward in time.

anterograde amnesia AMNESIA, ANTEROGRADE.

anterograde degeneration DEGENERATION (1).

anterolateral system One of the two main ascending neural systems for somatic sensation (the other is the DORSAL COLUMN MEDIAL LEMNISCAL SYSTEM). Its pathways originate in cells of the dorsal horn, cross at the spinal level and ascend in lateral columns. They carry information about pain, temperature and some touch, and function in perception, arousal and motor control.

anthropo- Combining form meaning *man* or *relating to man*.

anthropocentrism The point of view that *Homo sapiens* lies at the centre of things. The species analogue of *egocentrism*.

anthropoid Lit., in the form of a man. Used of the great apes.

anthropology Lit., the study of mankind. Depending upon who is doing the defining, anthropology may include archaeology, linguistics, psychology, sociology and smatterings of biology, anatomy, genetics and comparative literature. Most practitioners tend to segment the discipline into CULTURAL *ANTHROPOLOGY and PHYSICAL *ANTHROPOLOGY.

anthropology, cultural The subdiscipline within anthropology concerned primarily with the study of CULTURE and the complex social structures which make up communities, societies and nations. Originally the field focused upon nonliterate societies, particularly the non-Western, although this limitation no longer applies. syn., *social anthropology*.

anthropology, physical The subdiscipline within anthropology concerned primarily with the study of man from a biological and evolutionary perspective. Strong focus is on measurement, classification and comparative analysis of various racial, geographical and ethnic groups, and the evolutionary relationships between these biological factors and physical and cultural environments. Occasionally called *somatic anthropology*.

anthropology, social In Great Britain, the preferred synonym for CULTURAL *ANTHROPOLOGY.

anthropometry Lit., measurement of man. The area of PHYSICAL *ANTHROPOLOGY concerned with measuring and classifying the human physical form.

anthropomorphism Attributing human characteristics to lower organisms or inanimate objects. The anthropomorphic fallacy is most often committed by those unsophisticated in animal research. The tendency to say that a rat that is consuming a food pellet is 'enjoying itself' or that a cat receiving lateral hypothalamic stimulation is experiencing 'pleasure' is almost irresistible, but it can be misleading. One should be careful not to imbue nonhumans with what may be species-specific human characteristics.

anthroponomy A term put forward some years ago by Walter S. Hunter as a replacement for *behaviourism*. Hunter was such a staunch behaviourist that he even once suggested that the term *psychology* be abandoned since its connotations were too mentalistic. He was not taken seriously in either case.

anthropophagy Cannibalism.

anthroposemiotics SEMIOTICS.

anti- Common prefix meaning *against*, *opposing*, *counteracting*, *reversing*. var., *ant-*.

antiaging This term has become a modern-day buzz word to characterize any of a host of therapies, drugs, surgeries, diets, cosmetics and exercise programmes that claim to slow and even reverse the aging process. The term itself is something of an oxymoron; you cannot slow the aging, at best you can modify the effects. Few of the touted procedures have much empirical support other than the obvious ones, good nutrition, physical exercise, a well-balanced and active mental life and fortuitous genes.

antianxiety drugs An umbrella label for several classes of drugs that are prescribed for the reduction of anxiety. Included are the BENZODIAZEPINES such as CHLORDIAZEPOXIDE, CLONAZEPAM and DIAZEPAM, the muscle-relaxant derivative MEPROBAMATE, sedatives such as the BARBITURATES, and BUSPIRONE, which was first introduced as an ANTIPSYCHOTIC DRUG. Currently the most useful and most often prescribed are the benzodiazepines. While these drugs are called antianxiety drugs (or *anxiolytics*), there is little evidence that they directly relieve anxiety. Rather their primary action is to produce muscle relaxation and sedation through acting on the central nervous system. In some texts the term MINOR *TRANQUILLIZERS may still be used to refer to these drugs. For reasons outlined under that term, this is no longer recommended.

antibodies Proteins that recognize the proteins that mark invading micro-organisms (see ANTIGENS) and attack and kill them.

anticathexis Lit., against CATHEXIS. Thus: **1** An action that blocks cathexis, that prevents investment of psychic energy. **2** An action that maintains the repression of a cathection. The process presumed to carry this out is the reversal of emotional 'charge', turning love into hate or hate into love. Also called *countercathexis*.

anticholinergic Pertaining to a substance or agent which inhibits, impedes or blocks cholinergic action. That is, one which blocks impulses in the CHOLINERGIC NERVES.

anticholinergic drugs A class of drugs that interfere with the release of ACETYLCHOLINE and compromise the functions of parasympathetic neural pathways. The term tends to be reserved for drugs such as the naturally occurring ATROPINE and SCOPOLAMINE and the synthetics like BENZTROPINE and PROCYCLIDINE. All act on MUSCARINIC RECEPTORS and are used primarily to relieve the symptoms of muscular rigidity that occur in disorders like PARKINSON'S DISEASE. Other compounds such the TRICYCLICS and some ANTIPYSCHOTICS also have anticholinergic effects and are occasionally classified as such.

anticipation A preparatory mental SET in which one is primed for the perception of a particular stimulus.

anticipation error ERROR, ANTICIPATION.

anticipation method A technique for studying serial learning in which the subject is required to provide (anticipate) the next succeeding item of a list while viewing any particular item.

anticipatory aggression AGGRESSION, ANTICIPATORY.

anticipatory anxiety Loosely, anxiety about becoming anxious. It is common in individuals with anxiety disorders and can lead to the development of AGORAPHOBIA.

anticipatory attitude change The shift in an attitude that accompanies knowing that one is about to be exposed to a persuasive argument. When the topic is one the person

regards as important, a shift further toward the extreme pole is commonly seen. When it is relatively minor or unimportant, there is rarely much of an ATTITUDE CHANGE.

anticipatory images In Piaget's theory, images that allow one to envisage transformations even if they have never been experienced. For example, adults can easily image a wastepaper basket suddenly sprouting wings and flying upside down. Piaget felt that children under roughly 7 years of age were unable to produce such images, being limited to *reproductive images*, which can be formed only with direct experience of the object or event being imagined.

anticipatory regret REGRET, ANTICIPATORY.

anticipatory response Any response that precedes the stimulus designed to evoke or elicit it; any response that occurs before it should.

anticipatory schema SCHEMA, ANTICIPATORY.

anticonformity The tendency to reject pressure to conform. Unlike INDEPENDENCE (4), in which the connotation is that the individual is motivated by personal beliefs and opinions different from those put forward by the group, *anticonformity* is reserved for cases in which the individual reacts negatively to external pressures no matter what they are. Also called *counterconformity*.

anticonvulsants ANTIEPILEPTIC DRUGS.

antidepressant drugs A general pharmacological classification of drugs used in the treatment of depressive disorders. There are four main groups of drugs: the MONOAMINE OXIDASE (MAO) INHIBITORS, the TRICYCLIC COMPOUNDS, the SELECTIVE SEROTONIN REUPTAKE INHIBITORS and the MIXED-FUNCTION *ANTIDEPRESSANT DRUGS. The last of these are the most recently developed and are sometimes referred to as 'second generation' antidepressants. Some older classification systems included the *amphetamines* as antidepressants, although these are now more commonly grouped with the STIMULANTS; others include LITHIUM because of its use in the treatment of *bipolar disorder*. It is worth noting that while these drugs rapidly modify the concentrations of important BIOGENIC AMINES at critical synapses in the brain, their therapeutic effects are typically not felt for several weeks.

antidepressant drugs, mixed-function
Loosely, any of the ANTIDEPRESSANT DRUGS that function by modifying more than one neurotransmitter system. Those in current use affect the presence of both NOREPINEPHER-INE and SEROTONIN.

antidiuretic hormone VASOPRESSIN.

antidromic (neural) conduction The passing of a neural impulse in the reverse direction, from axon to the dendrites.

antiepileptic drugs A general category of drugs used to control seizures in disorders such as epilepsy. Interestingly, some (e.g. *clonazepam, carbamazepine*) are also used prophylactically to prevent the mood swings of *bipolar disorder* and other *mood disorders*. Also known as *anticonvulsant drugs*.

antiface In studies of face perception, a visual display of a human face that has been distorted so that it has the opposite features of the original, relative to an average face of the same gender and ethnicity. For example, the antiface of a person with a small mouth would have a large mouth, one with a wide nose would have a narrow one, etc.

antigens Protein markers that identify infectious micro-organisms to the IMMUNE SYSTEM, allowing it to develop ANTIBODIES.

antihistamine Lit., any substance or agent which inhibits or blocks the effect of *histamine*. Antihistamines are of some use in controlling rashes and allergic reactions caused by release of histamine and are helpful to sufferers of hay fever. They are also used occasionally as mild sedatives because they tend to produce drowsiness in most (although not all) persons.

anti-intraception A tendency to be opposed to that which is subjective, imaginative, humanistic. It is regarded as a characteristic of the AUTHORITARIAN PERSONALITY.

anti-language Language intended to be incomprehensible to anyone outside the group that speaks it, e.g. thieves' cant and cockney rhyming slang.

antimania drugs Drugs used for the treatment of *hypomania* and *bipolar disorder*. The drug of choice here is one of the *lithium* compounds. Note that, despite the label *antimania*, there is evidence that these drugs also help in preventing the depressive aspect of manic depression. See MOOD-STABILIZING DRUGS.

antimetropia A condition in which the two eyes have differences in refractive power. To a certain extent everyone is antimetropic; the term, however, is reserved for cases in which the differences are dramatic, e.g. one eye is myopic and the other hyperopic.

anti-Müllerian hormone A peptide hormone secreted by foetal testes. As the name suggests, it prevents the MÜLLERIAN SYSTEM from developing. Since the Müllerian is the default system, without this hormone a foetus will become female.

antinomy A logical contradiction or inconsistency of the most basic kind, where two (or more) separate principles lead to mutually incompatible conclusions: both 'A' and 'not A' are implied as being true. See, and compare with, PARADOX.

antiobsessional drugs A group of drugs used to reduce the symptoms of OBSESSIVE-COMPULSIVE DISORDERS. Included are CLOMIPRA-MINE, FLUOXETINE and FLUVOXAMINE. Interestingly, these drugs are all also used as antidepressants although their action here appears to be independent of their antidepressant effects; other antidepressants do not ameliorate the obsessive-compulsive symptoms.

antipraxia Characteristic of functions, processes or (in medicine) symptoms which are antagonistic to each other.

antipredator behaviour A general term for a variety of devices that prey species have evolved for protecting themselves from predators. Among them are camouflage, group defence, evasion, repellent odours or tastes, and mimicry.

antipsychotic drugs An umbrella label for several categories of drugs that are prescribed in cases of psychotic disorders. Included are the PHENOTHIAZINES and related THIOXANTHINES, the BUTYROPHENONES, the INDOLONES, and the generally less effective RAUWOLFIA ALKALOIDS. Generally speaking all of these drugs function to alleviate symptoms; they do not cure the disorders for which they are prescribed. They ameliorate the confused states, disturbed thinking and erratic affect of various psychoses and produce a general quietude, a slowing of responsiveness to external stimuli and a lessening of attentiveness without major changes in wakefulness or arousability. They also have a number of side effects that can be troublesome, such as muscular disorders, tremors, dry mouth, hypotension and various toxic allergic reactions. In this connection, see TARDIVE DYSKINESIA. In some texts the term MAJOR *TRANQUILLIZERS may still be used to refer to some of these drugs. For reasons outlined under that term, this is no longer recommended. Also known as *neuroleptics* (although see that term for nuances).

antipsychotic drugs, atypical A group of ANTIPSYCHOTIC DRUGS including CLOZAPINE and RISPERIDONE, that produce fewer extrapyramidal side effects (see EXTRAPYRAMIDAL SYNDROME) and are less likely to cause TARDIVE DYSKINESIA. They are DOPAMINE antagonists but also appear to block the effects of other neurotransmitters, specifically SEROTONIN. While developed primarily for use in schizophrenia and other delusional disorders, they appear to be effective as adjuncts in treatment of nonpsychotic conditions like OCD. Also called *second-generation antipsychotics*.

antisaccade SACCADE.

antisocial Descriptive of behaviour which is disruptive and harmful (or potentially so) to the functioning of a group or society. Contrast with ASOCIAL and PROSOCIAL.

antisocial personality disorder A personality disorder marked by a history of irresponsible and antisocial behaviour beginning in childhood or early adolescence (typically as a CONDUCT DISORDER) and continuing into adulthood. Early manifestations include lying, stealing, fighting, vandalism, running away from home, and cruelty. In adulthood the general pattern continues, characterized by such factors as significant unemployment, failures to conform to social norms, property destruction, stealing, failure to honour financial obligations, reckless disregard for one's own or others' safety, incapacity to maintain enduring relationships, poor parenting, and a consistent disregard for the truth. Also noted as an important feature is a glibness accompanied by a lack of remorse and a lack of, or lessened, ability to feel guilty for one's actions. Other labels that

have been used over the years to capture this syndrome include PSYCHOPATHY, PSYCHOPATHIC PERSONALITY and SOCIOPATHIC PERSONALITY.

Anton's syndrome ANOSOGNOSIA.

antonym test A verbal test in which the subject is given a word and must supply its antonym as quickly as possible.

anulus ANNULUS.

anus The opening of the rectum, the lower outlet of the alimentary canal.

anvil INCUS; AUDITORY *OSSICLES.

anxiety 1 Most generally, a vague, unpleasant emotional state with qualities of apprehension, dread, distress and uneasiness. Anxiety is frequently distinguished from FEAR by its being often (*usually* say some, *always* insist others) objectless, whereas fear assumes a specific feared object, person or event. **2** In theories of conditioning, the term is used to connote a secondary (or conditioned) drive that functions to motivate avoidance responding. Thus an avoidance response is assumed to be reinforced by a reduction in anxiety. **3** In Freudian theory, anxiety is treated as 1, with the additional assumption that it acts as a signal that psychic danger would result were an unconscious wish to be realized or acted upon. **4** In existentialism, the emotional accompaniment of the immediate awareness of the meaninglessness, incompleteness and chaotic nature of the world in which we live. See ANGST. There is an interesting temporal issue involved in these several uses. In the first two, anxiety is treated as a consequent emotion, a learned reaction which results from a particular state of affairs. In 3, it is regarded as an anticipatory reaction the origins of which lie at the level of unconscious conflict. In 4, it has neither of these elements, being treated instead as a pure, immediate outcome of 'being-in-the-world'. There are many compound terms that are built on this one. Some follow, others are found under the alphabetic listing of the modifying term.

anxiety disorder A cover term for a variety of maladaptive syndromes which have severe anxiety as the dominant disturbance. Included are GENERALIZED ANXIETY DISORDER,

PANIC DISORDER, PHOBIC DISORDER and POST-TRAU-MATIC STRESS DISORDER.

anxiety disorder, social A group of disorders marked by anxiety about performing in social settings, e.g. PUBLIC-SPEAKING *ANXIETY. See SOCIAL *PHOBIA, a common synonym, despite the fact that these disorders often do not display the morbid fear associated with true phobias.

anxiety disorders of childhood or adolescence A general category of mental disorders occurring in childhood or adolescence all of which have inappropriate anxiety as the primary feature. Included are AVOIDANT DISORDER OF CHILDHOOD OR ADOLESCENCE, OVER-ANXIOUS DISORDER and SEPARATION-ANXIETY DISORDER.

anxiety equivalent A psychoanalytic term for the physical symptoms which substitute for conscious awareness of anxiety, e.g. racing heart, trembling, light-headedness, sweating, rapid breathing. The term is not used for these sympathetic reactions when the individual is conscious of being anxious.

anxiety fixation A psychoanalytic term for anxiety in later life which is hypothesized to derive from earlier experiences.

anxiety, free floating The kind of vague, nebulous anxiety associated with the GENER-ALIZED ANXIETY DISORDERS. Also called, in older writings, *neurotic anxiety.*

anxiety hierarchy A series of related situations, acts or events (or mental images of these) which are ranked according to their anxiety-involving properties for an individual. They are used in desensitization techniques in behaviour therapy.

anxiety-induction therapies Any of a group of psychotherapeutic techniques based on the increase in anxiety as a precursor for eventually reducing it. All are based on the assumption that confronting the client with the source of their anxieties will ultimately prove effective when the feared negative consequences fail to materialize. Two main procedures are used here, FLOODING and IMPLOSION. Also known as *exposure therapies.*

anxiety, moral In psychoanalysis, anxiety which derives from the prohibitions of the superego. Compare with NEUROTIC *ANXIETY (2).

anxiety neurosis A subclass of anxiety disorders characterized by recurrent periods of intense anxiety. Usually included in this category are PANIC DISORDERS, GENERALIZED ANXIETY DISORDERS and OBSESSIVE-COMPULSIVE DISORDERS. The term is rarely used these days. Also called *anxiety state.*

anxiety, neurotic **1** FREE-FLOATING *ANXIETY. **2** In psychoanalysis, anxiety that derives from id impulses. Used more or less synonymously with INSTINCTUAL ANXIETY. Compare this meaning with MORAL *ANXIETY.

anxiety object A psychoanalytic term for the object upon which one symbolically displaces anxiety originally caused by other factors.

anxiety, persecutory PARANOID ANXIETY.

anxiety, public-speaking A SOCIAL *ANXIETY DISORDER marked by a fear of making a speech or presentation in public.

anxiety reaction GENERALIZED ANXIETY DISORDER.

anxiety, realistic Appropriate anxiety, that experienced to a legitimate threat. Such anxiety is adaptive as it marshals resources to deal with the circumstances.

anxiety-relief response A term coined by behaviour therapists for a learned operant response that can be used to reduce or relieve feelings of anxiety. The technique is to associate the response (usually saying out loud or thinking a word like 'calm' or 'relax') with the cessation of a painful stimulus (such as an electric shock). With the response now connected to a feeling of relief it can (at least in principle) be used in other anxious moments or circumstances.

anxiety sensitivity Chronic excessive sensitivity to the occurrence of ANXIETY (1) accompanied by a relative inability to tolerate anxiety when it occurs. ant., *tolerance of anxiety.*

anxiety, state See TRAIT *ANXIETY.

anxiety, tolerance of See ANXIETY SENSITIVITY.

anxiety, trait Anxiety owing to personality characteristics (*traits*) of an individual. The term is due to C. P. Spielberger, who distinguished it from *state anxiety*, which is a reaction to particular features of situations.

anxiolytic amnestic disorder SEDATIVE, HYPNOTIC OR ANXIOLYTIC AMNESTIC DISORDER.

anxiolytics ANTIANXIETY DRUGS.

anxiolytic withdrawal SEDATIVE, HYPNOTIC OR ANXIOLYTIC WITHDRAWAL.

anxiolytic withdrawal delirium SEDATIVE, HYPNOTIC OR ANXIOLYTIC WITHDRAWAL DELIRIUM.

anxious-ambivalent attachment See ATTACHMENT.

anxious-avoidant attachment See ATTACHMENT.

apanthropy An aversion to society or human companionship.

apareunia Inability to have sexual intercourse. The term is used for organic, 'mechanical' problems such as vaginal obstructions.

apathy Indifference, unresponsiveness, displaying less interest or reactivity to a situation than would normally be expected. adj., *apathetic* or (occasionally) *apathic*.

aperiodic reinforcement (schedule) A general term for reinforcement that is irregular or intermittent; any SCHEDULE OF *REINFORCEMENT other than continuous reinforcement is classified as *aperiodic*. Also called *intermittent reinforcement*.

aperture 1 Generally, an opening or orifice. **2** In any optical system, the opening through which light passes, e.g. the pupil of the eye.

Apgar score After Virginia Apgar, an American physician, a scaled score of a newborn's physical condition based on five measures (heart rate, respiration, muscle tone, colour and reflexive responsiveness). Usually an Apgar score is taken one minute after birth and again four minutes later.

aphagia Lit., the absence of eating. A condition in which the organism ceases ingestion of solid foods, assumed to result from a lesion in the LATERAL HYPOTHALAMUS. Compare with HYPERPHAGIA and distinguish from ANOREXIA NERVOSA.

aphakia Literally, without a lens. A condition in which the lens of the eye is missing or

has been removed, as in the common treatment for cataracts. The aphakic eye sees blues more vividly and is more responsive to very short-wavelength light, which is normally absorbed by the lens.

aphasia A general term covering any partial or complete loss of language abilities. The origins are always organic, namely a lesion in the brain. There are literally dozens of varieties of aphasia, and the classification systems and the symptoms of each variety are constantly being revised. Some classification systems are based on the (presumed) cortical locale of the lesion, others upon the general sensory and/or motor functions which are impaired, and still others on the particular linguistic skills that are lost. There is, not surprisingly, little agreement on the synonymity of the various specialized terms that are in use. The entries that follow give the most commonly used terms and the synonyms that seem warranted for each.

aphasia, acousticoamnestic Aphasia marked by diminished ability to understand and remember words and severe problems processing long sentences. It is typically associated with temporal lobe lesions.

aphasia, anomic An aphasia presumed to be due to lesions of the angular gyrus. The dominant symptom is a severe loss of the ability to name objects, i.e. lexical selection is badly impaired. Also known as *amnesic aphasia* and *nominal aphasia*.

aphasia, ataxic A general term for an aphasia characterized by loss of ability to articulate. Used similarly to MOTOR *APHASIA.

aphasia, auditory A form of aphasia in which the patient is unable to comprehend the meaning of spoken words. Also known as *word deafness* or *pure word deafness*, although these terms are misleading since the patient is not deaf. Of course, calling it an *aphasia* is also misleading since patients with the disorder are not aphasic and speak normally.

aphasia, Broca's A type of aphasia presumed to be due to damage to BROCA'S AREA. The aphasic who receives this diagnostic label typically produces little speech and that which is produced tends to be slow, very poorly articulated and generated with considerable effort. Usually, function words, inflectional endings and other 'dispensable' elements are dropped, giving the speech a *telegraphic* quality. Interestingly, such patients can usually comprehend spoken and written language normally or nearly normally, although in the motor form writing is also impaired. Also called *motor aphasia, expressive aphasia* or, on occasion, *nonfluent aphasia*. See discussion under MOTOR *APHASIA.

aphasia, conduction An aphasia presumed to be due to lesions which interrupt the nerve fibres connecting Broca's and Wernicke's areas (see ARCUATE FASCICULUS). The typical symptom here is difficulty in repeating a sentence just heard, although frequently there is also impairment of comprehension and some difficulty in articulation.

aphasia, developmental A term occasionally and incorrectly used for any of the syndromes properly called DEVELOPMENTAL LANGUAGE DISORDERS. Aphasia refers to *loss* of language; children in this category are those who fail to develop language properly.

aphasia, global A form of aphasia so named because language abilities are disrupted on a global scale. Generally presumed to be due to lesions in both Broca's and Wernicke's areas.

aphasia, jargon Aphasia marked by incoherent speech. Individual words tend to be pronounced properly but used in semantically inappropriate ways and syntax is garbled. Many regard it as a type of WERNICKE'S *APHASIA.

aphasia, mixed transcortical An aphasia caused by lesions involving the entire border zone of the frontal-parietal-occipital lobes. The language loss is usually total and the patient may only be capable of repeating words (*echolalia*) and show no other language competence. Also called, ambiguously, *isolation of speech syndrome*.

aphasia, motor A form of aphasia characterized by a partial or complete loss of the ability to produce articulate speech. Often, a particular variety of BROCA'S *APHASIA is termed motor aphasia. In principle, motor aphasias result from lesions of cortical tissue responsible for the motor functions of speech while Broca's aphasia is caused by lesions in Broca's area. However, the proximity of these areas in the brain makes such

distinctions academic. See also ANARTHRIA, used more generally for disturbances in articulation.

aphasia, optic A neurological condition marked by an inability to name visually presented objects. The condition differs from associative aphasia in that the patient knows the meaning of the stimulus (e.g. he or she may mime putting on a boot when shown one) but cannot produce the name (i.e. say 'boot'). Also called *anomia*.

aphasia, primary progressive A FRONTO-TEMPORAL *DEMENTIA marked by a gradual deterioration in language and speech functions but, unlike many other dementias, without any accompanying decline in general cognitive functions.

aphasia, syntactic A form of aphasia characterized by the loss of the ability to connect words properly so that the basic rules of syntax are adhered to. Also called *cataphasia*; see also, but distinguish from, AGRAMMATISM.

aphasia, transcortical A general label for an aphasia caused by a lesion that is outside of the perisylvan language centres: that is, outside of Broca's and Wernicke's areas. There are several forms here, *mixed, motor* and *sensory*.

aphasia, transcortical motor A nonfluent aphasia similar in many respects to BROCA'S *APHASIA with intact comprehension. The lesion, however, is anterior to Broca's area in the frontal lobe.

aphasia, transcortical sensory A fluent aphasia with dysfunctions of comprehension. The lesion is usually in the junction of the parietal, temporal and occipital lobes.

aphasia, traumatic A general term for any aphasia resulting from a head injury.

aphasia, Wernicke's A form of aphasia presumed to be due to lesions in WERNICKE'S AREA. Typically, the patient articulates normally, even fluently, but the speech tends to be 'empty', without coherency and full of lexical selection and grammatical errors. Comprehension of both written and spoken language is also impaired, as is the ability to repeat phrases. Also known as *receptive aphasia, sensory aphasia* and *fluent aphasia*.

aphemia Generally, loss of the ability to

speak. The term may be used as a strict synonym for MOTOR *APHASIA; some authors use it more broadly to cover impairments which are *functional* in origin (i.e. nonorganic). The former is preferred, the latter merely confusing.

aphonia Inability to produce the voiced speech sounds which use the larynx. Typically, the term is reserved for conditions that are not produced by brain lesions but due to any of a number of other factors, e.g. damage to peripheral nerves, laryngitis or functional disturbances.

aphoresis Lack of energy, weakness, poor endurance.

aphrasia Generally, inability (or refusal) to produce normal, fluent speech. The term is reserved for nonorganic syndromes; contrast with APHASIA.

aphrenia Lit., without mind. Used loosely in some older psychiatric writings for a loss of normal, conscious functioning.

aphrodisiac Generally, anything that stimulates sexual desire.

aphthenxia Generally, inability to speak owing to spasms in the muscles that control speech.

aplasia Generally, failure of an organ or body part to develop normally.

Aplysia californica A rather unappealing sea slug that has become a favourite of neurophysiologists. Its relatively simple nervous system is well known, and examination of changes that take place in it over time have led to insights into the biomolecular processes that underlie learning and memory.

apnea APNOEA.

apnoea Cessation of breathing. Typically temporary in nature and usually observed either immediately or soon after a period of heavy, deep breathing, which suggests that it is caused by a reduction in the stimulation of the respiratory centre because of lowered carbon dioxide levels. Although associated with several diseases it is also observed in perfectly healthy individuals during deep sleep, particularly the aged and the very young. It is believed by many to be a common cause of SUDDEN INFANT DEATH SYNDROME. var., *apnea*.

apo- Prefix denoting *away* or *separate*.

apokamnosic Easily fatigued.

apolepsis Cessation of function, used generally.

apomorphine A morphine derivative which acts as a central-nervous-system depressant. In low doses it blocks dopamine autoreceptors; in high doses it also blocks the postsynaptic receptors. It also acts on the brain's vomiting centre, making it an emetic, especially since when administered by injection it is not ejected with the vomit.

apopathic behaviour A general term for any behaviour influenced by or even requiring the presence of other persons, although not specifically directed at them. 'Showing off' is the classic example.

apoplexy Generally, an acute, abrupt loss of consciousness and subsequent motor paralysis caused by brain haemorrhage, embolism or thrombosis. This meaning is obsolete. If the term is used today it is applied strictly to pituitary haemorrhages.

apoptosis Literally, cell death; specifically, the natural loss of extraneous cells during development.

a posteriori Latin for *from what comes after*. Used to describe an inductively developed hypothesis or argument, i.e. one developed by inferring cause from a known set of facts.

***a posteriori* fallacy** The fallacious conclusion that event B was caused by event A made on the grounds that an after-the-fact analysis of one's data showed that B did indeed occur after A (*post hoc, ergo propter hoc*, 'after this, therefore because of this'). This fallacy, like all others, is a logical one: A may really have caused B but a retrospective analysis is not sufficient to show this. The fallacy typically occurs when a researcher does a bit too much DATA SNOOPING.

***a posteriori* test** Any statistical procedure that is introduced after the data have already been collected and examined. Typically carried out because interesting trends have emerged in the data that call out for examination. See also POST HOC TESTS.

apparatus 1 Most commonly in psychology, any device or instrument designed to facilitate running an experiment. **2** In physiology, any group of organs, parts and tissues which are functionally coordinated. Here, qualifiers are always used, e.g. vocal apparatus refers to the full set of structures and organs for producing sounds.

apparent motion MOTION, APPARENT.

appeal 1 Any action which serves to stimulate emotions or action in others. **2** The underlying value or incentive contained in a message or action.

appearance–reality task A task used with young children designed to explore their understanding of reality. In this task a child is shown and asked to identify objects that appear to be one thing but are actually something else, e.g. a rock made of painted sponge, an egg made from chalk. See also FALSE-BELIEF TASK.

appeasement behaviour In comparative studies and ethology, any behaviour of an animal which terminates an attack on it by another animal of the same species. See SUBMISSION (2).

apperception 1 In the original sense, dating back to Leibniz (1646–1716), a final, clear phase of perception characterized by recognition, identification or comprehension of what has been perceived. Several other historically prominent philosophical and psychological theorists have used the term with slight variations on this basic meaning. **2** For J. F. Herbart (1776–1841), the fundamental process of acquiring knowledge, wherein the perceived qualities of a new object, event or idea are assimilated with and related to already existing knowledge. He referred to the previously acquired knowledge as *apperceptive mass*. In some form or another, this basic notion that learning and understanding depend upon recognizing relationships between new ideas and existing knowledge is axiomatic of nearly all educational theory and practice. **3** W. Wundt (1832–1920) used the term in a somewhat similar fashion to refer to the active mental process of selecting and structuring internal experience, the focus of attention within the field of consciousness. Rarely used today although the concepts embodied in it are captured by other terms such as SELECTIVE ATTENTION.

apperceptive agnosia AGNOSIA, APPERCEPTIVE.

apperceptive mass APPERCEPTION (2).

appersonation A psychotic delusion in which one assumes the identity of another. Distinguish from the nontechnical term IMPERSONATION, which does not imply a delusion on the part of the individual.

appestat Loosely the area(s) in the hypothalamus assumed to play an important role in the control of appetite.

appetite 1 The term comes directly from the Latin for a *longing for*. This sense is carried over into most uses in psychology. Generally, motivational systems which are called *appetitive* are those that derive from normal physiological functioning, e.g. hunger, thirst, sex. The occasional tendency to limit the term to food and eating is inaccurately restrictive. Moreover, much contemporary usage implicitly reflects the notion that appetites may be learned or modified through experience. One may speak of developing an appetite for unusual foods or uncommon sexual preferences. **2** In some older writings, particularly those of McDougall's school of *hormic psychology*, an INSTINCT. But see that term for difficulties in meaning and usage.

appetite suppressant Any of several classes of drugs that suppress appetite and are used for weight control and obesity. Most are stimulants such as the amphetamines and related drugs (e.g. *phentermine, sibutramine*) that lower the reuptake of epinephrine, serotonin and dopamine. None have been shown to produce long-term weight loss without an accompanying nutritional and exercise programme. Also called *anorectants*.

appetitive See APPETITE (1) and APPETITIVE BEHAVIOUR.

appetitive behaviour Collectively, all those behaviours involved in searching for, obtaining and consuming a desired object (see APPETITE (1)). While the object is often food, the term is not restricted to this meaning and references to the sequence of behaviours surrounding sexual activity or drug-seeking as appetitive are common – with 'consuming' taking on metaphorical meaning when needed. Similarly, CLASSICAL CONDITIONING using 'positive' unconditioned stimuli such as food is termed *appetitive conditioning* and the food itself will be referred to as an *appetitive stimulus*.

appetitive conditioning APPETITIVE BEHAVIOUR.

appetitive stimulus APPETITIVE BEHAVIOUR.

applied psychology An umbrella term applied to all those subdisciplines within psychology that seek: (a) to apply principles, discoveries and theories of psychology in practical ways in related areas such as law, education, industry, marketing, opinion polling, sport; and/or (b) to discover basic principles that can be so applied. There is a subtle difference between these two approaches: one basically exploits what is known, the other strives for additional knowledge and is motivated by the aim of practical application.

applied research RESEARCH, PURE AND APPLIED.

apport The hypothesized moving of an object to a particular place by paranormal means. See PARAPSYCHOLOGY.

appraisal theory A general label for any of several theories of coping behaviour that emphasize the role of factors such as evaluating the nature of a given situation (e.g. how threatening is it?), determining whether or not the situation is controllable, and assessing one's abilities to make effective responses (SELF-EFFICACY).

apprehension 1 Etymologically the word derives from *prehension*, the act of seizing or of grasping. Hence, by extension, apprehension is the mental, conscious, 'grasping' of the nature of a stimulus or an event. Apprehension is generally treated as a rather primitive, immediate act (see APPREHENSION SPAN) and distinguished from COMPREHENSION, which involves greater reflection and interpretation. **2** By further extension, a vague fear or anxiousness about possible future occurrences. Here the notion is that one is 'seized' or 'enveloped' by a feeling of unease.

apprehension span The maximum number of objects or events that can be perceived in a single short exposure. It can be measured by having the subject report either the number of objects exposed or their identity. See also ATTENTION SPAN and SUBITIZE.

apprehensiveness A relatively mild sense of anxiety about forthcoming events, an uneasiness about future happenings.

approach–approach conflict CONFLICT, APPROACH–APPROACH.

approach–avoidance conflict CONFLICT, APPROACH–AVOIDANCE.

approach gradient The increased tendency of an organism to approach a desired goal as it gets closer to that goal. This gradient is assumed to be less steep than the *avoidance gradient*; that is, as one gets near them, positive goals do not increase in desirability as rapidly as negative goals increase in nondesirability. See CONFLICT et seq.

approach response Any movement toward an object or goal. *Movement* here may mean literal, physical movement toward a physical object or figurative, cognitive, affective movement toward a way of thinking or feeling about a person, idea, etc.

appropriateness of affect AFFECT, APPROPRIATENESS OF.

approximation conditioning A synonym for SHAPING.

appurtenance Kurt Koffka's term for the manner in which the various elements of a perceptual field are seen as coordinated and belonging together so that the display is perceived as an integrated whole.

apraxia From the Greek, meaning *without action*. Hence, partial or complete loss of the ability to perform purposive movements. The term is only used when other functions seem to be normal. That is, the individual is unable to carry out particular movement schemas even though motoric functions, perception and comprehension are intact. Apraxia is a general term and is invariably modified so that the type and form of the disability is specified, although usage is annoyingly inconsistent (e.g. the syndrome defined below under *ideational apraxia*, is occasionally referred to as *ideomotor apraxia*). adj., *apraxic, apractic*.

apraxia, akinetic A form of apraxia characterized by an inability to carry out spontaneous movements.

apraxia, amnesic (or **amnestic**) A form of apraxia characterized by an inability to carry out a sequence of movements upon request. The problem in most cases is faulty memory: the patient cannot remember the instructions about later movements when the time comes to perform them.

apraxia, buccofacial An apraxia marked by an inability to carry out voluntary movements involving the face, lips and tongue on request. Also called, more simply, *facial apraxia* or *oral apraxia*.

apraxia, callosal A LIMB *APRAXIA caused by damage to the anterior *corpus callosum*.

apraxia, constructional An apraxia characterized by a deficit in the ability to draw pictures or objects or assemble objects from other elements such as building blocks. It is caused by lesions in the right hemisphere, usually the right parietal lobe.

apraxia, facial BUCCOFACIAL *APRAXIA.

apraxia, ideational Improper use of objects owing to an inability to identify them correctly or to conceptualize their appropriate functions.

apraxia, ideokinetic A form of apraxia characterized by an inability to carry out a series of ordered movements. The patient may be capable of performing each separate act but the sequential order is confused.

apraxia, ideomotor A form of apraxia characterized by an inability to execute a single, complex movement properly. The patient performs inappropriate movements in the course of action.

apraxia, left parietal A LIMB *APRAXIA caused by damage to the posterior lobe of the left hemisphere.

apraxia, limb Apraxia characterized by (a) movements of the wrong part of a limb, (b) incorrect movements of the correct part of a limb, or (c) correct movements of a limb but in an inappropriate order. Occasionally the term IDEOKINETIC *APRAXIA is used for symptoms (a) and (b) and IDEOMOTOR *APRAXIA for (c).

apraxia, motor A general term for any of several forms of apraxia involving an inability to carry out planned acts; e.g. IDEOMOTOR *APRAXIA and IDEOKINETIC *APRAXIA.

apraxia, ocular An apraxia in which the patient is unable to maintain fixation so that the eyes wander back and forth between objects.

apraxia, optic An apraxia marked by a deficit in the ability to link an object with its functions. Patients have difficulty in tasks as simple as sewing a button on a sleeve, becoming confused about the functions of each object and the order in which the task needs to be carried out.

apraxia, oral BUCCOFACIAL *APRAXIA.

apraxia, sympathetic A LIMB *APRAXIA caused by damage to the anterior lobe of the left hemisphere.

a priori Latin for *from what comes before*. Hence, of reasoning, developed deductively, as, for example, a hypothesis formed on the basis of definitions previously formed or principles previously assumed.

a priorism The doctrine that the mind comes equipped with INNATE IDEAS and that, as a result, genuine knowledge independent of experience is possible. Contrast with EMPIRICISM. var., *apriorism*.

a priori (or **planned**) **test** A statistical procedure used in lieu of an overall significant analysis of variance, allowing one to test for significance of individual comparisons. Such a test can, in principle, be used only when the experimental hypotheses indicate that particular effects can be expected to be manifested in the data independent of overall effects. Compare with A POSTERIORI TEST.

aprosexia Inability to concentrate on things. The problem may result from sensory or mental deficiencies.

aprosodia A disorder of speech marked by loss of the ability to use properly the various PROSODIC FEATURES, such as stress, tonal shifts, cadence and emotional gesturing. There is a suggestion that it is associated with lesions in the right (or nondominant) hemisphere. *Sensory* and *motor* forms are distinguished if the disorder presents as primarily one of perceiving or producing prosodic features. Mild forms are called *dysprosodia*.

aptitude Generally, potential for achievement. The term is used with the connotation that a person displays an aptitude for something by virtue of a measurable, present ability which is interpreted as indicating that one may make, with some confidence, a prediction that the person's performance will increase markedly with additional training. The reason for phrasing this explanation in such convoluted fashion is that tests of aptitude are, in reality, tests of performance and interest; the distinction in usage comes from the notion of making a prediction about future achievements. See ABILITY and ACHIEVEMENT for further discussion.

aptitude, special APTITUDE TEST.

aptitude test Generally, any test designed to measure potential for achievement. Various types of aptitude test are often distinguished, namely *special*, *general* and *multiple*. Special-aptitude tests are those designed to measure potential for a restricted, single capacity, such as mechanical, clerical or musical aptitude. General-aptitude tests are broad-based tests designed to determine potential in relatively nonspecific domains; intelligence tests are general-aptitude tests. Multiple-aptitude tests are test batteries in which a number of factors are assessed. These classifications should be viewed pragmatically: special tests are only relatively special (e.g. the finger-dexterity test is a 'special' test for a specific aptitude but is clearly an aspect of a more general sensorimotor aptitude); and general tests are only relatively general (e.g. general intelligence tests are routinely factor-analysed into more specific components, such as verbal, quantitative, analytical, spatial). Multiple tests may, of course, be as 'special' or 'general' as the subtests which make up the full test battery.

aqueduct of Sylvius The canal in the midbrain running from the posterior end of the third ventricle to the fourth ventricle. Also called *cerebral aqueduct*.

aqueous humour The watery liquid in the anterior and posterior chambers of the eye between the cornea and the lens.

arachnoid membrane The web-like (hence the name) middle membrane covering the spinal cord and brain.

Arago phenomenon The relative insensitivity to light of the very centre of the visual field at very low levels of illumination.

arational NONRATIONAL.

arbitrary metric METRIC, ARBITRARY.

arborization Interlacing, branching. Used to describe neural networks, particularly those in the brain, that display tree-like conformations.

arbor vitae Latin for *tree of life*. Used of: **1** The tree-like outline seen in longitudinal sections of the cerebellum; **2** The branching ridges of the cervix.

arche- Combining form meaning *beginning*, *onset*.

archetypal form PRIMORDIAL IMAGE.

archetype 1 Generally, an original model, the first formed, the primordial type. **2** In Jung's characterization of the psyche, the inherited, unconscious ideas and images that are the components of the COLLECTIVE UNCONSCIOUS. Although Jung hypothesized the existence of many archetypes, several were presumed to have evolved sufficiently to be treated as distinct systems; see e.g. ANIMA, ANIMUS, PERSONA, SELF (6), SHADOW.

archicerebellum The phylogenetically oldest part of the cerebellum involved primarily in balance and eye movements. Inputs come from the inferior and medial vestibular nuclei and outputs return to the vestibular system creating a feedback loop that is critical in maintenance of balance. Also called *vestibulocerebellum*.

archicortex The phylogenetically oldest part of the cerebral cortex, specifically those components with only three distinct cell layers. It is involved in olfaction, is considered part of the limbic system and plays a role in emotions.

Archimedes spiral A simple line drawing of a spiral. It is used in the study of MOTION AFTEREFFECTS.

architectonic Systematic, well structured, orderly. Used primarily in neurophysiology to refer to the orderly structure of neural pathways and centres.

architecture 1 As borrowed from the science of building and design, a term used metaphorically for the overall configuration of a neurological structure, usually the brain or part thereof. **2** By extension, the overall composition of mental or behavioural functions, e.g. *cognitive architecture*. Note that the original term carries a sense of design and creation of structures; in contemporary neurobiology and psychology this connotation has been stripped away. adj., *architectural*, ARCHITECTONIC.

arc sine transformation A transformation which, when applied to data expressed in proportions, has the effect of minimizing differences between proportions near 0 and 1 and maximizing those near 0.5. Thus, the STANDARD *DEVIATIONS of two sample distributions of proportions are made more nearly equal, permitting the use of *t tests* without violating assumptions concerning homogeneity of variance.

arcuate fasciculus A major fibre pathway connecting WERNICKE'S AREA with BROCA'S AREA. Damage to the neurons in the pathway leads to CONDUCTION *APHASIA.

arcuate nucleus 1 A hypothalamic nucleus containing the cells which produce the hypothalamic hormones. **2** Any of the several groups of cells in the PYRAMIDS of the medulla. Neural tracts from the face and tongue terminate here and the nuclei play a role in facial somatosensory experience.

area The general dictionary meaning (circumscribed space, bounded domain) forms the conceptual basis for all specialized uses, namely: **1** A region of the cerebral cortex which can be geographically, histologically, or functionally distinguished from surrounding regions; see e.g. BROCA'S AREA. **2** The region under the curve of a distribution; or, more specifically, the region under the curve as specified by any two points along the x-axis. This area will contain a determinable number of cases (for frequency distributions) or a determinable proportion of cases (for probability distributions). **3** A field of study, e.g. the area of cognitive psychology.

area diagram A graphic method of presenting data in the form of a figure (most often a circle) divided into sections the size (area) of which is proportional in each case to the quantity represented. The familiar pie chart is a good example.

area postrema An area in the lower portion of the brain that is intimately involved in vomiting. Interestingly, the BLOOD–BRAIN BARRIER here is rather more permeable than in most other places, allowing relatively easy access of toxins to the vomiting centre so that the expulsion of the ingested poisons may be initiated.

area sampling SAMPLING, AREA.

area under the curve AREA (2).

areola 1 The pigmented area surrounding the nipple of the breast. **2** The part of the iris immediately enclosing the pupil of the eye.

argot A formal term meaning slang; specifically, a specialized slang which reflects the common and unique experiences of a particular group. Originally, the term was reserved for the language of criminal groups; now it is more widely used, and references to the 'scientist's argot' are found. See also JARGON.

argument constraints In linguistics, constraints imposed by the semantic entailments of verbs, adjectives, adverbs, etc., which must be satisfied for a phrase or sentence to make sense. For example, colour names require that the 'argument' be a physical thing; a verb like 'think' requires that the agent be a sentient creature; an adverb like 'angrily' entails an actor capable of emotions, etc. Violations of these constraints yield ANOMALOUS SENTENCES.

Argyll–Robertson pupil A dysfunctional pupil in which the normal reflexive contraction to light is missing, although the pupil still contracts normally during accommodation. The symptom is common in syphilitic *locomotor ataxia* and various forms of paralysis.

aristogenics An occasional synonym for EUGENICS

Aristotelian Of or pertaining to the doctrines of the 4th-century BC Greek philosopher. Aristotle argued that man is a rational animal endowed with an innate capacity for attaining knowledge from sense perception, and that knowledge is the result of deduction of universals and principles from perceptual information and not the 'recovering' of innate ideas, as Plato maintained. The term is also used to refer to Aristotle's methodology, which exhibits parallels to his psychological theory. He advocated the use of close observation and accurate classification of natural phenomena. Hence, the term is often used as a synonym for *empirical*. However, Aristotle also formalized a system of deductive propositional logic, so the term is also frequently used to refer specifically to this particular form of logic. At the most general level, the term can be taken to indicate the principle of careful deduction of knowledge, be it scientific or personal, from systematic observations of natural events.

Aristotle's illusion The misimpression that a single object is actually two objects when touched in the following manner: cross two fingers of one hand and have someone touch a marble or similar object to the two fingertips. Note that it is the 'outside' of each finger being touched, the source of the illusion.

arithmetic disorder, developmental A label for a syndrome among children characterized by a significantly lower performance in arithmetic achievement than one would expect from standardized tests, age, school, IQ, etc.

arithmetic mean MEAN, ARITHMETIC.

arithmetic series A series which increases or decreases by a constant factor, e.g. 2, 4, 6, 8, 10, 12,... Compare with GEOMETRIC SERIES.

arithmomania Lit., number madness. A compulsive, morbid fascination with counting objects, events, etc. It is seen in some SAVANTS.

Army Alpha and Beta Tests Two general tests of intelligence developed for use in screening recruits for the US Army in World War I. These tests were among the first large-scale, group-administered intelligence tests developed by psychologists. The Alpha was a standard examination that drew heavily on verbal skills; the Beta was a *performance test* designed for illiterates and recent émigrés to America whose English was poor.

aromatherapy An INNOVATIVE THERAPY based on the (dubious) assumption that the use of particular aromatic oils can improve psychological well-being. Aromatherapy sessions include massage and relaxation, and emphasize stress reduction, the real sources of whatever psychological improvement occurs.

arousal 1 Generally, a dimension of activity or readiness for activity based on the level of sensory excitability, glandular and hormonal levels and muscular readiness. **2** In physiology, a heightened state of cortical functioning. Cortical structures are 'aroused' by the stimulation from sensory receptors mediated through lower brain structures such as the reticular formation. Because of the breadth of usage and the generality of meaning, the term is typically used with qualifiers, e.g. cortical arousal (as above), sexual arousal, etc.

arousal theory THEORIES OF *EMOTION.

array 1 Generally, a display of scores, data, stimuli, etc. **2** More specifically, such a display arranged in tabular form. The table may be one-way (usually with scores ranked in order of magnitude), two-way (usually with scores arranged in columns and rows according to magnitude) or n-way, depending on the number of dimensions represented in the array.

arrest Generally, a stoppage, a cessation of the function, motion, development, etc. of a process. The term is used widely in discussions of physiological, medical, cognitive and emotional processes and its meaning is generally specified by context, e.g. *arrest of emotional development, cardiac arrest*.

arrhythmia Lack or disruption of normal rhythm; irregularity.

arrow (head) illusion MÜLLER–LYER ILLUSION.

arterio- Combining form denoting *artery* or *arterial*.

arteriosclerosis A general label for a variety of pathological conditions involving hardening, thickening and loss in elasticity of blood vessels, especially arteries. See also ATHEROSCLEROSIS.

arteriosclerotic dementia MULTI-INFARCT *DEMENTIA.

arteriovenous malformation A congenital knot of veins and arteries. If intact they cause no symptoms, but haemorrhages in the brain can cause a variety of cerebral dysfunctions.

arthritis Inflammation of a joint.

arthro- Combining form denoting *joint* or *articulation* of structures at a joint.

articular Pertaining to articulation or to the joints.

articulate 1 vb. To join together. 2 vb. To enunciate clearly. 3 adj. Well joined, properly constrained. Articulate speech is well formed, properly pronounced and meaningful; articulate movement is well coordinated and smooth.

articulation 1 Production of speech sounds by complex movements of the vocal organs, the *articulators*. Hence, this meaning refers specifically to the production of consonants and diphthongs, those phonetic elements in speech which require movements of the tongue, jaw, lips, pharynx, etc. Vowels are strictly 'steady state' phonetic elements and typically not considered part of articulation. This fine distinction, however, is not always made nor worried about outside highly technical writings. 2 The manner of connection of bones at a joint. 3 By extension, the joining together of separate elements of a complex system into a coordinated structure. This meaning is used in a variety of applied contexts such as education, organizational psychology, etc. 4 In GESTALT PSYCHOLOGY, the degree of complexity of a structure.

articulation disorder, developmental A general label for the failure of a child to develop appropriate and consistent ARTICULATION (1). Most frequently observed with the late-occurring speech sounds, e.g. *r*, *l*, *ch*, *sh*, *th*. Distinguish from DYSARTHRIA. Also called *phonological disorder*.

articulatory store A hypothesized memory system whereby auditory (and perhaps even visual) inputs are stored in a form that reflects their articulatory properties. Contrast with ACOUSTIC STORE, whereby the hypothesized mechanism is based on sensory systems for receiving sounds.

artifact Generally, any object made or modified by people. var., *artefact*.

artifact, cultural An artifact that has a culturally defined form and function.

artifact, experimental Any extraneous, uncontrolled element in a study that compromises the interpretation of the results.

artifact, statistical An incorrect or misleading inference due to a bias in collection or analysis of data, or the numbers themselves (taken collectively) which lead to this misleading inference.

artificial grammar GRAMMAR, ARTIFICIAL.

artificial intelligence (AI) 1 The interdisciplinary field, combining research and theory from cognitive psychology and computer sciences, which is focused on the development of artificial systems that capture and/or represent human-like thinking or 'intelligence'. 2 A manufactured intelligence that actually carries out human-like thinking and understanding. John Searle has made the distinction between 1 and 2 by calling the first 'weak AI' and the second 'strong AI'. For whatever it's worth, virtually no one in psychology, philosophy or the computer sciences has any problems with weak AI. It is seen as a natural consequence of attempts to build formal theories of human thought. On the other hand, there are many objections to even the possibility of strong AI. For more on this issue, see TURING'S TEST and CHINESE ROOM. Compare with COMPUTER SIMULATION, in which the intelligence is in the programmer of the computer and not the machine itself.

artificialism A PIAGETIAN label used for the tendency to view the world as having been created by people and hence to conclude that naturally occurring phenomena (the stars, the sun, flowers, rain) are the result of human action. Characteristic of the strongly egocentric view of the child in the PREOPERATORY STAGE. Vestiges of artificialism can be found in the myths and folk legends of many (perhaps even all) cultures.

artificial language LANGUAGE.

artificial pupil A device which controls the amount of light falling on the eye. The simplest is a pinhole; more elaborate ones have finely calibrated adjustable apertures.

artificial selection The process of selecting particular organisms for special breeding. Compare with NATURAL SELECTION.

artisan's cramp A muscle spasm caused by extended effort of the small muscles of the hand in tasks requiring fine motor coordination; 'writer's cramp'.

art therapy Therapy based on the use of artistic activities and materials. Used commonly with children where painting, sculpture and theatre are used to allow the child to express emotions. With adults it tends to be used as an adjunct to other therapeutic techniques and the focus is more on symbolic elements involved in the resolution of emotional conflicts and the solving of personal problems.

asapholalia Poorly articulated speech, mumbling.

ascendance A tendency to assume a leadership role in social interactions and groups. Ascendance is thought by some to lie at one pole of a dimension, the other end being represented by SUBMISSION. vars., *ascendence*, *ascendancy*.

ascending–descending series The kinds of series of stimuli used in the METHOD OF *LIMITS: see MEASUREMENT OF *THRESHOLD for description.

ascending pathway or tract Generally, any AFFERENT neural pathway, one that carries information from the periphery to the brain.

asceticism A way of living based upon voluntary abstention from sensual, physical pleasures and emphasizing simplicity and self-discipline. The ascetic usually professes to be focusing upon a higher moral/religious value system.

Asch situation A term used for the situation studied extensively by Solomon Asch in his investigations of conformity. The subject is one member of a group of people who are asked to make judgements about various stimuli (e.g. which of two lines is longer). Unknown to the subject, all other members of the group are stooges who deliberately agree that the erroneous answer is the correct one. Such circumstances allow for the assessment of the degree to which individuals succumb to group pressure to conform or maintain independence in their judgement. Also known as *Asch conformity experiment*.

ascribed role ROLE, ASCRIBED.

ASD AUTISTIC SPECTRUM DISORDER.

-ase Combining form used in the naming of an enzyme by attaching the suffix to the name of the substance it acts on.

asemasia ASYMBOLIA.

asemia ASYMBOLIA.

asexual 1 Literally, without sex or lacking sexuality. 2 Characterizing reproduction without the union of two sex cells. Compare here with SEXUAL REPRODUCTION.

'as if' A marvellous example of how specialists can take two perfectly ordinary, high-frequency words and convert them into a technical term with a welter of obscure, dense meanings and usages: 1 A variety of scientific thinking in which one formulates a coherent hypothesis and proceeds with one's explorations or experimentations on the presumption that it is true. The hypothesis so formed is often called the 'as if' hypothesis. 2 A philosophical point of view based on the notion that many of the most fundamental and useful principles of science are, in fact, hypothetical and as yet unproven. Science, of necessity, functions 'as if' they were valid. 3 Adler, influenced by this philosophical position, extended the domain of the term to the ways in which one's personality develops. The 'as if' became, for Adler, the presumption that one's striving for superiority had actually been achieved. See here GUIDING *FICTION. 4 In the study of children's play, the term is commonly used as a label for games of make-believe and fantasy.

asitia An aversion to food.

ASL AMERICAN SIGN LANGUAGE.

asocial 1 Without regard to society or social issues. This meaning is used to describe situations, events, behaviours or people which operate independently of (although not in opposition to – see ANTISOCIAL) social values and customs. An asocial person is one who is withdrawn from society. 2 Lacking in sensitivity to social customs. This meaning is closer to that of *antisocial* because the connotation is that such insensitivity can be potentially harmful to a group or society. See also NONSOCIAL, UNSOCIAL.

asomatognosia A denial of parts of one's own body. Commonly seen in cases of unilateral NEGLECT, when the patient has no problem identifying, say, their right arm while studiously denying that their left arm is theirs. When pressed they may claim that it is 'yours' or simply that they 'do not know' whose arm it is.

asonia TONE DEAFNESS.

aspartate ASPARTIC ACID.

aspartic acid An amino acid suspected of being a neurotransmitter. Because it is so widely distributed in the brain it has been difficult to localize its primary pathways. Also known as *aspartate*, its ionized form.

Asperger's syndrome (or **disorder**) An AUTISTIC SPECTRUM DISORDER, characterized by abnormalities of social interaction, particularly difficulty in reading body language and facial expressions, problems with changing tasks, preference for predictability of events and repetitive and stereotyped interests and activities, but without delay or retardation in language and cognitive development. Some authorities question whether it is a distinct syndrome or merely an instance of mild AUTISM (2).

asphalgesia Lit., self-pain. A feeling of burning or pain when touching a neutral object.

asphyxia Lit., lack of a pulse. Used, however, for the decrease in oxygen and increase in carbon dioxide produced by any interference with normal respiration.

aspiration 1 Desire, hope, aim; the goal(s) toward which one strives. **2** Breathing in. **3** The act of drawing something in or out by suction.

aspirational reference group REFERENCE GROUP, ASPIRATIONAL.

aspiration, level of Quite literally, the level to which one aspires. Operationally defined, a standard set by a person by which success or failure can be personally gauged. Compare with and distinguish from LEVEL OF *ACHIEVEMENT.

assault 1 A violent attack on a person. The form is usually used of physical attacks but the phrases *verbal assault* and *psychological assault* have become common. **2** Any invasive medical procedure carried out (illegally) without first obtaining the patient's permission.

assay To examine by test or trial. Hence, the analysis of any complex subject (e.g. a chemical substance, a drug) to determine its components.

A–S scale MEASUREMENT OF *AUTHORITARIANISM.

assertive behaviour facilitation ASSERTIVENESS TRAINING.

assertiveness training A general label for a variety of therapeutic techniques commonly used in the treatment of disorders that are characterized by a lack of assertiveness, such as DEPENDENT PERSONALITY DISORDER and SCHIZOID PERSONALITY DISORDER, and as a general training programme designed to teach persons how to assert themselves in our rather intimidating world. Also called *assertive behaviour facilitation*, although this term is used by some for only one of the various procedures, namely that based upon the use of assertive models whose behaviour the client learns to mimic.

assessment 1 Generally, any process that evaluates, rates, ranks or judges some feature of something, someone or some collection of things or individuals. **2** More specifically, PSYCHOLOGICAL *ASSESSMENT. **3** In evolutionary psychology, sizing up an organism in terms of its potential as a mate.

assessment, psychological Loosely, collecting information or data that allows for the assessing of an individual or individuals in terms of their psychological functioning. This definition is hopelessly broad but accurate. A wide variety of instruments are in routine use from standardized tests to psychometric instruments, from questionnaires to interviews, from physiological and medical work-ups to behavioural observations. All were developed to enable the making of recommendations, decisions and predictions about how individuals will function in particular settings and to carry out research on these topics.

assets–liabilities technique A therapeutic procedure in which the client compiles two lists of his or her behavioural and personality characteristics, one containing traits regarded as being of value (assets) and the other listing traits seen as personal liabilities. The technique is commonly used in behaviour therapy as a way of specifying goals for the client.

assignment therapy Moreno's term for a technique used in group therapy. After a sociometric analysis of the persons involved (see SOCIOMETRY), individuals are assigned to particular small groups based on an assessment of which particular collections of persons they can be expected to interact with so as to derive maximum therapeutic advantage.

assimilation The basic meaning is *to take in, absorb* or *incorporate as one's own*. A term that entails such broad connotations has proven hard to resist. In all of the following special usages this general sense is reflected to at least some degree. **1** In physiology, the absorption and conversion of food. **2** In Hering's theory of vision, the anabolism of photochemicals in the retina. **3** In Herbart's theory, when new ideas were incorporated into the existing *apperceptive mass* they were said to have been assimilated. **4** In Piaget's approach to development, the application of a general schema to a particular person, object or event. See here the accompanying Piagetian term ACCOMMODATION (3). **5** In early approaches to the study of memory, assimilation was proposed as a 'law' of memory whereby novel objects or events had to become incorporated into the existing cognitive structure before they could be remembered. **6** In standard psychodynamic approaches, certain pathologies, handicaps or simply unpleasant facts are often said to be assimilated when they are incorporated, in a tolerable way, into one's experiences. The proper antonyms for this meaning are *repression* and *suppression*. **7** In Jung's theory, the process of altering objects, events or ideas to fit the needs of the individual. **8** In Thorndike's theory, a term applied to situations in which an animal used a previously learned response in a new situation when there was sufficient commonality between the two. **9** In phonetics, the process by which two phonemes acquire common characteristics or become identical. **10** In sociology, the merging of groups or individuals with disparate backgrounds or identifications into one group with common identity. The process may be one-way, when one group or individual is absorbed by the other, or a mutual blending of the two. There are probably other usages in psychology but it seems clear that the term is already suffering from information overload. Some special uses in phrases follow.

assimilation-contrast theory A theory of attitude change based on the assumption that attitudes are modified by changes in the relationship between the originally held position, the opinion articulated by the person attempting to effect the change and the credibility of the source of the new attitude. Depending on these three factors, the person either will form a contrast with the source's opinions and not change (or even perhaps move in the opposite direction) or will assimilate the new attitude.

assimilation, generalizing In Piaget's theory, ASSIMILATION (4) based on a child's ability to notice the similarities among objects and to incorporate them into general classes and categories. It follows the development of RECOGNITORY *ASSIMILATION.

assimilation, law of An obsolete term for the notion that when in a novel situation one will behave in a manner similar to the way one did in similar circumstances encountered previously.

assimilation, reciprocal In Piaget's theory, the ASSIMILATION (4) of two schemas into each other such that both continue but each is modified by the assimilated components of the other. The interrelated development of visual and motor schemas is assumed by Piagetians to derive from this process.

assimilation, recognitory In Piaget's theory, ASSIMILATION (4) based on a child's ability to detect differences between objects and to make discriminative responses to them based on these differences. It follows the primitive REPRODUCTIVE *ASSIMILATION and is succeeded in turn by the more sophisticated GENERALIZING *ASSIMILATION.

assimilation, reproductive In Piaget's theory, the most basic form of ASSIMILATION (4), based on a child repeating the same reaction to a stimulus, object or environmental situation whenever it occurs. For example, grasping an object each time it appears allows, according to the theory, the child to assimilate its various features and properties. It is followed by RECOGNITORY *ASSIMILATION.

assimilative illusion A general label for any illusion in which the pragmatic, functional or emotional context within which the physical stimulus is embedded leads to an illusory misperception. The classic example is the child who, frightened by the dark, misrepresents objects in a room as monsters or threatening beasts. The term derives from the notion that the physical stimulus becomes incorporated into the emotional or cognitive scheme and so is interpreted in an illusory fashion.

assimilative learning ASSIMILATION (8).

association 1 Most generally, any learned, functional, connection between two (or more) elements. Identifying precisely what these elements are (e.g. ideas, acts, images, stimuli and responses, memories) and specifying the mechanisms underlying their connection (see here ASSOCIATIVE LAWS) is a theoretical exercise that has occupied many a philosopher and psychologist for many a year. See ASSOCIATIONISM for discussion of some of these. **2** The bond or the connection itself implied by meaning 1. In the heyday of an associately based behaviourism most theories of learning were couched in terms of *bonds* or *associations* between stimuli (S) and responses (R), or S–R connections. **3** A particular psychological experience evoked by a stimulus or event; for example, you are given the word 'sex' and a sequence of associations emerges. This meaning is embraced by 1 and is usually denoted by qualifiers, e.g. CONTROLLED *ASSOCIATION, FREE *ASSOCIATION. **4** In statistics, the degree to which changes in one variable are accompanied by changes in another. It is quite common in correlational analyses to speak of the *association* between statistically correlated variables. Note, finally, that the long and tortured history of usage of the term has spawned an enormous number of specialized uses. Most of those that have played or still are playing a role in psychology are listed below with the qualifiers most commonly used.

association areas The areas of the brain where the 'higher mental processes', such as thinking and reasoning, are assumed to occur. In general, those areas of the cortex which do not show clear motor or sensory function are assumed to be association areas. Most frequently cited are the frontal and parietal lobes.

association, backward A connection between one item of a list in a serial-learning task and an item or items that precede it. Backward associations are assumed to be weaker than FORWARD *ASSOCIATIONS. In either case, however, the more remote the association, the weaker the connection. See REMOTE *ASSOCIATION.

association by contiguity ASSOCIATIVE LAWS.

association, constrained A general term for any association procedure in which the stimuli the subjects are given or the types of responses allowed are limited. That is, any association other than FREE *ASSOCIATION.

association, controlled A technique used in both clinical and experimental work by which precise instructions are given to put boundaries on the kinds of associations given to stimuli by the client or subject. See e.g. ANTONYM TEST. It is a form of CONSTRAINED *ASSOCIATION.

association cortex ASSOCIATION AREAS.

association, direct An association between two items that is not mediated by other items or mnemonic devices.

association, forward A connection between one item of a list in a serial learning task and an item or items that follow it. Forward associations are assumed to be stronger than BACKWARD *ASSOCIATIONS.

association, free Any unconstrained association made between ideas, words, thoughts, etc. In a *free-association test* the subject is given a word and asked to reply with the first word that comes to mind. It has been used in such diverse areas as cognitive psychology to explore topics like meaning, syntax and implicit memory, and in psychoanalytical investigations and therapeutic procedures, where it mostly serves as a projective device to explore the client's unconscious.

association, immediate Generally, the first, short-latency (see LATENCY) response to a stimulus. An association which is *not* immediate may be either (a) one which is the second, third, etc., association in a chain or (b) one with an uncharacteristically long latency. The former is occasionally termed a *mediate association* (distinguish from REMOTE *ASSOCIATION); the latter has no generally accepted term but most psychotherapists consider such associations to be important revealers of underlying psychological conflicts and defences.

association, induced Any idea, image or word which results from a selected word presented to a subject; i.e. the first response to a stimulus in an ASSOCIATION TEST.

associationism A label usually attached to a philosophical/psychological doctrine that asserts that higher-order mental or behavioural processes result from the combination (association) of simpler mental or behavioural elements. Rather than representing an identifiable school of thought, associationism is more of a general principle which has served as the foundation for a variety of specific theories. Its roots can be traced back to the epistemology of Aristotle, who, in an essay on memory, proposed the three 'relations' between elements which lead to associations: similarity, contrast and contiguity.

Associationism really has two historically important lines, one philosophical, the other scientific. The philosophical is best represented by the British Empiricists (Locke, Berkeley, Hume, the Mills, etc.). With their strong antinativist bias they were in need of powerful principles by which complex mental life could be explained by appeal only to experience. Hobbes was the first to suggest that Aristotle's 'relations' could serve as an associationistic model of human cognition. The associationistic approach survived the many variations and points of disagreement between successive Empiricists and reached its highest level of development with Hartley and the Mills (father and son).

The scientific approach began with the first experimentation on memory by Ebbinghaus in 1885. The appeal to data to validate associationist doctrine continued through Pavlov's studies on conditioned reflexes and Thorndike's work on 'connectionism' and became, finally, the foundation on which Watson built behaviourism.

This orientation differed from the earlier philosophical approach in several ways. First, the primitive elements which became connected were no longer 'ideas' or 'sensa-

tions' but operationally defined stimuli and responses. Second, where the focus previously was on the rationalist analysis of associations already formed – a kind of 'armchair' introspectionism – it was now on how the associations were formed. Thus, *learning* became one of the most intensely researched areas in psychology. Third, mentalistic phenomena, available mainly through introspection, were no longer acceptable as legitimate data; attention shifted instead to objectively measurable behaviour. While no school has ever called itself 'associationist', the principle has proven to be one of the most enduring theoretical mechanisms. The basic notions of associationism have re-emerged in the cognitive sciences under the related term CONNECTIONISM (2).

association neuron INTERNEURON.

association, paradigmatic/syntagmatic In a free-association test, a *paradigmatic association* is any response that is related to the stimulus word by some semantic link, e.g. replying *table* to *chair*, *boy* to *girl*, or *black* to *white*. A *syntagmatic association* is any in which the response is a word that can syntactically follow in a sentence or a phrase, e.g. replying *runs* to *girl*, or *cloud* to *white*. Children tend to give syntagmatic associations, adults paradigmatic.

association, remote Any FORWARD or BACKWARD *ASSOCIATION between one item in a serial list and a nonadjacent item. Remote associations played an important role in Hull's (failed) attempt to explain the SERIAL-POSITION EFFECT.

association/sensation ratio The (roughly estimated) ratio of the size of the ASSOCIATION AREAS of the cortex to the size of the sensory areas. Although it has been used by some as a basis for comparing the learning capabilities of different species, conclusions drawn from such a measure should not be taken too seriously.

association test (or **experiment**) A generic label for any procedure, clinical or experimental, based on the presentation of a stimulus (usually, but not necessarily, a word) and having the subject respond with an association (usually, but not necessarily, a verbal one).

association time 1 The response time in an

ASSOCIATION TEST; the time it takes for the subject to respond to a stimulus. See also RESPONSE *LATENCY. **2** The time it takes for an association to be formed. The time in 1 is relatively easy to measure, that in 2 is not, the reason being that 1 concerns a strictly overt behaviour while 2 involves an internal, covert mental process. Over the years various techniques have been developed to try to deal with this issue; they range from the early work of Donders (see SUBTRACTION METHOD) to more recent studies with EEGs (see ELECTROENCEPHALOGRAM) and EVOKED POTENTIALS. In many modern writings the term *association time* is frequently eschewed in favour of any of a number of others, such as *retrieval time*, *reaction time* or *verification time*, depending upon which type of response is under examination.

associative agnosia AGNOSIA, ASSOCIATIVE.

associative bond The hypothetical link between the elements in an association.

associative-chain theory An early behaviourist theory of complex behaviour which argued that each of the several components in a sequential action was linked associatively to the preceding component so that the full act was 'chained off' in a smooth series of elementary acts. The theory is so simplistic that it is almost embarrassing to realize that it was once taken seriously: imagine regarding an uttered sentence as no more than a chain of words or a Bach partita as merely an associatively linked series of notes!

associative facilitation An obsolescent term for the facilitation of new associations by previously established ones.

associative illusion A general label for a large class of illusions all of which are produced by interactions between parts of the stimulus such that particular aspects of the display are misperceived. See e.g. PONZO ILLUSION.

associative inhibition 1 The inhibition of an established association by a new one. It can occur through either the acquiring of a new response to the old stimulus or learning to associate a new stimulus with the old response. Note that the use of the word *inhibition* here implies that the link between the associated elements has been weakened; the term *associative interference* is frequently used to avoid expressing any presumption about underlying bonds and instead to connote simply that some process is interfering with the retrieval of the old response. **2** A process assumed to be operating when new associations are unusually difficult to establish because of previously learned associations. See also BLOCKING and OVERSHADOWING.

associative interference ASSOCIATIVE INHIBITION (1).

associative laws A cover term for a number of older empirical and theoretical generalizations about the manner in which associations are formed. These include *contiguity*, the assumption that things which occur together in space and time will become linked with each other; *repetition* (or *frequency*), which assumes that elements which occur together often are likely to be associatively linked; *similarity*, whereby stimuli with similar referents are assumed to become associated with each other; *recency*, which assumes that the more recently formed associations are easiest to use or remember; *vividness*, in which unique, compelling associations are stronger than less vivid ones; *contrast*, in which things that differ from one another in compelling ways tend to be associated with each other; and *succession*, in which serial factors are assumed to be important in ordering associative chains. Dubbing them 'laws' was, in essence, wishful thinking. They are rather poorly formed for true laws and, as contemporary psychologists are all too aware, they do not carry much explanatory power. Most of them derive from the early ASSOCIATIONISM of philosophers and were not founded on hard experimental data. Nevertheless, they do have an often compelling intuitive validity, and the sophisticated student of psychology can see how many of these principles have re-emerged in other forms in studies of cognitive psychology, social psychology and dynamic psychology.

associative learning LEARNING, ASSOCIATIVE.

associative memory MEMORY, ASSOCIATIVE.

associative play PLAY, ASSOCIATIVE.

associative shifting Thorndike's notion that if a particular response can be maintained while the stimulus environment is gradually shifted (by adding new elements, removing old ones, etc.), the response will eventually be made to an entirely novel stimulus.

associative strength The (assumed) strength of the bond between a stimulus and a response. Defined thus, strength is a theoretical variable that can be measured in terms of the frequency with which the response is made to the stimulus, the resistance of the response to interference, memory for the response, etc. Although the term, theoretically, has broad applications it is used almost exclusively in verbal learning and conditioning studies.

assortative mating MATING, ASSORTATIVE.

assumed mean MEAN, ASSUMED.

assumed role ROLE, ASSUMED.

assumption The standard dictionary reveals the obvious: an assumption is something taken for granted, a supposition. However, it is important to note that the term is a very general one and that there are various specialized classes of assumptions. To wit: an AXIOM represents an assumption which is not subjectable to either proof or disproof but rather is universally accepted as given. In logic and mathematics, for example, axioms are accepted as self-evident for the sake of studying the consequences that can be deduced from them. A POSTULATE, on the other hand, is a principle the apparent truth of which is not universally accepted as self-evident. Instead, the postulate is adopted within the confines of a particular theory because it seems logically sound to do so, or because the postulate leads to a directly testable conclusion. The postulate, however, is still fundamentally an assumption since it is not a logical deduction within the theory and is not directly subjected to proof or disproof.

When the assumption (or, more properly, the proposition) is susceptible to proof or disproof by logical analysis, the proper term is THEOREM. Theorems, strictly speaking, are not assumptions: they are logical deductions from assumptions (axioms) and serve properly only within the confines of well-formed theories. However, not infrequently one is confronted with tentative explanations of data or as yet undemonstrated potential principles which are 'assumed' to be true. When such an assumption is stated in such a way as to be empirically evaluated or tested, it is properly called a HYPOTHESIS. In short, assumptions are things not to be taken for granted.

astasia Inability to sit upright or to stand owing to severe impairment of motor coordination. Astasia and *abasia* (a similar problem seen in walking) are often observed together, and an *abasia–astasia syndrome* has been noted that is essentially functional in origin.

astereognosis Partial or complete lack of ability to recognize objects by touch; a form of AGNOSIA.

astereopsis Lack of depth perception.

asthenia Generally, weakness, disability, lack or loss of strength. In physiology and medicine the most common usage of the term is with respect to weakness originating in muscular or cerebellar diseases. In studies of personality and affect, it usually refers to a general sense of debilitation, depression and inhibition.

asthenic type 1 A general label for a person who is chronically exhausted, displaying low energy levels, proneness to fatigue and a general lack of enthusiasm for life. **2** In Kretschmer's old classification system, a lean, slender body type which he believed was associated with a predisposition to schizophrenia.

asthenopia Lit., weakness of the eyes. A condition in which there is tiring of the eyes caused by a fatiguing of the extraocular muscles.

asthma A general term for any of several varieties of bronchial disorders characterized by a spasm of the upper respiratory system with difficult, laboured breathing caused by the spasmodic constriction of the bronchial tubes or the congestion of the tubes by the swelling of the mucous membranes. Asthmatic attacks often accompany allergic reactions but can also be precipitated by irritants in smoke and pesticides and exacerbated by stress and anxiety.

astigmatism An irregularity or defect in the curvature of the lens of the eye which produces distortions in the light falling on the retina. Generally correctable by the use of cylindrical lenses.

astrocytes GLIA.

astroglia GLIA.

astrology A pseudoscience, of interest mainly for insight into human gullibility, based on the belief that the stars (some of them!) have an influence on human personality or behaviour. The fallaciousness of astrology has been further underlined by modern statistical analysis and demonstrable errors in its purported astronomical basis. Most psychologists are led to the conclusion that the stars have about as much impact on our behaviour as we have on theirs. See also PARAPSYCHOLOGY.

asylum An obsolescent term (from the Latin for *sanctuary*) for any institution for persons unable to care for themselves.

asymbolia A partial or complete loss of the ability to comprehend the meaning of symbols. The loss may be specific to one domain (e.g. AMUSIA) or it may be widespread so that symbols of any kind, linguistic, musical, graphic or mathematical cannot be comprehended. Generally regarded as a form of APHASIA. vars, *asemasia, asemia*.

asymmetrical distribution SKEWNESS.

asymmetry Lacking in SYMMETRY. Used widely of bodies, organs, structures, distributions, logical relations, personal relationships, etc. when there is a lack of correspondence between the two sides. See SYMMETRY for various nuances of meaning and usage.

asymptomatic Lit., without symptoms. Generally used when an individual is known through lab tests or other techniques to have some disorder or disease despite the lack of overt physical or behavioural symptoms.

asymptote 1 Mathematically, the limit of the curve of a mathematical function, the line which the curve approaches but never reaches. 2 Behaviourally, the steady state of behaviour reached after no further changes in performance are detectable. Strictly speaking this latter usage is not correct since theoretically (i.e. according to meaning 1) an asymptote is never actually attained.

asynchrony Lack of coordination between events in time. Usage is generally restricted to situations in which synchrony is expected or normal. var., *asynchronism*.

asyndetic Disjointed, disconnected. Asyndetic speech is characterized by disjointed ideas strung together without grammatical regularities; asyndetic thought lacks connections between ideas and propositions. Both are common in schizophrenia. n., *asyndesis*.

asynergia Partial or complete loss of coordination between the muscle groups involved in complex motor acts. Typically, the responses required are made in a series rather than as a coordinated 'whole'. The disability is seen in cases of cerebellar disease or injury. var., *asynergy*.

ataque de nervios A CULTURE-SPECIFIC SYNDROME found in Latino cultures. Symptoms include uncontrollable shouting and trembling, attacks of crying, a feeling of heat rising in the chest and verbal or physical abuse aimed at others. Precipitating factors are stressful events, typically in the family, such as divorce, death or an accident involving a family member.

ataractic 1 adj. Tranquil, imperturbable. n., *ataraxia*. 2 n. A tranquillizing drug.

atavism 1 Reappearance of an earlier genetic characteristic not manifested in the immediately preceding generations; see REVERSION (2). Atavisms are significant occurrences since they show that genetic potential can survive for remarkably long periods of time without phenotypic displays. 2 The reappearance of a primitive form of behaviour. In this use of the term, the link with genetics made by meaning 1 is loose and may be missing altogether.

ataxia 1 Partial or complete loss of coordination of voluntary muscular movements. 2 Somewhat metaphorically, loss of coordination between emotions and thoughts; see MENTAL *ATAXIA. adjs., *ataxic, atactic*.

ataxia, intrapsychic MENTAL *ATAXIA.

ataxia, mental An abnormal lack of correspondence between thoughts or ideas and the expression of emotions. The term is generally reserved for cases that indicate a lasting discoordination in people whose behaviours are frequently at odds with their emotions, although an acute form can be induced by highly stressful situations. A good example is the pained laughter of many subjects in obedience-to-authority experiments while they were 'administering' possibly lethal shocks to other persons. See here OBEDIENCE. Also called *psychic ataxia, intrapsychic ataxia*.

ataxia, optic An ataxia characterized by a deficit in the ability to reach for objects under visual guidance. Also called *visuomotor ataxia*.

ataxia, sensory Ataxia caused by dysfunction in afferent pathways. Motor coordination is disrupted because of disturbances in conduction of sensory nerves, especially those responsible for proprioception.

ataxia, static Ataxia in which the lack of coordination results in a loss of the ability to maintain a normal standing position.

ataxic aphasia APHASIA, ATAXIC.

ataxic dysarthria DYSARTHRIA, ATAXIC.

ataxic speech A halting speaking pattern in which every syllable is stressed equally and typically followed by a pause. The normal prosodic features of intonation and stress are missing. Also called *scanning speech*.

ataxic writing Severely discoordinated writings.

atelia The maintenance of childish traits and characteristics into adulthood.

atelo- Combining form denoting *incomplete* or *imperfect*. Used typically with respect to developmental factors.

atherosclerosis A form of *arteriosclerosis* in which there is an accumulation of fatty substances in the blood vessels, obstructing them and impairing circulation.

athetosis A disability characterized by slow, twisting, snake-like movements, particularly in the arms and fingers. A variety of causes are known including encephalitis, hypoxia and damage to the basal ganglia.

athletic type One of Kretschmer's body types (see CONSTITUTIONAL THEORY) characterized by a well-proportioned, balanced physique.

athymia 1 Lack of feeling or emotional affect. 2 Absence of the thymus gland or absence of its secretions.

atmosphere effect An obsolescent term for the general-context effect in which the overall circumstances (i.e. the atmosphere) affect behaviour. When the term was first used it referred to the appearance of habits acquired in one context in a similar but inappropriate context, e.g. the inadvertent crossing of themselves by devout Catholics when entering a large imposing building such as a courthouse. The general notions connoted by the term are now carried by CONTEXT EFFECTS.

atomism 1 The general philosophical position that phenomena are best understood when broken down into their most elementary components. The term has a mildly derogatory flavour and is used mainly by critics of the position; proponents generally prefer ELEMENTARISM. 2 In sociology and social psychology, the approach to the study of a group or society that argues that all social phenomena must be viewed as the sum of the influences of the individuals that comprise the group. This position is rarely defended these days.

atonia Lack of muscle tone. vars., *atony*, *atonicity*.

atonic seizure A generalized seizure marked by a sudden loss of muscle tone. Also called *drop attack*.

ATP ADENOSINE TRIPHOSPHATE.

at risk Characterizing individuals, most often children and infants, who are more likely to develop disorders or dysfunctions owing to particular existing conditions. Children considered to be 'at risk' are those manifesting one or more of a collection of various factors, such as neurological SOFT SIGNS, low birth weight, a low APGAR SCORE, poor muscle tone, and any of several parental factors like a mother's drug or alcohol abuse.

atrium Any cavity or sinus; a chamber.

atrophy A wasting away of tissue caused by disease, old age or injury. Generally refers to muscle tissue; DEGENERATION (1) is the preferred term for neural tissue.

atropine (sulphate) An alkaloid derived from belladonna (the plant deadly nightshade). It is a respiratory and circulatory stimulant and counteracts parasympathetic stimulation. Hence, it relaxes nonvoluntary muscles and inhibits secretions by acting as a false transmitter preventing acetylcholine action. Local application in the eye causes pupil dilation and is used commonly in ophthalmological examinations. var., *atropin*.

attachment 1 Generally, a binding affection, an emotional tie between people. The usual connotation is that this kind of emotional relationship is infused with dependency: the persons rely on each other for emotional satisfaction. **2** In developmental psychology, an emotional bond formed between an infant and one or more adults such that the infant will: (a) approach them, especially in periods of distress; (b) show no fear of them, particularly during the stage when strangers evoke anxiety; (c) be highly receptive to being cared for by them; and (d) display anxiety if separated from them. See here ATTACHMENT BEHAVIOUR. **3** A tendency on the part of infants to form the kind of bond described in 2. The distinction between meanings 2 and 3 is needed because some authors treat attachment as an innate potential while others view it as a particular pattern of behaviour and make no presumptions concerning its genotypic foundations. **4** In anatomy, the connections by which tissues are joined to other bodily parts (usually muscle to bone).

attachment behaviour Bowlby's term for the behaviour of an infant with regard to the adult(s) with whom it has formed an ATTACHMENT (2). The essential feature of this behaviour is that the infant will seek out the adult (usually the mother) and behave so as to maintain maximally close contact. As Bowlby uses the term such behaviour is not merely a reaction to separation but a natural response to any distress or uncertainty.

attachment styles Quite literally, the particular styles of ATTACHMENT (1 or 2) established between any two individuals. The term originally emerged in the studies of parents and toddlers but is now used generally, although occasionally authors will refer to 'adult attachment styles' to prevent confusion. The *secure* style characterizes individuals who seek and are comfortable with social interaction and intimacy. The *ambivalent/resistant insecure* style characterizes those who both seek and reject intimacy and social interaction. The *avoidant insecure* style characterizes individuals who tend to avoid interaction and intimacy. Note that these two forms are also referred to as *anxious-ambivalent* and *anxious-avoidant* attachment, respectively, to mark the fact that anxiety is a common feature. In adulthood, the avoidant style is often bifurcated into a *dismissive* style in which social-emotional connections are avoided because others are devalued, and a *fearful* style in which one avoids connections because of fear of rejection. Attachments are viewed as consistent patterns of thinking, feeling and behaving in interpersonal situations. Since the conceptual focus here is on 'consistency' some argue for a *disorganized* type noted by a lack of consistent patterns of social behaviour.

attack 1 Sudden onset of a disease or a symptom. Usually used of major disorders in which the abrupt manifestation is dramatic and serious, such as epilepsy and cardiovascular disease. **2** Overt, aggressive action. Here the term covers both the physical and verbal varieties.

attack, quiet-biting PREDATORY ATTACK.

attensity A now obsolete term used by Titchener to refer to the clearness of a sensation which he hypothesized was important in attracting one's attention.

attention 1 A general term referring to the selective aspects of perception which function so that at any instant an organism focuses on certain features of the environment to the (relative) exclusion of other features. Attention may be conscious in that some stimulus elements are actively selected out of the total input, although, by and large, we are not explicitly aware of the factors which cause us to perceive only some small part of the total stimulus array. **2** The paying of particular notice to the behaviours and demands of another, usually of children or other relatively helpless persons who require that one attend to their needs. **3** (obs.) Titchener's term for a state of mental clarity in which one aspect of mind is more vivid than others.

attentional blink A brief pause in sensory

processing that occurs 200 to 800 msec after presentation of a stimulus. New stimuli presented during this interval are not likely to be perceived, possibly because the central nervous system is occupied in perceptual analysis of the first stimulus.

attentional capture CAPTURE.

attention decrement In social psychology, the tendency of people to pay less attention to information that is presented later in a given session. Good propagandists understand this principle implicitly and typically get the important points out early in a message.

attention-deficit disorder (ADD) ATTENTION-DEFICIT HYPERACTIVITY DISORDER.

attention-deficit disorder with hyperactivity (ADDH) ATTENTION-DEFICIT HYPERACTIVITY DISORDER.

attention-deficit hyperactivity disorder (ADHD) A disorder characterized by hyperactivity, attentional deficits and impulsivity. A *combined type* is often distinguished from an *inattentive type*. In the latter, there is a marked tendency for the child to withdraw from social settings and to pay little attention to events taking place in the environment with the hyperactive mode often missing or rarely manifested. In the combined form, the hyperactivity and impulsivity are present along with the lack of attention. Although ADHD is first manifested in childhood, it may not be diagnosed until later in life. It is a fairly common disorder and over the years various terms have been used for it and for disorders occasionally thought to be related. Included here are descriptive terms such as *attention-deficit disorder (ADD)*, *hyperkinesis*, *hyperkinetic syndrome* and *hyperactive child syndrome*, as well as others that imply some organic dysfunction such as *minimal brain damage*, *minimal cerebral dysfunction* and *minor cerebral dysfunction*. Also called *attention-deficit disorder with hyperactivity (ADDH)*.

attention, focal 1 (obs.) In Titchener's terms, the highest *attention level*. 2 More commonly, those aspects or objects of a perceptual field to which one is devoting attention.

attention level The extent to which one is attending to a stimulus. Historically, the term was used by the structuralists with a rather precise set of levels identified, ranging from the total nonattentiveness of an unconscious person to the vivid clarity of focal attention. Today the term is used without any real specification of levels or steps; rather it connotes a dimension of how much of one's attention is invested in or being attracted by a particular task or stimulus.

attention, margin of The 'edge' of one's attention. The term is used phenomenologically to refer to those components of a stimulus which the individual is only vaguely aware of or only poorly perceives. See FRINGE CONSCIOUSNESS and FRINGE OF CONSCIOUSNESS.

attention reflex The change in pupil size when attention is fixed on something. Also called *Piltz's reflex*.

attention-seeking Generally, descriptive of any behaviour engaged in for the purpose of securing the attention of others. Used with respect to the various devices children employ, particularly those which would otherwise prove maladaptive (although more than a few adults are pretty good at this little game).

attention span 1 Technically, the number of objects or separate stimulus elements that can be perceived in a single short presentation. See here APPREHENSION SPAN, SUBITIZING. 2 The amount of time that a person can continue to attend to one type of input. Meaning 2 is strictly nontechnical.

attenuation Lit., making thin. Thus, attenuating any stimulus means to reduce its strength, intensity, volume or value; an attenuator is any device which functions to attenuate a stimulus.

attenuator model A label for any of several models of selective attention which hypothesize a 'mental attenuator' that reduces the intensity of stimulus inputs not attended to. In the COCKTAIL-PARTY PHENOMENON, for example, the unattended messages are not completely shut out but rather attenuated so that a familiar or important piece of information, like one's name, 'gets through'. See also FILTER THEORY.

attic child A child raised in isolation, often

locked away in an attic by parents or guardians. See also FERAL CHILD for more details.

attitude Psychology regularly gets itself into stormy definitional waters, never more so than when a term like this one is used to denote a concept of fundamental importance in human behaviour and when the domain of reference turns out to be much more complex than the original neologists ever imagined. **1** Originally the term derived from the Latin *aptitudo* meaning *fitness*. Hence, an attitude rendered one fit to engage in the performance of some task. **2** In medical parlance, meaning 1 was (and still is) reflected by using *attitude* to refer to bodily position or posture, especially with regard to the positions of the limbs. **3** In ethology and comparative psychology meaning 2 was slightly extended to cover the idea of intended action, so that a crouching animal might be described as being in an 'attack attitude'. (So far so good, but subtleties are creeping in.) **4** In traditional personality and social psychology the term took on, for the first time, an explanatory role rather than merely a descriptive one. That is, an attitude was viewed as: Some internal affective orientation that would explain the actions of a person. This meaning is basically an extension of the idea of *intention* noted in 3, but contemporary usage generally entails several components, namely: *cognitive* (consciously held belief or opinion); *affective* (emotional tone or feeling); *evaluative* (positive or negative); and *conative* (disposition for action). There is considerable dispute as to which of these components should be regarded as more (or less) important. Cognitive theorists usually maintain that the underlying belief is fundamental, behaviourally oriented theorists focus on the conative (indeed, on occasion, quite extremely – see 5), while most other researchers consider a combination of the affective and evaluative components as critical. Exactly how the term is used in modern psychological literature thus depends largely on the theoretical tilt of the writer. **5** A response tendency. Here the notion is that the concept needs to be rescued from the fuzziness of 4, the way to do this being to operationalize it and regard attitudes as things which can only be inferred from observed behaviours. It was a nice try but, predictably, this meaning has all but disappeared. The connotation of these meanings has shifted over the years on the question of whether attitudes are fixed qualities or flexible and dependent on context. Early theorists tended to view them as relatively inflexible and characteristic of persons; most current researchers treat them as flexible and modifiable by the DEMAND CHARACTERISTICS of particular settings.

attitude change This phrase has come to stand as a label for a rather intensely investigated area of social and personality psychology. It covers a number of theories concerning the processes by which individuals can be persuaded to modify their attitudes. The theories reflect a rather overwhelming diversity of attitudes on the part of psychologists about the processes involved; a look at the discussion under ATTITUDE (4) will give a hint of this variety.

attitude change, negative and positive An attempt at changing the attitude of another may work, or it may, on occasion, have a reverse effect, changing the attitude but in a direction opposite to that intended. The former is called *positive* change; the latter *negative* change (or sometimes, the BOOMERANG EFFECT).

attitude cluster **1** A number of attitudes held by a person that are interrelated and distinct from other attitudes. **2** A set of related attitudes in a population of people that show strong covariance. Technically, high (or low) scores on one attitude within a cluster are accompanied by high (or low) scores on the others. Or, nontechnically, there is agreement across people. Note that 2 does *not* imply 1. For example, attitudes toward fiscal conservatism tend to cluster with attitudes toward sexual expression and victimless crimes in sense 2, but an extreme libertarian will display two distinct attitude clusters on these and related issues in sense 1.

attitude scale Any device designed to reveal a person's attitudes. They are usually paper-and-pencil tests in which the person agrees or disagrees with certain statements that have pre-established scale values. The individual's responses are assumed to reflect the way in which he or she would behave in specific situations – although, admittedly, there has been considerable dispute among specialists as to the degree of correspondence between the assessment of people's attitudes using these scales and the ways in which they actually behave in real-world circumstances. A number of specialized forms of attitude scale exist; see e.g. LIKERT SCALE, THURSTONE-TYPE SCALES.

attitudinizing Conscious outward manifestation of particular attitudes for the impact they have upon others in social settings; 'putting on airs'.

attraction 1 A characteristic of an object, activity or person such that it evokes approach responses from other objects or persons. **2** A tendency to approach an object, activity or person. Meaning 1 places the 'force' in the desired object: 'Marilyn Monroe held great attraction for many men.' Meaning 2 places it in the desirous person. 'Many men felt an attraction toward Marilyn Monroe.' It seems pretty clear that any sensible analysis of the psychology of attraction must appreciate that both aspects interact in complex, dynamic ways.

attribute 1 n. A perceived elementary or fundamental quality of a stimulus. The important thing to note here is that the attributes of a stimulus are psychological not physical: they are relatively invariant and represent whatever remains constant in changing stimulus conditions. For example, the attributes of colour are hue, saturation and brightness. **2** n. A defining characteristic of a thing. Concepts may be defined as particular clusters of attributes; see discussion under DISTINCTIVE FEATURE. **3** n. (obs.) In Titchener's structuralism, the fundamental characteristics of all sensations, which, as he specified them, were *quality*, *intensity*, *duration* and, for some sensations, *extensity* and *clearness*. **4** vb. To describe or impute, particularly to ascribe a particular trait or characteristic to a person. See here ATTRIBUTION THEORY.

attributional style An individual's style of assigning attributions concerning the good and bad events that occur in life. See also ATTRIBUTION THEORY and LOCUS OF CONTROL.

attribution, dispositional In Harold Kelley's ATTRIBUTION THEORY, a distinction was made between attributions based on personal, internal factors and those based on external, environmental factors. The former were called *dispositional*, the latter *situational*.

attribution error, fundamental A tendency of people observing the actions of another to interpret those actions as signs of or as resulting from an internal disposition or trait. It is regarded as an attribution *error* because making such an interpretation almost always underestimates the impact of the external environment and places too much responsibility for the behaviour on the individual's internal traits or tendencies. Some consider the term 'error' too strong, and prefer the term *correspondence bias*, indicating that there is a bias toward seeing a correspondence between people's behaviours and their true selves. It should be noted that there are significant cultural differences in the extent to which the effect is displayed. See ATTRIBUTION THEORY.

attribution of causality The theory, due to F. Heider, that a person's perceptions of the behaviour of another are determined largely by what he or she attributes the causes of that person's behaviour to. Specifically, the attribution is made either to *internal* personal causes or to the *external* action of the environment, or to some combination of the two. Thus, the argument goes, we evaluate the behaviour of others on the basis of perceived motives and intentions. Heider's work formed the conceptual basis of the more general approach known as ATTRIBUTION THEORY.

attribution of emotion A phrase commonly used to describe the theory of emotion put forward by S. Schachter, which argues that the experiencing of emotion is due to both the physiological activation level and the individual's cognitive interpretation of physiological changes.

attribution, situational DISPOSITIONAL *ATTRIBUTION.

attribution theory A general theoretical perspective in social psychology concerned with the issue of social perception. The act of attribution is one in which a person ascribes or imputes a characteristic (or trait, emotion, motive, etc.) to oneself or to another person. Thus, the term represents not so much a formal theory but a general approach to social psychology and personality theory in which behaviour is analysed in the light of this concept. Its roots go back to the GESTALT notion that information acquired through the past experiences of the observer plays an important role in processing new inputs. Modern attribution theory derives from the ATTRIBUTION OF CAUSALITY arguments of Heider and seeks to explain the manner in which people attribute characteristics and traits to people. In capsule form the theory maintains that the following sequence occurs in social situations: a person observes another engaging in some behaviour, makes an inference about that individual's intentions based on the perceived actions, then attributes some underlying motivating trait to the person which is consistent with the behaviour. There are many variations on this theme, including SELF-PERCEPTION THEORY, in which one's own conceptions of self are handled within this theoretical framework. For more discussion see PERSON PERCEPTION.

attrition From the Latin, meaning *a wearing away*. Hence: **1** Any loss of material through friction. **2** A decline in a population over time. The term has an interesting usage pattern which reflects a basic lack of concern over the precise cause of the loss. For example, fewer persons graduate from a university than enter it and the loss is usually noted as 'through attrition', with the connotation that somehow the inexorable laws of probabilities are operating.

atypical Generally and literally, not typical, not conforming to statistical expectations concerning the majority of cases under consideration. The term is common: **1** In statistical analyses to characterize scores which deviate markedly (usually two or more STANDARD *DEVIATIONS) from the measure of central tendency (usually the *mean*). **2** In descriptions of special individuals who differ in some fashion from the norm, e.g. disabled persons, gifted children, etc. Note that in this usage there is no evaluative connotation. **3** In the psychiatric literature as a label for a syndrome or disorder which does not quite fit the standard diagnostic category. For example, a person classified as displaying a dysthymic disorder (disturbed emotional expression) but with periods of up to two or three months of normal affect will be labelled an *atypical* dysthymic. This usage is a tacit admission of ignorance about making particularly difficult diagnoses. The term

enjoys wide use in psychology as a modifier of other mechanisms, syndromes, disorders and so forth. Some follow here, others can be found under the alphabetic listing of the main term; the meaning of most others is obvious.

atypical antipsychotic drugs ANTIPSYCHOTIC DRUGS, ATYPICAL.

atypical disorder Loosely, a psychiatric disorder where the patient exhibits unusual or uncharacteristic symptoms. The term is a rough synonym of NOT OTHERWISE SPECIFIED. Note, in the standard nosology, virtually every recognized disorder has an atypical version.

Aubert–Fleischl paradox A perceptual phenomenon whereby a moving stimulus seems to move more slowly when the observer fixates on the stimulus than when he or she fixates on the background.

Aubert–Förster phenomenon If two objects of different physical sizes are placed at different distances from the observer such that both subtend the same number of degrees of visual arc, the physically closer one can be recognized over a greater area of the retina than the physically more distant one.

Aubert phenomenon If a single vertical straight-line stimulus is presented to an observer the line will be perceptually displaced as the observer tilts his or her head.

audibility limits AUDIBILITY RANGE.

audibility range The full range of auditory stimuli which can be heard by the average adult subject. Full specification of this range is a complex task since the auditory system is not uniformly sensitive to all frequencies. However, the following rough outline will suffice: along the frequency (pitch) dimension the range is from about 20 Hz to 20,000 Hz, with maximum sensitivity in the neighbourhood of 1,000–4,000 Hz and a diminution in sensitivity to higher- and lower-pitched tones.

audible Detectable by the ear. Used of auditory stimuli that are above the threshold for the average person.

audience effects SPECTATOR EFFECTS.

audile VISILE.

audi(o)- Combining form meaning *hearing* or *related to hearing*.

audio analgesia Diminished sensitivity to pain produced by loud sounds.

audiogenic Pertaining to any phenomenon produced by or caused by sound.

audiogenic seizure Convulsions produced by long-term exposure to intense, high-pitched sound.

audiogram A graphic representation of a person's absolute auditory threshold. A complete audiogram shows thresholds for each ear for a number of different frequencies encompassing the normal range of hearing.

audiogyral (or **audiogravic**) **illusion** Misperception of the location of a sound source following disruption in bodily orientation, e.g. by being tilted, being made to think one has been tilted or being rotated rapidly.

audiology Originally, the study of hearing with emphasis on assessment, evaluation and treatment of hearing disorders. In recent years it has expanded considerably to include speech pathologies and disorders of balance resulting from middle ear disease, as well as the development of sophisticated hearing aids and cochlear prostheses.

audiometer A device for measuring hearing acuity. The standard procedure in audiometry is to evaluate the amount of hearing loss relative to established norms. The loss is generally expressed in decibels, meaning the number of decibels above the norm which were required for the individual being tested to just detect each test frequency.

audiometry The science of testing hearing.

audiometry, averaged electroencephalic A procedure for testing hearing in nonresponsive children (very young, autistic, severely retarded, etc.). It is based on the evaluation of changes in the electroencephalogram made by the perception of sounds and does not require any behavioural response from the subject.

audit Periodic review of a patient or of a pattern of patient care.

audition The broad area of study encompassing the psychological, physiological and psychophysical aspects of sound in organisms; specifically, studies of the mechanisms of hearing. Although many writers adhere to the convention that audition is a *sense* and hearing is a *process* many others do not. Hence, for combined terms not found here, see HEARING et seq.

audition, chromatic A form of SYNAESTHESIA in which colour sensations are evoked by auditory stimuli. Also called *coloured audition* and *coloured hearing*.

audito-oculogyric reflex Reflexive turning of the head and eyes in the direction of a sudden or alarming sound.

auditory Relating, in a general way, to the sense of hearing. Several related terms with more limited meanings are: ACOUSTIC, which is used for the physical descriptions of sound; HEARING, which is more properly used to refer to the full process rather than just the sensory aspects; AURAL, which is limited to the ear itself; OTIC, which is limited to the receptor cells; and TONAL, which is used to refer to the properties of auditory stimuli.

auditory acuity ACUITY, AUDITORY.

auditory agnosia AGNOSIA, AUDITORY.

auditory aphasia APHASIA, AUDITORY.

auditory attributes (or **dimensions**) TONAL ATTRIBUTES.

auditory canal The passage from the external ear to the eardrum, also known as the *external auditory meatus*.

auditory evoked potential EVOKED POTENTIAL.

auditory flicker FLICKER, AUDITORY.

auditory image IMAGE, AUDITORY.

auditory localization The perceptual determination of the point in space from which a sound emanates. The primary cues for localization depend on: (a) the fact that the ear closest to the sound source will receive the stimulation a short period of time before the other ear; (b) the head casts a 'shadow' which partially blocks out sound so that the ear closest to the source receives a more intense stimulus; and (c) the two ears receive different phases of the sound wave.

auditory masking MASKING.

auditory-musical intelligence MULTIPLE INTELLIGENCES THEORY.

auditory nerve VESTIBULOCOCHLEAR NERVE.

auditory ossicles OSSICLES, AUDITORY.

auditory pathways Collectively, those ascending and descending neural fibres that run between the hair cells of the inner ear and the auditory projection areas in the temporal lobe.

auditory phi (phenomenon) An analogue of the PHI PHENOMENON, a form of apparent motion produced by presenting two sounds in distinct locations with the appropriate time gap between them.

auditory (projection) areas The regions in the temporal lobes of the cortex where the ascending auditory pathways terminate.

auditory space The sense of the physical space surrounding one as perceived through sound. See AUDITORY LOCALIZATION.

auditory span The APPREHENSION SPAN for auditorily presented stimuli.

auditory spectrum SPECTRUM, AUDITORY.

auditory type Synonym for *audile*; see discussion under VISILE.

Aufgabe German for *task*. The term was used primarily by the early Würzburgers (see WÜRZBURG SCHOOL) to capture the notion that each particular task or set of instructions for performing a particular task carries with it a cluster of constraints which invite the use of particular processes. Although today the term is rarely used, the concept is important and is embodied in a variety of other terms, including *set*, *determining tendency* and *functional fixedness*.

augmentation principle In Kelley's ATTRIBUTION THEORY, the tendency to attribute especially strong motivations to an actor known to have carried out some action under conditions of high risk or when major constraints have been imposed.

aura A subjective experience that frequently precedes an epileptic seizure or an impending migraine headache. The aura may occur any time from a few hours to several seconds prior to onset. With migraines it usually consists of a variety of sensory-based hallucinations, e.g. flashes of light. With seizures it may have a variety of manifestations, including a sense of fear or strangeness, inappropriate feelings of familiarity (see DÉJÀ VU) or unusual sensations.

aural Of or pertaining to the ear. See AUDITION, AUDITORY et seq.

aural harmonic A harmonic produced within the auditory mechanism itself.

aural microphonic COCHLEAR MICROPHONIC.

Austrian school A group of early empirical psychologists led by the theologian-philosopher-psychologist Franz Brentano. They laid emphasis upon *acts* or processes of mind rather than upon the *contents*, as stressed by those who followed Wundt. The group evolved into the *Würzburg school* and served as an anticipator of the Functionalist system. See also ACT PSYCHOLOGY.

authoritarian Pertaining to the method of control by subjugation to authority, in which a clear social hierarchy exists and a single individual makes decisions and prescribes procedures.

authoritarian atmosphere K. Lewin's term for the general sociopolitical climate established when a group is led by a person who uses autocratic, authoritarian techniques. Compare with DEMOCRATIC ATMOSPHERE, LAISSEZ-FAIRE ATMOSPHERE.

authoritarian character AUTHORITARIAN PERSONALITY.

authoritarianism 1 A sociopolitical system based upon the subjugation of individual rights to the authority of the state and its leader(s). **2** An attitude or trait characterized by the belief that there should be strict adherence and obedience to authority. Here the term is applicable either to those who are in authority or to those subservient to authority. See AUTHORITARIAN PERSONALITY.

authoritarianism, measurement of Various scales were developed during the 1940s and 1950s to assess the hypothesized aspects of the authoritarian personality. They were: (a) the A–S scale (for anti-Semitism); (b) the E scale (for ethnocentrism); (c) the P–E–C scale (for politico-economic conservatism); and (d) the F scale (originally for fascism, later called anti-democracy).

authoritarian leader LEADER, AUTHORITARIAN.

authoritarian personality A term descriptive of one who desires an authoritarian social system, particularly one who seeks obedience, subordination and servile acceptance of authority. Such a person tends to be very obeisant toward those in authority over him or her and demanding of such obedience from those over whom he or she has authority. The term does not ordinarily refer to the person(s) in authority. Also called *authoritarian character*.

authority 1 Institutionalized and legal power as manifested within a social system. 2 The individuals who wield such power. Sociologists and social psychologists distinguish various forms of authority; a few main types follow. See also POWER.

authority, charismatic Authority due primarily to the extraordinary characteristics of an individual. It is uniquely different from other forms of authority in that the power arises outside of legitimate institutions.

authority, legal 1 Authority specifically established by law for the purpose of controlling and regulating social functions. Also called *rational-legal authority*. 2 Authority specifically established by the rules of an organization.

authority, nonlegitimate Authority achieved through coercion and force and maintained by systems of reward and punishment.

authority, rational Authority due primarily to the expert knowledge or abilities of an individual. Such authority lies outside factors such as personality or social class and is usually limited to the particular domain within which the expertise is displayed; a car mechanic will not necessarily be an authority on neurosurgery, and vice versa.

authority, traditional Authority which derives legitimacy and power from social and cultural traditions.

autism 1 From the roots *aut = self*, and *–ism = orientation or state*. Generally, any tendency to be self-absorbed to the extent that one's thoughts, feelings and desires are governed by one's internal apprehension of the world. The connotation is that such a condition is pathological; the internal states are not typically consonant with reality but are viewed in terms of fantasies and dreams, illusions and delusions rather than with an external reality shared by others. 2 A condition manifesting a cluster of dysfunctions similar to those outlined in meaning (1) that typically appear early in childhood. Most (although not all) cases are accompanied by severe cognitive deficits, particularly those associated with top-down, executive functions. Scores on standard IQ tests are typically below normal with up to 70% of cases scoring below 70 and as high as 40% scoring below 50. Repetitive motor activities like rocking, finger flicking or odd posturing are often seen. Typically there is reduced attention span although, paradoxically, some autistic children show amazing attentional capacities for particular games or activities. Others display a variety of odd ways of responding to the environment, usually including a fascination with inanimate objects and an insistence on routine, order and sameness. The hallmark of the disorder in any of its many and varied manifestations is a deficit in social functioning which, in the more severe cases is accompanied by diminished or even absent language skills. Occasionally the condition will be called *infantile autism* to mark its typically early onset. Because the disorder is manifested in such a wide variety of ways, the term AUTISTIC SPECTRUM DISORDER (ASD) is often used in the technical literature although the shortened form *autism* still dominates common usage. 3 Originally used by E. Bleuler for *schizophrenia*. This usage is not recommended.

autism, infantile Because AUTISM (2) typically appears early in life, often before language skills emerge, this term is an occasional synonym.

autism, socially shared Gardner Murphy's term for the tendency for groups to collectively elaborate and perpetuate beliefs for which there is no objective reality.

autistic Pertaining to AUTISM (1 or 2).

autistic disorder The term in the *DSM* for the PERVASIVE *DEVELOPMENTAL DISORDER discussed under the entries for AUTISM and AUTISTIC SPECTRUM DISORDER.

autistic fantasy A defence mechanism whereby the individual reacts to conflict and stress by engaging in excessive day-dreaming rather than appropriate task-oriented action and thought.

autistic spectrum disorder (ASD) A general label for any of a variety of disorders that emerge during childhood and manifest symptoms of AUTISM (1, but esp. 2). The very existence of this umbrella label implies what most contemporary researchers and clinicians suspect, that AUTISM is not a singular disorder and that the term itself is used as a kind of 'junk box' label that includes a number of disorders including ASPERGER'S SYNDROME and PERVASIVE *DEVELOPMENTAL DISORDER. In addition, children diagnosed with ASD will often vary quite dramatically in intelligence and in social and language skills, with many high-functioning autistics and Asperger's cases showing perfectly normal intelligence.

autistic thinking **1** Generally, thinking governed by internal wishes and desires irrespective of external real-world factors. **2** Thinking manifested by (or, better, inferred to be occurring in) an individual with autism.

aut(o)- A prefix meaning *self-initiated, self-directed* or *oriented toward the self*. Many combined terms using this prefix are self-explanatory, e.g. *autoanalysis* is self-analysis, *autocompetition* is competition with one's previous performances, etc. Terms that are less autoexplanatory follow.

autobiographical memory MEMORY, AUTOBIOGRAPHICAL.

autocathartic Descriptive of self-initiated behaviours which have cathartic value for the person (see CATHARSIS). Autobiographical writing often has such an effect.

autocentric Within the self. Occasionally used of the senses of smell and taste.

autochthonous From the Greek, meaning *from the land itself*; hence, used to refer to events originating from within an organism (relatively) independently of outside influences. For example, appetites such as hunger or thirst, obsessions, insights and ideas, have all been termed *autochthonous* at one time or another. Some clinicians characterize schizophrenia in this way, since so much schizophrenic behaviour seems to spring from within the person so affected. Compare with ALLOCHTHONOUS.

autochthonous gestalt An organized perception or other experience in which the integrating factors are self-produced rather than identifiable in the stimulus.

autochthonous variable VARIABLE, AUTOCHTHONOUS.

autoclitic A category of verbal behaviour proposed by Skinner in his analysis of language. Autoclitics represent a class of utterances intended to suggest verbal behaviour that is based upon the speaker's own role and dependent on other verbal behaviour. 'I am tempted to add…' or 'I agree with…' are classic examples. See TACT and MAND.

autoeroticism Lit., self-initiated eroticism. Although masturbation is the classic example of an autoerotic act, the term is also used for a variety of other behaviours and thoughts which have sexual elements, including fantasies, dreams, etc. var., *autoerotism*.

autoerotism AUTOEROTICISM.

autogenic Self-originated, self-initiated. See also AUTOGENOUS.

autogenous Usually a synonym for AUTOGENIC. However, it also overlaps in meaning with ENDOGENOUS (or ENDOGENIC), although without carrying the physiological connotations of that term.

autographism DERMOGRAPHIA.

autohypnosis Self-induced hypnosis.

autoimmune diseases Generally, diseases that result when the body's own cells are attacked by the IMMUNE SYSTEM. Such diseases often occur following infections, and it is suspected that the immune system somehow becomes sensitized to one of the body's natural proteins and attacks tissue containing it as though it were an invader. Rheumatoid arthritis, lupus and multiple sclerosis are autoimmune diseases.

autoinstructional device PROGRAMMED INSTRUCTION, TEACHING MACHINE.

autokinesis **1** Voluntary, self-initiated movement. **2** Movement resulting from stimuli that originate within the organism, e.g. movement produced by proprioceptive stimuli. **3** More metaphorically, a shift in cognitive or perceptual set brought about by internal, subjective factors.

autokinetic effect A type of apparent motion in which a small, objectively stationary spot of light in an otherwise dark environment appears to move about. The movement may cover as much as 20° of the visual field (i.e. upwards of 40° measured from point of origin) and is apparently not due to eye movements. Also called the *autokinetic illusion* or *phenomenon*.

automatic **1** Self-operating, capable of functioning without external control. **2** Without reflection or thought, spontaneous, involuntary. **3** By extension, machine-like.

automatic anxiety PRIMARY ANXIETY.

automaticity In cognitive psychology generally, the property of a process that it takes place largely independently of conscious control and of attention. In the classic example, the laborious, deliberative process of first learning how to drive a car gradually becomes replaced by the automatic operations of a well-practised driver who no longer needs to pay close attention to what he or she is doing. The behaviour is said to have become *automatized*.

automatic process AUTOMATICITY.

automatic speech **1** Speech delivered without conscious reflection on what is being said. Readily observed with extremely well-learned material, as with counting or saying the alphabet. **2** Speech which emerges devoid of conscious control. It is observed in some psychoses, in advanced senility and, occasionally, in highly emotional states.

automatic writing **1** Writing produced while attending to content and not to the actual process of writing itself. **2** Writing while one's attention is totally devoted to some other task. In experiments on automatic writing the subject's hand is hidden behind a screen to prevent him or her seeing what is being written. For what it's worth, Gertrude Stein did research on automatic writing while at college (and some of her critics say she never abandoned the technique).

automatism Any act performed automatically; that is, without conscious thought or reflection. The term is primarily used in reference to such undirected behaviour as is seen in PSYCHOMOTOR *EPILEPSY. Occasionally it is used to refer to reflexes and well-learned or habitual acts, although such usage is not recommended.

automatism, sensory Illusions or hallucinations produced by extended focusing on an object.

automatization The development of AUTOMATICITY.

automatograph Any device for measuring and recording involuntary movements.

automaton A machine that acts like a human being. The term is used primarily in studies of COMPUTER SIMULATION and ARTIFICIAL INTELLIGENCE.

automorphic perception The tendency to perceive others as similar to oneself. The term is reserved for instances when obvious differences are overlooked or misperceived.

autonoetic memory See NOETIC *MEMORY.

autonomic **1** Self-controlling or self-regulating. **2** Independent. **3** Spontaneous.

autonomic arousal disorder A SOMATOFORM DISORDER characterized by persistent or recurrent symptoms (other than pain) that can be attributed to autonomic arousal. The systems or organs typically affected include the cardiovascular (common symptoms include palpitations and fainting), respiratory (hyperventilation), gastrointestinal (vomiting, diarrhoea), urogenital (dysuria) and the skin (flushing, blushing).

autonomic balance The normal coordinated functioning between the parasympathetic and sympathetic divisions of the autonomic nervous system.

autonomic nervous system (ANS) A major division of the nervous system with two principal subdivisions, the *sympathetic* and the *parasympathetic*. The system is called 'autonomic' because many of the functions under its control are self-regulating, i.e. autonomous. The sympathetic division, anatomically, forms a fairly coherent system (see diagram on page 79). Its neurons originate in the thoracic and lumbar regions of the spinal cord (hence it is also called the *thoracolumbar system*) and synapse with the sympathetic

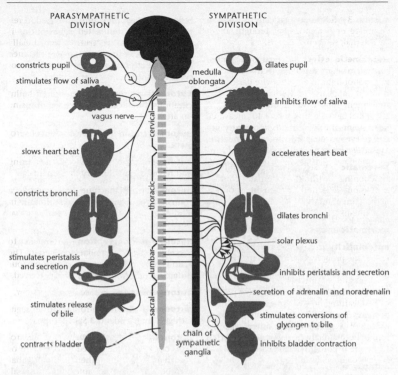

PARASYMPATHETIC DIVISION

SYMPATHETIC DIVISION

constricts pupil

stimulates flow of saliva

medulla oblongata

inhibits flow of saliva

vagus nerve

cervical

slows heart beat

constricts bronchi

thoracic

lumbar

sacral

dilates pupil

accelerates heart beat

dilates bronchi

solar plexus

stimulates peristalsis and secretion

inhibits peristalsis and secretion

secretion of adrenalin and noradrenalin

stimulates release of bile

stimulates conversions of glycogen to bile

contracts bladder

chain of sympathetic ganglia

inhibits bladder contraction

Autonomic nervous system

chain of ganglia (also called the *paravertebral ganglionic chain*). Depending upon the specific fibres in question, they either ascend or descend with the chain and exit elsewhere, synapse directly in the chain or pass through it to synapse with other ganglia on their way to their target organ. Taken as a whole, the sympathetic division serves 'arousal' functions, as shown in the figure.

The parasympathetic division has two distinct parts. Some fibres originate in the nuclei of the cranial nerves above the sympathetic division and others in the sacral region of the spinal cord below it. The parasympathetic division is involved in digestion and the maintenance of functions that conserve and protect bodily function (see figure) and is dominant during quiet, restful periods. Most (but not all) internal organs are served by both divisions of the ANS. Generally, the actions of the two divisions are

antagonistic, the sympathetic serving when catabolic processes (those involving energy expenditure) are called on, and the parasympathetic when anabolic (those involving energy build-up) are needed. However, pure antagonistic functioning is not the whole picture: the two divisions are interactive and 'cooperative' in many ways – for example, during extreme emotion when involuntary discharge of bladder and bowel may occur, or, in the male, during sex, when erection (parasympathetic) is followed by ejaculation (sympathetic).

autonomous Controlled from within, internally directed, self-regulatory. ant., *heteronomous*.

autonomous complex Jung's term for any complex which evolves unconsciously but, with the passage of time, wends its way into consciousness.

autonomy Independence.

autonomy, functional Gordon Allport's term for the tendency of a motive or motivating force to become independent from the original, primary drive that initiated it.

autonomy, group The characteristic of a group to remain relatively independent of, or outside, societal pressures.

autopagnosia An inability to name body parts. Patients with this disorder, which is caused by lesions to the left *parietal lobe*, cannot point to their elbow or knee or other body part when asked to, cannot indicate body parts on others (including manikins), and cannot name body parts when they are pointed to. Also called *somatopagnosia* and *autotopagnosia*, the condition is a form of AGNOSIA.

autophilia NARCISSISM.

autoplasty A process by which one's internal psychological system is developed. Autoplastic changes are changes in oneself. Contrast with ALLOPLASTY.

autopsychic Descriptive of psychological processes when the primary reference point is in the individual, e.g. delusions are autopsychic. Contrast with ALLOPSYCHIC.

autopsychosis A generic term for a psychotic condition in which the primary symptoms are displayed as disordered ideas concerning the self.

autopsy, psychological A psychological profile developed after an individual's death. The data consist of retrospective analyses of the individual's behaviour patterns prior to death collected by reviewing writings and letters and by interviewing family, friends, co-workers, etc. Such autopsies are usually carried out after suicides and in suspicious cases in which it is not clear whether death was accidental or self-inflicted.

autoreceptor A receptor molecule on a *neuron* that responds to the *neurotransmitter* that the neuron itself secretes.

autoshaping Automatic *shaping* of an operant response by pairing a stimulus with reinforcement such that the organism is attracted to the *manipulandum*. For example, a pigeon in a *Skinner box* has a light turned on

behind the 'key' (a small plastic disc) every time food is presented. After several dozen such pairings, the pigeon will 'automatically' begin to peck at the key whenever the light comes on even though it has never been specifically reinforced for key pecking.

autosome Any of the paired chromosomes, except for the sex (X and Y) chromosomes.

autosuggestion Lit., self-suggestion. The term comes from a system of self-improvement developed by Émile Coué, which was very popular in the 1920s and 1930s. The heart of Coué's rather simplistic system was contained in the phrase 'Every day in every way I am getting better and better', which he counselled people to repeat 20 to 30 times a day.

autotelic Characteristic of or pertaining to traits and behaviours which are intimately concerned with an individual's purposes and goals, especially those which are self-protective or self-defensive.

autotopagnosia AUTOPAGNOSIA.

auxiliary 1 adj. Providing support or assistance; helping. **2** adj. Additional, supplementary. **3** adj. Secondary, subsidiary. **4** n. In linguistics, a word with no full meaning of its own but which serves grammatical functions in combination with other words, e.g. conjunctions, prepositions, auxiliary verbs.

auxiliary ego In J. L. Moreno's theory, a person who takes on the role of representing and expressing another person's needs, desires, purposes, etc. Specifically, in a *psychodrama*, one who takes on the role of another person in such a way. For example, the role of the client's father is taken on by the client, but in a manner which reflects the way in which the client sees his or her father.

auxiliary inversion In linguistics, a form of interrogative in which the verbal auxiliary precedes the nominal element, e.g. 'Did she win the race?' Auxiliary inversions yield YES-NO QUESTIONS.

auxiliary solution Karen Horney's term for a type of NEUROTIC SOLUTION used to handle, partially or temporarily, conflicts. An auxiliary solution, in Horney's framework, is conceptually similar to a DEFENCE MECHANISM in that the conflict is not necessarily permanently resolved.

availability 1 In physiology, the extent to which a needed substance is present in a usable form for the tissues under consideration. 2 In studies of memory, the degree to which a particular piece of information can be retrieved from memory. 3 A COGNITIVE *HEURISTIC in which a decision-maker relies upon knowledge that is readily available rather than examining other alternatives or procedures. Although a useful heuristic, it can often lead to erroneous answers to questions or mistaken solutions to problems. For example, when asked whether more words in English begin with the letter r or have r as the third letter, virtually everyone answers 'begin with', despite the fact that there are roughly twice as many words with r in the third position. The error is caused by the fact that words beginning with r are readily available in memory whereas those with r in the third position are not.

average 1 A term which may refer to any one of three measures of CENTRAL TENDENCY, the (arithmetic) *mean*, the *median* or the *mode*. In general, when used without further explanation it refers to the mean. 2 Nontechnically, ordinary, typical, representative.

average deviation DEVIATION, AVERAGE.

average error ERROR, AVERAGE.

average error, method of MEASUREMENT OF *THRESHOLD.

averages, law of 1 The principle that, in the long run, the mean (average) of an extended series of observations may be taken as representing the best estimate of the 'true' value. This generalization is based on the assumption that, with unbiased sampling, the errors that occur will be distributed equally below and above the mean and, hence, cancel each other out. 2 By extension (assuming either a unimodal symmetrical distribution or a very large number of observations), the principle that the mean value will occur more frequently than any other value. 3 In popular terms, the principle that sooner or later it will all catch up with you.

aversion 1 Originally, a turning away. 2 Nowadays, a repugnance or dislike for something, an internal negative reaction. This meaning is reflected in a number of combined terms, e.g. CONDITIONED *AVERSION.

aversion, conditioned A learned AVERSION (2); specifically, an acquired syndrome in which an organism learns to avoid a particular food because of a conditioned aversion response to its smell or taste. The reaction can be formed in a single trial during which consumption of a novel food is followed by nausea and sickness, even when the toxic reaction itself is not experienced for some hours after eating. The key to conditioning here is that the original association must be with an internal, digestively linked stimulus, either the smell or the taste of the food substance, and the aversive outcome must be associated with an alimentary function such as nausea. It is a particularly interesting phenomenon because it can be formed over such a long interval of time; in all other forms of classical conditioning the optimal interval is of the order of half a second. Also known by a virtual blizzard of other terms including *conditioned flavour* (or *food*, or *taste*) *aversion* (or *avoidance*), *learned flavour* (or *food*, or *taste*) *aversion* (or *avoidance*), and any of the above without the qualifier *conditioned* or *learned*. Also found are terms like *bait shyness*, *toxicosis* and, simply, the *Garcia effect* (after the psychologist who did much of the early work). Note that in a parallel phenomenon a *preference* for a once neutral stimulus is conditioned.

aversion therapy A general term for any of a number of behaviour-modification techniques which use unpleasant or painful stimuli in a controlled fashion for the purpose of altering behaviour patterns in a therapeutic way. The use of such procedures has been primarily restricted to such disorders as alcoholism and drug abuse (and, in a few questionable cases, ego-dystonic homosexuality), and, generally speaking, has not been very successful.

aversive behaviour A general term used to describe the study of behaviour under conditions of noxious stimulation. Usually it covers the three major phenomena of *escape learning, avoidance learning* and the effects of *punishment*. Actually, the term is something of an anomaly for there is nothing aversive about the behaviour: the interest is in the behaviour which occurs under conditions which are aversive.

aversive control In studies of learning, a

general term used to characterize any situation in which behaviour has been brought under control by unpleasant or painful consequences, e.g. *escape learning*.

aversive racism RACISM, AVERSIVE.

aversive stimulus Any stimulus which appears to have noxious properties. Usually identified operationally as any stimulus to which an organism will learn to make some response so as to escape or avoid it, or as any stimulus which when presented contingent upon a response will produce a lower rate of that response or a cessation of it altogether. This very 'behavioural' definition derives from the simple fact that the term was coined by behaviourists and is used almost exclusively by them.

avocalia AMUSIA.

avoidance–avoidance conflict CONFLICT, AVOIDANCE–AVOIDANCE.

avoidance gradient The increased tendency of an organism to avoid a nondesirable goal as it gets closer to it. This gradient is assumed to be steeper than the *approach gradient*, i.e. negative goals increase in nondesirability with increased proximity more rapidly than positive goals increase in desirability.

avoidance learning (or **conditioning**) A type of instrumental or operant learning in which the subject must learn to make some response to avoid a noxious or aversive stimulus. In the typical avoidance-learning experiment there is a stimulus (e.g. a tone) which signals that the noxious stimulus (e.g. an electric shock) will be forthcoming unless the subject makes the appropriate response. If the response is made in time the noxious stimulus does not occur. The assumed reinforcer of such behaviour is anxiety reduction. Note that avoidance may be either *active*, when a specific response must be overtly made, or *passive*, when the subject must refrain from making a response which will produce the aversive stimulus.

avoidance response Any 'movement' away from an object or a goal. The notion of 'movement' may encompass anything from overt, physical locomotion away from some object or a metaphorical, covert shift in thoughts, opinions or beliefs.

avoidance rituals E. Goffman's term for the variety of social devices we use to keep social distance between ourselves and others, to maintain a certain formality in social interactions and to preserve individuality. Avoidance rituals and PRESENTATIONAL RITUALS together make up what Goffman called DEFERENCE BEHAVIOUR.

avoidant disorder of childhood or adolescence An anxiety disorder in children characterized by persistent and inappropriate shrinking from contact with strangers so severe that it interferes with normal social functioning in peer relationships. In the most recent edition of the *DSM* the disorder is classified as a SOCIAL *PHOBIA.

avoidant/insecure attachment ATTACHMENT STYLES.

avoidant-personality disorder A personality disorder characterized by a hypersensitivity to rejection that is so extreme that the individual avoids contacts with others and shies away from forming relationships unless given strong guarantees of uncritical acceptance. There is typically low self-esteem, a tendency to devalue personal accomplishments and inappropriate distress over personal shortcomings – all accompanied by a desire for affection and acceptance.

avolition Lacking in initiative; the inability to start and persist in goal-directed activity.

awareness 1 An internal, subjective state of being cognizant or conscious of something. **2** Alertness, consciousness. The term has a long history which has found it being used to refer to a wide range of subjective phenomena, from* simple, primitive detection of very weak stimuli to deep understanding of complex cognitive and affective events. Although it seems clear that the mental processes involved in being 'aware' of the presence of a dim light are fundamentally different from those involved in being 'aware' of the underlying psychodynamic factors which motivate action, the same term is used to cover them all.

awareness, learning without This phrase is often used in discussions of various learning phenomena in which a person is not 'aware' of their behaviour or the changes taking place in their behaviour. There are a number of experimental situations in which learning appears to take place without awareness, such as presentation of stimuli under low illumination, concept-formation experiments in which the concept is not easily verbalized, and verbal conditioning studies. It is safe to say that the issue is a highly controversial one, and just what each investigator means by 'awareness' is not always clear. For example, a psycholinguist who argues that a person is not aware of having learned the grammatical rules of language means something very different from a psychoanalyst who says that a client is not aware of acquired unconscious attitudes. See also IMPLICIT *LEARNING.

awareness, levels of This phrase emerged because of the recognition that the parent term, AWARENESS, had accumulated such a wide range of meanings and connotations that confusion was inescapable. Those who use the phrase maintain that a variety of levels of awareness exist, ranging from total lack of awareness of events (unconsciousness) to a highly tuned sensitivity to happenings in the environment. A number of more or less synonymous terms are also found, including *states of awareness, levels of consciousness, states of consciousness*.

awareness, unconscious An oxymoronic term blissfully on its way out of the psychologist's lexicon since it is so clearly a contradiction in terms. Preferred synonyms are IMPLICIT and TACIT.

axes Plural of AXIS.

axial Pertaining to an AXIS, situated in or along an axis.

axial amnesia AXIAL *DEMENTIA.

axial line Any line running along an AXIS of the body. Most commonly, the main, *cephalocaudal* axis.

axiom A proposition the truth of which is considered self-evident. Axioms are not susceptible to proof or disproof. In logical-theory construction the axioms form the fundamental, primitive elements upon which the whole theory rests. Differentiate from POSTULATE, in which the truth is not accepted as self-evident and needs to be considered within a chain of reasoning. See the discussion under ASSUMPTION. adj., *axiomatic*.

axis 1 A straight line which serves as a reference about which a structure, a figure or its parts may rotate or be conceptualized as rotating. This sense underlies the use of the term: in anatomy, where bodies, organs and their parts may be described with respect to one or more axes; in optics, where lenses may be characterized in terms of lines or passages of light; in chemistry, where arrangements of atoms and molecules are given relative to axes which define planes by which they are defined; etc. **2** In geometry, one of two (or more, depending on the number of dimensions under consideration) lines which are set to meet each other at a point and which can be used as a reference system to specify the location of any other point. The most commonly used system of axes is the CARTESIAN COORDINATES. **3** An underlying dimension, a class of information which may be used to group or to organize data. This meaning is an extension (and a loosening) of 2 above and is used in ways similar to FACTOR or DIMENSION.

axis I–V In the *DSM* system of psychiatric classification there are five axes, each designated by a Roman numeral. Axis I notes clinical syndromes, II developmental and personality disorders, III physical disorders and conditions, IV the severity of psychosocial stressors, and V global assessment of functioning.

axo- Pertaining to AXIS or to AXON.

axoaxonic synapse A synapse of a terminal button of the axon of one neuron upon the axon of another.

axodendrite A neural projection (or *process*) given off by an axon of a neuron.

axodendritic synapse The synapse of a terminal button of the axon of one neuron upon a dendrite of another.

axon A nerve-fibre projection (or *process*) leading from the cell body of a neuron which serves to transmit action potentials from the cell body to other adjacent neurons or to an effector such as a muscle. var., *axone*.

axonal transport The mechanism by which the molecules that participate in the process of synaptic transmission are distributed from the site of synthesis in the cell body to the axon terminal buttons. Compared with AXOPLASMIC TRANSPORT, it is a rather rapid process, roughly 400 mm per day.

axon hillock The area of a neuron where the axon rises from the soma. It has a lower threshold of excitation than the rest of the axon and an action potential can be readily produced there.

axoplasmic transport The process by which the soluble enzymes within a cell body move to the axonal terminals. Compared with AXONAL TRANSPORT, it is very slow, between roughly 1 and 3 mm per day.

axosomatic synapse A synapse of a ter-minal button of the axon of one neuron upon the cell body (the *soma*) of another.

axotomy Severing of an axon.

azaspirones A group of ANTIANXIETY DRUGS that function as SEROTONIN agonists. They have fewer side effects than the BENZODIAZE-PINES and are less likely to become drugs of abuse. However, the therapeutic effects often take up to two or three weeks so they aren't particularly useful for acute anxiety episodes. The prototype drug here is BUSPIRONE.

azygous Not paired, single.

B

babble Infant vocalizations, presumably produced without any meaning intended. As babbling gradually begins to include sounds typical of the speech environment and to be used for communication, various qualifiers are used, e.g. *directed babbling, controlled babbling*, etc. It is worth noting that even the profoundly deaf infant will babble for the first few months of life in a manner difficult to distinguish from that of normal-hearing infants.

Babinski reflex An upward extension of the toes upon stroking the sole of the foot. A normal reflex in infants up to about 1 year but a symptom of certain classes of organic disorders after that.

Babkin reflex In the newborn, a reflexive opening of the mouth in response to pressure on the palms.

baby blues See POSTPARTUM BLUES.

baby talk A basically silly term with two opposing denotations: **1** The speech *of* very young children. **2** The speech of adults and other children *to* very young children. See CHILD-DIRECTED SPEECH.

background 1 A person's collective experiences in life as they pertain to some task or job. **2** The total environmental setting preceding an event. **3** Any second sensory stimulus, as in 'background music'. **4** The set of objects and surfaces in the rear of a visual stimulus, the largely undifferentiated portion that contains no figure. See FIGURE–GROUND.

backpropagation In connectionist (or neural network) models with additional (or *hidden*) units, the process by which mismatches between input and output are corrected by having the error in the output units propagated back to the input units. Often simply referred to as 'backprop'. This may not be the clearest of definitions but the models can be quite mathematically complex. For more on these issues, see CONNECTIONISM (2), HEBB RULE, NETWORK MODELS and related entries.

backward association ASSOCIATION, BACKWARD.

backward conditioning An experimental conditioning procedure in which the conditioned stimulus (CS) follows the onset of the unconditioned stimulus (UCS) rather than preceding it. There is some dispute as to whether conditioning can occur with this arrangement. Contrast with DELAY, SIMULTANEOUS and TRACE CONDITIONING.

backward masking MASKING.

bad In psychoanalysis, the unpleasant, feared or malevolent aspects of an object. Thus, the 'bad mother' is the image of the punishing, love-withholding, persecuting mother.

bait shyness A particular instance of CONDITIONED *AVERSION.

balance Any state in which all opposing forces are equalized is said to be 'in balance'. The term is descriptively useful in aesthetics, the study of social interactions, investigations of emotional states, the maintenance of upright posture, etc.

balanced bilingualism BILINGUALISM, UNBALANCED.

balanced scale Any scale (or test or questionnaire) in which items with any potential source of bias are balanced. For example, half of the items may be presented as 'true' and half as 'false', or, in the case of Likert-type scales, half have the 'positive' or 'most agree' pole on the left side of the page and half have this pole on the right side.

balance theory A general theory of attitudes and attitude change due originally to F. Heider. The main assumption is that a person will seek to resolve or relate attitudes that are 'out of balance' with each other. Often used broadly as a label for a number of theories that put forward explanations of human behaviour in terms of the re-establishment of some form of psychological balance, e.g. theories based on COGNITIVE DISSONANCE or on PSYCHOLOGICAL *REACTANCE.

Baldwin effect An evolutionary mechanism put forward in the 1890s by James Mark Baldwin. It hypothesized a mechanism through which an increased capacity to learn new skills could be inherited and was proposed as a way of reconciling LAMARKIAN-ISM with DARWINISM. Baldwin's proposal was controversial the day it was announced and continues to be so. Originally called *organic selection*, it is also known as *Baldwinian evolution* and *ontogenic evolution*

Baldwin's figure/illusion A horizontal line with a box at each end. Large boxes make the line look shorter than small boxes, creating the illusion.

Balint's syndrome A neurological disorder characterized by three primary symptoms – OPTIC *ATAXIA, OCULAR *APRAXIA and SIMULTANAG-NOSIA – each of which is a disorder of spatial perception. The syndrome is caused by bilateral damage to the parieto-occipital region of the brain.

ballism A motor disorder (i.e. a *dyskinesia*) characterized by violent flailing movements. It is due usually to damage to one of the subthalamic nuclei associated with the BASAL GANGLIA. When only one side of the body is affected it is called *hemiballism*. Also known as *ballismus*.

ballistic Pertaining to or characteristic of the motion of projectiles. The eye movements known as *saccades* are often referred to as ballistic movements because the eye seems to 'throw itself' to its next fixation point. Such movements are easily seen in normal reading of printed materials.

band score See CONFIDENCE INTERVAL.

bandwagon effect A social phenomenon wherein people feel pressured to conform with a particular attitude or opinion when it is perceived as being held by a majority of persons in their group or society. This phenomenon can lead to the state known as PLURALISTIC IGNORANCE.

bandwagon technique A propaganda device in which it is claimed that a majority of people hold a position or belief so as to persuade others to adopt that position or belief.

bandwidth In acoustics: **1** The frequency range of a sound signal. **2** The frequency range of an instrument or device which responds to a sound signal. **3** In studies of information transmission and communication, a measure of the rate at which information can be transmitted.

baraesthesia (or **baraesthesis**) The sense of pressure or weight. var., *baresthesia*.

baragnosis An inability to provide accurate estimates of the weights of lifted objects. Usually a result of lesions of the parietal lobe. ant., *barognosis*.

Bárány test (or **method**) A test of the VES-TIBULAR APPARATUS in which the subject is rapidly rotated for some seconds and the resulting pattern of NYSTAGMUS is observed.

barbiturate abuse Generally, chronic, pathological use of barbiturates or similarly acting hypnosedatives to the point when the individual cannot stop or reduce the dosage, is intoxicated throughout the day and experiences disturbed and impaired social/occupational functioning as a result.

barbiturate amnestic disorder SEDATIVE, HYPNOTIC or ANXIOLYTIC AMNESTIC DISORDER.

barbiturates A large group of drugs classified as HYPNOSEDATIVES used as aids for sleeping, as anaesthetics and in the symptomatic treatment of epilepsy. Generally, barbiturates depress the activity of all excitable cells, although since the brain is particularly sensitive to them the therapeutic doses in use have negligible effects on other tissues. Barbiturate-induced sleep appears superficially normal but *REM sleep* (see SLEEP) is known to be significantly reduced. Depending on dosage, the effects range from mild sedation, through hypnosis and general anaesthesia, to coma and ultimately death. As with other drugs which depress central-nervous-system activity, the effects are magnified by alcohol, and alcohol–barbiturate poisoning is a significant cause of death both accidental and deliberate. Barbiturates can be divided into three classes, depending on speed and duration of action. The long-acting include *phenobarbital* and *mephobarbital*. These take effect slowly (approximately one hour after ingestion) and last roughly 8–12 hours. The intermediate-acting (15–30-minute onset time, 3–5-hour duration) include *pentobarbital*, *secobarbital* and *amobarbital*. The ultra-short-acting (1–2-second onset, 15–30-minute duration) include *thiopental* and *methohexital*. The long-term use of all barbiturates leads to TOLERANCE as well as both psychological and physiological DRUG *DEPENDENCE. These drugs, particularly the long-acting varieties, are sometimes classified as ANTIANXIETY DRUGS. See here SEDATIVE, HYPNOTIC, OR ANXIOLYTIC WITHDRAWAL.

barbiturate withdrawal SEDATIVE, HYPNOTIC or ANXIOLYTIC WITHDRAWAL.

barbiturate withdrawal delirium SEDATIVE, HYPNOTIC or ANXIOLYTIC WITHDRAWAL DELIRIUM.

bargaining Collectively all of those processes used by two or more persons or groups in their attempts to settle the give-and-take involved in a transaction between them. Buried in this definition are a host of critical variables which affect the bargaining process, such as expected outcomes (e.g. MINIMAX), gain and loss factors (see PAYOFF MATRIX) and personality factors (e.g. INTERNALIZATION, FACE-SAVING).

bar graph (or **chart** or **diagram**) A pictorial representation in which frequency, cost or some other attribute is represented as a bar. The length of the bar is proportional to the frequency or value represented. HISTOGRAMS and PARETO CHARTS are examples of bar graphs.

Barnum effect This term honours the master entrepreneur, showman and charlatan P. T. Barnum, best known for his aphorisms 'There's a sucker born every minute' and 'Something for everyone.' The eponymous effect is named after the latter and refers to the fact that a cleverly worded 'personal' description based on general, stereotyped statements will be readily accepted as an accurate self-description by most people. This principle is behind the fakery of fortune-tellers, astrologers and mind-readers and has often contaminated legitimate studies of personality assessment. Paul Meehl is credited with coining the term; in early research the effect was called the *fallacy of personal validation*.

bar(o)- Combining form meaning *weight, pressure*.

barognosis Antonym of BARAGNOSIS.

baroreceptor Specialized receptors that respond to changes in barometric pressure. Found primarily in the blood vessels and the heart.

barotaxis An automatic orienting response to a pressure stimulus as displayed, for example, by fish species that swim with (or against) water currents.

barotitis Inflammation of the ear caused by sudden shifts in barometric pressure. It is a not uncommon outcome of an aeroplane flight, especially if one has an upper respiratory infection which constricts the Eustachian tube and prevents normal adjustment of the ear to pressure shifts.

Barr bodies Spots at the edge of the nucleus of cells from individuals with more than one X chromosome. They are found in normal females (XX) but are missing in those with TURNER'S SYNDROME. They are also observed in abnormal males, e.g. those with KLINEFELTER'S SYNDROME. Because a Barr body is made up of a condensed mass of CHROMATIN, it is often called a *sex chromatin*.

barrier Any impediment or block that restrains or inhibits an organism from reaching a goal. Barriers may be physical features of the external environment or, more metaphorically, cognitive, emotional or behavioural limitations.

bar(y)- Combining form meaning *weighty, heavy, dull*.

baryecoia Partial deafness, hardness of hearing.

baryglossia Lit., thick tongue. Hence, slow, thick speech.

barylalia Indistinct 'thick' speech, poor articulation.

baryphonia Difficulty in producing articulate speech. var., *baryphony*.

basal 1 Of primary importance. **2** Pertaining to the base of a thing.

basal age AGE, BASAL.

basal forebrain A complex region of the ventral area of the forebrain. It houses a host of neural structures that are cholinergic and others that use GABA and glutamate. They project to various regions of the cortex, the thalamus, amygdala, hypothalamus, brain stem and hippocampus. Not surprisingly, they are involved in a variety of functions including arousal, cognition, motivation and emotion.

basal ganglia Three large, subcortical nuclei consisting of the *caudate nucleus*, the *putamen* and the *globus pallidus*. These nuclei are linked with several associated structures and pathways including the *subthalamic nucleus*, the *red nucleus*, the *substantia nigra* and the *nigrostriatal bundle* and are occasionally referred to collectively as the *extrapyramidal system*. The basal ganglia are intimately involved in the initiation and control of movement. Lesions in any of the associated structures or the inhibitory and excitatory connections they form with the spinal chord, the thalamus, the cortex and with each other have been implicated in a variety of disorders including PARKINSON'S DISEASE, HUNTINGTON'S DISEASE, TOURETTE'S SYNDROME and SYDENHAM'S CHOREA. Recent research also implicates the basal ganglia in IMPLICIT* LEARNING and PROCEDURAL *LEARNING.

There are various conventions for labelling parts of the basal ganglia. The putamen and caudate nucleus, because they share similar cell types, are collectively referred to as the *neostriatum*. The putamen and globus pallidus, because their overall configuration is lens-shaped, are occasionally called the *lenticular structure*. The globus pallidus is often labelled the *pallidum* and occasionally the *paleostriatum*. In some texts, the *amygdala* will also be included because of its anatomical proximity but, functionally, it is part of the *limbic system*.

basal metabolism rate (BMR) Measured in calories, this is the minimum energy output needed for minimum bodily functioning. The BMR is calculated by evaluating minimum heat production while the subject is at rest some 16 or so hours after eating.

base line 1 The abscissa. **2** BASE RATE. When 2 is the intended meaning, the spelling is usually as one word, *baseline*.

basement effect CEILING EFFECT.

base rate Generally, the normal frequency of occurrence of any response, statistic or other measure per unit of time. Base rates are used as foundations against which to evaluate effects of specific manipulations. For example, in assessing a new reading curriculum one would compare the new reading scores against the base rate prior to its introduction; in explorations of the occurrence of a disorder like schizophrenia in particular cultures, comparisons must be made against the base rate of the disorder across all cultures.

base-rate fallacy The tendency, when making decisions, to ignore the base rate at which events occur. It is surprisingly common; e.g. lotteries survive because people believe they have a much higher chance of winning than the base rate indicates; more people are afraid to fly than drive despite the much higher base rate of death on the roads than in the skies.

bashful bladder (syndrome) PARURESIS.

basi-, baso- Prefixes denoting *base* or *walking*.

basic Pertaining to a base, *fundamental*, *foundational*; occasionally, *primitive*.

basic anxiety Horney's term for a child's feelings of helplessness and isolation. These are assumed to arise from anything that interferes with or disrupts security. This concept is the primary one in Horney's theory of personality development. The strategies that the individual develops to deal with basic anxiety become the fundamental components of personality.

basic conflict Horney's term for the fundamental conflicts that emerge when NEUROTIC NEEDS are discoordinated. In her system, needs are classified into three groups: those involving movement toward people, away from people, and against people. A basic conflict will emerge if needs from two or three of these groups are activated simultaneously.

basic (level) category NATURAL *CATEGORY (2).

basic mistrust BASIC TRUST.

basic need Generally and loosely, any need based on primary, physiological factors; any need vital for survival. See BASIC NEEDS.

basic needs In Maslow's theory of personality, the primary human needs, including those which are physiologically based, like food, water and avoidance of pain (see FUNDAMENTAL NEEDS), and those which are psychologically based, such as security, affection and self-esteem (see INTERMEDIATE NEEDS). These needs are also termed *deficiency needs* or D-needs, on the assumption that if the object of need is absent a person will seek to make up for the deficiency. Maslow also assumed that basic needs have a priority hierarchy such that some take precedence over others; e.g. when there is no food there is little concern for self-esteem. See also META-NEEDS, NEED HIERARCHY.

basic rest-activity cycle (BRAC) A cycle approximately 90 minutes long in which the body's alertness waxes and wanes. The cycle is controlled by cells in the caudal brain stem. During sleep the BRAC controls the cycles of REM and SLOW-WAVE *SLEEP. See also BIOLOGICAL CLOCK.

basic skills In education, those skills deemed fundamental for further education and essential for learning other subjects; most commonly included are reading, writing and arithmetic.

basic trust The early development of a sense of fundamental trust in the environment. The concept is fundamental in Erik Erikson's theory of psychosocial development: the first life crisis occurs during the first year and a half, during which the presence of a loving, reliable and responsible caretaker leads to the development of a sense of security and basic trust in the environment, whereas unreliable, uncaring and irresponsible caretakers lead to the development of anxiety, suspicion and *basic mistrust*. See STAGES OF MAN.

basilar membrane A delicate membrane in the cochlea of the inner ear on which the ORGAN OF *CORTI is located. It varies in width, stiffness and mass along its length from the base (near the stapes) to the apex. Different portions of the membrane vibrate to different frequencies. The pattern of vibration is central to pitch perception, with the narrow end nearest to the stapes showing maximum displacement to high-pitched tones and the broad apex showing maximum displacement to low-pitched tones. See also THEORIES OF *HEARING.

basket cell A type of interneuron found in the outer layer (the molecular layer) of the cortex of the cerebellum.

basket endings Sensory receptors in the skin. Found at the base of individual hairs, they respond to movements of the hair.

basolateral group The phylogenetically newer part of the AMYGDALA.

Batesian mimicry MIMICRY.

bathy- Combining form meaning *deep*.

bathyaesthesia Deep sensitivity. Used for sensitivity in body parts under the skin, in muscles, internal organs, etc. var., *bathyesthesia*.

bathyanaesthesia Loss of deep sensitivity. var., *bathyanesthesia*.

battered Abused, beaten subjected to severe stress. Usage is occasionally extended to include psychological abuse as well as physical. The term is found in a host of phrases referring to battered children, battered women and to the psychological syndromes that can accompany such abuse (e.g. CHILD ABUSE).

battered child BATTERED.

battery (of tests) TEST BATTERY.

battle fatigue A term introduced during World War II for what was known earlier as *shell shock* and is now called COMBAT FATIGUE or POST-TRAUMATIC STRESS DISORDER. See also GROSS *STRESS REACTION, of which it is an example.

Bayes's theorem A mathematical expression of the various conditional probabilities of various events that gives the probability that a particular event (A) is a result of one (X) of a number of mutually independent events ($B, C, D, ... Z$) which might have produced A. The theorem is a mathematical prescription for estimating the probability that a hypothesis is true taking into account the conditional probabilities of several other mutually independent events that may (or may not) be true. It has been used as a model of attitude formation and choice behaviour since it provides a mathematical rule for deciding how one's prior opinion or choice(s) should optimally be modified in light of new evidence.

Bayley Scales of Infant Development
One of the most commonly used of the DEVELOPMENTAL SCALES for assessing the status of infants and young children. The current version is normed on children aged 1 to 42 months and uses five scales: motor, cognitive, language, adaptive behaviour, and social-emotional. The test is usually called 'the Bayley' for short.

beat A periodic fluctuation heard when two tones of slightly different frequency are sounded at the same time. The number of beats per second corresponds to the difference in Hz between the two frequencies. See also COMBINATION TONE, DIFFERENCE TONE.

Beck Depression Inventory (BDI) A self-report inventory developed by Aaron T. Beck, the American psychiatrist who is generally regarded as the father of COGNITIVE THERAPY, and based on a series of key aspects of behaviour and emotion with regard to which the subject selects the statement or statements that apply. For example, the subject selects one (or more) of four statements concerning decision-making that range from 'I make decisions about as well as I ever could' to 'I can't make decisions at all any more.' The scale is not intended to diagnose true depression, but can be used to screen for depression or to assess changes in affective state over time.

bedlam Originally derived from the Middle English pronunciation of the Hospital of St Mary of 'Bethlehem' ('be*d*lem'): **1** An asylum for the mentally disturbed. **2** Any raucous, noisy place or situation.

bedwetting ENURESIS.

behaviour A generic term covering acts, activities, responses, reactions, movements, processes, operations, etc.; in short, any measurable response of an organism. There has been a long (and agonizing) tradition of

attempting to put some set of coherent limits on the boundaries of denotation of this term. Doubtless, much of this derives from a well-meant but basically hopeless attempt to define psychology as 'the science of behaviour', a definitional gesture that has resulted in a fascinating kind of futility. The problem has been that as the range of phenomena included within the domain of psychology has increased there has been a need to expand the boundaries of what can be legitimately called 'behaviour'.

A quick overview of the history of the discipline reveals that, in general, which activities get included in the class of things called 'behaviours' depends on whether and how they are measurable. For example, strict behaviourists in the tradition of Watson and Skinner tend to include only those responses which are overt and objectively observable. Thus, they would exclude covert mental constructs of consciousness like schemas, ideas, strategies, memories and images (except as they are manifested in overt behaviour). Such an approach, however, leaves out much of what seems essential to an understanding of human behaviour and few psychologists today feel comfortable with such a rigid definition of behaviour. A more moderate compromise position is that taken by the so-called neobehaviourists, who permit the inference of internal states, intervening variables, hypothetical constructs, mediational processes and the like. Still behaviourist in their overall approach, such theorists insist that postulating these covert 'behaviours' is only legitimate when they can be linked with measurables. Still more flexible in their definition of behaviour are those inclined toward a cognitive or mentalistic approach. Here the essence of a 'behaviour' is its mental representation rather than the overt, measurable behavioural act. From this perspective the actions and processes of mind are included as aspects worthy of examination. For example, language is studied here with reference to underlying knowledge of rules of grammar, and the knowledge itself is the critical feature, not the overt utterances that people may be observed to produce.

Finally, there is the long-standing dispute as to whether or not physiological, neurological processes qualify as 'behaviour'. Here the same kind of historical pattern can be discerned. So long as these internal operations were relatively coherent and specifiable (e.g. muscle actions, reflex arcs, glandular secretions) early theorists felt comfortable calling them behaviours. But as the scope of investigation has expanded to include the detailed study of such things as electroencephalography, imaging techniques and the relationships between particular neurotransmitters and specific neural pathways, the issues have certainly become less clear. Indeed, it is not uncommon to see phrases like 'the behaviour of the brain is what causes the mind'. Here, clearly neurocortical action is included under the denotational umbrella of 'behaviour'.

What we have here is a conflict between, on one hand, the deep-felt need to keep psychology objective and precise and, on the other, the desire to extend its domains into cognition and neurophysiology. The casualty has been, of course, the term *behaviour* itself. It is used today in a manner that reflects the theoretical point of view of its user and can no longer be said to have a clear denotative domain, although this is not necessarily a bad thing. See also BEHAVIOURISM. var., *behavior*.

behavioural Pertaining to behaviour. Most typically used to characterize or refer to an analysis (theoretical or empirical) carried out on the basis of objective behaviour. Contrast with DYNAMIC; compare with STRUCTURAL. var., *behavioral*.

behavioural assessment (or diagnosis) A general procedure for diagnosing and evaluating psychological disorders by focusing on direct observation and self-reported measures of adaptive (or nonadaptive) functioning. The critical feature which distinguishes this approach from the traditional dynamic or analytical approaches is that interpretive or indirect-assessment techniques are not used.

behavioural clinic CLINIC, BEHAVIOURAL.

behavioural (or emotional) contagion CONTAGION, BEHAVIOURAL.

behavioural contract In BEHAVIOUR THERAPY, a technique in which a contract, typically involving the members of a family, is developed that stipulates responsibilities

that the client has and the privileges that he or she is permitted given their fulfilment.

behavioural contrast A phenomenon first reported by G. S. Reynolds. In certain two-choice discrimination situations he found that increases in response rate to one stimulus (S_1) produced decreases in response rate to the other stimulus (S_2) and vice versa. In the typical experiment the introduction of a different schedule of reinforcement for S_1 to either increase or decrease response rate to S_1 produced an opposite (contrasting) change in response rate to S_2.

behavioural-directive therapy Generally any of a variety of behaviour therapies that share the assumption that neurotic or maladaptive behaviours can be objectively treated independently of the rest of the client's personality. The term is used by some as synonymous with BEHAVIOUR THERAPY; others use it as the cover term with behaviour therapy considered as but one form of the behavioural-directive therapies.

behavioural dynamics Loosely, the underlying dynamic structure of motives which, in the psychodynamic approaches, are assumed to be ultimately responsible for observed behaviours of people.

behavioural ecology ECOLOGY, BEHAVIOURAL.

behavioural economics An interdisciplinary approach to economics that borrows heavily from psychology and sociology. While neo-classical economics is based on the assumption that people act rationally, behavioural economics is founded on the assumption that they act like people. That is, they tend to make economic and financial decisions using COGNITIVE *HEURISTICS rather than idealized models of rational action.

behavioural genetics The interdisciplinary science focusing on the study of the relationship between genetics and behaviour. This definition uses few words but marks an enormously complex field of endeavour which involves the many techniques of genetic analysis and the scientific analysis of the full range of behavioural manifestations of species.

behavioural homology HOMOLOGOUS (2).

behavioural integration INTEGRATION, BEHAVIOURAL.

behavioural intention THEORY OF *REASONED ACTION.

behavioural medicine A medical speciality based, in large measure, on the integration of research findings, methods and theory from the social sciences and the more traditional biological, anatomical approaches. It has its roots in earlier work on the *psychosomatic* aspects of disease but is a much more vigorously interdisciplinary and open approach to the interactions between mind and body and their impact on disease and health.

behavioural momentum A Skinnerian term for resistance to any change in the schedule of reinforcement, including extinction.

behavioural science Loosely, any science that studies the behaviour of organisms, including psychology, sociology, social anthropology, ethology and others. Occasionally used as a synonym for *social science*.

behavioural sink The disorganized and aberrant environment that some theorists feel is an outcome of severe overcrowding. The original studies that led to the coining of the term were carried out with rats and mice, which were kept in very crowded cages for extended periods of time. Current thinking on CROWDING counsels against extrapolating these findings to human societies.

behavioural teratogens TERATOGEN.

behaviour analysis 1 Within the Skinnerian behaviourist tradition, breaking down complex behaviours into their functional parts. **2** A general label for approaches to applied psychology and psychotherapy that focus on the objective, behavioural aspects. See also BEHAVIOURAL ASSESSMENT.

behaviour control Skinner's term for the classic behaviourist notion that all actions are caused by the contingencies of reinforcement and stimulation.

behaviour determinant In Tolman's learning theory, any variable which is causally related to (i.e. determines) behaviour.

behaviour disorder Any aberrant or maladaptive pattern of behaviour that is sufficiently severe to warrant the attention of counsellors or therapists. The term is preferred over any number of others previously used in this fashion, e.g. *neurosis*. See DISORDER for a discussion of the changing patterns of usage.

behaviour disorders of childhood A general psychiatric label for a number of disturbed behaviour patterns found in children and adolescents. Syndromes in this group are less severe than psychoses but considered to be serious enough to warrant therapy. Behaviours commonly cited here are delinquency, overaggressiveness, frequent running away from home, stealing, etc.

behaviour episode A term used (rather loosely) for a 'unit' of behaviour, a sequence of actions which has some reasonably well-defined beginning and ending.

behaviourism That approach to psychology which argues that the only appropriate subject matter for scientific psychological investigation is observable, measurable behaviour. Although flirtations with such a position go back to Hobbes, it was with John B. Watson in the 1910s (see WATSONIAN) that true behaviourism was born. In his polemical reaction to the subjectivism of introspectionism, Watson maintained that a proper scientific approach was one that limited behaviour to specific peripheral muscular and glandular responses and regarded consciousness and mental states as epiphenomena. This point of view is often dubbed *radical behaviourism* to distinguish it from other, more moderate orientations (e.g. NEOBEHAVIOURISM). B. F. Skinner championed a nuanced, although equally radical version (see SKINNERIAN). Whereas Watson's approach focused on acts themselves, a perspective that attracted Watson to the work of I. P. Pavlov, whose Russian version of behaviourism was oriented toward physiology and reflexive actions (see PAVLOVIAN), Skinner's approach was rather pointedly concerned with the *effects* that acts have on the environment. By shifting the focus in this fashion Skinner circumvented (or attempted to circumvent) the problems associated with the determination of exactly what a BEHAVIOUR is (see that term for discussion).

In addition to these points of view, various other positions are sufficiently close to them to have been (occasionally without their defenders' agreement) represented as forms of behaviourism. Included here are Clark L. Hull's neobehaviourist approach (see HUL-LIAN) and Edward C. Tolman's purposive psychology (see TOLMANIAN).

Behaviourism (in any of these guises) was largely an American pastime. Europeans who got involved in the disputes tended to be those with a more philosophical back-ground, such as Gilbert Ryle who, in his attempts to push behaviourism as far as it could go, also helped to reveal its limitations.

Today most psychologists feel uncomfort-able with radical behaviourism: there seems to be something unsatisfying about excising the causal role of internal, covert or mental processes in explanations of what it is people do (see COGNITIVE PSYCHOLOGY, COGNITIVE SCI-ENCE). Yet, in a sense, since all agree that what people *do* is the ultimate test, we still carry the vestiges of behaviourism no matter what general paradigm we may work within. This reflects the point of view of those who like to argue that we are all *methodological behaviourists*.

behaviourist One who espouses the theor-etical and methodological positions of BEHA-VIOURISM.

behaviouristic Pertaining to BEHAVIOURISM. Distinguished from BEHAVIOURAL.

behaviour method Generally, the approach to the study of psychological pro-cesses that relies strongly on the analysis of overt behaviour and rejects mentalistic analyses. The term is typically reserved for those who favour this kind of focus but wish not to be affiliated with the specific pos-ition of BEHAVIOURISM.

behaviour modification The process of changing (modifying) a person's behaviour. The term is generally used synonymously with BEHAVIOUR THERAPY.

behaviour problem A person, usually a child or adolescent, whose behaviour is per-sistently antisocial; that is, a behaviour prob-lem is a person who exhibits PROBLEM BEHAVIOUR.

behaviour rating Generally, any descrip-tion or characterization of the overt, observ-able behaviour of a specific subject in a particular situation. The term is restricted to reports which deal only with behaviour (who did what, to whom, when, etc.) and not with interpretations of possible under-lying motives or personality traits or the like.

behaviour sampling SAMPLING, BEHAVIOUR.

behaviour setting The general, ecological milieu within which behaviour takes place.

behaviour therapy That type of psycho-therapy which seeks to change abnormal or maladaptive behaviour patterns by the use of extinction and inhibitory processes and/or positive and negative reinforcers in classical and operant conditioning situations. The focus is on the behaviour itself rather than on an analytical or dynamic analysis of underlying conflicts or other root causes. The argument put forward by the behaviour therapists derives from the tenets of beha-viourism: in a nutshell, behaviour derives from contingencies of reinforcements and particular responses made in the presence of stimulus situations. Hence, behavioural disorders are assumed to result from 'unfor-tunate' contingencies in the life of the indi-vidual leading to the acquisition of maladaptive behaviours. There is no need to explore underlying conflicts; effective therapy should aim at modification of the behaviour(s) that the client currently mani-fests. A large array of specific therapeutic pro-cedures and modification techniques exists; e.g. ASSERTIVENESS TRAINING, DESENSITIZATION TECHNIQUE, IMPLOSION THERAPY, RECIPROCAL INHIB-ITION, TOKEN ECONOMY. See also COGNITIVE BEHAVIOUR THERAPY, in which the client's thoughts, imagery and ideation are also regarded as important elements.

being-beyond-the-world Within existen-tialism, the notion that one has responsibil-ity for the possibility of going beyond the (limited) momentary realities of one's exist-ence. Failure to fulfil (or to attempt to fulfil) this potentiality is, in existential analysis, a prime component of feelings of guilt. See and compare with BEING-IN-THE-WORLD.

being-in-the-world The generally accepted translation of Heidegger's term *Dasein*. It is used primarily within the exist-entialist framework, where it represents the central idea of that philosophy, that one's totality is given by the immediate and inev-itable phenomena which comprise the reality of the moment. This phenomenological world is conceptualized as comprising (a) the biological and physical (the *Umwelt*), (b) the human and social (the *Mitwelt*) and (c) the personal (the *Eigenwelt*). See and compare with BEING-BEYOND-THE-WORLD. See also EXISTEN-TIALISM, EXISTENTIAL THERAPY.

bel DECIBEL.

belief Generally used in the standard dictionary sense of an emotional acceptance of some proposition, statement or doctrine. See also ATTITUDE, OPINION.

belief-induced analgesia ANALGESIA, BELIEF-INDUCED.

belief systems CONCEPTUAL SYSTEMS.

belief–value matrix Tolman's term for an organism's learned expectations (beliefs) about the values of objects in the environment and the roles they play with respect to behaviour.

belladonna (alkaloids) See ATROPINE and SCOPOLAMINE.

belle indifférence, la French for *sublime indifference*. Used of various psychiatric conditions in which the patient seems blithely and inappropriately unconcerned about his or her disabilities. Most commonly seen in CONVERSION DISORDERS.

Bell–Magendie law The principle, first announced by Bell in 1811 and later (1822) by Magendie, that the ventral roots of the spinal nerves are motor in function and the dorsal roots are sensory. Incidentally, it is Magendie who really deserves credit for this finding. Bell's earlier work was rather poorly done and his conclusions wrong; in fact, he had it back to front, claiming that the ventral roots were sensory and the dorsal motor.

bell-shaped curve A nontechnical term for the NORMAL *DISTRIBUTION.

belongingness 1 One of E. L. Thorndike's supplementary principles of learning which assumes that stimuli are more likely to become associated if they are related to each other in some fashion. A good example of this principle is the phenomenon of *learned taste aversion* (see CONDITIONED *AVERSION). **2** In social psychology and sociology, the feeling of inclusion in or acceptance by a group. **3** The generalization that an array of stimulus elements is more likely to be perceived or reacted to as a whole if the elements 'belong' to each other in some recognizable fashion.

Bem Sex Role Inventory A *self-report inventory* developed by S. Bem for measuring the extent to which an individual identifies with the positive characteristics associated with traditional masculine (e.g. athletic, dominant) and/or feminine (e.g. affectionate, gentle) Western sex roles. The inventory also produces an *androgyny scale*, which reflects the extent to which the testee balances between identifying with the classic masculine and classic feminine traits.

Bender Gestalt Test A test developed in the 1930s by L. Bender. Although there are a number of administrative variations available, the typical procedure is to present the testee with nine relatively simple standard designs and ask him or her to copy them. The results are interpreted on the basis of the quality of the reproductions, the manner of organization of each copy and the pattern of spatial errors made. Bender originally conceptualized the test as a maturational test for use with children and as a device for exploring regression or retardation and detecting possible brain damage. Today it is used predominantly for detection of organic cerebral damage. The name of the test derives from the fact that Bender was an advocate of GESTALT psychology and used Gestalt principles in the construction of the test. Also called *Bender Visual Motor Gestalt Test*.

beneffectance The tendency to interpret events in ways that make one's own position or actions seem more favourable, to take credit for things that turned out successfully but to share or even deny responsibility for things that were failures.

Benham's top A disc, half black, half white, with four sets of three curved lines drawn on the white half. When rotated the disc demonstrates a visual anomaly: although itself colourless, colours can be observed. When it is rotated in one direction the colours appear in spectral order from centre to edge, when it is rotated in the opposite direction the order of colours is reversed.

benign Characteristic of a condition with a

good prognosis; one which is nonprogressive and with a hopeful outcome. The term is used for both physical and psychological conditions. Contrast with MALIGNANT.

Benzedrine AMPHETAMINES.

benzodiazepines A major group of ANTIAN-XIETY DRUGS, including *diazepam* and *loraze-pam*, which have tranquillizing effects and help to reduce the experience of anxiety. They work by activating the benzodiazepine receptors so that they increase the sensitivity of the GAMMA-AMINOBUTYRIC ACID (GABA) receptors with which they are coupled. Benzodiazepines are most effective against generalized anxiety disorders and have little or no effect on *panic disorder, obsessive-compulsive disorders* or *phobic disorders*.

benztropine An ANTICHOLINERGIC DRUG used to ameliorate the side effects of some ANTIPSY-CHOTIC DRUGS and as an adjunct in treatment of PARKINSON'S DISEASE.

bereavement The emotional reactions felt following the death of a loved one. The symptoms can resemble a full depressive syndrome (e.g. poor appetite, insomnia), but generally resolve without treatment.

berdache 1 Originally, a North American Indian who assumes the manner of dress, lifestyle and sex roles of a member of the opposite sex. **2** More loosely, a TRANSVESTITE.

Bernoulli distribution BINOMIAL *DISTRIBU-TION.

Bernoulli trial Any trial or situation with two mutually exclusive and exhaustive possible outcomes; e.g. head/tails in a coin flip. A series of Bernoulli trials yields a BINOMIAL *DIS-TRIBUTION.

Bernreuter Personality Inventory Developed in 1931, it was an early, important personality test. It is rarely used today.

best fit GOODNESS OF *FIT, LEAST-SQUARES PRIN-CIPLE.

bestiality Sexual behaviour between humans and animals. ZOOERASTY, ZOOPHILIA.

beta (β) adrenoreceptors Receptors that bind NOREPINEPHRINE. One type ($β_1$) produces a more rapid and forceful heartbeat; the other ($β_2$) relaxes smooth muscle, dilates blood vessels and airways and relaxes uterine muscles. See also ALPHA ADRENORECEPTORS.

beta (β) amyloid A protein found in large amounts in the brains of Alzheimer's patients and in many cases of Down syndrome. Both the NEURITIC PLAQUES and NEURO-FIBRILLARY TANGLES that are hallmarks of Alzheimer's contain excessive accumulations of β-amyloids.

beta blocker A drug that blocks the uptake of norepinephrine and epinephrine at BETA ADRENORECEPTORS. They slow heart rate, reduce cardiac muscle activity and cause constriction of smooth muscle in the bronchial tubes. Also called *beta adrenergic blockers*. Primarily used for hypertension, they have some value in treating social phobias and reducing tremors.

beta endorphin The most potent of the known ENDORPHINS.

beta error ERROR (TYPE I and TYPE II).

beta motion MOTION, BETA.

beta response In classical eyelid conditioning, a response that occurs shortly after presentation of the conditioned stimulus but anticipatory to the unconditioned stimulus. It is assumed that this is the 'true' conditioned response. Contrast with ALPHA RESPONSE.

beta rhythm (or **wave**) A pattern of electrical activity of the brain characteristic of the normal, awake, active person. On an EEG (ELECTROENCEPHALOGRAM) it is a wave of somewhat lower amplitude but higher frequency (roughly 17–25 Hz) than the ALPHA RHYTHM.

between-group variance VARIANCE, BETWEEN-GROUP.

between-subjects design A research design in which different groups of subjects are run under different conditions. Compare with WITHIN-SUBJECTS DESIGN.

Betz cells Large motor neurons in the precentral gyrus of the frontal lobe of the cerebral cortex and in the motor cortex. They are involved in mediation of voluntary motor activity.

Bezold-Brücke effect Changes in perceived hue with changes in luminance. Specifically, yellowish reds and yellowish greens are perceived as yellower with increases in illumination and bluish reds and bluish greens appear more blue. Purer reds, yellows, greens and blues do not show this effect.

bi- Prefix denoting *both, two, double, twice.*

bias 1 An inclination toward a position or conclusion; a prejudice. **2** A statistical sampling error: a *biased sample* is one that is not representative of the population about which inferences are to be made. **3** Any systematic factor in an experimental situation that introduces error. **4** As borrowed from *signal detection theory*, any preference for one choice or response over others, such as the often observed tendency to select 'heads' over 'tails' in coin-flipping. **5** In testing, any aspect of a test which yields differential predictions for groups of persons distinguishable from each other by a factor which, in principle, should be irrelevant to the test. For example, an IQ test which predicted different success rates for blacks and whites with the same measured IQ would be biased in this sense. Needless to say, such a testing bias would render a test useless. **6** A lack of fairness. Often used with qualifiers to specify the type of bias, e.g. INTERVIEWER BIAS, RESPONSE BIAS, VOLUNTEER BIAS.

biased sample (or **sampling**) BIASED *SAMPLING.

bidirectional activational models In the study of PATTERN RECOGNITION, models in which elements are activated and inhibited by both BOTTOM-UP and TOP-DOWN PROCESSING operations.

Bidwell's ghost PURKINJE AFTERIMAGE.

bifactor method A procedure in *factor analysis* which extracts a principal factor first and then extracts other factors. The first factor is one which loads on all the subtests and, hence, is taken by some to represent a general factor; the factors extracted later load on isolated clusters and are regarded as of secondary importance.

Big Five FIVE FACTOR THEORY.

bilabial A speech sound produced by bringing the lips together, e.g. [b] in *bat*, [m] in *mat*.

bilateral Having two sides; pertaining to

both left and right sides. The general construction of the anatomy and nervous system of most organisms displays *bilateral symmetry*: the left and right sides are more or less mirror images.

bilateral transfer TRANSFER, BILATERAL.

bilingual 1 adj. Characteristic of one who is able to speak two languages with approximately equal fluency. **2** n. A bilingual person, in sense 1. See BILINGUALISM for discussion of definitional problems.

bilingual, compound (and **coordinate**) See discussion under BILINGUALISM.

bilingualism The simple definition, fluency in two languages, leaves much unspecified that needs specification. One problem is that what qualifies as 'fluency' is left dangling. Usually the user of the term will specify whether the persons under consideration are bilingual on the basis of some criterion such as reading/writing skills, speaking ability, translating between the languages, etc. A second important issue concerns the conditions under which the two languages are learned. According to a commonly used system of classification, a person who acquires both languages in the same context (e.g. a home where both are spoken interchangeably) is called a *compound bilingual*, while one who learns each language in a different setting (e.g. one at home, the other at school) is a *coordinate bilingual*.

bilingualism, additive BILINGUALISM when the second language is acquired after the first is well established and generally functions to improve the person's ability to use language, especially in carrying out cognitive processes. Contrast with SUBTRACTIVE *BILINGUALISM.

bilingualism, balanced UNBALANCED *BILINGUALISM

bilingualism, subtractive BILINGUALISM when the acquisition of the second language appears to diminish the individual's ability to use language, especially for thinking. Contrast with ADDITIVE *BILINGUALISM.

bilingualism, unbalanced BILINGUALISM when the individual is considerably more fluent in one of the two languages than the other. When there is roughly equal fluency in the two languages the term *balanced bilingualism* is used.

bimodal Characteristic of any frequency distribution that has two points or scores that share the property of having the greatest number of cases; that is, a distribution with two MODES. The two modes need not have exactly the same frequency: there need only be two points reasonably remote from each other that show a clear concentration of scores.

binary-choice Characterizing any situation with two choices, one of which must be made.

binary number system A number system with only two digits, 1 and 0. It is used extensively in information theory and computer sciences. As the normal decimal system is coded so that each displacement to the left means multiplication by ten, here each displacement means multiplication by two. The following are the decimal–binary equivalents for 1 to 10: 1 = 1; 2 = 10; 3 = 11; 4 = 100; 5 = 101; 6 = 110; 7 = 111; 8 = 1000; 9 = 1001; 10 = 1010.

binaural 1 Of, or pertaining to, the functioning of both ears simultaneously so that the same input reaches both ears at the same instant. **2** More generally, pertaining to two ears. Compare with DICHOTIC.

binaural beat BINAURAL SHIFT.

binaural fusion FUSION, BINAURAL.

binaural ratio The ratio between the physical intensities of sound at the two ears.

binaural shift The perception that when each ear is presented with one of two tones of slightly different frequency under properly controlled conditions the point in space where the sound is localized shifts back and forth. The rate of shift is controlled by the frequency difference. Also called *binaural beat*, which is slightly misleading since BEAT generally does not involve spatial localization.

binaural time difference The differences in time of arrival and in intensity of a sound reaching both ears. Such differences are the major cues for sound LOCALIZATION. Also called, simply, *binaural difference* (without the *time*) since the intensity difference is not necessarily entailed by the temporal factors.

binding Loosely and generally, linking, connecting, joining, cohering. Hence: **1** In neurophysiology, any of the variety of processes by which drugs or neurotransmitters link with target sites on postsynaptic neurons. **2** In social psychology, the processes by which individuals come together to form groups. **3** In perception, the manner in which the several elements of a percept come to be seen together. **4** In psychoanalysis, an occasional synonym for CATHEXIS.

binding problem A conundrum that has bothered many for a long time. How is it that we link or 'bind' the various elements of complex displays? For example, what is it in our neural architecture that allows us effortlessly to bind up all the several aspects of an object – its colour, shape and movement patterns – so that they are perceived as belonging to the object and not to other aspects of the environment? If you don't think this is a *big* problem you haven't thought about it enough.

binding site That region of the postsynaptic receptor where neurotransmitters or drugs attach.

Binet (or **Binet–Simon**) **Scale** The first scale of intelligence for schoolchildren, issued by A. Binet and T. Simon in France in 1905, revised by them in 1908, and revised again in 1911 with the addition of a set of age norms. The Binet Scale is significant because it was the first of the mental tests to focus on the higher mental functions of cognitive capacity rather than on the more primitive operations of sensory abilities, reaction times, discrimination, etc. It has been revised many times and adapted for many different cultures, the most thorough revision being that of L. M. Terman at Stanford University. Still, the scale's origins are honoured in its name, and casual reference to a 'Binet' is laboratory jargon for the popular *Stanford–Binet Scale* of intelligence.

binge eating BULIMIA NERVOSA.

binge-eating disorder An eating disorder marked by binge eating and related distress similar to that seen in BULIMIA NERVOSA but without self-induced vomiting and purging.

binocular Of or pertaining to the simultaneous functioning of both eyes.

binocular cue Any visual cue for depth perception that requires both eyes, e.g. *retinal disparity*. Compare with MONOCULAR CUE.

binocular disparity DISPARITY, RETINAL.

binocular fusion BINOCULAR RIVALRY.

binocular perception PERCEPTION, BINOCULAR.

binocular (or retinal) rivalry A perceptual phenomenon that occurs when the proximal stimuli to the two retinae cannot be resolved into a single percept. The effect may be produced, for example, by presenting a field of blue to one eye and a field of yellow to the other eye. The resulting perception is an irregular alternation from the inputs of the two eyes so that the subject sees first blue, then yellow, then blue, etc. When the subject can resolve the two different inputs into a single percept (which, of course, is the normal state of affairs) the term *binocular* (or *retinal) fusion* applies.

binocular vision VISION, BINOCULAR.

binomial 1 n. An algebraic expression containing two terms. The binomial expansion is the binomial raised to an arbitrary power, or e.g. $(p + q)^n$. As the value of n increases, the binomial increasingly approximates the normal distribution. **2** adj. Characteristic of a thing with two forms.

binomial distribution DISTRIBUTION, BINOMIAL.

Binswanger's disease A form of dementia associated with untreated hypertension. The dementia is highly variable but typically progressive. It is classified as a vascular dementia marked by subcortical demyelination usually in the temporal and occipital lobes.

bio- Combining form meaning *life* or indicating a *relationship to life* or the *living*.

bioacoustics A hybrid field of study borrowing from zoology, biology, physics and psychology which investigates the ACOUSTIC communication systems of nonhuman species.

biochemical antagonism ANTAGONISM, DRUG.

biocybernetics An area of research concerned with the relationships between consciousness and biological functioning. The main interest is in the ways in which people may become aware of and ultimately learn to control biological events which normally are not within the scope of consciousness (e.g. alpha waves, blood pressure). *Cybernetics* refers to the frequent use of computers or other devices to provide feedback to the subject about these biological events. See BIOFEEDBACK. See also CYBERNETICS.

bioecological model Urie Bronfronbrenner's model of child development that conceptualizes development as occurring within a series of nested factors ranging from the most proximal to the most distal. The proximal factors (often called the *microsystem*) comprise the child and the caretakers and have the most immediate impact on development. The distal factors (the *macrosystem*) include cultural laws and norms and exert their effects through factors such as health and educational services, neighbourhood values, and parents' economic resources. Also called *ecological systems theory*.

bioenergetics 1 Originally, the study of energy transfer between living systems. **2** A form of psychotherapy derived from the theories of Wilhelm Reich. Contemporary advocates of the bioenergetic approach have, by and large, rejected Reich's *orgone* hypothesis but have retained the focus on organismic function and its relationship to emotional stability and well-being. See also BIOFUNCTIONAL THERAPY.

bioethics A field of study concerned with issues of ethics and values as they relate to medicine and related sciences such as biology, physiology and psychology.

biofeedback Information feedback about bodily function. Most biofeedback is mediated through normal sensory channels; e.g. if you close your eyes and hold your arm out, *kinaesthetic* feedback informs you of its position and allows you to make adjustments to perform a task. Biofeedback from an outside source can also be used to enable an organism to modify its functioning. For example, when EEG (ELECTROENCEPHALOGRAM) feedback is provided people can maintain some degree of control over their alpha waves. Similar manipulations have been performed with heart rate, blood pressure, blood flow in the extremities, etc. Note that some have taken to using the term as though it meant the direct control of internal, autonomic functions and activities. It should not be used in this fashion. It is merely a descriptive term for the process of providing an organism with information about its biological functions. See BIOFEEDBACK THERAPY. See also BIOCYBERNETICS, FEEDBACK.

biofeedback therapy The use of BIOFEEDBACK in a fashion that has a therapeutic function, as, for example, in developing a programme for a person with hypertension to lower their blood pressure.

biofunctional therapy A cover term for any psychotherapeutic approach that operates on the assumption that bodily functions are primary and that the mental and psychosocial components are secondary. Although pure biofunctional approaches are few (see e.g. BIOENERGETICS, ORGONE THERAPY), many, more eclectic, approaches, particularly those of the HUMAN POTENTIAL MOVEMENT, incorporate some aspects.

biogenesis Loosely, the origin and subsequent evolution of the living.

biogenic 1 Characteristic of or pertaining to processes by which living things give rise through reproduction to other living things. **2** Characteristic of or pertaining to aspects of behaviour which are biological or organic in origin.

biogenic amine hypothesis The general hypothesis that imbalances in the physiology and metabolism of several of the BIOGENIC AMINES are critical components in the pathogenesis of various psychotic disorders. The amines most suspect are the catecholamines *norepinephrine* and *dopamine* (see CATECHOLAMINE HYPOTHESIS and DOPAMINE HYPOTHESIS) and an indoleamine, SEROTONIN. While an intriguing working hypothesis, in this simple form it cannot be correct. For one, it fails to account for the various complex components of psychological disorders which include alterations in mood, sleep cycles, sexual function, appetite, temperature control and cognitive functioning. Even more problematical is the fact that the drugs used to treat these disorders (see e.g. ANTIDEPRESSANT DRUGS) rapidly change

amine levels although their therapeutic effects may not be felt for weeks.

biogenic amines Several groups of amines that are of particular interest because of their role in neural functioning, including the CATECHOLAMINES, the INDOLEAMINES and HISTAMINE.

biological clock A hypothesized biochemical mechanism that is responsible for the control of the behavioural systems which show periodicity. See e.g. BIORHYTHM and CIRCADIAN RHYTHM. Actually, the notion that each organism possesses a single biological clock that monitors the environment and controls all biorhythms is most certainly an oversimplification: it seems clear that there are multiple control systems operating for various functions. Also called *endogenous clock*.

biological memory MEMORY, BIOLOGICAL.

biological motion MOTION, BIOLOGICAL.

biological predisposition Very loosely, a disposition that can be traced back to biological factors. It is used most often for evolved tendencies to behave in particular ways or learn particular responses quickly and efficiently. For example, fear of enclosed spaces is common but not fear of knives, despite the fact that many cut themselves often but few have been locked in a closet. Presumably, humans evolved a biological predisposition to avoid enclosed, dangerous places but not sharp artefacts. Compare with HEREDITARY PREDISPOSITION.

biological psychiatry An approach to psychiatry that emphasizes the biological, physical and neurological aspects of behavioural disorders and focuses on psychopharmacological treatment.

biologic rhythms BIORHYTHMS.

biologism The use of biological principles as a basis for describing and explaining human behaviour. The term is never used by those who engage in such a theoretically oriented exercise: it is employed disparagingly by the critics of this approach.

biomedical therapy (or **treatment**) An umbrella term used to cover any form of psychotherapy based on biological techniques. Included are the various forms of drug therapies, electroconvulsive shock therapy and psychosurgery.

biometry (or **biometrics**) The use of mathematical and statistical procedures for the study of organisms.

biomimetics Literally, *copying biology*. Hence, an interdisciplinary field of study that uses computer simulations, mathematical models and robotics to mimic and model the structural features and behaviours of organisms.

biomusicology A field of study that explores the biological foundation of music, its creation and appreciation. One of the more intriguing findings is that those species that use music (birds, whales, us) tend to use similar patterns of tonality and structure.

bionics The study of living systems with emphasis on the construction of artificial systems that simulate their functions and characteristics.

bionomics Synonym for ECOLOGY.

biopsychology PSYCHOBIOLOGY.

biopsychosocial model 1 In psychopharmacology, a model that maintains that drug dependencies are the result not just of pharmacological effects but of a complex of interacting elements involving the reinforcing elements of drugs, cue effects contributed by environmental and social factors, conditioned drug effects and the need to avoid various aversive consequences of drugs. 2 In clinical work, a theory of schizophrenia that argues that the disorder results from severe cognitive and social stresses associated with particular neurological changes in genetically vulnerable individuals.

biorhythms A general label covering all forms of periodicity of biological systems. The most intensely studied are the daily or CIRCADIAN RHYTHMS, although many biological functions show a period other than a daily one, e.g. menstrual cycles, bird migrations, protective-colouring changes, etc. In recent years the term has become 'contaminated' by the emergence of a pseudoscience of the same name. Using the so-called 'biorhythm method' its practitioners claim to be able to predict a person's performance on a task on any given day, on the basis of a chart of their biorhythms from their day of birth. An utter lack of supportive evidence for these claims has, predictably, had little impact on public acceptance, but it has led researchers to cast about for a new label for their field, CHRONOBIOLOGY being the most recent candidate recommended. See also BIOLOGICAL CLOCK.

biosocial Characteristic of those features of behaviour that are a result of interactions between social and biological factors. The classic example is sexual behaviour.

biosphere 1 The portion of the earth that supports life. 2 The environment, particularly when it is characterized and described as an ecosystem, a domain for the support of life. 3 A. Angyal's term for the holistic entity containing the individual and the total environment. In his *organismic* theory the biosphere included the whole person, encompassing the biological, psychological and sociological aspects. 4 A small-scale, contained, self-sustaining ecosystem.

biostatistics 1 VITAL STATISTICS. 2 The use of statistical procedures and techniques in the study of living organisms.

biotope An ethological term used to describe an area with an overall similar environment. Within any given biotope there may be a variety of habitats or more restricted, specialized environments.

biotransformation Generally, any alteration in a substance within the body.

biotransport TRANSPORT.

biotype 1 The genetic constitution of an organism. 2 By extension, a group of organisms with a shared complex of genetic factors.

biperiden A drug with ANTICHOLINERGIC properties used in Parkinson's disease and to lessen the Parkinson-like side effects of long-term use of ANTIPSYCHOTIC DRUGS.

bipolar Lit., having two poles. 1 The term is used broadly, so the notion of 'pole' here can be taken in several ways. It can be used rather precisely to denote the end point(s) on a well-specified dimension, or it can be applied somewhat more loosely to two processes or branches of something, or two more-or-less opposed reactions to a person or an event. Hence: 2 In the study of personality, descriptive of traits which are expressible as opposite ends of a single dimension. For example, dominance and submission are considered to be bipolar traits in that they are clear and independent opposites. Note, however, that superficially opposite traits like leadership and followership are generally not called bipolar since good leaders are often good followers, thus the 'negation' of one does not imply the other. **3** In neurophysiology, a shortened form of BIPOLAR CELL (or NEURON).

bipolar affective disorder BIPOLAR DISORDER.

bipolar cell (or **neuron**) Any neuron with two extensions or processes (axon and dendrite) running in opposite directions from the cell body. Almost always sensory in nature, they are found extensively in the retina, where they form connections between the receptors and the ganglion cells. See also UNIPOLAR CELL, MULTIPOLAR CELL.

bipolar disorder A major MOOD DISORDER in which manic episodes occur. Although, in the classic form, both manic and depressive poles are manifested, the diagnosis can be made without the occurrence of a depressive episode. Several subtypes are distinguished and marked *manic*, *depressed* or *mixed* depending on the currently presenting symptoms; see the following entries for details. Also known as *bipolar affective disorder* and, in some older texts, *manic depression* and *manic-depressive disorder*. In the most recent texts, owing to the identification of BIPOLAR II DISORDER, it is often referred to as *bipolar I disorder*. It is treated with a variety of mood stabilizing drugs that include *lithium*, any of several antiepileptics (e.g. *carbamazepine*) and the atypical antipsychotics. These mainly treat the mania and delay or prevent relapses. Bipolar depression usually responds to combinations of mood stabilizers and antidepressants. The depression that occurs in bipolar disorder is typically not responsive to antidepressants used alone.

bipolar II disorder A mood disorder in which, unlike the classic BIPOLAR DISORDER, the mood swings are between intense depression and HYPOMANIA rather than full-blown MANIA (2). It usually responds well to mood stabilizers such as *lithium*.

bipolar disorder, depressed A type of bipolar disorder in which there has been at least one manic episode but the current presenting (or most recent) symptoms are those of a MAJOR *DEPRESSIVE EPISODE. The condition responds well to a combination of *antidepressant drugs* and *mood stabilizers*. Despite the presenting symptoms, antidepressants alone are not particularly effective.

bipolar disorder, manic A type of bipolar disorder in which the most recent extreme affective disturbance has been a manic episode. See MANIA (2).

bipolar disorder, mixed A type of bipolar disorder in which the full symptomatic picture of manic and depressed episodes is seen either intermixed or alternating every few days, or in which the depressive symptoms predominate although some manic components are observed.

bipolar disorder, rapidly-cycling A version of bipolar disorder in which the shifts between poles are 'rapid', that is, at least four such episodic switches occur within a year. A switch may be either to the opposite pole or to a remission lasting at least two months.

bipolar rating scale RATING SCALE, BIPOLAR.

BIRG Pronounced 'burge', this acronym stands for 'bask in reflected glory'. It refers to the act of boosting one's self-esteem by emphasizing one's identification with the accomplishments of an in-group. The classic example of BIRGing is the way everyone on a college campus seems to wear their school-name T-shirts and sweatshirts on the day after a big sporting victory.

birth control A very general term applied to any procedure or practice used to control the number of conceptions and births. It is not synonymous with *contraception*, but the latter is included as one method of birth control along with, among others, the intrauterine device (IUD) and abortion. Moreover, some authors also use the term to refer to procedures and techniques for planning and facilitation of conception and birth. See CONTRACEPTION for further discussion.

birth cry The reflex crying which accompanies the beginning of natural respiration immediately following birth.

birth defect Generally, any congenital

abnormality. The term is used to cover defects which are genetic (e.g. *phenylketonuria*) as well as those that are a result of environmental factors (e.g. defects caused by the mother's ingestion of harmful substances during gestation).

birth injury Any injury sustained by an infant during birth; distinguish from BIRTH TRAUMA (1).

birthmark A congenital disfiguration; e.g. a *naevus*.

birth order The chronological order of birth of children in a given family. There are small but real correlations between birth order and several other factors such as IQ, eminence and socioeconomic success, with the first-born generally showing a mild advantage.

birth, preterm Birth before the completion of the full, normal gestation period, i.e. prior to the 37th week of pregnancy. See also PREMATURE INFANT, which is defined more in terms of development than of chronology.

birth rate The number of live births per 1,000 people in the total population. Usually given per year.

birth trauma 1 As argued primarily by Otto Rank, the original and pervasive assault upon the psyche occasioned by being summarily expelled from the comfort of the womb into a hostile, nongratifying world. Rank went on to argue (unconvincingly) that all anxiety neuroses stem from this universal experience. Note, however, that, despite the failure of most theoreticians to be convinced by Rank's thesis, it is still true that many of those with a psychoanalytic orientation assume that the sudden assault of the real world upon the previously protected foetus has lasting effects. The difficulty of such a position is that since everyone is subjected to the same experience it is impossible to establish its true impact on development. **2** BIRTH INJURY.

bisection, method of Bisection simply means cutting into two parts. Hence: **1** In neurophysiology, the technique of severing one or more of the commissures of the brain to produce a split-brain preparation. **2** In psychophysics, see the discussion under METHODS OF *SCALING.

biserial correlation CORRELATION, BISERIAL.

bisexual 1 n. HERMAPHRODITE (2). **2** n. One whose sexual preferences include members of both sexes. **3** adj. Characteristic of 2. **4** Occasionally, a synonym for *ambisexual*. This usage is no longer recommended because of the much more common meanings 1 – 3. In many older texts, the state of bisexuality (2 and 3) is also called *amphigenous inversion*.

bistability Characterizing any situation in which two stable states exist, each of which can be occupied successively. The condition is found widely. In perception, REVERSIBLE *FIGURES like the Necker cube display bistability; in biophysics, it is seen in cells whose MEMBRANE POTENTIALS change abruptly from one state to another in an all-or-nothing fashion; in neurology, it characterizes certain *cell assemblies* with only two states, low-frequency and high-frequency firing.

bistable percept See BISTABILITY.

bit A contraction of the words 'binary digit' meaning a 'piece' of information sufficient to reduce the alternatives in a choice situation by one half. Hence, if you have four alternatives and are provided with information that eliminates two of them, you have received one bit of information.

bite bar A rigid plate which a subject can bite down on firmly so that the head is held steady. Bite bars are commonly used in visual research so that the subject does not move his or her head about needlessly and the experimenter has control over where in the visual field a stimulus is presented.

bitemporal hemianopsia Loss of vision in the outside halves of both visual fields. The disorder typically results from damage to the OPTIC CHIASM, most often caused by pituitary tumours that compress the fibres in the chiasm.

bitter A sharp, astringent and mostly unpleasant taste associated with various alkaloids, some salts and vitamins and found in various common foods including arugula, watercress, quinine and coffee. One of the five primary qualities of TASTE (2), it is assumed to have evolved as a mechanism to prevent poisoning since many toxic substances taste bitter.

bivariate Pertaining to conditions in which there are exactly two variables.

bivariate association Any statistical relation between two variables, e.g. *product moment correlation*.

black In vision, an achromatic sensation represented as the lower limit in the lightness dimension along the white–grey–black continuum. The percept black, however, is often a relative phenomenon. An object will appear black when it is subjected to low light levels while surrounded by a relatively brightly illuminated background. The same stimulus may appear to be a neutral or even light grey if this pattern is reversed.

Black American English A label commonly used for the dialect of American English spoken by many Americans of African descent. The term needs to be used with considerable care. While there is an identifiable dialect here with its characteristic patterns of pronunciation, a few syntactic devices not found in other dialects and, of course, a substantial number of specific semantic and idiomatic usage patterns, it is simply not the case that all American Blacks use it. Moreover, there are a number of other regional dialects in the USA, particularly in the South, which have similar dialect features. When used by the experts, the term usually relates to the particular linguistic patterns observed among Black Americans from large urban centres, where the divergences between this dialect and the so-called STANDARD ENGLISH spoken by the remainder of that particular geographical unit are most evident. Finally, it must be emphasized that there is no evidence whatsoever that suggests that Black English is in any way deficient in communicative or expressive function. There is no disagreement on this point among scholars (despite some unfortunate erroneous statements to the contrary by the uninformed). Also called *African-American Vernacular English*.

black box A term derived from physics, where it was used to stand for a model of the functioning of any complex system based on the hypothesizing of constructs, mechanisms and procedures internal to the system. The basic notion here is that when one cannot know precisely what is inside a system causing it to function in the way it does, one treats it as though it were an impenetrable 'black box' and makes inductive interpretations about its internal properties. The black box then becomes a model of the system and a representation of it that can, in theory, account for how the system functions given the various inputs to it and the observed outputs from it. The use in psychology is obvious: merely let the complex system under examination be an organism. Note that the black box is never empty: it is populated, often richly, with structures, constructs, operations and the like. Some – usually behaviourists who have an aversion for hypothesizing internal mechanisms, or for what Skinner called 'spurious physiologizing' – have called their approach *black box psychology*. This, of course, is a misuse of the original meaning of the term. See here EMPTY ORGANISM.

blackout 1 Generally, temporary loss of consciousness. **2** The amnesia experienced by some severe alcoholics when they have no memory of a period of time during which they were extremely intoxicated. Such alcoholic blackout periods can be up to several days in duration.

blame avoidance (need) H. Murray's term for, quite literally, the need to avoid blame, a motive for acting in a socially accepted manner so as to avoid censure, disapproval, punishment, etc. Note that Murray, for completeness, also hypothesized a *blame escape need* for a motive which operates when one has not succeeded in avoiding blame and is impelled to flee a situation (physically or psychologically) to escape further censure.

blame escape (need) BLAME AVOIDANCE (NEED).

blank trial 1 A trial in an experiment in which some irregular stimulus conditions are introduced. It serves to keep the subject from making automatic responses and to keep attention focused on the task at hand; see e.g. CATCH TRIAL **2** A trial in an experiment in which reinforcement or information feedback is not forthcoming.

-blast(o)- Combining form meaning *primitive cell, bud, germ*.

bleen See GRUE.

blending Generally: **1** In perception, any process in which the various components of a complex display are combined and integrated. More specifically: **2** In reading, the synthesizing of the phonetic elements of a word into the full word. For example, a child may be taught to read a word like 'bat' by blending the sounds of the phonetic elements 'buh-ah-tuh'. This process is more than simply uttering the elements rapidly; it involves layering and integrating them into a single syllable 'bat'. **3** The process of combining the facial elements of two or more different emotions, such as displaying an anger face that also shows the raised upper lip that is characteristic of disgust. Such *blends* presumably reflect the component emotions experienced. **4** In evolutionary biology, the mixing of traits that appear to be combinations of features in the parental phenotypes.

blind 1 Lacking in vision, without sight. See BLINDNESS in this sense. **2** Without awareness, e.g. BLIND ANALYSIS.

blind alley A passage or arm of a maze that is a dead end; also called a *cul-de-sac*.

blind analysis Generally, any analysis carried out without knowledge about conditions or information that might lead to biases in interpretation. In a blind clinical diagnosis a psychologist or psychiatrist would proceed without knowing the results of any other diagnosis that may have been made; a blind analysis of test protocols would be carried out without knowledge of the person from whom they were taken. For extensions of this basic notion see DOUBLE-BLIND.

blindness This term is often misused in that it is thought to refer to complete lack of vision. Strictly speaking, there is a continuum of visual acuity and the point at which a person is considered blind is usually a legal issue. The standard generally adopted is when visual acuity is less than 20/200 after correction or the visual field is restricted to 20° of arc or less. However, the term is used broadly to refer to any of an array of disorders, including a variety of highly specific defects such as loss of vision in one area of the visual field, loss of sensitivity to particular hues, diminished ability to see in low illumination, etc. The causes are equally varied and may include dysfunctions from the most peripheral, such as occlusion of the lens, to the most central, such as neurological damage in the visual cortex.

blindness, cortical (or **cerebral**) Blindness resulting from a brain lesion.

blindness, functional Loss of vision in the absence of any known organic dysfunction. Also called *psychogenic, hysterical* or *psychic blindness*.

blindsight L. Weiskrantz's term for 'sight', or, better, 'visually guided behaviour', that is influenced by stimuli that fall within blind areas (see SCOTOMA) of the visual system. In such cases the patient displays the capacity to respond to visual stimulation that he or she is not conscious of seeing.

blind spot The small spot on the retina that is insensitive to light. It is at this point that the neural fibres leave the eyeball to form the optic nerve; there are no photoreceptors here. The blind spot is located in the horizontal plane about 12–15° of arc toward the nose from the *fovea*. Also called the *optic disc*.

blink reflex Reflexive closing of the eyelid induced by a bright light, a sudden noise, a puff of air, etc. It has been extensively studied in classical conditioning investigations.

blob A region in the primary visual cortex containing neurons that are sensitive to specific wavelengths. Part of the PARVOCELLULAR SYSTEM, it was given its peculiar name because when stained it appears as a blob.

block 1 Most generally, any obstruction or barrier which prevents a process from occurring. The term is used broadly to cover physical barriers which impede flow through a passage (e.g. arterial block), biochemical agents which prevent neural transmission (e.g. nerve block or neural block), and psychogenic barriers (e.g. emotional blocks). **2** An abrupt cessation in the flow of a process. Usage here is generally restricted to processes such as speech and thought. See BLOCKING (1). **3** A failure of memory in which the retrieval of information is somehow thwarted; see e.g. TIP-OF-THE-TONGUE STATE. **4** A group or sequence of trials in an experiment.

block design An experimental design in which subjects are distributed into distinct groups, called blocks, so that each is representative of the population. Each block of subjects then undergoes particular experimental manipulations. The name for this design comes from the practice in agricultural research of dividing a large area into subplots, or blocks.

block design, randomized A BLOCK DESIGN procedure where the several subjects in each group are randomly assigned to different manipulations.

block-design test Any performance (i.e. nonverbal) test using coloured blocks or tiles with which the subject is required to match or copy given designs.

block diagram HISTOGRAM.

blocking 1 Generally obstructing or inhibiting of a process of thought or language. Most people experience it as a kind of *lacuna*, an absence of processing. 2 In conditioning, a circumstance in which, if an association is first formed between two stimuli (x and y), then later a compound stimulus ($x + z$) is associated with y, the association between z and y tends not to be learned; that is, it is 'blocked' by the previously established link between x and y.

block sampling SAMPLING, BLOCK.

blood–brain barrier A selectively permeable guard between the circulating blood and the brain which functions by preventing some substances from reaching the brain. The barrier is thought to consist partly of cells making up the walls of the capillaries in the brain. Astrocytes (a type of GLIA) are hypothesized to function as 'directors' of the growth of capillaries so that they form especially narrow openings which act as the barrier. The blood–brain barrier is selective in that some substances cross it while others do not, and it is not uniform throughout the system; see e.g. the AREA POSTREMA, where the barrier is more permeable than most other places.

blood-injection-injury type phobia SIMPLE *PHOBIA.

blood oxygen level dependent BOLD.

blue The PRIMARY *COLOUR experienced when the normal eye is stimulated by light of approximately 470–475 nm.

blue (colour) blindness TRITANOPIA.

blue-yellow (colour) blindness DICHROMACY.

blunder blip ERROR RELATED NEGATIVITY.

blunted affect A disturbance in AFFECT characterized by sharply reduced intensity of emotional expression.

B-lymphocytes SPECIFIC *IMMUNE REACTIONS.

BMI BODY MASS INDEX.

BMR BASAL METABOLISM RATE.

body 1 Generally, in physical or anatomical terms, the principal part of a thing: the primary, central portion of an organism, the soma of a cell, a coherent organized collection of tissue, an organ, a small structure within a larger one, etc. 2 In metaphysics, the material substance of an individual. See here MIND–BODY PROBLEM. Many combined terms in psychology expressing these meanings are found; some use *body* as the base (e.g. *body type*), while many others use either the Latin form, *corpus*, or the Greek form, *soma*.

body-build index Eysenck's measure of body type based on the ratio between one's height and chest circumference. Those within the 'normal' range are called *mesomorphs*, those a standard deviation or more above the mean, *leptomorphs*, and those a standard deviation or more below, *eurymorphs*. See also the discussion under CONSTITUTIONAL THEORY.

body dysmorphic disorder A SOMATOFORM DISORDER characterized by preoccupation with an imagined defect in appearance. The most common complaints involve skin spots, wrinkles, excessive hair (typically facial) and shape of the nose. Occasionally the term *dysmorphophobia* is used, although it is not recommended since the disorder is properly not a phobia.

body image (or **concept**) The subjective image one has of one's own body, specifically with respect to evaluative judgements about how one is perceived by others and how well one is adjusted to these perceptions. Some use the term only in relation to physical appearance, others include judgements concerning body functions, movement, coordination, etc. Disturbed or inappropriate body image is an aspect of many neurotic disorders; see e.g. ANOREXIA NERVOSA, of which it is a hallmark symptom.

body integrity identity disorder A rare disorder characterized by an obsessive desire to have one (or more) limbs amputated. The limb is always perfectly normal but the desire can be utterly compelling. Little is known about the aetiology of the syndrome.

body language The system whereby information about feelings and emotions is communicated through nonverbal channels involving gestures, body position, facial expressions and other *paralinguistic* devices. See e.g. KINESICS, NONVERBAL COMMUNICATION.

body mass index (BMI) An index commonly used in studies of obesity and *body image* to provide an objective measure of weight relative to height. The BMI is a somewhat controversial measure, as its accuracy in relation to actual body fat composition can be distorted by a number of factors, including level of fitness, bone density and ethnicity. The index is calculated by dividing weight in kilograms by height in meters squared. When imperial measures are used (pounds, inches), the index is multiplied by 703. Also called *Quételet index*.

body memory MEMORY, BODY.

body type SOMATOTYPE.

Bogardus Social Distance Scale See SOCIAL DISTANCE SCALE.

bogus pipeline PIPELINE TECHNIQUES.

BOLD An acronym for *b*lood *o*xygen *l*evel *d*ependent. In fMRI (FUNCTIONAL MAGNETIC RESONANCE IMAGING), the BOLD response represents the rate at which particular cortical areas are using oxygen, a measure that reflects their degree of neural activity.

bond 1 n. Generally, a connection or link between things. Hence: **2** n. The hypothetical link between a stimulus and its associated response, the so-called *associated bond* or *S–R bond*. **3** An emotional connection between persons. Used here of adults as well as children; see e.g. ATTACHMENT, PAIR-BONDING. **4** A force which binds atoms or molecules together. **5** The biochemical or biomechanical link between a transmitter substance and its receptor site on a neuron. vb., *to bond* or *to bind*.

bonding Generally, the forming of a relationship; more specifically, that of a parent to an infant.

bone conduction The transmission of vibrations through the bones of the skull. A bone-conduction test indicates whether sound is mediated without conduction through the ossicles of the middle ear. It enables an audiologist to determine whether a hearing loss is due to defective conduction in the outer or middle ears or to nerve damage in the inner ear.

bone-fide pipeline technique PIPELINE TECHNIQUES.

Bonferroni correction A statistical adjustment that corrects for the increase in making a TYPE I *ERROR that occurs when multiple *t* tests are carried out. Basically, for each of *n* *t* tests, the significance level used becomes 1/ *n* times what would normally be employed.

boomerang effect A shift in attitude which not only goes against what was intended but actually in the opposite direction. It is a not uncommon outcome of excessive and insensitive attempts to dissuade persons from prejudices they hold. Also called *negative attitude change*.

bootstrap This term is generally used to describe operations in which one uses existing knowledge or information to develop more powerful routines which are then themselves used in similar fashion, so that the system 'lifts itself by its own bootstraps'. Although no organism or machine can literally bootstrap itself, the term is used metaphorically in cognitive psychology and artificial intelligence to characterize theoretical procedures in which the system (organic or mechanical) 'builds' useful structures for more powerful procedures than were originally programmed (genetically or artificially) into it.

borderline adj. **1** Of or pertaining to cases that are difficult to classify because they lie near a boundary that separates categories. **2** In testing, descriptive of any score that falls between one and two standard deviations from the arithmetic mean.

borderline intelligence A term introduced in an attempt to specify the level of intellectual capacity differentiating those capable of functioning normally and independently in the world from those in need of some form of institutional assistance. The term specifically refers to individuals who are right at the division between these two classes. Occasionally it is used 'quantitatively', by citing IQs in the 70–84 range as defining this level. Also called *borderline mental retardation*; see MENTAL RETARDATION.

borderline personality disorder A PERSONALITY DISORDER in which the individual chronically lives 'on the borderline' between normal, adaptive functioning and real psychic disability. Usually such a person is identified by any of a number of instabilities; for example, interpersonal relations tend to be unstable, affect shifts dramatically and inappropriately, self-image may be disturbed, displays of anger and temper are common, impulsive acts which are self-damaging, such as gambling or shoplifting, are frequent.

borderline schizophrenia SCHIZOPHRENIA, BORDERLINE.

Boston Diagnostic Aphasia Examination (BDAE) A test designed to evaluate the loss of language and related functions typically associated with left hemisphere damage. It is often administered along with supplemental tests, such as the BOSTON NAMING TEST.

Boston Naming Test (BNT) In its current form, a test consisting of line drawings of various objects, from the common to the obscure, for which the patient is asked to provide the names. It is often used supplementary to the BOSTON DIAGNOSTIC APHASIA EXAMINATION.

bottleneck theory Any of several models of INFORMATION PROCESSING based on the assumption that as the amount of information that needs to be processed increases, a 'bottleneck' develops and performance drops off.

bottom-up A spatial metaphor used to characterize systems and operations that proceed from relatively simple, concrete elements toward those with more abstract, symbolic features. Used widely. See, for example, DIRECT PERCEPTION for a bottom-up model of perception, IMPLICIT *LEARNING for a cognitive acquisition mechanism that

behaves in a similar manner and INDUCTION (1) for an analogous process in logical analysis and problem-solving. Compare with TOP-DOWN.

bottom-up processing Generally, processing that operates in a BOTTOM-UP fashion. Raw, unanalysed stimuli come in at the 'bottom' of a hierarchy of operations and the information works its way 'up' to more abstract, cognitive representations. Compared with TOP-DOWN PROCESSING, bottom-up processing is fast and automatic and takes place largely without conscious control or even awareness of the functions. Also called *data-driven processing*.

bouffée délirante In the French psychiatric nosology, an acute psychotic disorder with symptoms similar to those used of SCHIZOPHRENIFORM DISORDER (the *DSM* term) and ACUTE POLYMORPHIC PSYCHOTIC DISORDER (the *ICD* category).

Boulder model SCIENTIST-PRACTITIONER MODEL.

boulimia BULIMIA NERVOSA.

boundary Generally, a demarcation that separates two domains. Hence: **1** In social psychology, any abstract limit that represents the points of psychological separation between individuals and groups. Knowing what side of a social boundary one is on plays a significant role in determining acceptable behaviours. This meaning developed from Kurt Lewin's early FIELD THEORY where boundaries were viewed as divisions between regions of the LIFE SPACE. **2** In psychotherapy, a metaphoric line that determines acceptable behaviour on the part of the therapist (rules on touching clients) and marks topics that are off-limits (the therapist's personal life). **3** In vision a locus of points in a display that marks the separation of objects. Boundaries are treated in vision as edges and are elaborated by FEATURE DETECTORS in visual RECEPTIVE FIELDS. **4** In linguistics, the auditory events in the speech stream that mark the separation of words.

bounded rationality RATIONALITY, BOUNDED.

bound energy A psychoanalytic term applied occasionally to the ego's energy supply. The notion of being 'bounded' derives from the metaphoric role of the ego as being reality-directed and neither wasteful nor frivolous with its energy.

bound morpheme MORPHEME.

bouton terminal French for TERMINAL BUTTON.

bow motion (or **movement**) MOTION, BOW.

bow-wow theory THEORIES OF *LANGUAGE ORIGINS.

BRAC BASIC REST-ACTIVITY CYCLE.

brachy- Prefix meaning *short*.

brachycephalic Having a disproportionately short head. See CEPHALIC INDEX.

brachymetropia Nearsightedness; see MYOPIA.

brady- Prefix meaning *slow*.

bradyacusia Poor hearing. The term is misleading: there is nothing 'slow' about the individual's hearing (SEE BRADY-).

bradyaesthesia A general term for any reduced perceptual functioning. var., *bradyesthesia*.

bradyarthria Abnormally slow and hesitating speech.

bradyglossia An abnormal slowing of speech.

bradykinesia Slowness of motor movements.

bradylalia Slowness of speech.

bradylexia Abnormally slow reading. The term is reserved for cases in which the slowness is deemed not to be due simply to overall low intellectual functioning. See also DYSLEXIA.

bradyphrenia Abnormally slow cognitive functioning. Often observed in cases of extensive diffuse cortical impairment but may also be found in Parkinsonism and in patients with frontal lobe damage.

braidism An occasional synonym for *hypnotism*, from the name of the English surgeon James Braid.

braille (or **Braille**) A touch-based writing and reading system in which patterns of raised dots are used to represent letters and numerals. Named after its developer, the blind French educator Louis Braille.

brain Simply, that part of the central nervous system encased within the skull. The functions of the various parts of the human brain, which has been accurately called the single most complex object in the known universe, are defined and discussed under separate entries dealing with individual parts of the brain.

brain centre Any one of a number of areas in the brain in which there are complex interconnections between afferent and efferent fibres. The term has two distinguishable uses. It is used to refer to explicit and identifiable structures, such as the hypothalamus, and also to refer to hypothetical groups of neurons assumed to control a particular function, such as the speech centre.

brain death Said to have occurred when standard electroencephalographic (EEG) data indicate that key components of the brain are no longer functioning. Proposed in recent years as the best one for the determination of death, largely because sophisticated life-support systems can keep other organs (e.g. heart, lungs, kidneys) functioning, meaning previously used criteria, such as lack of breathing or undetectable pulse, can no longer serve as reliable indicators of death.

brain injury (or **damage**) Generally, loosely and indefinably vaguely, any injury to the brain. The cerebral damage can result from physical blows, lesions, toxic agents, anoxic or hypoxic episodes, infections, inflammation, seizures, metabolic insufficiencies, strokes, aneurysms or surgical procedures. See TRAUMATIC BRAIN INJURY (TBI).

brain lesion Any damage to brain tissue produced by injury, disease, surgery, etc. See LESION.

brain potential The electrical potential of the brain, or the electrical activity of the brain (see here ELECTROENCEPHALOGRAM). Although the term is often used colloquially to mean intellectual potential, it is not used in this sense in the technical literature.

brainstem That part of the brain that is left when both the cerebrum and cerebellum are removed.

brainstorm A sudden insightful idea, usually accompanied by a compelling emotional reaction.

brainstorming A group problem-solving technique in which everyone sits around and lets fly with ideas and possible solutions to the problem at hand.

brainwashing Any systematic attempt to change an individual's ideas, attitudes, beliefs and behaviours. The term derives from a Chinese colloquialism and it became a focus of considerable study after the experiences of prisoners of war. Whether such emotional and cognitive 'laundering' has lasting effects, particularly after the person has returned to their original environment, is open to question.

brainwaves Spontaneous electrical discharges of the brain as recorded by an EEG. See ELECTROENCEPHALOGRAM.

Brawner decision A legal decision regarding the use of an INSANITY DEFENCE in the USA. It states: 'A person is not responsible for criminal conduct if at the time of such conduct as a result of mental disease or defect he lacks substantial capacity either to appreciate the wrongfulness of his conduct or to conform his conduct to the requirements of law.' Compare with MCNAGHTEN RULE, DURHAM RULE and ALI DEFENCE.

Brazelton Scale NEONATAL BEHAVIOURAL ASSESSMENT SCALE.

breakthrough In psychotherapeutic work, a progressive quantum step in a client's attitudes, reactions, behaviours, feeling of self, etc. The term is generally reserved for such changes when they occur after long periods of no progress.

breast In classical psychoanalytic writings, the term refers to both the anatomical part and to a symbolic representation of it in the mind. In the latter (and psychoanalytically interesting) sense the breast becomes the focus of oral wishes, the source of psychic nutrition, the object which satisfies needs. In short, it becomes the mother but without the personhood of the real mother.

breathing related sleep disorder APNOEA.

bregma The juncture in the skull where the sagittal and coronal sutures meet.

bricolage Ingenuity in patching together

impromptu techniques or objects to attain a goal or solve a problem. The term is French and an individual inventive in such a manner is called a 'bricoleur'. The key here is improvisation and breaking of FUNCTIONAL FIXEDNESS.

brief depressive disorder, recurrent A *mood disorder* characterized by recurrent MAJOR *DEPRESSIVE EPISODES that are relatively short-lived (i.e. less than two weeks in duration).

brief psychotherapy A general term used to cover any psychotherapy which is specifically designed to be relatively short in duration. Most such therapeutic programmes are quite goal-oriented and their aims are typically well specified, e.g. eliminating a particular phobia.

brief psychotic disorder An acute psychotic disorder with the defining feature that the duration is of no more than two weeks. The diagnosis is made when the patient shows normal adaptive functioning prior to onset and when the episode is precipitated by an identifiable and serious psychologically stressful event. Also called *brief reactive psychosis*.

brief reactive psychosis BRIEF PSYCHOTIC DISORDER.

brightness 1 The dimension of a colour that locates it on the black–white continuum. Compare with HUE and SATURATION. Sometimes the term *lightness* is used synonymously. **2** The perceived intensity of any visual stimulus dependent on the amplitude and wavelength of the light. Note that different subjective brightnesses are produced by different colours having the same physical intensity; see e.g. BEZOLD-BRÜCKE EFFECT, PURKINJE EFFECT, SPECTRAL SENSITIVITY. **3** A subjective quality of tone. See TONAL BRIGHTNESS. Occasionally called *brilliance*, especially in older writings. **4** A relatively high degree of intelligence – a distinctly nontechnical usage.

brightness adaptation ADAPTATION (1).

brightness constancy The tendency for a visual stimulus to be perceived as having the same brightness under widely divergent conditions of illumination despite the fact that the different conditions deliver different amounts of physical energy to the eye. See CONSTANCY.

brightness contrast 1 The relative brightness of two stimuli. 2 The effect of modifying the perceived brightness of a stimulus by the prior or simultaneous presentation of another stimulus. See CONTRAST.

bril A subjective unit of the perceived brightness of a light. The bril scale is established by equating the subjective value 100 bril with the physical value of 1 millilambert and then plotting brighter and dimmer illuminations relative to this anchor point.

brilliance 1 BRIGHTNESS, TONAL BRIGHTNESS. 2 A nontechnical term for extremely high intelligence or creativity.

Briquet's syndrome A rather loosely defined behaviour disorder characterized by vague feelings of unease and poorly articulated, indefinite complaints. See SOMATIZATION DISORDER.

British empiricism EMPIRICISM.

Broca's aphasia APHASIA, BROCA'S.

Broca's area A cortical area involved in the processing of language functions. For virtually all right-handed individuals it is located in the inferior frontal gyrus of the left hemisphere; for the left-handed it is still generally in the left hemisphere although on occasion it is found in the corresponding area on the right. The area was named after the French surgeon Paul Broca, who reported in 1861 that many aphasic patients had lesions in this area. Today it is generally acknowledged that this is not 'the' speech centre: many different areas of the brain have been implicated in language behaviour, of which Broca's area is only one. See e.g. WERNICKE'S AREA.

Brodmann's areas A system for mapping the cortex based on the 'architecture' of the cellular structure. While, as of this writing, well over 200 physiologically distinct areas in the brain have been identified, Brodmann's original (1909) system demarcated 52 areas differentiated from each other on the basis of histologically distinct features. Despite more recent work showing the inadequacy of Brodmann's original maps and the fact that there is not always correspondence between Brodmann's areas and functional

areas established by other mapping techniques, his is still the most commonly used classification system.

broken home A strange term used for a family in which one of the parents is absent owing to death, divorce, desertion, etc. The word *broken* entails the notion of malfunctioning; the coiner of this term was obviously injecting an unwarranted judgement about single-parent homes.

Bruce effect A phenomenon first observed in mice by Hilda Bruce in which the termination of a pregnancy is brought about by substances in the urine of a virile male mouse other than the one which impregnated the female. Having thus eliminated the offspring of the first male, the animal may now impregnate the female himself and thus increase the likelihood of passing his own genes on to future generations.

Brunswik faces A series of schematic faces made up of simple lines for the eyes, nose and mouth. They have been used largely in perceptual and cognitive studies of discrimination and categorization.

Brunswik ratio A way of expressing any perceptual constancy, developed by Egon Brunswik. The easiest example to understand is size constancy: a subject stands in one place viewing a standard stake placed some distance away and is asked to judge which of a series of variable stakes is the same size as the standard. The amount of size constancy is given by the ratio $P - R/C - R$, where R = relative retinal size (angle of vision subtended on the retina), C = objective physical size and P = perceived or judged size. Similar ratios are used for other constancies. When the logarithm of the values is used, the formula is called the *Thouless ratio*.

brute force A problem-solving technique by which all possible alternatives are attempted or all possible paths to a solution are followed. Brute-force techniques are usually last resorts when HEURISTICS are not known or do not exist.

bruxism Grinding of the teeth, especially during sleep.

buccal Pertaining to the mouth or cheek.

buccofacial apraxia APRAXIA, BUCCOFACIAL.

buffer items FILLER (MATERIAL).

buffer (store) A term borrowed from computer science and often used to refer to a limited-capacity memory store in which information is held temporarily while being processed.

bug A problem in a process, an error in a program. The term comes from computer sciences; see DEBUG.

buggery Slang for anal intercourse. See SODOMY (1).

bulb 1 Any expansion of an organ, vessel, neural process, etc. 2 An obsolete term for the MEDULLA OBLONGATA.

-bulia Combining form meaning *will*.

bulimia nervosa An eating disorder characterized by repeated episodes of 'binge' eating followed by misuse of laxatives and self-induced vomiting. In the classic syndrome tremendous amounts of high-calorie foods can be eaten rapidly and with little chewing. Episodes are usually associated with depression and followed by guilt and self-deprecation. Surprisingly, bulimia is frequently found in conjunction with *anorexia nervosa*. var., *boulimia*.

bundle hypothesis A label that was used derisively by Gestalt psychologists for the structuralist argument that a complex percept is no more than the sum of (a 'bundle' of) its several stimulus elements.

Bunsen–Roscoe law The principle that the absolute threshold for vision is a multiplicative function of the duration and intensity of the stimulus. The law holds reasonably well for short durations of up to about 50 msec. An example of TEMPORAL *SUMMATION in that the effect of a stimulus summates over time.

buprenorphine A drug that has both OPIATE agonist and antagonist properties. It was introduced as an analgesic and later used in the treatment of heroin addiction owing to its ability to moderate the euphoric impact of opium-based compounds.

bupropion A MIXED-FUNCTION *ANTIDEPRESSANT DRUG that inhibits the reuptake of dopamine and norepinephrine and has nicotinic antagonistic properties. It is used as an adjunctive drug in treatment of depression and ADHD and in smoking cessation. It has fewer side effects than most antidepressants although there is suggestion of an increased risk of seizures.

burst 1 Generally, any sudden increase in responsiveness. 2 In operant conditioning, the rapid output of responses after a period of relative quiescence typically found under certain schedules of reinforcement, e.g. *fixed-interval schedules*. 3 In electrophysiology, the rapid firing of a stimulated nerve fibre.

buspirone The prototypical AZASPIRONE drug used in the treatment of anxiety.

butaperazine One of the PHENOTHIAZINE DERIVATIVES used in the treatment of schizophrenia.

butorphanol A synthetic opiate with both antagonist and agonist properties used primarily as an analgesic, particularly in the treatment of migraine headaches.

butyrophenones A group of ANTIPSYCHOTIC DRUGS (e.g. *haloperidol*), similar in action and effect to the PHENOTHIAZINES.

buzz word Colloquial for any word or term which is instantly responded to with a predictable, emotional reaction.

bystander (intervention) effect The more people present when help is needed, the less likely any one of them is to provide assistance. Once thought to be a symbol of the dehumanizing urban environment, the effect is now known to be quite general. It occurs largely because of two simple cognitive effects. The more people about, the more likely it is that each will assume that someone else will provide the assistance and, when no one acts, to believe that help is, in fact, not needed. See also ALTRUISM, HELPING BEHAVIOUR.

byte A number of binary digits (see also BIT) taken together as a coordinated unit. The term was introduced in a half-joking manner (many bits make up a *bite* – and this spelling is also found), but it has stuck as a useful term in computer sciences and information theory.

C

C **1** Constant. **2** CONTROL GROUP. **3** Centigrade.

c **1** Correction factor. **2** In studies of the HERITABILITY of traits, the proportion of *phenotype* variance that is attributable to the shared or common environment of the study pairs. Also denoted as ce or c^2. Occasionally capitalized.

CA CHRONOLOGICAL *AGE.

CA1, CA2, CA3, and CA4 fields Major subdivisions of the HIPPOCAMPUS. The CA1 and CA3 fields have been most carefully studied, especially with regard to their role in memory. The designation 'CA' comes from *cornu ammonis* (or *Ammon's horn*), which the hippocampus is also called.

cable properties In neurophysiology, the collective properties of axonal transmission of a neural impulse. Such properties are represented basically as passive conduction of the current in decremental fashion along the length of the axon (or cable).

cachexia Lit., bad condition. Generally, any state of ill health, malnutrition, physical wasting-away.

cachinnation Inappropriate, hysterical laughter.

cac(o-) Combining form meaning *bad, diseased, degenerate*.

cacoethes Generally, a bad habit or propensity.

cacogeusia A neurological condition in which ordinarily palatable foods produce a disgusting, putrid taste.

cacosmia An abnormal neurological condition in which normally pleasant or neutral smells are experienced as foul and disgusting.

caffeine An alkaloid found in various common foods including coffee and chocolate. Its stimulating effects are produced by its ability to block the activity of *phosphodiesterase*, an enzyme that destroys secondary messengers at cerebral synapses, thus increasing the activity of many neurons and producing arousal and wakefulness. There is also evidence that caffeine activates *dopaminergic* neurons. Caffeine, despite its routine consumption, is actually a fairly powerful drug and its use is a psychologically significant element of a number of clinical disorders, as the following entries point out.

caffeine-induced anxiety disorder Quite literally, clinically significant anxiety caused by consumption of caffeine. Generally classified as a SUBSTANCE-INDUCED DISORDER, in some cases the anxiety can be strong enough to be confused with a panic attack.

caffeine-induced disorders A general label for any of several clinical disorders related to the consumption of caffeine. Included are CAFFEINE INTOXICATION, CAFFEINE-INDUCED ANXIETY DISORDER and CAFFEINE-INDUCED SLEEP DISORDER.

caffeine-induced sleep disorder Clinically significant disturbances of sleep caused by caffeine. The typical presenting symptom is insomnia.

caffeine intoxication A state of nervousness, anxiety, insomnia and PSYCHOMOTOR AGITATION. In sensitive persons as little as 250 mg (roughly 2–3 cups of coffee or 3–5 cups of tea) is sufficient to produce these effects. Also called *caffeinism*.

caffeine withdrawal A syndrome caused by abrupt cessation of caffeine consumption following prolonged daily use. Typical symptoms are marked fatigue, dysphoria usually in the form of mild depression, nausea and headaches.

CAH CONGENITAL ADRENAL HYPERPLASIA.

CAI COMPUTER-ASSISTED INSTRUCTION.

calcarine cortex The cortical area surrounding the CALCARINE FISSURE. Also called STRIATE CORTEX – see that term for more detail.

calcarine fissure The fissure or sulcus on the medial surface of the occipital lobe of the cortex which divides the medial portion of the lobe into superior and inferior portions. The primary visual sensory area is located in the CALCARINE CORTEX.

California infant scale(s) Now called, after their designer, the BAYLEY SCALES OF INFANT DEVELOPMENT.

California Psychological Inventory (CPI) A self-report inventory originally derived from the MMPI (MINNESOTA MULTIPHASIC PERSONALITY INVENTORY). It consists of several hundred 'yes–no' questions and yields scores on a number of scales including self-acceptance, self-control, socialization, achievement and dominance.

California Verbal Learning Test (CVLT) A neuropsychological test used for detecting memory deficits, especially those involving language.

callosal apraxia APRAXIA, CALLOSAL.

callosectomy, callosotomy COMMISSUROTOMY.

callosum CORPUS CALLOSUM.

caloric nystagmus NYSTAGMUS, CALORIC.

CALP COGNITIVE ACADEMIC LANGUAGE PROFICIENCY.

calyx An eggcup-shaped dendritic process in which another cell is embedded.

camera Latin for *vault*; a chamber, room, cavity, box, etc. In anatomy, an internal body chamber; in experimental research, a specially constructed chamber, e.g. *camera inodorata*, an odour-free enclosure for studying smell.

campimetry The measurement of the visual field.

canal A narrow channel or tube, a passage-way. A term used more or less synonymously with a number of others, e.g. *groove, duct, foramen, tract*, etc.

canal, central A thin canal in the centre of the spinal cord filled with cerebrospinal fluid.

canalization **1** Generally, narrowing, restricting. A thing or process is said to be canalized if its range of manifestation is diminished, particularly to the point where only one of the many possible alternatives is observed. **2** In G. Murphy's theory, a culturally determined narrowing of preferred ways of satisfying drive states. **3** In neurology, the hypothesized process whereby a neural pathway becomes traversed more easily with increasing use. **4** In evolutionary genetics, the notion that a particular epigenetic capability or behaviour pattern will continue to be manifested in the face of less than optimal environments, or, if disturbed or interrupted by extreme conditions, be fairly easily restored when conditions are made appropriate once more.

cancellation tests Any of a number of tests used in the diagnosis of various neurological conditions. The patient attempts to cancel or cross out specific targets in a complex array. For example, patients with attentional deficits tend to make omission errors, those with particular forms of acquired dyslexia have problems with linguistic materials, while neglect patients only cancel out targets on one side of the array.

candela A measure of the intensity of a light. The internationally accepted standard is defined by a complex set of physical parameters; experientially, a 100 watt incandescent bulb emits about 120 candelas.

candle An obsolete unit of luminance measured at the source of light. The intensity of light on a given surface was presented in terms of foot-candles; that is, the intensity of one candle at 1 ft (0.3 m) distance. See CANDELA. See also LUX.

cannabis (sativa) *Cannabis* is the name of a genus of plants. The *sativa* variety is the most common and is cultivated legally for hemp and limited medical uses and illegally for its various psychoactive products, which are known by a wide variety of names including hashish, marijuana (var., marihuana), charas, bhang, ganja, dagga and just plain cannabis – in addition to an ever-increasing number of slang terms. The active ingredients are tetrahydrocannabinols (THC), the primary one being an isomer, delta-9-tetrahydrocannabinol, which has been synthesized and is known to produce central-nervous-system effects. The range of effects of the drug is quite wide and is dependent on dosage, the setting in which it is taken, the psychological and physical make-up of the individual and whether other substances such as alcohol are taken at the same time. There is considerable debate over the short- and long-term effects of cannabis. There is little evidence of DRUG *TOLERANCE and no substantial data to support charges of a DRUG *DEPENDENCE, although a psychological dependence can emerge in frequent users, and high doses can produce CANNABIS INTOXICATION. See THC for more detail.

cannabis intoxication A pattern of maladaptive psychological and behavioural changes, including motor dysfunctions, euphoria, anxiety, impaired judgement and a sense of time slowing, that accompany cannabis use. Several physical signs may also occur, including tachycardia, dry mouth and increased appetitie.

Cannon–Bard theory THEORIES OF *EMOTION.

cannula A small hollow tube which can be inserted into tissue for the purpose of administering chemical preparations or removing fluids for analysis. Its most common use is in the study of brain tissue, when the ultrathin tube is inserted into the organism's brain and the action of specific chemical substances can be systemically evaluated.

canon 1 Any working principle or formula. However, not every formula or heuristic gets to be labelled a canon; the term is generally reserved for important, fundamental principles that seem likely to lead to meaningful truths. See e.g. LLOYD MORGAN'S CANON. 2 A model or standard, or a body of models or standards. See CANONICAL.

canonical Used generally as derived from CANON (2); that is, characterizing or relating to elements or events which are ordered or structured according to some principle or model.

canonical correlation CORRELATION, CANONICAL.

capacity 1 Generally, a synonym of ABILITY. 2 In computer sciences and cognitive science, the amount of information which a given system can handle; see e.g. CHANNEL CAPACITY, STORAGE CAPACITY. 3 Absorbing or holding power, as in *electrical capacity*. 4 Volume, as in *vital capacity*.

Capgras syndrome A DELUSIONAL MISIDENTIFICATION DISORDER which manifests as a belief that that 'doubles' have replaced persons whom one knows. The term is reserved for cases of fairly severe psychiatric disorders, although similar delusions have been observed in patients with REDUPLICATIVE *PARAMNESIA.

capillary From the Latin, meaning *hair-like*. 1 A minute blood vessel. The capillary system connects the arterial and venous systems. 2 A minute lymph duct through which exchange of nutrients and waste from blood tissue takes place.

capsaicin A chemical in the fruit and seeds of pepper plants that irritates free nerve endings in the mouth and skin. It is of interest in psychology because it produces a secondary analgesic effect and because of the strong individual and cultural differences in its use in cuisine.

capture Short for *attentional capture*. A process wherein a feature of a stimulus display immediately attracts or 'captures' one's attention. Movement, particularly in the periphery of the visual field, works extremely well.

carbamates A group of drugs that function as ACETYLCHOLINESTERASE inhibitors. They appear to slow the progression of various dementias and have fewer side effects than other compounds with similar action.

carbamazepine An antimania drug used to treat BIPOLAR DISORDER, particularly when the patient cannot tolerate the side effects of *lithium*. It also is used to treat seizures that originate in the medial temporal lobes.

carboxyl group A molecule made up of two oxygen atoms and one hydrogen atom bound to a carbon atom (COOH). See AMINO ACID.

cardiac Pertaining to the heart.

cardinal From the Latin for *important*; primary, central, fundamental.

cardinal characteristic (or **trait**) A personality characteristic that is highly descriptive and singularly identifying for a particular individual.

cardio- Prefix meaning pertaining to the heart.

cardiogram A shortened form of ELECTRO-CARDIOGRAM.

cardiovascular Pertaining to the heart and the blood vessels of the circulatory system.

card-sorting task (or **test**) Any task in which the subject is required to sort cards according to some principle or rule. Some are simple sensory/motor tasks in which sorting is carried out according to a specific instruction ('triangles in one pile, circles in the other'); others are more complex, including tasks in which the subject must figure out the rules that determine the correct sorting, e.g. WISCONSIN CARD SORTING TEST.

caregiver 1 Generally, anyone involved in any of the phases of health care. It may apply to one who identifies illness, helps prevent it, treats or rehabilitates patients, etc. The term is generally applied to community workers, paraprofessionals, orderlies, etc. but may also refer to trained clinical psychologists or physicians. **2** A parent or other adult who provides childcare, a CARETAKER.

caretaker A general term for anyone who is intimately involved in the raising of a child. The term is used broadly and may include parents, other members of an extended family, a governess, etc.

carnal Pertaining to the flesh. Occasionally used literally, but more often as a euphemism for *sexual*.

carotid artery The artery that serves the rostral (i.e. anterior, or frontal) portions of the brain.

carpal Pertaining to the wrist.

carpal age AGE, CARPAL.

carpentered environment Any physical setting that has been built by humans according to architectural plans that do not follow natural physical forms. Most buildings are built with an eye to square corners, straight lines, even doorways, and hence fulfil this definition. In the study of perception, particularly in cross-cultural and anthropological studies, it is argued that such environments are unnatural and give rise to inappropriate percepts.

carphenazine A PHENOTHIAZINE DERIVATIVE used to treat schizophrenia.

CART Abbreviation of *cocaine and amphetamine-regulated transcript*. It is a naturally occurring neurotransmitter found in the arcuate nucleus of the hypothalamus. It plays a role in eating with high levels inhibiting food intake.

Cartesian Pertaining to the theories and discoveries of the great French mathematician and philosopher René Descartes (1596–1650). The positions represented are a strong form of *dualism*, with mind (or soul) being nonmaterial and indivisible and body being material and divisible; body is mechanical and to be understood through physical and mathematical study, mind through rational means. The *rationalism* which characterized Descartes's point of view led him to articulate a variety of a priori or innate ideas, including those of self, God and perfection. Descartes's philosophical perspective, ignored by psychologists for the most part during the behaviourist decades, has recently, with the renewed interest in the philosophy and psychology of mind, come under fresh scrutiny, although it should be clear that his perspective still doesn't have many adherents.

Cartesian coordinates A system for locating any point in plane space relative to two axes set at right angles. Developed by René Descartes, it forms the basis for the standard graphing techniques to represent data. The horizontal line is denoted as the x-axis and the vertical as the y-axis. They cross at right angles at the origin, or zero point, and the position of any arbitrary point is given by its value on each axis.

cary(o)- Variant of KARY(O)-.

case 1 Generally, any instance or occurrence of a thing, such as a particular event, a characteristic instance or a disease. **2** An individual who displays a characteristic, or a patient who has a disorder or a disease.

case-based reasoning A form of ANALOGICAL REASONING in which knowledge obtained from working on an earlier situation (case) is used to solve a new problem.

case study (or **history**) An account of a single individual in which a detailed record is compiled including personal history, background, test results, interviews and the like. Research using case studies is common when other approaches are not possible, as when an unusual psychiatric case is presented or when a unique or rare type of brain injury occurs. See, for example, ANNA O. and HM.

caseworker Any health-related professional or paraprofessional who handles individual cases over an extended period of time, often across multiple settings. It is the comprehensiveness of supervision that distinguishes the caseworker from others in the field.

caste 1 A closed hereditary social stratum or class which controls to a considerable degree the marital possibilities, prestige, available occupations, etc. of its members. Some authors restrict the term to the formalized system in India, others use it for any such rigid stratification system. Occasionally qualifiers are appended to specify the type of caste system, e.g. *colour* or *racial caste, religious caste*. See also SOCIAL CLASS. **2** In the social insects, any specialized (functionally and/or structurally) set of individuals. The honey bee with its three castes (queens, workers, drones) is the classic example.

castrate CASTRATING, CASTRATION.

castrating Term used more in the popular literature than in the technical to refer to individuals whose aggressive, dominating style of interacting undermines others and deprives them of opportunities to take the initiative. It is most frequently used of women with regard to their manner of interaction with males but this restriction is not mandated by the strict meaning of the term. CASTRATION (especially 4).

castration 1 From the Latin for *pruning*, the surgical removal of the male gonads, the testes. **2** By extension, the removal of the female gonads, the ovaries. **3** In the classical psycho-analytic literature, the (symbolic) removal of the male external genitalia, especially the penis. See here CASTRATION ANXIETY, CASTRATION COMPLEX. For meaning 1 *orchiectomy* is an occasional synonym; when nonhumans are under consideration, *geld* is often used. For meaning 2 *ovariectomy* is a synonym, and, for animals, *spay*. Note that while castration is certainly an effective method of birth control, it should be distinguished from *vasectomy* (in males) and *salpingectomy* (in females), which are surgical procedures for sterilization that do not interfere with normal hormonal processes, as does castration. **4** Metaphorically, the removal of some prized or precious 'possession', usually a pattern of behaviour or personality, such as initiative or personal power, not a physical object. See CASTRATING.

castration anxiety A psychoanalytic term for the anxiety resulting from real or imagined threats to one's sexual functions. It refers to symbolic threats, not specific threats to one's physical genitals (CASTRATION (3)). It is used in the context of meaning 3 of the base term and hence refers not to specific threats to one's physical genitals but to symbolic threats. Although originally the term was applied only to males, whose fear surrounds the loss of masculine erotic function, it can in principle be applied to females; see CASTRATION COMPLEX.

castration complex In classical psychoanalytic theory, the fear associated with loss of one's genitals. In males the complex is supposedly manifested as anxiety surrounding the possibility of loss, in females as the guilt over having already experienced the loss. The original position with regard to males has, of course, been critiqued rather severely but is still, generally speaking, a part of the standard psychoanalytic theory; the position with regard to females has been so vigorously attacked that it is rarely taken seriously any longer.

castration, hormonal Typically the term CASTRATION (1 and 2) refers to a surgical procedure. When the qualifier is used it is meant to refer to those forms of hormonal treatment that bring about the same biological and behavioural changes but without surgical intervention. Also called *chemical castration*.

CAT 1 COMPUTERIZED AXIAL TOMOGRAPHY. **2** CHILDREN'S APPERCEPTION TEST.

cata- From the Greek, meaning *down*. Also used as a prefix to indicate *from, against* and, on occasions, *in accordance with* or *repeating* (the latter sense is found in speech and language pathologies). vars., *cath-, kata-*.

catabolism 1 Generally, the breaking down of living things or body structures. **2** The expenditure phase of METABOLISM. Contrast with ANABOLISM.

catalepsy 1 The rigid maintenance of a body position over extended periods of time. **2** FLEXIBILITAS CEREA or CATATONIC WAXY FLEXIBILITY. See also CATATONIA and CATATONIC *SCHIZOPHRENIA.

catalexia A tendency to repeat inappropriate words during reading.

catalyst In chemistry any substance that affects a chemical reaction but itself remains unaltered. The term now enjoys wide usage and in psychology generally refers to any person or set of stimulus conditions that influences some social or cognitive process. Note that the requirement that the catalytic agent itself remain unchanged by the involvement is often missing in contemporary usage.

catamnesis The medical history of a patient from the time when first seen by a physician or a therapist, or from the onset of a disability. Compare with ANAMNESIS.

cataphasia SYNTACTIC *APHASIA.

cataplexy A sudden loss of muscle tone resulting in the individual collapsing 'like a sack of potatoes'. It may result from a sudden emotional shock or a stroke and is an occasional symptom in narcolepsy, where it appears to be due to the person suddenly going into REM SLEEP, one of the characteristics of which is muscle flaccidity.

catastrophe theory A mathematical theory developed by René Thom which attempts to formalize the nature of abrupt discontinuities in functions. For example, the dog that suddenly and without warning attacks a person, or the precipitate onset of many 'nervous breakdowns' in seemingly undisturbed persons. The theory has been subjected to vigorous criticisms concerning the mathematics and its applicability. The jury is still out.

catastrophic reaction Kurt Goldstein's term for extreme agitation or anxiety following a cerebral injury. It is more common with left hemisphere lesions than with right and tends to be manifested when the patient is confronted with situations that make their limitations obvious.

catastrophic thinking The act of greatly overestimating the likelihood and severity of negative events; e.g. thinking that one will never recover from a bad love affair, or imagining people burned or houses destroyed when seeing smoke. When excessive in frequency, severity or self-focus, this type of thinking raises the risk of depression and anxiety disorders, particularly *panic disorder*. Also called *catastrophizing*.

catathymic amnesia EPISODIC *AMNESIA.

catatonia Muscle rigidity. It is a common symptom of CATATONIC *SCHIZOPHRENIA and can be manifested in a variety of ways including catatonic *negativism* characterized by the patient assuming odd postures and resistance to efforts to move his or her limbs, a catatonic *excitement* marked by frantic, purposeless activity or a *stupor* where there is little motor activity and a near total withdrawal.

catatonic excitement CATATONIA.

catatonic negativism CATATONIA.

catatonic posturing CATATONIA.

catatonic rigidity CATATONIA

catatonic schizophrenia SCHIZOPHRENIA, CATATONIC TYPE.

catatonic stupor CATATONIA.

catatonic waxy flexibility A condition in which the patient's limbs can be moved or moulded into any position, which they will then maintain often for extended periods of time. The term comes from the fact that when the limbs are being moved they feel as though they are made of wax. Called *flexibilitas cerea* in some older texts.

catch trial A trial in a signal-detection experiment in which the signal is not actually present. A positive response in such a trial is termed a FALSE ALARM. See SIGNAL DETEC-

TION THEORY. The original German term here was *Vexierversuch*, meaning *hoax trial*.

catecholamine hypothesis A hypothesis about the possible biochemical basis of schizophrenia. In simple terms the assumption is that excessive build-up of the *catecholamines* (especially *dopamine* – see DOPAMINE HYPOTHESIS) in particular synaptic clefts in the brain is responsible for the symptoms of the psychosis. Evidence in support comes from the observation that chronic use of amphetamines produces a 'model' paranoid schizophrenic psychosis and that substances that function to mildly increase the level of the amines (e.g. MAO inhibitors, tricyclic compounds) have antidepressant effects.

catecholaminergic Of neurons and neural pathways in which the neurotransmitter secreted is one of the CATECHOLAMINES.

catecholamines A group of BIOGENIC AMINES that includes EPINEPHRINE, NOREPINEPHRINE and DOPAMINE, all of which are known to play significant roles in nervous-system functioning.

categorical **1** Relating to a CATEGORY. **2** Absolute, independent of other things. Psychological terminology, especially in studies of perception and cognition, almost always carries meaning 1; more philosophical usages frequently carry 2.

categorical perception The perception of individual stimuli as belonging to a particular category of stimuli rather than as unique, identifiable events. It is most easily observed in the tendency to hear the acoustic variations within a *phoneme* class as all representing the same sound; that is, not to perceive the differences between these variations. Such categorical perception is pronounced when the stimuli are stop consonants (e.g. /b/ versus /p/) but can also be observed in nonspeech continua such as plucked versus bowed strings.

categorical scale NOMINAL *SCALE.

categorical syllogism SYLLOGISM.

categorization The process of forming a CATEGORY (1). See also CONCEPT et seq. especially CONCEPT FORMATION AND LEARNING.

category **1** In modern psychological terminology, especially in theories of cogni-

tion, this term is used in ways which derive from the extensive concern with its meaning in philosophy. The common notion here is that a category is somehow like a CONCEPT, a class, a group, or even a system. That is, for example, if there exists the category 'lion', this carries with it the existence of a mental *concept* 'lion' in the mind, a theoretical *class* of objects which belong in it, an actual *group* of lions, and a *system* or set of decision rules about which objects belong in the category and which do not. It should be fairly obvious that a term with connotations like these is going to enjoy (or suffer from) rather extensive and varied usage. Some authors use it as though it refers to a specific, real-world class which, at least in principle, can be identified and defined perhaps by a list of distinguishing features (lions are mammals, felines, predators, have four legs, sleep a lot, etc.); others use it as though it refers to the mental representation of a class in the mind of the knowing person (i.e. the image or idea of a lion); still others prefer to treat the term in a pragmatic fashion and let patterns of behaviour or usage dictate category boundaries ('lion' is a distinct category distinguishable from, say, 'house cat', since the sentence 'My lion spends every evening on my lap purring' is somewhat unlikely to refer to a real-world situation). For more on these issues and usage patterns see related terms such as CONCEPT, PROTOTYPE and REPRESENTATION. **2** In older philosophical writings, a basic mode of thought or being. Aristotle used it for the ten classes which he felt could provide a complete inventory of all things knowable; for Kant it represented the divisions of understanding beginning with quantity, quality, relation and modality. **3** In statistics, any division or grouping of data according to specific quantitative criteria.

category, basic (-level) NATURAL *CATEGORY (2).

category estimation METHODS OF *SCALING.

category, natural **1** A category which exists in relation to the natural, biological and anatomical structure of the perceiver. For example, colours are natural categories in this sense since all people with a normal, intact visual system respond to the visual spectrum in roughly the same fashion. Even though a person's language may not have separate words for 'red' and 'orange' they will discriminate between them in the same fashion as a speaker of English. **2** A category represented by things that occur naturally in the real world and which share particular features or are reacted to in similar ways, e.g. 'furniture', 'bird', 'sport'. Note that those who prefer to use the term only in sense 1 use the term *basic category* or *basic-level category* for sense 2.

category, superordinate A CATEGORY (1) characterized by being somewhat abstract and containing within it a number of basic-level categories. Examples abound, *sin* encompasses many specific forms of sin, *animal* subsumes a host of specific animals. The psychologically interesting features of superordinate categories are that, (a) the members are diverse and superficially distinct ('flatworm' doesn't share many physical features with 'lion' but both are unquestionably members of the same category 'animal') and (b) the differences among them are fewer and less significant than those between members of separate categories ('lion' and 'flatworm' are more similar to each other than either is to 'chair').

catelectrotonus A state of increased excitability of a neuron, nerve or muscle in the region of the cathode (negative pole) when a current is passed through it.

catharsis From the Greek, meaning *purification, purging.* **1** In psychoanalytic theory this meaning was borrowed to refer to the release of tension and anxiety resulting from the process of bringing repressed ideas, feelings, wishes and memories of the past into consciousness. **2** Lay usage has broadened the meaning a bit and one often sees the term used to refer to any satisfying emotional experience. See also ABREACTION.

cathexis From the Greek, meaning *retention, holding.* In psychoanalytic theory, the investing of libidinal energy in an activity, an object or a person. Thus, one sees references to goals as being cathected, or to the EGO as an object of a cathection. Freud conceptualized cathexis as a kind of psychic analogue of an electric charge and often the terminology used reflects this: the language of cathexis uses expressions like 'charge' and 'current', and these things are said to 'flow' and become 'bound' to objects, and even to

'reverse charge' (*anticathexis*). vb., *cathect.* var., *cathection.*

cation A positively charged ion. See ANION.

CAT scan COMPUTERIZED AXIAL TOMOGRAPHY.

cauda equina The collection of spinal roots that runs through the lower third of the spinal column below the point where the spinal cord itself ends.

caudal 1 Pertaining to the tail or a tail-like structure. **2** Inferior in position.

caudate nucleus A tail-shaped mass of subcortical grey matter. One of the components of the BASAL GANGLIA, along with the *lenticulate* (or *lentiform*) *nucleus*, it forms with the *corpus striatum*. It is involved in the inhibitory aspects of the voluntary control of movement, and impaired caudate function is associated with Parkinson's disease.

causalgia THERMALGIA.

causality A term for what is essentially a philosophical issue, denoting the abstract quality that links the occurrence of an event or state with the prior occurrence of a previous event or state such that the latter is deemed contingent upon the former. Because the term is philosophical and refers to an abstract relation it is sometimes distinguished from CAUSATION, which is preferred in psychological parlance.

causal texture An old philosophical notion resurrected and streamlined during the 1940s and 1950s by both E. C. Tolman and E. Brunswik. The essential notion is that every event in the environment is linked to every other event. The degree of dependence may run from the infinitesimal and negligible to absolute causal dependency. An important component of this hoary idea is that the dependencies are not viewed as certain or deterministic but rather as probabilistic or stochastic.

causation A basically empirical principle which states that for whatever effects are observed there was a cause that preceded them. The principle of causation (or cause and effect) is asymmetric and unidirectional. In *simple* causation, where there is a single known or knowable cause, it functions as the necessary and sufficient conditions of the effect observed; in *multiple* causation, where there may be several distinguishable causal factors for a particular observed effect, the issues of sufficiency and necessity are weakened. Multiple causation is the modal case in the social sciences.

cautious shift CHOICE SHIFT.

CCC CONSONANT TRIGRAM.

ceiling effect The term *ceiling* is used to refer to the maximum score on a test or a limit on the performance of some task. The term *ceiling effect* is taken to refer to: **1** In testing, the limitation on a testee's scores as he or she approaches this theoretical upper bound. **2** In studies of behaviour, the failure to observe any improvement in performance owing to the fact that the subject is already performing at maximum capacity. Actually, this usage is a bit misleading since the real meaning here is *lack of an effect* (of learning or instruction or whatever) *due to the existence of a ceiling*. The converse is called a *basement effect* or a *floor effect*. **3** In pharmacology, the maximum dose of a drug that will produce the desired effect.

celeration Event frequency per unit of time, e.g. number of responses per minute per day. The term is mainly used in behavioural analyses.

cell 1 In biology, the structural unit of plants and animals. **2** In statistics, a compartment in an array or matrix.

cell assembly A hypothetical group of neurons in the brain assumed to become functionally interrelated and organized into a complex 'closed circuit' by repeated stimulation. Cell assemblies were the central component of the model of neural circuitry introduced by the Canadian psychologist Donald O. Hebb in an effort to account for particular perceptual phenomena. Hebb's theory was one of the first attempts to model the complexities of the brain and has been one of the more influential. The notion of a cell assembly is a central element in modern CONNECTIONISM (2) and in models of cortical function based on neural NETWORK MODELS (2).

cell body The integral 'life support' component of a neuron. The cell body (or *soma*) contains the nucleus and other sup-porting structures. If it is damaged the whole neuron dies.

cellular Pertaining to, derived from or composed of cells.

cen(o)- *Common, frequent.* var., *coen(o)-*.

cenogamy A rarely practised form of marriage whereby two or more men and two or more women unite into a single marital unit. Also called *group marriage*.

censor CENSORSHIP.

censorship 1 In psychoanalytic theory, the joint functioning of the ego and superego to accept or reject ideas, impulses, wishes, etc. emanating from the unconscious. The term *censor* was first applied by Freud in his early writings to the hypothetical agency that distorted dreams and controlled repression. As the theory evolved, the notion of the censor became the basis for the development of the notion of the superego. For this reason *censor* has typically been used to stand for some hypothetical entity, while *censorship* has referred to a set of operations. Whether the entity which carries out these functions is actually called the *censor* depends on who is doing the writing and when. **2** Any arbitrary regulation of the publishing, communicating or promulgating of information and ideas.

cent A unit of pitch defined as $\frac{1}{1200}$ of an octave.

center CENTRE.

centesis Puncturing of a cavity.

centi- Prefix denoting one hundredth ($\frac{1}{100}$).

centile 1 Any one of the points on a ranked distribution of scores each of which contains one hundredth of the scores. Thus a centile rank of 55 means that the score representing the rank is higher than 55% of all the scores in the distribution. Note that this is equivalent in meaning to *percentile*. **2** Less commonly, one of the 100 classes that makes up a population. To appreciate the difference between meanings 1 and 2, note that it makes no sense in the context of 1 to refer to a centile rank of 100 since such a score would have to be higher than all the scores, including itself. But it does make sense to refer to a centile rank of 100 in the context of 2 since this would mean the top classification of the distribution of scores.

central 1 Pertaining or referring to something in the middle, or in the main portion of a body or a structure. 2 Pertaining to some fundamental or important thing. Meaning 1 is generally contrasted with *peripheral* or *distal*, meaning 2 with *secondary* or *derivative*. The term occurs in a large number of combinatory forms, some of which are semantically obvious; others are given in the following entries.

central canal The narrow tube filled with cerebrospinal fluid that runs the length of the *spinal cord.*

central conflict In K. Horney's theory of personality, the psychic conflict between one's REAL *SELF and one's IDEALIZED *SELF.

central deafness CEREBRAL *DEAFNESS.

central dyslexia DYSLEXIA, CENTRAL.

central executive In Baddeley and Hitch's model of WORKING *MEMORY, the component that modulates and exercises control (see here EXECUTIVE FUNCTIONS) over the EPISODIC BUFFER, PHONOLGICAL LOOP and VISUO-SPATIAL SKETCHPAD.

central fissure (or **sulcus**) The fissure of the cerebral cortex that separates the motor cortex (the *precentral gyrus*) from the sensory cortex (the *postcentral gyrus*). The pre- and postcentral gyri mark the division between the frontal and parietal lobes of each hemisphere. Also called the *fissure of Rolando.*

central inhibition INHIBITION, CENTRAL.

centralism An old term for the point of view that behaviour can only be understood and explained through appeals to brain processes and brain function. Usually contrasted with another old term, PERIPHERALISM.

central-limit theorem In nonmathematical terms: as the size of any sample of scores becomes arbitrarily large, the sampling distribution of the mean approaches the normal distribution. This theorem gives an intuitive insight into why the normal distribution is so important in statistics, since any sample will eventually approach normality provided enough data are collected. The rate at which the normal distribution is approximated is surprisingly rapid for most of the populations that are investigated in psychology.

central nervous system (CNS) That component of the NERVOUS SYSTEM composed of the brain, the spinal cord and their associated neural processes.

central nucleus A nucleus in the amygdala, this receives sensory information from the primary sensory cortex, the association cortex and the thalamus. It projects fibres to the hypothalamus, midbrain, pons and medulla and is involved in coordinating the various components that make up the expression of emotional responses.

central route to persuasion ELABORATION LIKELIHOOD MODEL.

central tegmental tract A noradrenergic system that arises in the medulla and the pons of the brainstem and projects to the hypothalamus. Also called the *ventral noradrenergic bundle.*

central tendency The tendency for the scores in any distribution to cluster around some central point which then can be taken to represent the 'average' or most 'typical' score in the distribution. The three DESCRIPTIVE STATISTICS that are most commonly used as measures are the ARITHMETIC *MEAN, the MEDIAN and the MODE.

central trait theory Solomon Asch's view that the particular personality characteristics (or *traits*) that an individual displays are of special importance in how we view that person. Asch also argued that context plays an important role in determining how any particular trait is interpreted.

central vision VISION, CENTRAL.

centration (or **centring**) DECENTRATION.

centre 1 n. The midpoint of a body, organ or other structure. 2 n. A collection of nerve cells within the central nervous system that controls or mediates a particular process, activity or function. There are a large number of such structures: those that are germane to psychology are listed under the qualifying term. 3 vb. To focus on a particular aspect of a stimulus, to concentrate on a specific element or feature of something. See DECENTRATION. var., *center.*

centre clipping PEAK CLIPPING.

centrencephalic 1 Localized in a (relatively) precise area in the brain. 2 Located near or in the centre of the brain. Note, these two meanings are vaguely contradictory.

centre-surround receptive field A hypothesized RECEPTIVE FIELD whose signals are processed by a collecting ganglion cell or cortical neuron such that the neuron will respond only if the stimulation in the centre of the sensory field is different from that in the surrounding portion. For example, a 'centre-on/surround-off' cell will fire only if the centre of its field is stimulated while the outer area is not.

centroid method A factor-analysis technique in which the correlation matrix is represented mathematically on the surface of a sphere. The first axis of rotation is passed through the centre of the sphere, while the other axes are initially set at right angles to the first (i.e. they are orthogonal to or independent of it) but are then rotated to reveal the various factors.

cephalalgia Lit., pain in the head; a headache.

cephalic Pertaining to the head.

cephalic index First used in physical anthropology, this index is expressed as the ratio of the length of the head to its breadth x 100. Except in pathological cases the resulting nomenclature (*dolichocephalic* = long head, *mesocephalic* = moderate head, *brachycephalic* = short head) is without any real significance and without correlation with normal or abnormal behaviour. Note, if the measurements are taken on the bare skull the index is called *cranial* rather than cephalic.

cephal(o)- Combining form meaning *head*.

cephalocaudad (or -**al**) **development** The hypothesized principle that growth (especially embryological) and behaviour development follow a sequence that begins at the head and extends toward the tail end. Generally included in the hypothesis is *proximodistad* (or -*al*) development, which is the tendency for growth and behaviour development to proceed from the body toward the extremities.

CER (or **cer**) CONDITIONED EMOTIONAL RESPONSE.

cercal receptor A pressure-sensitive receptor on the abdomen of some insect species, often studied in research on the evolution of the nervous system. pl., *cerci*.

cerebellar Pertaining to the CEREBELLUM.

cerebellar gait A lurching, unsteady gait that resembles that of an inebriated person. It is associated with widespread cerebellar dysfunction although it is also seen in cases with localized lesions in the *vermis*.

cerebellar peduncles Three myelinated tracts that connect the cerebellum to the brainstem.

cerebellum The Latin diminutive form of CEREBRUM, thus, lit., little brain. The cerebellum is the primary structure in the hindbrain and is involved in muscle coordination and the maintenance of body equilibrium. The cerebellum is particularly important in initiating and controlling very rapid motor sequences of the limbs, movements that occur so fast that they cannot be modulated by sensory feedback. Classic examples in humans are hitting a baseball and returning a serve in tennis. Other species with rapid motor responses, such as birds and monkeys, have well-developed cerebellums.

cerebral Pertaining to the CEREBRUM. Used metaphorically and nontechnically for *intellectual, smart*.

cerebral aqueduct AQUEDUCT OF SYLVIUS.

cerebral blindness BLINDNESS, CEREBRAL.

cerebral commissure COMMISSURE.

cerebral cortex The surface covering of grey matter that forms the outermost layer of the CEREBRUM. In evolutionary terms it is the most recent neural development and its approximately 9 to 12 billion cells are responsible for primary sensory functions, motor coordination and control, mediating most of the integrative, coordinated behaviours, and, most important, the so-called 'higher mental processes' of language, thinking, problem-solving, etc.

cerebral dominance DOMINANCE, CEREBRAL.

cerebral hemispheres The two symmetrical (at least superficially – histologically they are known to be distinguishable in a variety of ways) hemispherical halves of the CEREBRUM.

cerebration 1 Neurological action of the cerebrum. 2 Metaphorically, thinking.

cerebrocerebellum NEOCEREBELLUM.

cerebrospinal fluid Lymph-like fluid filling the ventricles of the brain, the central canal of the spinal cord and all other areas in the skull and spinal canal not given over to solid tissues and blood vessels. Its functions are not completely understood. It clearly has a role in cushioning the brain against injury from shocks, it assists in transport of nutrients and appears to play a role in homeostasis and metabolism of cells in the central nervous system.

cerebrotonia One of the three classic components of temperament assumed within CONSTITUTIONAL THEORY (see that entry for details).

cerebrovascular accident STROKE (2).

cerebrum The largest and most prominent structure of the brain. It consists of two hemispheres separated by the longitudinal fissure, below which are the three cerebral commissures connecting the two halves. The inner core is composed of white matter made up of myelinated fibres and the grey basal ganglia; the outer covering (the cerebral cortex) is made up entirely of grey matter. The human cerebrum consists of perhaps 15 billion cells and is the latest brain structure to have evolved. It is involved in processing and interpretation of sensory inputs, control over voluntary motor activity, consciousness, planning and executing of action, thinking, ideating, language, reasoning, judging and the like; in short, all of those functions most closely associated with the so-called 'higher mental functions'.

ceremony A socially or culturally dictated sequence of acts with symbolic significance as defined by a culture's traditions. A ceremony is generally considered a somewhat larger and more elaborate event than a RITUAL; in fact, ceremonies are said by some to be composed of several rituals.

certifiable A forensic (legal) term for someone who, in the opinion of medical or psychological experts, is in need of some form of treatment, guardianship or institutionalization. See also SECTIONED.

ceruminous deafness DEAFNESS, CERUMINOUS.

cerveau isolé ENCÉPHALE ISOLÉ.

cervix The neck of any organ or body part, particularly of the womb. adj., *cervical*.

ceteris paribus Latin for 'other things being equal'.

C fibres FREE NERVE ENDINGS.

CFF (or cff) CRITICAL FLICKER FREQUENCY.

CFS CHRONIC FATIGUE SYNDROME.

CFT COMPLEX FIGURE TEST.

chained schedule SCHEDULES OF *REINFORCEMENT.

chaining (or chained responses) General terms referring to the linking together of a sequence of behaviours. The initial response in a chain provides a set of cues which becomes associated with and thus elicits the next response, and so on, such that the full sequence is 'chained off'.

challenge In *psychopharmacology*, to administer a therapeutic dose of a drug to observe its effects. For example, the expression 'scopolamine-challenged subjects' refers to subjects given a moderate-to-high dose of scopolamine.

challenged A loose designation of an individual with any of a variety of disorders, disabilities or dysfunctions. Originally a nontechnical term, it is wending its way into the formal literature, as in phrases like 'arithmetically challenged' for someone with *dyscalculia*.

chance A term that must be used carefully. It has at least two distinct meanings: 1 An event occurring within a given system that is caused by factors lying outside of that system. Thus, in any psychological experiment, some data will be due to manipulations of the independent variables and some will be 'due to chance'. This does not mean that these are random data but merely data for which the causes lie outside of the experiment. Similarly, it may be 'chance' that a tree fell on your car and not somebody else's but this does not eliminate causal factors. **2** An event that is random in nature and determinable or describable by the use of probability theory. Even in this sense events are not regarded as wholly causeless but merely as caused by multitudinous independent and interdependent factors that are essentially unknowable; e.g. the sequence of heads and tails in successive coin flips or the exact position of any gas molecule in a large room. Lay language often confuses chance with 'accident' or 'luck'. Such usages are popular but strictly nontechnical.

chance differences In statistical analyses, any differences due to random factors. Contrast with CONSTANT *ERROR and with BIAS.

chance error ERROR, CHANCE.

chance-half correlation CORRELATION, SPLIT-HALF.

chance variation In genetics, a variation that has no clearly identifiable antecedents. Darwin made this concept a central assumption in the process of evolution by natural selection.

chancroid A venereal disease characterized by the eruption of a sensitive, inflamed ulcer in the genital area. The infection may spread to the lymph nodes, penis (or vulva) or anus but is localized in these areas. Treatment is usually with antibiotics.

change blindness The failure to notice a change in a scene. The effect is easily elicited by presenting two successive photographs with a change in the second; e.g. three people wearing hats are in the first photo but in the second, one of them has removed her hat. The change is rarely noticed. The implication is that to perceive something it is not enough to simply 'look' at it, we must also attend to it. See also CHOICE BLINDNESS, INATTENTIONAL BLINDNESS.

change of life Nontechnical term for MENOPAUSE.

change-over delay (COD) A SCHEDULE OF *REINFORCEMENT used with concurrent operants which allows a response to be reinforced only after a certain amount of time has elapsed since the last change-over from the other response.

channel As borrowed from *information the-*

ory, a complete system for transmitting a signal, from its input phase to its final output phase. The channel generally operates on the basis of some code or language which relates the input and output in systematic ways. The term has become popular in psychology because it is possible to view an organism as a channel, its receptors being the locus for the input and its responses the locus for the output. Further, any subsystem of an organism, such as its visual system or a memory system, may be similarly viewed.

channel capacity The maximum amount of information (measured in *bits*) that any channel can carry.

chaos theory A theory imported from the mathematics of nonlinear systems that some have attempted to apply to the behaviour of complex systems such as the weather and human beings. One of the mathematical approaches used in DYNAMICAL SYSTEMS (THEORY).

character 1 The original Latin meaning was an inscription or marking which differentiated some one thing from others for identification purposes. Although this meaning is still appropriate, the preferred synonyms here are *trait* or *characteristic*. As the psychological use of the term evolved it came to mean: **2** The sum total or integration of all such markings (traits) to yield a unified whole which reveals the nature (the 'character') of a situation, event or person. Freudian theory further emphasized this use by the introduction of terms like *anal character*. Today it is much more common to find the term PERSONALITY (especially 3) used with essentially this meaning.

character analysis 1 Wilhelm Reich's term for his form of psychoanalysis. Unlike the classical Freudian approach, Reich focused less on specific symptoms and more on character or personality. The analysis itself was based on dealing with the client's CHARACTER DEFENCES. **2** An occasional synonym for DIDACTIC *ANALYSIS.

character armour W. Reich's term for an individual's system of defences.

character defence Generally, any personality trait that functions primarily to fulfil some unconscious defensive purpose.

character disorder Lit. and loosely, a disorder of CHARACTER (2). The term was used originally in reference to individuals who displayed pathological vacillation. Today, it serves as a general label for persons who chronically and habitually engage in maladaptive behaviours, who are inflexible, restrict their own opportunities for growth and usually manage to function in ways that evoke unpleasant reactions from those around them.

characteristic Some individualistic feature, attribute, etc. that serves to identify and 'characterize' something. Generally used synonymously with TRAIT in discussion of personality.

characteristic feature DISTINCTIVE FEATURE (3).

character neurosis K. Horney's term for any long-standing neurotic syndrome manifested first in childhood.

characterology Obsolete term for: **1** The general study of personality. **2** The study of personality through physical characteristics; see here CONSTITUTIONAL THEORY. Note, however, that constitutional theory, although lacking in validity and power, was a theory in what was at least a respectable science; characterology, on the other hand, was a pseudoscience which focused on irrelevant features such as hair colour, complexion, nose shape and cranial configuration.

character trait In most usages this term is an unnecessary redundancy: *trait* alone will suffice. However, psychoanalysts occasionally use the full term to refer to behavioural tendencies which are inherited (or at least presumed to be).

charismatic authority AUTHORITY, CHARISMATIC.

Charpentier's bands FECHNER'S COLOURS.

Charpentier's illusion Any of several different illusions studied by the French physician Augustin Charpentier. One involves misestimating weights (SIZE–WEIGHT ILLUSION), another the illusory movement of stationary lights (AUTOKINETIC EFFECT), and a third the illusion that held objects are relatively smaller (or larger) than they actually are following the squeezing of standard sized objects.

Charpentier's law A descriptive generalization that holds for visual stimuli at THRESHOLD projected on the fovea: $aI = k$, where a is the area of the image, I is the intensity of the stimulus and k is a constant.

chatterbox effect COCKTAIL PARTY SYNDROME.

cheese effect A potentially serious side effect of MONOAMINE OXIDASE INHIBITORS. Foods such as cheese, yogurt, wine and some nuts and fruits containing pressor amines can cause sympathetic reactions in patients taking these drugs, leading to dangerously high blood pressure levels and heart rates.

chemesthesis The faculty for sensing chemical solutions other than through taste and smell. Receptors are widely distributed, occurring primarily in the exposed moist surfaces of the mouth, throat, nose and eyes. The sense is subtly linked with the perception of pain and how separate they are is still an open question. Distinguish from CHEMICAL SENSE(S). Also called *common chemical sense*.

chemical antagonism DRUG *ANTAGONISM.

chemical castration See HORMONAL *CASTRATION.

chemical cosh UK slang term for the use of drugs for control purposes in total institutions to pacify or restrain violent or uncooperative detainees, with or without their consent.

chemical sense(s) Those sensory systems responsive to chemical stimuli; namely, SMELL (or olfaction) and TASTE (or GUSTATION). Distinguish from CHEMESTHESIS.

chemical transmission Generally, the transmission of information between neurons. The four kinds of chemical involved, NEUROTRANSMITTERS, NEUROMODULATORS, HORMONES and PHEROMONES, are used to control the behaviour of individual cells, whole organs or entire organisms. The first three operate within an organism, the last between organisms.

chemo- Combining form meaning *pertaining to chemicals* or *chemical action*.

chemoreceptor Those sense organs responsive to chemical action. Differentiate from *chemical sense*, which refers to the whole modality, while chemoreceptors are the actual receptors such as the taste buds.

chemotherapy **1** In medicine generally, any technique based on drugs or chemicals, as in the treatment of cancer. **2** In psychotherapy, DRUG THERAPY.

cherry picking Lab slang for selecting only particular findings to report from a large data base. It is occasionally done semi-legitimately to isolate particular findings for further analysis. More often it is just another way to lie with statistics. See DATA SNOOPING, a similar statistical gambit that lends itself to both use and abuse.

chi (χ) A Greek letter used in many formulas and statistical tests. See CHI-SQUARE.

Chicago school FUNCTIONALISM (2).

chicken game A variation of the PRISONER'S *DILEMMA game, in which mutual selection of the competitive response produces the most severe penalty (or lowest reward) for both players.

child A person between either **1** birth and maturity, **2** birth and puberty or, according to some, **3** infancy and puberty. The last is preferred; see CHILDHOOD.

child abuse Generally, any form of physical or psychological mistreatment of a child by parents or guardians. The most common form involves severe and repeated physical injury (contusions, broken bones), although many will also consider as abuse other forms of mistreatment such as starvation, locking the child away in attics or closets, burning with cigarettes or other hot objects, sexual assault (see SEXUAL ABUSE) and emotional and psychological degradation. See CHILD NEGLECT for a distinction.

child analysis Psychoanalysis of a child.

child development A subdiscipline within the field of CHILD PSYCHOLOGY. The key word is *development*; it denotes that the focus is on aspects of physiology, cognition and behaviour that show qualitative and quantitative change as a child passes from birth to maturity. Some use the term to reflect an emphasis on growth and maturation and a concomitant de-emphasis on learning. This bias is not universally shared and most use it to cover maturation, learning and the critical inter-actions between them. See also DEVELOPMENTAL PSYCHOLOGY.

child-directed speech The speech of adults to young children. Such speech is different from adult-to-adult speech in important ways. Utterances are shorter, less syntactically complex, contain very few fragmentary or ungrammatical sentences and have sharply restricted lexical selections. Interestingly, older children also use it when talking to the very young. The term is not used for the sing-song style of speaking used with infants, pets or other cute creatures. Also called MOTHERESE, although see that entry for reasons why this is not recommended.

child-guidance clinic CLINIC, CHILD-GUIDANCE.

childhood **1** n. Usually, the period between infancy and adolescence. See CHILD. **2** adj. Pertaining to this period. Used frequently in psychiatry and clinical psychology to characterize the form of a disorder observed in children, e.g. CHILDHOOD *SCHIZOPHRENIA.

childhood disintegrative disorder A serious disorder of childhood in which there is apparently normal development for at least the first 2 years of life, followed by significant loss of previously acquired skills in such areas as language, social skills, bowel or bladder control and sensorimotor coordination. There are problems differentiating this disorder from AUTISM, although it appears to have a worse prognosis. Also known as *Heller's syndrome, dementia infantilis* and *disintegrative psychosis*.

childhood, disorders of A commonly found shorthand expression for the full, formal, psychiatric diagnostic category *disorders first evident in infancy, childhood or adolescence*. The category includes a number of disorders of particular kinds, as follows: (a) disorders found at other points in the life of a person, such as *schizophrenia* and *affective disorders*, but which are given special designation as *childhood disorders* when they are first detected prior to adulthood being reached; (b) PERSONALITY DISORDERS, when they are diagnosed prior to age 18; and (c) a number of other disorders that typically emerge during infancy, childhood and adolescence, such as MENTAL RETARDATION, CONDUCT DISORDER, some

EATING DISORDERS and the DEVELOPMENTAL DISORDERS (*pervasive* and *specific*). See each of these for details.

childhood schizophrenia SCHIZOPHRENIA, CHILDHOOD.

child neglect Maltreatment of children that takes the form of omitting actions normally associated with optimal development. Examples are improper attention to health, clothing, education and emotional caring and support. The term is generally not extended to cases in which poverty or other environmental factors make provision of such actions impossible. Distinguish from CHILD ABUSE.

child psychology Generally taken as the most neutral umbrella term for the interdisciplinary science that studies the child in any of a large number of systematic ways. The actual approach taken by any given child psychologist may differ dramatically from that taken by another. It may be focused either on the normal and adaptive or on the abnormal and pathological; it may be applied or pure in its orientation; it may be concerned with motivation and emotion, with socialization, cognition, learning, or, indeed, any of the processes of psychology generally. The field is actually defined and delimited simply by the articulation of age boundaries: any processes observed occurring within the range from infancy to adolescence are 'fair game'. See also CHILD DEVELOPMENT and DEVELOPMENTAL PSYCHOLOGY.

Children's Apperception Test (CAT) A variation on the THEMATIC APPERCEPTION TEST (TAT) designed for use with children.

children's culture KIDS' CULTURE.

chimera 1 In genetics, an individual possessing two (or more) cell types resulting from an *in utero* fusion of two distinct zygotes. **2** Any organism composed of tissues from more than one organism of different species. **3** A mythological creature, a monster made up of the parts of several animals. **4** In perception, a compound stimulus created by combining elements from a variety of different images. Chimeric faces are used in a variety of research settings. **5** By extension, a foolish fantasy.

Chinese Room This term designates a thought experiment developed by John Searle. In this mythical room sits a person – let's call her Maxine – who knows no Chinese but is equipped with a set of complex instructions that tell her how to manipulate Chinese characters from one form into another. On a regular basis a set of Chinese characters appears in her 'in-box'. Maxine obediently consults her instructions, which tell her how to produce particular sequences of Chinese characters to each of the inputs. She then sends these new sequences back through the 'out' slot. If the instructions Maxine is working with follow the rules of syntax of Chinese, from the point of view of a native Chinese speaker outside the room she will appear to know Chinese perfectly. But, of course, she doesn't. Nor does Maxine plus her instructions equal understanding. In fact, there is no understanding anywhere in the room. It is Searle's point that although the Chinese Room appears to satisfy TURING'S TEST, it actually fails to truly represent human intelligence. Searle maintains that this is a compelling argument against the possibility of *strong AI*. Others, of course, are not so convinced. See ARTIFICIAL INTELLIGENCE.

chir(o)- Combining form meaning *hand*.

chi-square (χ^2) A statistical test of differences between independent samples using frequency data, or between a sample and some set of expected scores. The test is based on differences between observations and expectations: $\chi^2 = \Sigma(O_i - E_i)^2/E_i$, where O_i represents each of i observed scores and E_i each of i expected scores. There are actually a number of different chi-square tests, although all are based on the same general principle; for example, by using a theoretical model to determine the expected scores the test becomes a test of GOODNESS OF FIT. See also CHI-SQUARE *DISTRIBUTION.

chloral hydrate A nonbarbiturate SEDATIVE first synthesized in the 1830s. It was the first sleep aid developed and, while it produces fewer disruptions of sleep patterns than other compounds (particularly the BARBITURATES), its toxicity has limited its use.

chlordiazepoxide A commonly prescribed ANTIANXIETY DRUG of the BENZODIAZEPINE class. Trade name Librium.

chlorpromazine A PHENOTHIAZINE, it was

first used to reduce presurgical anxiety before its ANTIPSYCHOTIC properties were discovered in the 1950s. Within a few years it revolutionized treatment of schizophrenia and acute mania and ushered in the era of psychopharmacological approaches to psychiatric disorders. It is rarely used today because of a host of side effects including EXTRAPYRDAMIDAL SYNDROME and TARDIVE DYSKINESIA.

chlorprothixene A THIOXANTHENE used in the treatment of schizophrenia.

choice blindness A failure to notice that a stimulus chosen earlier is, in fact, not the one that is currently before them. It is surprisingly easy to demonstrate. An individual is asked to select a person they would prefer to work with from photos of two people, say one with blond hair and one with brown. Later they are presented with the other photo as their new co-worker. Surprisingly often they fail to realize that this is not the person originally chosen. See also CHANGE BLINDNESS, INATTENTIONAL BLINDNESS.

choice experiment A general label used for any of a number of basic experimental designs in which the subject is required to select one among two or more responses depending on which one of two or more stimuli was presented. The subject may be working under a *time set*, in which the response must be made as quickly as possible, or under an *accuracy set*, for which speed is relatively unimportant. See also REACTION TIME and the various forms of that term.

choice point 1 Generally, any set of circumstances in which a choice among several alternatives is required. **2** Specifically, the physical point in a maze where the subject may take any one of two or more paths.

choice reaction CHOICE EXPERIMENT.

choice reaction time REACTION TIME, CHOICE.

choice shift A general term covering the various kinds of changes in the choices made by a group of persons when compared with the average or typical sentiments about the choices of the separate individuals. In some conditions a *risky shift* is observed, when the group decides to choose a more radical, riskier course of action than the individuals, taken separately, would have selected; in others a *cautious shift* is seen,

when the group takes a more conservative stance than separate individuals favour.

choking A tendency for an athlete to perform poorly when pressure is increased, as at a critical juncture in a game. Originally a slang term, it has been adopted in the technical literature. Factors that play a role are attentional focus (concentrating on one's body and actual physical movement is usually counterproductive) and emotional tone (high levels of anxiety do not bode well).

cholecystokinin A hormone found in the intestines and in the brain that has been implicated in the control of eating behaviour. High concentrations suppress eating.

choleric Irritable, touchy, easily angered.

choline An amine widely distributed in bodily tissue. It is an essential component in normal fat and carbohydrate metabolism. It is a precursor of ACETYLCHOLINE (ACh); derived from the breakdown of fats it is taken into neurons, where, in the presence of choline acetylase, ACh is produced.

cholinergic Of neurons and neural pathways which, when stimulated, release ACETYLCHOLINE, or for which acetylcholine is the transmitter substance.

cholinesterase Generally, any enzyme that functions by breaking down choline esters; see e.g. ACETYLCHOLINESTERASE.

cholinesterase inhibitors A class of drugs that block the action of CHOLINESTERASE and thereby increase the amount of choline esters such as ACETYLCHOLINE in the brain. Recent evidence suggests that they can slow the progression of cognitive dementias such as those seen in ALZHEIMER'S DISEASE.

Chomskyan Pertaining to or characteristic of the theories of linguist, philosopher and political commentator, Noam Chomsky (b. 1928). For more detail on his highly influential approach to psycholinguistics, see LAD and TRANSFORMATIONAL *GRAMMAR. vars., *Chomskian, Chomskean.*

chorda tympani A group of afferent fibres that carries part of the neural input from the taste receptors in the tongue. It is part of the VIIth cranial nerve.

chorea Any neurological disorder marked by muscular twitching and jerky, involuntary movements, particularly of the arms, legs, trunk, neck and face, e.g. Huntington's chorea, Sydenham's chorea. Interestingly, choreic movements, like those in other involuntary movement disorders, subside during sleep.

choreiform movement Nonrepetitive, dance-like movements with a random, irregular quality.

choreoathetosis Combination of CHOREA (usually of the trunk and limbs) and ATHETO-SIS (usually of the face, tongue and hands), seen in cerebral palsy and Huntington's disease.

choroid coat (or **membrane**) A delicate pigmented coat of tissue that surrounds the eye (except, naturally, in the front, where the cornea admits light). It backs the retina, protecting it from stray, reflected light.

chrom(a)- Combining form meaning *colour*. var., *chrom(o)-*.

chroma 1 In the Munsell colour system, the dimension that corresponds with *saturation*, the 'purity' of a colour. 2 The quality of any visual stimulus that differentiates it from grey.

chromaesthesia 1 Generally and literally, a form of SYNAESTHESIA in which nonvisual stimuli produce the experience of colour sensations. 2 More specifically, the experiencing of colour with auditory stimuli. Meaning 2 is usually intended, hence *coloured hearing* and *coloured audition* are used as synonyms. var., *chromesthesia*.

chromatic adj. Referring to the hue and saturation dimensions of visual stimuli as opposed to the black–white (or *achromatic*) dimension.

chromatic aberration ABERRATION, CHROMATIC.

chromatic adaptation 1 A decrease in sensitivity to a colour stimulus with prolonged exposure. Under conditions of optimal fixation (e.g. the *fixed image* technique) saturation decreases until only a neutral grey is left. 2 Modification in the perceived hue and/or saturation of a light stimulus resulting from prior viewing of a light of different hue and/or saturation.

chromatic audition AUDITION, CHROMATIC.

chromatic colour Since *colour* is used in reference to the whole visual spectrum, including the black–white (or *achromatic*) dimension, this term is used for specific reference to the other two dimensions – hue and saturation – of a visual stimulus. A chromatic colour is one which cannot be placed in the black–grey–white series.

chromatic contrast COLOUR CONTRAST.

chromatic dimming When the brightness of a fixated chromatic stimulus is abruptly lessened the observer experiences dramatic decrease (or 'dimming') in saturation, so much so that occasionally the complementary colour momentarily appears.

chromatic induction INDUCED COLOUR.

chromaticity The aspect of a colour stimulus given by its dominant wavelength (hue) and its purity (saturation) taken together. Also called *chromaticness*.

chromaticness CHROMATICITY.

chromatic valence A relative measure of the hue-producing effectiveness of a chromatic stimulus. When two such stimuli are mixed so that the result is perceived as grey, they are, by definition, equal in their chromatic valence.

chromatin A mix of nucleic acids (including DNA) and protein found in chromosomes and cell nuclei. The name comes from the fact that it stains with appropriate dyes. The term *chromatin positive* refers to the presence of *sex chromatin* (see BARR BODIES) which marks the cell as from a female, and *chromatic negative* which refers to its absence and means the cell is from a male.

chromatopsia An abnormal condition in which a chromatic quality is 'added' to stimuli. Achromatic (colourless) objects are seen as having colour and everything coloured has additional tint to it. It results from taking certain drugs and may occur following exposure to intense visual stimulation. Also called *chromopsia*.

chrom(o)- CHROMA-.

chromopsia CHROMATOPSIA.

chromosomal aberrations Variations in either the number of chromosomes or the location of genetic material on chromosomes. See CHROMOSOMAL ALTERATIONS and CHROMOSOMAL ANOMALIES.

chromosomal alterations Processes by which rearrangements among chromosomes occur. Three well-documented processes are: *inversion*, in which the bands within a particular chromosome become rearranged; *translocation*, in which two chromosomes fuse; and *reciprocal translocation*, in which there is an exchange of a DNA segment between two chromosomes. Such alterations are assumed to play a role in evolution.

chromosomal anomalies Anomalies or abnormalities involving either loss of one chromosome or the addition of one or more. A number of specific abnormalities are known to occur with some frequency; see e.g. FRAGILE X SYNDROME for an instance of a weak chromosome, TURNER'S (or 45, X) SYNDROME for an instance of a missing sex chromosome, and KLINEFELTER'S (or 47, XXY) SYNDROME and DOWN SYNDROME (trisomy 21) for instances of an additional chromosome.

chromosome A microscopic body in the nucleus of a cell which is conspicuous during mitosis. The term literally means *coloured body* and chromosomes were so named because they stain deeply with basic dyes. Chromosomes carry genes, the basic hereditary units. Each species has a constant, normal number of chromosomes. There are 46 in human somatic cells, arranged in 23 pairs; the ovum and sperm contain 23 each, one from each pair. Of this 23, 22 are the *autosomes* and 1 is the sex chromosome (either X or Y). In fertilization the 23 chromosomes from the male unite with the 23 from the female. The X chromosome is the 'female determining' chromosome, the Y the 'male determining'. Normal female somatic cells are XX, normal male are XY; normal female ova are X, normal male sperm either X or Y. An XX embryo will be female, an XY male.

chronaxie A value that expresses the sensitivity of a nerve to stimulation. It is measured by first determining the threshold of the nerve, the amount of direct current which if applied indefinitely would just excite it. This value is then doubled and the amount of time this current must be applied before the nerve responds is the chronaxie. var., *chronaxia*.

chronic Generally, long-term, drawn out, extending over a long period of time. Thus, a chronic disease is one in which the symptoms are long-lasting, a chronic experiment one carried out over an extended period of time. Compare with ACUTE (3 and 4).

chronic affective disorder CYCLOTHYMIC DISORDER and DYSTHYMIC DISORDER.

chronic brain disorder (or **syndrome**) Any disorder resulting from extensive, long-lasting brain damage such as those caused by syphilis, brain tumours, strokes, drugs, etc. The most common are those due to alcohol abuse and Alzheimer's disease.

chronic (drug) tolerance TOLERANCE, CHRONIC.

chronic fatigue syndrome (CFS) A syndrome characterized by tiredness that is unrelated to exertion and unrelieved by rest. Memory deficits and other cognitive problems are often cited as other symptoms. While some regard CFS as a well-defined, identifiable disorder, there is certainly nothing close to unanimity. For example, some claim that many cases are misdiagnoses of Guillain–Barré syndrome, an autoimmune disease marked by peripheral demyelination, while others cite fibromyalgia syndrome as the true underlying problem. Both of these disorders have symptoms that overlap with those of CFS. Others maintain that it is not a distinct disorder at all but a diffuse psychopathological condition linked with depression and perhaps elements of a social phobia. Given the lack of agreement, the term should be used with great care, if at all.

chronic pain PAIN, CHRONIC.

chronic preparation PREPARATION, CHRONIC.

chronic progressive encephalopathy of boxers DEMENTIA PUGILISTICA.

chronic tic disorder TIC DISORDERS.

chronic undifferentiated schizophrenia CHRONIC *SCHIZOPHRENIA.

chron(o)- Combining form meaning *time*.

chronobiology A cover term for the study of biological rhythms, biological clocks, circadian rhythms, etc.; in short, any regular pattern of behaviour that displays periodicity falls within the scope of this hybrid science. Some use BIORHYTHMS synonymously, but see that term for details.

chronograph Any device that records and presents graphic records of time intervals.

chronological age AGE, CHRONOLOGICAL.

chronometric Lit., of time measurement. A term most often used to characterize the time course of cognitive operations. For example, continuously increasing the complexity of a task along a known dimension will systematically increase the time it takes subjects to perform the task, yielding a chronometric analysis of the processes involved. For an example of how this technique is used see SUBTRACTION METHOD.

chronometrics, mental The measurement of the real time for the carrying-out of mental processes. See CHRONOMETRIC.

chronoscope Any device for measuring time intervals.

chronotaraxis Inability to identify the time, the day of the week or, in severe cases, even the season of the year.

chunking A term first suggested by George A. Miller for the organization process whereby distinct 'bits' of information are collected together perceptually and cognitively into larger, coordinated wholes, or 'chunks'.

-cide Suffix meaning *killer* or *act of killing*.

cilia 1 Eyelashes. 2 Hairlike processes projecting from the surface of various cells (e.g. in the bronchi). sing., *cilium*.

ciliary muscle The smooth muscle that controls ACCOMMODATION (2). It is attached to the lens of the eye so that when it contracts the lens is thickened and when it relaxes the lens is flattened, for close-up and distant vision respectively.

cingulate cortex The outer layer of the CINGULATE GYRUS.

cingulate gyrus The cortical part of the limbic system that lies along the lateral walls of the groove that separates the two cerebral hemispheres and just above the *corpus callosum*. It has been shown to be involved in emotional behaviour, in hoarding and in the acquisition and retention of avoidance responses.

cingulotomy A form of PSYCHOSURGERY in which fibres in the CINGULUM BUNDLE and overlying cingulate cortex are destroyed. It is used primarily with intractable cases of obsessive-compulsive disorder and, on occasion, for patients with chronic pain syndromes or refractory depression.

cingulum bundle A group of axons that connects the cingulate and prefrontal cortex with the limbic cortex of the temporal lobe. Cutting this bundle has been used as a psychosurgical technique in severe cases of *obsessive-compulsive disorder*.

circadian From the Latin *circa* meaning *about* and *dies* meaning *day*, pertaining to the 24-hour day.

circadian hour CIRCADIAN TIME.

circadian peak and trough The points during the 24-hour cycle when body temperature hits its high (peak) and low (trough). Although there are large individual differences, most people's troughs occur at around 4–6 pm and 4 am. Their peaks are usually around 8–10 am and pm.

circadian rhythm *Circadian* comes from the Latin *circa*, meaning *about*, and *dies*, meaning *day*. Hence, rhythms with an approximately 24-hour cycle are called circadian. Any rhythm with an approximately 24-hour cycle.

circadian rhythm sleep disorder SLEEP-WAKE SCHEDULE DISORDER.

circadian time Time as marked by the period of a full circadian cycle in an organism that is allowed to 'free run' (that is, the organism is maintained in a constant environment without the normal day/night or light/dark cycle). The standard model maintains that in most species the cycle will drift from the 24-hour day to one of roughly 25 hours, although recent evidence suggests this might not be as universal an effect as once thought. Nevertheless, in the technical literature circadian time is based on a 25-hour day and a *circadian hour* is one of roughly 62.5 minutes.

circuit, reverberating REVERBERATING CIR-CUIT and CELL ASSEMBLY.

circular behaviour Generally, behaviour which stimulates like behaviour. Laughter in one person stimulates laughter in another which further increases laughter in the first. The terms *circular response* and *circular reaction* are used as synonyms by many but see CIRCULAR REACTION for a special meaning in Piagetian theory.

circular reaction 1 CIRCULAR BEHAVIOUR. **2** In Piagetian theory, an action that can be repeated, e.g. grasping. Piaget assumed that circular reactions are important for making adaptations during the sensorimotor stage. He differentiated *primary* circular reactions from *secondary* and *tertiary*; the primary are derived from reflexes and are centred on the infant's own body, the secondary involve repetitive manipulation of objects, and the tertiary are characterized by repetition with variations that reflect adaptations to different objects, for example picking up a pencil one time and a ball the next.

circular reasoning Empty reasoning in which the conclusion rests on an assumption the validity of which is dependent on the conclusion. The apocryphal story of the instinct theorist is illustrative: when asked why all the sheep in an open field clustered together he replied, 'Because all sheep have a gregarious instinct.' When pressed as to how he knew they had this instinct he answered, 'It's obvious, just look at them all clustered together in that open field.' The futility of this kind of reasoning is in direct proportion to the amount of energy invested in it.

circum- Combining form meaning *around*.

circumlocution Literally, *talking around something*. A manner of speaking in which particular topics or subjects are not specifically mentioned, but are 'talked around'. It is often found in patients with ANOMIAS who are compensating for an inability to recall specific words and, non-clinically, in politicians.

circumplex A circular chart that represents elements or variables in relationship to one another. Those that are arrayed directly across the circle are negatively related to one another; those adjacent to one another are strongly related, and those set at right angles to each other are unrelated.

circumstantiality A psychiatric term for a manner of speaking that is inappropriately indirect and 'circular'. The speaker tends to talk all around the real topic and delays excessively in dealing with the things under discussion. Compare with TANGENTIALITY.

circumstriate cortex PRESTRIATE CORTEX.

circumvallate papilla LINGUAL PAPILLA.

circumventrical system A group of structures around the third ventricle (hence the name) that is suspected of being the area where osmometric and volumetric signals (see THIRST et seq.) are integrated. Drinking, salt intake and the secretion of VASOPRESSIN are thought to be controlled here.

CIS bias COLLECTIVE INFORMATION SAMPLING BIAS.

11-cis retinal RHODOPSIN.

citalopram A SELECTIVE SEROTONIN REUPTAKE INHIBITOR used as an ANTIDEPRESSANT DRUG. Trade name Celexa.

civilian catastrophe reaction A situational personality disorder brought about by the extreme stress of a major disaster such as an earthquake, a plane crash or a flood. See here GROSS *STRESS REACTION. The symptoms include helplessness, regression and partial amnesia, and are similar to those seen in POST-TRAUMATIC STRESS DISORDER.

CL (and **CLalt**) COMPARISON LEVEL.

clairaudience The hypothesized extrasensory perception of a distant sound. See PARAPSYCHOLOGY.

clairvoyance The hypothesized extrasensory perception of a distant object or event. See PARAPSYCHOLOGY.

clan SIB (2).

clang association An association in a verbal task in which two words or other stimulus items become linked because of acoustic similarity.

clarification A technique used in nondirected therapy whereby the therapist provides a summary of what the client says, focusing on and clarifying its meaning.

class There are several specialized uses of this term; all carry the basic notion that a class is a grouping, an aggregate or a category of some kind. **1** In logic, any category of things or events which share common properties or features that can serve as distinctions segregating those things or events from others. **2** In sociology, a synonym for SOCIAL CLASS. **3** In education, a group of students taught together as a unit. **4** In statistics, any of the divisions resulting from a subdividing of a ranked distribution of scores.

class-free test CULTURE-FREE TEST.

classical An adjective which, when applied to a theory, method or point of view, carries the implication that the theory, etc. (a) set the standards for the field and formed the basis for later developments and elaborations, and/or (b) is a bit antiquated and probably wrong.

classical conditioning 1 An experimental procedure in which a CONDITIONED STIMULUS (CS) that is, at the outset, neutral with respect to the *unconditioned response* (UR) is paired with an *unconditioned stimulus* (US) that reliably elicits the unconditioned response. After a number of such pairings the CS will elicit, by itself, a *conditioned response* (CR) very much like UR. In Pavlov's classic experiments the neutral CS was a bell, which was paired with a food US that reliably produced a UR (salivation). After some trials the bell itself was sufficient to produce a flow of saliva, the conditioned response. **2** The learning that takes place in this type of experimental procedure. Perhaps the best way to think of classical conditioning is that it is a set of circumstances under which responses of an organism established by natural selection come under the control of a new stimulus – provided this new stimulus (the CS) has some predictive value for the occurrence of the US. See here RESCORLA-WAGNER THEORY. See also INSTRUMENTAL CONDITIONING, LEARNING, OPERANT CONDITIONING and related entries.

classical psychoanalysis CLASSICAL THEORY.

classical theory Within psychoanalysis, since there have been so many variations of psychoanalytic theory developed over the years, this term has come to stand for the 'pure' form of the theory as put forward by Freud and developed by his disciples without major modification of the basic theoretical framework. Also referred to as *classical psychoanalysis*. See here FREUDIAN.

classification 1 The process of categorizing things or events into mutually exclusive classes. **2** The result of such a process.

Classification of Mental and Behavioural Disorders (CMBD) The section of the World Health Organization's INTERNATIONAL CLASSIFICATION OF DISEASES that deals with the nosology of mental disorders. See also DIAGNOSTIC AND STATISTICAL MANUAL for the system approved by the American Psychiatric Association.

classification test 1 Generally, any test in which the subject is requested to sort the stimulus materials into classes. **2** Specifically, a test designed to facilitate the process of classifying persons for some reason, e.g. for putting them into particular instructional programmes.

class inclusion 1 Generally, the notion that if class A is part of the larger class B, all members of class A are members of class B. **2** In PIAGETIAN theory, a child's ability to reason simultaneously about the whole and about the parts of which it is composed.

class interval The range of scores in a CLASS (4) in a frequency distribution.

class limits The upper and lower bounds of a class interval.

clean Laboratory jargon for things which are neat and consistent. Most commonly used of experimental data. Note that through one of those quirks of language the antonym here is not *dirty* but *noisy*; see NOISE (3).

clearness The original meaning of the term was that proposed by the structuralists: an elementary attribute of phenomenological experience. A clear sensation or a clear image was one which was in the centre of attention and stood out vividly from the background. The structuralists, in their search for phenomenological consistency, characterized both perceptual and cognitive processes in similar ways. The notion of clearness is still valid today in both of these areas but the connotations are different. In perception, *clearness* is the degree to which perceived objects appear definite, distinct and with well-defined boundaries. In cognition, it refers to that which is coherent and understandable.

cleft 1 n. A fissure. **2** adj. Split, divided.

cleft palate A congenital fissure or gap in the palate (roof of the mouth). Minor clefts involve only the soft palate; serious clefts extend forward through the hard palate, the gum ridge and upper lip.

Clérambault's syndrome An erotic delusion that one is loved by an older, influential person, often a famous or powerful person in society. See SIMENON'S SYNDROME.

Clever Hans The most famous of the Elberfeld horses of Germany. Hans seemed to be able to perform rather startling mental tasks such as addition, square roots and multiplication and even spelling words. It was ultimately discovered by the German psychologist Oskar Pfungst in 1907 that the horse was actually performing his apparent mental gymnastics by responding to subtle cues provided by the asker of each question or to his trainer Wilhelm von Osten. Hans's technique was to 'count' out an answer by stamping his foot the required number of times. He 'knew' when to stop by taking his cue from unconscious and extremely subtle changes in body position and breathing pattern on the part of the humans around him. The term *Clever Hans effect* (or *phenomenon*) has come to stand for any situation in which one unconsciously controls the results of a study or the behaviour of others by subtle, implicit communication. See also EXPERIMENTER BIAS, ROSENTHAL EFFECT. Also commonly known by the original German name, *der kluge Hans*.

cliché A response provided in a *projective test* so common or popular that it provides little or no insight into the respondent. For example, describing one of the Rorschach inkblots as 'an angry animal' reveals mainly that the respondent is not particularly imaginative.

client A term preferred by many as a replacement for *patient* in clinical psychology. Originally it was reserved for nondirective therapies such as Carl Rogers's *client-centred* approach, but it is now used by many others who wish to move clinical approaches in psychology away from the medically oriented model of aberrant behaviour. See also ANALYSAND for another, slightly differently motivated, replacement term for *patient*.

client-centred therapy A form of psychotherapy developed by Carl Rogers. The therapist is nondirective and reflective and does not interpret or advise except to encourage or clarify points. The operating assumption is that the client is the most able to deal with personal problems and the best course for the therapist is to offer a nonjudgemental, accepting atmosphere within which to explore and work them out. Also occasionally known as *nondirective therapy*, although that term may be used to encompass approaches not specifically associated with the Rogerian point of view.

climacteric MENOPAUSE.

clinic The original meaning derives from a Greek word denoting *pertaining to a bed*. Obviously this sense no longer holds; in fact, contemporary usage is restricted to organizations or places where patients or clients can walk in. Thus: **1** A place where persons come for individual work-up, diagnosis and/or treatment. In this general sense the term covers both the physical and the psychological. Hence, qualifiers are usually affixed so that the focus of the clinic is clear; e.g. BEHAVIOURAL *CLINIC, CHILD-GUIDANCE *CLINIC, OUTPATIENT *CLINIC. **2** The organization itself, including the building and its staff. **3** A short course or demonstration with either educational or quasi-therapeutic aims. Many have counselled against this usage but their advice has gone unheeded and 'smokers' clinics', 'speed-reading clinics' and the like abound.

clinical **1** adj. Generally, pertaining to a CLINIC, in any of the meanings of that term. **2** Characterizing an approach to personality and psychotherapy that focuses on the individual as a whole rather than seeking for general principles or doing normative studies. **3** Pertaining to medical or other therapeutic practice that relies heavily on intuitive and subjective judgements of the clinician. **4** Characterizing an approach to research which is based on observation (sometimes rather informal, sometimes highly systematic) of a relatively few subjects in natural situations. Often contrasted with the so-called *experimental* approach, which emphasizes highly controlled studies using large numbers of subjects. See CLINICAL METHOD, CLINICAL *PREDICTION.

clinical group(ing) Basically, psychiatric

nosology, the classification of persons according to symptoms displayed.

clinical interview Loosely, a synonym of CLINICAL METHOD, especially (3). When used as a synonym of meaning (1), the inclusion of therapeutic procedures implied in that term are not necessarily present.

clinical method 1 A general cover term for all those methods and procedures of diagnosis, classification and treatment of diseases and other disorders. **2** An approach to the study of psychological phenomena (disordered as well as normal) based on personal, intuitive, subjective analyses. See CLINICAL (3 and 4) and CLINICAL *PREDICTION. **3** In Piaget's terminology, a method of data collection based on quasi-natural interaction with a child in which the experimenter presents some object or task to the child or asks the child particular questions. The child is permitted to respond freely and the experimenter 'takes up' on the responses and moves on to other tasks or asks additional questions. Piaget's term here reflects his recognition that this data-gathering method has much in common with a psychiatric interview. Distinguish from CLINICAL TRIAL and CLINICAL STUDY. See also CLINICAL INTERVIEW.

clinical pain PAIN, CLINICAL.

clinical prediction PREDICTION, CLINICAL.

clinical psychology The area of psychology concerned with aberrant, maladaptive or abnormal human behaviour. Within the vast umbrella of clinical practices are diagnosis, evaluation, classification, treatment, prevention and research. Although recent years have reflected a trend toward the empirical approach, in which the clinician draws on the findings and methodology of the researcher, clinical psychology still largely reflects its historical lineage, which is predominantly medical in orientation. However, to appreciate the enormous range available to the practising clinician (and, even more bewilderingly, to the person seeking psychotherapy), a few of the more recognized and widely practised therapies should be consulted: BEHAVIOUR, DRUG, CLIENT-CENTRED, COGNITIVE-BEHAVIOURAL, ENCOUNTER, GESTALT and GROUP therapy, PSYCHOANALYSIS (various forms), etc.

clinical significance Characterizing an

effect that is unusual or noteworthy in that it plays a significant role in a person's life. The term enjoys wide currency and may be found referring to a patient's symptoms, the manner in which one's performance differs across tasks, the differences between a given individual and a reference group or, by extension, differences between groups. Distinguish from STATISTICAL SIGNIFICANCE in that an effect can be statistically reliable but not of clinical interest. For example, scoring a few points higher on a test of verbal ability than nonverbal might be detected by a statistical test, but is unlikely to have an effect on one's life and would not be termed 'clinically significant'.

clinical study TRIAL (3).

clinical trial TRIAL (3).

clinical type Any individual case in which the symptoms and behaviours conform to one of the many identifiable syndromes of clinical psychology and psychiatry.

clinic, behavioural Any clinic that specializes in behaviour therapy.

clinic, child-guidance A clinic specializing in the psychological problems of children.

clinic, outpatient A clinic specializing in individuals who are not currently hospitalized or institutionalized.

clitoris The highly sensitive structure of erectile tissue that forms part of the female external genitalia. The clitoris develops from the same primordial structures as the penis and, not surprisingly, plays an important role in sexual stimulation and orgasm.

cloaca theory The 'theory' often believed by children that birth takes place through the anus. Not unexpectedly, psychoanalytic theory makes much of this simple but understandable confusion on the part of an unsophisticated child.

clock In operant conditioning, a stimulus some dimension of which varies with time. Thus, expressions like 'FI + clock' mean that the subject is being reinforced on an FI schedule of reinforcement in the presence of some stimulus which is being used to mark time since the last reinforcement. For more detail, see SCHEDULES OF *REINFORCEMENT.

clomipramine An ANTIDEPRESSANT DRUG in

the category of TRICYCLIC COMPOUNDS. It is also used as an ANTIOBSESSIONAL DRUG and has proved effective in treating OCD.

clonazepam One of the BENZODIAZEPINES used as an ANTIANXIETY DRUG. Its main advantage is that it is one of the most potent drugs in this group; its primary drawback is that it is slow-acting and takes several hours to reach peak efficiency. It is also used in the treatment of epilepsy.

clone From the Greek for a cutting taken for the purpose of propogation. Hence: **1** n. A group of cells which are descended from a single cell. **2** n. All of the descendants, taken collectively, produced asexually from a single ancestor. **3** vb. To produce either of the above.

clonic Pertaining to CLONUS.

clonic spasm SPASM.

clonus Rapid, involuntary contraction and relaxation of a muscle. Contrast with TONUS.

closed adoption Adoption in which neither the biological nor the adopting family has information about the other. The adopted child is not permitted to have any contact with, and in some cases is given no information about, his or her biological parents. Also called *confidential adoption*. Compare with OPEN ADOPTION.

closed class words A category of words in a language that does not easily allow for new entries. They typically are items that have grammatical roles in the language (see FUNCTION WORD) and include articles, prepositions and determiners.

closed-head injury Any injury to the head that is nonpenetrating. Such injuries can be, and often are, rather serious since severe cerebral damage can occur even though the skull has not been penetrated. See also, TRAUMATIC BRAIN INJURY.

closed instinct INSTINCT, CLOSED.

closed question Any question that an individual must answer by selecting one or more of a set number of alternatives. Compare with OPEN-ENDED QUESTION.

closed system A system, actual or theoretical, that is bounded off from other systems and operates, or is conceptualized as operating, without externally imposed additions or changes.

closure, law of GESTALT LAWS OF ORGANIZATION.

clouding (of consciousness) A perceptually and cognitively confused state.

clozapine An ATYPICAL *ANTIPSYCHOTIC DRUG. Unlike most such drugs, it has minimal *extrapyramidal* effects, its primary site of action is the *nucleus accumbens* not the *neostriatum*, and it is much less likely to produce Parkinsonian side effects (e.g. TARDIVE DYSKINESIA).

cloze procedure A procedure for studying reading processes. One or more words are deleted from a prose passage and the subject is required to fill in the blanks.

clue A hint, a stimulus that guides behaviour. Occasionally used as a loose synonym for CUE.

cluster **1** In factor analysis, a group of variables which have higher correlations with each other than with other variables. **2** More generally, any group of objects or events which seem, subjectively, to belong together, to form a natural group.

cluster analysis A general label for a variety of mathematical techniques for determining the underlying structure in complex data. Cluster analyses are similar in some respects to factor analyses in that both involve the search for unitary elements (either *factors* or *clusters*) that account for the variability observed in the data.

clustering The tendency to group objects, words, pictures or ideas into clusters which 'belong together' in some subjective way. The effect is seen most clearly in experiments on the free recall of long lists of words in which subjects recall the list with the related words grouped together.

cluster suicides Multiple suicides occurring close together in time in a limited geographical area. They most commonly involve disturbed adolescents and are suspected of having an element of contagion, one well-publicized suicide triggering others. See WERTHER SYNDROME.

cluttering Rapid, often incoherent speech characterized by eliding words and syllables.

CMBD CLASSIFICATION OF MENTAL AND BEHAVIOURAL DISORDERS.

CNS (or **cns**) CENTRAL NERVOUS SYSTEM.

CNS depressants Broadly, any drug that has a depressive impact on the functions of the central nervous system. The term covers a wide variety of compounds including, among others, ALCOHOL, ANTIANXIETY DRUGS, BARBITURATES, HYPNOTICS, OPIATES and SEDATIVES and is used for all even though they differ in mode of action, site of primary neurological impact and underlying biochemistry. All, however, share several properties. At the lowest effective doses they depress the inhibitory centres; with increasing dosage levels they produce wide-ranging neuro-inhibitory effects so that cognitive functions are compromised, reaction times are slowed and emotions are damped. At higher levels all are toxic and depress respiration, heart rate and can induce unconsciousness, coma and death.

CNS stimulants Broadly, any drug that functions to stimulate the central nervous system. The term is used for a host of compounds including, among others, AMPHETAMINES, CAFFEINE, CATECHOLAMINES, COCAINE and NICOTINE, despite the fact that they differ in the manner of action, the site of primary neurological impact and underlying biochemistry. However, they share a number of characteristics. At low doses all produce alertness, wakefulness and increased energy. With increases in dosage levels they produce strong feelings of well-being and confidence. At higher levels all have serious side effects including agitation, panic, hallucinations and paranoia.

co- Combining form meaning *along with*, *joint* or *equally*.

coacting group GROUP, COACTING.

coalition In social psychology, an alliance formed for the purpose of gaining a particular objective such as increased resources, power or influence. Because coalitions focus on specific gains that could not be achieved with smaller numbers, the term carries the connotation that the group is temporary and the alliance unstable.

coarctated Pressed together, narrowed.

Used occasionally of behaviours or functions that are inhibited or constricted.

cocaine (hydrochloride) An alkaloid obtained from the coca leaf. It has anaesthetic properties when applied locally, and stimulating and mood-elevating effects when taken internally by ingestion, injection or inhalation. Both DRUG *DEPENDENCE and DRUG *TOLERANCE develop with continued use. Cocaine acts by blocking the reuptake of dopamine. Long-term abuse is associated with a toxic psychosis similar to that seen with amphetamines.

cocaine and amphetamine-regulated transcript See CART.

coccyx The small bone at the base of the spine in humans and tailless apes. It is formed from four fused rudimentary vertebrae.

cochlea The coiled, snail-shaped (hence its name) structure in the inner ear which contains the receptor organs of hearing. In humans it has 2 turns, the base is quite broad and it tapers as it coils. The cochlea is a bony cavity containing three fluid-filled canals (the *scala vestibuli*, *scala tympani* and *scala media* or cochlear duct), each running virtually its full length. The canals are separated from each other by *Reissner's membrane* and the BASILAR MEMBRANE.

cochlear duct (or **canal**) COCHLEA.

cochlear implant An implant, consisting of an array of fine electrodes that is surgically inserted into the cochlea of the inner ear. It is linked to an external microphone and a signal processor so that different regions of the *basilar membrane* are stimulated by sounds of different frequencies. Such devices can restore at least partial hearing to the deaf, often to the point where they can understand speech and even use a telephone.

cochlear microphonic A set of electric potentials that are generated by the hair cells of the inner ear and can be recorded from the cochlea. The waveform is similar to that of the acoustic input, sufficiently so that if the cochlear microphonic of a rat's inner ear is amplified and fed through ordinary speakers, one can understand words spoken to the animal. Also called the *Wever-Bray effect*.

cochlear nerve VESTIBULOCOCHLEAR NERVE.

Cochran Q test A nonparametric statistical test, an extension of the MCNEMAR TEST for use with more than two samples. It is useful for testing whether three (or more) sets of frequencies or proportions differ significantly from each other, and can be applied to data which are dichotomous (e.g. 'yes/no' or 'pass/fail').

cocktail-party phenomenon A term coined by C. Cherry to characterize the ability to attend selectively to a single person's speech in the midst of the competing speech of many others. The primary factors responsible for the effect are the context, the REDUNDANCY of speech, the physical location of the speaker and the pitch of the speaker's voice.

cocktail party syndrome Not actually a *syndrome* but a behavioural pattern best characterized as the propensity to talk endlessly about absolutely nothing. It is seen in a number of disorders, most notably WILLIAMS SYNDROME. Also called *chatterbox effect*.

coconsciousness Term used by M. Prince for the divided, coexisting consciousnesses seen in cases of multiple personality.

code 1 A set of rules or operations that transforms items, objects or data from one systematic form into another. **2** vb. To perform such a transformation. Thus, for example, the hearer of a sentence will code the sequence of physical, acoustic events into a meaningful form. For precision the term needs to be distinguished from *cipher*, meaning a simple system in which one symbol explicitly replaces another. *Code* (and its derivations) is reserved for the modification of the items so that they are reorganized into different size units or even different numbers of units. To illustrate: a person who does not understand French will code a sentence in French merely in terms of its sounds or phones (indeed, the verb *code* probably shouldn't even be used); a fluent speaker of French will code it in terms of its syntax, semantics, pragmatics, etc. The operation of coding a stimulus input is known as *encoding*, the unscrambling of an already coded input is called *decoding*. Usage here is quite broad. Not only are linguistic messages characterized in this manner but other communicative exchanges are as well. For example, a person who facially expresses sadness is said to encode sadness; one who perceives sadness in someone's face is said to decode sadness. **3** A language or dialect form. See here CODE SWITCHING, ELABORATED CODE, RESTRICTED CODE. **4** By extension, any neural process whereby input stimuli are detected and transformed into a pattern of neural impulses. Used here essentially synonymously with TRANSDUCTION (2). **5** In medicine, a designation that determines the kind of procedures to be used in case of an emergency. A 'no code' designation here usually signals 'do not resuscitate'. **6** A set of standards or rules for conduct.

codeine An opium alkaloid derived from morphine. It has the usual analgesic and sedative properties of opiates and is commonly used in low doses as an analgesic and a cough suppressant.

co-dependency Quite literally, a mutual dependency such as that between two individuals each of whom is emotionally dependent upon the other. Also written without the hyphen.

code-switching The term *code* is used here in sense 3 of that word. Hence, the phrase can have several meanings: **1** The switching of levels of formality in language; e.g. a politician code-switches when moving from the 'back-room', where a political position is worked out, to the political podium, where the position is presented to the public. **2** The switching of dialects; e.g. by urban African-Americans who alternate dialects according to whom they are addressing. **3** The switching of languages, as commonly done by fluent bilinguals. **4** The switching of writing systems, as commonly done by people fluent in two or more writing systems. See GRAPHOLOGY (2).

code test A test in which a message in one form must be converted into a coded form by replacing each symbol with some arbitrarily determined equivalent, e.g. A = 1, B = 2, etc., and the participant then writes a message in the new form. Also called *coding* or *digit-symbol test*. A dedicated pedantic might note that these should all be called *cipher* tests since a direct one-to-one replacement is not a true CODE.

coding 1 Generally, the process of modifying or transforming a message from its input form into some other form. See the discussion under CODE (1 and 2). **2** The transformation of data from one form to another. **3** CODE TEST.

coefficient Lit., produced together. Hence: **1** In chemistry, a figure that indicates the number of molecules of a substance in a reaction. **2** In mathematics, a constant factor by which other values are to be multiplied. **3** In statistics, a value that expresses the degree to which some relationship between factors is to be found. This meaning is most commonly found in combined forms, e.g. *correlation coefficient*. In this volume coefficients are listed by name.

coefficient of correlation CORRELATION COEFFICIENT.

coefficient variation COEFFICIENT OF *DISPERSION.

coenaesthesia Lit., common feeling. Hence, the normal collective sense of being alive, of being aware. vars., *coenesthesia, cenesthesia*.

coen(o)- CENO-.

coexposure In EPIDEMIOLOGY, linked exposure to two or more environmental factors that influence medical and/or psychological health.

cognition A broad (almost unspecifiably so) term which has been traditionally used to refer to such activities as thinking, conceiving and reasoning. Most psychologists have used it to refer to any class of mental 'behaviours' (using that term very loosely) with underlying characteristics of an abstract nature involving symbolizing, insight, expectancy, complex rule use, imagery, belief, intentionality, problem-solving and so forth. While the term is typically applied to mental activities in the general sense, individual thoughts, ideas or pieces of knowledge are also sometimes referred to as cognitions. See COGNITIVE PSYCHOLOGY and COGNITIVE SCIENCE.

cognitive academic language proficiency (CALP) The overall proficiency of a student in the language of instruction, particularly when the native language is different from that used in school. It's worth noting that children will often appear fluent

in the new language but have not (yet) developed the specific language skills needed to succeed academically.

cognitive analytic therapy A form of therapy that blends elements of PSYCHOANALYSIS with the more focused approach of COGNITIVE-BEHAVIOUR(AL) THERAPY.

cognitive-appraisal theory THEORIES OF *EMOTION.

cognitive architecture The overall structural features (the ARCHITECTURE) of the cognitive functions of a system. The term is used loosely. The 'system' may be the components of a computer program designed to simulate human cognition (the original use) or it may be the human brain whose neurostructural characteristics are being represented. It's a nice term; don't abuse it.

cognitive-behaviour(al) therapy An approach to psychotherapy based originally on BEHAVIOUR THERAPY and consistent with its basic tenets. Its novel aspect involves the extension of the modification and relearning procedures to cognitive processes such as imagery, fantasy, thought and self-image. Proponents of the approach argue, not unpersuasively, that what the client *believes* about the things he or she does and about the reasons for them can be as important as the doing of them.

cognitive complainers Elderly individuals who complain about cognitive and memory problems but who show no detectable memory loss on standard tests. There are suspicions that such individuals may be at risk of developing ALZHEIMER'S DISEASE.

cognitive contour SUBJECTIVE *CONTOUR.

cognitive derailment A term used loosely in clinical settings to refer to the tendency for thoughts and associations to follow one another in illogical and unpredictable ways. This tendency is often seen in schizophrenic disorders. Also called *cognitive slippage*.

cognitive development Loosely, the growth of cognitive functions. While strictly speaking the term can be applied to any individual, it is almost always used for the emergence of cognitive functions in infants and children. The connotations are neutral with regard to whether particular development is due primarily to a biological unfolding of innate capacities or to the acquisition of knowledge through experience.

cognitive dissonance An emotional state set up when two simultaneously held attitudes or cognitions are inconsistent or when there is a conflict between belief and overt behaviour. The resolution of the conflict is assumed to serve as a basis for attitude change, in that belief patterns are generally modified so as to be consistent with behaviour.

cognitive dissonance theory Leon Festinger's theory of attitude change based on the notion that we are motivated to adjust our attitudes to relieve COGNITIVE DISSONANCE. Also called *dissonance theory*.

cognitive ethology An interdisciplinary field encompassing the work of ethologists, psychologists and zoologists that focuses on the exploration of the mental life of animals, with special attention to their behaviour in their natural environments.

cognitive heuristic HEURISTIC, COGNITIVE.

cognitive impairment disorders An umbrella term covering those disorders the primary symptoms of which include impaired cognitive functioning, e.g. DELIRIUM, DEMENTIA and AMNESIA.

cognitive impenetrability Zenon Pylyshyn's term for those characteristics of perceptual function that take place unaffected by such 'top-down' processes as expectations, prior knowledge or context. No one doubts the existence of such effects in low-level or 'early' perception (see e.g. SUBJECTIVE *CONTOUR); the issue is how far 'up' the perceptual system processes are impenetrable.

cognitive map A term coined originally by E. C. Tolman to describe his theoretical interpretation of the behaviour of an animal such as a rat learning its way round a maze. Tolman argued that the animal was developing a set of spatial relationships – a cognitive 'map' – rather than merely learning a chain of overt responses. Evidence from experiments on *place learning* and *latent learning* was cited as supportive. The notion of a spatial representation that is the mental analogue of a real map seems fairly obvious. All one need do is close one's eyes and answer the question 'How many windows are in my home?' to appreciate the phenomenological reality of an image-like 'map' of the physical layout.

cognitive marker R. Ornstein's term for a representation of an individual mental event such as a thought, an image, an impression, etc. He argued that the passage of subjective time was related to the number of such markers, which, he argued, is why it seems to take longer to drive to a new location than to an old one; you notice more specific details on the former because they are novel.

cognitive neuroscience The broad approach to cognitive psychology that emphasizes the study of the neurological factors that underlie cognitive function. It is richly interdisciplinary involving research with humans and animals, clinical populations and normal participants. It utilizes various methods from scanning techniques to sophisticated computational modelling and searches for answers to basic scientific questions as well as cures and preventative measures for cognitive disorders. Also called *neurocognition*.

cognitive operations OPERATIONS, COGNITIVE.

cognitive psychology A general approach to psychology emphasizing the internal, mental processes. To the cognitive psychologist behaviour is not specifiable simply in terms of its overt properties but requires explanations at the level of mental events, mental representations, beliefs, intentions, etc. Although the cognitive approach is often contrasted sharply with the behaviourist approach it is not necessarily the case that cognitivists are antibehaviouristic. Rather, behaviourism is viewed as seriously incomplete as a general theory, one which fails to provide any coherent characterization of cognitive processes such as thinking, language and decision-making. To get a feeling of the general issues and problems within the area see ATTENTION, CONCEPT FORMATION, INFORMATION PROCESSING, MEMORY (et seq.), PSYCHOLINGUISTICS, etc. It is safe to say that contemporary psychology is overwhelmingly cognitive in nature and virtually every area of study, from classical conditioning to organization behaviour, from physiological to social psychology, and from neuroimaging to clinical psychology, has been infused with an overlay of cognitive theory and interpretation.

cognitive rehabilitation Any systematic programme of therapy following brain injury. Some programmes focus on restoration of lost or impaired function, others on the acquisition of compensatory mechanisms, and still others on more holistic approaches that involve vocational training and involvement of family and individual counselling.

cognitive reserve The hypothetical reservoir of brain plasticity that allows one to retain or recover cognitive functions typically lost due to age or neurological impairment. The term is used most often as descriptive of individuals with dementias like ALZHEIMER'S DISEASE who show less decline in function despite widespread neural pathology. The exact neural mechanisms are unknown, but behavioural studies show that education, intelligence and physical exercise are all positive factors.

cognitive restructuring In cognitively oriented therapies, a technique where the client learns to RESTRUCTURE (1) those thought patterns, images and beliefs that are self-defeating and modify them so that they become self-affirming and adaptive.

cognitive schema SCHEMA.

cognitive science The name given to the cluster of disciplines that study the human mind. It is an umbrella term which covers a host of once disparate approaches, such as cognitive psychology, epistemology, linguistics, computer sciences, artificial intelligence, mathematics and neuropsychology.

cognitive slippage COGNITIVE DERAILMENT.

cognitive style The characteristic manner in which cognitive tasks are approached or handled. Several dimensions have been identified along which individuals' cognitive styles can be shown to differ. See specifically LEVELLING, FIELD DEPENDENCE (AND) INDEPENDENCE and REFLECTIVITY–IMPULSIVITY.

cognitive therapy The form of psychotherapy developed by Aaron T. Beck based on the notion that the way in which an individual structures and interprets his or her experiences determines his or her mood

and subsequent behaviour. Seeing and thinking negatively are argued to cause negative feelings and behaviours; changing the manner in which an individual conceptualizes things lies at the heart of the therapeutic procedure. The approach and term are Beck's; similar orientations go under the more general heading COGNITIVE-BEHAVIOUR THERAPY.

cognitive unconscious A general term used to cover the variety of mental processes and functions that take place largely independently of consciousness or awareness. Included are IMPLICIT LEARNING, IMPLICIT MEMORY, INCUBATION (3) and SUBLIMINAL *PERCEPTION. Note that some authors also regard many of the psychoanalytic processes as belonging under this umbrella term.

cognize To know; occasionally, to think.

cogwheel rigidity A kind of ratchet-like resistance to joint movement often seen in Parkinson's disease.

Cohen's d See d (1).

Cohen's kappa (κ) An index of the extent to which two raters (or rating systems) are in agreement.

cohesiveness (or cohesion) The standard dictionary meaning is generally intended in psychology: a tendency to stick together or to be united either physically or logically. The term enjoys wide use in reference to social groups, concepts in education, items in a learning task, elements of a perceptual field, etc.

cohort Originally the term cohort referred to an ancient Roman military unit consisting of from 300 to 600 soldiers. It is more commonly used now, however, to refer to: **1** Very generally, any group or band of persons. **2** In demography, a number of persons all possessing a common characteristic; for example, a group of children born in the same year. **3** In ethology, a number of organisms of a given species which function together as a group.

cohort effect An effect or phenomenon the cause of which is attributable to the adventitious properties of a COHORT (2). For example, in developing nations a skill such as literacy shows strong cohort effects.

coition COITUS.

coitus Heterosexual, vaginal intercourse culminating in the introduction of semen into the female reproductive tract. Thus, *coitus interruptus* is coitus interrupted by the male withdrawing from the vagina prior to ejaculation. SEXUAL INTERCOURSE is a common synonym but consult that term for some distinctions; *coition* is generally used synonymously also but is occasionally reserved for the process in general rather than the actual act; *copulation* is a fairly pure synonym.

coitus interruptus Lit., interruption of coitus. See WITHDRAWAL (1).

coke Street slang for *cocaine*.

cold 1 A sensation evoked by any stimulus that is below normal skin temperature (roughly 32°C, 89°F). Note that the sensation of cold is a relative one and depends on the adaptation level of the skin. An object that is at 26°C (80°F), which ordinarily feels cool to the touch, can be made to feel warm if the hand is held in 21°C (70°F) water for a minute or so before touching the object. The equivalent effect occurs with stimuli warmer than normal skin temperature: they can be made to feel cool by adapting the skin to relatively warm water. Contrast with WARMTH. **2** Loosely, characterizing actions, processes and functions that are passive, calm and calculating as in 'cold' cognition (e.g. carrying out calculations), perceiving 'cold' colours (e.g. greens and blues) and experiencing 'cold' emotions (e.g. contempt), although note that the term COLD EMOTION is also used with a different meaning. Contrast with HOT.

cold emotion The agitated physical state experienced with some stimulating drugs (e.g. epinepherine). The bodily conditions mimic those of emotional arousal but there is a lack of true affective experience.

coldness Lack of emotionality; often specifically used of sexual feeling. See the discussion under FRIGIDITY.

cold pressor stress (CPS) A common experimental stress-induction procedure in which the subject immerses a hand in icy water for as long as it can be tolerated.

cold spot A point on the skin where a punctate stimulus that is below adaptation level of the skin will evoke a sensation of cold. It was first thought that such cold spots were due to specific 'cold receptors' in the skin, but subsequent microscopic study has failed to discover any precise relationship between specific nerve fibres and specific sensations.

cold turkey Slang for the process of terminating a physiological DRUG *DEPENDENCE by abruptly ceasing to take the drug with no support from other drugs. Depending on the severity of the dependence and the form of drug involved, such a process can be a most trying experience. This is particularly true in the case of opiates, amphetamines, alcohol and nicotine.

collateral 1 adj. From the Latin for 'together, in parallel'. Also used of objects that are situated side by side, off to one side and, by extension, subsidiary. **2** In personality and behavioural assessment, characterizing an independent source of information. An informant's report may be called a *collateral report* as may material gathered from other sources such as workups, imaging techniques or biochemical assays. **3** n. In kinship studies, a nonlinearly related kin member, e.g. a cousin, uncle or aunt. **4** n. In neurophysiology, a COLLATERAL FIBRE.

collateral fibre A branching fibre from the axon of a neuron. In some neurons, particularly those in the cortex, collateral fibres return to the region of the cell body. Such recurrent collateral fibres act as inhibitors, so that the cell cannot be refired for a time.

collective consciousness GROUP MIND.

collective guilt GROUP SUPEREGO.

collective hysteria MASS HYSTERIA.

collective information sampling (CIS) bias The tendency of groups to focus on and discuss facts and issues familiar to all members rather than exchanging information known only by one or a few members.

collective unconscious Jung's term for that aspect of the unconscious shared by all. Also called the *racial unconscious*, this was assumed by Jung to be inherited and transpersonal and, in his conceptualization, to consist of the residue of the evolution of our species. Its components were termed *archetypes*.

collectivism A set of beliefs and/or behaviours in which the rights of the group are given priority over the rights of its individual members. Contrast with INDIVIDUALISM (2).

colliculus From the Latin for *little hill*, any of four prominent collections of neural tissues of the *corpora quadrigemina* in the brainstem. The anterior pair are called the *superior colliculi* and are part of the visual system. In lower vertebrates they represent the sole system; in higher vertebrates they are not as important as the direct retinal-geniculate-cortex system and serve mainly as visual reflexes to moving stimuli. The posterior *inferior colliculi* are part of the auditory system, and the auditory fibres pass through them on the way to the mediate geniculate nucleus and the auditory cortex.

colour The subjective sensation associated with light. Colour experience depends on three components of the physical energy: *wavelength*, *purity* and *intensity*. Wavelength corresponds to the psychological attribute of HUE (or what the layman would call 'colour'), purity to SATURATION and intensity to BRIGHTNESS. See these terms for details of meaning and usage. Note that the adjective CHROMATIC is used to refer to stimuli that are analysable into all three of these attributes and ACHROMATIC for stimuli that only have the brightness attribute. In layman's terms, the former have 'colour', the latter are 'black and white'.

colour adaptation CHROMATIC ADAPTATION.

colour agnosia Loss of the ability to recognize colours while retaining normal colour vision. See AGNOSIA.

colour amnesia Loss of memory of the colour of familiar objects. For example, a person may forget that apples are red or green. The term is used only in cases of patients who retain normal colour vision.

colour anomia Loss of the ability to name colours while retaining normal colour vision and the ability to name objects. See ANOMIA.

colour antagonism COMPLEMENTARY *COLOUR.

colour attribute Any of the visual qualities of hue, saturation and brightness.

colour blindness Any one of a complicated variety of congenital defects in vision that

renders a person unable to distinguish two or more colours that normal individuals can distinguish easily. Although there is a form of total colour blindness (see ACHROMATOPSIA and MONOCHROMACY), it is quite rare and most colour-blind individuals distinguish many wavelengths. The most common variety is *dichromacy*, whereby the colours experienced can be described by using only two hues (i.e. the *dichromat* can match any given sample using only two wavelengths in mixture, the trichromat with normal colour vision needs three). The vast majority of dichromats confuse reds and greens; blue–yellow dichromacy is rare. Colour blindness is a sex-linked genetic trait and is far more frequent in males than females, with approximately 1 in 15 men showing some defects but only about 1 in 100 women.

colour circle A schematic representation of the visible spectrum showing the dimensions of hue and saturation. Hue is given by the position on the circle and saturation by the distance from the centre, as in the accompanying figure.

WAVELENGTHS (in nm)

EXTRA SPECTRAL HUES

colour, complementary Any of two colours that can be additively mixed to produce an achromatic grey. Schematically, the hues of complementary colours are found at opposite points on the COLOUR CIRCLE. See COLOUR MIXING and THEORIES OF *COLOUR VISION. Also known as *antagonistic colour*.

colour constancy The tendency for a colour to look the same under wide variation in viewing conditions.

colour contrast The influence of the colour of the surrounding medium on the perceived colour of an object. Best demonstrated by the enhancement of two complementary colours side by side. For example, if blue and yellow fields are juxtaposed a *simultaneous contrast* occurs, whereby, at the border, both colours appear more intense. *Successive contrast* can also be experienced by fixating on one colour for a time, then looking at its complementary. Also called *chromatic contrast*.

colour deficiency COLOUR BLINDNESS.

coloured audition CHROMATIC *AUDITION.

coloured hearing CHROMATIC *AUDITION.

coloured noise PINK *NOISE.

Coloured Progressive Matrices Test See PROGRESSIVE MATRICES TEST.

colour equation A description of the results of a colour match in which the subject adjusts the amounts of each of three primary colours needed to match a test colour. The equation is usually in the form $c(C) \equiv r(R) + g(G) + b(B)$, where the lower-case letters indicate the number of units and the upper-case letters indicate the colours, with C standing for the test colour, R for red, G for green and B for blue. Note that $\equiv$ is typically used here rather than = because the equation represents subjective equivalence.

colour, film A colour seen as nonsubstantial, without contour and indefinitely localized. Film colours do not feel as if they 'belong' anywhere and are rarely experienced in the real world. The sky on a very clear day comes reasonably close. Compare with SURFACE *COLOUR, COLOUR MIXING.

colourimeter Any device or instrument for measuring colour.

colourimetry The specification and measurement of colour. The science of colourimetry is based on the notion that all possible colours of visual stimuli can be specified in terms of but three properly chosen variables. These are the three PRIMARY *COLOURS (1) which, when mixed in the correct proportions, subjectively match the target stimulus.

colour memory MEMORY, COLOUR.

colour mixing Lit., the mixing of colours. It is important to distinguish between two basic types of mixing: light or 'film colour' and paint or 'surface colour'. Mixing of lights is an additive process whereby the resulting hue is an interaction of the mixed hues. Mixing of paints is a subtractive process whereby the resulting hue is the one not absorbed by the surface. Thus, mixing yellow and blue light produces grey or white, mixing yellow and blue paint produces green. In psychology the term is almost always used to refer to the mixing of lights, and the mixing is accomplished by presenting two (or more) colour stimuli to the same portion of the retina in any of several ways, such as simultaneous projection, rapid succession or alternation.

colour pyramid COLOUR SOLID.

colour shades Colours with brightnesses darker than middle or neutral grey. Compare with COLOUR TINTS.

colour solid An extrapolation of the COLOUR CIRCLE to include the dimension of brightness (or lightness) so that any colour may be given as a unique point in the solid depending on its combination of hue, saturation and brightness. Note that the colour solid may be presented as either a double cone or a double pyramid. The pyramid form is favoured by many since the four PRIMARY COLOURS (2) form the corners. The two forms are shown opposite.

colours, primary **1** Any three colours (or, more properly, *hues*) no two of which if mixed will produce the third. In this sense there is a very large number of sets of primaries; they are not identified as specific wavelengths but by their relationships to each other and the principles of colour mixing. **2** As based on introspection, the optimum, purest colour experiences – those that appear to an observer as being made up of but a single hue and which cannot be subjectively broken down into other components. Here, four primaries are found: *blue* at approximately 475 nm, *green* at roughly 510 nm, *yellow* at 585 nm and *red*, which is extraspectral and requires a little blue light to get rid of a slight yellowish tinge, at roughly the complement of 495 nm.

Meaning 1 is the one commonly presented in standard general texts in psychology; meaning 2, however, is the one that is accepted in the technical literature on colour vision. If 1 is the intended meaning, the proper term for 2 is *unique hues*.

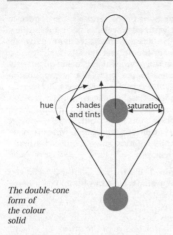

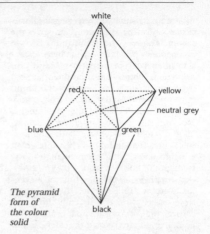

The double-cone form of the colour solid

The pyramid form of the colour solid

colour surface A plane section of the COLOUR SOLID taken at a right angle to the perpendicular. It represents all the hues and saturations at a given brightness level.

colour, surface A colour seen as belonging to or lying on an object. Surface colours are localized and 'substantial', part of the real world. Compare with FILM *COLOUR, COLOUR MIXING.

colour tints Colours with brightnesses lighter than middle or neutral grey. Compare with COLOUR SHADES.

colour triangle A schematic diagram in the shape of an equilateral triangle (usually) with the apices representing the red, green and blue primaries. The enclosed area represents all the colours possible through mixing these.

colour value In the Munsell system of colours, the dimension corresponding approximately with brightness.

colour vision, theories of Any of several theoretical models that seek to characterize and explain the basic phenomena of colour vision, of which there are a number: (a) the existence of primary colours; (b) the existence of complementary colours and their appearance in contrast effects and afterimages; (c) the laws of colour mixing; and (d) the various symptoms of the different kinds of colour blindness. The two best-known attempts at a systematic theoretical

explanation of these are the Young–Helmholtz theory (also known as the trichromatic theory, or trireceptor theory) and the Hering theory (or opponent process theory).

The Young–Helmholtz theory assumes three types of colour receptors. Although each type is assumed to respond to all wavelengths, they have different spectral sensitivities, so that one is more sensitive to long wavelengths (reds), one to medium wavelengths (greens) and one to short wavelengths (blues). All other colours are assumed to be perceived as combinations of these, so that the perception of yellow, for example, is characterized as being due to the simultaneous stimulation of red and green receptors and their integration in the visual neural pathways and the visual cortex. The theory accounts nicely for the laws of colour mixing, although it has some difficulty with the other basic phenomena. In particular, the theory cannot easily explain the fact that dichromats who confuse red with green see yellow. It also has difficulty explaining complementary colour afterimages.

The Hering theory, since updated by Hurvich and Jameson and known as the opponent process theory, assumes three sets of receptor systems: red–green, blue–yellow and black–white. Each system is assumed to function as an antagonistic pair. As in the Young–Helmholtz theory, each of the receptors (or receptor pairs) is assumed to be sensitive to light of all wavelengths but with maximum sensitivity to wavelengths of particular kinds. The assumption that gives the theory its power is that stimulation of one of an opponent pair not only produces excitation of that receptor system but also produces an inhibitory effect on the other; red light stimulates the red receptors and simultaneously inhibits the green. The theory accounts well for all of the phenomena, including the colour-contrast and colour-blindness data, which are bothersome to the Young–Helmholtz theory. At present it is regarded as a better approximation to the true state of colour vision. Note, however, that any theory of colour vision must eventually deal with the fact that the retina processes visual stimuli differently from the cortical and subcortical visual centres. This point is important because the careful examination of the retina has turned up only three types of cone pigments and they correspond rather nicely with the spectral absorption curves derived from the Young–Helmholtz theory. It seems likely that (to force a gross oversimplification) retinal receptors act as per the Young–Helmholtz theory and the signals are then recoded into the opponent process form by higher-level neural systems.

Finally, be it noted that there have been other candidates for a theory of colour vision. See here LADD–FRANKLIN THEORY, RETINEX THEORY. The former is not taken seriously for it has many problems; the latter is taken seriously but it is so very different in kind from the others that many researchers are simply not clear how to evaluate and test it.

colour, volume Colour seen as filling a three-dimensional space. It is perceived as organized and transparent and 'bulky'.

colour weakness A term sometimes used in place of COLOUR BLINDNESS, particularly since most colour-deficient individuals have a lesser (i.e. weaker) ability to distinguish colours, not no ability at all.

colour wheel A simple device for mixing colours by rotating a wheel (usually a disc) the surface of which is covered with coloured paper or plastic. By varying the area covered by any colour a variety of mixing effects can be obtained. The mixing obtained this way is termed *retinal mixing*. Occasionally, the term is used (incorrectly) as a synonym for COLOUR CIRCLE.

colour zones The retina is not uniformly sensitive to all wavelengths, and the differentially sensitive areas are termed colour *zones*. For the normal eye all colours can be seen in the *fovea*, which is made up entirely of cones. In the middle zone around the fovea, blues, yellows and the full range of achromatics are perceived, primary red and green are experienced as grey, and the other reds and greens have a blue or yellow tinge. In the periphery of the retina (which is made up entirely of rods) there is only achromatic experience.

column 1 In statistics, a vertically arranged series of numbers. **2** In physiology, a nerve which extends longitudinally in the central nervous system or a series of *cerebral cortex* neurons that are stacked in an organized fashion one on top of the other.

com- Combining form meaning *with*, *jointly*. var., *con-*, occasionally *col-*.

coma An abnormal state of deep stupor with total absence of consciousness and loss of all voluntary behaviour and most reflexes. The term is reserved for cases resulting from injury, disease or other trauma.

comatose In a coma or a coma-like state.

combat fatigue A form of POST-TRAUMATIC STRESS DISORDER or GROSS *STRESS REACTION that occurs subsequent to involvement in military action. The term is no longer used in the technical literature. var., *battle fatigue*, *combat neurosis*.

combination tone A subjective tone produced by the simultaneous sounding of two or more tones. Combination tones are formed in the auditory system itself (probably by the mechanical, physical properties of the cochlea) and are not present in the physical stimulus. If two tones are sounded, for example 1,000 and 1,200 Hz, three types of combination tones will be heard: a *difference tone* of 200 Hz; a *summation tone* of 2,200 Hz; and a series of descending tones produced by a complex relationship between the two original tones.

commensalism A symbiotic relationship between two organisms of different species. See SYMBIOSIS.

commissive A class of SPEECH ACTS in which the speaker places him- or herself under obligation to do something or carry through with something; e.g. promises are commissives.

commissural fibres The neural tracts of a COMMISSURE that connect corresponding regions on the two sides of the central nervous system.

commissure Generally, any transverse band of neural fibres passing over the midline in the central nervous system and connecting corresponding regions on each side. The two major pathways that shunt information back and forth between the hemispheres are the CORPUS CALLOSUM and the ANTERIOR COMMISSURE.

commissurectomy COMMISSUROTOMY.

commissurotomy Generally, the severing of a commissure. Usually, the reference is to the CORPUS CALLOSUM, the large commissure that links the two hemispheres of the brain and, occasionally, to the smaller ANTERIOR COMMISSURE. See SPLIT-BRAIN TECHNIQUE. Also known by a host of other names including *commissurectomy*, *callosectomy*, *callosotomy* and *corpus-callosotomy*.

commitment The process whereby an individual judged to be dangerous either to him- or herself or others or to be incapable of functioning without psychiatric assistance is admitted into a psychiatric treatment programme. The process may be involuntarily carried out in so far as the individual is concerned, in which case it becomes a forensic (legal) matter, or it may be voluntary, when the person judges him- or herself to be in need of treatment.

commitment theory In SOCIAL and EVOLUTIONARY PSYCHOLOGY, the theory that individuals will engage in immediately self-sacrificing actions for some long-term benefit or goal.

common chemical sense CHEMESTHESIS.

common factors In psychotherapy, those factors that promote success, independent of the specific type of therapy, e.g. expectation of positive change, focused attention and empathy.

common fate The Gestalt principle that aspects of a perceptual field that function

or move in similar manner tend to be perceived together.

common sense 1 In the Aristotelian sense, the capacity to comprehend the qualities of an object through use of the other senses. 2 In Thomas Reid's revival of this basic idea the focus was on the ability to apprehend qualities common to all the senses (time, space, numerosity). 3 Beliefs, opinions, practical understanding of things shared by the 'common man'. 4 Colloquially, good, reasoned judgement.

common trait A trait found in all persons in a particular society or culture.

communication 1 Broadly speaking, the transmission of something from one location to another. The 'thing' that is transmitted may be a message, a signal, a meaning, etc. In order to have communication both the transmitter and the receiver must share a common code, so that the meaning or information contained in the message may be interpreted without error. See also CHANNEL, CODE, INFORMATION THEORY. 2 The message or the actual information transmitted. There is a tendency on the part of some writers to use communication as synonymous with LANGUAGE. This is a mistake and the reasons for keeping these terms distinct are given under that term.

communication disorders An umbrella category for disorders of speech and language. Included are EXPRESSIVE LANGUAGE DISORDER, MIXED EXPRESSIVE–RECEPTIVE LANGUAGE DISORDER, PHONOLOGICAL DISORDER and STUTTERING.

communication unit Communications theory usually structures a communication system into an ensemble of elements called a 'unit'. It consists of a transmitter (or sender) which encodes a message, a communication channel through which the message travels and a receiver which receives and decodes the message.

communitarianism 1 COLLECTIVISM. 2 A set of beliefs and behaviours in which the rights and freedoms of the individual members are balanced with the rights of the group to which they belong.

community A settlement of people concentrated in one geographical area. The defining feature of a community is a 'self-consciousness' on the part of each member that the group is a social unit and that he or she shares group identification with the others.

community psychology An applied branch of psychology in which the practitioner works in a variety of ways with a community. It may include therapy-like interactions with community members but is more often oriented toward improving the quality of life.

comorbidity The simultaneous existence of two or more diseases or disorders.

companionate love LOVE, COMPANIONATE.

comparable forms FORMS, COMPARABLE.

comparable groups GROUPS, COMPARABLE.

comparative judgement Quite literally, any judgement about a stimulus made relative to (in comparison with) some other stimulus. A common procedure in *scaling* experiments, in which a standard stimulus is often used against which all other stimuli are judged.

comparative psychology A subdiscipline of psychology concerned with the investigation of the behaviour of various species of animal with an eye toward the drawing of comparisons (similarities and distinctions) between them. The approach draws on such areas of psychology as learning theory and on other disciplines, including ethology, physiology, genetics and evolutionary biology.

comparison level (CL) In *social psychology*, the average overall level of personal interaction that an individual expects to find in a relationship. People with high CL expect to have rewarding and fulfilling relationships with others. According to the full analysis here there is also a 'CLalt', or 'comparison level for alternatives' (i.e. other people), which, if higher than the CL, leads a person to be less committed to his or her current relationship.

comparison stimulus STANDARD (especially 2).

compartmentalization 1 Generally, the isolation of various of one's thoughts, feelings and beliefs from each other, particularly ones that would be in conflict otherwise. 2 K.

Horney used the term to describe a sense of disconnectedness that comes from the excessive use of compartmentalization (1) as a defence mechanism to shield one from the anxiety and tension that such inconsistencies produce.

compatibility 1 Generally, suitability for mixing without producing unfavourable results; characterizing a harmonious coexistence. In psychopharmacology, the term is used in this sense to describe various drug combinations, and in social and personality psychology to characterize particular kinds of interpersonal interactions. 2 In logic, any noncontradictory relation between two statements, principles or propositions.

compatible 1 Able to exist in harmony. 2 CONGRUENT.

compensating error ERROR, COMPENSATING.

compensation 1 Generally, any act or process that functions to make up for, counterbalance or offset the effects of previous acts or processes. 2 In Freudian theory, a defence mechanism that counterbalances deficiencies and covers up personal shortcomings associated with them, thereby preventing them from reaching consciousness. 3 In Adlerian theory, the primary psychological mechanism through which individuals deal with feelings of INFERIORITY. Compare here with OVERCOMPENSATION. 4 In the neurosciences, the recovery of function following neural damage, specifically to the central nervous system, either by growth of new neural tissue or having the functions of damaged structures subsumed by other tissue.

compensatory movement (or **reflex**) Any movement that functions to restore normal body position or equilibrium.

compensatory trait TRAIT, COMPENSATORY.

competence 1 Generally, ability to perform some task or accomplish something. 2 In forensic psychiatry, COMPETENT. 3 In the study of language and psycholinguistics, the embodiment of the deep, abstract rules of a language. The distinction is made here between competence and PERFORMANCE. A theory of the former would be a theory of linguistic knowledge and grammar, of what an idealized mature speaker-hearer of a language *could* say and understand; a theory of the latter would be a theory of behaviour, of what real speaker-hearers actually do say and how utterances of others are understood.

competent In forensic psychiatry, a designation used of a person who has been judged mentally capable of standing trial. The usual criteria for being declared competent are: (a) the person understands the nature of the charges and the legal consequences of adjudged guilt; and (b) the person is able to assist in his or her defence.

competition RIVALRY.

complement Generally, that which completes something.

complementarity The presumed tendency for people to seek out others who have qualities that they lack or that complement their own.

complementary colour COLOUR, COMPLEMENTARY.

complementary instincts In psychoanalysis, instincts that lie at opposite ends of some dimension. The classic examples are Freud's *eros* and *thanatos*.

complete learning method An experimental procedure in which the subject works with the material until one complete errorless trial is achieved.

completion test Any test in which the individual is given parts of items and must complete them, e.g. a fill-in-the-blanks test.

complex 1 Antonym of *simple* or *elementary*. **2** n. A constellation of emotionally toned ideas or dispositions. Meaning (1) is pronounced with the emphasis on the first syllable in the UK but on the second in the US. When meaning (2) is intended, the emphasis is always on the first syllable. Psychoanalytic theory has scattered various complexes liberally throughout its literature (e.g. Oedipus, Electra, inferiority). Although intended primarily as descriptive devices, they have gradually come to have pathological connotations because of the dominant theme that complexes are often repressed and in conflict with other behaviours. The term, however, should not necessarily convey pathology and it should be used carefully because it will often be misinterpreted.

complex cell See SIMPLE CELL.

complex figure test (CFT) Any of several tests in which the participant is asked to reproduce a complex line figure. The most commonly used is the Rey–Osterrieth, shown here. Any of the CFTs can be administered in either a copy or a recall form with varying recall intervals used. All are used in investigation of various neurological disorders.

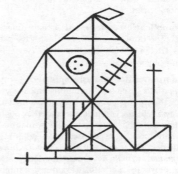

complex indicator A Jungian term for one or more responses in a word-association test that indicate the existence of a repressed complex. Such response characteristics as stammering, unusually long or short response latencies, highly improbable associates and blushing are often taken as complex indicators.

complex partial seizure The type of seizure seen in PSYCHOMOTOR *EPILEPSY. Note that some now use this term as a distinct diagnostic category replacing psychomotor epilepsy.

complex reaction time REACTION TIME, COMPLEX.

complex tone COMPOUND *TONE.

compliance Generally, yielding to others. Hence, many writers restrict this term to the overt behaviour of one person that conforms to the wishes or the behaviours of others. That is, they use it to imply there is no notion that the compliant person necessarily believes in what he or she is doing. See CONFORMITY for more on this point. Compare with PRIVATE ACCEPTANCE.

compliant character K. Horney's term for a person who displays neurotic self-effacement, deference and inappropriate yielding.

Horney regarded such people as displaying a *neurotic compliance.*

complication 1 Generally, any secondary factor or set of factors that functions to increase the complexity and intractability of a situation. 2 In medicine, a second disease or syndrome superimposed on one already present. 3 In older psychology texts, a combining of sensory experience from two or more senses.

complication experiment An experimental procedure the data from which gave rise to Titchener's LAW OF *PRIOR ENTRY (see this entry for details).

componential analysis/approach Any approach based on determining and analysing the component parts that are assumed to play a role in a complex phenomenon. Such approaches have proven useful in semantics, where meaning is assessed by ascertaining the defining features of words (e.g. *bachelor = unmarried, male, adult*) and the affective sciences where emotions are examined as interactions of several components (*appraisal, action, physiological factors, culture*).

componential subtheory See TRIARCHIC THEORY OF INTELLIGENCE.

component instinct PARTIAL INSTINCT.

component systems theory DYNAMIC COMPONENT SYSTEMS THEORY.

composite A unitary experience or whole made up of elements belonging to several other experiences. The common compound terms *composite figure, composite image, composite trait,* etc. are all self-explanatory.

compos mentis Latin for *of sound mind.*

compound bilingual BILINGUALISM.

compound conditioning CONFIGURATIONAL LEARNING.

compound eye A type of eye found in many insects and crustaceans. Rather than a single focusing unit (lens) and projection surface (retina), it contains many individual optical systems (*ommatidia*) each with its own lens and photosensitive elements. The large compound eye of *limulus* (the horseshoe crab) has been the object of considerable study and the source of discoveries about visual systems in general.

compound reaction time COMPLEX *REACTION TIME.

compound stimulus Generally, any complex stimulus made of more than one basic element. For example, in animal conditioning, the simultaneous presentation of a tone and a light would function as a *compound stimulus.* See BLOCKING.

compound tone TONE, COMPOUND.

comprehend 1 To understand, with the implication that the understanding is deep and thorough. 2 To combine several ideas or principles under a central theme.

comprehension The act of understanding a thing. The most common uses of the term are in education and psycholinguistics, and, perhaps surprisingly, it is used in both contexts with similar connotations. To say that a student *comprehends* a principle entails assumptions about the state of a student's knowledge concerning the material 'containing' the principle; a similar statement holds for a person who *comprehends* an utterance. Most contemporary cognitive psychologists argue that this comprehension process has two distinct and interlocking components: a *construction* process whereby an interpretation of the material is built up, and a *utilization* process whereby the interpretation is matched to other knowledge so that the information can be used to answer questions, deal with new situations, follow instructions, etc. Note that some authors differentiate between *comprehension* and *understanding*, regarding the former as more concrete and dealing with specifics and the latter as more abstract and connoting a deeper and more symbolic cognitive act (see here UNDERSTANDING (1 and 3)). This distinction is, however, ignored by most theorists, who use the two terms more or less synonymously.

comprehension test 1 In cognitive assessment, any test designed to gauge comprehension of everyday functioning and evaluate understanding of common-sense situations or principles. Typical items ask questions like 'Why do people live in houses?' or 'Why do people read books?' 2 In the study of reading, any test designed to assess understanding of material read.

comprehensive solution In K. Horney's

theory, a form of NEUROTIC SOLUTION in which one comes to view oneself as being the idealized self.

compromise formation In psychoanalysis, a pattern of reacting to a conflict such that elements of both components of the conflict are expressed. Classical theory regards it as a kind of fusion between the repressed impulse and the repressing agency.

compulsion 1 Behaviour motivated by factors that compel a person to act against his or her own wishes. **2** The psychological state in which one feels so compelled. **3** The underlying compelling force itself. Differentiate from an OBSESSION, the focus of which is more on thoughts and feelings than on behaviour, and from an IMPULSE, in which the compelling quality is more sudden and satisfiable. The term *compulsion* usually carries connotations of repetitiveness and irrationality. Strictly speaking, a compulsion may be either endogenous (from within) or exogenous (from without) but the former is the usual meaning intended; COERCION or *constraint* typically serve for the latter. See also IMPULSE CONTROL DISORDER, OBSESSIVE-COMPULSIVE DISORDER.

compulsive 1 Characterizing a COMPULSION. **2** Characterizing a person with a COMPULSIVE CONDUCT DISORDER or displaying a COMPULSIVE PERSONALITY DISORDER.

compulsive conduct disorder A behaviour disorder characterized by a pronounced tendency to engage in repetitive, compulsive acts. See OBSESSIVE-COMPULSIVE DISORDER.

compulsive disorder Loosely, any maladaptive behaviour marked by an irresistible drive. See IMPULSE-CONTROL DISORDER for general information and specific entries (e.g. gambling, alcohol, eating, hoarding) for details.

compulsiveness 1 Originally, the tendency to repeat specific motor acts. **2** More broadly, any tendency for repetitive behaviour both affective and cognitive as well as motor. See also IMPULSE-CONTROL DISORDER, OBSESSIVE-COMPULSIVE DISORDER.

compulsive personality disorder A personality disorder characterized by compulsive behaviours, e.g. excessive frugality, obstinacy, cleanliness. Also called *anankastic*

personality. See also COMPULSION and OBSESSIVE-COMPULSIVE DISORDER.

computational metaphor The term refers to the use of computers as models of human functioning and to the extended notion that human cognition is a computational process as opposed to, say, an analog process. See also ARTIFICIAL INTELLIGENCE and COMPUTER SIMULATION.

computational models Roughly, any of a large class of formal models of cognitive function that are based on the notion that 'cognition is computation'. These models are all based on the so-called *computational metaphor* and assume that the essential features of human thought can be captured by the sequence of computations the brain carries out in performing cognitive functions. Included are PARALLEL DISTRIBUTED PROCESSING MODELS and neural network models based on CONNECTIONISM (2).

computer-administered tests A general term for any test that has been adapted so that it can be administered and scored by a computer.

computer-assisted instruction (CAI) Generally any use of computers to facilitate teaching techniques. See PROGRAMMED INSTRUCTION, TEACHING MACHINE.

computerized axial tomography (CAT) A noninvasive technique for examining soft tissue, most commonly the brain. A narrow X-ray beam is passed repeatedly through the tissue (for a full brainscan 180 separate scans are made). A computerized system analyses the pattern of absorption at each point, which yields the data for full visualization. In a CAT-scan of the brain one can produce a visual representation of important structures including grey matter, the cerebrospinal fluid-filled cavities, blood vessels and any abnormalities such as tumours or lesions. Also called, simply, *computerized tomography* or *CT-scan*. See SCAN for more information and cross-references to other procedures.

computer simulation Quite literally, the use of a computer to simulate something. Generally the 'something' is human thought or behaviour; that is, one attempts to program a computer to behave in a manner that is analogous to thought processes or behaviour. In such research the computer itself is relatively unimportant; the critical element is the program, which is literally a theory of the behaviour under examination. For example, the General Problem Solver (GPS) program solves and fails to solve problems in a manner that are similar to humans; hence, it simulates human cognition and can be taken as a theory of human problem-solving. Note that the GPS does not solve just any old problem handed to it; it is not an intelligent beast in that sense. To appreciate this distinction see ARTIFICIAL INTELLIGENCE.

COMT gene Short for catecho-O-methyltransferase, it is a gene that codes for the enzyme that moderates production of DOPAMINE and NOREPINEPHRINE. There are two variants (known as *val* and *met*), one inherited from each parent. The *val/val* version has been linked with slightly poorer performance on executive tasks that involve the frontal lobes and recent work suggests an association with schizophrenia in that individuals with this double *val* variant show increases in midbrain dopamine with greater frontal lobe activity while those with the *met* version show the opposite pattern. See DOPAMINE HYPOTHESIS for more on the links between dopamine and schizophrenia.

con- Variation of COM-.

conation That aspect of the mental processes having to do with volition, striving, willing. The term was used historically to represent a basic mental faculty (along with *affection* and *cognition*) and is rarely heard today.

concatenation A general term referring to the stringing or linking together of items into a chain. Thus, a sentence may be spoken of (albeit a bit simplistically) as a concatenation of words.

concaveation Bringing a nonpregnant female animal into contact with young of the species. It can, under the appropriate conditions, produce an approximation to the chain of behaviours associated with parenting, including even lactation in females who have had previous pregnancies.

conceive From the Latin, meaning *to take into oneself*: **1** To become pregnant. **2** To form an image, idea or opinion. **3** To apprehend or understand. By extension of these: **4** To have or think of a concept.

concentration-camp disorder A disorder observed in many of those who survived the concentration camps of the Holocaust. Generally regarded as a special form of POST-TRAUMATIC STRESS DISORDER, it is notable for the relative prominence of SURVIVOR GUILT.

concept 1 A complex of objects all of which share some attribute(s) or property(ies). **2** The internal, psychological representation of shared attributes. Strictly speaking, the term should only be used in sense 2 since it is the mental representation that *is* the concept and it is the mental representation that is ultimately responsible for behaviour with regard to the outside world. There are assuredly things in the world which are chairs, but the concept of *chair* is 'in the head', not the world outside. However, one can get away with meaning 1 on the grounds that in order for a concept to get *into* the head there must be a complex of objects which reflect the properties that are cognitively represented. In psychological parlance concepts are often ranged along a concreteness–abstractness continuum, on which something like *chair* is regarded as highly concrete, i.e. easily identified, easily imaged and (relatively) easily categorized and classified, while something like *government* is regarded as highly abstract, i.e. not easily identified, poorly imaged and (relatively) resistant to simple categorization. For more on these problems (which are of legendary difficulty in both philosophy and cognitive psychology) see CATEGORY and related terms.

concept acquisition Generally, the process whereby one learns, i.e. acquires, a new concept. See the discussion under CONCEPT FORMATION AND LEARNING.

concept discovery A term generally used for the process whereby one discovers which of several previously learned concepts is the proper one for a given situation. In practice, problems arise in actual usage; see the discussion under CONCEPT FORMATION AND LEARNING.

concept formation and learning These terms are often used synonymously to refer to the process of abstraction of a quality, property or set of features that can be taken to represent a concept. However, there is considerable latitude in actual usage. For example, some authors restrict *formation* to the actual acquisition of a concept and use *learning* for the conditions under which one must learn how to apply a concept that is already known or formed. Accordingly one would study, for example, the *formation* of the concept 'round' in a child while examining how the child *learns* to apply it by responding differently to things which are round and things which are not. If the reader finds this a bit confusing (and the astute reader will, for there are good reasons for arguing that the senses of 'round' here are not differentiable), it should be noted that the literature in cognitive psychology abounds with terms which have been introduced to refer to whatever it is that is going on here: *concept acquisition, concept development, concept discovery, concept identification, concept use, concept attainment, concept construction* and *concept induction* are probably the more frequently used. Complicating matters further is the growing use of CATEGORY for CONCEPT and CATEGORIZATION as yet another synonym for concept learning. The reason for this free-flowing use of synonyms and near synonyms is that several interrelated cognitive processes are involved in human conceptual 'behaviour'. To wit: (a) those of the actual induction operations whereby one comes to know a concept symbolically; (b) those of the forming of the underlying mental representation of a concept itself; (c) those which are part of the distinguishing of various concepts from each other; and (d) those of the selection process whereby one discovers which of various concepts is appropriate for use in a particular situation. There is precious little agreement about terminology here and the most useful counsel is read carefully and reflect critically. It is recommended that *concept acquisition* serve for (a), *concept discovery* or *concept identification* serve for (c) and *concept use* for (d). All other terms should wither away through lack of use. There is no simple term for (b), which is really quite all right because no one understands the process anyway.

concept identification Lit., the identification of a concept. The term is generally used in relation to experiments in which the relevant concept is already known to the subject (e.g. 'round' in an adult) and what needs to

be learned is the identity of this concept as the critical one as opposed to some other. See also the discussion under CONCEPT FORMATION AND LEARNING.

conception 1 Most generally, the mental process of thinking, of conceiving or of imagining. **2** More specifically, the mental process of forming a concept. **3** A mental attitude concerning some thing. **4** The fertilization of an ovum by a sperm. The use of the same term for the creation of both a thought and a life is no etymological accident; it derives from the earliest attempts of the ancients to understand these processes by taking the *epigenetic* point of view for both forms of creation.

conception age AGE, CONCEPTION.

conceptual systems O. J. Harvey's term for the kinds of systematically applied processes which he hypothesized underlie the contents of an individual's beliefs. They range from concrete and rigid systems of the authoritarian through more abstract and integrated systems characterized by self-confidence and flexible perspective-taking.

conceptual tempo A person's preferred pace or rhythm in carrying out cognitive tasks. See REFLECTIVITY–IMPULSIVITY.

concept use CONCEPT FORMATION AND LEARNING.

concomitant variation *Concomitant* describes something that accompanies something else (often, but not always, with the connotation of being subordinate). The full term has two meanings: **1** A correlation; a change in one variable that accompanies change in another. **2** A principle of inductive inference used originally by Mill that states that when two things vary together they are probably either related to each other or to a third common factor. Both usages are neutral on the question of a true causal relation between factors.

concordance Generally, agreement, harmony. The term is used freely to refer to factors or phenomena that are coordinate, e.g. the degree to which a twin pair share similar traits or diseases.

concordance, coefficient of (W) An estimate of the degree of association among two or more sets of rankings. The coefficient, usually abbreviated *W*, is an index of the divergence of the observed agreement in rankings from the maximum possible agreement. It is also known as *Kendall's coefficient of concordance*.

concrete 1 Specific, precise, represented by some particular exemplar. The opposite of ABSTRACT (1). **2** Practical, useful.

concrete intelligence INTELLIGENCE, CONCRETE.

concrete operations A set of cognitive operations cited by Piaget as characteristic of the thought of a child during the CONCRETE OPERATORY STAGE. A variety of behaviours are assumed to reflect these operations and all are characterizable as ways of logically grouping and relating information about the world. As such, they are logical and yet still tied to the physical (concrete) world and to physical (concrete) actions. Distinguish from FORMAL OPERATIONS.

concrete operatory stage (or **level** or **period**) In Piagetian theory, the stage of cognitive functioning following the PREOPERATORY STAGE and preceding the FORMAL OPERATORY STAGE. It is generally assumed to begin around the age of 6 with the establishment of CONSERVATION and to end around age 12 with the beginning of abstract thinking, which marks the start of the formal operatory period.

concrete operatory thought The cognitive operations that exemplify the CONCRETE OPERATORY STAGE.

concurrent schedules SCHEDULES OF *REINFORCEMENT.

concurrent validity VALIDITY, CONCURRENT.

condensation In psychoanalytic theory, a hypothesized process whereby two or more images or elements combine to form a single composite image. The resulting 'condensed' image is assumed to carry the symbolic meaning of the separate images. It is regarded as an essential unconscious process best exemplified in dreams.

condition 1 n. An antecedent (either logical or empirical) that needs to be present for some outcome to occur. Conditions are classified as being *necessary* and/or *sufficient* (e.g. being warm blooded is a necessary condition

for an animal to be classified as a mammal but it is not sufficient). **2** n. Generally and loosely, any state of any system or individual organism. Although this meaning is etymologically neutral, the term is often used in clinical writing to refer to a diseased or disordered state. **3** vb. To bring about the process of CONDITIONING, in any of the senses of that term. **4** vb. Loosely and colloquially, to modify or change the circumstances of a system or an organism. This meaning is best avoided in the technical literature although it can be found in research on motor skills and athletics.

conditional probability PROBABILITY, CONDITIONAL.

conditional positive regard POSITIVE REGARD.

conditional reflex Pavlov's original term for what is more commonly called CONDITIONED RESPONSE. *Response* came to replace 'reflex' as a more general and neutral term and *conditioned* resulted from an early translator's error. Some researchers are going back to using the *-al* form here and many studies of classical conditioning now refer to a *conditional response*.

conditional response CONDITIONAL REFLEX.

conditioned In studies of CONDITIONING: **1** Descriptive of a response that has, through the proper presentation of conditioning procedures, been made dependent on a once-neutral stimulus. **2** Characterizing the once-neutral stimulus that now elicits a conditioned response. **3** By extension of 1 and 2, descriptive of a laboratory subject reliably displaying a conditioned response. **4** Generally, dependent upon something else, *conditional*.

conditioned aversion AVERSION, CONDITIONED.

conditioned avoidance (response) Any conditioned response which anticipates and prevents (or 'avoids') the occurrence of a noxious event. The reinforcement for such behaviour is assumed to be the reduction of anxiety or fear that follows successful avoidance.

conditioned emotional response (CER) Generally, any emotional reaction which has been acquired through conditioning procedures. Almost always used to refer to emotions with negative components, most often anxiety.

conditioned escape (response) Any conditioned response which terminates (thus allowing 'escape' from) a noxious stimulus.

conditioned flavour (or food) aversion (or avoidance) CONDITIONED *AVERSION, TOXICOSIS.

conditioned inhibition The suppression of a conditioned response by the simultaneous presentation of another stimulus (usually denoted as CS – CS⁻ to differentiate it from the conditioned stimulus, CS + CS⁺) which is not associated with the unconditioned stimulus (the US).

conditioned preference A process whereby a preference for a once-neutral stimulus is established. It operates in a fashion analogous to that of CONDITIONED *AVERSION (see that entry for details).

conditioned reflex The early Russian physiologists who first studied conditioning preferred to use this term rather than the now more common term *conditioned response*, owing to the fact that most of the behaviours which they worked with were reflexive in nature, such as the production of saliva in response to the placing of food in the mouth. See the discussion under CONDITIONAL REFLEX for other nuances of usage.

conditioned reinforcer REINFORCER, CONDITIONED.

conditioned response (CR or Rc) Lit., any response which is learned or altered by conditioning. In classical conditioning, the CR is a response that comes to be elicited by a previously neutral stimulus; in operant conditioning, it is a response that has been followed by a reinforcer. Convention has it that the term should be reserved for the classical conditioning situation only, but not all writers follow this.

conditioned stimulus (CS or Sc) Any stimulus that, through conditioning, comes to evoke a conditioned response. The CS is an originally neutral stimulus that develops its eliciting power through pairing with an unconditioned stimulus. This term is used in classical conditioning only; in operant conditioning one generally refers to a *discri-*

minative stimulus that sets the conditions for the operant response to be made.

conditioned suppression A reduction or suppression in responding in the presence of a previously neutral stimulus. The suppression is produced by pairing the neutral stimulus with a noxious stimulus. For example, if a one-minute tone is repeatedly followed by a shock, the subject will come to suppress responding for the full minute that the tone is on.

conditioned taste aversion (or avoidance) CONDITIONED *AVERSION, TOXICOSIS.

conditioning A generic term for a set of empirical concepts, particularly those that specify the conditions under which associative learning takes place. Often divided into two separate types: *classical conditioning* (or *Type S* or *respondent* or *Pavlovian*) and *operant* (or *Type R* or *instrumental* or *Skinnerian*). The basic difference between the two is that in classical conditioning the outcome of a trial (the unconditioned stimulus, or US) always occurs regardless of how the subject responds, e.g. Pavlov's dogs received food whether or not they salivated. In operant conditioning the outcome of a trial (the reinforcer) is contingent upon the subject making a specified response, e.g. Skinner's pigeons were not given food unless they pecked the key the requisite number of times under the proper stimulus conditions. The terms *classical* and *operant* conditioning, however, are often used in two ways: (a) to refer to a set of experimental procedures (indeed, this is how they were used above); and (b) to refer to two distinct types of learning that are assumed to occur under the two experimental procedures. The first use is operational, the second is theoretical.

The traditional view used to be that classical conditioning was a kind of primitive, reflex-like process that was elicited from an organism by an appropriate pairing of CS and US, while operant conditioning was seen as based on volitional behaviour emitted by an organism. However, phenomena such as AUTOSHAPING, BLOCKING (2), and SENSORY PRECONDITIONING plus the wide acceptance of the RESCORLA–WAGNER THEORY, show that classical conditioning, this most basic of processes, has previously unsuspected complexities and subtleties. Consequently, in the contemporary literature, the term *conditioning* tends to be used to refer not to a process but to an operation; specifically, to the arrangement of contingencies among events and the behavioural consequences brought about by such contingencies. Operationally, classical conditioning is subsumed by STIMULUS–STIMULUS *LEARNING (SS) contingencies, as between the CS and the US, and operant conditioning by response-stimulus (RS) contingencies, as between the organism's response and the environment's stimulus feedback. There are numerous specialized forms of conditioning, some of which are given below; others may be found under the heading of the modifying term.

conditioning by successive approximations SHAPING.

conditioning, excitatory A general term in classical conditioning for situations in which a positive correlation exists between the conditioned stimulus and the unconditioned stimulus, so that increases in responding in the presence of the conditioned stimulus are observed. Contrast with INHIBITORY *CONDITIONING, in which decreases in responding are found.

conditioning, inhibitory A general term in classical conditioning for situations in which there is a negative correlation between the conditioned stimulus and the unconditioned stimulus, so that decreases in responding in the presence of the conditioned stimulus are observed. Compare with EXCITATORY *CONDITIONING.

conduct disorder(s) A general psychiatric classification encompassing a variety of behaviour patterns in which the person affected repetitively and persistently violates the rights, privileges and privacy of others. Various subtypes have been proposed over the years, some based on differing degrees of socialization, on whether or not aggressive tendencies exist, and on whether or not the displays are confined to the family setting or more widely manifested.

conduction 1 The transmission of a neural impulse from one location to another. **2** The mechanical transmission of sound waves through the eardrum and the ossicles.

conduction aphasia APHASIA, CONDUCTION.

conduction deafness DEAFNESS, CONDUCTION.

conductivity 1 Generally, the electricity-conducting capacity of a substance. **2** Specifically the electricity-conducting capacity of a neuron or nerve.

cones The photoreceptors in the retina that mediate colour vision. They are most densely packed in the fovea and thin out toward the periphery. Cones have higher thresholds than RODS and function primarily in photopic or daylight vision. Three different cone *opsins* (photopigments) are found in the human retina, each with its own characteristic *spectral sensitivity curve*; the visual system uses the information from these three types of cones to produce colour vision.

confabulation Generally, making up details or filling in gaps in memory. There are three distinct uses: **1** The commonly observed cognitive process whereby one adds or elaborates on partial memories so that they make sense. It may be consciously controlled or take place implicitly. **2** The process whereby such additions or elaborations occur as part of a neurological condition. It is often seen in cases of NEGLECT and ANOSOGNOSIA and can be characterized as 'honest lying' based on a failure to edit memory retrievals which are clearly false or absurd. **3** In psychoanalysis, a DEFENCE MECHANISM in which inaccuracies and fabrications are introduced to protect an individual from the anxiety that would be created by accurately recalling earlier events.

confederate In some experiments in social psychology not all the 'participants' are real subjects. Frequently a psychologist is interested in the effects of social or peer-group pressure, and to ensure control over this pressure some of the participants may be confederates (i.e. stooges) of the psychologist who are instructed to act in certain ways to influence the real subjects. See, for example, the discussion under CONFORMITY.

confidence 1 Trust; belief in a person's trustworthiness. This is the meaning intended in most social and personality psychology contexts. **2** Assuredness, self-reliance. This meaning applies in the context of the examination of choice behaviour, signal detection, problem-solving and the like when an individual's confidence that he or she has detected a signal, made the proper choice, found the correct solution, etc. is a factor of considerable importance. In such experiments participants are frequently required to estimate their degree of confidence on some numbered scale for each response made. **3** In the phrase, *in confidence*, a secret matter; an agreement that information so passed is not to be divulged. See PRIVILEGED COMMUNICATION.

confidence interval An interval or range of values within which the theoretical probability of an event may be specified. The wider the interval the higher the confidence, and vice versa. For example, we may say with almost complete confidence that 'John's IQ is between 50 and 150'; as we narrow the interval our confidence decreases, so that we would not be very confident in stating 'John's IQ is between 99 and 101.' The confidence interval is generally given in standard deviation units around the mean (for a group) or an obtained score (for an individual).

confidence limits The limits outside of which an event is not expected to occur by chance with more than some specified probability. They mark the *confidence interval* and are usually given in standard units around the mean. Also called *fiducial limits*.

confidential adoption CLOSED ADOPTION.

confidentiality The characteristic of being kept secret; an intimacy of knowledge shared by a few who do not divulge it to others. The term is most commonly used with respect to the legal and ethical issues which, in principle, protect this contract of trust, particularly as regards information passed during psychiatric or psychological therapy. The phrase *confidential communication* is the legal term used to cover such material.

configuration **1** Generally, a particular arrangement of objects, machines, people, stimuli, etc. See SYSTEM (especially 3). **2** In perception, the term is used in ways very similar to the term GESTALT. The connotation here is that the essential nature of an arrangement is the coordinated whole and not the several objects, people, etc. of which it is composed. Occasionally the phrase *configurational ten-*

dency is used to refer to the tendency to respond to the full, organized arrangement.

configurational learning (or **conditioning**) Learning (or conditioning) in which the conditioned stimulus is a compound stimulus (e.g. a light and tone presented together). After extensive training, a conditioned response is only obtained to the full compound stimulus, or the 'configuration'; the separate elements (i.e. the light or the tone alone) produce no responding. Compare with OVERSHADOWING. Also known as *compound learning* (or *conditioning*).

configurational tendency CONFIGURATION (2).

configuration-superiority effect A class of perceptual and cognitive effects in which entire well-defined stimuli are more easily identified and processed than any of their component parts when seen in isolation. For example, in the WORD-SUPERIORITY EFFECT a whole word is identified more easily than any of its letters. While these effects have a paradoxical feel to them because the identity of the full configuration seems to require processing of its several parts, NETWORK MODELS (1) give a good theoretical account. Also called *configural-superiority effect*.

confirmation A theoretical construct developed by E. C. Tolman for the fulfilment of an EXPECTANCY. In this sense the term provides a theoretical base for the notion of reinforcement since, according to Tolman, confirmation of an expectancy is the basic reinforcer of behaviour.

confirmation bias The tendency to seek and interpret information that confirms existing beliefs. It is seen both in social situations, where information that disconfirms one's beliefs is often ignored or misinterpreted, and in cognitive tasks like problem-solving, where people frequently test hypotheses that, if true, confirm already held beliefs rather than entertain hypotheses that would disconfirm those beliefs.

conflate **1** To fuse two different meanings or concepts. **2** Occasionally, CONFOUND. This meaning is misleading and not recommended.

conflict An extremely broad term used to refer to any situation in which there are mutually antagonistic events, motives, purposes, behaviours, impulses, etc. The following entries describe the classic conflict situations and the various kinds of conflicts that are theorized to exist.

conflict, actual A presently occurring conflict. In psychoanalysis, such conflicts are assumed to derive from *root conflicts*.

conflict, approach–approach A conflict resulting from being drawn toward two equally desirable but mutually incompatible goals. The conflict is generally resolved when one gets closer (physically or metaphorically) to one of the two goals, since desirability typically increases with proximity. See APPROACH GRADIENT.

conflict, approach–avoidance A conflict resulting from being both drawn and repelled by the same goal. This type of conflict is particularly difficult to resolve in that with distance the goal appears more desirable than fearful whereas with proximity its aversive qualities tend to dominate, causing withdrawal, which, of course, leads to an increase in the goal's perceived positive features relative to the negative ones. A classic example is the conflict experienced on being offered a job with a rise in salary but a substantial increase in workload.

conflict, avoidance–avoidance A conflict resulting from being repelled by two undesirable goals when there are strong pressures to choose one or the other. It is a particularly unpleasant situation which prompts one to select the 'lesser of two evils'. When the conflict is intense a person may simply 'leave the field' and refuse to choose between the alternatives.

conflict, double approach–avoidance A variation on the simple APPROACH–AVOIDANCE *CONFLICT, in which each of two goals has both positive and negative aspects. A typical example is the conflict felt by a person on a diet faced with a delicious, calorie-rich chocolate cake and a carrot which, for all its nutritional value, still tastes like a carrot.

conformity Generally, the tendency to allow one's opinions, attitudes, actions and even perceptions to be affected by prevailing opinions, attitudes, actions and perceptions. There are at least three distinct subtypes: (a) *behavioural*, i.e. the tendency to 'go along with the group', to attempt to act in ways consistent with the majority; (b) *attitudinal*, i.e. the tendency to change an attitude or belief in response to pressure from others, which may or may not result in behavioural change; and (c) *personality trait*, i.e. the tendency for an underlying characteristic of an individual's personality to change under the influence of (a) or (b).

confound In experimental work, to fail to separate two variables with the result that their effects cannot be independently ascertained. If in an experiment on memory and age all the older participants are female and all the younger are male, then sex and age are 'confounded' and the memory data cannot be properly interpreted. Contrast with CONTROL, which is what is missing when variables are confounded.

confrontational techniques In psychotherapy, the use of direct efforts to force individuals to face their shortcomings and failures. They emerged from the extension of techniques used in ENCOUNTER GROUPS with difficult clients such as long-term drug users and prison inmates. The data suggest that they are not particularly effective; their primary impact is to produce resistance among the participants.

Confucian values LONG-TERM ORIENTATION.

confusion (confusional state) DELIRIUM.

congenital Present at birth. The term is not necessarily synonymous with INNATE or HEREDITARY. A congenital condition may be due to factors other than heredity, e.g. *fetal alcohol syndrome* or retardation produced by the mother contracting German measles early in pregnancy.

congenital adrenal hyperplasia (CAH) A syndrome in which the adrenal cortices are unable to produce cortisone as normal and release excess adrenal androgens instead. Females with CAH are born with masculinized external genitalia; males have normal genitalia. CAH can be controlled with regulated doses of cortisone, allowing normal sexual and reproductive functions to develop on schedule. Surgical repair may be needed to feminize the genitalia of girls.

congenital toxoplasmosis TOXOPLASMOSIS.

congruence principle The generalization

that it is easier to search memory for a match than a mismatch. Most easily seen in experiments in which a subject must determine whether or not each of several test stimuli is a searched-for target. Reaction times are far faster for the positive cases (the matches) than for the negative (the mismatches).

congruent Harmonious, concordant. The degree to which the various elements of a situation are congruent or not can have a significant impact on the use of EXECUTIVE FUNCTIONS. For some classic examples see FLANKER EFFECT and SIMON EFFECT. ant., *incongruent*.

congruent attitude change In social psychology, a change in an attitude in the direction of the attitude already held by the individual.

congruent retinal points Two points, one on each retina, that are projections of the same point in the external stimulus configuration. Distinguish from IDENTICAL RETINAL POINTS and contrast with DISPARATE RETINAL POINTS.

congruity theory A theory of attitude change that focuses on attitudes about the source and the content of a message. If an individual has positive or negative feelings toward both, the message is congruent and attitudes are not changed. However, if one feels positive toward one but negative toward the other, there is strong motivation to change either one's opinion of the speaker or one's attitude toward the message.

conjoined twins Twins joined at birth. The term replaces the unfortunate *Siamese twins*, which can still be found in nontechnical writings.

conjoint measurement Measurement wherein that which is being measured is composed of two or more components each of which affects the thing measured. Many psychological variables are conjoint, e.g. preferences, beliefs, utilities. For example, one's preference for a particular car may be made up of its style, cost, economy, handling, etc. An increase in cost could shift preference dramatically even though the other factors remained constant.

conjugal paranoia DELUSIONAL DISORDER, JEALOUS TYPE.

conjugate movement Coordinated movement, as of the two eyes.

conjugate reinforcement SCHEDULES OF *REINFORCEMENT.

conjugation Coupling, joining.

conjunctiva Mucous membranes that line the eyelid and the corners of the eyeball.

conjunctival reflex Reflexive closing of the eyelid to stimulation of the cornea or the conjunctiva. Also called *corneal reflex*.

conjunctive concept A concept defined by the mutual presence of two or more aspects. In a concept-identification experiment using various coloured shapes as stimuli, a conjunctive concept might be 'red *and* round'. See DISJUNCTIVE CONCEPT and RELATIONAL CONCEPT.

conjunctive motivation H. S. Sullivan's term for a striving to achieve a permanent, satisfying harmony in the many diversities of life. Compare with DISJUNCTIVE MOTIVATION.

conjunctive schedule SCHEDULES OF *REINFORCEMENT.

conjunctive task A type of group task in which the performance of the group as a whole is dependent upon the performance of the weakest member. A performance by a small musical group is an example of a conjunctive task. Compare with ADDITIVE TASK and DISJUNCTIVE TASK.

connate Appearing at or shortly after birth. See CONGENITAL.

connection Generally, any link or relation between two 'things'. The 'things' may be stimuli, responses, ideas, thoughts or images, neural actions, emotions, etc. The term is used promiscuously throughout all of psychology.

connectionism 1 E. L. Thorndike's term for his early associationistic theory of learning. **2** In cognitive psychology, an approach to the study of cognitive processes based on the assumption that a system (such as a brain) operates as though it were composed of a network of *nodes*, each of which will have at any point in time a certain level of activation. Each of these nodes is assumed to be interconnected with other nodes at different levels of the system in either an excitatory or an inhibitory manner, so that activating one node will have particular effects on the others. The whole network is assumed to be dynamic in that, so long as inputs are fed to it, it will keep adjusting the levels of activation and the strengths of the various interconnections between the nodes. Connectionist models have proven to be quite powerful and when expressed as computer models (COMPUTER SIMULATION, ARTIFICIAL INTELLIGENCE) have provided intriguing insights into human memory, learning and neurocognitive functioning. Theories based on these principles are also referred to as *associationist models, parallel distributed processing (PDP) models* or *neural network models*.

connector (neuron) A neuron that lies between and connects two other neurons or a receptor and an effector. Also called an INTERNEURON.

connotative meaning MEANING, CONNOTATIVE.

consanguine Having the same forebear. Usually restricted to one, two or at most three generations back, i.e. parents, grandparents, great-grandparents. A consanguine marriage is one between relatively close relatives.

consanguinity Genetic relatedness.

conscience A reasonably coherent set of internalized moral principles that provides evaluations of right and wrong with regard to acts either performed or contemplated. Historically, theistic views aligned conscience with the voice of God and hence regarded it as innate. The contemporary view is that the prohibitions and obligations of conscience are learned; indeed, Freud's characterization of the SUPEREGO was an attempt to provide an account of its origins, development and manner of functioning. See also MORAL DEVELOPMENT.

conscientiousness In the FIVE FACTOR MODEL, the broad personality disposition that determines the degree to which one is careful, precise, thoughtful and responsible in one's actions.

conscious 1 adj. Generally, characterizing the mental state of an individual who is capable of (a) having sensations and perceptions, (b) reacting to stimuli, (c) having

feelings and emotions, (d) having thoughts, ideas, plans and images, and (e) being aware of (a) to (d). Note that when the term is applied to nonhuman organisms, there is considerable dispute as to just which of the processes under (d) can be said to be included, although those under (c) will be considered present for all but the most primitive species. Differentiate the state of *being conscious* from the condition of *having* CONSCIOUSNESS (particularly 2 and 3). **2** n. In psychoanalytic theory, the aspect of mind that encompasses all that one is momentarily aware of. This usage is generally marked by the use of the definite article, as in 'the conscious', and is differentiated from the PRECONSCIOUS and the UNCONSCIOUS.

consciousness 1 Generally, a state of awareness: a state of being CONSCIOUS (1). This is the most general usage of the term and is that intended in a phrase such as 'he lost consciousness'. **2** A domain of mind that contains the sensations, perceptions and memories of which one is momentarily aware; that is, those aspects of present mental life that one is attending to. See ATTENTION. **3** That component of mind available for INTROSPECTION. This meaning is found in the older writings of structuralists and other introspectionists as well as in modern discussions conducted on the assumption that knowledge held in consciousness is knowledge that is available for recall and can be communicated to others. **4** In psychoanalysis, the CONSCIOUS (2).

The term has a distinctly chequered history. At times it has represented the central focus of psychology (see STRUCTURALISM) and at others been banned from the psychologist's lexicon as representing nothing more than the epiphenomenal flotsam of bodily activity (see BEHAVIOURISM). The ongoing fascination with it, however, stems from the compelling sense that consciousness is one of the defining features of our species, if not *the* defining feature; that to be human is to possess not only self-awareness but the even more remarkable capacity to scan and review mentally that of which we are aware. Many authorities treat consciousness not as a 'thing' but as representing a continuum. While they regard the introspectively poignant form that humans manifest as lying at one pole, they view the mental lives of other species as not different in kind from ours. If this seems a tad wrong-headed, it shouldn't. It is exactly the way in which contemporary psychology treats related topics, such as MEMORY.

As a topic for a scientific psychology consciousness is in clear resurgence, mainly within the areas of cognition, language and neuropsychology and the interdisciplinary approaches of the cognitive sciences and the philosophy of mind. Much of the contemporary focus is on the issue of just which of our cognitive processes such as memory and learning are open for conscious inspection and which are not. See here IMPLICIT *MEMORY and IMPLICIT *LEARNING.

consensual eye reflex The reaction of both pupils when only one eye is exposed to a change in light intensity.

consensual reflex CONTRALATERAL REFLEX. Generally, any reflex observed on the opposite side of the body from the place stimulated.

consensual validation 1 The use of agreement between two or more persons as providing evidence for the validity of a phenomenon. See CONSENSUAL *VALIDITY. **2** In H. S. Sullivan's theory, the principle that the socially valid meanings of symbols and ideas derive from a coherent consensus among the members of a community. From Sullivan's point of view, normal development is the process of changing from individualistic meanings to socially shared meanings.

consequent 1 An event or phenomenon which occurs following some other event such that it 'invites' the inference that it was caused by that event. **2** In logic, the conclusionary proposition, the so-called 'then' clause. See ANTECEDENT.

consequentialism See DEONTOLOGY.

conservation A term introduced by Piaget for the understanding that quantitative aspects of a set of materials or other stimulus display are not changed or affected by transformations of the display itself. The key notion here is that one who is a 'conserver' is one who recognizes that the critical quantitative properties are not altered by arbitrary transformation or other modifications of the situation. The amount of fluid in a jar is not changed by pouring it into differently shaped containers, the number of objects in a row is not changed by altering their spatial arrangement, the mass of a quantity of clay is not changed by rolling it into many little balls, etc. Conservation, like other cognitive operations, is assumed by Piagetians to be attained only at a certain developmental stage; it is usually taken as the strongest evidence that a child is at the CONCRETE OPERATORY STAGE. In its 'pure' form conservation is considered to be a singular cognitive operation, the recognition that quantity is preserved no matter what transformations are applied so long as nothing is added and nothing taken away. However, it appears that various applications of this principle by the child require different amounts of experience; typically conservation of number is observed before conservation of length, and conservation of weight and volume appear later still. See DÉCALAGE.

conservatism In political theory, the point of view that defends the status quo, that maintains that the *conservative* position is to be defended.

conservative 1 adj. In social/political terms, descriptive of any point of view or proposal that argues that change is to be resisted, that current modes of functioning should be maintained. **2** n. One who adheres to this point of view.

conservative statistic Any statistic that tends to underestimate. See e.g. SCHEFFÉ TEST.

consistency Occasional synonym for RELIABILITY.

consistency theories A general label for theories of attitude change that maintain people strive for consistency between actions and beliefs. The underlying assumption is that a lack of consistency is psychologically uncomfortable, so that when a person behaves in a manner inconsistent with a belief, he or she is motivated to change something to re-establish consistency. Such theories include BALANCE THEORY, CONGRUITY THEORY and COGNITIVE DISSONANCE THEORY.

consolidation Loosely, the various neurophysiological processes assumed to take place following the acquisition of new knowledge or the learning of new behaviours. The processes involve temporally graded neural changes that fix or 'consolidate' the mental traces rendering them relatively robust and long-lasting. The exact operations in the nervous system that account for consolidation are not known but are hypothesized to involve any of several possible mechanisms, including (a) modifications in the ease with which neurotransmitters affect neighbouring neurons, (b) alterations in the amount of particular neurotransmitters in critical neural pathways, and (c) increases in the number of synaptic connections that are made between neurons. There are good reasons for suspecting that sleep, particularly REM and Stage-4 NREM, play a role in at least some forms of consolidation. Some authors also use the term as a kind of neurological metaphor for the transition from SHORT-TERM *MEMORY to LONG-TERM *MEMORY.

consonant Any speech sound produced by partial or complete closure at some point in the vocal tract accompanied either by audible friction or by a sudden release of air. Consonants include *plosives*, *fricatives*, *nasals*, *laterals* and *glottal stops* (or *catches*). Contrast with VOWEL.

consonant trigram Any meaningless, unpronounceable combination of three separate consonant such as JBK or QKZ. Such CCCs (as the term is often abbreviated) are used in studies of memory, perception, verbal learning, etc. when it is desirable to keep the meaningfulness dimension to a minimum. Compare with NONSENSE SYLLABLE.

conspecific An ethological term for another organism of the same species as the organism under consideration. Compare with ALLOSPECIFIC.

constancy The tendency for perceived objects to give rise to the same (or quite similar) perceptual experiences even though there may be wide variations in the conditions of observation – that is, variations in both the DISTAL STIMULUS (the objects themselves) and the PROXIMAL STIMULUS (the energy impinging on the receptors). Essentially all perceptual qualities display constancy to some extent; see, e.g. BRIGHTNESS CONSTANCY, COLOUR CONSTANCY, SHAPE CONSTANCY.

constancy hypothesis The hypothesis that strict isomorphism holds between the proximal stimulus and the sensory experience. The hypothesis, in principle, assumes a total lack of any effect due to the context within which the observations take place. The hypothesis is really a 'straw man' erected for easy demolition by the Gestaltists (who took the opposing position of CONSTRUCTIVISM) and attributed to structuralists and behaviourists a position they never actually defended. A modern and more defensible variation on the basic idea is embodied in Pylyshyn's notion of COGNITIVE IMPENETRABILITY.

constancy of internal environment HOMEOSTASIS.

constancy of the IQ 1 The extent to which there is test–retest reliability in IQ. **2** By extension, the extent to which IQ tends to remain constant over the years. The term, however, is widely used to refer to a general theoretical model of the underlying basis of intelligence. Test–retest reliability quotients tend to be reasonably high and there is evidence that measurements remain fairly constant over years, which some have, erroneously, taken to be evidence of genetically endowed intelligence. However, it is important to appreciate that constant IQ is also critically dependent on the kinds and constancy of environments people are raised in and the kinds and constancy of educational and instructional experiences they have. See INTELLIGENCE for more on this issue.

constancy of the organism HOMEOSTASIS.

constant Basically, something that does not vary (as in statistical or mathematical terms) or is not permitted to vary (as in experimental controls).

constant error ERROR, CONSTANT.

constant stimuli, method of MEASUREMENT OF *THRESHOLD.

constellation 1 Generally, any reasonably well-organized matrix of associations, ideas, images, effects, etc. **2** Specifically, in psychoanalysis, a nonrepressed set of coordinated, emotionally charged ideas.

constituent IMMEDIATE CONSTITUENT.

constitution Generally, the genotypic endowments of a person as expressed in the phenotype. Used broadly by some to cover both physical and psychological aspects; used more narrowly by others with a focus on the physical. In the several early attempts to construct a CONSTITUTIONAL THEORY, the emphasis was on the physical constitution as the important determinant of the cognitive, social and affective traits that are learned.

constitutional theory Any of several theories of personality that focused on those aspects of a person that are inherent, particularly those attributes of morphology and physiology that are organic, genetic and relatively stable, and their relationships with psychological and behavioural characteristics. Three theories stand out: (a) Galen's, which was based on four basic types – *sanguine, melancholic, choleric* and *phlegmatic*; (b) Kretschmer's, with three basic types – *pyknic* (stocky), *asthenic* (slender) and *athletic* (muscular) – and one mixed type – *dysplastic* (disproportioned); and (c) Sheldon's, which hypothesized three fundamental constitutional types – *ectomorphic* (thin), *mesomorphic* (muscular) and *endomorphic* (fat).

Galen's theory was based on the ancient presumption of bodily humours as controllers of the psyche, and not surprisingly is the least sophisticated. Kretschmer's was founded on psychiatric observations and sought to relate body type to propensity for particular mental disorders. He argued that the asthenic was prone to schizophrenia, the pyknic to manic-depression and the athletic to sanity. There is little or no evidence to support Kretschmer's claims. Sheldon's theory is the most sophisticated of the three, based as it was on more modern findings in the structure of embryonic cellular tissue. Moreover, Sheldon sought a general theory of personality, not merely a psychiatric one. He argued there were three primary components in physique: *endomorphy* (heavy, poorly developed bones and muscles), *mesomorphy* (strong, well-developed bones and muscles), and *ectomorphy* (thin, light bones and muscles); and three primary components in temperament: *viscerotonia* (loving, comfortable, sociable), *somatotonia* (adventurous, vigorous, physical) and *cerebrotonia* (restrained, self-conscious, fearful). Sheldon's attempts to uncover correlations between the three body types and the three personality types was a noble effort which reflected a touch of validity, but as a unified theory of personality it was a failure. See also PERSONALITY (especially the discussion of *type theories*) and SOMATOTYPE.

constitutional types CONSTITUTIONAL THEORY.

constrained association ASSOCIATION, CONSTRAINED.

construct 1 n. The least confusing way to use this term is to treat it as a rough synonym of *concept*, at least in so far as both are basically logical or intellectual creations. Essentially one infers a construct whenever one can establish a relationship between several objects or events. In common use is the notion of a *hypothetical construct*, where the process is not presently observable or objectively measurable but is assumed to exist because it (hypothetically) gives rise to measurable phenomena. The EGO is a hypothetical construct in this sense. **2** n. In testing, a quality or a trait; see here CONSTRUCT *VALIDITY.

constructional apraxia APRAXIA, CONSTRUCTIONAL.

construction need H. Murray's hypothesized need to produce, to build things.

constructivism 1 In perception, a general theoretical position that characterizes perception and perceptual experience as being constructed from, in Gregory's words, 'fleeting fragmentary scraps of data signalled by the senses and drawn from the brain's memory banks – themselves constructions from snippets of the past'. The essence of all constructivist theories is that they view perceptual experience as more than a direct response to stimulation. They view it instead as an elaboration or 'construction' based on hypothesized cognitive and affective operations. Contrast with the theory of DIRECT PERCEPTION. **2** In social psychology, *social constructivism* approaches the study of social psychological topics from a similar philosophical stance. Social constructivists argue for some extreme but interesting positions, including the notion that there is no such thing as a knowable objective reality. Rather, they maintain, all knowledge is derived from the mental constructions of the members of a social system.

construct validity VALIDITY, CONSTRUCT.

consultant Generally, any expert brought in to provide advice and counsel.

consultation In medicine and clinical psychology, diagnosis and treatment plan arrived at through the combined efforts of two or more clinicians.

consultation-liaison psychiatry A psychiatric speciality that is concerned with the overall functioning of a health-care system.

consumer Clearly, one who consumes. The consumer in psychology, particularly social psychology and industrial psychology, is viewed as one who is the recipient and user of services and goods. This notion goes beyond simply treating a consumer as the purchaser of a head of lettuce; a consumer is also one who is a client in psychotherapy, a student in a university, a citizen in a society, and, indeed, he or she may also be a victim of the functions, operations and decisions of organizations in society. The term, obviously, is used rather broadly.

consumer psychology A branch of applied psychology that explores the principles that underlie the consumption of goods and services in a society. Sometimes known as *consumer research*, it examines applied topics such as marketing, the impact of advertising, and brand loyalty. It is also concerned with the scientific study of complex psychological processes, such as choice behaviour, decision-making, multidimensional scaling, preference formation and conscious and unconscious motivation.

consummatory response (or **act**) The behaviourist's term for the final response in a behaviour chain, the one which terminates in a frequently occurring sequence. Eating, drinking and copulating are all examples.

consummatory stimulus A stimulus that elicits a consummatory response.

contact 1 Generally, any face-to-face interaction between two or more people. 2 Within the contexts of Gestalt therapy and biofunctional therapy, a rich, fulfilled 'relationship'. It may be between a person and his or her bodily processes, between two individuals, between the several aspects of a group interaction, etc. The frequency with which we read, hear or meet people who have 'made contact' with themselves has unfortunately converted a useful phrase into something of a boring cliché.

contact comfort A term introduced by Harry Harlow to characterize the satisfying feeling that comes from making contact with soft, comfortable objects. The desire for contact comfort is common in many species and is particularly prevalent among the primates. It is known to be an important aspect of early development and for the establishment of normal mother–infant ties.

contact desensitization A variation of the DESENSITIZATION TECHNIQUE in behaviour therapy in which the therapist maintains physical contact with the client to help in lowering anxiety and facilitating the procedures.

contact hypothesis At its core, simply the hypothesis that direct face-to-face contact between members of conflicting social groups can, under certain conditions, reduce prejudice and hostility between the groups. Much of the research work has focused on specifying the conditions that are likely to produce this desirable effect.

contagion, behavioural (or **emotional**) Spread of an activity or a mood through a group. A classic example is group fainting – one child may faint while dissecting a frog in a biology lesson, promptly followed by numbers of others.

contamination The general meaning derives from the Latin for *to render impure*. Hence, **1** Any experimental or methodological situation in which one allows previous knowledge, uncontrolled variables, information concerning the expectations of the study, etc. to interfere with the proper collection and interpretation of the data. For example, a clinician searching for a hereditary basis for schizophrenia who knew that someone else in a patient's family already had the disorder would very likely have his or her diagnostic judgement 'contaminated' by this knowledge and tend to interpret any signs of a disorder as schizophrenia. **2** A process whereby substances, objects, foods and even persons become 'tainted' because of contact with some highly undesirable substance, object, food or person. For example, many people will consider an entire plate of food as 'contaminated' if a fly lands on one small corner of the plate.

contempt An emotional reaction to the perception of some thing, action or being that it is unworthy or inferior. Considered to be a *cold emotion*, its facial expression is presumed to be a unilateral lip curl, although there is little scientific evidence of a unique behavioural or facial expression.

contempt–anger–disgust triad hypothesis The proposal that these three emotions are: (a) elicited by violations of moral codes; (b) inform moral judgements; and (c) form the basis of human societies. The model assumes that violations of individual rights elicit anger, of social order and duty, contempt, and those of divinity and purity, disgust.

content **1** adj. With the accent on the second syllable, satisfied with things the way they are. **2** n. With the accent on the first syllable, that which is contained in something else. This meaning is very broad and used to refer to the sensations, images, thoughts, etc. of mind, the particular items or questions in a test, the material expressed in a dream, the elements of a communicated message, etc. Hence, it is usually accompanied by a qualifier, as the following entries show.

content-addressable store A term used in theoretical models of memory, particularly those manifested as computer simulations. The notion is that at least some components of human memory may be characterized as a set of storage registers for holding information, each with an 'address' that gives its 'location' in memory and the 'contents' of the store.

content analysis A general term covering a variety of methods for analysing a discourse, message or document for varying themes, ideas, emotions, opinions, etc. Most such analyses consist of sophisticated counting schemes in which the frequency of particular words, phrases, affective expressions and the like are determined.

content, latent and manifest These terms derive from depth psychology and are used to distinguish between those aspects of a 'message' that are overt, consciously intended and expressed, and found clearly represented in the material (i.e. they are *manifest*), and those aspects that are pre-

sumed to underlie the manifest content but are repressed and hence not consciously or overtly represented (i.e. they are *latent*). The message here may be considered broadly, and dreams, narratives, writings, etc. can be the topic of examination, although DREAM CONTENT is the most common and usually what is intended.

content psychology Occasional label for the approach of the early structuralists who were primarily concerned with the use of introspection to examine the contents of consciousness.

content validity VALIDITY, CONTENT.

content word Any word that has semantic content or meaning. Nouns, verbs, adjectives and adverbs are all content words. Contrast with FUNCTION WORD.

context **1** Generally, those events and processes (physical and mental) that characterize a particular situation and have an impact on an individual's behaviour (overt and covert). **2** The specific circumstances within which an action or event takes place. **3** In linguistics, the surrounding words, phrases and sentences that are components of the meaning of any given word, phrase or sentence.

context effects A cover term for those behavioural effects that result from the particular context within which a stimulus is presented or a response is made. No behaviour, no thought, no dream – in short, nothing any organism can ever do – can take place in a physical or psychic vacuum. Context effects are necessarily ubiquitous. This is at once a most trivial and most profound statement: ignoring its obvious truth has led more than a few well-meaning theorists to grief. The trick for the scientist is to discern just which context effects are significant and worthy of accounting for and which are negligible.

context specific learning LEARNING, CONTEXT SPECIFIC.

context theory A theoretical point of view maintaining that all behaviour must be analysed within the context in which it occurs, that to interpret any act independently of context will ultimately be misleading. Also called *contingency theory*.

contextualism CONTEXT THEORY.

contextual subtheory See TRIARCHIC THEORY OF INTELLIGENCE.

contiguity A state of close proximity or association, either in space or in time, of two or more events.

contiguity principle 1 Originating with Aristotle, the notion that contiguity between two events is both the necessary and the sufficient condition for a dynamic association between them to be formed. The years have brought many a vigorous criticism of this seemingly straightforward principle. The necessity of contiguity is challenged by simple memory processes whereby one can recall a previous event and associate it with a contemporary one. The natural rebuttal here is to note that the act of retrieval effectively makes the two events contiguous in the mind – but that somewhat robs the principle of explanatory power, since all associative operations must be contiguous within the individual and nothing is gained by invoking the principle. See here REDINTEGRATION. The sufficiency question has been challenged by the principle of reinforcement, which maintains that simple contiguity is not enough for an associative bond to be formed but rather must be accompanied by some reinforcing or rewarding event to 'cement' the link. The standard reply here is to turn the argument back on itself by pointing out that there is no satisfactory theoretical characterization of just what a reinforcer is, nor what makes or fails to make any arbitrary event function as one. See here REINFORCE-MENT. 2 In learning theory, the notion that a response made in the presence of a stimulus will be learned simply by virtue of the spatiotemporal contiguity between the two. See here CONTIGUITY THEORY.

contiguity theory A theory of learning usually associated with E. R. Guthrie. The position he articulated was the ultimate learning theory in terms of parsimony for it had but one principle, that of contiguity. Specifically, the last response to occur in the presence of a stimulus was assumed to be learned. All learning was assumed to be one-trial and all-or-none; the gradual improvement in performance usually observed was argued to be the result of the fact that most behaviours are made up of many complex responses and most stimuli are rather complicated affairs, and so many individual S–R connections were needed for effective behaviour. Praised for its elegance and widely tested and debated during the heyday of behaviourism, it has been since abandoned as a viable theory.

continence Self-restraint with respect to: 1 retention of urine, faeces and other bodily discharges; 2 sexual impulses.

contingency 1 In logic the characteristic of a proposition such that it does not have to be true or does not have to hold. 2 By extension, an event is said to be contingent on another if there exists some demonstrable relationship between the two such that the occurrence of one tends to be accompanied by the occurrence of the other. A contingency, stated thus, is a statistical circumstance and may be defined simply as the degree to which the values of one variable are related to the values of another variable. However, there is a strong tendency to use the term with the connotation that the relationship is more than fortuitous, that it is causal and that the occurrence of the second event is dependent (or 'contingent') upon the prior occurrence of the first. Note that 2 does not contradict 1; the second event (or proposition concerning it) need not occur by itself nor hold in isolation but only in conjunction with the first.

contingency coefficient A statistical measure (based on CHI-SQUARE) of the strength of association between two variables.

contingency contract In behaviour therapy, a contract drawn up between therapist and client so that it is clear precisely which behaviours the client must produce in order for reinforcements or rewards to be received.

contingency management The execution of a specific type of CONTINGENCY CON-TRACT in which the client is paid in either money or redeemable vouchers for verified abstinence from an undesirable behaviour or verified engagement in desirable behaviour.

contingency table A two-way table presenting the cross-tabulations of frequencies of occurrences of the categories of events listed in the columns and rows.

contingency theory See CONTEXT THEORY.

contingent aftereffect Any AFTEREFFECT where the visual experience in one dimension (e.g. colour) is contingent on another dimension (e.g. orientation), e.g. MCCULLOUGH EFFECT.

contingent reinforcement (or **reward**) REINFORCEMENT, CONTINGENT.

continuant In phonetics, a distinctive feature for distinguishing the sounds of a language. Continuants 'continue' over time (e.g. all vowels and certain consonants such as [r, l, th, s, z]), noncontinuants are characterized by a stoppage of the air flow (e.g. [p, t, b]).

continuation GOOD CONTINUATION and GESTALT LAWS OF ORGANIZATION.

continuity A characteristic of a system or a process such that it displays continuous, successive gradations. The term is used very generally to refer to physical variables, mental states, social systems, etc. which display uninterrupted changes. See CONTINUUM.

continuity, principle of The notion that objects travel in continuous paths and do not shift position without traversing intermediate points – even if those intermediate points are obscured from sight. Infants display an understanding of this principle at about 6 months.

continuity theory A theory of learning that maintains that associations are formed and gradually strengthened with each reward or reinforced response. Actually it is not so much a distinct theory as a general theoretical principle assumed in a variety of models of the learning process. Contrast with ALL-OR-NONE *LEARNING.

continuous Characterized by uninterrupted changes, without breaks or steps – or with steps infinitesimally small and thus not detectable. Thus, *continuous scales* are those in which the function measured is assumed to be continuous even though the measuring system is broken down into discrete units, as with height, weight, etc. Similarly for continuous series, continuous variables and so forth. Contrast with DISCRETE.

continuous reinforcement SCHEDULES OF *REINFORCEMENT.

continuum 1 Most generally, any uninterrupted series of changes, any continuous, gradually changing sequence of values. 2 In mathematics, a variable with a continuous underlying metric such that for any two values there exists a third value between them. 3 Somewhat less formally, any variable capable of being represented as a continuous series. In psychological work, such continua are typically represented by polar labels; e.g. the pleasantness dimension runs from unpleasant to pleasant, with all intermediate points existing in principle.

contour The outline of a figure or object. The term is used metaphorically in that the outline exists only in so far as there is a marked difference in brightness, texture or colour between two adjoining places in the visual field. The line of demarcation is strictly psychological.

contour, subjective A contour perceived where there is none in the physical stimulus but only the requisite conditions for its inference by the viewer, as in the figure on p. 168. Also known as *anomalous, cognitive* and *illusory contours*.

contra- Combining form meaning *against* or *opposite*.

contraception The term used for any of several methods of birth control which prevent the fertilization of an ovum by a sperm cell. See BIRTH CONTROL.

contract, psychological The unwritten set of expectations that exists between the persons in a relationship, the members of a group, the people who work for an organization, etc. The term is used most often in industrial/organizational psychology, where it covers the levels of performance that each member of an organization is expected to reach and each member's own expectations with respect to salary advancement, benefits, perquisites, etc. Moreover, such nebulous components as the quality of life, job satisfaction and personal fulfilment are implicitly a part of the psychological contract.

contracture Relatively permanent contraction of a muscle due either to a spasm (usually temporary) or an abnormal paralytic condition (often permanent).

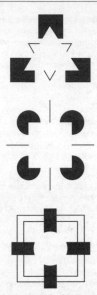

Several examples of subjective contours

contradictory 1 n. In logic, either of two propositions which cannot both be true and cannot both be false; that is, if one is true the other is necessarily false, and vice versa. See and compare with CONTRARY. **2** adj. Descriptive of an interaction or discourse containing contradictions.

contralateral Pertaining to the opposite side. Contrast with IPSILATERAL.

contralateral reflex Any reflex occurring on the opposite side of the body from that stimulated. Also called *consensual reflex* and *crossed reflex*.

contrary In logic, either of two propositions which may both be false but cannot both be true. For example, the proposition 'All lexicographers are mad' has as a contrary 'No lexicographers are mad', and both are (probably) false. However, the first proposition has a CONTRADICTORY, 'Not all lexicographers are mad', and either this or the second proposition must be true.

contrast A marked difference between two stimulus conditions revealed by bringing them together. The contrast may be *simultaneous*, in that the events or stimuli are pre-

sented together in time and space, or it may be *successive*, in that one event follows the other in close succession. Simultaneous contrasts are generally more striking. Such effects are observed in a large number of stimulus dimensions. Descriptions of these are listed under the main term, e.g. COLOUR CONTRAST.

contrast effect A disproportionate increase in a response with an increase in incentive. That is, if an animal is bar-pressing for 1 g of food reinforcement and is suddenly shifted to 5 g it will characteristically respond at a higher rate than a comparable animal that has been receiving 5 g reinforcements all along. There is also a corresponding negative effect. Also known as the *Crespi effect* after the psychologist who did the initial research on it.

contrast, principle of The associationistic principle that observing or thinking about a particular quality tends to produce recall of its opposite.

contrasuggestibility A tendency (seemingly possessed by all children) to take a position counter to or opposite to one which has been suggested.

contrectation 1 Generally, to touch with the hands. **2** Specifically, sexual fondling and caressing.

control 1 The exercise of the scientific method whereby the various treatments in an experiment are regulated so that the causal factors may be unambiguously identified. The essence of the term is one of exclusion in that the scientist seeks to eliminate the effects of irrelevant variables by 'controlling' them, leaving only the experimental variable(s) free to change. **2** Manipulation; the ability to modify and change behaviour by systematic use of appropriate reinforcements and punishments. This is the sense of the term in the behaviourist tenet that one of the basic goals of psychology is the *control* of behaviour.

control experiment An experiment designed to replicate and solidify the findings of a previous study by specifically evaluating the effects of a variable that was not (or was only partially) controlled in the original.

control group (or **condition**) A group (or

condition) in an experiment that is as closely matched as possible to the experimental group (or condition) except that it is not exposed to the independent variable(s) under investigation.

controlled analysis Psychoanalysis in which the analyst is a trainee and is carefully supervised by a qualified analyst.

controlled association ASSOCIATION, CONTROLLED.

controlled sampling SAMPLING, CONTROLLED.

controlled variable INDEPENDENT *VARIABLE.

control, statistical When irrelevant factors are beyond direct experimental control it may be necessary to allow for their effects by making mathematical corrections of the actual data. Such corrections are referred to as statistical controls since they do not enter into the analysis until the data are subjected to statistical evaluations.

control strategy Loosely, any technique designed to control the behaviour of another. It is most often used for those employed by adults to change problematic behaviour of a child. Sometimes called *control practices*.

control variable VARIABLE, CONTROL.

convenience sampling SAMPLING, CONVENIENCE.

conventionality 1 Acting according to standard social practices. 2 A personality characteristic manifested by a tendency to adhere strongly to social conventions. Conventionality is viewed by many as a component of the AUTHORITARIAN PERSONALITY.

conventional level of moral development MORAL DEVELOPMENT.

convergence 1 Generally, the property of tending toward a particular point. Used of several elements or components of a system that are oriented in a coordinated manner at a specific locale. Hence: 2 In perception, the turning of the eyes inward to focus on an object that is being viewed binocularly. As a binocular cue for depth perception it is most effective with objects relatively close to the observer. Compare with DIVERGENCE. 3 In neurophysiology, the coming together

of several neural processes on a single neuron or on a neural pathway or neural centre.

convergent evolution Evolution of similar forms and structures in genetically unrelated species as a reaction to similar lifestyles or environmental factors. See ANALOGUE (2).

convergent thinking THINKING, CONVERGENT.

convergent validity VALIDITY, CONVERGENT AND DISCRIMINANT.

conversational maxims H. P. Grice's term for those basic principles of conversation that speakers normally adhere to in order to optimize communication. He identified four such: (a) *quantity* – do not provide too much (nor too little) information; (b) *quality* – do not say that which you know to be false, be genuine; (c) *relation* – be relevant; and (d) *manner* – be orderly, brief and nonobscure. The terms *conversational postulates* and *cooperative principle* are rough synonyms, although they are typically used in a more general sense, encompassing all the maxims.

conversational postulates CONVERSATIONAL MAXIMS.

converse In logic, a proposition derived by conversion (reversing the terms) of another proposition.

conversion The standard meaning is the transformation of something from one state to another. Hence: 1 The dramatic shift from one set of beliefs to another, especially religious beliefs. PRIVATE ACCEPTANCE is an occasional synonym. 2 The transformation of a psychological maladjustment into physical forms (see CONVERSION DISORDER). 3 The shift of a set of scores from one scale to another. 4 The interchanging of the terms in a proposition.

conversion disorder A SOMATOFORM DISORDER characterized by the 'conversion' of a psychic conflict into somatic form. The symptoms can vary widely and blindness, deafness, paralysis, seizures, mutism, loss of balance, anaesthesia and a host of other dysfunctions have all been recorded. The resulting functional disorder may appear superficially to have physical or physiological causes but may frequently follow no known organic system (see e.g. GLOVE ANAESTHESIA). The presenting symptoms are not feigned and not under conscious control. Also called *conversion reaction, conversion hysteria* or *hysterical neurosis, conversion type*.

convolution A fold of the cerebral cortex, a GYRUS. Convolutions are marked as the areas between the sulci or fissures.

convulsant Any agent that produces a convulsion.

convulsion A general, molar, extensive seizure with involuntary muscular contraction and relaxation. Contrast with SPASM, which is small and localized, and with CLONUS, which is a slow, rhythmic contraction.

convulsive disorders A general cover term for a class of pathological conditions in which convulsions are a common symptom. Included are Jacksonian epilepsy, psychomotor epilepsy and other centrencephalic seizures, all of which are demonstrably brain disorders with characteristic EEG patterns. Not included are various other conditions which may display seizures as symptoms.

convulsive therapy A generic label for a number of psychotherapeutic procedures based on the artificial inducing of a convulsion. The use of convulsive therapy derived from the observation that epilepsy and schizophrenia rarely co-occur – a classic case of the fallacious inferring of cause and effect from correlation. Such procedures seem to have no effect on schizophrenic symptoms, although some are of value in certain cases of depression. For details on specific convulsive therapies see ELECTROCONVULSIVE SHOCK THERAPY and INSULIN THERAPY.

co-occurrence COVARIATION.

Coolidge effect The phenomenon that the males of many species will show high continuous sexual performance for extended periods of time with introductions of new, receptive females. The name for the effect derives from an old and very bad joke about the American president Calvin Coolidge, which space limitations prevent telling here.

cooperative learning LEARNING, COOPERATIVE.

cooperative play PLAY, COOPERATIVE.

coordinate 1 vb. To organize or arrange objects, events, concepts, etc. according to a prescribed or harmonious pattern. 2 n. One of the dimensions by which a point is located in space. 3 adj. Equal in rank or value as compared with being *subordinate* or *supraordinate*.

coordinate bilingual BILINGUALISM.

coordinate morality ARCHETYPAL FORM.

coordination Generally, harmonious interrelated functioning of the several elements of a system, as in motor coordination or hand–eye coordination.

coping strategies Conscious, rational ways of dealing with the anxieties and challenges of life. The term is used for those strategies designed to deal with the source of the anxiety; e.g. a student anxious about a forthcoming examination copes by studying especially long hours for it. Compare with DEFENSIVE STRATEGIES, which are directed at the anxiety itself rather than its source.

copro- Combining form meaning *faeces, filth, excrement*, etc. A creative person can find no end of uses for this prefix. Existing technical ones are given in the following entries.

coprolagnia COPROPHILIA (2).

coprolalia 1 Generally, excessive use of verbal obscenities. 2 A verbal tic disorder consisting of repeating vulgarities, or often simply the initial part of a vulgarity, as frequently seen in TOURETTE'S SYNDROME.

coprophagia Lit., eating faeces.

coprophilia 1 An unusual interest in faeces. 2 A PARAPHILIA, in which sexual arousal and pleasure are obtained from faeces. Also called *coprolagnia*.

copulation COITUS.

copulin A vaginal pheromone isolated in rhesus monkeys which stimulates the male to copulate. The level of secretion is highest at the time of ovulation, thereby maximizing the likelihood of impregnation.

cord Occasional shorthand for *spinal cord*.

core gender (or **sex**) **identity** A term used in psychoanalytic models of sexual development to refer to the early sense of self as male or female. This identification is assumed to occur in the second year of life.

core knowledge KNOWLEDGE, CORE.

corium The 'true' skin, the layer lying directly below the epidermis. Hair follicles, sweat glands and smooth muscle fibres all lie in it.

cornea The transparent outer layer of the eye covering the iris and the pupil. The cornea is completely free of blood vessels and functions as a refractor of light.

corneal reflection technique A procedure whereby one may make a detailed analysis of eye movements by photographing the movements of light reflected off the cornea.

Cornelia de Lange syndrome A congenital syndrome characterized by mental retardation, short stature, skeletal abnormalities and a variety of facial features including a small, rounded head, bushy, confluent eyebrows and a sharply upturned nose. Aetiology is unknown, although a hereditary basis is suspected.

Cornell technique Another name for GUTT-MAN SCALING. Occasionally called *Guttman–Cornell technique*.

cornu ammonis HIPPOCAMPUS.

corollary A proposition that follows naturally from something else, needing no additional proof. Contrast with THEOREM, which does require proof.

coronal In phonetics, a distinctive feature characterizing sounds produced with the blade of the tongue raised slightly (e.g. *t* in *top*); in noncoronals the tongue remains in a neutral position (e.g. *p* in *pop*).

coronal section SECTION (2).

corporal Bodily. Hence, corporal punishment is physical punishment to the body.

corpora quadrigemina Four prominent elevations on the dorsal surface of the midbrain. The anterior pair (also called the *superior colliculi*) mediate visual reflexes, the posterior pair (*inferior colliculi*) contain auditory centres. See COLLICULUS for more detail.

corpus 1 A body or a principal part of a body or organ. **2** In studies of language, the set of words, sentences and other linguistic forms that a language learner is exposed to. pl., *corpora*.

corpus callosum The great commissure of the brain, the band of myelinated fibres that serves interconnecting functions between the two cerebral hemispheres, located at the floor of the longitudinal fissure. The corpus callosum transfers information from one hemisphere to the other; it is through it that the 'left brain' knows what the 'right brain' has seen, felt, heard, etc. and vice versa. Severing the callosum produces a SPLIT BRAIN.

corpuscle 1 Generally, any small round body. **2** An encapsulated sensory nerve ending. See e.g. PACINIAN CORPUSCLE.

corpus luteum A progesterone-secreting endocrine structure that develops within a ruptured ovarian follicle. See MENSTRUAL CYCLE for more detail.

corpus striatum From the Latin for *striated body*. That portion of the forebrain containing the CAUDATE NUCLEUS, LENTICULAR NUCLEUS and INTERNAL CAPSULE.

correction 1 Generally, any specific manipulation that counters the effects of error. Hence: **2** In statistical analysis of data any transformation or manipulation of scores that minimizes errors of observation, chance or other factors. **3** In vision, the use of lenses to correct for refractive errors of the eye. **4** In social/criminological terms, altering an individual's behaviour to bring it into conformity with society's norms; prisons are often called (perhaps euphemistically) *correctional institutes*.

correction for chance CORRECTION FOR GUESSING.

correction for continuity A statistical correction required in the use of some statistical tests when the actual data are from a discrete distribution but the test assumes an underlying continuous distribution.

correction for guessing Adjustment of the scores on a test by subtracting from the number of correct answers the number that presumably could have been answered correctly by pure chance or by simple guessing. Also called *correction for chance*.

corrective 1 n. Generally, any procedure that produces a correction. **2** n. In pharmacology, any drug that modifies the action of another drug. **3** adj. Pertaining to such a drug or its action.

correlate 1 n. Any of two variables or factors which are systematically related to each other; that is, they 'co-relate'. **2** n. A principle or an argument that is strongly indicated by some other principle or argument. This meaning is a loose way of connoting in non-formal situations what is meant by *corollary*; e.g. 'It is a correlate of computer simulation work that theories will be formally testable.' **3** vb. To place a thing in a situation where it is in a known relation to another thing. **4** vb. To calculate a CORRELATION COEFFICIENT.

correlated Descriptive of a relationship between variables such that they show a non-zero correlation coefficient, i.e. they reveal some reliable statistical dependency on each other.

correlation 1 In statistics, a relationship between two (or more) variables such that systematic increases or decreases in the magnitude of one variable are accompanied by systematic increases or decreases in the magnitude of the other(s). The existence of such a statistical relationship is traditionally used as a basis for making predictions about the expected magnitude of one variable given the known magnitude of the other(s). The stronger the relationship (i.e. the further from zero the obtained correlation coefficient), the greater the confidence in the accuracy of prediction. **2** Somewhat more loosely, any relationship between things such that some concomitant or dependent changes in one (or more) occur with changes in the other(s). Note that in both of these usages one properly withholds the presumption of causality between the variables. Correlations are statements about concomitance; they may suggest, but do not necessarily imply, that the changes in one variable are producing or causing the changes in the other(s). **3** In physiology, the overall processes by which the various bodily processes occur in coordinated relation to each other. Distinguish from NEUROLOGICAL *CORRELATION.

correlational statistics STATISTICS, CORRELATIONAL.

correlation, biserial (r$_{bis}$) A correlation in

which one variable is measured on a graduated or many-valued scale and the other is dichotomous or two-valued; for example, the correlation between the pass–fail rate on a course and scores on an academic aptitude battery.

correlation, canonical A measure of the relationship between two sets or groups of variables. The technique is based on calculating a core (or *canonical*) value for the several variables in each set. A classic example would be finding a correlation between several indices of community violence (one set) and a number of measures of child functioning (the other set). Also called *canonical analysis*.

correlation, chance-half CORRELATION, SPLIT-HALF.

correlation cluster A group of variables all of which have higher positive correlations with each other than with other groups of variables or single variables. Such a cluster is taken as evidence of the existence of a *factor* in *factor analysis*.

correlation coefficient A number that expresses the degree and direction of relationship between two (or occasionally, more) variables. The correlation coefficient may range from −1.00 (indicating a perfect NEGATIVE *CORRELATION) to +1.00 (indicating a perfect POSITIVE *CORRELATION). The higher the value, either negative or positive, the greater the concomitance between the variables. A value of 0.00 indicates no correlation: changes in one variable are statistically independent of changes in the other. A large number of statistical procedures exist for determining the correlation coefficient between variables, depending on the nature of the data and the methods of collection. The PRODUCT-MOMENT *CORRELATION is the most commonly used, and when the terms *correlation coefficient* or, simply, *correlation* are found without qualifiers they may be taken to mean this particular measure. Other forms of correlation are usually clearly identified.

correlation, curvilinear Generally, any correlation in which the rate (or rates) of change of the variables is nonlinear. See CURVILINEAR *REGRESSION. Also called *nonlinear correlation* and, on occasion, *skew correlation*.

correlation, direct An occasional synonym for POSITIVE *CORRELATION.

correlation, first-order A PARTIAL *CORRELATION in which the influences of only one variable are held constant.

correlation, fourfold point PHI COEFFICIENT.

correlation, indirect (or **inverse**) Occasional synonyms for NEGATIVE *CORRELATION.

correlation, intraclass A measure of the degree to which two or more raters' judgements show INTERRATER *RELIABILITY. There are several procedures in use, all of which, unlike most other methods, can be used with more than two raters.

correlation, Kendall rank (and **Kendall partial rank**) KENDALL TESTS.

correlation, linear Any correlation in which unit-sized changes in one variable are associated with unit-sized changes in another; that is, the *regression line* is a straight line. Most statistical procedures for obtaining a correlation coefficient are based on this assumption of linearity.

correlation matrix MATRIX, CORRELATION.

correlation, multiple (**R**) The relationship between one (dependent) variable and two or more (independent) variables. A multiple correlation coefficient yields an estimate of the combined influence of the independent variables on the dependent.

correlation, negative A correlation in which increases in one variable are associated with decreases in another or in which large values in one variable are associated with small values in the other. The coefficient has negative values between 0 and −1.00. Also called *inverse* or *indirect correlation*.

correlation, neurological A hypothesis that there is a direct correspondence between each distinct mental or behavioural act of an organism and a particular set of unique neurological events.

correlation, nonlinear CURVILINEAR *CORRELATION.

correlation, part SEMIPARTIAL *CORRELATION.

correlation, partial The resulting correlation between two variables after the effects of one or more other related variables have been removed.

correlation, Pearson product-moment PRODUCT-MOMENT *CORRELATION.

correlation, perfect A correlation in which every change in one variable is matched by an equivalent change in another; the correlation coefficient here is either +1.00 or −1.00. (Don't hold your breath looking for one of these in the social sciences.)

correlation, phi PHI COEFFICIENT.

correlation, point-biserial A correlation in which one variable is measured on a continuous scale and the other is dichotomous or two-valued. Contrast with BISERIAL *CORRELATION, which is used when one scale is graduated but not continuous.

correlation, positive A correlation in which increases in one variable are associated with increases in another; or in which large values in one variable are associated with large values in the other, and small with small. The correlation coefficient has positive values between 0 and +1.00. Also called, on occasion, *direct correlation*.

correlation, product-moment (**r**) The most commonly used method of measuring a correlation between two quantitative variables that are related in a linear fashion. The early work on the mathematics of the procedure was done by Karl Pearson, and it is often called the Pearson product-moment correlation, or simply the Pearson correlation. It is a *parametric* test and, as such, is based on the usual parametric assumptions. The *product-moment*, which is the foundation of the correlation, is the mean (or the sum) of the products of the deviations of each score from the mean of each variable.

correlation, rank-difference RANK-ORDER *CORRELATION.

correlation, rank-order A correlation which is based on the ranks of the scores on the two variables. It is derived from the Pearson product-moment correlation and is the most widely used *nonparametric* correlation. It is often called the *rank-difference correlation* because the critical factor in the calculation of the coefficient is the difference between the ranks on the two variables. Occasionally called *Spearman rank-order correlation*.

correlation ratio A measure of the extent to which a given regression line departs from linearity.

correlation, semipartial A type of MULTIPLE *CORRELATION in which one variable is partialled out but only from one of several other variables. Also called *part correlation*.

correlation, simple 1 Any correlation based on only two variables, as contrasted with *multiple correlation*. 2 Any linear correlation, as compared with a *curvilinear correlation*.

correlation, skew CURVILINEAR *CORRELATION.

correlation, Spearman rank-order RANK-ORDER *CORRELATION.

correlation, split-half The correlation between the scores on two halves of a test. See SPLIT-HALF *RELIABILITY.

correlation, spurious A correlation that results not from any direct relationship between the variables under assessment but from their relationships to a third variable (or fourth, or more) that has no connecting relationship with them. For example, there is a significant positive correlation between the number of letters and corresponding letter names that a child knows when entering school and his or her success in reading. However, specific teaching of this information to children during preschool years has proven ineffective in later reading instruction. The correlation is spurious: the critical factor is not knowing letters and their names but being raised in homes in which intellectual activity is prized, which almost invariably leads to the alphabet being taught as a matter of course.

correlation table A two-way tabulation of the relationship between the values of two variables. The scores on one variable are given in the row headings, the scores on the other in the column headings, and the intersection cells show frequency for the corresponding values on each. Such tables are useful in the preparation and presentation of correlational analyses.

correlation, tetrachoric (r$_t$) A correlation

based on two variables each of which is expressed as a dichotomy (two-valued). The tetrachoric, however, is based (mathematically) on the assumption that both variables are continuous and normally distributed but only expressed, for the purposes in hand, as dichotomous.

correspondence bias The tendency to see an individual's behaviour as corresponding to an internal disposition or trait. The term is often used interchangeably with FUNDAMENTAL *ATTRIBUTION ERROR.

correspondent inference theory A theory of attribution based on the notion that while the CORRESPONDENCE BIAS tends to be the preferred attribution for an actor's behaviour, it is adjusted to the extent that the actor is seen as having little choice and/or is engaging in socially desirable behaviour. Note that this theory seeks only to explain single observed instances. For a theory of multiple observations over time, see COVARIATION MODEL OF ATTRIBUTION.

corresponding retinal points Usually: 1 A synonym for CONGRUENT RETINAL POINTS. Unfortunately, on occasion: 2 A synonym for IDENTICAL RETINAL POINTS.

cortex From the Latin, meaning *bark* or *rind*. It is used to refer generally to the outer layer of tissue of any organ and specifically, and most commonly, to the CEREBRAL CORTEX. pl., *cortices*.

cortex, association ASSOCIATION AREAS.

cortex, motor MOTOR AREAS.

cortex, sensory SENSORY AREAS.

Corti, organ of ORGAN OF CORTI.

cortical Pertaining to a cortex, usually, although not exclusively, the CEREBRAL CORTEX. The following entries give some idea of the ways in which the term is used.

cortical blindness CEREBRAL *BLINDNESS.

cortical centre A cortical area or region which serves as a terminal point for incoming sensory nerve fibres or as an origin for motor fibres.

cortical control Control *of* subcortical centres *by* cortical ones; not vice versa.

cortical deafness CEREBRAL *DEAFNESS.

cortical dominance See the discussions under DOMINANCE (especially 5, 6, 7) and CEREBRAL DOMINANCE.

cortical induction Cortical activity in one area resulting from activity in an adjoining area.

cortical inhibition Inhibition or blocking of neural impulses by a cortical centre.

corticalization The gradual subsuming of control of behavioural and psychological processes by the cerebral cortex. Corticalization can be seen as an evolutionary process; it increases with ascent up the phylogenetic scale, its most prominent manifestation being in the primates. See ENCEPHALIZATION.

cortical processes Those processes mediated by cortical tissue. The term is frequently used as a synonym for *voluntary* or *conscious* processes. A phrase such as 'cortically mediated response' can be read as 'voluntary response'.

cortico- Combining form meaning CORTICAL.

cortico-basal ganglionic degeneration A PARKINSON-PLUS SYNDROME characterized by postural abnormalities, apraxia and rigidity. General cognitive deficits similar to those seen in Parkinsonism are also present. Also known as *corticostriatonigral degeneration*.

corticoid CORTICOSTEROID (HORMONES).

corticomedial group A group of nuclei that make up the phylogenetically older part of the *amygdala*. They receive sensory information about the presence of *pheromones* and send it to the *forebrain* and the *hypothalamus*.

corticospinal pathway A complex neural pathway arising in the *cortex* (mainly in the primary motor area) and terminating in the ventral grey matter of the *spinal cord*. The axons that make up the *lateral corticospinal tract* cross over in the medulla and synapse on spinal motor neurons and interneurons that control movements of the arms and hands. Those that make up the *ventral corticospinal tract* cross over near the terminal point in the spine and control movements of the muscles of the trunk.

corticospinal tract CORTICOSPINAL PATHWAY.

corticosteroid (hormones) Any of several steroid hormones that are produced in the cortex of the adrenal glands. Included are the GLUCOCORTICOIDS such as CORTISOL and the MINERALOCORTICOIDS such as ALDOSTERONE. Corticosteroids are important elements in the body's reactions to stress; they also modulate immune responses, help in regulation of inflammation and have important metabolic functions.

corticosterone A CORTICOSTEROID (HORMONE) produced by the cortex of the ADRENAL GLANDS; it influences metabolism of the carbohydrates and of sodium and potassium.

corticostriatonigral degeneration CORTICO-BASAL GANGLIONIC DEGENERATION.

corticotrophic hormone ADRENOCORTICOTROPHIC HORMONE.

cortin An extract of the adrenal cortex; it contains several active steroids, e.g. *corticosterone*.

cortisol A CORTICOSTEROID (HORMONE) that is intimately involved in the body's reaction to stress. It suppresses the immune system, has anti-inflammatory properties, increases blood pressure and elevates blood sugar levels. Abnormally high levels due to long-term chronic stress are associated with muscle wasting, hyperglycemia, and damage to cells in the hippocampus resulting in memory loss. Cortisol undergoes natural diurnal regulation; highest levels occur in the morning and drop off throughout the day, hitting their lowest point during sleep.

cortisone A CORTICOSTEROID (HORMONE) similar to CORTISOL. In synthetic form it is a useful anti-inflammatory drug for arthritis, bursitis and some skin conditions.

cost-benefit analysis As borrowed from economics, the computation of potential costs and benefits of a particular action. The assumption is that people engage in a hasty computation when faced with daily decisions, particularly in situations that call for altruistic acts. For example, upon seeing a young parent struggling up steps with a stroller an observer might weigh the benefits of feeling good after helping against the costs of the effort and being late for work.

costly punishment PUNISHMENT, COSTLY.

Cotard's syndrome A delusional disorder marked by any one of a series of delusions ranging from being convinced that one has lost organs or other body parts to believing that one has no soul or is, in fact, dead. In extreme cases, the patient fulfils the ultimate existential moment and is convinced that he or she does not exist. It is rarely seen outside of severe psychoses such as schizophrenia and bipolar disorder although it has been observed in patients with lesions of the non-dominant temporal-parietal cortex.

co-twin control An experimental procedure whereby hereditary factors can be controlled. One member of a pair of identical twins is subjected to an experimental treatment while the other is not.

counselling A generic term that is used to cover the several processes of interviewing, testing, guiding, advising, etc. designed to help an individual solve problems, plan for the future, etc. Clinicians who specialize in guidance in marital problems, drug abuse, vocational selection, community work, etc. are often called *counselling psychologists*. var., *counseling*.

counselling, marriage MARITAL THERAPY.

counter- Combining form generally meaning *opposed* but with two different connotations: (a) *against*, as in *countersuggestion* or *counteract*; and (b) *complementary* or *reciprocal*, as in *counterpart*.

counter 1 n. An agent or instrument that counts things, e.g. clocks count seconds. **2** n. In operant conditioning, a stimulus one dimension of which varies with the number of responses that a subject has made. This systematic variation essentially 'counts' responses and, if the organism attends to it, it functions as a source of information about its behaviour. **3** An agent or process that functions in an opposing manner, one that counters the actions of another agent or process. vb., *to counter*.

counteraction need H. Murray's term for a need to overcome failure, to strive forward after defeat.

counterbalancing An experimental procedure for controlling irrelevant factors. A good example is fatigue: if a subject is to perform two tasks, *x* and *y*, the order of running

would be counterbalanced so that fatigue factors were spread equally across both *x* and *y*. To wit: one half of the subjects would perform task *x* first and one half task *y* first. If the experiment were run so that all subjects performed *x* first, it would not be possible to tell whether *y* was more difficult than *x* or merely that the subjects were getting tired.

countercathexis ANTICATHEXIS.

countercompulsion A compulsion adopted to counter the effects of another compulsion.

counterconditioning An experimental procedure whereby a second, incompatible response is conditioned to an already conditioned stimulus. For example, a rat trained to press a bar in the presence of a light may be counterconditioned to turn a wheel when the light comes on. The general principle here lies behind many of the procedures used in behaviour therapy in which the modification of the client's behaviour consists of training up new responses to stimuli that are incompatible with the old ones. For example, DESENSITIZATION is basically conditioning a relaxation response to a stimulus that once evoked anxiety.

counterfactual A contrary-to-fact conditional statement or hypothetical instance which, for any number of reasons, cannot be subjected to empirical evaluation. Some counterfactuals may be beyond technology (e.g. 'If the sun's energy were diminished by 10%, life on earth could not exist'), others lie outside of ethical considerations (e.g. 'If we do not inoculate, millions will die'), while others still are historical hypotheticals (e.g. 'If Hitler had become a successful artist, World War II would not have occurred'). Counterfactuals play an important role in the evaluation of theories since they lead one to examine the formal structure of theoretical explanations to see which counterfactuals could be viewed as supportive and which fail to provide support. See MENTAL *EXPERIMENT.

counterfeit role ROLE, COUNTERFEIT.

counterformity ANTICONFORMITY.

counteridentification In analytic psychotherapy, a form of COUNTERTRANSFERENCE that occurs when the therapist identifies with the client as a reaction to the client's identification with the analyst.

counterintuitive 1 Generally, characterizing propositions that violate currently held beliefs or depart from common sense. The proposition may turn out to be correct; the sense of violation stemming from the fact that the assumptions were wrong. More than a few important scientific proposals appeared to be counterintuitive at first (e.g. Einstein's theories). **2** Of statements that violate normal semantic, physical and folk assumptions, as in expressions like 'walking dead', or in references to floating rocks or cats who wink knowingly at you. Here, the possible truth value is missing.

counterinvestment In psychoanalytic theory, the attachment of an overt feeling that is counter (or opposite) to a supposedly repressed one, such as displaying love when one unconsciously hates (or, for that matter, showing hate when one loves). The difficulty encountered with this notion is how to know what the 'real' emotion is. Projective tests are thought by many to reveal the deep, unconscious motives, but there are problems: see PROJECTIVE TECHNIQUES for a discussion.

counterphobic character A psychoanalytic term for the type of person who regularly engages in and derives pleasure from behaviours and activities that 'normally' would be regarded as dangerous and anxiety-provoking.

countershock phase The second part of the alarm reaction stage in the GENERAL ADAPTATION SYNDROME.

countersuggestion 1 Generally, a suggestion designed to overcome or 'counter' a previously made suggestion. **2** In Piagetian research, a suggestion made to a child that counters or contradicts something the child has previously said or claimed is true. The purpose is to evaluate how robust the child's belief is and to determine how the child will defend his or her belief against the countersuggestion.

countertransference 1 In psychoanalysis, the analyst's displacement of affect (i.e. TRANSFERENCE) onto the client. **2** More generally, the analyst's emotional involvement in the therapeutic interaction. In the former

sense countertransference is a distorting element in a psychoanalysis and can be disruptive; in the latter sense it is considered benign and, by some, inevitable.

counterwill O. Rank's term for, quite simply, the ability to say 'no'. For Rank this represented the key concept in the development of a healthy personality. Note, this resistance of will covers both external pressures from others and internal impulses.

count/mass noun distinction The linguistic distinction between entities that are discrete, individuated and countable (e.g. trees, computers, plates) and those that are not (water, salt, honey). Languages (like English) that mark this distinction have rules for pluralization and article use. The distinction is important in the debate about whether features marked in speech reflect or influence the learning of *natural categories* and in theories of child language acquisition. Also called *mass/count noun distinction*.

couples therapy The terms *marital therapy*, *marriage therapy*, *marriage counselling* and the like all imply that a couple should be married in order to seek advice and help with their relationship. This term has been introduced to reflect the reality that many persons who are in long-term relationships not graced by state or church are also in need of therapy.

couvade (*coo-vahd*) The experiencing of the rigours of pregnancy and childbirth by the father. The turmoil of the male is quite real and indicative of the effectiveness of psychosomatic phenomena. While it exists as a custom in some societies, it also occurs spontaneously in all.

covariance Lit., covariation. Changes in one variable accompanied by changes in another. This coordinated variance is expressed by $\Sigma xy/N$, where x and y are deviations of each score from the means of each variable and N is the number of cases.

covariate Any variable that is controlled for by statistically subtracting out its effects by the use of ANALYSIS OF COVARIANCE or MULTIPLE REGRESSION.

covariation A relationship between objects or events such that they systematically vary together in ways that lead to the conclusion that they are causally linked. Distinguish from *co-occurrence*, the connotation of which is only that the events occur together. To appreciate the importance of this distinction see CORRELATION (1, 2) and RESCORLA–WAGNER THEORY.

covariation model of attribution A theory of attribution designed to explain how social perceivers attribute observed behaviour when they have multiple observations to draw on. According to H. Kelley, who first proposed the model, people rely on the observed covariation between the hypothesized cause and the observed behaviour. In particular, people rely on *consensus information* (to what degree do other people behave the same way in this situation?), *distinctiveness information* (to what extent is this behaviour by this actor only elicited by this situation?) and *consistency information* (to what extent does this actor–situation pairing always result in this behaviour?).

cover memory SCREEN MEMORY.

covert Covered, disguised, hidden. The term is most often used to refer to processes that cannot be directly observed, such as imagery or thought.

covert desensitization See DESENSITIZATION PROCEDURE.

covert extinction A technique in behaviour therapy whereby the client imagines that reinforcements are no longer forthcoming for the behaviour that is to be extinguished.

covert reinforcement A technique in behaviour therapy whereby the client imagines reinforcers occurring for the behaviours that are desired. Usually used with anxiety disorders, the client imagining the rewards of successfully coping with the anxiety-producing situation.

covert speech SUBVOCALIZATION.

CP 1 CEREBRAL *PALSY. **2** In linguistics, a clause. **3** In pragmatics, the *cooperative principle*. See CONVERSATIONAL MAXIMS.

CPI CALIFORNIA PSYCHOLOGICAL INVENTORY.

CPT CURRENT PROCEDURAL TERMINOLOGY.

CR 1 CONDITIONED RESPONSE. **2** CRITICAL RATIO.

cranial Pertaining to the CRANIUM.

cranial capacity The volume of the CRANIUM.

cranial division The uppermost part of the parasympathetic division of the AUTONOMIC NERVOUS SYSTEM.

cranial index CEPHALIC INDEX.

cranial nerves The 12 nerves that enter and leave the brain directly rather than through the spinal cord (SEE SPINAL NERVES). They are numbered and individually named:
I *Olfactory*: smell; afferent from olfactory receptors.
II *Optic*: efferent controlling vision; afferent from retina.
III *Oculomotor*: efferent to eye muscles; all external muscles except oblique and rectus.
IV *Trocular*: oblique muscles of eye.
V *Trigeminal*: efferent and afferent serving face, nose and tongue.
VI *Abducens*: efferent to rectus muscles of eye.
VII *Facial*: efferent to facial muscles; afferent from taste buds, anterior part of the tongue.
VIII *Vestibulocochlear*: afferent serving hearing and balance. Also called *auditory-vestibular* or, simply, *auditory*.
IX *Glossopharyngeal*: efferent to the throat; afferent from taste buds, posterior part of the tongue.
X *Vagus*: afferent and efferent serving heart, lungs, thorax, larynx, pharynx, external ear and abdominal viscera.
XI *Spinal accessory*: afferent and efferent serving neck muscles.
XII *Hypoglossal*: efferent to tongue muscles.
For more detail, see the separate entry for each nerve.

cranial reflex Any reflex mediated directly by one of the cranial nerves. Distinguish from SPINAL REFLEX.

cranio- Combining form meaning *pertaining to the cranium* or, more loosely, *the skull*.

craniometry Study of the skull, with emphasis on measurement.

craniosacral division Occasional synonym for the parasympathetic division of the AUTONOMIC NERVOUS SYSTEM.

cranioscopy PHRENOLOGY.

cranium That portion of the skull enclosing the brain.

crash Slang term for 'coming down' from an amphetamine- or cocaine-induced 'high'. The experience occurs only after extended use and typically involves feelings of anxiety, tremors, heightened irritability and depression.

creatinine A by-product of muscle metabolism used as a proxy measure for muscle mass in health psychology studies of healthy adults. It is also used medically to assess kidney function.

creationism A point of view derived from theological considerations that argues that life and the existence of species, particularly *Homo sapiens*, are the result of a specific creative act handicrafted by a supreme being. There actually are several creationist points of view, ranging from the fundamentalist, which depends on the literal interpretation of the Bible, to somewhat more 'liberal' perspectives, which allow for some Darwinian-type evolutionary processes for lower species but view man as separate from these non-spiritual mechanistic organisms. The most recent candidate is 'intelligent design' which argues that Darwinian mechanisms may operate once things got started, but that some form of supernatural intelligence was required to first create life. See DARWINISM, EVOLUTION and EVOLUTIONARY THEORY.

creative intelligence See INTELLIGENCE, CREATIVE and TRIARCHIC THEORY OF INTELLIGENCE.

creative synthesis The philosophical principle that when several elemental components are organized or coordinated the resulting synthesis has properties and characteristics that are fundamentally different in kind from those of the separate components viewed independently. See also EMERGENTISM, HOLISM, SYNTHESIS.

creative thinking CREATIVITY. Compare with CRITICAL *THINKING.

creativity A term used in the technical literature in basically the same way as in the popular, namely to refer to mental processes that lead to solutions, ideas, conceptualization, artistic forms, theories or products that are unique, novel, appropriate and useful. See also DIVERGENT *THINKING, INSIGHT (3, 4).

credibility Believability. In studies of PERSUASION the credibility of the source of a statement is an important variable; persons with high credibility, not surprisingly, have more persuasive impact than those with low credibility. adj., *credible*.

credulity A disposition to believe too readily or on the basis of too little evidence. Distinguish from CREDIBILITY.

creole In studies of language, a PIDGIN that has become the dominant verbal communication system for a people and acquired its own native speakers. This process is called *creolization*. Typically, the term gets dropped at this point for the name of the new language, unless it has become part of the language's name, as in Haitian Creole. The process of *decreolization* refers to the loss of features within a creole due to increased contact with one of its original pidgin ancestors and a reconvergence with that language.

Crespi effect CONTRAST EFFECT.

cretinism A congenital condition caused by a deficiency in thyroxin and characterized by severe lack of physical growth and mental retardation. Secondary symptoms include rough dry skin, patchy coarse hair, late and erratic dentition, and an enlarged, protruding tongue.

Creutzfeldt–Jakob disease (CJD) A neurological disorder marked by abnormal posture, spastic paralysis of the limbs with tremor and rigidity, disturbed vision and a devastating, rapidly progressing dementia not unlike that seen in ALZHEIMER'S DISEASE. It is caused by prions (virus-like objects lacking nucleic acids), which are also responsible for bovine spongiform encephalopathy, known colloquially as mad-cow disease.

crf Abbreviation for *continuous reinforcement*; see SCHEDULES OF *REINFORCEMENT.

crib death SUDDEN INFANT DEATH SYNDROME.

cri du chat (*cree-doo-shah*) A chromosomal abnormality resulting in mental retardation, microcephaly, dwarfism and a laryngeal abnormality which gives the affected infant a cry that sounds like a cat crying (hence the name of the syndrome).

criminal psychopath 1 A term for an individual whose illegal acts stem from uncontrollable psychological problems such as those seen in IMPULSE-CONTROL DISORDERS. **2** A person with ANTISOCIAL PERSONALITY DISORDER who commits illegal acts as part of the disorder. The first meaning is no longer used in the technical literature; the second is rare but still found. Both, however, are common in nontechnical writing. Also called *criminal sociopath*.

criminal responsibility A legal term relating to the state of mind of a defendant at the time of the crime and the question of whether he or she could distinguish right from wrong and hence be held personally responsible for the criminal actions taken.

criminal type An antiquated term for a type of individual who repeatedly engages in criminal actions and who, according to some unreconstructed Lombrosians, may possess a constitutional predisposition to do so.

criminology A hybrid science – a blend of law, sociology, psychology and medicine – that studies crime, criminals and penology.

crisis From the Greek for *turning-point*, hence: **1** Any inflection point in the course of events. Strictly speaking, a crisis can be either a sudden improvement or a sudden deterioration. **2** In medicine, the turning-point in a disease. **3** Any sudden interruption in the normal course of events in the life of an individual or a society that necessitates re-evaluation of modes of action and thought. A general sense of a loss of the normal foundations of day-to-day activity is the dominant connotation of the term and is broadly applied. For example, an individual is said to undergo a psychological crisis when abrupt departures from normality occur, such as the death of a loved one or the loss of one's job. **4** By extension, in the philosophy and history of science the term is used with similar connotations to refer to circumstances in which the presently accepted principles of a science are directly challenged and found wanting. Note that in all of these usages there is an accompanying sense that a crisis is something that is uncontrollable, that it must be allowed to run its course. pl., *crises*.

crisis intervention **1** Any short therapeutic-like effort to deal with the circumstances following a local disaster, a hurricane or fire, a family crisis or the like. Such interventions typically reduce the likelihood of POST-TRAUMATIC STRESS DISORDER. **2** A type of psychotherapy that focuses on acute, critical situations such as drug overdoses, suicide attempts and profound depressive episodes. Often these are handled over the telephone or through drop-in centres staffed by paraprofessionals.

crisis rites Ceremonies performed at times of crisis. Sociologists and anthropologists usually cite examples – for instance, rain dances in response to droughts – from so-called 'primitive' cultures. Modern industrialized democracies also have them, e.g. voting in the opposition party whenever the economy goes sour. In both cases the rites are ineffectual. See SUPERSTITIOUS BEHAVIOUR.

crista **1** Generally, any crest-like structure like those found in mitochondria. **2** More specifically, the organ in the ampulla of each SEMICIRCULAR CANAL containing the hair cells that respond to movements of the endolymph set up by angular rotation of the head. pl. *cristae*.

criterion **1** Generally, a standard against which a judgement, evaluation or classification can be made. More specifically: **2** A level of performance that is set as a goal by which progress is judged. This meaning is common in studies of learning and memory, which set a criterion and take it as representative, e.g. one complete errorless run through all items. **3** In signal detection theory, an internal cut-off point along the dimension of neural activity below which the response 'no signal' is made and above which the response 'signal' is made. For details see SIGNAL DETECTION THEORY. **4** In statistics, the dependent variable. pl., *criteria*; adj., *criterial*. **5** In psychometrics, the information that is used to judge the properties of an assessment procedure. For example, in CONTENT *VALIDITY the criterion is the judgement of experts regarding the content of the assessment.

criterion group A group of selected individuals whose scores on a test may be used to evaluate the test scores of others and to assist in determining the validity of the test. For example, a group of professional musicians might serve as the criterion group for a test of musical aptitude.

criterion score A score on the dependent variable that is predicted on the basis of hypotheses concerning the effects of the independent variable. See also COEFFICIENT OF *VALIDITY for discussion of how criterion scores are used in the determination of the validity of a testing instrument.

criterion variable VARIABLE, CRITERION.

critical 1 Pertaining to or characteristic of criticism. This meaning, particularly when applied in philosophically oriented work, implies that the approach taken to the work being criticized is *unbiased*, that the critic is attempting to review the work without prejudice. **2** Characteristic of sceptical, fault-finding reviews. This meaning, closer perhaps to lay usage, connotes an unfavourable analysis and assessment. **3** Pertaining to CRISIS in any of the meanings of that term. **4** Characteristic of a judgement or decision that is of great importance, of something that is *crucial*.

critical bandwidth In audition, the range of frequencies that interact in special ways within the ear. The term has a variety of extremely technical uses that go beyond the scope of this volume; the interested reader should consult a text on audition or hearing.

critical flicker frequency (cff) The point at which a flickering stimulus is no longer perceived as periodic but shifts to continuous. The cff increases with increases in intensity. Also known as *critical flicker, critical fusion frequency, flicker fusion point* or *flicker fusion frequency*.

critical lure See LURE.

critical period A period of time, biologically determined, during which an organism is optimally ready for the acquisition of specific responses. The best-known example is the critical period for *imprinting* in certain species of duck, which is a 'window' of a few hours following hatching. If imprinting does not occur in the critical period it can never be learned and the duckling will not develop normally. See also SENSITIVE PERIOD.

critical ratio (CR) The ratio of the difference between two statistics to the standard error of the difference. The CR is a special case of the T TEST.

critical region REGION OF REJECTION.

critical thinking THINKING, CRITICAL.

Crocker–Henderson system A system for representing the psychological components of smell using four basic odours: fragrant, acid, burnt and caprylic ('goat'). It was not terribly successful in accounting for psychophysical data; the more complex systems of Henning and Zwaardemaker give better characterizations.

Cronbach's alpha A measure of the internal reliability of the items in a test or on a questionnaire. It ranges from 0 to 1.0 and reflects the extent to which the items are measuring the same thing. For example, if all respondents who say 'no' endorse the first item on a scale to the maximum degree also endorse the remaining scale items to the maximum degree, the alpha for this scale is 1.0.

cross adaptation ADAPTATION, CROSS.

cross conditioning Incidental conditioning that occurs to an irrelevant stimulus that adventitiously occurs simultaneously with an unconditioned stimulus.

cross-cultural method A quasi-experimental method used in social psychology, sociology, anthropology, etc. for evaluating cultures on several different cultural dimensions, such as child-rearing practices, literacy and language use. The patterns of scores of the various cultures are then compared. The primary purpose of this type of research is not so much comparison of different cultures *per se* as it is comparison of various practices in different cultural settings.

cross-culture test CULTURE-FREE TEST.

cross-dressing Wearing clothes of the opposite sex; see TRANSVESTIC FETISHISM.

crossed reflex A reflex on the contralateral (opposite) side of the body from that stimulated. See CONSENSUAL REFLEX, CONTRALATERAL REFLEX.

cross fostering Generally, the rearing of young by nonbiological parents. As an experimental procedure it is often used with animals in an effort to tease apart genetic and environmental characteristics. For example, it turns out that wild rats raised by laboratory-bred tame rats are far less aggressive than littermates left with biological parents. Cross-fostering that occurs in adoptions can be used as a basis for making retrospective analyses of similar contributions of heredity and environment in various disorders.

cross-impact matrix method A statistical procedure for making estimates about future trends and events. It is a refinement of TREND ANALYSIS and projects possible future occurrences probabilistically by extrapolating from known data. The heart of the procedure is the synthesizing of predictions made using a variety of other methods (hence the name). See also DELPHI METHOD.

crossing over In genetics, the exchange of genes between two chromosomes. The exchange occurs between corresponding loci on homologous chromosomes during meiosis.

cross-modal Involving more than one perceptual modality or system. In cross-modal *discrimination* (or *transfer*), one can pick an object out of a visual display when one has merely touched it previously. In cross-modal *integration*, signals from two different modalities are blended and one perceives a compromise between the two; e.g. MCGURK EFFECT. Also called *cross-modality*.

cross-modal discrimination/integration See CROSS-MODAL.

cross-modality matching METHODS OF *SCALING.

cross-parent identification A child's identification with the parent of the opposite sex.

cross-section SECTION (2).

cross-sectional method An approach to research often used in developmental, clinical and social psychology when large groups of subjects are studied at one point in time (also called the *synchronic method*). Contrast with the LONGITUDINAL (or *diachronic*) method, used when the behaviour of individual subjects is followed over an extended period of time.

cross tolerance TOLERANCE, CROSS.

cross validation A procedure for further evaluating the validity of a test by administering it a second time to a new sample of individuals selected from the same population as the first time.

crowd A large but temporary gathering of persons with a common interest or focus. Note that the notion of temporariness is lost when the terms CROWDING or OVERCROWDING are used.

crowding 1 An area of study in social psychology dealing with the impact of numbers of individuals on behaviour. While it is clear that the characteristic behaviours that human beings (and other animals) exhibit are affected by the sheer size of the group they are in or the population density of the community within which they live, the manner in which these variables affect behaviour are extremely complex. The aberrant behaviours initially reported by early researchers (see BEHAVIOURAL SINK) are not always found and, from the psychological perspective, for simplicity's sake, it is more reasonable to think of crowding as that situation in which achieved privacy is less than desired privacy. Also called *overcrowding*. **2** Teuber's term for the result of the shifting of language function to the right hemisphere from a damaged left hemisphere which accompanies lesions that occur early in life. Such a shift is typically associated with diminished performance in visual-spatial abilities, which Teuber argued came about because the right hemisphere's normal functions were now being 'crowded' out by the newly assumed linguistic role. **3** A tendency to attempt to copy many stimuli in a space intended for one. Seen in various neurological disorders, such as NEGLECT.

crucial experiment From the Latin *experimentum crucis* (which is sometimes used), this term refers to any experiment the outcome of which will definitely and unambiguously establish the truth or falsity of a proposition or hypothesis. Alas, in science generally and in psychology specifically, the *experimentum crucis* is nearly always an illusion, for a new conundrum always seems to be lurking behind the data.

crude In statistics: **1** Characterizing data not yet analysed or transformed; see RAW. **2** Approximate; a crude statistic is an estimated or approximate statistic.

crude score RAW *SCORE.

crutch Generally, any supportive device. Specifically: (a) a physical device, e.g. to assist in walking; (b) a cognitive *heuristic*, e.g. a MNEMONIC, for facilitating the learning and memorizing of material; or (c) a DEFENCE MECHANISM whereby an affliction, real or imagined, is used to rationalize failure or inadequacy.

cryptaesthesia Lit., hidden sensations. A cover term in parapsychology for all forms of extrasensory perception. See discussion under PARAPSYCHOLOGY. var., *cryptesthesia*.

crypt(o)- Prefix meaning *hidden, secret, occult*.

cryptogenic epilepsy EPILEPSY, CRYPTOGENIC.

cryptography The study, development and utilization of codes. The term is properly used to refer to artificially developed systems for transmitting messages secretly. Distinguish from CODE.

cryptomnesia Lit., hidden or unconscious memory. Generally, ideas and thoughts that are often apparently creative and novel but are really memories of past experiences and events that the individual does not (consciously) recall. See IMPLICIT *MEMORY. Also called *source amnesia*, although this term is not recommended for this meaning.

cryptophasia Lit., secret speech. Specifically, the peculiar communication codes occasionally observed in pairs of twins and some pathological cases. They are not true, novel languages as many at first assumed but unsystematic variations on a natural language. Also called *idioglossia*.

cryptorchidism A condition in which one (unilateral) or both (bilateral) testicle(s) is/are undescended.

crystallized intelligence INTELLIGENCE, CRYSTALLIZED.

CS 1 CONDITIONED STIMULUS. **2** CODE SWITCHING.

CSF CEREBROSPINAL FLUID.

CT scan COMPUTERIZED AXIAL TOMOGRAPHY.

cue 1 That aspect of a stimulus pattern that may be used in making a discrimination between that stimulus and any other; an identification mark, a clue. **2** A signal that guides (or 'cues') behaviour. It may be either a part of the experimental stimulus, in which

case it marks the occasion for an operant response, or part of a response in the form of some feedback from having made it, when it serves as a cue for another response. Both meanings have verbal forms in which signals or stimuli that function in these ways are said to 'cue' behaviour or 'cue' a process, and adjectival forms in which the processes so engaged are said to have been 'cued' (see here, CUED *RECALL).

cued panic attack A PANIC ATTACK that is so tightly associated with a particular situation that just imagining the situation can trigger an attack.

cued recall See RECALL, CUED.

cue function The functional role of a stimulus as a guide to or evoker of behaviour. See FUNCTIONAL *STIMULUS.

cue reversal REVERSAL *LEARNING.

cue validity VALIDITY, CUE.

cul-de-sac BLIND ALLEY.

cult Any group of individuals with a common core of beliefs and rituals viewed as unacceptable by the dominant surrounding culture. Cults are cohesive and require strong commitment in belief and action from adherents. They are often, but not always, religious in nature but their practices, philosophies and values are invariably at odds with mainstream society. The term as used has a distinct negative connotation. Compare with SECT.

cultural Pertaining to culture. The term, in its general sense, is used in many combined forms, some of which follow here, others of which follow the entry for CULTURE. For those not listed in either of these places, see SOCIAL et seq. or, as a last resort, GROUP.

cultural absolute ABSOLUTE, CULTURAL.

cultural adaptation ADAPTATION (2).

cultural anthropology ANTHROPOLOGY, CULTURAL.

cultural artifact ARTIFACT, CULTURAL.

cultural assimilation ASSIMILATION.

cultural blindness The disposition to view the events of the world through the values and norms learned in one's own culture; the inability to be aware of or sensitive to the view that those of different cultures may have of events and relations between persons. Basically, a synonym of ETHNOCENTRISM.

cultural determinism 1 Generally, the point of view that human behaviour is primarily shaped and controlled by cultural and social factors. 2 More specifically, the point of view that culture, transcending as it does the lives of particular persons, must be approached as an object of scientific study independent of the individuals who make it up at any point in time; e.g. the notion that culture is *superorganic*.

cultural drift The gradual shifting of the values and norms of a culture over time. The changes that produce it are typically small and may go quite undetected until they accumulate and the shift in orientation becomes apparent.

cultural-familial mental retardation MENTAL RETARDATION, CULTURAL-FAMILIAL.

cultural integration INTEGRATION, CULTURAL.

cultural items Those items in a test which clearly reflect specific aspects of a particular culture and which will favour persons with the appropriate learning experiences. See CULTURE-FREE TEST.

cultural lag 1 CULTURAL RESIDUE. 2 CULTURE LAG. Note that these two usages have rather different references.

cultural monism The social philosophical perspective that maintains that ethnic, racial and religious minorities should be assimilated into the dominant culture. Advocates of this view maintain that internal strife is less likely with a monistic system than with cultural PLURALISM (4).

cultural norms The rules or standards of conduct of a society that specify certain behaviours as appropriate and others as inappropriate. Generally included in a set of cultural norms are rewards and punishments typically meted out for conforming to or violating them.

cultural parallelism PARALLELISM, CULTURAL.

cultural pluralism PLURALISM (4).

cultural psychiatry An approach to psychiatry that reflects sensitivity to the cultural history of the client. Various behaviours that

are regarded as disorders in one culture may well be normal, accepted patterns of activity in another.

cultural relativism The position that one cannot evaluate, interpret or judge phenomena properly unless they are viewed with reference to the culture in which they originated. The view extends from cultural products such as music, art, literature and industry to broad concepts like *cultural norms*, *mores* and *ethics*. In general, the operating principle is that the customs of one culture can never be validly judged inferior or superior to those of another.

cultural residue Aspects of a culture that are maintained despite the fact that whatever utilitarian functions they originally had have been lost through technological or attitudinal changes. Typically such *survivals* (as they are often called) are preserved for decorative use. Sometimes also called *cultural lag(s)*.

cultural transmission The process of learning through which the values, standards, norms, etc. of a culture are passed on to succeeding generations. See also ACCULTURATION (1) and SOCIALIZATION.

culture 1 The system of information that codes the manner in which the people in an organized group, society or nation interact with their social and physical environment. In this sense the term is really used so that the frame of reference is the sets of rules, regulations, *mores* and methods of interaction within the group. A key connotation is that culture pertains only to nongenetic transmission; each member must *learn* the systems and the structures. 2 The group or collection of persons who share the patterned systems described in 1.

culture area A geographic region within which common cultural patterns are prevalent. Typically, such an area contains subcultures that have their own distinctive elements, although all reflect the shared characteristics.

culture-bound syndrome CULTURE-SPECIFIC SYNDROME.

culture complex An integrated, structured pattern of cultural traits and activities that functions as a coordinated unit within a society. Examples run the gamut from the football (soccer) complex in many European and South American countries to the rice-growing complex in many Southeast Asian countries.

culture conflict 1 The conflict that occurs when a person or a group is confronted with two or more contradictory cultural standards or practices both of which are partially acceptable and over which there are conflicting loyalties. **2** The actual conflict between groups over such divergent standards and practices. Meaning 1 is that usually intended, the conflict being that *within* the person(s) confronted with the problem.

culture contact Generally, any form of interaction between persons of two distinct cultures that results in mutual modification of the cultures through reciprocal assimilation of traits.

culture-epoch theory The largely discredited theory that holds that (a) all cultures evolve through a series of stages (or 'epochs') and that (b) each individual develops in a manner which mirrors this sequence. For more discussion on this general viewpoint see RECAPITULATION THEORY.

culture-fair test CULTURE-FREE TEST.

culture-free test A test designed to be, as far as possible, free of any particular cultural bias so that no advantage is derived by individuals of one culture relative to those of another. Such tests generally eliminate or severely underplay language factors and other skills that may be closely tied to a particular culture. A variation is the *class-free test*, which is designed to be fair across socioeconomic classes within a given culture. There is considerable doubt about whether such tests are or ever can be made to be truly fair to all persons independent of culture. Also called *culture-fair test*.

culture island A self-contained community with its own distinct culture surrounded by a larger culture. Classic examples are the Amish agricultural communities in the United States and the Roma in Europe.

culture lag Those aspects of a culture that can be observed to be changing less rapidly than others. Compare with CULTURE LEAD.

culture lead Those aspects of a culture that can be observed to be changing more rapidly

than others. In a sense, a lead is an anticipatory change, a shift within a culture that can be interpreted as a preparatory adjustment. Compare with CULTURE LAG.

culture pattern 1 Occasional synonym for CULTURE COMPLEX. **2** The dominant aspects of a culture.

culture shock The emotional disruption often experienced by persons when they pay an extended visit to or live for some time in a society that is different from their own. The typical manifestations are a sense of bewilderment and a feeling of strangeness, which may last for a considerable length of time depending on the individual and the disparateness of the new culture from the original, familiar one.

culture-specific syndrome Any pathological behavioural syndrome specific to a particular culture. See e.g. Southeast Asian KORO and Eskimo PIBLOKTO. Note that there are questions as to whether these disorders are really specific to particular cultures. The *ICD-10*, for example, considers them to be local variants of anxiety, depressive or somatoform disorders. Also called *ethnic psychosis* or *culture-bound syndrome*.

culture trait A very flexible term indeed, used most commonly to denote the simplest significant components of any culture. However, in the hands of different writers, it may serve to stand for any number of things; e.g. a culture-bound material implement such as a cocktail glass, a functionally coordinated set of physically diverse implements such as all the varieties of container for alcoholic beverages, a social interaction such as a cocktail party, or a belief or attitude such as being pro or con cocktail parties. Thus the notion of a trait being a 'simple' component is very much dependent on the level of analysis undertaken. See also CULTURE COMPLEX and MEME.

culturgen A term coined by E. O. Wilson and C. J. Lumsden to denote the basic individual unit of a culture. The concept emerges as a central one in SOCIOBIOLOGY, in which the choice between alternative culturgens (e.g. the acceptance or rejection of incest, to use one of the sociobiologist's favourite cases) is seen as a critical element in the evolution of culture.

cumulative **1** Generally, characterizing anything reached by successive additions. **2** In statistics, a method of summing a series of scores in which each successive score is added to the sum of all preceding scores.

cumulative frequency curve A graphic representation of a series of scores summed cumulatively. Generally the scores are arranged in order of increasing magnitude so that the curve reveals their functional relationship. If the underlying distribution is normal, the curve is an OGIVE.

cumulative frequency distribution DISTRIBUTION, CUMULATIVE FREQUENCY.

cumulative recorder A device used frequently in operant research which automatically plots responses against time. The organism's response rate is given by the slope of the curve; the higher the rate, the steeper the slope.

cumulative scaling method GUTTMAN SCALING.

cuneate nucleus (or **cuneus**) A group of neurons located in the lower medulla that relays neural impulses from the upper trunk and arms to the somatic sensory areas of the brain; the first synaptic junction in the pathway.

cupula A gelatinous body in the ampulla of the SEMICIRCULAR CANALS in which the hair cells of the CRISTA are embedded.

curare (*kyu-rah-ree*) The common name for d-Tubocurarine, a chemical substance found in certain South American plants that causes paralysis in striated muscles. Curare acts by blocking cholinergic transmission at the myoneural junction by competing with acetylcholine at the receptor sites.

cure **1** A return to health. **2** Any procedure or treatment that restores health. Compare with HEAL.

curiosity The tendency to seek the novel. Some psychologists regard it as an innate propensity in many species, others are sceptical. Part of the difficulty is in distinguishing between what is entailed by curiosity and what is entailed by simple exploration of one's environment.

Current Procedural Terminology (CPT) A coding system developed by the American Medical Association for identifying procedures in medicine, psychotherapy and evaluation. Unlike diagnostic systems like the DSM or the ICD, the CPT does not provide a classification system; it is concerned with the actual services rendered or procedures carried out. When health-care systems are billed for services, the CPT is used to specify the procedures used.

curse-of-knowledge **1** The tendency to assume that one's own knowledge is shared by others. Here, it can be a contributing factor in the breakdown of communication between parties. **2** The inclination to think in particular ways based on highly developed, sophisticated knowledge. Here, it can result in a failure of innovation and a lack of cognitive flexibility. Both usages focus on a distinctly ironic feature of increased knowledge and understanding.

curve **1** Any line the position of which is given with reference to a set of coordinates. **2** In statistics, a collection of points described by an equation. **3** More generally, a line given to represent a series of values of one or more variables. Strictly speaking, a curve may be straight.

curve fitting **1** Any of a number of procedures for obtaining a smooth, regular curve that accurately 'fits' or characterizes a given set of data. They may be freehand approximations (called 'eyeballing') or mathematically rigorous procedures, e.g. GOODNESS OF *FIT and LEAST-SQUARES PRINCIPLE. **2** A slightly derogatory expression used of theoreticians who play fast and loose with the values of the parameters of equations that are taken as theoretical representations of data. The implication is that someone who is 'merely curve fitting' is juggling parameters in an unjustifiable manner so as to make the theoretical curves fit the data.

curve, normal NORMAL *DISTRIBUTION.

curvilinear Pertaining to a nonrectilinear curve, i.e. a line which is not straight.

curvilinear correlation CORRELATION, CURVILINEAR.

curvilinear regression REGRESSION, CURVILINEAR.

curvilinear relationship Any relationship

between two variables that when plotted produces a curved line.

customary, prevailing and reasonable (CPR) fees A set of principles for establishing fees for psychological services based on assessments of prevailing standards. CPR fees are used by insurance companies and governments for reimbursement for services provided.

cutaneous Pertaining to or affecting the skin itself or the skin as a sense organ.

cutaneous pain ACUTE *PAIN.

cutaneous rabbit A rather engaging illusion. Three tappers are placed on the arm, one on the wrist, one near the elbow and one on the upper arm. While the arm is resting, a series of rapid taps is delivered at the wrist, followed by two taps near the elbow and three on the upper arm. The experience, and it is quite compelling, is of a small animal running up one's arm. In an alternative procedure, rapidly alternating taps at two points on the skin can elicit a phantom 'hop' between these two points.

cutaneous sense Any sense the receptors for which lie in the skin, immediately below it, or in the external mucous membranes. Included here are touch, pressure, temperature (warm and cold), pain, and the common chemical senses. Occasionally called *dermal sense*.

cutoff See CUTOFF *SCORE.

cutting Clinical slang for a pathologically-motivated act of self-mutilation, particularly the slashing or cutting of the arms seen in those with BORDERLINE PERSONALITY DISORDER.

CVA Abbrev. for *cerebrovascular accident*; see STROKE (2).

CVC (trigram) NONSENSE SYLLABLE.

CVLT CALIFORNIA VERBAL LEARNING TEST.

cybernetics A discipline developed largely through the work of Norbert Wiener and the name of which is derived from the Greek word for *steersman*. It is primarily concerned with control mechanisms and their associated communications systems, particularly those which involve feedback of information to the mechanism about its activities. As it has developed over the years cybernetics has become multidisciplinary, involving, among others, engineering, computer sciences, psychology, biology and sociology. In fact the blend of fields has been so effective that the term itself has fallen out of use and, in the popular literature, has come to be associated with the mere computational.

cycle 1 A recurring series of events. **2** A complete vibration of a sound or light wave.

cycle per second (cps) A measure of the frequency of a vibrating stimulus. The term is 'officially' obsolete and has been replaced by HERTZ (HZ).

cyclic adenosine monophosphate In the activation of *receptors*, a second messenger that operates in the production of postsynaptic potentials and in the mediation of the effects of peptide hormones. Also called *cyclic AMP*.

cyclic AMP CYCLIC ADENOSINE MONOPHOSPHATE.

cyclic disorder CYCLOTHYMIC DISORDER.

cyclic GMP CYCLIC GUANOSINE MONOPHOSPHATE.

cyclic guanosine monophosphate A second messenger similar in form and function to CYCLIC ADENOSINE MONOPHOSPHATE only with *guanosine* substituted for *adenosine*. Also called *cyclic GMP*.

cyclic nucleotide An umbrella term for those compounds such as CYCLIC ADENOSINE MONOPHOSPHATE and CYCLIC GUANOSINE MONOPHOSPHATE that function to mediate the intracellular effects of a variety of neurotransmitters.

cyclopean eye A hypothetical eye in the median plane between the two real eyes that can be represented as a theoretical coordinate of the eyes.

cyclopean stimulus In visual perception, a display that is brief and provides a 'snapshot' view to the observer. The term tends to be used primarily in studies of motion detection in which the observer is presented with a rapid series of brief displays (cyclopean stimuli) rather than a continuous streaming display.

cyclophoria Abnormal rotation of the eyeball due to weakness in the oblique muscles; a form of HETEROPHORIA.

cycloplegia A paralysis of the ciliary muscle which controls the pupil of the eye, resulting in a dilated pupil even under high light levels.

cyclothymic disorder A MOOD DISORDER characterized by cyclical mood swings. Distinguish from BIPOLAR DISORDER, in which the range of emotions is much more extreme. *Cyclothymia* is used as a psychiatric label only when there has been an extended disruption in affect (usually 2 years or more); it is not meant to apply to acute emotional reactions. Also called *cyclic disorder*.

cyesis Pregnancy.

-cyte Suffix denoting *cell*.

cyt(o)- Prefix denoting *cell*.

cytoarchitectonics (or **cytoarchitecture**) Lit., the study of the ARCHITECTURE (1) (the organization and patterns) of the cells within the cerebral cortex.

cytogenetics A branch of the study of heredity specializing in the structure and function of chromosomes and genes.

cytogenic gland Any gland that produces cells: the sex glands, lymph nodes, spleen.

cytogenic syndrome Any condition marked by a variety of physical and behavioural symptoms caused by some abnormality in the size, number or shape of the chromosomes, e.g. KLINEFELTER'S SYNDROME, TURNER'S SYNDROME.

cytology Science concerned with the study of the formation, structure and function of cells.

cytoplasm The protoplasm of a cell outside of the nucleus.

cytosine One of the four nucleotide bases which make up DEOXYRIBONUCLEIC ACID and RIBONUCLEIC ACID.

cytotoxic Destructive of, or toxic to, cells. Cytotoxic agents are substances that destroy cells or inhibit their multiplication.

D

D **1** In Hull's theory, DRIVE. **2** In statistics generally, a DIFFERENCE *SCORE. **3** In statistics specifically, a crude measure of dispersion of a distribution of scores given by the difference between the 10th and 90th percentiles.

d **1** A measure of EFFECT SIZE, expressed as the difference between two means divided by the standard deviation of the population. Also called *Cohen's d*. **2** Deviation of a score from a measure of central tendency, usually the mean. **3** A difference score representing the two ranks of an individual on two separate tests.

d' A measure of the sensitivity of an observer to some stimulus 'event'. The notion of an 'event' here is interpreted broadly. It may be the occurrence of a simple stimulus, the occurrence of a stimulus that differs in some fashion from another stimulus, a part on an assembly line that has a flaw, a shadow on a chest X-ray, etc. In SIGNAL-DETECTION THEORY *d'* is an index of how sensitive an observer is to a stimulus independent of criteria for responding, pay-offs for being right or wrong, the probabilities of the stimuli actually being presented and any instructional set that may be given to the subject. It is thus an index for the 'ideal' observer. Pronounced '*d*-prime'.

DA Abbreviation for **1** DOPAMINE. **2** DEVELOPMENTAL AGE.

dactology Manual sign language.

-dactyl- Word element meaning *pertaining to the finger* and, by extension, *toe*.

Daltonism Red-green colourblindness. Named after John Dalton, an English chemist who had it and first described it. See DICHROMACY.

damping Diminution in the amplitude of a wave.

dance therapy The use of the physical and aesthetic aspects of dance as a therapeutic medium. It is most commonly used with disturbed children.

dark adaptation The process of adjustment of the eyes to low intensities of illumination; the shift from the *photopic* system to the *scotopic* system. Total dark adaptation for the originally brightly illuminated eye requires approximately 4 hours, although the process is largely complete after about 30 minutes. The cones adapt first, completing the process in about 7 minutes, while the rods continue their adaptation for the full 4 hours. The point where the shift to photopic vision occurs is often called the *rod-cone break*. The totally dark-adapted eye is over one million times as sensitive as the normally illuminated eye.

dark light Not light at all, rather a level of spontaneous activity in the receptors of the eye which, under the proper conditions, can be phenomenologically real and detected as a sense of light.

Darwinian algorithms In EVOLUTIONARY PSYCHOLOGY, domain-specific adaptations that have evolved for very specific operations. An oft-cited example is face recognition.

Darwinian fitness FITNESS (2).

Darwinism The theory of evolution due to Charles Darwin (1809–82). The fundamental tenet of Darwinism is the principle of natural selection, whereby the variations in form displayed by the members of a species have differential survival values. Those variations that are 'adaptive' in the struggle for survival are the ones most likely to enable those possessing them to live and, if they confer reasonably high *Darwinian fitness*, to be passed on to their possessors' offspring. This process gradually gives rise to diverse forms, leading ultimately, through selective adaptation to specific econiches, to the emergence of new species. Note that the term denotes a gradualist position; theories which emphasize a saltatory process in which new species are assumed to emerge in a relatively short period of geological time, are properly not called Darwinian, nor are theoretical models such as the Lamarckian hypothesis of inheritance of acquired characteristics. The currently accepted Darwinian-based model is often called *neo-Darwinism*. See EVOLUTION and EVOLUTIONARY THEORY.

Dasein Translated literally from the German the term means *to be* (*sein*) *there* (*da*). However, it is generally rendered in English as BEING-IN-THE-WORLD.

Daseinanalyse The original German for what is now generally known as *existential analysis* or *existential psychology*. See DASEIN, EXISTENTIALISM and EXISTENTIAL THERAPY.

DAT Abbreviation for **1** *dementia of the Alzheimer's type*, see ALZHEIMER'S DISEASE. **2** DIFFERENTIAL APTITUDES TESTS.

data **1** The body of evidence or facts gathered in an experiment or study. *Data* is the plural form of *datum*. **2** In perception and cognitive psychology, stimuli that have been sensed, experienced. See DATA-DRIVEN PROCESSING for an example of this usage.

data-driven processing In *cognitive psychology*, processing that is determined primarily by the input stimuli, the data. See BOTTOM-UP PROCESSING for more detail.

data snooping Laboratory jargon for rummaging through one's data looking for statistically significant effects without an a priori rationale. The 'significant' findings that emerge from such operations are likely to be spurious and due merely to random fluctuations, particularly when the database is large or the number of factors high. To a certain extent such *fishing expeditions* are carried out by nearly all researchers but the responsible course is to use any adventitious findings as heuristics for future experimentation and not to report them as robust effects based

on the original study. Compare and contrast with A POSTERIORI TESTS and A POSTERIORI FALLACY.

datum Singular of DATA.

Daubert criteria The standard for the admissibility of scientific evidence in US federal courts. The evidence must be presented by an approved expert who has knowledge of the field and stature in the eyes of scientific peers; it must be falsifiable (see FALSIFICATIONISM) and have withstood empirical tests.

day blindness HEMERALOPIA.

day-dreaming Mental meandering, fantasizing, etc. while one is awake. Some distinguish day-dreams from sleeping dreams by arguing that, among other obvious factors, wishes are not hidden, disguised or repressed in the waking variety.

daylight vision PHOTOPIC VISION.

day residue In the study of dreams, the fragments of recent experiences during waking hours that emerge as dream images.

dB (or **db**) Abbreviation for DECIBEL.

DBT DIALECTAL BEHAVIOUR THERAPY.

de- Prefix meaning: **1** *down, away from*; **2** *apart from, undone*.

deafferent Referring to the removal of neural pathways that mediate *afferent* (i.e. *sensory*) information from the periphery to the central nervous system.

deaf-mute A person who can neither hear nor speak. The often-heard slang expression 'deaf and dumb' for such persons is, owing to the dual meaning of *dumb*, inaccurate as well as insulting and should be avoided.

deafness A continuum of hearing impairment ranging from partial to total (or *profound*, as it is often called). Like blindness, deafness is often erroneously thought to be an all-or-nothing affair. Also like blindness, it can be due either to genetic defects, injury or cortical disorder, or to a variety of anatomical/physiological factors. Deafness can be quite specific, so that only certain ranges of hearing (e.g. high-pitched tones) may be affected. Specialized forms follow.

deafness, cerebral Any form of deafness caused by brain lesions. Several other terms are used when there are good reasons for identifying the locus of the lesion, e.g. *cortical deafness* for lesions in the cortex, *central deafness* for damage to the auditory centre in the brain.

deafness, ceruminous The technical term for hearing loss due to build-up of earwax.

deafness, conduction A form of deafness due to some abnormal condition that interferes with the mechanical conduction system that transmits vibrations from the middle ear to the auditory receptors of the inner ear. It may result from damage to the eardrum, pathological changes in the bones of the middle ear or inflammation in the inner ear.

deafness, congenital Lit., deafness existing at the time of birth. The term is applied generally, including to cases due to genetic as well as environmental factors.

deafness, functional 1 Psychogenic deafness; loss of hearing in the absence of any known organic dysfunction. **2** Deafness due to a breakdown in the normal functioning of some aspect of the auditory system. These two meanings are at odds with each other; 1 is preferred (SEE FUNCTIONAL DISORDER).

deafness, hysterical Obsolete term for FUNCTIONAL *DEAFNESS (1).

deafness, nerve Deafness resulting from any neurological impairment of the auditory receptors in the cochlea or the auditory nerve. Usually contrasted with CONDUCTION *DEAFNESS.

death Put simply (but inadequately), the point at which an organism ceases to be alive. Before modern medical support devices, death was determined by the inability of an individual organism to keep *itself* alive. With sophisticated physiological support, the criteria most frequently cited have to do with cerebral functioning (i.e. BRAIN DEATH). The issues here are not simple or easy; they involve more than the merely biological and touch upon essential questions, ethical, philosophical and theological.

death feigning A response to threatening situations in which an organism goes into a state of *tonic immobility* and appears to be dead. Recovery is rapid and complete after the threat passes. Also called *thanatomimesis*. See INJURY FEIGNING.

death instinct THANATOS.

death wish The hypothesized motivational syndrome that causes affected individuals to repeatedly put themselves in life-threatening situations. The term is used more in popular writings than scientific, although some liken it to Freud's notion of THANATOS.

debility Generally, weakness in function, loss of ability. Used commonly of organic and motor functions, occasionally of cognitive functions.

debriefing Telling the subject of an experiment what it was about and, when necessary, revealing any deception or withholding of information that may have been a necessary element in the study. This latter aspect is sometimes called *dehoaxing*. Occasionally, a debriefing may contain questions designed to elicit the subject's perception of what was going on in the experiment.

debug Laboratory jargon (borrowed from computer sciences) meaning to detect, identify and correct an error in a program, a research project, a logical argument, a complex piece of equipment, etc.

deca- Combining form meaning *multiplied by ten; ten times.*

décalage This term, which translates from the French as, roughly, *discontinuity* or *slippage* (among other meanings), is found primarily in Piagetian approaches to the study of cognitive development. According to a strict Piagetian approach, cognitive development proceeds in distinct stages, therefore when a child moves to a higher level of cognitive functioning all the concepts based on the new level ought to appear at roughly the same time. *Décalage* is a collective term for all forms of nonsynchronous appearance of concepts, of which there are three main kinds: (a) *horizontal décalage* – the failure of the various aspects of a single cognitive operation to emerge together, as, for example, when a child shows conservation of number but not of mass (see the discussion under CONSERVATION); (b) *vertical décalage* – transformations in a particular concept (e.g. number, causality) with shifts to new cognitive stages; and (c) *oblique décalage* – the simultaneous enrichment of existing structures and preparations for later stages. The latter two present no real problem for Piagetian theory;

the first does, and it is not clear whether horizontal *décalages* reflect differences in task difficulty, differences in the formation of cognitive structures or perhaps erroneous classifications of the behaviours.

decathexis Withdrawal of CATHEXIS.

decay 1 Generally, a wasting away, a gradual deterioration. **2** In the study of memory the term is used as a biological metaphor to characterize the (presumed) gradual degradation and/or disintegration of neural traces. When one refers to a 'decayed' memory trace the implication is that somehow the neural underpinnings of the memory have 'faded' like an unfixed photograph. Presumably, decay can be prevented by the neurological process of CONSOLIDATION. See also FORGETTING.

deceleration ACCELERATION.

decentring (or **decentration**) In Piagetian theory, **1** Transition from an early stage of development during which a child has seen things as 'centred' on his or her own body and actions (see EGOCENTRISM) to a more mature stage in which the child perceives the environment as 'decentred' and his or her body and actions assume their objective relationships with other objects and events. Several decentration periods are assumed to take place, with respect to action, to representation and to cognition. **2** The perceptual or cognitive ability to break frame, to step outside of the sharp demands of a physical stimulus; e.g. *conservation* of volume occurs when a child is able to break away from 'centring' on the height of a liquid in a container and take into account other aspects of the situation (the width of the container, the fact that no one has added or subtracted any liquid, etc.) that provide compensation and balance distortions produced by the more primitive 'centring' process.

deception 1 Generally, action or speech designed to mislead another. **2** In ethology, patterns of behaviour in animals that suggest a similar function. Note that the term is not applied to 'hard-wired', inflexible patterns of action such as DEATH FEIGNING, but to circumstances in which an animal acts in a manner that suggests it is intentionally trying to mislead another animal. The classic example is one chimpanzee acting as though something interesting is taking place under a bush and

when another goes to look the first steals the food of the second. There are many who doubt the existence of deception in any species other than our own where it is, alas, ubiquitous.

decerebrate 1 vb. To remove the cerebrum, typically by transacting the *brainstem*. **2** adj. Of an organism which has been subjected to decerebration or which behaves as though it has been.

decerebrate rigidity A term coined by C. S. Sherrington for the exaggerated muscle tone of limb extensors in cats which had been subjected to a transection of the brain stem between the superior and inferior colliculi of the midbrain.

deci- Combining form meaning *one tenth*, *divided by ten*.

decibel (dB) A unit of measurement generally used to express sound intensity. It is always given as a ratio between pressures (physical forces), and one must specify the standard used as the reference. The generally accepted system uses 0·0002 dynes/cm^2 for sound measurement, which corresponds roughly to the average human threshold for a 1,000 Hz tone. The intensity of any given tone is thus expressed by:

$$dB = 10 \log_{10} I_1/I_2$$

where I_1 is the intensity under consideration and I_2 is the standard. Since the relationship is logarithmic, increments in decibels are reflected by geometric increases in intensity. At a distance of 5 ft (1.5 m) a human whisper is roughly 20 dB, normal conversation 60 dB, a pneumatic drill about 100 dB and the pain threshold for a broad-spectrum sound (like rock music) about 120 dB. Note, however, that the decibel is not only a measure of sound intensity; it is also, literally, 1/10th of a *bel*, a unit used occasionally in electrical and light measurement. Since the measure is a ratio of two energies, it is not logically restricted to sound pressure but may also be used of other physical continua.

decile One of nine points which divides a distribution of ranked scores into equal intervals. Each interval thus contains one tenth of the scores.

decision-making 1 Loosely, the process of

choosing. **2** In cognitive psychology, the subfield that investigates how various organisms (often, but not exclusively, adult humans) make choices when presented with various alternatives.

decision theory A label for any theory that seeks to describe and explain decision-making. Approaches vary from the highly formal, mathematical approaches based on game theory and probability theory to the more informal, intuitive theories which deal with beliefs, attitudes and other subjective factors. The range of study that falls under this label is quite wide and includes problem-solving, choice behaviour, utility theory, game economic theory and the like.

declarative A SPEECH ACT in which one tells someone something, i.e. one makes a *declaration*. The function of a declarative is to bring about a new set of circumstances. A classic example is 'You're fired.'

declarative knowledge KNOWLEDGE, DECLARATIVE.

declarative learning LEARNING, DECLARATIVE.

declarative memory MEMORY, DECLARATIVE.

de Clérambault's syndrome PSYCHOSE PASSIONNELLE.

decode (decoding) CODE.

decompensation 1 Lit., failure to compensate. **2** In psychiatry, a failure of one's defence mechanisms, usually leading to exacerbation of one's condition.

deconstructionism A point of view originally articulated by Jacques Derrida in the form of an approach to textual analysis. At its core, Derrida's argument is based on the proposition that all terms used in text presuppose and invariably suppress opposing concepts. Maleness presupposes and suppresses femaleness; reason, passion; secularity, the theological; and so forth. The power of the original arguments emerged from the likely truth that most texts, including those in psychology, did, indeed, contain such socially, politically and philosophically sensitive construals and that 'deconstructing' them to note and revise their entailments was a good thing. Alas, when taken to its (logical?) extreme, deconstructionism turns into an obfuscatory exercise that ends up disputing the possibility of rational inquiry and of a knowable reality.

decontextualization Interpretation of a text, a discourse, a dream, etc. based entirely on the literal meaning of the material; i.e. an interpretation that takes no account of the *context* within which the material occurs. Compare with RICH INTERPRETATION.

decorticate The state of being without a cortex (meaning, almost invariably, the cerebral cortex). Certain classes of behaviour requiring little or no functioning of the 'higher mental processes' are sometimes referred to as decorticate activities. Occasionally the term is used of species that do not have a neocortex, e.g. avians.

decorticate rigidity Marked bilateral rigidity in the arms and legs associated with bilateral dysfunctions in the cerebral cortex.

decrement In general, any decrease in anything can safely be referred to as a decrement. The term is used of behavioural performances, of knowledge, of memory, etc.

decussation The crossing over of neural pathways from one side of the nervous system to the other, especially in the midbrain. Owing to the contralateral innervation of many body–brain relations, the locus of decussation is often of interest.

deduction Reasoning that begins with a specific set of assumptions and attempts to draw conclusions or derive theorems from them. In general, it is a logical operation which proceeds from the general to the particular. Deductive inference is, in and of itself, an abstract process which requires no verification other than logical consistency. The proof of the pudding is in the appropriateness and demonstrability of the theorems and conclusions which are deduced. Contrast with INDUCTION. Both forms of reasoning have come under close study in psychology, particularly in how they relate to concept formation and problem-solving.

deep 1 Generally, below the surface, as in anatomical descriptions of underlying organs and tissues. **2** Characteristic of sensations arising in muscles, internal organs, the viscera. **3** Profound, dealing with the underlying abstract properties of things as opposed to their superficial forms. See DEPTH OF PROCESSING. **4** In acoustics, pertaining to low-pitched tones. **5** In vision, pertaining to richly saturated colours. **6** In psychoanalysis, characteristic of material that the client brings to the analysis that derives from early life experiences or from experiences that have been repressed. See DEPTH ANALYSIS, DEPTH PSYCHOLOGY.

deep alexia ALEXIA, DEEP.

deep cerebellar nuclei Quite literally, a set of nuclei located deep within the *cerebellum* that receive and transmit information between themselves and the cerebellar cortex.

deep dyslexia DYSLEXIA, DEEP.

deep interpretation RICH INTERPRETATION.

deep pain CHRONIC *PAIN.

deep reflexes Reflexes in underlying tissue. The 'knee jerk' is a good example; it is elicited by a tap on the patellar tendon.

deep sensitivity (or **sensibility**) Sense of pressure, the receptors for which are in deep subcutaneous layers of the skin or in muscles.

deep structure In linguistics, particularly transformational grammar, a layer of meaning that underlies the 'surface' layer of a sentence as given by the actual words. To take a classic example: the two sentences 'John is easy to please' and 'John is eager to please' have similar surface structures – proper noun, verb, adjective, infinitive. Yet they have different deep structures as can be shown by attempting to put each of them into equivalent passive forms. The first becomes the acceptable 'It is easy to please John' while the second becomes the anomalous 'It is eager to please John', indicating that the 'real' subjects of the two original sentences in the deep structure are different. Compare with SURFACE STRUCTURE.

Deese paradigm An experimental method introduced by James Deese in which a series of semantically related words are presented (e.g. *dream, rest, bed, pillow*). In a later memory task participants often falsely remember a related general word (in this case, *sleep*) as being in the list. Also called Deese, Roediger, McDermott paradigm.

defect 1 A flaw, an imperfection. **2** A failure

to function owing to such. Distinguish from *deficit* and derived terms, in which the connotation is that there is a *lack* of something rather than a flaw.

defective 1 adj. Imperfect, structurally incomplete, nonfunctional. **2** n. A person so characterized. The most common usage pattern in older writings was to refer to persons who were below average intelligence. A number of terms were coined, *mental defective, high-grade defective* and *low-grade defective* among the least charming. These have all but disappeared from the technical literature; their demise from the lay language would not be mourned. See MENTAL RETARDATION.

defeminizing effect Quite literally, the effect, in the developing foetus, produced by the presence of ANTI-MÜLLERIAN HORMONE, which prevents the development of the female anatomical characteristics controlled by the MÜLLERIAN SYSTEM.

defence 1 Broadly speaking, any action that any organism takes to protect itself. Hence: **2** In medicine, a resistive reaction to a disease, or a learned pattern of behaviour that protects one from possible injury or disease. **3** In clinical psychology and psychiatry, any of a number of reactions that one learns and uses unconsciously to protect one's internal psychic 'structures' (such as the *ego* or *self*) from anxiety, conflict, shame, etc. Meaning 3 is borne by a variety of combined forms, each with its own referential nuances. See e.g. DEFENCE MECHANISM, DEFENCE REACTION, DEFENSIVE STRATEGY, NEUROTIC *DEFENCE. var., *defense*.

defence mechanism A term applied to any enduring pattern of protective behaviour that functions to provide a defence against the awareness of that which is anxiety-producing. The word *behaviour* here needs some clarification. For many writers it denotes some overt pattern of action or some way of thinking or feeling that functions by circumventing or modifying whatever it is that evokes feelings of anxiety or threat. For many others, particularly those with a psychoanalytic bent, the overt behaviour is treated as merely a manifestation or symbol of some underlying intrapsychic process – which they take to be the true defence mechanism. These theorists use *defence reaction* for the overt behaviour. It should be clear, though, that no matter which nuance is intended everyone seems to agree that the term should be reserved for processes (or behaviours) that are unconsciously motivated, unconsciously acquired, and developed to protect the self or ego from unpleasantness of many kinds. Literally dozens of defence mechanisms have been hypothesized; some of the more commonly cited are *repression, regression, rationalization* and *projection*.

defence, neurotic Roughly speaking, psychoanalytic theory divides defence mechanisms into those that are *neurotic* and those that are *normal*. As every clinician knows, the difficulty with defence mechanisms is that while they may function as effective protectors of self in some of life's situations, they often prove counterproductive in others. Hence, no matter how one chooses to view them, they can always lead to psychological disorders or, to use the classical term, to a *neurotic breakthrough*. Although various authors differ on classification here, generally all of the defence mechanisms, save successful *repression* and *sublimation*, are regarded as *neurotic* defences on the grounds that sooner or later they almost inevitably lead to maladaptive ways of dealing with the world.

defence reaction DEFENCE MECHANISM.

defence reflex Any reflexive, involuntary response to a stimulus, e.g. an eye blink to an oncoming object, limb retraction from a hot surface.

defensive attribution SELF-SERVING BIAS.

defensiveness 1 An excessive sensitivity to criticism. Used here with the connotation that the criticism is not merely absorbed in hurt silence but reacted to in a defensive way. In this sense, some use the term as referring to a personality trait or characteristic. **2** A particular manner of behaving which functions to protect one from anxiety, embarrassment or unease, e.g. refusing to answer certain kinds of questions about oneself or one's actions.

defensive strategy A general term for any of a number of strategies that people use to defend themselves from anxiety. It is similar in notion to DEFENCE MECHANISM in that defensive strategies are designed unconsciously to deal directly with anxiety itself rather than

its source. For example, a student anxious about a forthcoming examination spends the evening in a pub, drinks heavily, forgets to set the alarm clock and sleeps through the appointed hour. Compare with COPING STRATEGIES.

deference behaviour E. Goffman's term for a large variety of social behaviours that function to keep social intercourse smooth and civil. The term derives from the fact that such behaviours operate basically by conveying respect for and appreciation of people. See PRESENTATIONAL RITUALS and AVOIDANCE RITUALS for Goffman's two major classes of deference behaviours.

deference need H. Murray's term for the need to defer to a leader or superior.

deficiency Generally, a lack of something, a condition in which some important element is missing. Distinguish from DEFECT, where the connotation is that there is a failure owing to a flaw or improper arrangement of parts.

deficiency needs 1 Generally, any homeostatically based need system such as hunger or thirst. **2** Maslow used the term in his theory of personality in a somewhat broader fashion to characterize his hypothesized level of BASIC NEEDS. In his sense, not all deficiency needs are based on physiological homeostasis; also included are various social and interpersonal needs.

deficit DEFECT.

defining feature DISTINCTIVE FEATURE (3).

definition A marking of the boundary between two classes or groups. Figures that stand out well are said to have good definition, words the meanings of which are well articulated and clearly distinguishable from others are said to be well defined, etc.

definitions Terminological precision is a giant bore when you're in love and positively tedious for a poet. In science, however, it is a high goal and the ambiguity so powerful in good poetry can be the source of monstrous confusion if allowed to slip in undetected. In the attempt to reach for clarity of meaning and use, a large number of definitional devices have been developed. Some of them are rather straightforward, some quite elaborate. The following are the more commonly used procedures for 'marking the boundaries of meaning' of terms in science:

(a) *Nominal:* a definition of a term made by simply supplying a name for a set of observations or events. Often such definitions are but shorthand expressions for cumbersome descriptions; e.g. *IQ* was once defined as 100 times the ratio of mental age to chronological age. When new terms are introduced in a science, particularly before their appropriateness or relevance have been evaluated, they are usually introduced by providing a nominal definition.

(b) *Formal:* a definition by specification of the features or characteristics that all members of the class, category or concept under consideration have in common and that can be used to distinguish that class, category or concept from any other. Formal definitions are useful once one understands the properties of the definiendum; e.g. *bachelor* is formally defined as unmarried, adult, male.

(c) *Real:* a definition that attempts to get at the 'real' nature of the term being defined. It usually carries with it a theoretical connection between several observations or events; e.g. *frustration* as an emotional reaction resulting from being thwarted or prevented from reaching a goal. Here, the validity and relevance are open to test.

(d) *Enumerative:* defining a class by (one hopes) exhaustively listing all of its members. This is a bit of a cheat and although it works to clarify meaning in the case of a small class it most assuredly has its limits.

(e) *Operational:* a definition based on the set of operations that produced the thing defined; e.g. *hunger* as a state of affairs resulting from food deprivation. Abstract and hypothetical concepts lend themselves nicely to this type of definition.

(f) *Reduction sentence:* a definition that carries with it a statement about antecedents and consequents; e.g. *anxiety* might be defined as follows: 'If a person is given an anxiety test then he or she is defined as anxious if and only if his or her score is in the top 10%.' Note that the definition is in sentence form, that antecedent conditions (the test) and consequences (the score) are specified, and that the sentence may be reduced to logical notation if needed. This kind of definition is useful in dealing with complex, theoretical notions.

The preceding are the more commonly used 'legitimate' varieties. Two other forms are also rather common, although they are distinctly unsatisfactory:

(g) *Tautological:* here one 'defines' a term by using synonyms or variants of the term itself. This dictionary abounds with these but then again so does every other and we won't apologize; after all, a fingernail is a nail on a finger.

(h) *Circular:* a definition which uses a 'circle' (or 'cycle') between two (or more) terms which are used to 'define' each other; e.g. *hormone* as a substance produced by an endocrine *gland* and *endocrine gland* as a producer of hormones. Precious little is gained by 'short cycles' of this kind; oddly though, *long* cycles can prove rather illuminating, and as a *reductio ad absurdum* every dictionary is a very long cycle of circular definitions.

The problem of definition is not a simple one and it certainly won't succumb to lexicographical legerdemain. It is, in fact, one of the deepest of philosophical conundrums and has resisted all manner of analysis. Ideally, one needs a metalanguage within which to express one's definitions of terms in the target language. For many areas of science, mathematics and/or logic serves as the metasystem; for the social sciences we must be content for the nonce with an elaborate 'bootstrapping' operation in which each term in the lexicon is defined by other terms which themselves are defined elsewhere. In this volume we have tried to balance precision with pragmatics; terms are defined 'properly' when possible and usage patterns are laid out where mandated. Analytical philosophers may not approve of this style but our aim is to improve and refine communication among practitioners and students of psychology and related areas of science; gentle criticisms concerning specific failures to do this should be sent to the publisher or the authors.

deflection A defence mechanism that functions by diverting attention or awareness away from the object or situation that arouses anxiety.

defusion FUSION (2).

degenerate 1 n. The standard dictionary definition is usually something like, 'one who deviates markedly from a social norm, particularly in the area of sexuality'. In actual usage the term has a distinctly negative connotation and is, moreover, differentially applied according to gender. For example, a sexually active woman may be so labelled but not a sexually active man – so long as he avoids young boys. adj., *degenerate*. **2** vb. To deteriorate, to decline in function or standards. In this sense the term is applied to mental, moral or biological processes or structures. See DEGENERATION.

degeneration 1 In physiology, deterioration of neural tissue caused by injury or lack of critical chemicals. Contrast with ATROPHY. If individual neurons are examined, two kinds of degeneration can be observed. Severing an axon or destroying the cell body will cause the distal part of the axon to degenerate rapidly; this is called *anterograde* degeneration. If the axon is severed some distance from the cell body, the proximal part of it will also degenerate but more slowly since it still receives nutrients from the cell body; this is called *retrograde* degeneration. **2** Deterioration of moral standards. See DEGENERATE (1).

degraded stimulus Any stimulus that has been modified so that it is more difficult to perceive. In formal terms, one says that the *signal-to-noise ratio* has been lowered. A stimulus may be degraded by erasing part of it, embedding it in noise, masking it, putting it out of focus, lowering the volume or intensity level, etc.

degrees of freedom (df) A mathematical concept used to express the fact that in statistical operations there are limits to the values that one is free to choose given particular constraints on the situation. The limit is determined by the number of observations, events or data points one has, minus the number of constraints. The easiest way to understand this is with a simple example: consider a distribution of five scores with mean $\bar{X}$. The last number in the distribution is completely determined by the first four and the value of the mean. That is, one is 'free' to choose the first four numbers, but given them and the mean the last number is fixed in value. In this case $df = 4$, which is the number of observations, 5, minus the one constraint, the mean.

In statistical operations such as *t* tests and analyses of variance, the power of a test

depends, in part, on the degrees of freedom. This makes sense intuitively, since as the number of degrees of freedom increases one expects variability to increase. However, when an experimental effect is real and variability is low, the power of the test is increased. For example, the *t* test with $df = 1$ requires a $t = 6.31$ for significance, while with $df = 10$ only a $t = 1.81$ is required.

dehoaxing DEBRIEFING.

dehydroisoandrosterone A natural androgen produced by the adrenal cortices and found in males and females. Compared with *testosterone* it has extremely low biological potency.

deindividuation The loss of one's sense of individuality. The classic example is what often occurs in mobs when the separateness of each person is lost in the surge of the crowd and individual choice is submerged in mob action. Compare with ANONYMITY.

deinstitutionalization Moving the location of mental health care from an institution to a community-based programme.

Deiters' cells Supporting cells in the ORGAN OF CORTI.

deixis A term used to refer to the context-boundedness of language. The deictic aspects of a linguistic message are those elements that refer to time, space and the interpersonal components. Purely deictic segments in English are 'here/there', 'this/that', 'before/after/now', etc. Deixis, of concern to philosophers for some time, has become a topic of interest in developmental psycholinguistics, with the focus on how children acquire these subtle aspects of language.

déjà vu French for *already seen*. The term is applied to a rather compelling illusion of familiarity with a scene that is actually new. The phenomenon is thought by some to be due to a response to cues in the new situation that are common to old, roughly similar, experiences; others believe it to be due to a kind of momentary neural 'short circuit' which causes the impression of the scene to arrive at the memory store (metaphorically speaking) before it has registered in the sensorium. There is some evidence for the latter view since frequent *déjà vu* experiences are symptomatic of certain kinds of brain damage. There are several *déjà* experiences, – others include *déjà pensé* or already thought and *déjà entendu* or already heard – all of which are usually classified as PARAMNESIAS.

de Lange syndrome CORNELIA DE LANGE SYNDROME.

delay conditioning An experimental conditioning technique in which the onset of the unconditioned stimulus (US) occurs some time after the onset (although prior to the termination) of the conditioned stimulus (CS). For most conditioned responses, the optimal delay between CS onset and US onset is 0.4 to 0.5 seconds. Contrast with BACKWARD CONDITIONING, SIMULTANEOUS CONDITIONING, TRACE CONDITIONING.

delayed instinct INSTINCT, DELAYED.

delayed matching to sample MATCHING TO SAMPLE.

delayed reaction (procedure) An experimental procedure in which the subject responds to a stimulus some time after it has been removed from sight. For example, the subject watches while the stimulus object is hidden but is not allowed to search for the object until a delay period has expired. It is a difficult task for young children and many animals; success is assumed by some to reflect the existence of symbolic capacity.

delayed reinforcement (procedure) Generally, any situation or experimental procedure in which the presentation of the reinforcer is delayed until some time after the response has been made.

delayed response A term used to characterize the major event in the DELAYED REACTION PROCEDURE.

delayed sleep-onset insomnia INSOMNIA, DELAYED SLEEP-ONSET.

Delboeuf illusion See EBBINGHAUS ILLUSION.

delinquent Generally, anyone who commits a crime or who violates a legal code. However, the term is almost always used of a juvenile offender, for which the defining age is set by local legal statute (typically around 16 to 18 years).

delirium A disoriented condition with clouded consciousness, often accompanied by hallucinations, illusions, misinterpretations of events and a generally confused quality with reduced capacity to sustain attention to things in the environment. Delirium is frequently of fairly rapid onset (often after a head injury or seizure) but may also develop slowly over time, particularly if metabolic factors are responsible. It is currently classified in psychiatry as an *organic mental syndrome* and several varieties are known, classified usually by cause.

delirium of persecution A term occasionally applied to those cases of delirium that have a compelling fearfulness and hallucinations of being threatened as their dominant symptoms. Distinguish from DELUSIONS OF PERSECUTION.

delirium, substance-related A large number of drugs, when abused, can produce a clinical delirium. In some cases it is brought on by large doses (e.g. of amphetamines), in others it follows a period of repeated abuse (e.g. of phencyclidine or PCP), while in others still it occurs as a withdrawal syndrome after extended abuse (e.g. alcohol-withdrawal delirium).

delirium tremens An acute DELIRIUM, with all of its characteristic symptoms, that is associated with excessive alcohol abuse. The definition is pretty straightforward but usage patterns can be rather confusing. Some writers have used the term (and its slang abbreviation, *the DTs*) as though the syndrome were caused by alcohol consumption, which is true but only in a misleading manner. The proper usage is for a delirium the onset of which follows, usually by a day or two, the *cessation* of alcohol intake after many years of alcohol abuse. To eliminate this confusion the former syndrome is now called ALCOHOL HALLUCINOSIS (of which, incidentally, a true delirium is not a symptom) and the latter is known as ALCOHOL-WITH-DRAWAL DELIRIUM.

Delphi method A procedure for predicting future events based on the pooling of judgements made by a number of experts. The procedure is named after the Greek oracle of Delphi.

delta (Δ) A notation used to refer to a change in the value of some variable or factor. Usually presented in abbreviated form with the thing that is changing; e.g. ΔR is a change in the level of responding, ΔS a change in the level of the stimulus, ΔI a change in intensity, etc.

delta motion (or **movement**) MOTION, DELTA.

delta rule In connectionist modelling (see CONNECTIONISM (2)), a procedure that allows for complex links to be formed between elements. It is a more powerful technique than the HEBB RULE because it is based on having the network (see NETWORK MODELS) compare the desired (final) outcome pattern with the current, actual pattern and make appropriate changes. Such mechanisms are referred to as *supervised* rules.

delta waves Electroencephalographic (EEG) signals of low frequency (1–3 Hz) and high amplitude (approximately 150 mV). Delta waves are characteristic of a person in deep sleep.

delusion A belief that is maintained in spite of argument, data and refutation which should (reasonably) be sufficient to destroy it. Care should be taken in the use of the term – one person's delusion may be another's salvation. Also note that the term is not typically used when one's culture or subculture subscribes to the belief. Distinguish from HALLUCINATION and ILLUSION. With respect to the various forms of psychiatric disorders involving delusions, the official terminology has shifted in recent years. For example, the term *delusions of grandeur* has given way to *delusional disorder, grandiose type* and *delusions of persecution* to *delusional disorder, persecutory type*. Terms currently recommended by the *DSM-IV* and the ICD-10 are given below, along with those found in older texts.

delusional disorder An umbrella term for any mental disorder that has as a significant symptom some form of delusion. Note that terminology has shifted several times in recent years, particularly in North America. While the entries that follow use 'type' as a tag for particular forms of delusions, not all nosologies use this format. A diagnosis of *delusional disorder, erotic type* in one system may be listed as *erotic delusional disorder* or *erotic delusion* in another.

delusional disorder, erotic type A delusional paranoid disorder characterized by the belief that a famous or highly regarded person is in love with one. Also called *delusional disorder, persecutory type* and, more simply, *erotic delusion*.

delusional disorder, grandiose type A delusional disorder which typically takes the form of believing that one has some great but unrecognized talent or insight. Distinguish from MEGALOMANIA.

delusional disorder, jealous type A delusional disorder characterized by the belief, without reasonable cause, that one's mate is unfaithful. In the classic form, the most minute piece of 'evidence', such as a thread or disarrayed clothing, may be used to justify the belief. Also known as *conjugal paranoia*.

delusional disorder, persecutory type The classic form of DELUSIONAL (PARANOID) DISORDER. The individual suffers from a cluster of delusions, usually involving the malign intentions of others. They may feel that others are out to 'get' them, that they are being cheated, conspired against, maligned, spied on and so forth. The oft-used term *paranoid delusion* is no longer recommended when characterizing the symptoms of this disorder, being instead reserved for cases of PARANOID (TYPE) *SCHIZOPHRENIA, which involves delusions of grandiosity and jealousy as well as persecution. See also PARANOIA.

delusional disorder, somatic type A cover term for delusions that involve: (a) the whole body image, as in *anorexia nervosa*, sufferers of which feel fat despite being emaciated; or (b) parts of the body, as in the case of a patient who believes that some part of his or her body is missing (see ORGANIC *DELUSIONAL SYNDROME) or imagines that various bodily parts do not function properly, or that he or she emits a foul odour from the skin, mouth, rectum or vagina.

delusional jealousy DELUSIONAL DISORDER, JEALOUS TYPE.

delusional misidentification disorder (or **syndrome**) An umbrella term for any DELUSION whose dominant characteristic is the belief that some person(s), object or location has somehow been changed or modified. When they have a singular focus, they are called MONOTHEMATIC *DELUSIONS. Classic examples are CAPGRAS SYNDROME, FREGOLI SYN-

DROME, INTERMETAMORPHOSIS and SUBJECTIVE DOUBLES.

delusional (paranoid) disorder An umbrella term for the various forms of paranoid disorder characterized primarily by one or more persistent, nonbizarre delusions with a paranoid flavour. Apart from the delusions and their ramifications, the individual's behaviour is not abnormal in any pronounced fashion. The term is used only when there is no evidence of any other mental disorder. See also PARANOIA.

delusional speech The speech typical of one with a delusion. Seen most commonly in delusions of grandeur, when allusions to personal influence, power, accomplishments, etc. are common, and in delusions of persecution, when the language is rich with paranoia, suspiciousness, accusations, etc.

delusional syndrome, organic A delusional disorder due to a known organic factor. The term is used broadly to include those disorders brought on by drug abuse (see SUBSTANCE-RELATED *DELUSION) and those that result from epilepsy, brain lesions or other diseases that affect the central nervous system. This diagnostic category is no longer listed in the *DSM*. See discussion under ORGANIC (5).

delusion, monothematic Any delusion with a single underlying topic, e.g. CAPGRAS SYNDROME, FREGOLI SYNDROME.

delusion, nihilistic Any delusion marked by a sense of nonexistence. It may be of the self, parts of the self, or the world. Cases of DELUSIONAL DISORDER, SOMATIC TYPE may also be termed nihilistic when they involve the sense of nonexistence of the body or of a body part.

delusion of being controlled A delusion in which the person experiences feelings, impulses, thoughts and actions as though they were imposed by some external force or some other person.

delusions of grandeur DELUSIONAL DISORDER, GRANDIOSE TYPE. Also called *grandiose delusion*.

delusions of persecution DELUSIONAL DISORDER, PERSECUTORY TYPE.

delusions of reference Delusion in which one interprets remarks or references which are neutral or intended for others as having negative significance for oneself. Everyone has a bit of this (see IDEAS OF REFERENCE), but the term itself is reserved for pathological cases.

delusion, substance-related A general label for any of a variety of delusional disorders that result from either extended abuse or single high doses of a drug. A large number of substances are known to produce delusions of various kinds, including alcohol, amphetamines, various hallucinogens, marijuana and cocaine.

delusion, systematized A singular delusion that is marked by multiple elaborations involving other delusions, all of which are traced, in the mind of the individual, back to a single event or theme.

demand 1 n. A requirement, an imperative need. Often used in this sense to refer to either internal or external states that have motivating properties, e.g. nutritional demands or family demands. **2** adj. Characterizing or describing properties of situations that invite or even require particular kinds of behaviour from individuals. See e.g. DEMAND CHARACTERISTICS.

demand character A Gestalt term for those characteristics of a stimulus situation that invite particular modes of reaction to it. See AFFORDANCE, which is used in similar ways.

demand characteristics 1 Those features of an experimental setting that bias the subject to behave in particular ways, that invite from the subject a particular interpretation of the study and recruit particular kinds of behaviour. When used in this fashion the term refers to confounding features in a study that contaminate the results. See EXPERIMENTER BIAS for one kind. **2** More generally, the qualities of a particular experimental setting that simply, by their nature, invite certain kinds of behaviour. For example, memory experiments that use nonsense syllables characteristically 'demand' of a subject the use of various mnemonic devices. Here the notion of bias is not connoted; these are features that, by virtue of their properties, are typically associated with one or another behaviour pattern. **3** By extension, any social setting which, by its very nature, establishes a set that carries with it behavioural 'demands'.

Note that some authors use the term only to refer to the qualities and properties of the situation (as in the above); others, however, use it to refer to the feelings, expectations and desires of the individual in such settings. Those who use it in the latter sense typically use *task demand* or *environmental demand* in the former. See also SET (2), which some use as a cover term for all of these effects.

demand feeding SELF-DEMAND (SCHEDULE OF) FEEDING.

dementia Generally, a loss of intellectual capacity to the extent that normal social and occupational functions can no longer be carried out. The term is reserved for multifunctional disorders characterized by the loss of memory, reasoning, judgement and other 'higher mental processes'. Typically, alterations in personality and modes of social interaction accompany these cognitive deficits. Some authors use the term only for progressive syndromes, with the connotation of irreversibility; others are neutral on prognosis. Usually the writer is clear on this point. The contemporary approach to the dementias is to treat them as *organic mental syndromes* and to use a qualifying term to identify the suspected cause. See following entries.

dementia, AIDS Dementia associated with the direct involvement of HIV in the brain. Usually not observed until the later stages of AIDS, the symptoms include apathy, loss of ability to concentrate, memory impairments and diminished performance on tasks associated with frontal-lobe functions.

dementia, alcoholic Dementia observed in the last stages of severe, chronic alcoholism. It is characterized by poor judgement, diminished cognitive ability, lack of interest in personal hygiene, flattened affect and, significantly, an anterograde amnesia (see KORSAKOFF'S SYNDROME). See AXIAL *DEMENTIA.

dementia, axial Dementia marked by severe anterograde amnesia resulting from damage to the midline (i.e. axial) brain structures, including the thalamus, hippocampus, mammillary bodies and fornix. The classic form is KORSAKOFF'S SYNDROME, seen after extended chronic alcoholism. See ALCOHOLIC *DEMENTIA.

dementia, fronto-temporal Any of several presenile, neurodegenerative disorders that affect primarily the frontal and temporal lobes of the brain. The first symptoms are usually changes in personality and, in most cases (e.g. PICK DISEASE) followed by loss of language, memory and other cognitive functions. Unlike ALZHEIMER'S DISEASE, these dementias typically emerge between the ages of 40 and 60 years but, like Alzheimer's show a progressive, unrelenting deterioration. Also spelled *frontotemporal* and occasionally called *frontal and temporal lobe dementia* or simply *frontal dementia* (esp. in European publications). The terms FRONTAL-LOBE SYNDROME and ORGANIC *PERSONALITY SYNDROME will also, although not always appropriately, be found referring to these and similar disorders.

dementia infantilis CHILDHOOD DISINTEGRATIVE DISORDER.

dementia, multi-infarct Dementia due to significant cerebrovascular disease. The disorder is not uniformly progressive but proceeds in distinct steps, with a loss in only some intellectual functions early in its course, resulting in a patchy deterioration. The disorder is a result of multiple and often extensive localized cortical lesions, and, in addition to intellectual deterioration, a variety of neurological signs are symptomatic, e.g. weakness in the extremities, exaggeration of deep reflexes, dysphagia, hypertension and other vascular abnormalities. Also called *arteriosclerotic dementia*, *psychosis with cerebral arteriosclerosis* and VASCULAR *DEMENTIA (see that term for more detail).

dementia naturalis An obsolete term for extreme mental retardation.

dementia of the Alzheimer's type (DAT) ALZHEIMER'S DISEASE.

dementia, organic Loosely, any dementia caused by a lesion or brain injury. This diagnostic category is no longer listed in the DSM. See discussion under ORGANIC (5).

dementia paralytica PARESIS.

dementia praecox The original, although

now obsolete, term for schizophrenia; the literal meaning is *premature dementia.*

dementia, presenile Specifically, a dementia with onset prior to age 65. The criterion here is quite arbitrary but is generally accepted by diagnosticians.

dementia, primary degenerative A form of dementia characterized by gradual and progressive deterioration. It is typically associated with old age (see SENILE *DEMENTIA) and usually leads to death within 5 to 10 years. The disorder is strongly associated with widespread cerebral atrophy.

dementia pugilistica A chronic dementia caused by multiple concussions. Symptoms include memory loss, speech impairment, unsteady gait, tremors and episodes of confusion and depression. As the name suggests, it is commonly observed among boxers, so much so that in many recent texts it is referred to as *chronic progressive encephalopathy of boxers.* Known nontechnically as *punch-drunk.* See TRAUMATIC BRAIN INJURY.

dementia, semantic A form of progressive dementia marked by the loss of knowledge of and diminished memory for the meanings of words. Nonsemantic perceptual and motoric functions are largely unaffected.

dementia, senile A general term for any dementia associated with the aged. Senile dementias are of the primary degenerative type and are associated with a variety of causes, including *Alzheimer's disease, Pick's disease* and certain vitamin deficiencies and cerebrovascular pathologies. Obsolete synonyms are *senile psychosis, geriatric psychosis* and *geriopsychosis.*

dementia, vascular A term recently proposed to replace MULTI-INFARCT *DEMENTIA to reflect the fact that this disorder is due largely to diminished cerebral blood flow.

democratic atmosphere K. Lewin's term for the general sociopolitical climate established when a group is led by a person with democratic values and a free exchange of ideas and open discussion of issues are encouraged. Contrast with AUTHORITARIAN ATMOSPHERE and LAISSEZ-FAIRE ATMOSPHERE.

demography The study of human populations – in their structures, distributions, geographic locations, increases and decreases over time, etc. Although demography began with examination of vital statistics, it is now a rich, multi-discipline science embracing such areas of study as fertility, marriage, education, social class, race, ethnicity, distribution of wealth and resources, epidemiology, crime and population migration and has borrowed heavily from biology, ecology, economics, sociology and psychology.

demonology 1 A legitimate area of study of folklore and cultural myths concerned with demons and spirits. **2** A pseudoscience which claims to study demons and spirits as real entities. See PARAPSYCHOLOGY.

demonomania The delusion that one is possessed by a demon or spirit.

demonstration 1 Formally, the presentation of a proof of a theorem. **2** Less formally, a compelling presentation of an effect which functions to make a point. Many 'experiments' in science are really demonstrations, in that they are designed not so much to test a hypothesis as to show that a particular interpretation of a phenomenon is correct. The Gestalt psychologists used this technique masterfully. **3** A pedagogic technique whereby the teaching is by presentation of examples and illustrations.

demyelination Literally, the loss of MYELIN, the fatty sheath surrounding the axons of many neurons. It is a component of various disorders, including multiple sclerosis and Guillain-Barré syndrome, but can also be caused by viruses and various toxins. Occasionally spelled *demyelinization.*

dendrite Any of the richly branching, tree-like processes attached to the cell body or SOMA (1) of a *neuron.* Dendrites function as the receiving end of a neuron and are stimulated by *neurotransmitters,* which flow across the SYNAPSE from the terminal buttons of other (presynaptic) neurons on to the DENDRITIC SPINES.

dendritic 1 Generally, tree-like, branching. **2** Specifically, pertaining to dendrites and their structure and function.

dendritic spike An ACTION POTENTIAL that is observed in the dendrites of many PYRAMIDAL CELLS.

dendritic spine A small bud-like outgrowth on the surface of a dendrite. Dendritic spines synapse with the terminal buttons of presynaptic neurons.

dendrodendritic synapse   A *synapse* between the *dendrites* of two *neurons*.

denervation   Removal of the nerve supply to an organ or other tissue. Note that 'removal' here is intended loosely; one may merely sever or otherwise render nonfunctional neural pathways without literally removing the nerves.

denial   A DEFENCE MECHANISM that simply disavows or denies thoughts, feelings, wishes or needs that cause anxiety. The term is used purely for unconscious operations that function to 'deny' that which cannot be dealt with consciously.

denotative meaning   MEANING, DENOTATIVE.

density   **1** Generally, the degree to which the elements or parts of a display or complex stimulus are grouped together. **2** More specifically, in statistics, the extent to which the various data points lie proximate to the regression line. See here REGRESSION (2). **3** In audition, a dimension of experience characterized by the degree to which a tone sounds 'compact' or 'thin'. **4** In demography, the number of persons per unit area, i.e. *population density*.

dental   A speech sound produced by placing the tongue against the teeth, e.g. /θ/, the unvoiced 'th' in *thin*.

dental age   AGE, DENTAL.

dentate gyrus   A part of the HIPPOCAMPAL FORMATION that receives inputs from the ENTORHINAL CORTEX and projects to an area within the HIPPOCAMPUS itself. See these terms for more detail.

dentate nucleus   One of the DEEP CEREBELLAR NUCLEI. It plays a role in the control of skilled, rapid movement.

deontology   In moral reasoning, the principle that decisions and actions are properly made according to fundamental moral principles. This position is typically contrasted with *consequentialism*, where decisions are based on the outcomes. To see the distinction consider what the truly moral action should be if a runaway train is about to kill five people walking on the tracks but you can

throw a switch to send it to another spur where there is only one person who would be killed.

deoxyribonucleic acid (DNA)   A large, complex molecule made up of four nucleotide bases (*adenine, guanine, cytosine* and *thymine*) and a 'backbone' of a sugar molecule (specifically, *2-deoxy-D-ribose*, hence the name). The nucleotide bases are arranged in pairs down the centre of the double-helix-shaped molecule, forming the specific arrangement which carries the genetic code determining the functioning of every cell. The code is based on sequences of 3 nucleotide base-pairs, with each sequence specifying one of 20 amino acids. Since there are 64 possible combinations there is considerable flexibility in the arrangement and more than enough to code any given protein's sequence of amino acids. Each of the chromosomes in the nuclei of all cells is made up of DNA; it is, thus, the chemical basis for all heredity and the carrier of all genetic information. See also RIBONUCLEIC ACID (RNA).

dependant   A person in a relationship characterized by dependence on others or on a substance. var., *dependent*.

dependence   **1** In statistics, a relationship between variables such that changes in one are accompanied by changes in another. Note that in this sense the term connotes a causal link between the variables. Occasionally an author may wish to use the term while remaining neutral on cause and effect; in such cases the phrase *statistical dependence* is used, 'statistical' suggesting that 'true' cause and effect has not been determined. **2** In social psychology, excessive reliance on others for support, opinions, beliefs, ideas, etc. **3** In psychopharmacology, DRUG *DEPENDENCE. var., *dependency*.

dependence, drug   In recent years this term (and its shorthand form, *dependence*) has come to be favoured over *addiction* and *habituation* in scientific writing. Put in simplest terms, an individual is said to have developed dependence on a drug or other substance when he or she has a strong, compelling desire to continue taking it. Note that this desire may derive from a wish either (a) to experience its effects or (b) to avoid or escape the aversive experiences produced by its absence (see here WITHDRAWAL SYMP-

TOMS). Dependence on a drug may in origin be largely psychological (see PSYCHOLOGICAL *DEPENDENCE) or physiological (see PHYSIO-LOGICAL *DEPENDENCE). See also SUBSTANCE DEPENDENCE.

dependence, physiological Drug dependence produced by alterations in physiological states resulting from repeated administrations of the drug. The characteristic that marks such dependence and differentiates it from PSYCHOLOGICAL *DEPENDENCE is that severe physiological dysfunctions emerge if the drug is suddenly discontinued or if an antagonist is administered. The opiates and the barbiturates both produce such dependence with prolonged use. The term is preferred over the once widely used *addiction* and *drug addiction*. Also referred to as *physical dependence*.

dependence, psychological Drug dependence characterized by a rather pervasive drive to obtain and take the substance. This term is usually defined by exclusion; i.e. it is used for any dependence on a drug the action of which does *not* produce fundamental biochemical changes such that continued doses of the drug are required for normal functioning. PHYSIOLOGICAL *DEPENDENCE covers these other cases. Drugs like marijuana are commonly cited as likely to produce psychological dependence with habitual use. The term is preferred over the previously common *drug habituation*.

dependency 1 In social and personality psychology, the reliance to a higher degree than normal of one person on another (or others) for emotional, economic or other support. **2** A characteristic of an individual in such a dependent state; a lack of self-reliance. See DEPENDENCE (2), with which it is often used synonymously.

dependency, chemical DEPENDENCE, DRUG.

dependency, morbid K. Horney's term for an extreme, neurotic surrender of self to another such that one person becomes pathologically reliant on another for things social and emotional.

dependency needs A loose cover term for 'vital' needs, those required for normal functioning. Used for both the physical/biological (food, water, warmth, shelter) and the psychological (affection, love, security).

dependent Characterizing DEPENDENCE or DEPENDENCY in any of the meanings of those terms.

dependent personality disorder A personality disorder characterized by such extreme passivity that the individual affected allows others to take over responsibility for his or her life. Such individuals are typically lacking in self-confidence, unsure of their abilities and willing to allow decision-making in all matters to be taken over by others. Also called *passive-dependent personality* and, especially in older writings, *asthenic personality*.

dependent variable VARIABLE, DEPENDENT.

depersonalization The thought or feeling that the self as normally experienced no longer exists. In EXISTENTIALISM the focus is on the sense that one is a mere cog in a blundering, dehumanized social machine. In contemporary psychiatry and clinical psychology the focus is on more discrete perceptions such as one's body feeling alien or the sense that one is viewing oneself from a distance. Fleeting thoughts and perceptions such as these are common and normal. However, they are regarded as constituting a *depersonalization disorder* or (in older texts) *neurosis* if severe, pervasive or prolonged. Depersonalization is often accompanied by DEREALIZATION. Compare with DISSOCIATION, which is a more general term.

depersonalization disorder (or **neurosis**) DEPERSONALIZATION.

depolarization In neurophysiology, a reduction in the electrical potential of a neuron from its normal resting potential of roughly -70 mV. Very small stimuli produce relatively minor and transient depolarizations; with larger stimuli, those sufficient to depolarize the membrane beyond approximately -60 mV, the neuron 'breaks away' and depolarization becomes complete even to the point of reversing the charge so that the inside of the axon approaches $+40$ mV. This discharge is called the ACTION POTENTIAL. See also ALL-OR-NONE LAW (1).

depressed Loosely descriptive of any organism or system functioning at less than normal levels. It most often refers to persons suffering from DEPRESSION, but is also used of neurological processes whose operations are diminished by damage or drugs and even of groups of individuals whose social functions are compromised by external or internal forces.

depressed bipolar disorder BIPOLAR DISORDER, DEPRESSED.

depression 1 Generally, a mood state characterized by a sense of inadequacy, a feeling of despondency, a decrease in activity or reactivity, pessimism, sadness and related symptoms. In this sense depressions are quite normal, relatively short-lived and (damnably) frequent. **2** In psychiatry, any of a number of MOOD DISORDERS in which the above characteristics are extreme and intense. Depression in this sense may be a symptom of some other psychological disorder, a syndrome of related symptoms that appears as secondary to another disorder, or a specific disorder itself. Note that many psychiatrists regard ANHEDONIA (a general lack of interest in the pleasures of life) as a defining characteristic of depression – even to the point of regarding it as sufficient for a diagnosis independent of the individual complaining of being depressed. Contemporary approaches to depression tend to emphasize the underlying neurophysiological components as much as the more traditional psychological and social factors. See here ANTIDEPRESSANT DRUGS and related entries. The following entries describe many of the major varieties of depressive disorder. Others are found elsewhere under the modifying term.

depression, agitated A depression in which the individual displays psychomotor agitation as a dominant symptom. The overt symptoms are irritability, excitability and restlessness.

depression, endogenous Depression resulting from 'internal' factors, both physiological and psychological. The term is used clinically when there is no *apparent* precipitant, although many prefer not to use it at all on the grounds that it implies that there are *no* precipitating events. Compare with REACTIVE *DEPRESSION.

depression, exogenous See REACTIVE *DEPRESSION.

depression, major A MOOD DISORDER

marked by a severe and extended MAJOR *DEPRESSIVE EPISODE.

depression, neurotic 'Ordinary' severe depression. A mildly out-of-date term used as a cover for any depression that is not a PSYCHOTIC *DEPRESSION, i.e. one which does not entail a loss of contact with reality.

depression, psychotic Severe depression in which the individual loses contact with reality and suffers from an array of impairments of normal functioning.

depression, reactive Depression resulting from events occurring in one's life. *Depression* is used here in a clinical sense and connotes that the affective reaction is inappropriate given the events themselves, thus differentiating the meaning of the term from that of *grief*. See also the discussion under DEPRESSION. Also called *exogenous depression*. Compare with ENDOGENOUS *DEPRESSION.

depression, retarded Depression characterized by psychomotor retardation as the dominant symptom. The individual tends to be lethargic, laconic and slow to initiate action.

depression, unipolar A MAJOR *DEPRESSIVE EPISODE. The qualifier *unipolar* is used for cases in which the depressive episodes recur without the appearance of the manic phase that is observed in the classic form of BIPOLAR DISORDER.

depressive 1 n. One suffering from a DEPRESSION (2). **2** adj. Characterizing depression.

depressive anxiety A psychoanalytic term for anxiety provoked by a sense of fear concerning one's own hostile feelings toward others. The usage here derives from the oft-stated (but, frankly, unproven) notion that 'depression is hostility turned inwards'.

depressive disorder A category of MOOD DISORDERS marked by either single or recurrent MAJOR *DEPRESSIVE EPISODES without a history of MANIA (2). See also DEPRESSION.

depressive disorder, minor A *mood disorder* characterized by periods of depression but lacking the full range of symptoms that mark a MAJOR *DEPRESSIVE EPISODE.

depressive episode, major In psychiatry, a DEPRESSION (2) with all of the classic symptoms of ANHEDONIA, sleep disturbances, lethargy, feelings of worthlessness, despondency, morbid thoughts and, on occasion, suicide attempts. The term is reserved for cases in which there is no known organic dysfunction.

depressive neurosis DYSTHYMIC DISORDER.

depressive personality disorder A disorder marked by pervasive, low-level depressive thoughts and behaviours. Moods are dominated by gloominess, unhappiness and pessimism. Affected individuals often have low self-esteem and feelings of guilt but, interestingly, often see themselves as merely realistic.

depressive spectrum A syndrome of a diagnosed DEPRESSION (2) along with a family history of alcoholism and/or one of the AFFECTIVE DISORDERS.

depressogenic Loosely, characterizing anything that increases the likelihood of DEPRESSION.

depressor nerve Specifically, a branch of the vagus (Xth cranial) nerve that functions to lower blood pressure. Often, however, one will find any nerve that reduces motor or glandular function referred to as a *depressor*.

deprivation Strictly speaking the term refers to the loss of some desired object or person and is used to mean either the act of removing the object or person or the state of loss itself. There is also a curious technical usage, as in phrases like '48-hour food deprivation' and '85% of normal body weight deprivation'. In such cases the term refers to an experimental procedure in which the hunger drive or nutritional need state of an organism is controlled by specifying (operationally) the level of deprivation.

deprivation, relative The perception that you, or members of your in-group, have less than you deserve, or less than some relevant comparison group. In studies of aggression, this idea was proposed to explain the fact that aggression toward others sometimes arises in a group that is, objectively speaking, not particularly deprived. The key here is that the deprivation is perceived, and that the state of deprivation is relative to that of some other group or to what was expected.

deprogramming A nontechnical term used to refer to efforts to retrain people who have joined obscure, fanatical groups to live in society again. The assumption is that some groups, using techniques of isolation and peer pressure, 'programme' people to their values and way of life, and in order to readapt to normal life and values such people must be 'deprogrammed'. The term is slowly dropping out of use.

depth analysis Psychoanalysis is often called depth analysis since the assumption is that it probes deep below the well-defended conscious level of mind to the underlying dynamic factors that presumably motivate a person.

depth of processing In cognitive psychology, a coding dimension that runs from the superficial to the abstract. The further along this dimension a stimulus is processed, the greater the 'depth'. For example, the stimulus 11 may be processed as two straight lines, as a number that rhymes with another number, as a number between 10 and 12, or as the only 2-digit prime number with both integers the same. Each level here represents a deeper, more abstract analysis than the preceding. According to most contemporary analyses of human memory, the greater the depth to which a stimulus is processed, the more likely it will be stored in memory for later recall. See also SHORT-TERM *MEMORY and LONG-TERM *MEMORY. The variable itself is often referred to as *levels of processing* or occasionally, *LOP*.

depth perception Quite literally, the perception of depth, viewing the world in three dimensions. There are two standard usages here: one refers to the distance of objects from the viewer, the other to the three-dimensionality of objects themselves. Depth perception is an old and still intensely pursued topic in experimental psychology. To get a feeling for the kinds of issues that occupy researchers, see PERCEPTION et seq.

depth psychology A generic term used to cover any psychological system that assumes that explanations of behaviour are to be found at the level of the unconscious. Freudian and Jungian theories are the classic examples, and many authors use the term as a rough synonym for psychoanalysis.

derailment A disorder of thought manifested by erratic shifting of topics, frequent *non sequiturs* and inappropriate hesitations. A common symptom in schizophrenia, it is assumed due to a LOOSENING OF ASSOCIATIONS. The term is often modified to specify the type of derailment, e.g. *cognitive derailment, volitional derailment*.

deranged Loosely and largely nontechnically, disturbed or disoriented. Used with regard to cognitive, intellectual abilities.

derealization An alteration in the perception of the environment with the sense that somehow one has lost contact with external reality. A common component of DEPERSONALIZATION.

dereistic Pertaining to the use of fantasy, imagination or day-dreaming. In pathological cases, i.e. those in which contact with reality is seriously weakened or lost, it serves as a rough synonym for *autistic*.

derivation 1 That which is the result of a formal set of inferences, the outcome of a deductive process. **2** The deductive process itself.

derivative 1 n. That which is not original, a thing developed, deduced or obtained from something else. **2** adj. Secondary, acquired from something else. **3** adj. In psychoanalysis, characterizing behaviours that emerge from unconscious conflicts disguised or distorted so as not to produce anxiety.

derived Developed out of, transformed from, acquired from, adapted from, etc. The term has a number of combinatory forms; the following are representative of usage.

derived need A need developed from or learned by close association with a primary need. See e.g. ACQUIRED *DRIVE.

derived property In Gestalt theory, a property of a stimulus due to the characteristics of the whole situation of which it is a part.

derived scale Any scale that is a result of a transformation from another scale.

derived score Any score that is a result of a transformation from another score, e.g. the *z-score*.

derma 1 Loosely, the skin. **2** Specifically, the layer of skin just below the outermost (epidermal) layer.

dermal sense CUTANEOUS SENSE.

dermatitis Generally, any inflammation of the skin. Several varieties are known, usually associated with specific causes such as allergic reactions to particular substances. However, there is evidence that in some cases psychosomatic factors lead to a predisposition and/or exacerbation of many forms. There is also a suggestion that other forms are autoimmune reactions.

dermatome An area of skin innervated by the fibres of a single dorsal root. For example, there are 12 spinal roots for the thoracic area and there are also 12 (in cases, partly overlapping) dermatomes on the chest and trunk area of the body, each corresponding to one of the spinal roots.

dermographia Lit., skin writing; hence, a condition in which tracings made on the skin are followed by marked reddening of the area. Also called *autographia*.

dermooptical perception Lit., seeing with the skin. The term is used in PARAPSYCHOLOGY for the hypothesized (but undemonstrated) ability to 'see' with one's skin, e.g. to detect the colours of objects by touching them.

Descartes, René CARTESIAN.

descending pathway or tract Generally, any EFFERENT neural pathway, one that carries information from the brain out to the periphery.

description 1 A full, complete and accurate (to the extent that such is possible) characterization of a situation based on careful observation. In the philosophy of science, description is generally held to be a necessary precursor of EXPLANATION. **2** In introspection, reporting psychological processes in a 'pure', uninterpreted fashion.

descriptive grammar GRAMMAR, DESCRIPTIVE.

descriptive principle The principle that the basic goal of behavioural science is accurate description in terms of relations between observed events such that prediction of and control over behaviour may be achieved. The principle represents, at least on the surface, a nontheoretical stance, since attempts at developing causal laws and explanations are to be resisted. In its pure form, Skinnerian behaviourism reflects this principle.

descriptive psychiatry A term generally used of any system of psychiatric diagnosis based on the relatively straightforward descriptions of overt, observable symptoms. Usually contrasted with the *dynamic* schools, in which diagnosis is based on underlying, covert psychic factors.

descriptive statistics STATISTICS, DESCRIPTIVE.

descriptive unconscious PRECONSCIOUS.

desensitization Generally, any decrease in reactivity or sensitivity. Used for: (a) reactions to simple stimuli, e.g. a sudden noise will produce a dramatic startle response the first time but after successive presentations within a short time the reaction diminishes and disappears; and (b) more global emotional reactions. See DESENSITIZATION PROCEDURE and compare with HABITUATION.

desensitization procedure A clinical technique used in behaviour therapy designed to produce a decrease in anxiety toward some feared object or situation, i.e. to desensitize a patient. It is particularly useful in treating phobias and other behaviour problems based on anxiety. The basic technique consists of exposing the patient to a series of approximations to the anxiety-producing stimulus under relaxed conditions until finally the anxiety reaction is extinguished. For example, a child's fear of fire engines may be gradually overcome by exposing the child first to pictures of fire engines, then to toy models, etc. When the procedure is implemented in a 'real world' setting where the client actually experiences the anxiety-provoking events, it is often called *in vivo desensitization*; when the procedure is done using imagery in a neutral setting (like a therapist's couch) it will be called *covert desensitization*. Also called *systematic desensitization*.

desexualization 1 Generally, any procedure that results in the removal of sexual significance from something. *Removal* here is used rather loosely and may refer to any of a number of processes: *sublimation*, concealment, *counter conditioning*, etc. **2** Occasionally, the act of *castration*.

design 1 Any plan or schema for action. The connotation is that there is forethought, that the nature and structure of some plan has been well articulated and reasoned through. See EXPERIMENTAL *DESIGN. **2** A purpose or goal.

design, experimental The overall plan of an experimental investigation. An entire area of experimental psychology is concerned with various ways to design studies to maximize precision and analysability and to minimize ambiguity and confusion. Topics considered are: selection of experimental participants, assignment of these to conditions, choice of controls, administration of treatments, recording of data, etc. It should be noted that usually experiments are designed with reference to the type of statistics one wishes to use or the kind of questions one may legitimately ask of one's data. Quite frequently the kind of statistical analyses one may perform are dependent on the particular experimental design used. See also CONTROL.

design, factorial A common type of experimental design in which levels of one treatment are varied over all the levels of another treatment. For example, if one wishes to study the effects of different levels of deprivation (say, levels A and B) and different amounts of training (say, levels 1 and 2) on some process such as learning in a laboratory rat, then the levels of deprivation will be varied factorially over the levels of training, resulting in four groups of subjects: A1, A2, B1, B2.

desipramine A TRICYCLIC COMPOUND used as an ANTIDEPRESSANT. It retards the reuptake of norepinephrine. Previously used for a variety of behavioural disorders, it has been largely replaced by compounds with fewer side effects.

desmopressin A synthetic analogue of VASOPRESSIN with stronger antidiuretic action and less hypertensive effects.

destruction method A method used in physiological research whereby the functions of particular areas of the nervous system are studied by surgically destroying them or removing them. The inference is that the resulting behaviour is a function of the remaining undestroyed tissue. See also ABLATION, EXTIRPATION.

destrudo In psychoanalysis, the energy for the hypothesized death instinct, THANATOS.

desynchronization 1 Generally, any disruption of synchrony. **2** In EEG recordings, the disruption of alpha rhythm seen when attention is directed to a stimulus. See ALPHA BLOCKING.

desynchronosis A mismatch between the time one is accustomed to and the time of one's present location; in short, a fancy term for *jet lag*.

detached affect A psychoanalytic term for affect which has been removed (i.e. detached) from the painful, anxiety-producing idea or thought with which it was originally associated. In Freud's view, all obsessions resulted from the *reattachment* of such affect to some other, originally neutral, idea or thought.

detached character K. Horney's term for a type of personality characterized by an emotional remoteness, a self-assured form of detachment and a lack of concern for the feelings of others.

detachment 1 Generally, a sense of emotional freedom; the lack of feeling of emotional involvement in a problem, in a situation, with another person, etc. **2** In K. Horney's theory, a defence mechanism that functions by preventing one from forming emotionally intimate ties with others, resulting in a neurotic, emotional aloofness with a lack of empathy and sensitivity for others. *Neurotic* in this context can present a bit of a problem since on occasions a perfectly reasoned and rational choice may be made, depending on the circumstances, to engage in the process of emotional detachment. In such cases the designation *neurotic* is inappropriate.

detection theory SIGNAL DETECTION THEORY.

detection threshold THRESHOLD (esp. 1).

deterioration Progressive loss of function. Used in various combinations involving muscular, emotional, intellectual, judgemental, neuronal, etc. functions.

deterioration index The inverse of the HOLD INDEX.

determinant Any causal or antecedent condition or agent. This seemingly straight-forward term is used in a most confusing array of combined terms by many authors when they seek to characterize the particular causes of particular patterns of behaviour. The terminology here is certainly well intended but generally rather unsatisfying. To wit: *organismic* determinant is frequently used for causal factors presumed to arise 'within' an organism, *genetic* for those determinants deemed hereditary, *environmental* for those judged to be purely (or at least predominantly) in the external environment, *situational* for momentary determinants of particular acts, *personal* for those argued to derive from personality traits or characteristics, etc. The difficulty, of course, is that one can rarely (if ever) unambiguously determine the locus of the determinants of behaviour in this manner; *caveat lector*.

determinant, dream In the psychoanalytic approach to dream analysis, a psychic factor that is judged to be significant in giving a dream an essential quality.

determinants, constitutional Those aspects of a person's general physical and physiological make-up that are regarded (by some theorists) as important factors in personality. For more detail see CONSTITUTIONAL THEORY.

determination 1 From the Latin for *limiting*. Hence, the establishment of limits or boundaries. Often used with the connotation that the analysis is quantitative, and the determinations are precise; e.g. the stimulus conditions in a psychophysical experiment are said to receive precise *determination*. **2** By extension, the reaching of a conclusion, the making of a decision. **3** By further extension, a personality trait characterized by a tendency to push onward toward one's goal despite barriers and hardships.

determination, coefficient of That proportion of the variance of the dependent variable attributable directly to the actions of a specified independent variable. The complement of this statistic, the variance *not* resulting from that independent variable, is called the *coefficient of nondetermination*.

determiner 1 Generally, a cause, an antecedent condition, that results in some particular outcome; a DETERMINANT. **2** In linguistics, a generic term covering articles (*a, an, the*), possessives (*his, theirs, Mary's,* etc.), demonstratives (*this, that*) and a variety of other forms all of which are normally used before attributes in noun phrases.

determining set SET (2).

determinism Very loosely, the doctrine that assumes that every event has causes. In classical mechanics it was assumed that were one to know the position and momentum of every particle of matter at one instant in time, then one could, in principle, know their position and momentum at any other point in time future. Such a position is the ultimate in 'hard' (or *nomological*) determinism. This particular view was 'softened' somewhat with the development of quantum mechanics, in which the deepest knowable levels of cause and effect appear to be probabilistic in nature, shifting the notion of perfect prediction to probabilistic prediction. In psychology the debate is somewhat less cosmic and considerably less well defined. It generally revolves round the existentialist's and humanist's insistence on a measure of 'free will', with which a person can remain outside the ever-probing tentacles of the behavioural and cognitive sciences. The debate, however, is probably an empty one. If one wishes to study behaviour and the mind scientifically it must be assumed that the things one does have causes and that they are ultimately knowable. The question is really whether there is some 'thing' called *free will* which stands outside scientific analysis of cause and effect or whether it is (merely?) a particular mental/affective state which itself plays a role in the causation of behaviour. Most contemporary social scientists, if they think about the issue at all, take a position that can best be described as 'uncomfortable pragmatism'. That is, in their day-to-day work they treat their subjects as probabilistically determined, chalk up what they cannot predict accurately to as yet unknown factors of causation (and perhaps a variation of the uncertainty principle) and prefer to think of themselves as actually operating according to their own free choice independently of a crass determinism that diminishes their sense of their own humanity.

detour problem An experimental setting that requires subjects initially to move away from a goal in order to obtain it eventually. Detour problems require a certain level of cognitive functioning to solve and are difficult for infants and most animals. The problem was first introduced by the Gestalt psychologists under the German term *Umweg Problem*.

detoxification The process of treatment using rest, fluids and changes in diet to restore proper physiological functioning following disruption by overuse of drugs.

detumescence Subsidence of swelling. Used commonly to refer to the subsiding of the erectile tissue of the genital organs (penis and clitoris) after erection.

deuteranomaly A visual condition in which there is a slight diminution in sensitivity to green wavelengths.

deuteranopia The more common of the two forms of DICHROMACY; it is characterized by a lowered sensitivity to green light. The term comes from the Greek *deuteros* meaning *second*, and the theory is that this form of colour blindness is produced by a deficiency in the green-light-absorbing pigment (green being the second primary). Compare with PROTANOPIA.

devaluation A defence mechanism whereby one attributes exaggerated and inappropriate negative qualities to oneself or others.

development 1 The sequence of changes over the full lifespan of an organism. This is the meaning first introduced into psychology; the area of 'developmental' psychology in the early decades of the 20th century referred to the study of the full lifespan, from birth to death. Today the tendency is to use the term more restrictively. See, for example, DEVELOPMENTAL DISABILITY and DEVELOPMENTAL *APHASIA, in which the age range is restricted to birth to adolescence. **2** Maturation. The connotation here is that the process is a biological one and largely dictated by genetic processes. This sense is probably the oldest and etymologically goes back to the Old French *desveloper* meaning to *unwrap* or *unfold*. Developmental processes of this kind are often contrasted with those that are the result of learning. See here the discussion under CHILD DEVELOPMENT. **3** An irreversible sequence of change. To some degree this notion of irreversibility is contained in meanings 1 and 2, but it is listed separately because of its significance in medicine and psychiatry, which refer to the *developmental course* of a disease or disorder, over which a number of distinct stages follow one upon the other. **4** A progressive change leading to higher levels of differentiation and organization. Here the connotation is one of positive progress, with increases in effectiveness of function, maturity, sophistication, richness and complexity. This sense is generally intended in phrases like *human development, social development, intellectual development* and *emotional development*. Note that the genetic connotations of meanings 2 and 3 are absent here; rather, the implication is that processes attributable to environmental factors (learning, nutrition, etc.) are responsible.

Clearly, we have a rather loose term on our hands here. And, as is so often the case with terms that reference processes of fundamental importance, it is applied very broadly. In almost any of the above senses, that which develops may be just about anything: molecular systems, bones and organs, emotions, ideas and cognitive processes, moral systems, personalities, relationships, groups, societies or cultures. Not surprisingly, there is a large number of specialized terms based on this one; the more commonly used follow.

developmental Generally, pertaining to DEVELOPMENT, in any of its senses. Note, however, that there is a tendency to denote a number of clinical syndromes and psychological disorders as *developmental* when (a) they occur only during childhood or (b) the occurrence during childhood is marked and significantly different from occurrence in adolescence or adulthood. Some of these disorders are given below, others can be found under the heading of the modifying word.

developmental coordination disorder A disorder characterized by marked impairment of motor coordination that is severe enough to interfere with academic achievement or normal living. The term is not used if the lack of coordination is due to a physical disorder or to mental retardation.

developmental delay An umbrella term

for a situation in which a developmental milestone is reached significantly later than the norm. The term is only used for delays exhibited by infants, toddlers and preschoolers. Typically modifiers are used to mark the specific form of delay.

developmental disability A general term for any significant handicap that appears in childhood or early adolescence (the criterion often stated is prior to age 18) and continues for the life of the individual.

developmental disorder, pervasive A class of childhood disorders characterized by a serious distortion of basic psychological functioning. The notion of distortion here is a general one and may involve social, cognitive, perceptual, attentional, motor or linguistic functioning. See e.g. AUTISM and ASD.

developmental disorders, specific A class of disorders that emerge during childhood characterized by disruption or delay in a specific area of perceptual or cognitive functioning that is independent of any other disorder. See e.g. DEVELOPMENTAL *ARITHMETIC DISORDER, DEVELOPMENTAL *LANGUAGE DISORDER. Note that in the latest edition of the DSM, these disorders are classified as either COMMUNICATION DISORDERS or LEARNING DISORDERS.

developmental level(s) Period(s) of life defined by age. The most common set of levels in use is:

birth to 1 year: infancy
1 year to 6 years: early childhood
6 years to 10 years: mid-childhood
10 years to 12 years: late childhood (or preadolescence)
12 years to 21 years: adolescence
21 years to 65 years: maturity
65 and upwards: old age.

developmental milestones Significant behaviours the appearance of which are used to mark the progress of development. Walking is a milestone in locomotor development, conservation in cognitive development, production of functional sex cells in sexual development, etc.

developmental norm(s) The average level(s) of performance on some task by a representative group of children at a particular age or developmental level.

developmental psychology Strictly speaking, the field of psychology concerned with the lifelong process of change. *Change* here means any qualitative and/or quantitative modification in structure and function: crawling to walking, babbling to speaking, illogical reasoning to logical, infancy to adolescence to maturity to old age, birth to death. When first articulated as a substantive subdiscipline in psychology by G. S. Hall around the turn of the 20th century, it was quite explicitly this kind of 'cradle-to-grave' field of investigation. However, it should be noted that most of the scientists who call themselves *developmental psychologists* are interested in childhood, indeed so much so that for many the term *developmental psychology* has become equivalent to CHILD PSYCHOLOGY. To clarify issues of terminology here various other labels have emerged for more specialized subdisciplines. *Lifespan psychology* is used by some for the original meaning, and chronologically narrower fields such as the *psychology of adolescence* and the *psychology of the aged* (see here GERONTOLOGY) are recognized.

developmental quotient (DQ) DEVELOPMENTAL *AGE divided by chronological age.

developmental scales A general label for any of a variety of tests and procedures for evaluating the developmental status of infants and preschoolers. Of necessity, all such scales are either performance tests or oral tests and, in general, must be individually administered. See e.g. BAYLEY SCALES OF INFANT DEVELOPMENT, GESELL DEVELOPMENT SCHEDULES.

developmental sequence A general term applicable to the order of appearance in any sequence of behaviours, growth of structures, series of functions, etc. that has a pattern characteristic of a given species.

developmental stage Any period of development during which certain characteristic behaviours appear. This definition is rather loose; see STAGE THEORY for details.

deviance Generally, any pattern of behaviour that is markedly different from the accepted standards within a society. The connotation is always that moral or ethical issues are involved, and the term is typically quali-

fied to indicate the specific form of deviance being referred to, e.g. sexual deviance.

deviate 1 n. Generally, one who differs markedly from the statistically established central tendency (loosely, the average) of a group. Note that, unlike 2 and 3, this meaning is evaluatively neutral. On the scale of intelligence, Einstein was a deviate in this sense. **2** n. One who differs markedly from accepted standards of practice in a group, especially standards of morality or ethics. See here DEVIANCE. **3** n. One whose sexual behaviours are considered inappropriate by general society; see the discussion under SEXUAL *PERVERSION. vb., *deviate*.

deviation Departure from some norm. The term is used to refer to such departures in behaviour, in attitudes and in statistics. In behaviour, it generally refers to disorders or clinical syndromes. In studies of attitudes, the reference is generally to patterns of attitude change. In statistics, it refers to the degree to which a score differs from some measure of *central tendency*, usually the mean.

deviation, average A measure of the variability of a sample of scores from the mean of the sample. It is given as the arithmetic mean of the differences between each score and the mean. It is rarely used; the STANDARD *DEVIATION is preferred.

deviation score A value giving the degree to which any single score deviates from the mean of all the scores in a sample. Generally denoted as x or d.

deviation, standard A measure of the variability of a sample of scores from the mean of the sample. It is given as $SD = \sqrt{[\Sigma(X_i - \bar{X})^2/N]}$, where $\bar{X}$ is the mean, X_i the ith score and N is the total number of scores. When N is less than about 25 or so, the SD is 'biased' in that it does not give a proper estimate of the true population SD, i.e. the SD of the population from which the sample under consideration was drawn. To correct for this bias with samples under 25, $N - 1$ is used in the denominator. The SD is the preferred measure of dispersion of a set of scores – along with the VARIANCE, which is SD^2. In general, when one is referring to the standard deviation of a sample of scores, the notation SD is used; when referring to the standard deviation of a full population or to a theoretical distribution, the Greek letter σ is used.

device Any instrument, piece of apparatus or cognitive procedure used for some specific purpose.

devolution 1 Reversal or undoing of evolution. **2** Degeneration, catabolism.

dexter From the Latin, meaning *right* or *favourable*. All terms so derived pertain to: **1** The right side of the body in general or the right hand specifically (*dextral, dextrality*); or **2** Skilfulness, particularly manual (*dexterity, dextrousness*). Contrast with SINISTER.

dexterity test Any sensorimotor test that requires both speed and accuracy of fine motor movement.

dextrad Toward the right side (of the body).

df Abbreviation for DEGREES OF FREEDOM.

dhat A CULTURE-SPECIFIC SYNDROME found in India. It is marked by anxiety and hypochondriacal concerns with semen, discoloration of urine and a feeling of weakness.

DI DELTA (Δ).

di- Prefix meaning *two*.

dia- Prefix meaning *within* or *through*.

diacritical marking system (DMS) A writing system developed to assist children in learning to read. The basic intent is the same as with the INITIAL TEACHING ALPHABET except that the normal visual patterns of the letters are kept intact and pronunciation cues are supplied by a system of diacritical marks.

diadic Pertaining to two; characterizing things which are paired or arranged in twos. var., *dyadic.*

diad, social A two-person group, a face-to-face encounter between two people. Long-range social interactions, such as those occurring over the telephone, are sometimes considered social diads. var., *social dyad.*

diagnosis The identification of a disease, disorder, syndrome, condition, etc. In clinical psychology the term is used in the same general sense as in medicine; i.e. classification and categorization are the central concerns. Thus, a person displaying a particular

form of aberrant behaviour may be diagnosed as having schizophrenia or bipolar disorder or some other specific psychological/psychiatric disorder. Unfortunately, such usage has at times obscured more than it has clarified. A diagnostic procedure of this kind is accurate only to the extent that specific diseases or syndromes in fact exist. The assumption always used to be that these diagnostic categories were as well defined as, say, pneumonia or measles; that is, clinical psychological and psychiatric diagnosis was based on the *medical model*. It is now generally recognized that such an assumption is not always tenable. To deal with the serious problem of inappropriate diagnosis more and more emphasis is placed on behaviour, on thought and on affect; in short, on those aspects of what a person does, thinks and feels which are deviant in terms of societal norms or which are counterproductive to living a normal life. The diagnostic emphasis in both psychiatry and clinical psychology has shifted in recent years from identifying and labelling a presumed underlying 'disease' or 'mental illness' to a more objective characterization of symptoms displayed. While this shift helped clarify some issues, it has left others unresolved. First, there is little focus on the severity of particular behaviours, thoughts or emotions. Is an individual who is immobilized by depression and displaying suicidal ideation suffering from the same disorder as one who shows a lack of energy and interest in life? Second, there has been little effort to order diagnostic classification systems by underlying neuropathology. This lack is understandable given the lack of knowledge about brain function and psychopathology but it implies that diagnostic classification systems will continue to be revised as insight is gained. Third, in some venues where private insurance payments have an impact on the practice of clinicians, the 'official' classifications (see DIAGNOSTIC AND STATISTICAL MANUAL) force particular diagnoses in order to qualify for coverage leading to circumstances where funding trumps proper practice.

diagnosis creep The tendency for a particular diagnosis to be made with increasing frequency as a disorder becomes more intensely studied and widely known. It results from: (a) more careful and accurate diagnostic techniques that reveal more true cases; and (b) a loosening of diagnostic criteria and a broadening of the boundaries of the disorder which produces an increase in false diagnoses.

diagnosis, differential Diagnosis aimed at distinguishing which of two (or more) similar diseases or disorders an individual has. The term has enjoyed considerable extension beyond the medical/clinical areas and is used for distinguishing between conditions of many kinds in social psychology and the study of personality.

Diagnostic and Statistical Manual **(I, II, III, III R, IV and IV-TR)** The full name is *Diagnostic and Statistical Manual of Mental Disorders*. The *DSM* (for short) is the official system of classification of psychological and psychiatric disorders, prepared and published by the American Psychiatric Association. The first version, *DSM-I*, was published in 1952, and subsequent revisions (*II, III, III R, IV and IV-TR*) appeared in 1968, 1980, 1987, 1994 and 2000 respectively. Along with the appropriate sections of the *ICD* (INTERNATIONAL CLASSIFICATION OF DISEASES) the *DSM* is the major guide to the classification, treatment and prognosis of psychological/psychiatric disorders. It should be clear from the simple fact that six editions have been published in 48 years that psychiatric nosology is hardly an exact science. Interestingly, during that period the number of identified disorders has grown from about 100 to more than 300 – a fact that should alert all users of the manual to the likelihood that social, cultural and even political factors play a role in the determination of the categories of psychiatry. Moreover, it should be made very clear that actual usage lags behind the mandated nomenclature; for example, since *DSM-III* there have been no psychiatric conditions that are officially classified as *neuroses* (the more neutral term *disorder* is used), although hardly a textbook exists on personality and/or abnormal psychology that does not use the term. In this dictionary every effort has been made to include all terms, even the ones no longer receiving the APA's imprimatur, particularly when they are still in wide use. *DSM-IV* and *DSM-IV-TR* are particularly noteworthy for their extreme specificity. Disorders are quite specifically defined and the emphasis is on beha-

viours, thoughts, feelings and desires that are counterproductive to the individual displaying them. There is a shift away from the identification of specific diseases or 'neuroses'. One important element of *DSM-IV* and *DSM-IV-TR* is the degree to which their terminology has been coordinated with that of the Classification of Mental and Behavioural Disorders in *ICD-10*. Previously these two classification systems had been developed independently and international terminological confusions were all too common. See DIAGNOSIS for more on this point. Note that the full name of the manual is rarely used; it is typically abbreviated to *DSM* plus the relevant number.

diagnostic interview A common procedure in clinical situations in which the client or patient is interviewed for the purpose of reaching some reasonable determination of the nature of his or her disorder and its aetiology and of planning a method of treatment.

diagnostic test A general cover term for any test or procedure used in an attempt to pinpoint the specific nature and (perhaps) origins of a disability or disorder. In psychological work the term is used in a somewhat misleading fashion since *diagnostic* here refers not to the identification of a disease or a syndrome but rather to the determination of the particular source of an individual's difficulties in a certain area. Most tests described as 'diagnostic' evaluate such skills as reading, language and sensorimotor coordination.

diagnostic value Quite literally, the value of a test in making a diagnosis; that is, its VALIDITY.

diagram 1 Generally, a schematic drawing that presents the essential features of some system. A diagram may represent either the proper physical relations between features in a spatial and/or temporal manner or it may present them in a symbolic and/or logical fashion. **2** Common shorthand form of SCATTER DIAGRAM. **3** An arbitrary sign used in a logographic writing system such as Chinese.

dialect A form of a natural language differing from the standard and usually spoken in a particular geographic region. The word *differing* here is tricky. A dialect is usually regarded as sufficiently distinct in pronunciation patterns, grammar, vocabulary and the use of idioms to be clearly detectable as a separate linguistic form, yet not so different as to be classified as a separate language. However, in practice, political and social issues often weigh more heavily than linguistic considerations. For example, the Mandarin and Cantonese 'dialects' of Chinese are not mutually intelligible, while the Norwegian and Swedish 'languages' to a considerable extent are. Clearly, geopolitical factors have led to the first two being classified as dialects of one language and the second two as separate languages. Compare with ACCENT.

dialectic 1 Of reasoning involving extensive deductive argument, particularly that aimed at the clarification of the meaning of concepts. The ancient dialectical approach involved the development of contradictions and their solutions as the means of elucidation. **2** Of the philosophy of Georg W. F. Hegel, which was based on the theory that reality develops through the interplay of thesis, antithesis and synthesis. For Hegel every action (thesis) produced a counterreaction (antithesis) and was inevitably followed by an integration of these opposites (synthesis). The *dialectical materialism* of Marx and Engels was greatly influenced by Hegel's principle.

dialectical behaviour therapy A form of psychotherapy developed by Marsha Linehan that synthesizes features of COGNITIVE-BEHAVIOURAL THERAPY and Buddhist MINDFULNESS in order to effect change. Called dialectical because it involves the therapist accepting the individual while helping the individual change and because it attempts to balance logical and affective components of experience, it appears to be effective with difficult cases such as BORDERLINE PERSONALITY DISORDER.

dialectical reasoning 1 In Aristotle's scheme, reasoning from the basis of commonly held, as opposed to demonstrably true, premises. **2** A form of reasoning in which opposites can be entertained as simultaneously true by finding a middle ground solution. Because philosophers of logic (correctly) object to the use of the term 'reasoning' for this second meaning, *dialectical thinking* is preferred.

dialectical thinking See DIALECTICAL REASONING (2).

dialectic(al) psychology Loosely, the theoretical stance that argues that conflict and change are the basic principles of life. Dialectics had its origins in Heraclitus and was further developed in philosophical and political forms by Hegel and Marx respectively. As a theory specifically concerned with change, it has found an audience in developmental psychology, where it has become associated with those theories that argue that development is a series or flux of transformations impelled by essential conflicts between a child's cognitive system and reality, or between coexisting cognitive components.

From this position, individuals are seen to transform their environments by action which, in turn, changes them. Thus, people develop through their own labour and action, the resistances they meet and the conflicts they engender. Major development changes (or 'dialectical leaps') occur when the day-to-day quantitative changes reach a critical number or mass. Piaget's position is often labelled dialectic.

dialysis The process of purifying a liquid by passing it through a membrane.

Diana complex A psychoanalytic term for the (assumed) repressed desire of a woman to be a man.

diaphoresis Profuse sweating.

diary method The study of an individual, usually a child, through a daily record of behaviour.

diaschisis Diminished neural activity in the regions of the brain surrounding the site of a lesion. It is caused by disturbances in the neural network connecting these areas with the site of the damage, which may be some distance apart, even in opposite hemispheres. The effects are usually transient and functions recover.

diastole The relaxing phase of the heart cycle.

diathesis An inherited predisposition to a particular disease or other condition. Usually the term is used with qualifiers specifying the disease or condition.

diathesis–stress hypothesis The generalization that many abnormal behaviour patterns are the result of an inherited susceptibility combined with a particularly stressful environment and a lack of learned skills for coping with the stress.

diazepam A commonly prescribed ANTIANXIETY DRUG of the BENZODIAZEPINE class. Trade name Valium.

dichaptic Simultaneous stimulation of two sides of the body, usually the hands, with different stimuli. The tactile equivalent of *dichoptic* and *dichotic*.

dich(o)- Combining form meaning *in two parts*.

dichoptic Stimulation of the two eyes with distinctly different stimuli. The visual equivalent of *dichotic*.

dichorhinic Stimulating each nostril with a different odorant.

dichorionic twins MONOZYGOTIC *TWINS.

dichotic Stimulation of the two ears with distinctly different stimuli. Contrast with BINAURAL (1) and DIOTIC. The auditory equivalent of *dichoptic*.

dichotomous variable A variable that can take just two values, e.g. male/female.

dichotomy Division or classification into two, not necessarily equal, parts.

dichromacy General term for any of several kinds of colour-vision deficiency. As the name suggests, dichromats can match any given sample hue using only two other wavelengths, as opposed to trichromats (those with normal colour vision – see TRICHROMACY), who require three. Two forms of dichromacy involve weakness in the perception of reds and greens (PROTANOPIA and DEUTERANOPIA); two others involve blues and yellows (TRITANOPIA and TETARTANOPIA – although the existence of the latter has not been firmly established). Over the years a number of terms have been used synonymously with *dichromacy*. They include *dichromatism*, *dichromatiopsia*, *dichromopsia*, *dichromia* and *dichromasy*. There are also various adjectival forms for each of the noun forms although, blissfully, only one term for an individual with the deficit: *dichromat*.

dichromacy, anomalous Either of the rare forms of DICHROMACY which involve colour deficiencies in the blue and yellow regions of the spectrum, i.e. *tritanopia* and *tetartanopia*.

dichromasy DICHROMACY.

dichromat An individual with any of the various forms of DICHROMACY.

dichromatism DICHROMACY.

dichromatopsia DICHROMACY.

dichromat, uniocular A person who has normal colour vision in one eye but is a *dichromat* in the other. Such persons are very rare but are extremely useful subjects in the study of colour vision.

dichromia DICHROMACY.

dichromopsia DICHROMACY.

Dick–Read method A natural childbirth technique developed in England during the 1930s. It is based on giving the mother physiological, anatomical and hygienic instruction along with training in relaxation and controlled breathing.

dictator game A game used in studies of BEHAVIOURAL ECONOMICS. One player (A) determines how much money in a specified pool to keep and how much to give to player B. Player B has no say and must take what is offered by the 'dictator'. Most people in A's situation, despite having total control over the distribution, offer a reasonable and occasionally generous amount to B. See also ULTIMATUM GAME.

DID DISSOCIATIVE IDENTITY DISORDER.

didactic Instructional, pertaining to teaching.

didactic analysis ANALYSIS, DIDACTIC.

didactic therapy THERAPY, DIDACTIC.

diencephalon A major subdivision of the forebrain consisting primarily of the *thalamus* and the *hypothalamus*.

diet The term derives from a Greek word meaning *way of living*. Thus: **1** Food substances and liquids normally consumed in day-to-day living. **2** Any specific programme of food intake prescribed for a particular reason, e.g. a low-cholesterol diet, a diet for a

diabetic. **3** Any diminished food-intake programme for the purpose of losing weight.

dietary neophobia A fear of new foods. It is
found in the young of many species who will
not eat an unfamiliar food until a parent has
consumed it and is not harmed by it. It is also
often observed in humans, especially among
children, who may exhibit a dislike of new
and different foods. Note that the use of *phobia* here is not quite right in that the fear is
not a phobic disorder but a pattern of behaviour that has adaptive value. Differentiate
from the simple term *neophobia*, which, despite being occasionally used synonymously,
is properly used for an irrational fear of new
things generally.

**difference associated with subsequent
memory (DM)** A pattern of neurological
activity in the brain associated with something remembered as compared with something forgotten. If the neural correlate (e.g.
an *event related potential*) observed when a
previously seen item is recognized is different from the one seen when an item is forgotten, the difference between the two is a
DM. There are also differences associated
with subsequent *illusory* memory (called
DIMs). These are observed when comparing
brain activity for accurate memories with
false memories, such as those obtained
using the DEESE PARADIGM. DMs and DIMs are
neurological snapshots of the *encoding* process.

difference limen THRESHOLD.

difference threshold THRESHOLD.

difference tone COMBINATION TONE.

Differential Aptitudes Tests (DAT) A battery of group-administered tests designed to
assess a variety of cognitive functions
thought to be important for academic functioning. It is used with those aged 13 years
and older.

differential conditioning Conditioning
produced by reinforcing responses made to
one of a set of stimuli while withholding
reinforcement from responses made to the
other(s). See DISCRIMINATION.

differential diagnosis DIAGNOSIS, DIFFEREN-
TIAL.

differential emotions theory See THEORIES
OF *EMOTION.

differential extinction Selective extinction of responding by withholding reinforcement for a particular response while
continuing to reinforce other responses.

differential fertility FERTILITY, DIFFERENTIAL.

differential growth GROWTH, DIFFERENTIAL.

differential inhibition A term coined by
Pavlov to describe the gradual elimination of
responding to stimuli which are similar to,
but discernibly different from, the original,
conditioned stimulus.

differential limen THRESHOLD.

differential psychology An approach to
the study of psychology that focuses on individual differences in behaviour.

differential rate reinforcement In operant conditioning, a term for a class of SCHED-
ULES OF *REINFORCEMENT in which the delivery
of reinforcement depends on the immediately preceding rate of responding. Included
here are *differential reinforcement of high rate
(drh)*, *differential reinforcement of low rate (drl)*
and *differential reinforcement of paced responses
(drp)*.

differential reinforcement REINFORCE-
MENT, DIFFERENTIAL.

**differential reinforcement of appropri-
ate behaviour** Quite literally, reinforcing
socially appropriate behaviour. It is used as a
behaviour modification technique whereby
praise and attention accompany prosocial
behaviours while socially inappropriate reactions and antisocial behaviours are ignored.

**differential reinforcement of high rate
(drh)** SCHEDULES OF *REINFORCEMENT.

**differential reinforcement of low rate
(drl)** SCHEDULES OF *REINFORCEMENT.

**differential reinforcement of other
behaviour (dro)** SCHEDULES OF *REINFORCE-
MENT.

**differential reinforcement of paced
responses (drp)** SCHEDULES OF *REINFORCE-
MENT.

differential response Any response made
selectively to one of several stimuli presented. See DISCRIMINATION.

differential scoring Analysing the results of a test battery by rescoring the responses along a number of different dimensions so as to extract measures along a number of variables.

differential stimulus DISCRIMINATIVE *STIMULUS.

differential threshold THRESHOLD.

differentiation 1 In embryology, a process whereby a group of initially similar cells generates a number of different kinds of cell. 2 In mathematics, the process of carrying out a differential. 3 In sociology, the process by which groups, roles, statuses, etc. develop within a society. In psychology proper there are three distinct uses: 4 In conditioning studies, whenever an organism must learn to make two or more different responses to two or more similar stimuli. The particular experimental conditions used dictate whether this set of circumstances is one of *response* differentiation or *stimulus* differentiation. 5 In perception, when a stimulus array changes from perceived homogeneity to perceived heterogeneity so that the various aspects of the array become distinguished. Here one speaks of learning to differentiate between stimulus conditions. Contrast this meaning with that of ENRICHMENT. 6 In OBJECT RELATIONS THEORY, the degree to which other people are seen as distinct from the self, with their own personality structures and motivations.

difficult child An infant or child who exhibits a temperament characterized by high activity, distractibility, intense negative affect, irregular daily patterns, aversion to novelty and change, and hypersensitivity to stimuli. An *easy child* is one with developmentally appropriate attention skills, positive affect, acceptance of change, and establishment of regular daily patterns. A *slow-to-warm-up child* is one who displays an aversion to change and novelty, low activity and expressivity levels, is easily overstimulated, resists changes and takes longer than average to 'warm-up' to novel settings. These terms emerged colloquially but are now found in the technical literature, particularly in studies of infant TEMPERAMENT.

diffraction Bending of light or sound waves round the edges of some object.

diffuse Scattered, spread, not localized. Used of thought or behaviour which is undifferentiated, uncoordinated or lacking direction, and of light that has no clear source.

diffusion 1 Generally, spreading. The connotation is that something found in one locale spreads and scatters through another. Hence: 2 Interpenetration of liquids or gases such that they become mixed. 3 The spreading of the effects of a localized stimulus through neighbouring tissues. 4 The scattering of light in the eye produced by characteristics of anatomical structures, principally the spherical aberrations of the lens. 5 In sociology, the spread of culture traits from one society to another or from one distinct group to another within the same society.

diffusion of responsibility RESPONSIBILITY, DIFFUSION OF.

diffusion tensor imaging A MAGNETIC RESONANCE IMAGING technique useful for imaging the white matter of the brain. Since the MYELIN that defines white matter diffuses water along axons, magnetic imaging can pick up the direction of water diffusion and hence the location of axon bundles and tracts in living tissues.

digital Pertaining to: 1 The figures in any given numbering system, e.g. 0–9 in the decimal system, 0–1 in the binary system. 2 The fingers and toes.

digit-span test A test of immediate or short-term memory. The subject is given a series of random digits and immediately recalls as many as possible. See SPAN OF *APPREHENSION and SHORT-TERM *MEMORY.

digraph Any two letters in a word that are pronounced as a single phonetic unit, e.g. *ch* in *church*.

digraphia The use of two or more (despite the 'di-' prefix) writing systems in daily life. Commonly seen in immigrant communities and countries such as Japan where multiple *graphologies* are used.

dihydrotestosterone An ANDROGEN produced from testosterone. It contributes to the development of the male external genitalia.

dilation Expansion, enlargement. var., *dilatation*.

dildo(e) An artificial penis.

dilemma A situation in which one is faced with two (or, colloquially, more) mutually exclusive or mutually incompatible alternatives from which to choose when neither can be taken as truly satisfactory. Dilemmas present a fertile domain for the study of choice behaviour and the manner in which people balance various positive and negative outcomes in making decisions. See the following entries for a few of the more intensely investigated circumstances.

dilemma, moral A situation in which one is confronted with two choices such that selecting one violates one set of moral precepts and selecting the other violates another. A classic case is that confronting a physician who is asked by a terminally ill patient in great pain to provide a fatal overdose of a drug so that the patient may die with dignity.

dilemma, prisoner's A game based on the classic detective-to-suspect situation. In the typical format each player (prisoner) is told separately that, although there is little direct evidence to convict him or her, there are two choices: confess or don't confess. If neither confesses, there will be a minor penalty for both; if both confess, there will be a relatively severe penalty for both; but if only one confesses, the prosecutors will 'go easy' on the confessor while 'throwing the book' at the other. In psychological studies the penalties are usually replaced by small rewards, and confessing or not by a choice between two responses, but the principle remains the same. If both subjects make response A, both receive a moderate reward, say 5p; if both select response B, both receive a very small reward (1p); but if one chooses A and the other chooses B, the one who chooses A receives a high reward (10p) while the other receives only a very small one or perhaps none at all. Not surprisingly, the game holds a particular fascination for psychologists because the outcome is always dependent on the choices of both players and on the degree of cooperation they display.

dilemma, social Any situation in which the immediate outcome or pay-off for an individual is high if that person 'defects' from social mores but the ultimate outcome for *all* persons is reduced if too many people

defect. Examples are ubiquitous and reflect many of the classic and profound ills of any large society. For example, if you keep your thermostat high your home remains warm, but if too many keep their thermostats high the fuel supply becomes exhausted and everyone freezes; also called *social trap*.

DIM DIFFERENCE ASSOCIATED WITH SUBSEQUENT MEMORY.

dimension Originally this term was applied to just three characteristics of physical space: height, width and depth. Now, however, it is used to refer to any well-defined quantitative series. Thus, one speaks of colour as having three dimensions (brightness, hue, saturation) or of a pure tone as having three (amplitude, frequency, phase). Moreover, the term has become increasingly common with reference to nonquantitative aspects of complex stimuli, so that references to *semantic dimensions* or *social dimensions* are often seen. Note that in these latter cases the dimensions themselves are frequently difficult to specify. A variety of sophisticated techniques have been developed to extract these dimensions from large databases; see e.g. MULTIDIMENSIONAL ANALYSIS, MULTIDIMENSIONAL SCALING.

diminishing returns Nontechnical phrase for negatively accelerated improvement. What is meant is that past a certain point each additional effort results in smaller and smaller amounts of progress; the gain is just not worth the effort.

dimming In perception, the enhancement of an afterimage by reducing the intensity with which the image is projected.

dimorphism Lit., having two forms or manifestations. Typically used to refer to species of which there are two distinguishable forms, as in juvenile and adult or male and female.

DIMS *disorders of initiating and maintaining sleep*; see INSOMNIA.

DIN colour system A colour-classification system used widely in Europe. It is based, like the Munsell colour system, on the three primary dimensions of hue, brightness and saturation.

ding-dong theory THEORIES OF *LANGUAGE ORIGIN.

diopter A unit for measuring the power of a lens for bringing parallel rays of light to a focus.

diopteric aberration SPHERICAL *ABERRATION.

diotic Stimulation of the two ears with the same stimulus. See BINAURAL (1). Contrast with DICHOTIC.

diphenylbutyl piperidines A subgroup of the *butyrophenones* used as ANTIPSYCHOTIC DRUGS primarily in the treatment of schizophrenia. The most common is *pimozide*. They are somewhat less effective in relieving the schizophrenic symptoms than the more frequently used PHENOTHIAZINES (e.g. *chlorpromazine*), but seem to have fewer side effects.

diphthong (*dif-thong*) Any speech sound in one syllable produced by gliding from one vowel to another, e.g. the *i* in *ice*.

diplacusis 1 Generally, hearing two tones when only one was presented. 2 Specifically, condition in which a person perceives a different pitch when a tone is presented to one ear from that perceived when an identical tone is presented to the other ear. When both ears are simultaneously stimulated a pitch somewhere between them is heard.

diplegia Paralysis of similar parts on both sides of the body, e.g. both arms or both legs.

dipl(o)- Combining form meaning *double*.

diploid number The normal number of chromosomes in the somatic cells of a particular species. In humans the diploid number is 46. The diploid number is twice the HAPLOID NUMBER.

diplopia Vision characterized by double images. The condition results from a failure to fuse properly the images from the two retinas. Contrast with POLYOPIA.

dips(o)- Combining form meaning *thirst*.

dipsomania Intense craving for alcoholic beverages. Distinguish from *alcoholism*; dipsomania occurs in widely spaced 'attacks' of relatively short duration.

direct 1 Straight, uninterrupted. 2 Unmediated by other processes, not enriched.

direct apprehension DIRECT PERCEPTION.

direct association ASSOCIATION, DIRECT.

direct correlation Occasional synonym for POSITIVE *CORRELATION.

direct dyslexia DYSLEXIA, DIRECT.

directed An occasional synonym for *goal-directed*. Used in phrases like *directed movement* (movement aimed coherently at some goal) and *directed thinking* (the kind of goal-oriented thinking involved in problem-solving).

directive A *speech act* in which the speaker tries to get the listener to do something for him or her. For example, 'Please close the door.' But see also INDIRECT DIRECTIVE.

directive therapy A general label for any psychotherapeutic approach that focuses and directs the client to change. Generally included are *hypnotherapy*, *rational emotive therapy* and some forms of *behavioural therapy*. Also called *active therapy*.

direct perception The central concept of the theoretical position about the process of perception put forward by J. J. Gibson. The argument is that perception consists of a cognitively unmediated, inferentially unenriched process whereby the properties of the distal stimulus are directly apprehended. Gibson's *bottom-up* position contrasts with other theories, which argue that other processes operate to organize, enrich and interpret the percept (see CONSTRUCTIVISM). Often the term *direct realism* is used to characterize Gibson's system, on the grounds that the ecologically important aspects of the environment are directly represented in that which is perceived. For more on this point see ECOLOGICAL VALIDITY.

direct realism DIRECT PERCEPTION.

direct reflex 1 Generally, any reflex occurring on the same side of the body as the stimulus. Contrast with CROSSED REFLEX. 2 Specifically, the prompt pupil-contraction response to a light shone in the eye.

direct scaling INDIRECT *SCALING.

dirhinia Of both nostrils. Dirhinic stimulation affects receptors in both nostrils simultaneously.

dirty halo effect TRAIT NEGATIVITY BIAS.

dis- 1 A prefix of Latin origin meaning *apart*, *away from*, *lack of*, *separation from*, *reversal*.

2 Variant of DYS-. Note, meaning 1 should be distinguished from 2 since the latter carries a distinctly negative sense absent in the former. Alas, spelling variations that violate these etymological roots abound, e.g. *disorder, disability*.

disability Generally, any lack of ability to perform some function; more specifically, a congenital impairment or loss of function through trauma, disease, etc. See DISABLED. In many locales there are also governmentally defined criteria. The one used in the US, for example, is 'inability to engage in any substantial gainful activity by reason of any medically determinable physical or mental impairment which can be expected to last or has lasted for a continuous period of not less than 12 months'.

disabled Characterizing one suffering from a *disability*. Because of the many negative connotations which have developed around the term *handicapped*, many prefer this term to refer to any individual who suffers from a condition that only superficially limits his or her functioning. A look at the entry DISABILITY, however, should alert the reader that the word *superficially* needs clarification. The notion entailed by the new usage is that the person may indeed suffer from a most severe (i.e. disabling) condition such as paraplegia but may nevertheless be quite capable of living a rich and fulfilling life provided that certain adjustments are made for the disabling condition such as the installation of ramps for wheelchairs, elevators, modified equipment on the job, etc.

disambiguation The act of determining the contextually appropriate meaning(s) of an ambiguous word, phrase or sentence or an ambiguous situation.

DISC1 Short for *disrupted-in-schizophrenia 1*, a gene whose actions have been implicated in the disturbed cognitive and emotional processes common in schizophrenia. Mutant forms of the gene (and there are several) appear to lead to abnormal brain development, specifically in the proteins responsible for the development and maintenance of critical neural systems.

discharge 1 The firing of a stimulated neuron. **2** The release of pent-up tensions. **3** The flowing-away of a bodily secretion, or the secretion itself.

discharge of affect Quite literally, the diminishing of experienced affect by displaying and expressing it. The term originated in psychoanalytic theory as part of the 'hydraulic' characterization of psychic energy but is now used more broadly. Distinguish, however, from CATHARSIS.

discipline The several shades of meaning of this term are captured by the following two primary usages: **1** n. Control of conduct, either of subordinates by a superior or of one's own conduct. Although one usually exercises discipline through the use of punishment, it is also possible to exert control by careful manipulation of positive rewards. Strictly speaking it is not correct to use *punishment* and *discipline* as synonyms; one may use punishment to discipline a child but the use of punishment does not necessarily imply that one is really disciplining the child. **2** n. A branch of knowledge or scholarship, e.g. the discipline of linguistics or of biology. Note that 2 derives from 1. Originally the term was used as a rough synonym for education, and receiving 'formal discipline' meant that one would develop discipline in particular subjects. vb., *discipline* (for 1).

disconnection syndrome Geschwind's term for any neurological syndrome caused by disruption of the transmission of information from one region of the brain to another. Geschwind's point was that many neurological syndromes (e.g. those involving the corpus callosum, and many of the aphasias, apraxias and amnesias) result not because a lesion disrupts function at a particular site, but because it interferes with pathways of communication between cortical areas.

discontinuity theory A theory of discrimination learning that maintains that learning cannot take place until the organism focuses on those aspects of the stimulus that are critical to the required discrimination. Superficially similar to *insight* learning, it belongs to the same general class of theories as ALL-OR-NONE *LEARNING.

discontinuous Not CONTINUOUS. Characteristic of variables or measures in which not all possible values are 'represented'. *Represented* is in inverted commas here because a variable or measure may be manifested as a series of discrete values which in fact represent a true underlying continuous scale; e.g. height is usually represented on a discontinuous scale in discrete units such as inches or centimetres, and perhaps quarters or tenths thereof, but the underlying scale is continuous and a person passes through all possible heights. Compare with a variable like *number of errors in a learning experiment*, which is truly discontinuous.

discontinuous variable DISCONTINUOUS.

discordance Generally, disagreement, disharmony. ant., CONCORDANCE.

discounting principle In Kelley's theory of ATTRIBUTION, a rule of thumb whereby people adjust their confidence in the causal attribution they have drawn for an event. Plainly stated, if there is more than one plausible cause for an event, you should not be totally confident that any one cause is the 'real' one. The more possible causes, the more discounting takes place.

discourse For want of a better definition, most speech-act theorists call any utterance longer than a sentence a discourse.

discourse analysis In linguistics and related disciplines, the analysis of 'units' larger than a sentence; e.g. in writing, an analysis of paragraphs, in speech, an analysis of turns at talking.

discrete Separate, distinct, individually identifiable, discontinuous.

discrete emotions theory The theory that humans have a number of distinct emotions that are biologically discrete and characterized by unique indicators and facial patterns. This perspective clashes with one that argues that emotions differentiate out of a general activation that lacks unique affective qualities. Note that the acknowledgement of biological substrata for emotions does not rule out the potency of the social environment in fostering, inhibiting or blending emotions. See THEORIES OF *EMOTION for more on these issues.

discriminability Properties of objects or events in the world that permit one to distinguish between them, to discriminate them one from the other. adj., *discriminable*.

discriminal dispersion The distribution of responses made in a discrimination experiment.

discriminant analysis A variety of REGRESSION (2) analysis that permits one to use continuous independent variables to place individual cases in categories on a dependent variable. For example, one could use variables such as grade point index and number of days absent from school to predict whether or not students will graduate on time.

discriminant validity CONVERGENT AND DISCRIMINANT *VALIDITY.

discriminated operant An operant the properties of which are defined by the stimulus conditions under which it typically occurs and (as is always the case in the study of operant behaviour) the effects that it has. A discriminated operant occurs in the presence of a DISCRIMINATIVE *STIMULUS.

discriminated operant conditioning DISCRIMINATION (1).

discriminating power The degree to which a test or any individual test item is capable of discriminating between criterial (see CRITERION) and noncriterial cases.

discriminating range RANGE, DISCRIMINATING.

discrimination Three meanings here, two technical and 'neutral', the third conceptually founded on the technical but alive with the ethical and moral connotations of politics, race, religion, etc. **1** In technical writing, the ability to perceive differences between two or more stimuli. It also may be looked upon as a class of experimental procedures called, collectively, *discrimination training procedures*. For example, in operant-conditioning experiments, responses in the presence of one stimulus (S^D) are reinforced but responses in the presence of another (S^Δ) are not. In classical conditioning, in the presence of one stimulus the CS (conditioned stimulus) and US (unconditioned stimulus) are paired (i.e. the CS is a 'true' CS – usually denoted as CS^+), but in the presence of another stimulus they are not (i.e. the CS here is not a true CS since it does not signal a US – it is usually denoted as CS^-). In the operant case such training leads to the emitting of responses in the presence of the S^D but not in the presence of the $S^Δ$. In the classical case it leads to elicitation of the CR in the presence of the CS^+ but not in the presence of the CS^-. In these examples the term is clearly being used to describe a training procedure whereby an organism learns to respond differentially to different stimuli. Note that the question of PERCEPTUAL *LEARNING (the organism's learning to detect the physical differences between the stimuli themselves) arises only indirectly. In most discrimination-training procedures an a priori assumption is made that the organism does perceive the differences between the stimuli but does not react differently toward them because it has never been reinforced for treating them differently. **2** In perception and psychophysics, the capacity to distinguish between stimuli. For more detail here, see THRESHOLD (2). **3** By extension, in social psychology and related areas, the unequal treatment of individuals or groups based on arbitrary characteristics such as race, gender, sex, ethnicity, cultural background, etc. Without going unnecessarily into the politics of this usage of the term it may be noted simply that a careful understanding of the technical meanings can produce considerable insight into the problem. See here PREJUDICE. vb., *discriminate* (for all senses).

discrimination reaction time REACTION TIME, DISCRIMINATION.

discriminative stimulus (S^D) STIMULUS, DISCRIMINATIVE.

disease Medically, any abnormal bodily condition. By extension, any abnormal psychological condition. The historical roots of the use of the term are traceable to the fact that the first efforts to deal with psychological disturbances came from those trained in medicine. The tradition is quite ancient and goes back to the 15th-century physicians who were called on to differentiate between those individuals who were suffering from diseases and those who were suspected of being witches. The legacy of this trend has been to regard psychological disturbances as diseases and to introduce various related phrases such as *mental illness* and *psychological sickness* into the field and to refer to the sufferer as a *patient*. Although no one disputes that biological dysfunctions underlie a

number of psychological and psychiatric disorders, under increasing pressure from those who take behavioural and/or cognitive approaches to problems of a clinical nature, the medical flavour of the terminology has been diminished in recent years. *Disorder* is generally preferred to *disease*; diagnosis deals more with behaviour and patterns of thought than with hypothesized disease-like syndromes; *client* is used by many in place of *patient*; etc. For more on this general point and the changes in terminology entailed, see DIAGNOSIS and related terms.

disease model A term used to characterize the medical approach to psychological disturbances. It is usually used by the more behaviourally oriented clinicians with an accompanying sneer and a tone of disdain. See the discussion under DISEASE for the reasons behind this attitude.

disequilibrium Antonym of EQUILIBRIUM.

disfluency Any nonfluent speech, e.g. stuttering.

disgust Literally, a bad taste. By extension, a negative emotional state that follows exposure to a stimulus that is unpleasant but not an immediate physical threat. Disgust involves active rejection of the stimulus. Although its origins are in taste and the spitting out of bitter foods, in adults disgust is often seen in reaction to social stimuli.

dishabituation Reappearance of a behaviour that had previously been habituated. See HABITUATION.

disinhibition 1 As originally used by Pavlov, this term refers to the removal of an inhibition by an extraneous stimulus. This process is easily seen during the extinction of a classically conditioned response: after a dozen or so trials of extinction of a salivary response the introduction of a sudden novel stimulus will evoke a significant conditioned response. Pavlov was supposed to have discovered the phenomenon serendipitously when an assistant slammed a door during the extinction phase of an experiment. **2** More generally, the lowering of inhibitions (particularly social ones) that occurs under the influence of some added factor. Alcohol and various other drugs function as disinhibitors in this sense, as does injury to certain portions of the *frontal lobes*.

disintegration Generally, loss or serious disruption of organization in some system. The term is used broadly and the system under discussion is usually specified, e.g. behavioural, moral, personality, cognitive.

disintegrative psychosis CHILDHOOD DISINTEGRATIVE DISORDER.

disjunctive concept A concept that is defined by the presence of any one of two or more aspects. In a concept-learning experiment using various coloured shapes as stimuli, a disjunctive concept might be something like 'red *or* round' so that any red or any round object would be considered correct. Compare with CONJUNCTIVE CONCEPT and RELATIONAL CONCEPT.

disjunctive motivation Sullivan's term for striving for only the temporary, seeking to achieve only limited or substitute goals. Compare with CONJUNCTIVE MOTIVATION.

disjunctive reaction time REACTION TIME, DISJUNCTIVE.

disjunctive syllogism SYLLOGISM.

disjunctive task A type of group task in which the performance of the group as a whole depends on the performance of the group's strongest member. A group of people trying to solve a difficult physics problem is a good example. If one person knows how to solve the problem, the group as a whole will solve the problem. Compare with ADDITIVE TASK and CONJUNCTIVE TASK.

dismissive style ATTACHMENT STYLES.

disorder Generally, and literally, lack of order, disruption of order once present. In this sense the term has become one of the most favoured in contemporary psychiatry and clinical psychology. In the contemporary nosologies, *disorder* has replaced *disease* and *neurosis* in the naming and labelling of all maladaptive and dysfunctional behaviours. Specific forms are listed here under the qualifying term.

disorganized Characterizing that which has lost, or had disrupted, its previous structure and functioning. Used commonly in clinical cases featuring disruption in behaviour, thought, affect, personality, etc.

disorganized attachment ATTACHMENT STYLES.

disorganized (type) schizophrenia SCHIZOPHRENIA, DISORGANIZED (TYPE).

disorientation Inability to orient oneself with regard to spatial, temporal and contextual aspects of the environment. Acute disorientation brought on by alcohol, drugs or dramatic alterations in one's circumstances is not uncommon and not abnormal; long-term progressive disorientation is a symptom of a variety of psychological and/or neurological disorders.

disparate retinal points Retinal points stimulation of which produces different spatial sensations. The phenomena of RETINAL *DISPARITY and DISPARATION are due to stimulation of disparate retinal points. Contrast with CONGRUENT RETINAL POINTS.

disparation When an object is either nearer or further away from the momentary point of fixation of the two eyes there is a difference between the images that fall on each retina, resulting in a blurred, double image. *Disparation* refers to the difference between the retinal images, not to the double image itself. One of the two images is usually suppressed, as can be observed easily if a finger is held in front of the eyes while they are focused on a distant object.

disparity, retinal The slight difference between the two retinal images when viewing an object. It is produced by the separation of the two eyes so that each is looking at the object from a different angle, and serves as the basis for stereoscopic vision. In normal viewing it functions as a binocular cue for depth perception. Also called *binocular disparity* and, in some older texts, *visual disparity*.

dispersion 1 In statistics, variability, spread. Indices of dispersion are measures which describe the VARIABILITY of any distribution of scores. In simplest terms, dispersion is the tendency for scores to depart from the CENTRAL TENDENCY. The magnitude of a measure of dispersion of a distribution tells something about the relative 'poorness' of the measure of central tendency as a representation of that distribution. Three measures of dispersion are used, RANGE, AVERAGE *DEVIATION and STANDARD *DEVIATION, the last being the overwhelming favourite in statistical analyses. See also VARIANCE. 2 Spreading out of the population of a group or family. See INBREED-ING AVOIDANCE.

dispersion circle The circle of light seen on looking at a single-point source.

dispersion, coefficient of An index of relative variability given by 100 times the measure of dispersion divided by the measure of central tendency. Usually the STANDARD *DEVIATION and the MEAN serve in this role. Also known as *coefficient of variability* or *coefficient of variation*.

displaced aggression AGGRESSION, DIS-PLACED.

displaced vision The variety of perceptual experiences produced by various modifications of the visual field brought about by wearing special lenses that alter incoming light. The effects run the gamut from dramatic displacements, as with reversing lenses which invert the entire visual world, to more subtle modifications, as with lenses that create 10° displacements, lenses with vertical or horizontal warps, lenses which produce chromatic aberrations, etc.

displacement 1 Generally and literally, the movement of an object from one place to another. An array of extensions of this simple meaning are in common use, to wit: **2** In behavioural terms, the substituting of one response for another, especially when the original response is blocked or thwarted; see here DISPLACED *AGGRESSION. **3** The transference of affect or wishes and desires from their original object or person to another object or person. Displacement, in this sense, is regarded as a *defence mechanism*. **4** In vision, ALLELOTROPIA.

displacement of affect AFFECT, DISPLACE-MENT OF.

display 1 In ethology, a species-specific behaviour pattern that functions to communicate specific information about the state of an animal. Displays are many and varied and function to communicate such states as aggressiveness, submission and receptivity to copulation. They are also used to deceive; see e.g. DEATH FEIGNING. **2** In experimental psychology, the presentation of a stimulus.

display rules In cultural and ethnographic studies, rules and structures within a particular culture or subculture that dictate the expression of emotions in certain situations. The term was introduced by Paul Ekman, who used it to emphasize the notion that, while there are certainly universal components to the expression of emotions, each culture has its own rules that dictate how they may be displayed.

disposition 1 Generally, an ordered arrangement of elements which stand in a particular relationship to each other such that certain functions may be carried out readily. This is the core meaning and arrives in straight translation from the Latin word for *arrangement*. By extension: **2** In the study of personality, any hypothesized organization of mental and physical aspects of a person that is expressed as a stable, consistent tendency to exhibit particular patterns of behaviour in a broad range of circumstances. In this sense, the many tendencies to act to which literally dozens of special terms have been applied as descriptive labels – *trait, ability, habit, set, instinct, drive, temperament, sentiment, motive, faculty,* etc. are all interpretable as dispositions. The theoretical problem that has spawned this terminological forest is the need to explain the regularity and consistency of behaviour (more or less) independently of variation and alteration in the environment. For a more detailed discussion of this problem, see PER-SONALITY. **3** A tendency to be susceptible. This meaning is common in psychiatric and clinical psychological writings, e.g. a disposition for schizophrenia. The term is often used in this sense with the connotation that the tendency is inherited, but this is not always defensible and often begs an important empirical question.

dispositional attribution ATTRIBUTION, DIS-POSITIONAL.

disrupted-in-schizophrenia 1 DISC1.

disruptive behaviour disorders An umbrella term for a variety of psychiatric disorders that have disruptive behaviour as a significant feature, including ATTENTION-DEFICIT HYPERACTIVITY DISORDER, OPPOSITIONAL DEFIANT DISORDER and the CONDUCT DISORDERS.

dissimilation Occasional antonym of ASSIMILATION.

dissmell 1 The reflex to avoid an unpleasant odour. **2** By extension, in DISCRETE EMOTIONS

THEORY an emotional state that results from exposure to an unpleasant but not immediately dangerous stimulus, and that causes withdrawal from or avoidance of that stimulus. Distinguish from *disgust* where the stimulus is forcibly rejected.

dissociated vertical deviation A visual condition in which the eyes are discoordinated in a vertical manner. It is associated with various neurological disorders.

dissociation 1 Used generally to characterize the process (or its result) whereby a coordinated set of activities, thoughts, attitudes or emotions becomes separated from the rest of a person's personality and functions independently. Mild forms are seen in COMPARTMENTALIZATION, in which one set of life's activities are separated from others, and in the amnesias of hypnosis and some emotional disorders. More extreme forms are observed in the DISSOCIATIVE DISORDERS. **2** H. S. Sullivan used the term to characterize the process whereby thoughts or memories that produce anxiety are cut off from consciousness. This *dissociative reaction* (as it is often called) is to be distinguished from schizophrenia on the grounds that each of the dissociated aspects maintains its integrity; the general disintegration and loss of contact with reality of the true schizophrenias is not observed.

dissociative amnesia AMNESIA, DISSOCIATIVE.

dissociative disorder A general cover term for those psychological disorders characterized by a breakdown in the usual integrated functions of consciousness, perception of self and sensory/motor behaviour. Generally included here are DEPERSONALIZATION DISORDER, MULTIPLE PERSONALITY and some forms of AMNESIA and FUGUE.

dissociative fugue FUGUE.

dissociative identity disorder (DID) The currently recommended term for what is generally known as MULTIPLE PERSONALITY. The argument behind the new designation is that it is not so much that there are separate and distinct 'personalities' present in this disorder, but rather that the patient functions as though his or her personal IDENTITY (1) no longer displays its normal integrity and is being manifested in two or more dissociated forms. While Hollywood screenwriters find

this syndrome irresistible, many authorities still doubt the existence of DID as a distinct syndrome.

dissociative trance disorder TRANCE DISORDER, DISSOCIATIVE.

dissonance theory COGNITIVE DISSONANCE THEORY.

distal Lit., distant, away. Hence: **1** In anatomy, referring to the farthest point(s) from the centre of the body, from the centre of an organ or from the point of attachment of an organ or other structure. **2** In perception, see DISTAL STIMULUS. Compare with PROXIMAL.

distal effect The outcome of any response that has some impact on the environment.

distal response Any response with DISTAL EFFECTS.

distal stimulus Lit., a stimulus away (distant) from the receptor on which it acts. In the study of perception one differentiates between: (a) stimuli that act directly upon a sensory receptor, e.g. light waves themselves as they impinge on the retina; and (b) stimuli that are in the external environment, e.g. the chair from which the light waves are reflected. The latter comprise the *distal stimuli*, the former the PROXIMAL STIMULI.

distance, psychological This term is used broadly and may refer to real, physical distance, as it functions psychologically, or to a mental dimension of separateness or dissimilarity between things. Thus: **1** In perception, the physical distance between a stimulus source and the receiving organism presented in terms of the psychophysical relations involved. **2** In social psychology, the degree of awareness between persons usually expressed as a statement about the amount of difficulty experienced when interactions occur. For refinements of meaning here see SOCIAL DISTANCE. **3** In graphic presentations of the outcome of factor analysis or of multidimensional scaling, a measure of the degree of similarity between data points. **4** In A. Adler's theory, a cover term for any of several psychic devices for coping with situations that could potentially reveal one's weaknesses or shortcomings. Adler identified four such techniques: *functional illness*, *indecision* or *hesitation*, *ceasing to try* and the *invention of false barriers*. **5** The deliberate maintenance of dispassion, a lack of emotional involvement. Here one speaks, for example, of a clinician maintaining psychological distance from his or her clients.

distance receptor Any receptor or receptor system that responds to stimuli arising some distance from the body. The eye, ear and nose are examples. Also called *tele[o]-receptor*.

distance vision VISION, DISTANCE.

distance zones Areas of PERSONAL SPACE, specifically zones within which different levels of intimacy are acceptable. There are, of course, many ways to taxonomize such zones; the following four are commonly specified: (a) *intimate* – out to about 18 in (45 cm) from the body; (b) *personal* – from the boundary of intimate out to about 4 ft (1·2 m); (c) *social* – from 4 to 12 ft (1·2 to 3·6 m); and (d) *public* – beyond about 12 ft (3·6 m). See also CROWDING.

distinctive feature 1 Generally, an attribute (i.e. feature) of some object or event that is critical in distinguishing that object or event from others (i.e. it is distinctive). The term enjoys wide currency in psychology and related disciplines. In most psychological parlance it is used loosely to refer to attributes of persons, places, events or concepts that help to differentiate them from other persons, places, events or concepts; e.g. a distinctive feature of a triangle is that it has three sides. 2 In phonetics, an aspect of a phoneme that distinguishes it from another. Here the features are always presented as binary pairs, i.e. each phoneme either possesses a feature (usually noted as +) or it doesn't (–). For example, *voicing* is a distinctive feature that distinguishes between the phonemes /s/ and /z/ as in *sue* and *zoo*: in *sue* the /s/ is '–voice' and in *zoo* the /z/ is '+voice'. 3 In the study of semantics attempts have been made to discover features which would permit the objective defining of words and concepts. Features which are critical elements of a term are often called *defining features* (e.g. 'having feathers' for *bird*); others that are typical of a word are known as *characteristic features* (e.g. 'flying' for *bird*). For details on these efforts see FEATURE MODEL, SEMANTIC FEATURE.

distorted room AMES ROOM.

distortion 1 Nontechnically, any twisting or contorting that alters the shape of something so that it is no longer faithfully represented. Hence: 2 In optics and perception, alterations in images produced by the characteristics of lenses. 3 In studies of memory, modifications in the information stored so that recall data display systematic errors. 4 In psychoanalysis, a defence mechanism that (presumably) functions to alter or 'disguise' dream content that would be unacceptable in nondistorted form.

distractibility 1 Quite literally, the capacity for being (easily) distracted. The term is used commonly of children, who are easily 'seduced' from the task at hand by another task, or even thought. 2 In a clinical sense, a pathological condition of mental functioning in which the person affected is cognitively so labile that attention is diverted by the most minimal stimulus, internal or external. It is observed in many anxiety disorders, in manic states and in schizophrenia.

distractor 1 Any event or stimulus which diverts attention. In studies of human memory distractors are frequently used in the exploration of *short-term memory*. The typical distractor technique consists of giving the subject a stimulus to commit to memory but then introducing another task that commandeers his or her attention and interferes with rehearsal and/or coding of the first stimulus. 2 A 'filler' item on a test; an item which is irrelevant to the things actually being tested. Such distractors help keep the test-wise subject from figuring out the focus and purpose of the test.

distractor technique DISTRACTOR.

distress–relief quotient (or **ratio**) A ratio of the number of verbal indicators of distress to the number of verbal indicators of relief in the statements of a client in psychotherapy. Occasionally used as a 'quick and dirty' method for assessing the amount of progress (or lack thereof).

distributed practice PRACTICE, DISTRIBUTED.

distribution Any systematic presentation of scores, data, etc. in such a way that the frequency or probability with which any one score or category of scores occurs is given. Distributions may be theoretical and expressed in formal mathematical terms, or they may be empirical and simply report the observed data. The following entries describe the distributions most often encountered in psychological research.

distribution, Bernoulli BINOMIAL *DISTRIBUTION.

distribution, binomial The theoretically expected probability distribution when random samples of size N are taken from a (Bernoulli) population containing exactly two categories or classes, e.g. coin tosses, gender. For example, the distribution of heads in a number of coin flips is the binomial distribution. The larger the sample size, the more the binomial approximates the normal distribution. Also called a *Bernoulli distribution*.

distribution, chi-square (χ^2) The distribution of the random variable χ^2. If random samples of size 1 are taken from a normal distribution with mean μ and variance σ^2, then $\chi^2 = (\chi_1 - \mu)^2/\sigma^2$, where χ_1 is the sampled score. As the sample size is increased, the distribution approaches the normal distribution. See CHI-SQUARE for more detail.

distribution, cumulative frequency Any listing of scores, observations or data according to ordered classes in which the total number of entries in each class includes all those cases falling in lower classes. The last class thus includes all of the data from the distribution. See CUMULATIVE CURVE.

distribution, F The theoretical probability distribution of the random variable F. If random samples of size N are drawn independently from a normal population each will generate a chi-square distribution with degrees of freedom = N. The ratio of two such chi-squares each divided by its degrees of freedom (df) is called an F ratio and follows the F distribution; i.e. $F = (\chi_1^2/df_1)/(\chi_2^2/df_2)$. The F distribution forms the mathematical base for the *analysis of variance* and is of extreme importance in statistical testing and inferential statistics.

distribution-free Characterizing a class of statistical operations that makes no assumptions about the theoretical distribution that may underlie the sample data. See NONPARAMETRIC STATISTICS.

distribution, frequency Any distribution based on a listing of the frequency of occurrence of the scores according to classes or categories. Thus, each set of classes is paired with a number that represents its observed frequency. Regardless of the method of presentation (bar graph, frequency polygon, frequency curve, etc.) any such display is called a frequency distribution. Compare with PROBABILITY DISTRIBUTION.

distribution, grouped frequency Similar to frequency distribution but the scores are classified according to intervals or groups of categories rather than to each possible measurement category. Usually used when either the frequencies are relatively low in individual categories or the number of possible categories is unmanageably large.

distribution, hypergeometric A variation of the binomial and multinomial distributions. Whereas these distributions assume either random sampling *with* replacement or infinitely large populations, the hypergeometric assumes sampling from a finite sample *without* replacement.

distribution, multinomial A generalization of the binomial distribution. It is the theoretically expected probability distribution when random samples are taken from a population containing more than two categories or classes.

distribution, normal The theoretically expected probability distribution when samples are drawn from an infinite population in which all events are equally likely to occur. The distribution is continuous for all values from $-\infty$ to $+\infty$; it is symmetrical and unimodal with mean, median and mode at the same value. Some warnings in dealing with the normal distribution: (a) It is specified only by its mathematical rule, it really never exists in nature but is only approximated (this is, of course, true for most of the other distributions as well, but the normal has a tendency to be reified more than, say, the hypergeometric). (b) Although the normal distribution curve has the familiar bell-shaped form, not every bell-shaped curve is a normal distribution. (c) Finally, the normal distribution is critically important in statistical theory and statistical testing since many statistical tests, in order to be used appropriately, assume that the data approximate normality – that is, it is assumed that the population from which they are drawn is a normal population. See also CENTRAL-LIMIT THEOREM, PARAMETRIC STATISTICS.

distribution, Pascal A probability distribution of the number of attempts necessary to obtain a particular number of successes; e.g. the number of flips of a coin it would take to get a total of, say, 10 heads.

distribution, Poisson A special, limited case of the binomial distribution. In particular, it is the theoretically expected distribution when the number of cases sampled is quite large but drawn from a relatively small population that is characterized by one of the two categories being relatively rare.

distribution, probability Similar to frequency distribution except that instead of pairing each class or category with the frequency with which it occurs it is paired with its probability of occurrence. Thus, while the sum of the frequencies in a frequency distribution must be N (or the total number of scores), the sum of the probabilities in a probability distribution must total 1·00.

distribution, ranked Any distribution of scores arranged according to ranks.

distribution, sampling Any distribution that results from taking samples of specified size from a population. See the discussions under SAMPLE, SAMPLING and related terms.

distribution, t The theoretical distribution of the random variable t. If random samples of size N are drawn from a normal population with mean μ, then $t = (\bar{X}-\mu)/(s/\sqrt{N-1})$, where $\bar{X}$ is the sample mean and s is the sample standard deviation. Thus, t is based on the ratio of a statistic to its standard error. The distribution of t approximates the normal with increasing N. The various t tests based on the distribution allow one to estimate the level of significance of a statistic of certain size obtained from a sample of given size. As such they are extremely important statistical tools in evaluating the degree to which a sample differs from a theoretical underlying distribution, or the degree to which two samples differ from each other. Also called *Student's distribution*.

distribution, uniform A distribution in which all classes have the same frequency or the same probability. Often called a *rectangular distribution* since the graph of such a distribution is a rectangle.

distributive analysis and synthesis The form of psychotherapy developed by Adolf Meyer. It involves a detailed examination of the client's past life (analysis) with the aim of forming a positive, constructive synthesis. The therapy is a strongly directive one with the therapist giving extensive guidance and direction.

disulfiram A drug used for treatment of alcoholism. It causes acetaldehyde, a breakdown product of alcohol, to accumulate in the blood, resulting in a variety of most unpleasant experiences including dizziness, nausea, vomiting, sweating and a throbbing headache. Its use is based on principles of conditioning that predict that the patient will associate the unpleasant experience with the alcohol (the drug has no effect if alcohol is not present) and develop an aversion to it (see here CONDITIONED *AVERSION for the model conditioning phenomenon). Its success rate in treating alcoholism is not high and one likely reason for the failure is that alcohol is not the unusual or novel stimulus that the conditioned aversion response requires for effective learning.

disuse, law (or **principle**) **of** One of E. L. Thorndike's original laws of conditioning. It states that a learned association will become weakened by lack of use.

disutility Basically, the opposite of *utility*, but with a wrinkle. In economics, game theory, choice behaviour, etc. one can speak about the UTILITY (especially 3) of an outcome fairly straightforwardly. However, it is not clear that disutility of a negative outcome will have the same subjective value (quantitatively speaking) as the equivalent positive outcome. That is, it is not clear that the disutility of losing $100 is subjectively as 'bad' as the utility of winning $100 is subjectively 'good'. See RISK AVERSION.

diuresis Secretion and passage of an unusually large volume of urine.

diuretic Any substance that causes increased secretion and passage of urine.

diurnal (cycle) *Diurnal* means pertaining to day or to the daylight hours; contrast with

NOCTURNAL. However, in the fuller term *diurnal cycle*, it has a more general meaning, being essentially synonymous with *daily*. Thus, an expression such as 'changes in blood pressure follow a diurnal cycle' really refers to changes over a full 24-hour period. See also CIRCADIAN, which, properly, is the term for such cycles.

divagation   Disorganized, incoherent speech.

divergence 1 Generally, the property of moving away from a central point or of lying in different directions. 2 In perception, the turning outward of the eyes as the point of focus is shifted away from the perceiver. It functions as a binocular cue for depth perception. 3 In neurophysiology, the branching and spreading out of the several processes of an individual neuron or the fibres of a neural pathway. Contrast with CONVERGENCE.

divergent thinking THINKING, DIVERGENT.

diversity   In social and organizational psychology, heterogeneity or variation within a group. In the technical literature the term is used loosely. There is little consensus on whether it should be restricted to variations in race/ethnicity, gender and age, or expanded to include education, ideology, skills and other characteristics. It also functions as a political code word to enhance sensitivity to issues of ethnicity, sexual orientation and physical disability.

dizygotic (DZ)   Pertaining to two zygotes. See DIZYGOTIC *TWINS.

DL   Abbreviation meaning *difference* (or *differential*); see THRESHOLD. The L stands for the Latin word *limen*, meaning *threshold*, originally introduced as the equivalent of the German *Schwelle*.

DM   DIFFERENCE ASSOCIATED WITH SUBSEQUENT MEMORY.

DMS   DIACRITICAL MARKING SYSTEM.

DNA   DEOXYRIBONUCLEIC ACID.

D-needs   BASIC NEEDS.

docile 1 Easily trainable, teachable. 2 Tractable, manageable.

doctrine   DOGMA.

dogma   A transliteration of a Greek word meaning *that which seems good*. It is used of beliefs that are fixed and firmly held, based on authority and accepted independently of facts and other empirical support. The most frequent usage is theological, but secular and quasi-scientific dogmas abound. The meaning of the term shades gently and often insidiously with that of *doctrine*. Strictly speaking, a doctrine is a teaching or a principle advocated and taught. The conceptual line usually put forward to distinguish between the two is, in principle, *empirical demonstration*. That is, doctrines are usually held to be authoritative statements promulgated with promissory notes that evidence will be forthcoming; dogmas are usually presented as true by fiat and no evidential basis for them is sought. *Doctrine*, which has more or less neutral connotations, is frequently used of extensive theoretical positions that go beyond the available data and invite support on the basis of the still-uncashed promissory note, e.g. Freudian doctrine, behaviourist doctrine. *Dogma*, in science, has clear negative connotations suggesting that a position is held not merely independently of data but actually in defiance of incompatible facts. In the give and take of doing science, one's opponent's doctrines are dogmas.

dolichocephalic   Having a long, narrow head. See CEPHALIC INDEX.

doll's eye reflex   A reflexive movement of the eyes in the opposite direction to the movement of the head.

dolour   Pain; usually physical, occasionally psychological.

dolourology   The study of the causes and treatment of pain.

domain 1 The subject matter of a science or a DISCIPLINE (2). 2 An area of functioning. Here, the usage is exceedingly broad. It may refer to the content of a problem or the nature of a process, be as limited as a class of problems to be solved or as inclusive as an entire area of functioning as in the *cognitive domain*.

domain generality   The extent to which a cognitive ability manifests itself across a wide range of problems. A classic example is a child who has grasped the principle of CON-

SERVATION and displays it in a variety of settings. Compare with DOMAIN SPECIFICITY.

domain specificity The extent to which a cognitive ability fails to be displayed across multiple domains, e.g. a child shows number CONSERVATION but not length or volume. Compare with DOMAIN GENERALITY.

domal sampling SAMPLING, DOMAL.

domepezil A NOOTROPIC DRUG used in cases of mild dementia. It inhibits ACETYLCHOLINES-TERASE and increases levels of acetylcholine in the brain, particularly in areas of the basal forebrain where such increases are thought to be related with memory functions.

dominance 1 From the Latin, meaning *ruling*. Hence, in the broadest sense, it refers to a relationship in which one thing is in a position of control over another. *Thing* here is meant to be taken loosely, as the specialized usages that follow show, and *control* may be taken to mean anything from physical control to temporal precedence, relative importance or, simply, preference. **2** In genetics, the quality through which one *allele* of a pair suppresses the expression of the other and thereby prevails in the *phenotype*. **3** In ethology, a tendency to exert control over the behaviour of other members of a group of *conspecifics*. See here DOMINANCE *HIERARCHY. **4** By extension of 3, a personality trait characterized by a tendency to seek and maintain control over other people. See here ASCEN-DANCE. **5** Preference of use, generally of one side of a bilateral anatomical structure. See EYE *DOMINANCE, LATERAL *DOMINANCE, HANDED-NESS. **6** Control of one structure or organ by another. This meaning is carried in phrases like *cortical dominance* or *cerebral dominance*. Note that a certain ambiguity exists here; the dominance may be of the brain over other parts of the central nervous system or it may be of one part of the brain over other parts. See here the discussion under CEREBRAL *DOM-INANCE. **7** HEMISPHERIC *DOMINANCE. See that term and CEREBRAL *DOMINANCE for further discussion of usage. adj., *dominant*.

dominance, cerebral The tendency of one cerebral hemisphere to be dominant in the control of bodily movement and speech. Some loose but defensible generalizations can be made here. In bodily movement the dominant hemisphere is contralateral; that

is, for left-handed individuals the right hemisphere is dominant and vice versa. See HAND-EDNESS for more detail. In control over speech and language, of those who are right-handed the vast majority are left-hemisphere dominant; of those who are left-handed a majority, although a considerably smaller one, are also left-hemisphere dominant. Note that the term *cerebral dominance* carries a subtle confusion in that it is easily mistaken to mean dominance of the cerebrum over something else. To avoid this many authors use other terms such as *hemispheric dominance*, which is literally more accurate anyway; see LATERALITY, which covers the full range of effects of brain–body 'sidedness' nicely; or DOMINANCE (see, especially, meanings 5, 6 and 7).

dominance, cortical See DOMINANCE (especially 5, 6 and 7) and CEREBRAL *DOMINANCE.

dominance, eye The tendency for one eye to be used in focusing on an object. In general, when one is scanning a visual field, as in reading, one eye dominates and 'leads' the other from focal point to focal point.

dominance, hemispheric See CEREBRAL *DOMINANCE. In the literature *cerebral dominance* is encountered more often than *hemispheric dominance*, although the latter is more precise.

dominance hierarchy HIERARCHY, DOMIN-ANCE.

dominance, mixed (cerebral) The contemporary 'received' view of hemispheric functioning is that each cerebral hemisphere plays a dominant role in particular cognitive and sensorimotor functions (see LATERALITY for explication). The phrase *mixed dominance* is used in cases in which there are reasons to suspect that the 'normal' clear distribution of lateral functioning is not present and one hemisphere does not consistently lead the other in control over particular behaviours.

dominance need H. Murray's term for the need to control others.

dominant Generally, displaying the characteristic of DOMINANCE in any of the meanings of that term. Note, however, that *dominant* may have any of four different antonyms depending on the sense of dominance that is intended. To wit: *recessive* for sense 2, *submissive* for 3 and 4, *nonpreferred* for 5 and *nondominant* for 6 and 7.

dominant trait DOMINANCE.

dominator A retinal ganglion cell that responds over the entire visible spectrum. Such cells do so in a nonuniform fashion and display peak sensitivity at particular wavelengths. Compare with MODULATOR.

Donders' method SUBTRACTION METHOD.

Don Juanism SATYRIASIS.

door-in-the-face technique A way of obtaining compliance whereby an individual initially requests something very large, so large that it will surely be denied, then de-escalates to a more modest request, which was the one originally desired. Compare with the FOOT-IN-THE-DOOR TECHNIQUE.

dopamine (DA) An important neurotransmitter, a *catecholamine* that has both excitatory and inhibitory functions depending on the pathway and the properties of the postsynaptic receptors. DA has been implicated in an astonishing array of functions including movement, attention, learning, the reinforcing effects of drugs and various neuropsychiatric disorders. Decreased DA in nigrostriatal pathways is associated with the rigidity, poor balance and akinesia of PARKINSON'S DISEASE. Imbalances in dopamine have also been implicated in schizophrenia (see DOPAMINE HYPOTHESIS), ATTENTION-DEFICIT HYPERACTIVITY DISORDER, and TOURETTE'S SYNDROME. It is a precursor of NOREPINEPHERINE and EPINEPHRINE. Note that several forms of DA have been discovered and may be identified by any of several notational systems, e.g. DA1, or D1 or D_1.

dopamine hypothesis The hypothesis that schizophrenia is associated with 'excessive activity' of the dopaminergic neurons of the limbic system. The 'excessive activity' could, in principle, result from any number of sources, increased production of dopamine and inhibition of reuptake of it being the most likely. The clinical effects of ANTIPSYCHOTIC DRUGS are intimately related to the blocking of DA (although the exact causal links here are still unclear). See DOPAMINE.

dopaminergic Characterizing or pertaining to pathways, fibres or neurons in which dopamine is a neurotransmitter.

Doppler shift (or **effect**) A shift in hue or pitch as the source of a stimulation moves relative to the observer. Approaching sources produce increases in frequency (hue shifts toward the blue, pitch toward higher tone); receding sources produce the reverse. The effect is most easily detected with moving sound sources.

dorsal From the Latin, meaning *to the back* or *to the rear*. Used as a directional term in physiology and anatomy. Contrast with VENTRAL. Note that in combined forms both *dorsal* and *dorso* are found.

dorsal column medial lemniscal system One of two main ascending neural systems for somatic sensation (the ANTEROLATERAL SYSTEM is the other), carrying information about touch, vibration and limb position. The dorsal columns are composed of axons from dorsal-root ganglion cells which ascend ipsilaterally to the medulla, cross over and ascend as the medial lemniscus (see here LEMNISCAL SYSTEM) to the thalamus.

dorsal lateral geniculate nucleus A nucleus within the LATERAL GENICULATE NUCLEUS from which pathways project to the primary visual cortex.

dorsal root SPINAL ROOT.

dorsal stream See V1.

dorsal tegmental bundle A noradrenergic system the cell bodies of which are in the locus coeruleus of the pons in the brainstem and the fibres of which project to the cerebral cortex, hippocampus, thalamus, cerebellar cortex and medulla.

dorsolateral column A fibre bundle in the *spinal cord* involved in opiate-induced ANALGESIA.

dorsolateral nucleus A thalamic nucleus that projects to the cingulate gyrus. Also called the *lateral dorsal nucleus*.

dorsolateral pathway A neural pathway that runs from the brainstem to the spinal cord and is involved in the control of the muscles used in movement of the forelimbs.

dorsolateral prefrontal cortex The upper, lateral part of the PREFRONTAL CORTEX. It functions in the control of WORKING •MEMORY and the handling of attentional resources. Neural damage here disrupts

EXECUTIVE FUNCTIONS, particularly in the control of attention.

dorsomedial nucleus A thalamic nucleus that receives input from the limbic system and other thalamic nuclei and projects to the prefrontal cortex. Also called the *medial dorsal nucleus*.

dosage 1 The amount of a medicine or other preparation prescribed to be given. **2** The administration of medicine in doses.

dose 1 n. The amount of a medicine or other preparation to be taken at one time. **2** vb. To administer in doses.

dose-related response curve A graph of the effect that a drug has depending on the size of the dose administered. Not surprisingly, it is rarely a simple monotonic function. Also called *dose-response curve*.

dot pattern Simply and literally, any arrangement of dots presented as a stimulus or part of one. They are used in studies of motion detection (the dots move in coordinated ways), categorization (dots form patterns) and induction (the dot patterns are based on rules).

dot probe task A procedure in which two stimuli appear briefly on a screen followed by a place-marker (like a dot) in one of the two locations. The subject is asked to identify the stimulus that occurred in that location.

double-alternation problem An experimental procedure that requires the subject to make the sequence of responses A–A–B–B.

double approach–avoidance conflict CONFLICT, DOUBLE APPROACH–AVOIDANCE.

double aspectism See MIND–BODY PROBLEM.

double bind A situation in which a person is confronted with a series of contradictory messages from a powerful or socially significant other. A classic case emerges when a child has a parent who has difficulty with close, affectionate relationships but cannot admit to such feelings. The parent communicates coldness and withdrawal when the child approaches but then reaches out with simulated love when the child pulls back from the coldness. The child is caught in a 'double bind' as no course of action proves satisfactory and all assumptions about how to act will be disconfirmed. The term was coined by Gregory Bateson who thought that such child-rearing patterns might underlie disorders such as autism or schizophrenia. There is no support for Bateson's theory but the double bind setting continues to be extensively studied.

double-blind An experimental procedure in which neither the participant nor the person administering the experimental procedures knows what are considered to be the crucial aspects of the experiment. It is commonly used to guard against EXPERIMENTER BIAS, DEMAND CHARACTERISTICS and the PLACEBO EFFECT. Double-blind procedures are used when it is feared that knowledge of what is expected of the participant will influence his or her performance, or when knowledge of what the experiment is about will influence the experimenter's interpretation of what the participant is doing. This kind of control is common in drug studies in which neither the participant nor the person administering the preparation knows whether they are using a drug or a placebo. The effects of the drug can then be separated from any preconceptions about what the drug is or is not supposed to do.

double-blind crossover A variation of the DOUBLE-BLIND technique whereby, as an added control, the conditions are crossed in the middle of the experiment. For example, in the course of a study of the effects of a drug those participants receiving the drug are switched over and administered the placebo and vice versa. In a properly designed study, neither the participants nor the person administering the drugs know who is in either group, or when (or even whether) the crossover occurs.

double dissociation A general term used of any procedure that enables a researcher to distinguish clearly between two functions or processes. Suppose, for example, a number of neurological patients show similarly poor performance in a visual-motor task. A clear double dissociation would occur if, in follow-up work, some of the patients showed normal performance on a visual test that had no motor component but poor performance on a motor test with no visual component, while others showed the reverse pattern. The term *multiple dissociation* is also used, especially in neurological work, when three or more procedures may be used to tease apart the component parts of a complex syndrome.

double-entry table A table in which scores are entered by column and row simultaneously, e.g. a *scatter diagram*.

double vibration (dv) An obsolete term for *cycle*. See discussion under VIBRATION.

double vision DIPLOPIA.

doubling An adaptive division of the self into two distinctive 'parts' that may function independently. The goal is to allow the doubled self to behave in ways that are unpalatable to the original. It was first documented in Nazi doctors and is seen in soldiers or guards who torture prisoners. It is not viewed as a clinical disorder and so should be distinguished from DISSOCIATED IDENTITY DISORDER.

downer Street slang for any drug that has relaxing, antianxiety effects. Generally included are the HYPNOTICS, MINOR *TRANQUILLIZERS and SEDATIVES.

Down syndrome A congenital condition characterized by a flat skull, stubby fingers, an unusual pattern of skin folds on the palms of the hands and the soles of the feet, epicanthic folds on the eyelids, a fissured tongue and often severe mental deficiency. The disorder is named after the British physician J. Langdon Down, who first described it in 1866. It is the single most common clinical condition with mental retardation as primary symptom and occurs in approximately 1 out of every 700 births. However, the mother's age is a critical factor: among mothers under 30 its incidence is just 1 per 1,000, among mothers over 45 its incidence is as high as 1 per 40. There are actually several variations of the syndrome. By far the most common (over 90% of cases) is that in which the infant has an extra 21st chromosome or part thereof, making a total of 47 chromosomes instead of the normal 46. For this reason, the name *trisomy 21* is often used. This condition is not a truly inherited disorder but due rather to faulty cell division. In the *mosaicistic* form, which is relatively rare (accounting for less than 2% of the cases), some cells have the extra 21st chromosome but some do not, indicating that the error occurred some time after ferti-

lization. In the *translocation* form the extra 21st chromosome is found attached to another chromosome, usually the 15th. Down syndrome is still occasionally referred to as *mongolism* (which was Down's term for it – he thought that development of the foetus had been arrested at the 'Mongolian' level of civilization and regarded the epicanthic folds as evidence of this). This term has, fortunately, dropped out of use, although it may still be seen in older texts. Also referred to as *Down's syndrome*.

dowsing In PARAPSYCHOLOGY, the unsubstantiated ability to locate underground water or other substances using two wires, a forked stick or other 'divining rod'.

doxepin A TRICYCLIC COMPOUND with anticholinergic properties introduced as an antidepressant. Its use is limited because it is so highly sedating although in low doses it can help manage neuromuscular pain.

***d*-prime** d'.

DQ DEVELOPMENTAL QUOTIENT.

drama therapy PSYCHODRAMA.

dream A lot of people have wrestled with this one; let's define it simply as 'imagery during sleep'. Dreaming appears to occur in many organisms and is intimately related to rapid-eye-movement (or REM) sleep.

dream analysis A technique originally used in psychoanalysis whereby the contents of dreams are analysed for underlying or disguised motivations, symbolic meanings or evidence of symbolic representations. In typical dream analysis the individual relates a dream and then free associates about it with the aim of deriving insight into underlying dynamics. Freud, quoting the old proverb 'Pigs dream of acorns and geese dream of maize', assumed that dreams were expressions of wish-fulfilment. However, according to the standard theory, since most wishes have been repressed, the deep meaning of dreams (DREAM CONTENT) has to be interpreted through a veil of censorship, disguise and symbolism. See also DREAM SYMBOLISM.

dream anxiety disorder A SLEEP DISORDER marked by repeated waking from sleep with detailed recall of frightening dreams. The dreams are marked by their vividness and often feature threats to survival and security.

Also known as *nightmare disorder*. Distinguish from SLEEP TERROR DISORDER.

dream content According to psychoanalytic theory the content of a dream is of two types: (a) *manifest* – that known to the dreamer, the 'surface' of the dream; and (b) *latent* – the deep, hidden aspects that presumably need to be interpreted before their meanings can be made clear. See also LATENT AND MANIFEST *CONTENT.

dream determinant DETERMINANT, DREAM.

dream ego Jung's term for a separate component of the ego which he felt was responsible for dreaming.

dream instigator DAY RESIDUE.

dream interpretation DREAM ANALYSIS.

dream, lucid A dream during which the person is aware of the act of dreaming and thus has the capacity to control the content of the dream. While most dreaming occurs during REM sleep, the term is also found referring to similar states that occur during non-REM periods.

dream-series method A technique for studying dreams. The individual keeps a dream diary (recording dreams upon awakening) until some 50 or more accounts have been accumulated. The full set is then examined for patterns, recurring themes, etc.

dream symbolism Within the various psychoanalytic approaches, the disguised expressions in dreams wherein one thing is a 'stand-in' or a symbol for something else. The usual interpretation is that the symbols are necessary for deeply repressed wishes to escape censorship. There are 'standard' interpretations for some commonly occurring dream symbols – towers, pencils, pistons and other entities which share functional, physical or linguistic similarities are almost universally taken as phallic symbols, while boxes, doorways and tunnels are vaginal. However, it is misleading to generalize blindly about the symbolic elements of dreams. If dream analysis is to be of value it needs to be carried out with a sensitivity to the dreamer's own life and to the manner in which the free associations to a dream unfold. 'Pop psychology' books on dream symbolism and meaning should be avoided.

dream-work Freud's term for the processes through which the latent content of a dream is transformed into the manifest content.

drh Abbreviation for *differential reinforcement of high rate*. See SCHEDULES OF *REINFORCEMENT.

drive A term with a plethora of usages, some quite precise, others very loose. Probably the clearest usage, and the one from which all others derive, is that which treats a drive as a motivational state produced by (a) deprivation of a needed substance such as food, a drug or a hormone, or (b) presence of a noxious stimulus such as a loud noise, excessive cold or heat or a painful stimulus. Note that the term, in this sense, refers to a hypothetical state of an organism and must be inferred either from controlled operations (deliberately depriving the subject of a needed substance) or from observations of the behaviour exhibited (e.g. choosing food over sex, or vice versa). Properly, one should differentiate between drive and need, in that *need* is used to describe states of deprivation and does not necessarily imply a motivational state. The standard view here is to treat need states as producing drive states, which motivate behaviour. Complications, to be sure, are lurking behind this conceptualization; see INCENTIVE for one of them.

drive, acquired (or **secondary**) Any drive the motivating properties of which are learned through association with a PRIMARY *DRIVE. The classic example is the human drive for money.

drive-arousal stimulus Any stimulus that serves to activate a dormant drive state. It may be either internal (thinking about a juicy, chargrilled steak) or external (the smell of the same).

drive, nonregulatory Any drive (such as sex) that serves functions other than those that maintain the consistent bodily states necessary for the survival of the individual organism. Compare with REGULATORY *DRIVE.

drive, primary Any drive that arises from an intrinsic physiological characteristic of an organism. Some are universal, such as the drives to obtain food and water, to reproduce, to avoid pain and to maintain a stable temperature; others are species-specific, such as the nest-building and imprinting drives.

drive reduction Literally, the reduction of a drive. See DRIVE-REDUCTION HYPOTHESIS for an early specialized use.

drive-reduction hypothesis A general principle that maintains that the goal of all motivated behaviour is the reduction or alleviation of a drive state. As used first by E. L. Thorndike and more importantly by Clark L. Hull, it became the theoretical mechanism through which reinforcement operated. That is, any event which served to reduce a drive state was assumed to reinforce (or increase the likelihood of) the response that preceded it. Contrast this usage with CONTIGUITY THEORY. For more on this general issue, see REINFORCEMENT.

drive, regulatory Any DRIVE (such as hunger or thirst) that functions so that an organism seeks out substances that serve to maintain consistent bodily states necessary for survival. Compare with NONREGULATORY *DRIVE.

drive specificity DRIVE STIMULI.

drive stimuli (S_D) The hypothesized efferent neural impulses resulting from a drive state. In Hull's later theory these were the stimuli the reduction of which was assumed to regulate reinforcement. Note that S_D was also assumed to display *drive specificity*, so that a drive stimulus was associated with the particular set of responses that reduced it.

drl Abbreviation for *differential reinforcement of low rate*. See SCHEDULES OF *REINFORCEMENT.

dro Abbreviation for *differential reinforcement of other behaviour*. See SCHEDULES OF *REINFORCEMENT.

dromomania An obsessive need to travel. Originally called the *vagabond neurosis*, the syndrome gets classified as a disorder only when the desire becomes maladaptive. Such individuals spend more than they can afford on travel, fantasize constantly about it and become so absorbed in travel that the rest of their lives suffer.

drop attack ATONIC SEIZURE.

drp Abbreviation for *differential reinforcement of paced responses*. See SCHEDULES OF *REINFORCEMENT.

drug abuse Improper use of drugs. The usual connotation is that of excessive, irresponsible and self-damaging use of psychoactive and/or addictive drugs. See SUBSTANCE ABUSE.

drug addiction DRUG *DEPENDENCE.

drug agonism AGONISM, DRUG.

drug antagonism ANTAGONISM, DRUG.

drug dependence DEPENDENCE, DRUG.

drug dependency insomnia REBOUND *INSOMNIA.

drug-dispositional tolerance TOLERANCE, DRUG-DISPOSITIONAL.

drug holiday A period of time during which a drug is discontinued.

drug-induced Parkinsonism PARKINSONISM, DRUG-INDUCED.

drug interaction The effects of two (or more) drugs taken together, when their combined effects are different from what would be produced by only one of them taken alone. For more details see DRUG *ANTAGONISM and DRUG SYNERGISM.

drug synergism A form of drug interaction in which there is an increase in the effectiveness of one or more of the drugs as a result of the presence of the other(s).

drug therapy Broadly, any approach to psychotherapy that treats behavioural and mental disorders with various psychoactive drugs, primarily mood stabilizers, antipsychotics, anxiolytics and antidepressants. The use of such compounds is a 'hot topic' in psychotherapy. Some maintain that, since many disorders stem from biochemical imbalances, they are an essential form of therapy; others argue that many, if not most, disorders are best treated without the use of powerful and occasionally toxic compounds. Most practitioners take a balanced position. They use drugs when called for but as an adjunct to more traditional therapies, not replacements for them. Also called *pharmacotherapy*.

drug tolerance TOLERANCE, DRUG.

D sleep SLEEP, D.

DSM Abbreviation for the DIAGNOSTIC AND STATISTICAL MANUAL. The *DSM*, which is the diagnostic guidebook of the American Psychiatric Association, has been revised several times; the current version is *DSM-IV-TR*, which appeared in 2000.

D system A group of serotonergic neurons (see SEROTONIN) with their cell bodies in the dorsal part of the RAPHE NUCLEUS. Interestingly, they do not appear to form synapses with other neurons but release serotonin diffusely. See also M SYSTEM.

DTI DIFFUSION TENSOR IMAGING.

DTs DELIRIUM TREMENS.

d-tubocurarine See CURARE.

dual-code hypothesis The generalization proposed by A. Paivio that human memory is composed of two coding systems, one based on a visual-imagery process and one on a verbal-coding process.

dual diagnosis Literally, the ascription of more than one diagnosis to an individual. The term is most commonly used when a person exhibits *substance abuse* along with an Axis I or II disorder (see AXIS I – V).

dualism Any of a number of philosophical positions which admit of two separate states of nature or two sets of fundamental principles in the universe. As originally promulgated by Plato, the distinction was between mind and matter. In contemporary debates the issue is usually divided along lines of mind and body. There can be a strong dualistic position whereby understanding the operation of one sphere has no bearing at all on an understanding of the other, or a softer form of dualism in which some distinctions between, say, mental and physical phenomena are accepted but without assuming that they are metaphysically different in any fundamental way. The classic forms of dualism are *interactive*, when mind and body are assumed to be separate but interacting, and *parallel*, when mind and body are seen as different manifestations of a complex organism and assumed to 'travel on separate but parallel tracks'. Descartes is usually cited as the strongest proponent of interactive dualism; the early structuralists like Titchener were vigorous defenders of the parallel position, which they often referred to as *psychophysical* dualism. See also MIND–BODY PROBLEM and MONISM.

dual personality MULTIPLE PERSONALITY.

dual-process models Generally, any model based on the assumption of two distinguishable processes or, by extension, two kinds of mechanisms, coding operations, emotional reactions, decision heuristics or, indeed, virtually any conceivable operation. Like their cousins, the TWO-FACTOR THEORIES, these models of cognitive, perceptual or emotional processing have been proposed to account for a host of functions and we hope future generations can resist their allure.

dual task procedure Loosely, any experimental process in which the participants have to carry out two tasks simultaneously. For example, they may be asked to respond as quickly as possible to a light that comes on while also keeping track of the number of tones that are sounding. Dual task procedures are commonly used in studies of divided attention.

dual threshold THRESHOLD, DUAL.

ductless gland GLAND.

dull normal An obsolete term for an individual with below average intelligence. See MENTAL RETARDATION for details on contemporary terminology.

dumb Mute, unable to speak.

dummy 1 Loosely, synonym of PLACEBO, used chiefly in Britain. 2 More specifically, a completely neutral placebo, one with no effect at all. Compare with ACTIVE *PLACEBO.

dummy variable A dichotomous variable that is coded 1 to indicate presence of an attribute and 0 to indicate absence.

Duncan Multiple-Range Test A POST HOC TEST used after an ANALYSIS OF VARIANCE has been run. It enables one to test which of the several mean differences are significant.

duplexity (or **duplicity**) **theory** The theory, now universally accepted as correct, which posits that there are two separate receptor mechanisms in the retina: the *cones*, which are colour-sensitive and used in high illumination (see PHOTOPIC VISION), and the *rods*, which are achromatic and used in low illumination (see SCOTOPIC VISION).

dura mater Lit., *hard mother*. The outermost of the three meninges covering the spinal cord and brain, and the toughest. See also ARACHNOID MEMBRANE and PIA MATER.

duration The standard dictionary meaning generally applies. The early introspectionists, however, spoke of *duration* as a subjective, unanalysable attribute of a sensation which was regarded as the basis for the experience of the passage of time.

Durham rule A legal principle regarding the use of the INSANITY DEFENCE. It states that 'an accused is not criminally responsible if his unlawful act was the product of mental disease or mental defect'. It was put forward in 1954 in the USA but is no longer accepted by the courts.

DV DEPENDENT *VARIABLE.

d.v. Abbreviation for *double vibration*. See VIBRATION for discussion.

dyadic DIADIC.

dyad, social SOCIAL *DIAD.

dynamic 1 Generally, characteristic of or relating to things that are in flux or are changeable. 2 More specifically, a label for systems of psychology that emphasize motivation (R. S. Woodworth always referred to his form of functionalism as *dynamic* psychology), those that focus on unconscious processes (Freud and Jung are both considered proponents of a dynamic approach) and those that emphasize complex fields of psychological force (Lewin's field theory is a good example). Contrast with STATIC and STRUCTURAL. See DYNAMIC SYSTEM.

dynamic component systems theory An approach to the study of the development of emotions that focuses on the interactions between appraisal and action in cultural contexts. See THEORIES OF *EMOTION.

dynamic constructivism The theory, popular in social and cultural psychology, that knowledge, beliefs and interpretive patterns are constructed and acquired within a social and cultural context. These epistemic systems are regarded as flexible and dynamic and can be activated or deactivated by particular environmental demands. Contrast with IDEALISM and REALISM.

dynamic equilibrium Generally, the state of a dynamic system in which, although shifting and changing, the overall pattern of forces or energy is in a stable, organized configuration.

dynamic psychology DYNAMIC (2).

dynamic system Any system in which the several elements are interwoven or interrelated in such a way that changes in one sector of the system have systematic effects on the rest of the system.

dynamic(al) systems (theory) An umbrella term for a variety of theoretical models that seek to explain human behaviour in terms of the dynamics of change over time. The approach is based on the assumption that all complex systems like those that support perception, cognition, judgement, social interaction, lifespan development (among many others) undergo lawful patterns of change over time and that 'time-sensitive' mathematical systems can capture this 'unfolding'.

dynamic unconscious UNCONSCIOUS (3(a), (b)).

dynamism 1 A mechanism of adjustment. The term is generally used in this sense with the connotation that it refers to a rather stable manner of behaving, the primary function of which is to fulfil drives and motives and to protect oneself from stress and discomfort. 2 By extension, H. S. Sullivan used the term to cover a variety of interpersonal relations that function in this manner.

dynamometer Any instrument for measuring strength of muscular response, usually hand-grip.

dyne A unit of force defined as that needed to accelerate 1 g of matter 1 cm per second.

dynorphins ENDOGENOUS OPIATES.

dys- Prefix meaning *faulty, ill, bad, difficult*. There are literally scores of technical terms that use it and doubtless more are coined every day. It is generally used to indicate (a) a particular function that has failed to develop normally (e.g. *dyslexia*) or (b) a function that has been disrupted (e.g. *dysmenorrhoea*). Frequently the meaning of a term can be derived from the root word, and to save space such terms are not included here; the less obvious ones follow, however. Occasional var., DIS-.

dysacousia 1 Inordinate discomfort caused

by loud noises. **2** Difficulty in hearing. Meaning 1 is the more common.

dysaesthesia Generally, inappropriate sensitivity, particularly to touch and pain. A cover term for any increased or decreased sensitivity as well as for other more specific syndromes (e.g. *formication*). var., *dysesthesia*.

dysarthria Generally, defective speaking, impaired articulatory ability, typically when the result of peripheral motor or muscular defects; compare with ANARTHRIA. A variety of subtypes are distinguished based either on the pattern of symptoms or on known neurological lesion. The more common are given below.

dysarthria, ataxic A dysarthria characterized by slurred speech caused by cerebellar lesions.

dysarthria, hyperkinetic A dysarthria associated with lesions in the basal ganglia and marked by speech with erratic, abnormal rhythms and accompanied by involuntary movements. Note that basal ganglia lesions are also associated with a *hypokinetic* version, characterized by slow, flattened speech.

dysarthria, hypokinetic HYPERKINETIC *DYS-ARTHRIA.

dysarthria, upper motor neuron A mild dysarthria associated with acute upper motor neuron lesions. These lesions cause a weakness in the muscles that control the tongue and in the lower facial muscles, which affects speech. The symptoms typically diminish over time.

dysbasia Difficulty in walking; a form of ATAXIA.

dysbulia 1 Lit., weakness of will. **2** Impaired thinking, inability to fix attention on something.

dyscalculia A learning disability in which a child of normal or above normal intelligence experiences inordinate difficulty in learning standard arithmetic. Distinguish from ACAL-CULIA. See also DEVELOPMENTAL *ARITHMETIC DISORDER.

dyschiria A general term for a variety of neurological disorders all of which share a dysfunction in the side of space opposite the site of the lesion, including such disorders as NEGLECT and SOMATOPARAPHRENIA.

dyschromatopsia A general term for any deficiency in colour vision. There are several variants: *dyschromia, dyschromopsia, dyschromacy*.

dyschronism Generally, disturbed time sense, particularly that caused by flight across 5 to 10 time zones, which maximally disrupts biological rhythms. See also DESYN-CHRONISM.

dysdiadochkinesia Difficulty in performing rapid alternating movements as with the fingers or hands. It is a good example of a neurological SOFT SIGN. When the ability is completely absent it is called *adiadochkinesia*.

dyseidetic Characterized by poor visual imagery.

dyseidetic dyslexia DYSLEXIA, DYSEIDETIC.

dysergasia Lit., inability to function properly. In psychology, a disorder characterized by hallucinations, irrational fears, disorientation, dream states and the like brought on by a cerebral nutritional deficit; occasionally caused by a toxic condition such as alcohol intoxication.

dysexecutive syndrome Loosely, a syndrome marked by disruptions in EXECUTIVE FUNCTIONS, including difficulty with new tasks, cognitive perseveration and problems initiating and inhibiting action. Whether this syndrome is distinct from several others with similar profiles such as FRONTAL-LOBE SYN-DROME, FRONTO-TEMPORAL DEMENTIA and ORGANIC *PERSONALITY SYNDROME is unclear.

dysfunction Broadly, generally and ubiquitously, any disruption in normal functioning.

dysgenic 1 Characterized by abnormal development due to genetic factors. **2** Pertaining to genetic factors that lead to abnormal development.

dysgeusia A condition characterized by a disruption of the sense of taste. In serious cases eating the most mundane foods can be an extraordinarily unpleasant experience.

dysgnosia A cover term for any impairment of intellectual functioning.

dysgraphia Inability to write properly or to express oneself through writing. It is regarded as a form of APHASIA and may be manifested in a variety of ways. Some dysgraphic patients lose the ability to write numbers but not letters, others can write uppercase letters but not lower, while still others can write only consonants, not vowels. Other forms of the disorder are more general and involve problems with phonological and/or orthographic representations.

dysgraphia, orthographic A form of dysgraphia characterized by correct spelling of regular words but not irregular ones. People with this disorder can sound out words normally, so are able to write nonsense if it is regular (e.g. they will spell 'grell' correctly), but they have difficulty with real words such as *cough*, which tends to come out as 'cawff'. The condition is usually associated with lesions in the inferior parietal lobe.

dysgraphia, phonological A form of dysgraphia characterized by an inability to sound out words and write them phonetically. People with this disorder can usually write familiar words normally by visualizing them but fail badly on unfamiliar words and on pronounceable nonwords. The condition is associated with damage in the superior temporal lobe.

dyshomophilia A psychosexual disorder in which the sufferer is severely distressed and rendered highly anxious by his or her sexually arousing fantasies about homosexuality. The individual's sexual preferences are not an issue here; the condition can emerge whether the person affected is exclusively homosexual or heterosexual or, indeed, even completely asexual. Compare with and distinguish from EGODYSTONIC *HOMOSEXUALITY.

dyskinesia Generally, an impairment of voluntary movement; specifically, abnormal movement patterns such tics, ballism, chorea or tremors, such as those seen in Parkinson's disease and tardive dyskinesia.

dyslalia Impaired speech due either to psychological (functional) causes or to defects in the peripheral speech organs. When the cause is brain damage APHASIA is the proper term.

dyslexia Basically and loosely, any reading disorder. However, there is a distinct lack of consensus among educators, psychologists and physicians on exactly how to character-

ize reading failures, particularly in terms of the aetiology of the condition, the cognitive and perceptual elements that must underlie it, and precisely how poor a person's reading ability should be in order to be classified as a case of dyslexia. When it occurs early in life, during the period when a child is attempting to learn to read, it is regarded as a LEARNING DISABILITY and often referred to as *developmental dyslexia*. Here the term is reserved for children who are significantly behind grade or intellectual level in reading and when there is no evidence of any generally debilitating disorder like mental retardation, major brain injury, severe emotional problems or cultural factors such as coming from a home where the language spoken is not the one used in the wider community. Compare this meaning with that of ACQUIRED *DYSLEXIA, which is used as a cover term for a host of reading disorders that result from neurological injury. Synonymous terms include *developmental reading disorder* and *developmental dyslexia*. In the UK *dyslexia* is often used as a cover term for both the developmental and the acquired forms. Given this pattern of confusing and overlapping usage, it should come as no surprise that many specialized terms are used to refer to specific subtypes of dyslexia. Some of those in common use follow. Distinguish from ALEXIA.

dyslexia, acquired A cover term for any DYSLEXIA in an individual who previously read normally. Several subclasses are recognized; some are listed below.

dyslexia, attentional An unusual form of ACQUIRED *DYSLEXIA marked by relatively normal reading of individual words but gross disruption of reading of words in text.

dyslexia, central Any ACQUIRED *DYSLEXIA attributed to impairments of the higher or more cognitively based functions associated with reading, including DEEP, SURFACE and PHONOLOGICAL *DYSLEXIA. Compare with PERIPHERAL *DYSLEXIA.

dyslexia, deep A form of ACQUIRED *DYSLEXIA marked by the occurrence of semantic errors in reading, e.g. deep dyslexics are likely to read *bird* as 'pigeon' or *cat* as 'dog'. They also typically have difficulty reading FUNCTION WORDS (such as articles, prepositions and conjunctions) and have more trouble with abstract words than concrete (*tree* is easier than *free*). The disorder has been observed in patients with a variety of injuries, most commonly large perisylvan lesions extending into the frontal lobes. It is also usually associated with GLOBAL and BROCA'S *APHASIA.

dyslexia, developmental Because there are several forms of ACQUIRED *DYSLEXIA, this term is occasionally used to distinguish the more common cases of children who have no identifiable neurological disorder but still experience difficulty in learning to read. See DYSLEXIA for more details.

dyslexia, direct A form of ACQUIRED *DYS-LEXIA in which the patient can read words aloud but not understand them.

dyslexia, dyseidetic A form of developmental dyslexia characterized by difficulty in reading words as 'wholes'. Children with this disorder tend to read very phonetically, sounding out every word and labouring over even the most common words. The term is roughly synonymous with SURFACE *DYSLEXIA although some reserve the latter for cases in which the disorder is acquired.

dyslexia, dysphonic A form of developmental dyslexia marked by weak phonological decoding skills. Children with this disorder tend to rely on whole-word identification and have difficulty reading novel, irregularly spelled words. The term is roughly synonymous with PHONOLOGICAL *DYSLEXIA although some reserve the latter for cases in which the disorder is acquired.

dyslexia, neglect A form of ACQUIRED *DYS-LEXIA often observed in patients with left-side NEGLECT, who have trouble reading because they are unresponsive to the left sides of words. Interestingly, the disorder has a lexical component; that is, a patient may read a word like *slipper* correctly but be unable to read the nonword *plipper*. Because left-side neglect is the key here, the same patient will usually be able to read the nonword *slipparge*.

dyslexia, peripheral Any ACQUIRED *DYS-LEXIA characterized by deficits in the processing of visual elements of the stimulus words. Compare with CENTRAL *DYSLEXIA.

dyslexia, phonological A form of ACQUIRED *DYSLEXIA marked by difficulties in learning to sound words out. Phonological dyslexics can learn to read using the WHOLE-WORD METHOD but have difficulties with new words or names they have not encountered before. Compare with SURFACE *DYSLEXIA and DYSPHO-NIC *DYSLEXIA.

dyslexia, surface A form of ACQUIRED *DYS-LEXIA marked by difficulties in recognizing and deriving the meanings from words. Surface dyslexics must sound out words carefully in order to read them; hence, they have difficulties with irregularly spelled words. Compare with PHONOLOGICAL *DYSLEXIA and DYSEIDETIC *DYSLEXIA.

dyslexia, word-form A variety of ACQUIRED *DYSLEXIA that essentially combines the symptoms of both *surface* and *phonological dyslexia*. Interestingly, those with this disorder can sometimes still read by laboriously spelling out each word. Also called *spelling dyslexia*.

dyslogia A deficiency in the ability to express ideas verbally.

dysmenorrhoea Painful menstruation. *Primary dysmenorrhoea* is used of the condition when it appears with the *menarche* (first period), *secondary dysmenorrhoea* when it develops later in life, usually because of uterine or pelvic pathology. var., *dysmenorrhea*.

dysmetria Inability to direct the range and force of voluntary movements. A symptom of some cerebellar lesions.

dysmetropsia Disturbance in the ability to visualize the size and shape of objects.

dysmnesia Generally, any impairment of memory. Occasionally, a cognitive dysfunction secondary to a memory disorder.

dysmorphophobia BODY DYSMORPHIC DIS-ORDER.

dysnomia ANOMIA.

dysorexia Generally, any disturbance in normal appetite; see e.g. ANOREXIA.

dysosmia Disruptions in the sense of smell.

dyspareunia A SEXUAL PAIN DISORDER marked by recurrent or persistent genital pain before, during or after sexual intercourse. The term is used for both men and women.

dysphagia An umbrella term for any abnormal eating pattern. Some authors restrict its application to eating disorders caused by neurological dysfunctions, others use it more generally. For specific forms see APHA-GIA, BULIMIA, HYPERPHAGIA and PICA.

dysphasia Loosely, any DEVELOPMENTAL *LAN-GUAGE DISORDER. Occasionally used as a syno-nym of APHASIA, which is not recommended (see DYS-).

dysphemia A speech defect caused by psy-chological factors.

dysphemism The use of an offensive or dis-paraging term in place of a more neutral one; the opposite of *euphemism*. Often used in pol-itical rhetoric as a form of persuasion, espe-cially during wars.

dysphonetic sequencing disorder A dys-lexia characterized by phonetic confusions and misperceptions of phonetic sequences.

dysphonia 1 A general term for any lan-guage dysfunction involving speech sounds or *phonation*. **2** A synonym for APHASIA, although this usage is not recommended. *Dysphonia* does not carry the specific conno-tation of *aphasia*, namely that language func-tions once existed and then were lost through neurological damage. See here DEVELOPMENTAL *LANGUAGE DISORDER, which is preferred as a synonym for 1.

dysphonia, puberum The change in voice in males during puberty.

dysphonic dyslexia DYSLEXIA, DYSPHONIC.

dysphoria Negative or uncomfortable affect, usually in association with anxiety, restlessness or depression. ant., EUPHORIA (1).

dysphrenia Obsolete term for any mental disorder.

dysplasia Any abnormal development of tissue; any abnormal growth.

dyspnoea Difficulty in breathing. var., *dys-pnea*.

dyspraxia Disorder involving difficulty with movement and coordination.

dysprosodia APROSODIA.

dysregulatory psychopathology Loosely, any disorder characterized by poorly regu-lated behaviours such as inappropriate aggression, excessive spending of money and a general lack of the ability to modulate

reactions to emotionally arousing stimula-tion.

dyssemia Impairment in sending or receiv-ing nonverbal social cues. Can include diffi-culty in decoding or encoding emotion, and in understanding personal space. Regarded as a symptom of a nonverbal LEARNING DISABIL-ITY (2).

dyssocial personality An obsolescent term for a personality disorder characterized by a seriously distorted sense of ethics and mor-ality.

dyssomnia A general label for a group of sleep disorders in which the primary disturb-ance is in the amount, quality or timing of sleep. Dyssomnias are generally regarded as psychogenic in origin and due primarily to emotional disturbances, high levels of stress, anxiety, etc. Examples are INSOMNIA, HYPER-SOMNIA, and SLEEP–WAKE SCHEDULE DISORDER. Compare with PARASOMNIA.

dysspermia Difficult or painful ejaculation.

dysstasia Difficulty in standing upright.

dysthymia Generally, despondency, depression. See DYSTHYMIC DISORDER.

dysthymic disorder A *mood disorder* char-acterized by a general depression, lack of interest in the normal, standard activities of living and a ubiquitous 'down in the dumps' feeling. *Dysthymia* is not meant to be used for cases of acute depression; it is only used for disruptions of normal affect lasting at least 1 year. Distinguish also from MAJOR *DEPRESSIVE EPISODE. Also called *depressive neurosis*.

dystocia Difficult labour.

dystonia Impaired muscle tone.

dystonic movement Slow, twisting bodily movement with interspersed periods of mus-cular tension.

dystrophy A general term for any condition produced by faulty nutrition or a metabolic dysfunction.

dysuria Painful or difficult urination.

DZ Abbreviation for DIZYGOTIC.

DZA (or DZa) Abbreviation for a set of dizy-gotic twins raised apart from each other.

E

E A multifunctional abbreviation used for: **1** Experimenter. **2** Experimental group. **3** Energy. **4** Error. **5** Within the theory of learning of C. L. Hull it is found in a veritable 'alphabet soup' of symbols used to refer to various theoretical constructs. A few of the more common are: $_sE_R$ = excitatory potential; $_sE_R$ = reaction potential (from generalization); $_s\bar{E}_R$ = effective reaction potential. The interested reader is referred to any of the older (1950s) standard texts of learning theory for fuller explanation of these and others; they are rarely used in contemporary work in learning.

-e- Alternative spelling to *-ae-* used in terms of Greek and Latin origin.

e² In studies of genetic influences, the portion of the variance that is attributable to environmental factors. An example would be differences in achievement between two identical twins due to each having different teachers in school. Sometimes capitalized. See ENVIRONMENTALITY.

ear Most generally, the organ of hearing. Three anatomical divisions make up the full organ. The outer ear consists of the *pinna* (what is, in general parlance, called the ear) and the external auditory *meatus* (or canal) up to the *tympanic membrane* (or eardrum). The middle ear contains the *ossicles*, the three bones which transmit vibrations of the tympanic membrane to the *oval window* on the *cochlea*. The middle ear is also connected to the *pharynx* via the *Eustachian tube*, which serves to equalize air pressure. The inner ear consists of the cochlea and the *semicircular canals*. Within the cochlea are the receptor cells for audition.

eardrum TYMPANIC MEMBRANE.

early 1 In developmental psychology, referencing a time somewhere toward the first few years of life. Exactly when 'early' ends is not always clear. In research on language development 'early' can be anywhere from 5 years to puberty; in memory research 'early' usually refers to recall of events that occurred before the age of 3; in emotional development and personality formation usage depends on the theoretical stance of the writer and can mean anything from 5 years of age to early adulthood. Note that *late* suffers from a similar pattern of ambiguous usage with reference to events that occur after some number of years of life have passed. **2** In perception and cognitive psychology, before something else as in EARLY-SELECTION MODEL.

early Alzheimer's disease MILD COGNITIVE IMPAIRMENT.

Early Learning Advisor (ELA) A computerized assessment and planning system based on the concept of the ZONE OF PROXIMAL DEVELOPMENT, used by some teachers to assess students and select appropriate educational goals and techniques in reading and writing. When the system is applied to the acquisition of reading and writing skills, it is called the *Early Literacy Advisor*.

early-selection model A model of SELECTIVE ATTENTION that assumes that items are selected for attention early in processing, soon after the sensory input has been received. Compare with *late-selection model* where the assumption is that attention is not focused on the item until later in processing, after it has been identified and categorized. The distinction between these two is not as clear as the proponents of each had hoped and, indeed, both kinds of processing take place depending on a myriad of factors.

easy child See DIFFICULT CHILD.

eating disorders A general term used to cover a variety of conditions characterized by serious disturbances in eating habits and appetitive behaviours. See e.g. ANOREXIA NERVOSA, BULIMIA NERVOSA, PICA and RUMINATION DISORDER OF INFANCY.

Ebbinghaus curve The classic forgetting curve for nonsense material. It shows a sharp drop in recall immediately after learning, followed by a slow, gradual loss of material. It was discovered by the early German psychologist Hermann Ebbinghaus.

Ebbinghaus illusion This illusion has several versions, all based on the principle of relative size. The most commonly found is the one shown here; both inner dots are the same size. Note, some credit this illusion to J. Delboeuf.

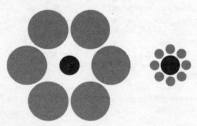

EBS ELECTRICAL BRAIN STIMULATION.

eccentric Lit., off-centre. The term is used occasionally to characterize persons whose peculiar behaviour is accompanied by success.

eccentric projection A term used occasionally to characterize the experience of a locus of stimulation as 'out there' in the world rather than at the receptors stimulated. Vision and hearing are the clearest examples; one is conscious of the external scene (the *distal stimulus*) and not the actual events that activate the sense (the *proximal stimulus*).

ECG ELECTROCARDIOGRAM.

echo- Combining form meaning *repetitive*.

echographia The compulsive writing of words and phrases heard. A graphic analogue of ECHOLALIA.

echoic The auditory analogue of ICONIC (see that term for discussion).

echoic behaviour Skinner's term for imitations of verbalizations of others.

echoic memory MEMORY, ECHOIC.

echokinesis ECHOPRAXIA.

echolalia The compulsive and apparently senseless repetition of a word or phrase just spoken by another person. Generally symptomatic of a functional disorder, although it is a frequent component of autism in which the sound 'repeated' may be a nonsensical invention of the individual and not necessarily one made by another. Also called *echophrasia*.

echolocation Lit., the location of objects in space by using the echoes of self-produced sounds. Some species (bats, cetaceans) have evolved this process to a high degree of precision.

echopathy A general term for any pathological mimicking of the speech, gestures, actions or mannerisms of others.

echophrasia ECHOLALIA.

echopraxia Pathological tendency to repeat gestures made by others; occasionally seen in schizophrenia of the catatonic type and in some patients with frontal lobe damage. Also called *echokinesis*.

eclectic Generally, not following any one system but selecting and using whatever is considered best in all systems. In experimental and theoretical work, an eclectic approach tends to be rather loose and informal, no one theoretical position being regarded as universally applicable; if there is any allegiance it is to the attempt to coordinate and reconcile differences between competing theoretical positions in the search for harmony, for synthesis. In clinical psychology and psychiatry, an eclectic therapist is one who uses whatever therapeutic procedures seem most applicable to the case. This may mean taking a psychoanalytic bent with one client but a more direct, behavioural approach with another.

ecmnesia Loss of memory for recent materials while retaining memory for more remote events; see ANTEROGRADE *AMNESIA.

ecological Pertaining to ECOLOGY.

ecological fallacy A logical *fallacy* in which conclusions about individuals are drawn based on data from groups. For example, crime rates tend to be higher in neighbourhoods with large numbers of the elderly, but it would be fallacious to conclude that the elderly are more likely to commit crimes.

ecological niche A position or function of an organism (or, more commonly, a species) in a particular environment.

ecological optics Basically, the notion of ECOLOGICAL VALIDITY applied to the study of visual perception. J. J. Gibson's theory of DIRECT PERCEPTION assumes such a process as central to vision.

ecological psychology A term used occasionally to refer to the approach to psychology that elaborates on J. J. Gibson's theory of DIRECT PERCEPTION.

ecological validity 1 A term originally coined by Egon Brunswik for the degree to which the distal and proximal stimuli covary. He conceived of the basic operation of perception as estimating the true, physical (distal) stimulus on the basis of the varying proximal stimulus values that actually impinge on the receptor systems. The higher the ecological validity of a proximal cue for a distal stimulus property, the more likely it is to be learned and used. The term is also used with this meaning in the context of the DIRECT PERCEPTION theory of J. J. Gibson. 2 Loosely, the validity that a principle discovered in a laboratory setting has outside that setting in the field, in the real world. 3 Somewhat more specifically, a form of CRITERION-RELATED *VALIDITY based on the degree to which results can be generalized from group to group. Norms established using university students might have low ecological validity when applied to blue-collar workers of the same age.

ecology 1 Broadly, the study of the relationship between organisms and their environments. The discipline is concerned with the complex interrelationships of the various plants and animals with each other and with the physical environment in which

they live. There are several subdisciplines in the field, dealing with plant ecology, animal ecology and human ecology. 2 In K. Lewin's theory, the study of those psychological factors that contribute to a person's LIFE SPACE. The term also has a variety of specialized uses reflecting either of the two basic meanings that appear in combined forms; some of these follow and others can be found following ECOLOGICAL.

ecology, behavioural A term used by some for the extension of the science of ecology into psychology. The focus is on the interaction (or, as the proponents of the approach prefer, the *transaction*) between the environment and the behaviours of the organisms in it. The orientation is strongly holistic and employs naturalistic observation as the primary research tool.

ecology, social The approach to ecology that emphasizes the interactions between individuals and their environment.

ecology, urban A field of study drawing on the researches of various other disciplines such as biology, sociology, psychology and geography. It focuses on the investigation of urban environments as 'natural' ecological systems.

economy, principle of PRINCIPLE OF *PARSIMONY.

ecosphere Those portions of the natural environment that are habitable by life forms.

ecosystem A relatively restricted ecological unit.

ecphoria 1. The establishing of a memory trace. 2 The activation and modification of a previously established memory trace. The term is rare in either sense. var., *ecphory.*

ECS ELECTROCONVULSIVE SHOCK.

Ecstasy See MDMA.

ecstatic state RELIGIOUS *TRANCE.

ECT Usually, 1 ELECTROCONVULSIVE THERAPY. Occasionally, 2 ELEMENTARY COGNITIVE TASKS.

ect(o)- Combining form from the Greek meaning *outside, external.*

ectoderm The outer layer of embryonic cellular structure that develops into the outer skin, the nervous system, the organs of special sense, the pineal gland and part of the pituitary.

ectogenous Characteristic of that which has its origins outside of the body. var., *exogenous*.

ectomorphy One of the three primary dimensions of body type (ENDOMORPHY and MESOMORPHY being the others) in Sheldon's CONSTITUTIONAL THEORY. An ectomorph is one whose physique is dominated by the embryonic ectodermal component, i.e. the outer skin and the nervous system. Hence, ectomorphic persons are thin with large skin surfaces relative to weight.

-ectomy Combining form meaning *removal*, specifically surgical removal.

ectopia Displacement or misposition, particularly of an organ or part thereof.

ectoplasm 1 The outermost layer of cell protoplasm. 2 In PARAPSYCHOLOGY, a hypothesized psychic substance said to emanate from the body of a medium in a trance during a séance.

eczema Any of several types of chronic DERMATITIS. The most common form is marked by heightened sensitivity to particular irritants. It has a familial component and is linked with other allergies such as hay fever and asthma.

edema Swelling of tissue due to injury or trauma. var., *oedema*.

edge Basically, a 'line' in the visual field on one side of which there is a detectable difference in some aspect of the stimulus compared with on the other. Note that as the term is used, there is no actual, literal line; the edge is merely the boundary between the two adjacent areas of the visual field.

Edipus complex OEDIPUS COMPLEX.

EDR Abbreviation for *electrodermal response*; see GALVANIC SKIN RESPONSE.

educable mentally retarded MILD *MENTAL RETARDATION.

education To *educe* means to draw forth, develop, elicit. Hence, the process of drawing something out, of making a connection, specifically of establishing a connection that reflects the fundamental relations between objects or events.

educational age AGE, EDUCATIONAL.

educational guidance GUIDANCE.

educationally subnormal (ESN) MILD *MENTAL RETARDATION.

educational psychology A subdiscipline of psychology concerned with theories and problems in education. Generally included within the province of the field are the application of principles of learning to the classroom, curriculum development and reform, testing and evaluation of aptitudes and abilities, socialization processes and their interaction with cognitive functioning, teacher training, etc.

educational quotient (EQ) The ratio of EDUCATIONAL *AGE to CHRONOLOGICAL *AGE times 100.

Edwards Personal Preference Schedule A self-report personality inventory consisting of 225 forced-choice items. The items have been selected to correspond to the 15 needs which Henry Murray has theorized are fundamental in human personality. Whether the test really measures what it sets out to is an unresolved issue but the test is interesting because of its attempt to circumvent biased responding due to social desirability – a factor which contaminates many personality tests.

EEG ELECTROENCEPHALOGRAM.

effacement See SELF-EFFACEMENT.

effect 1 n. An event that reliably follows another event, its cause. 2 vb. To bring about a state of affairs, to have an impact on something. 3 In statistics, differences between means that can be attributed to the independent variables in the study. If words in the middle of a list are learned less well than those at the beginning or the end, there is an *effect* of serial position on memory. There are MAIN EFFECTS (such as in this example) and *interaction effects* (see INTERACTION).

effectance Effectiveness; the capacity to cope with the environment, to be competent. In Adler's approach, an effectance *motive* is assumed, which functions by making a child feel a strong need to become competent so as to overcome feelings of inadequacy or inferiority.

effect, empirical law of See LAW OF *EFFECT.

effective habit strength In C. L. Hull's theory, the strength of a particular learned response as established by the collective reinforcement processes that have operated on it in the past.

effective reaction potential In C. L. Hull's theory, the REACTION POTENTIAL minus any inhibiting tendencies.

effective stimulus FUNCTIONAL *STIMULUS.

effective visual field That portion of the visual field in which there is relatively good acuity, e.g. where stimuli such as letters can be recognized.

effective weight WEIGHT (3).

effect, law of 1 Broadly and generally, the behaviourist principle that events in the world serve to select particular behaviours from the (infinite, or at least very large) pool of possible behaviours. Behaviours that lead to 'good things' are repeated, those that lead to 'bad things' are not. Behaviourists view the law of effect as a behavioural parallel to the principle of natural selection – the well-designed behaviours are selected from the pool of responses, their occurrence is made more likely, and the others are allowed to become extinct (see EXTINCTION). **2** In E. L. Thorndike's early theory, this 'law' took on singular importance. He saw the impact of reinforcement and punishment as among the core determinants of behaviour, arguing that the former 'stamped in' behaviours and the latter 'stamped' them out. As his theory evolved he introduced a number of variations to the basic principle including the *empirical law of effect*, which stated simply that any response followed by 'positive consequences' (i.e. reinforcements) became more likely to occur than one not so followed. He later termed this general principle the *weak law of effect* to contrast it with the *strong law of effect* which maintained that, in fact, the presence of some reinforcer was *necessary* for learning to occur. At one time he put forward a *negative law of effect* which was essentially the reciprocal of the empirical law, maintaining that negative consequences (i.e. punishers) diminished the probability of behaviour. He later 'repealed' this law on the grounds that punishment did not really 'stamp out'

behaviours, it merely made them less likely to occur. These, and other specialized 'Thorndikean' terms are rarely used today but are of significant historical interest. For more on related terminology, see PUNISHMENT, REINFORCEMENT and SUPPRESSION.

effect, negative law of See LAW OF *EFFECT.

effector Generally, a muscle or gland at the terminal end of an efferent neural process which produces the observed response.

effect size In statistics, quite literally, the size of an EFFECT (3). Tests of a null hypothesis may tell you that an effect is significant, but they do not tell you how large the effect is, and, of course, if *n* is large very small effect sizes can produce very large significance levels. Measures of effect size such as OMEGA SQUARED are based on the proportion of variance in the data that can be attributed to experimental variables and essentially tell you how many standard deviation units the group means are separated by.

effect, spread of To account for the phenomenon of GENERALIZATION, E. L. Thorndike proposed that the effect of 'satisfiers' or 'annoyers' spread to other stimuli present at the time of the response or to stimuli which are similar in nature to the originally reinforced or punished stimulus.

effect, strong law of See LAW OF *EFFECT.

effeminate Lit., female-like. The most common meaning, however, is descriptive or characteristic of a biological male who displays behaviour patterns which, in societal terms, are more closely associated with females. Note that some authors consider effeminacy to encompass physical as well as psychological/behavioural characteristics, although the tendency is to restrict usage to the latter. See also ANDROGYNY. Distinguish from HOMOSEXUAL; some effeminate men may indeed be homosexual but effeminacy itself is a poor predictor of sexual orientation.

efferent From the Latin for *carry away from*. Hence, in neurophysiology, the conduction of nerve impulses from the central nervous system toward the periphery (muscles, glands). Efferent neurons and neural pathways carry information to *effectors* and are commonly called *motor* neurons or pathways.

efficacy In Piagetian theory a very primitive cognitive experience whereby a young child assumes his or her emotions and feelings are responsible for events in the world. Contrast with SELF-EFFICACY.

effort 1 In loose physical terms, the work required to perform some action. However: **2** In psychology, the subjective sense of the amount of work required to perform some action, usually with the implications that (a) there is some resistance or barrier to be overcome in order to carry out the action and (b) the action carried out is voluntary.

effortful processes Processes that are dependent on conscious reflection and demanding of attentional and cognitive resources. Compared with AUTOMATIC PROCESSES, they are open to conscious inspection, require attentional focus and show considerable variability among individuals.

E–F scale A scale from the *Minnesota Multiphasic Personality Inventory* (*MMPI*) made up of 30 items and designed to measure attitudes toward ethnocentricity and authoritarianism (the *F* is for *Fascism*).

ego 1 From the Latin for *I*. Hence, the 'self' conceptualized as the central core around which all psychic activities revolve. This is the foundational meaning and is neutral as regards evaluative connotations and theories of personality. **2** One of the components in the Freudian tripartite model of the psychic apparatus (along with the ID and SUPEREGO). In the classical theory the ego represents a cluster of cognitive and perceptual processes including memory, problem-solving, reality-testing, inference-making and self-regulated striving, that are conscious and in touch with reality, as well as specific defence mechanisms that serve to mediate between the primitive instinctual demands of the id, the internalized social, parental inhibitions and prohibitions of the superego, and the knowledge of reality. In this conceptualization the ego serves as an executive who functions adaptively to maintain psychic balance. **3** The collected psychological processes that are concerned with SELF. In semi-technical and even some popular writings this is the meaning usually intended. It connotes a hypothetical entity with which an individual is overly concerned, a kind of psychological touchstone that serves as a basis for one's interests, values, attitudes, desires, etc. This is the meaning captured in terms like *egocentric, egoistic* and *egotistic*.

ego-alien EGO-DYSTONIC.

ego analysis A psychoanalytic term for a relatively short form of analysis which focuses on the integrative, positive ego functions rather than on the deeply repressed id functions.

ego anxiety In psychoanalytic theory any reaction resulting from threats to the ego; the anxiety caused by conflicts between id, ego and/or superego. In the classical theory, the genesis of all *ego defences* is found here.

ego block A very general term used for anything that is seen, in psychoanalytic terms, as preventing or inhibiting the full development of the ego.

ego, body Freud used this term to capture the notion that at its ultimate core the ego derives from the bodily sensations.

ego boundary A vaguely topological concept that implies that part of the normal ego development consists in establishing a boundary separating self from others. Presumably, anyone who identifies too readily with others at the expense of their own identity is lacking in ego boundary or has a weakly established ego boundary.

ego cathexis A channelling or focusing of libido on an object within the domain of the reality-oriented ego.

egocentric Pertaining to or characteristic of EGOCENTRISM.

egocentricity EGOCENTRISM.

egocentric speech Speech which derives from and serves purely internal needs and thoughts. See EGOCENTRISM.

egocentrism (or **egocentricity**) As the roots of the term suggest, the perspective in which one is preoccupied with the self and relatively insensitive to others. When used of adults the connotation is of self-absorption and self-centring. When used of children, particularly in the context of Piagetian theory, it pertains to speech and thought dominated by a child's own internal cognitions.

ego complex A term used by Jung to refer to

a group of emotional reactions toward or about oneself. Also called *self-sentiment*.

ego-control The construct that refers to one's characteristic manner of exerting self-control over behavioural and attentional impulses. Ideally, one displays a pattern of moderate and flexible self-control. Those who display excessive inhibition, relatively little change in interests and good delay of gratification are called *overcontrollers*; those who display spontaneity, fast tempo and unconventionality, *undercontrollers*.

ego defence The process of harnessing the libidinal energies of the id in defence of the ego. In general, all DEFENCE MECHANISMS may be characterized as ego defences.

ego depletion The reduction of the capacity for self-control and other effortful processes by the exercise of volitional self-control in the immediate past. The concept is based on the assumption that we have only limited capacity for effortful, volitional activity and that when this capacity is depleted, we see impairments in self-control and other processes that require active mental exertion.

ego development The gradual emerging awareness of a child that he or she is a distinct, independent person. Classical psychoanalysis assumes that the process is one in which the ego progressively acquires functions that enable the individual to master impulses and to learn how to function independently of parents. Erikson's STAGES OF MAN point of view regards the entire scope of life as understandable only from the perspective of stages of ego development. Piaget, on the other hand, handles the issue by focusing on cognitive development with considerably less emphasis on dynamic factors. There is precious little consensus here.

ego-dystonic Descriptive of wishes, dreams, impulses, behaviours, etc. that are unacceptable to the ego; or, perhaps more accurately, unacceptable to a person's ideal conception of self. Hence, an ego-dystonic idea is one that seems to have invaded consciousness, to have come from 'outside' the self. Contrast with EGO-SYNTONIC.

ego-dystonic homosexuality HOMOSEXUALITY, EGO-DYSTONIC.

ego erotism NARCISSISM.

ego failure A breakdown in ego function, specifically a failure to restrain id impulses so that they conform with the strictures of the superego.

ego function Usually this term refers to the primary role of the ego – to mediate between the id and the superego in ways that are responsive to society and self-protection. However, in the classical psychoanalytic perspective, absolutely anything a person can do is, strictly speaking, an ego function. This usage stems from a simple tautology since in the classical theory all functions are assigned to the ego.

ego ideal The ego's conception of positive ideals; in short, what a person would like to be or prefer to accomplish in terms of that which is positive and good. Generally a distinction is made between the *ego ideal* and the *superego* on the grounds that the former represents prescriptions for life, is modified through growth and experience, and behaviour that violates it produces shame; the latter represents proscriptions, is fixed at a young age, and behaviour in conflict with it evokes guilt.

ego instincts Collectively, all impulses for individual self-preservation. In Freud's early writings the ego instincts were distinguished from the id instincts, which were primarily sexual and reproductive. In his later writings this distinction became blurred because of the recasting of instincts as those for life (EROS) and those for death (THANATOS).

ego-integrative Tending toward integrating the ego; reaching for a point of coordination and harmony in life.

ego integrity The final stage of Erikson's STAGES OF MAN. It juxtaposes ego integrity and despair. Full ego integrity in this conception permits the acceptance of old age and one's ultimate death without despair.

ego involvement 1 A situation of committing oneself wholeheartedly to a task. **2** A situation wherein one determines that a particular goal or task is important to one's ego.

egoism In simplest terms, *self-interest*. Hence: **1** A label for the point of view that self-interest is at the base of all behaviour (contrast here with ALTRUISM). **2** The tendency to behave strictly or largely according to self-interest. Compare here with EGOTISM.

egoistic Conceited, self-serving, motivated by self-interest. See EGOTISTICAL for discussion of and comparison between these and similar and often confused terms.

egoistic suicide SUICIDE, EGOISTIC.

ego libido Libido invested in the ego. In psychoanalytic writings the term is sometimes used to refer to the psychic energy available for carrying out ego functions and sometimes used for self-love. Contrast with OBJECT LIBIDO.

egomania Pathological preoccupation with one's ego or, better, with one's self. See also discussion under -MANIA.

ego neurosis A theoretical classification in psychoanalysis that includes neuroses, such as functional paralyses, hysteria and memory loss, that are hypothesized to result from disruption of ego functions.

ego–object polarity The distinction between the self and that which is not-self. It is normally rather sharp, hence the notion of polarity. See EGO BOUNDARY.

egopathy A general term for the tendency to bolster one's own ego by inappropriate hostility and aggression toward others.

ego psychology 1 Generally, the psychology of the ego. That is, the examination of those developing structures and processes that are regarded as being within the purview of the ego; specifically included here are memory, language, judgement, decision-making and other reality-oriented functions. **2** A label for those variations of psychoanalytic theory that focus on the ego and its role in personality development.

ego-resilience RESILIENCE.

ego resistance A psychoanalytic term used to characterize resistance on the part of the patient (read, 'the patient's ego') to give up neurotic patterns of behaviour, to recognize repressed impulses and to abandon defence mechanisms.

ego strength Psychoanalytic theory characterizes the strength of the ego in terms of its share of available psychic energy. Theoretically, the stronger the ego the greater the resoluteness of character and, according to some, the more likely the individual will be able to withstand the slings and arrows…In the final analysis, psychoanalysts use the term in pretty much the same way as it is used in the common, nontechnical language.

ego structure A generic term used to characterize the pattern and organization of ego traits, functions, etc. Just what actual structure the ego can be said to have depends entirely upon the theorist under consideration.

ego-syntonic Descriptive of values, feelings and ideas that are consistent with one's ego, that feel 'real' and acceptable to consciousness. An ego-syntonic idea feels 'like it belongs'. Contrast with EGO-DYSTONIC.

ego-syntonic homosexuality HOMOSEXUALITY, EGO-SYNTONIC.

ego threat Generally, any danger to the ego's efforts to adapt to the demands of reality. In the psychoanalytic framework, those pressures and instinctual demands of the id that are perceived as incompatible with the constraints of reality and/or the superego's prohibitions.

egotic Pertaining to or characterizing the ego. The term is used by some authors because the other adjectival forms (*egoistic*, *egotistic*, *egotistical*) have taken on evaluative connotations that are distinctly negative.

egotism The tendency to regard oneself very highly, specifically to the point of having an annoyingly overblown opinion of oneself. Compare with EGOISM (2).

egotism, implicit A phenomenon in which individuals are unconsciously influenced in their decision-making by personal demographics such as their birth dates or letters in their names. Such effects are quite real; even when corrected for frequency effects, Johns are more likely to marry Joannes than Daphnes or Marys.

egotistic(al) Conceited, maintaining a high opinion of oneself. Note that this notion of conceit is shared with the term *egotistic* but the connotations of the two are different. *Egoistic* describes those who view themselves as at the centre of things and who have great concern for their own self-interest; *egotistic* refers to those who tend to have, in addition, an unrealistic and obnoxious sense of self-importance. One can be very egoistic yet have little in the way of egotism.

egotization A psychoanalytic term for the hypothesized process by which a mental process becomes part of the ego or self; i.e. the process by which it comes to be freed from id-based impulses of aggression and sexuality and becomes structured and reality-oriented.

ego trip A nontechnical term used broadly for any pattern of behaviour engaged in primarily for the purpose of boosting one's sense of self.

eidetic imagery From the Greek *eidos*, meaning *form* (usually taken to mean *form in the mind*), mental imagery that is vivid and persistent. The critical features of those with such imagery (called *eidetikers*) are: (a) that they continue to 'see' a representation of a visual stimulus some time after it has been removed; and (b) that they are 'seeing' a true visual image and not merely memory of the stimulus. A true eidetic image lasts for some time and hence is differentiated from an *icon* (see discussion under SENSORY INFORMATION STORE) and from an AFTERIMAGE. Eidetic imagery is more common in children (conservative estimates put its incidence at about 5 in 100) than in adults (in whom it is estimated to occur in less than 1 in 1,000, some authorities even putting it at less than 1 in a million).

eidetiker EIDETIC IMAGERY.

eigenvalue In FACTOR ANALYSIS, a quantification of the amount of variability in a set of VARIABLES (1) that is explained by an underlying FACTOR (4). Generally, eigenvalues less than 1 are taken to indicate that the factor is not explaining a notable amount of variance.

Eigenwelt This term is German for, and literally translated as, *self-world*, and is used in existentialism to refer to the relationship between each person and him- or herself. This concept, in isolation, makes precious little sense; its meaning, however, is easily appreciated when juxtaposed with its companion existentialist concepts *Mitwelt* and *Umwelt*. The former refers to a person's relationships with other persons, with a person's

contemporaries, and the latter to a person's relationship with the environment.

eighty–twenty (80–20) rule PARETO PRINCIPLE.

eikon ICONIC.

Einstellung German for *attitude* or *set*. Used to denote a kind of cognitive readiness for a particular stimulus or class of stimuli. For example, a subject in an experiment that has been using only auditory stimulus materials will establish such a set and will be startled by, and may not even correctly perceive, a visual stimulus if one is suddenly presented. See SET (esp. 2).

ejaculatio praecox PREMATURE EJACULATION.

ejaculatory incompetence The inability to ejaculate within the vagina during intercourse; in a sense, the reverse of *premature ejaculation*.

Ekbom syndrome RESTLESS LEG SYNDROME.

EKG ELECTROCARDIOGRAM.

ekphorize In psychiatry, to bring back the effect of a particular psychological experience.

ELA 1 ENGLISH LANGUAGE ARTS. **2** EARLY LITERACY ADVISOR.

elaborated code B. Bernstein's term for the speech mode adopted when one is speaking with persons from different backgrounds from oneself, persons with whom few assumptions can be made concerning shared background or common knowledge. Under such conditions discourse is relatively slow, words and phrases are carefully selected, and speech is elaborately planned. Compare with RESTRICTED CODE.

elaboration In cognition, any process whereby a particular memory of a stimulus is interpreted, elaborated, associated with other stimuli or in any other way 'fleshed out'. Although it seems fairly clear that such elaborative strategies are used by essentially everyone as aids to memory, there is considerable debate in the field as to whether it is reasonable to regard all of the knowledge in LONG-TERM *MEMORY as resulting from the use of elaboration. See also CONSTRUCTIVISM for more discussion on a similar point.

elaboration likelihood model A theory of

attitude change that assumes two routes to persuasion. In the central route, which is most likely to be used when both motivation and resources to process a message are high, the perceiver pays attention to the content of the message, thinking about and 'elaborating' on the arguments in it. In the peripheral route, which is more generally used when motivation and/or resources are low, the perceiver focuses on surface characteristics of the message, such as its length or the credibility of the source. This theory is useful in the study of attitude change, as it helps define under what conditions people are likely to pay attention to content over style.

elaborative rehearsal Rehearsing of information using ELABORATION. See also REHEARSAL.

Elberfeld horses A group of superbly trained horses in Germany, popular during the early part of the 20th century. The most startling was *der kluge Hans* (CLEVER HANS), who could seemingly perform complex mathematical problems, answer factual questions, spell, etc.

elder neglect NEGLECT (1) of the elderly. The term is reserved for cases where the individual is compromised in his or her ability to function and external care and support from responsible others is needed.

elderspeak An artificial manner of speaking that younger adults often use with the elderly. It is slow, with short sentences and a limited vocabulary. It's often used in the mistaken belief that all elderly persons are at least slightly demented and, unlike CHILD-DIRECTED SPEECH, which has similar features but is useful in language development, is usually a waste of time and embarrassing to all concerned.

elective mutism SELECTIVE MUTISM.

Electra complex OEDIPUS COMPLEX.

electrical brain stimulation (EBS) The application of a weak electrical current (usually in the form of a series of short pulses) to a specific locale in the brain. The technique is used in a variety of contexts, from neurosurgical procedures, in which it helps the surgeon determine the areas of the brain that need to be surgically removed and those that need to be protected, to experimental studies of the relationship between various

cerebral structures and the functions they control. Also called by a variety of other names including *electrical stimulation of the brain* (ESB) and *intracranial stimulation* (ICS).

electrical synapse Communication between cells that takes place electrically. While most SYNAPSES are chemical (see NEURO-TRANSMITTER), electrical forms of information exchange play a role in synchronizing cortical activity by allowing signals to spread rapidly across distant neural cell populations.

electric shock therapy (EST) ELECTROCONVULSIVE THERAPY.

electrocardiogram (ECG or EKG) A record of the activity of the heart made by recording the spreading electrical potential generated by the heart beat and putting it in graphic form. In addition to its obvious medical applications, ECG has been used as a measure of emotional arousal, of physical exertion, etc., and as such has served the role of dependent variable in studies of classical conditioning, emotionality and the like.

electroconvulsive shock (ECS) A brief electrical shock applied to the head that produces full-body seizure, convulsions and usually loss of consciousness. ECS is used in two distinct ways: (a) As a research tool to study (in animals) the neurophysiology of memory. Here the usual technique is to pass a current through the brain, producing RETROGRADE *AMNESIA (loss of memory for recent past events). There is considerable debate as to whether the technique functions by interfering with the process of CONSOLIDATION or whether it disrupts the retrieval of the memory. (b) As a therapeutic procedure for major depression; see ELECTROCONVULSIVE THERAPY.

electroconvulsive therapy (ECT) The use of electroconvulsive shock as a therapeutic procedure for psychiatric disorders. The technique consists of applying a weak electric current (20–30 mA) bilaterally to the temperofrontal region of the skull until a *grand mal* seizure results. The patient is sedated using an ultra-short-acting barbiturate, and a muscle relaxant is administered to minimize the intensity of the muscular reactions. ECT produces a period of drowsiness, temporary confusion and disorientation, and a variety of memory deficits, some of which the patient recovers over time, although gaps may remain indefinitely. Recent years have seen a significant drop in the use of this procedure in many large understaffed institutions, where it had been used primarily to produce docility in the patient threatened with it. Its only recognized therapeutic use is in the treatment of cases of severe depression that have proven unresponsive to ANTIDEPRESSANT DRUGS. Precisely why ECT has this antidepressant effect is still unknown. Also called *electroshock therapy* (*EST*); distinguish from ELECTROTHERAPY.

electroculogram ELECTRO-OCULOGRAM.

electrode Generally, any medium for transmitting an electric current to an object or for recording electrical activity from an object. Often which kind of electrode is in use is specified by appending qualifiers, e.g. *stimulating* or *recording*. Typically the medium is a metallic device, and in most psychological and physiological research the object is bodily tissue.

electrodermal response (EDR) GALVANIC SKIN RESPONSE.

electroencephalogram (EEG) A record of the changes in electrical potential of the brain. Electrodes are generally attached to (or occasionally just under) the scalp and the wavelike potentials are amplified and recorded. Detailed EEG analyses have revealed that the brain undergoes systematic changes in the kinds of potential exhibited during various activities. See, for example, ALPHA WAVE, DELTA WAVE. Note that the terms *electroencephalogram* and *electroencephalograph* are used virtually interchangeably; the field of study and use of the device is called *electroencephalography*.

electrolyte A substance which when in solution conducts an electrical current and is decomposed by its passage. Salts, bases and acids are all electrolytes.

electromyogram (EMG) A graphic record of the changes in electrical potential in a muscle.

electronarcosis The induction of unconsciousness by passage of an electrical current through brain tissue. See ELECTROCONVULSIVE SHOCK.

electronystagmography The recording of

NYSTAGMUS by detection of the electrical activity of the muscles of the eye.

electro-oculogram (EOG) A device for measuring eye movements by recording the electrical potentials of the muscles that control them. var., *electroculogram*.

electro-olfactogram (EOG) A device that records the electric potentials within the olfactory system. Also called *olfactometer*.

electroretinogram (ERG) A graphic record of the changes in electrical potential of the retina.

electroshock therapy (EST) ELECTROCONVULSIVE THERAPY.

electrotherapy Therapy using mild, brief electrical stimulation. The term is to be distinguished from *electroshock therapy* and *electroconvulsive therapy*, since the electrical charges used are of a nonconvulsive nature.

element Aside from the standard dictionary meanings this term has several specialized usages in psychology: **1** The early structuralists used it to refer to the basic unit of consciousness. It was used here in a manner analogous with its usage in chemistry. That is, the contents of consciousness were assumed to consist of combinations of a finite number of basic mental elements, just as all physical matter consists of combinations of a finite number of chemical elements. **2** In G. Kelly's social theory, it referred to an object abstracted out of the rest of the environment by use of a special construct. **3** In W. K. Estes's mathematical learning theory, it denoted a hypothesized unitary component of a stimulus. Estes's treatment of the term is best thought of as equivalent to the notion of a point in geometry: all space is made up of points, all stimuli made up of elements. In this conception, learning becomes the conditioning of stimulus elements to responses. adjs., *elementary* = simple; *elemental* = pertaining to an element, primary, basic. See also ELEMENTARISM and REDUCTIONISM.

elementarism A cover term for any atomistic philosophical position that maintains that complex phenomena can be understood only by reducing them down to their most primitive (i.e. elementary) parts. The structuralist school in psychology typified this position in that its proponents were searching for the elements of mental content. Similar schools of thought are represented by REDUCTIONISM and ATOMISM. Opposing are HOLISM and GESTALT.

elementary cognitive tasks A loose category of tasks including simple laboratory tests of short-term memory, word retrieval, categorization and decision-making. Unfortunately the abbreviation ECT is occasionally used for them.

elementary perceiver and memorizer (EPAM) An important early computer simulation model of rote memory developed by E. A. Feigenbaum.

elicit To draw forth, draw out. The term is used to refer to behaviour that is not spontaneously produced by an organism but is drawn out by the presentation of the appropriate stimulus. Thus, the term *elicited behaviour* becomes synonymous with *reflexive* or *resonant behaviour* and is viewed as that behaviour characteristically produced by classical conditioning. Compare with EMIT.

elimination disorders Disorders of childhood in which a child urinates (see ENURESIS) or defecates (see ENCOPRESIS) in inappropriate places. The term is only used if there is no evidence of organic disorders that might be causing the lack of control.

eliminative materialism A philosophical point of view that argues that concepts like 'mind' and 'consciousness' have already shown themselves to be less than useful and that we would be better off representing such mentalistic notions in the language of the neurosciences. In short, by focusing on the material, we can eliminate the need for the subjective.

ellipsis The omission of a word or words from a spoken or written message where the missing words are predictable or determinable from the structure of the sentence or from context. Some psychoanalysts regard the occurrence of ellipses as significant and a form of PARAPRAXIS.

elopement In psychiatry, the unauthorized departure of a patient from a psychiatric institution.

emasculation Literally, the loss of masculinity. It can be a physical loss such as CASTRA-

TION or it can refer to a more symbolic state where a male feels as though his sense of self as a man has been stripped away by the actions of others.

embedded figure A general class of ambiguous figures in which a particular shape is interwoven with a general pattern, making it difficult to detect. For example, of the following shapes the hexagon (on the left) occurs embedded within the triangle (on the right):

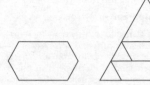

embedded-figures test A paper-and-pencil test that requires that the subject locate a simple figure embedded in a larger, more complex field (see above). It is used primarily as a device to evaluate FIELD DEPENDENCE.

embodied Generally, of or pertaining to the body. More specifically, of perceptions and cognitions that are influenced by real or anticipated body states and movements. The term is used to suggest that the manner in which stimuli or events are grasped or meaning extracted from them is dependent upon how an organism's sensorimotor capacities allow it to interact with these events as they occur in specific environmental niches. See EMBODIED COGNITION.

embodied cognition An approach to cognitive psychology that argues that cognitive systems and functions cannot be properly understood without taking into account the manner in which inputs are EMBODIED. The model emerged as a reaction to the computationalist approach (see COMPUTATIONAL METAPHOR, COMPUTATIONAL MODELS) where cognition is viewed as a kind of 'cold' process that takes place independent of feelings, emotions and other 'bodily' functions. For example, that a load feels heavier the longer one anticipates carrying it or that the distances that one must travel appear greater when one is fatigued suggests that simple computation of the physical properties of the input stimulus is insufficient to understand how it is being dealt with. The model's complexities are still being developed and are being extended to a variety of domains including development (early learning is viewed as largely acquiring skills that involve how one's body must be used), emotion (if people use the muscles that underlie smiling by having them say 'eeeee' they think jokes are funnier than if they use the muscles for frowning by having them say 'oooo') and metaphor (love is widely viewed as 'warm or hot' and as 'red').

embolalia   Meaningless babbling. var., *embololalia*.

embrace reflex MORO REFLEX.

embryo Generally, an organism in the earliest stages of prenatal development. In mammals, the organism during that period before it develops physical similarity to its mature form. In *Homo sapiens*, the organism during the period of about six weeks during which internal and external organs become differentiated. The embryonic period follows the germinal, which itself lasts about two weeks, during which time the fertilized ovum grows into a hollow sphere approximately 5 mm across. After the embryonic stage the term foetus is used.

emergent Descriptive of or characteristic of new or unexpected properties or qualities that emerge as a result of combinations or rearrangements of existing elements. The most prominent examples are *mind* and *consciousness*, emerging from complex neurophysiological and biochemical components. The critical aspect of an emergent property is that one could not predict it from its constituent parts. *Emergentism* is a philosophical position that stresses that objects and phenomena (particularly psychological ones) have emergent properties. Reference is also made to *emergent evolution* as a way of characterizing the appearance of novel phenomena.

emergentism EMERGENT.

emerging adulthood The developmental period in which people respond to the question 'Are you an adult?' with the answer 'In some ways yes, in some ways no.' Thus defined, it is the period succeeding adolescence during which full adult responsibilities are not yet assumed. In the West, this typic-

ally spans the early 20s, but there is a great deal of individual variation in duration and timing.

emesis Vomiting.

EMG ELECTROMYOGRAM.

emic–etic distinction By extension from the distinction between PHONEMIC and PHONETIC, a distinction between two different approaches to the study of human systems and phenomena. *Emic* approaches focus on behaviours and cognitions that are meaningful to the object of concern, be it an individual or, more commonly, a society. *Etic* approaches focus on developing more objective, scientifically-determined, observation-driven units of analysis. HERMANEUTICS can be characterized as an extreme *emic* approach, while BEHAVIOURISM is an extreme *etic* approach.

emission A discharge, a giving out or sending forth. Used broadly to cover bodily discharges, specifically semen during ejaculation, overt responses made by an organism (see here EMIT), messages output in communication, etc.

emission, acoustic A sound emitted by the inner ear. Actions in the *cochlea* cause a mechanical wave to travel back to the *tympanic membrane* that then produces a sound wave that can be heard with special instruments.

emit To produce, to send out. The term is used to refer to behaviour that is generated or produced by an organism within the context of an appropriate stimulus. Thus, the phrase *emitted behaviour* becomes synonymous with *operant behaviour* and is characteristic in free responding situations and in operant conditioning. Contrast with ELICIT.

emmenia Menstrual flow.

emmeniopathy Any menstrual disorder.

Emmert's law A generalization about the nature of negative afterimages that states that the perceived size of an image varies directly with the distance that it is projected. For example, an image will appear smaller if it is projected on a piece of paper fairly close to the subject than if it is projected on to a wall some distance from the viewer.

Note that the term *projected* is used metaphorically here.

emmetropia Normal vision in the sense that when the eye is at rest the light is refracted so that the focus is directly on the retina. Compare with the common refractive disorders of ASTIGMATISM, HYPEROPIA and MYOPIA.

emote To display emotion.

emotion Historically this term has proven utterly refractory to definitional efforts; probably no other term in psychology shares its combination of nondefinability and frequency of use. Most textbook authors wisely employ it as the title of a chapter and let the material presented substitute for a concise definition. The term itself derives from the Latin *emovere*, which translates as *to move, to excite, to stir up* or *to agitate*. Contemporary usage is of two general kinds: **1** An umbrella term for any of a number of subjectively experienced, affect-laden states, the ontological status of each being established by a label the meaning of which is arrived at by simple consensus. This is the primary use of the term in both the technical and the common language. It is what we mean when we say that *love, fear, hate, terror*, etc. are emotions. **2** A label for a field of scientific investigation that explores the various environmental, physiological and cognitive factors that underlie these subjective experiences.

There is little dispute over 1, other than a prevailing sense that it is unfortunate that a term of such importance is used in such loose subjective fashion. The confusing array of usages that confronts the psychologist comes from 2, where the 'definitions' that abound are really mini-theories about the underpinnings of emotions. Although they differ in the relative contributions assigned to each, nearly all contemporary theories of emotion recognize four classes of factors: (a) *instigating stimuli*: these may be exogenous (events in the world) or endogenous (thoughts, images); (b) *physiological and neurological correlates*: included here are general systems (central- and autonomic-nervous-system activities) as well as more specific patterns of action (e.g. thalamic-hypothalamic interactions, the role of the prefrontal cortex); (c) *cognitive appraisal*:

the personal significance of an event dictates to a considerable extent the emotions aroused, thus snarling tigers behind clearly strong cage bars do not result in fear, panic or flight; (d) *motivational properties*: emotional arousal is almost always viewed as playing a role in impelling activity. See MOTIVATION.

In addition to these recognized correlates of emotion, the term generally carries a number of other connotations: First, emotional states are normally regarded as *acute*. They are accompanied by relatively short-lived levels of arousal and desires to act; fear, joy, disgust, pity, love, etc. are regarded as relatively momentary conditions the experiencing of which motivates activity and then subsides. Indeed, in psychiatry many of the *affective disorders* are characterized by an inappropriate chronic experiencing of an emotional state. This sense of the term helps to distinguish it from a term like SENTIMENT. Second, emotions are regarded as intensely experienced states; the point here is to distinguish an emotion from a *feeling*. No one would argue that a fine line exists here; this is merely a terminological heuristic. Third, emotional states are often behaviourally disorganized. This is particularly the case with extreme states of rage, terror, grief and the like, in which an individual's behaviour may be erratic, chaotic and lacking in organization. Fourth, emotions are, to a certain extent, evolutionarily determined and reflect species-specific survival strategies of considerable genetic antiquity. This point is reflected most clearly in the work in evolutionary psychology, biology and ethology as it has affected psychological theory. Fifth, emotional reactions tend to be nonhabitual and to result from particular constraints of the environment and how it is appraised. The contrast to be recognized here is with other behaviours that are motivated by underlying biochemical actions like hunger and thirst, which typically are satisfied by relatively stereotyped, habitual behaviour patterns. This issue is related to the fact that emotional states are not cyclical or regular but are dependent on specific situations and how they are evaluated for their personal significance.

For more on the nuances of usage see the following entries: AFFECT, FEELING, MOOD, SENTIMENT.

emotional 1 Generally, pertaining to any aspect of emotion; characterizing states, processes, expressions etc. that carry the quality of emotion. **2** Characterizing an individual who is experiencing an emotion or one who displays a propensity for emotional reactions.

emotional anaesthesia A numbing of one's emotions, a diminished responsiveness to the outside world. Often seen in cases of POST-TRAUMATIC STRESS DISORDER.

emotional bias Basically a nontechnical term for any personal bias stemming from emotional causes; it is used with the connotation that the individual is not capable of making objective assessments because of this bias.

emotional blocking A general phrase used to refer to an individual's inability to perform complex mental tasks because of a highly intense emotional state.

emotional contagion BEHAVIOURAL (or EMOTIONAL) *CONTAGION.

emotional deprivation Any situation in which an individual is deprived of emotional reactions from others. It is used almost exclusively of children who are raised in situations lacking in love, affection and contact. See ANACLITIC DEPRESSION and MATURATIONAL DEPRIVATION SYNDROME.

emotional disorder Any condition in which emotional reactions are inappropriate for the situation presented. See AFFECTIVE DISORDER, the preferred term here.

emotional expression Very generally, any anatomical, muscular, physiological, behavioural reaction that accompanies a felt emotion and functions as the manner in which it is displayed. Note, some authors treat the expression of an emotion as distinct (or at least theoretically distinguishable) from the subjectively experienced emotion; others regard the expressive or emotive component as an integral aspect of the whole emotion; and still others consider it to be an evolutionarily selected signal to others about a motive to act in a particular way.

emotional indicator Any of a number of physiological measures which reflect the state of emotional arousal; see e.g. GALVANIC SKIN RESPONSE, I/E RATIO. Also called *emotionality indicator*, for reasons explained under EMOTIONALITY.

emotional instability A tendency to be emotionally labile, to display inappropriately abrupt and unpredictably extreme emotionality.

emotional intelligence INTELLIGENCE, EMOTIONAL.

emotionality Because of all the confusion surrounding the connotations of the term EMOTION many writers (primarily those with behaviourist leanings) favour this term. Their point is to try to avoid the surplus meanings of *emotion* by operationalizing the term. In this sense *emotionality* is defined in terms of behaviours that are observable and theoretically linked to the (hypothetical) underlying emotion. For example, in animal studies emotionality may be gauged by crouching, trembling, excess urination, defecation, etc. In humans such measures as heart rate, blood chemistry, breathing rate and galvanic skin response, may be used.

Note that this meaning of the term is actually not far removed from the ordinary sense in which it is used; i.e. to refer to the degree with which an individual reacts to emotive situations, with the connotation that such displays are often excessive given the circumstances. In both the behaviourist's technical sense and the layperson's common meaning the underlying notion is that it is the behavioural manifestations that are taken as the critical component in assessment of the emotion experienced.

emotionally unstable personality An obsolete psychiatric label for one who is emotionally labile, especially in the display of inappropriate reactions to minor stresses. See MOOD DISORDERS, the contemporary umbrella term for this and related disorders.

emotional maturity Loosely, the state in which one's emotional reactivity is considered appropriate and normal for an adult in a given society. The clear connotation in most cultures is one of self-control and the ability to suppress extreme emotional reactions.

emotional release A nontechnical term used interchangeably with CATHARSIS and/or ABREACTION.

emotional stability Used both technically and nontechnically to characterize the state of one who is emotionally mature, whose emotional reactions are appropriate for the situation and are consistent from one set of circumstances to another.

emotions, primary Those emotions that are thought of as 'direct' and unlearned. Paul Ekman, who did much of the early research, included anger, fear, sadness, disgust and happiness; others added surprise and contempt. While the list is still open to debate, all agree that primary emotions are innate and, hence, will be found in all cultures and expressed by similar facial expressions. Compare with SECONDARY *EMOTIONS.

emotions, secondary Emotions that are not found in all cultures and, hence, are assumed to be learned and dependent on social factors, e.g. jealousy, envy. Compare with PRIMARY *EMOTIONS.

emotion, theories of As the extended discussion under EMOTION suggests, the field of emotion is far from having received a satisfactory theoretical characterization. Nevertheless, a number of legitimate candidates for such a theory have been put forward over the years. They all tend to be complex and (with one exception) to involve both physiological and cognitive components, although the emphasis on each differs considerably from theory to theory.

(a) *James–Lange theory*: C. G. Lange was a Danish physiologist who proposed a theory of emotions so similar to William James's that both are given credit in the name, although the theory is essentially what James proposed in 1890. Letting James speak for himself (always a good idea): '… my theory is that the bodily changes follow directly the perception of the excitatory fact, and that our feeling of the same changes as they occur *is* the emotion.' Lange's position was similar, albeit he omitted the step on perception and concluded that the vasomotor (bodily) changes were the emotion. The theory has been subjected to rather telling criticism. The strongest objections were raised by Cannon (see below), who questioned the central role of the feedback from the peripheral organs.

(b) *Cannon–Bard theory*. This theory is due primarily to the work of the American physiologist Walter B. Cannon and is often referred to as the *thalamic* theory of emotion. In simplest terms it argues that the integration of emotional expression is controlled by the thalamus sending relevant excitation patterns to the cortex at the same time as the hypothalamus controls the behaviour. It was put forward as part of Cannon's critique of the earlier *James–Lange theory* (see above), which postulated that the sensory feedback controlled the emotional expression. This theory has also been subjected to rather telling criticism in the form of the following more recently developed theories.

(c) *Activation (or arousal) theory*. Not a true theory so much as a generalization about emotions. It is predicated on the assumption that emotions are not unique states but merely lie collectively at the extreme pole of a dimension of neurophysiological arousal or activation opposite the pole represented by coma and deep sleep. This generalization shows up as a component in several other theoretical conceptions of emotions, specifically the *cognitive-appraisal theory*.

(d) *Behaviouristic theory*. As one might expect, this point of view deals with all emotions as either unconditioned (i.e. innately given, species-specific) or conditioned (i.e. learned, acquired) responses. Both physiological and cognitive elements are regarded as unimportant, the focus being on objectively measurable manifestations of what behaviourists like to call 'emotional behaviour'. See here the discussion under EMOTIONALITY.

(e) *Cognitive-appraisal theory*. Here emotions are regarded as subjective states that are the product of an initially evoking stimulus, a set of accompanying physiological changes and a cognitive appraisal or interpretation of the situation as beneficial or harmful, good or bad, for the individual. The key notion here is the cognitive appraisal itself, the argument being that a single physiological arousal state can yield several, even antithetical, emotions depending on how the individual interprets the situation. See also MACLEAN'S THEORY OF EMOTION, PAPEZ'S THEORY OF EMOTION.

(f) *Differential emotions theory*. The theory assumes that there are a relatively small number of core emotions and that they act as motivators of behaviour. They are also seen as intimately linked with personality in that emotions are treated as building blocks for an individual's personality. The effect of the cognitive appraisal factor, important in other theories, is downplayed. Rather, each emotional condition is seen as becoming progressively differentiated as the person develops.

(g) *Dynamic component systems theory.* This approach incorporates many of the factors identified in other models but emphasizes the role that culture and social systems play in the development of emotional expression and experience as a child grows. While in some ways not a true theory, it is included here simply because any complete theory of emotions, their expression and experience and the dynamic manner in which they develop in childhood and over the full lifespan must, ultimately, take the role of cultural factors into account.

emotive Characteristic of a situation, event or other stimulus that elicits emotion.

emotive imagery Quite literally, imagery that evokes emotion. The term is most often used in behaviour therapy and cognitive-behavioural therapy for a procedure in which the client images emotion-arousing scenes while relaxed and in a comfortable, protective setting. The technique is based on Wolpe's notion of RECIPROCAL INHIBITION, in which the positive supportive setting inhibits the anxiety.

empathic disorders An umbrella term used for disorders, such as AUTISM and ASPERGER'S SYNDROME, which are marked by stunted social skills and inappropriate patterns of social interaction. There are suggestions that these disorders have a genetic basis and are probably caused by neurological damage in sensory areas in the brain.

empathy **1** A cognitive awareness and understanding of the emotions and feelings of another person. In this sense the term's primary connotation is that of an intellectual or conceptual grasping of the *affect* of another. **2** A vicarious affective response to the emotional experiences of another person that mirrors or mimics that emotion. In this sense there is the clear implication that an empathic experience is a sharing of the emotion with the other person. **3** Assuming, in one's mind, the role of another person. This meaning derives from 1, but differs slightly in that there is the added notion that empathy involves taking on the perspective of the other person. This meaning is common in the literature on moral development, in which some theorists argue that empathy with another is a prerequisite for the development of a moral code. **4** In H. S. Sullivan's theory of personality, an unverbalized, covert communication process whereby attitudes, feelings and judgements are passed from person to person without ever being publicly articulated. Sullivan's use of the term is quite broad and encompasses the more restricted connotations of the above meanings. See also SYMPATHY for more on the terminology of shared affect.

empathy-altruism hypothesis (or **model**) A model of helping behaviour which proposes that feeling empathy for a suffering person increases the likelihood that one will help that person, even when there is no direct reward for helping. In other words, we are likely to be altruistic to the extent that we feel empathy.

empirical An extremely common term in psychological parlance. It enjoys (or perhaps suffers from) a number of diverse and rather specialized meanings. It is used specifically as follows: **1** Relating to facts in general. **2** Relating to experience in general. **3** Descriptive of procedures carried out without explicit regard to any theory. **4** A general synonym for *experimental*. **5** Descriptive of any procedure based upon factual evaluations. **6** Pertaining to *empiricism*. Note that all of these usages are based on or relate directly to *data*, to their collection, analysis or evaluation. It is in this general sense that the term is most frequently used. Note that such usage places *empirical* in opposition (more or less) to RATIONAL.

empirical construct Any construct the existence of which is hypothesized or inferred on the basis of empirical evaluation, i.e. on the basis of observed facts and data. Although the term *construct* implies an essentially theoretical or hypothetical entity, the adjective *empirical* indicates the data are sufficiently consistent and convincing.

empirical equation EQUATION, EMPIRICAL.

empirical law LAW, EMPIRICAL.

empirical law of effect LAW OF *EFFECT.

empirical test The evaluation or assessment of a hypothesis or theory by appeal to data, facts and experimentation.

empirical validity VALIDITY, EMPIRICAL.

empiricism A broad-based philosophical position grounded on the fundamental assumption that all knowledge comes from experience. Historically, the empiricist tradition stems from the work of a number of British philosophers of the 17th and 18th centuries (Locke, Hume, Berkeley, Hartley). It is important to distinguish empiricism as a *theory* and empiricism as a *method*. As a theory the primary assumption is that knowledge results from experience and learning. In its extreme form (mind as *tabula rasa* or 'blank slate' at birth) it can no longer be seriously defended – the data on developmental stages, on cognitive growth, etc. clearly point to some degree of genetic predisposition for many behaviours. The contemporary empiricist position is akin to a mild form of scepticism and is best represented by what it is against: the positions put forward in A PRIORISM, NATIVISM and RATIONALISM. That is, the empiricist relies upon an as yet unworked-out theory of induction for the acquisition of knowledge and rejects any doctrine that argues that the human mind enters the world pre-equipped with ideas or concepts that are independent of personal experience.

As a method, empiricism advocates the collection and evaluation of data. In this sense the focus is on experimentation, and an empirical investigation is one guided primarily by induction from observation rather than by deduction from theoretical constructs. Although the theoretical issues are still hotly contested, particularly in contemporary cognitive psychology, it is safe to say that the empirical methods thoroughly dominate contemporary psychological investigation.

empty-chair technique A technique used in Gestalt therapy whereby the client projects the image of a person about whom he or she has unresolved feelings and engages in 'conversation' with the image.

empty organism A phrase often used derisively by opponents of behaviourism to characterize that approach's unwillingness to make inferences about internal states or to posit hypothetical constructs. See also, and distinguish from, BLACK BOX.

emulation The process of copying a pattern of behaviour. The term carries the connotation that the person doing the copying is attempting to achieve the same goals as the person he or she is emulating. Distinguish subtly from IMITATION, the implication of which is that it is the behaviour alone that is being mimicked without there necessarily being a particular goal beyond this.

enactive representation 1 Loosely, fairly primitive mental representation based on encoding motor action and movement. 2 In Jerome Bruner's theory of development, a form of mental representation based on action and movement and characterized by failure to distinguish between perception and action; for example, a child representing a 'full glass' as 'one that can spill'. As the child develops, an *iconic* (or *ikonic*) form emerges in which representations and images are intimately tied to perceptual forms. These mental representations typically continue through the preschool years and are succeeded by *symbolic representations* where the child can grasp and express ideas through the use of language and play. Often the underlying processes that accompany each form of representation will be called a 'mode' and references to an *iconic mode* or *symbolic mode* are commonly found.

enantiobiosis A relationship between organisms that is mutually antagonistic, the opposite of SYMBIOSIS.

enantiodromia Jung's term for the view that eventually all things become transformed into their opposites.

encapsulated nerve endings Structurally the opposite of free nerve endings, these are made up of a free nerve ending which penetrates a capsule of epithelial or muscular tissue and serve as receptors for certain kinds of stimulation. See PACINIAN CORPUSCLE.

encapsulation, psychological K. Lewin's term for any behaviour that prevents a person from experiencing a painful situation, such as refusing to read newspaper accounts of massacres or covering one's eyes when an accident is imminent.

encéphale isolé A surgical preparation produced by transection of the brainstem at the caudal end of the medulla just above the spinal cord. An *encéphale isolé* animal is paralysed but displays normal sleep–wake cycles. When the transection is further up, in the area between the superior and inferior colliculi (the *cerveau isolé* or *mid-collicular* transection), the animal is comatose. A cut made between these, the *midpontine* section, produces wakefulness.

encephalitis Inflammation of the membranes covering the brain, or of the brain itself.

encephalization The gradual subsuming of the control of function by the brain. As an evolutionary process it is manifested to a greater and greater degree as one moves up the phylogenetic scale. See also CORTICALIZATION.

encephal(o)- Combining form meaning *pertaining to the brain*.

encephalon Relatively rare term for the brain.

encephalopathy General term for any disease or dysfunction of the brain.

encode (encoding) CODE.

encoding specificity In cognitive psychology, the generalization that the initial encoding of learned material will reflect the influence of the context in which the learning took place. For example, learning a word like *jam* in the context *fruit-jam* typically leads to a diminished ability to recognize it when presented later in another context such as *traffic-jam*. See CONTEXT SPECIFIC *LEARNING.

encopresis Faecal incontinence, involuntary expulsion of faeces.

encounter group A small group which focuses on intensive interpersonal interactions (or encounters). The group usually has as its goals the removal of psychological barriers and defences, achieving openness, honesty and the willingness to deal with the difficulties of emotional expression. Group members are encouraged to deal with 'here-and-now' and to eschew intellectualization and personal history. Encounter groups and their use in psychotherapy began with the HUMAN POTENTIAL MOVEMENT.

encryption Within cryptography, the act or process of converting a message into a coded form; encoding.

enculturation The process by which an individual adapts to a new culture, eventually assimilating its practices, customs and values. See also ACCULTURATION and SOCIALIZATION.

end In the social sciences this term usually carries the connotations of a goal; an end is more than a mere terminus, it is that which is aimed at or desired, the result of purposeful striving.

end brain TELENCEPHALON.

end brush The delicate arborization of the ends of an axon.

end button TERMINAL BUTTON.

endemic Restricted to a particular geographical area. Used in EPIDEMIOLOGY; compare with PANDEMIC.

end foot TERMINAL BUTTON.

endo- Combining form meaning *within*, *inside* or *toward the inside*. var., *ento-*.

endocrine Used of glands that secrete hormones internally; that is, their secretions are distributed through the body by the bloodstream, the glands being ductless. Contrast with EXOCRINE and see the discussion under GLAND.

endocrine gland GLAND.

endocrinology The study of the body's internal secretions. The term is used broadly, and the investigations go beyond the endocrine glands to include internal secretions from any source.

endoderm The inner layer of embryonic cellular structures that develops into the digestive tract and the *viscera*.

endogamy Limiting marriage to within a social or cultural group such as a caste or clan. Contrast with EXOGAMY.

endogenous (or endogenic) Lit., originating from within. Used to refer to phenomena the origins of which are internal or within the body. When the genesis of a phenomenon is clearly physiological the term *somatogenic* is typically used; when it appears to be mental, the term preferred is *psychogenic*. Contrast with EXOGENOUS.

endogenous clock BIOLOGICAL CLOCK.

endogenous depression DEPRESSION, ENDO-GENOUS.

endogenous opiates A group of naturally occurring, opiate-like peptides produced by the brain or the pituitary, including the *endorphins*, *enkephalins* and *dynorphins*. They play important roles in the control of emotional behaviours such as those associated with pain, anxiety, fear and related affective states produced by pain. The binding sites are found in a variety of locations, including neurons in the PERIAQUEDUCTAL GREY and the LIMBIC SYSTEM.

endolymph The liquid found in the membranous canal of the semicircular canals of the inner ear.

endometrium The mucous membrane that lines the inner surface of the uterus.

endomorphy One of the three primary dimensions of body type (along with *ectomorphy* and *mesomorphy*) in Sheldon's CONSTITUTIONAL THEORY. An endomorph is one whose physique is dominated by the embryonic endodermal component, fatty tissues and the viscera. Hence, endomorphic persons are overweight, have poorly developed muscles and bones, and have a small skin surface area relative to weight.

endophasia 1 Internal speech. 2 Making the appropriate lip, tongue and jaw movements of speech but without producing any sound. Meaning 2 entails 1.

endophenotype A measurable factor, undetectable by visual inspection, that can serve as a marker along the pathway between a disease or syndrome and a genotype for it. Endophenotypes are clues to possible genetic underpinnings of the disease or syndrome; they can be neurophysiological, endocrinological, cognitive or behavioural. For example, slowed reaction times are regarded by many as an endophenotype for autism.

endopsychic Characterizing that which is in the mind.

end organ A general term for any sensory receptor.

endorphins ENDOGENOUS OPIATES.

end plate Often called a *motor end plate*, the terminus of a neuron that makes the functional contact with a muscle cell.

end-plate potential (EPP) The depolarization of the postsynaptic membrane caused by acetylcholine release by the terminus of the end plate. The EPP causes muscle fibres to fire and induces muscle contraction.

end-pleasure See discussion under FORE-PLEASURE.

end test POST-TEST.

enelicomorphism PEDOMORPHISM.

energization The allocation of activation, effort and arousal to a task.

energy One of those terms that have a reasonably precise definition in the physical sciences but lose their clarity when dragged into psychological jargon. The best that can be done here is to point out that the term is usually used as a rough equivalent of *strength* or *vigour* as descriptive of psychological activity.

enervation 1 Diminishing of energy, weakening. 2 The removal of a nerve. Distinguish from INNERVATION.

engineering psychology A branch of INDUSTRIAL/ORGANIZATIONAL PSYCHOLOGY that focuses on the interface between the person and the machine; that is, the study of the behaviour of individuals using tools, working with machines, etc. It also includes the design of machines so that they match the behavioural and cognitive capabilities of human operators.

English language arts In the United States educational system, the skills involved in reading, writing and speaking English, as well as the use of electronic media in English, are generally called by this all-encompassing term.

engram A postulated biochemical change resulting from external stimulation. The term was coined by the German biologist Richard Semon, who hypothesized the engram to be the biochemical manifestation of memory, the permanent alteration of neural tissue that represents what has been learned. The decades-old 'search for the engram' as a reified entity has so far been unsuccessful, and the term is used as a kind of biological metaphor for what must, in principle, exist somewhere in the brain. Note that it is used today also with the notion that each engram has a locus, but with the understanding, too, that the underlying neural correlates of memory are likely to turn out to be quite diffuse and widespread.

engulfment R. D. Laing's term for a form of anxiety that is experienced by insecure persons who view relationships with others as threats to their identity.

enkephalins ENDOGENOUS OPIATES.

enrichment 1 A term applied to some theories of perceptual learning that assume that perceptual processes go beyond a direct representing of the various aspects of the stimulus field. Gestalt theory, for example, hypothesizes the use of organizational tendencies which structure the input stimulation to give rise to percepts. Contrast with DIFFERENTIATION (5). 2 The construction of environments that are complex and provide optimal levels of stimulation, particularly to developing organisms or those acquiring skills. This meaning is common in rehabilitation medicine, organizational psychology, education and the study of learning.

entelechy 1 Realization, actuality. In this sense the term is used in specific contrast to *potential*, or that which is on the path to realization. 2 The 'vital force' proposed in the philosophy of VITALISM.

enteric nervous system The large neural system in the walls of the intestinal tract. Largely independent of the central nervous system, it controls motility, absorption, secretion and blood flow in the gut.

enteroceptor INTEROCEPTOR.

entitivity Donald Campbell's term for the degree to which a collection of coordinated individuals are seen by others as truly constituting a group and not merely an uninteresting aggregate of persons. Having common goals, physical closeness and psychological commonality are important features. Also called *entitativity*, which has entirely too many 't's'.

entity theory Loosely, any perspective that

argues that psychological qualities such as intelligence or personality are quantifiable and fixed. Such approaches are usually contrasted with *incremental theories* that treat these qualities as mutable processes and argue that behaviour reflects effort and opportunity.

ento- ENDO-.

entoptic Within the eye. Entoptic phenomena are visual experiences produced by factors within the eye itself, e.g. FLOATERS.

entorhinal cortex A part of the HIPPOCAMPAL FORMATION that serves as the major input and output communication link between association areas of the neocortex and the HIPPOCAMPUS. The area is specifically damaged in Alzheimer's disease.

entrainment Basically, a synchrony between two or more components in a system. This meaning is very general and is used in many contexts. It will be found applied to neural structures in the brain that function in coordinated ways, to people who live together who find their circadian rhythms becoming synchronized, and to mother–child dyads where voices and movements become coordinated.

entrapment In social and political psychology, the process whereby individuals and/or groups continue to increase their commitment to a policy that is clearly failing. Those involved become reluctant to relinquish their commitment since to do so is to proclaim that earlier analyses and allocations of resources were in error. Hence, the commitment is escalated to justify the previous poor judgement. The process is all too familiar.

entropy Formally, a mathematical measure of the disorganization or 'shuffledness' of a system. The term originally emerged from the study of heat and was first conceptualized as the portion of heat not available for doing work. It was within this context that the second law of thermodynamics stated that the entropy of a system never diminishes, that thermal equilibrium (death) is the end state of all isolated systems. Within psychology: 1 In cognitive theory it tends to be associated with *uncertainty*. That is, the greater the uncertainty about the outcome of any situation the greater will be the information contained in it and the greater will be the measure of entropy. In this context see the discussion under INFORMATION. **2** In psychoanalytic theory, the degree to which psychic energy is no longer available for use, having been invested in a particular object. Note that this distinctly metaphoric usage parallels the original thermodynamic conceptualization. **3** In social psychology, the amount of energy no longer available for producing social change and social progress. Here the metaphoric extension is rather extreme; it is simply unclear what form of energy is being referred to. The argument put forward is that increase of this 'social' entropy is responsible for the gradual decline and stagnation of a society or culture.

enuresis Incontinence, the involuntary passing of urine. Sometimes equated with bed-wetting, particularly when it occurs in young children, although the term applies to a broader class of phenomena.

environment The term comes from the Old French and translates roughly as *encircle*. Hence, the environment is that which surrounds. Clearly, this general meaning is going to invite a wide range of uses. Typically the term has a qualifier appended so that precisely what it is that is being surrounded is made clear. For example, the *cellular* environment consists of the tissue fluids that surround a cell; the *prenatal* (or *uterine*) environment is that enveloping the organism during gestation; an individual's *internal* environment consists of those physiological and psychological events occurring within him or her, etc. When the term is used without a qualifier it is generally taken to stand for the total physical and social surroundings of an individual organism. Note also that the term carries with it the connotation of influence, i.e. that which is part of a given environment of an organism is that which has some actual or potential role to play in the life of that organism. Hence, a city-council meeting in Cardiff would not be part of the environment of a New Yorker except in the most trivial and uninteresting sense. However, ultraviolet radiation, which one is utterly insensitive to as a stimulus event, would be considered part of each person's environment.

environmental agnosia LANDMARK *AGNOSIA.

environmental demand DEMAND CHARACTERISTICS.

environmental dependency syndrome A neurological disorder in which events and objects in the environment trigger inappropriate actions. It is a regarded as a disruption of EXECUTIVE FUNCTIONS.

environmental determinant DETERMINANT.

environmentalism A general term for a class of theoretical and philosophical schools that stresses the role of the environment in determining behaviour. Contrast with NATIVISM and HEREDITARIANISM, and see also HEREDITY–ENVIRONMENT CONTROVERSY.

environmentality The proportion of the variance of a particular *trait* in a population that can be traced to environmental factors. This term is preferred by those who feel that the term HERITABILITY invites researchers to focus too strongly on genetic factors and neglect the role of the environment on behaviour. Abbreviated as c^2.

environmental load theory Not so much a theory as an assertion that when information input reaches a critical level OVERLOAD occurs.

environmental psychology An interdisciplinary subfield in psychology that draws from the data and theories developed in a variety of areas including social psychology, sociology, ethology, political science, architecture and anthropology and turns them upon, as the name suggests, issues involving the complex interactions between people and their environments.

environment of evolutionary adaptiveness A term used in evolutionary psychology to reference the early environment of *Homo sapiens*. Generally, this environment is construed as posing survival challenges to groups of hunters and foragers, thereby having the potential to shape human nature through the actions of evolutionary mechanisms.

envy Generally classified as a special form of anxiety, envy is based on, as McDougall put it, 'a grudging contemplation of more fortunate persons'. Usually distinguished from JEALOUSY, which involves a third party, typically a loved one.

enzygotic Developed from the same ovum.

enzyme Any of a number of organic catalysts that produce chemical changes in other substances without being changed themselves. Enzymes are complex proteins found particularly in digestive processes that break down complex food substances into simpler compounds.

EOG 1 ELECTRO-OCULOGRAM. **2** ELECTRO-OLFACTOGRAM.

eonism An occasional synonym of TRANSVESTISM. The term comes from the Chevalier d'Eon, an 18th-century political adventurer who achieved some notoriety on account of his preference for women's clothing.

EP EVOKED POTENTIAL.

ep- EPI-.

EPAM ELEMENTARY PERCEIVER AND MEMORIZER.

ependyma The membrane lining the cerebral ventricles and the central canal of the spinal cord.

epi- Prefix designating *outside, above, apart from, in addition to*. var., *ep-*.

epicritic 1 Generally, pertaining to extreme, highly developed sensitivity, particularly cutaneous sensitivity. **2** In H. Head's system of cutaneous sensibility, one of the two divisions of the afferent neural system which mediated the finely tuned, delicate responses to warm, cold and light pressure stimuli. The other, the PROTOPATHIC, was assumed to be rather gross and undifferentiated and to be evolutionarily older. The neurological substrata of Head are no longer accepted but the sensitive discriminations he characterized are still called epicritic.

epidemic 1 In medicine, the rapid spread of an infectious disease through a population. **2** By extension, the rapid spread of a social/psychological phenomenon through a population; e.g. an epidemic of suicide occurred when the stock market crashed in 1929.

epidemiology A hybrid science with psychological, sociological, demographic and medical aspects that deals with the study of diseases, their distributions in populations and their environmental impact.

epidermis The outer layer of the skin.

epigenesis The notion that during development the complex morphological properties of an organism develop gradually out of an interaction between the prenatal environment and intracellular processes. Compare with PREFORMATIONISM.

epiglottis The thin valve-like structure of cartilage that covers the *glottis* and prevents food and drink from entering the *larynx*.

epilepsy An umbrella term for a number of disorders characterized by various combinations of the following: periodic motor or sensory seizures (or their *epileptic equivalent*) accompanied by an abnormal encephalogram (EEG), with or without actual convulsions, clouding of or loss of consciousness, and motor, sensory or cognitive malfunctions. A number of classification systems for the epilepsies have been proposed, some based on the aetiology of the disorder, some on the cortical locus of the abnormal discharge, others on the EEG pattern manifested, on the clinical form of the seizures themselves, on the severity of the seizures or on various combinations of some or all of these factors. The following entries present the most commonly diagnosed forms of epilepsy and give the standard clinical characterizations of each. The root term itself comes from the Greek, meaning *to seize* or *grasp*. Also called *seizure disorder*.

epilepsy, cryptogenic See IDIOPATHIC *EPILEPSY.

epilepsy, focal Epilepsy characterized by a relatively localized focus of the cortical dysfunction and manifested by similarly specific sensorimotor seizures. Also called *partial epilepsy*. Compare with GENERALIZED *EPILEPSY.

epilepsy, generalized Epilepsy characterized by diffuse, general seizures with an EEG pattern that reveals pathological activity over the entire surface of the brain. Compare with FOCAL *EPILEPSY.

epilepsy, idiopathic Epilepsy for which there is no known organic cause. Also called *cryptogenic epilepsy*.

epilepsy, Jacksonian motor A form of focal epilepsy characterized by seizures involving involuntary motor movements on the side of the body contralateral to the cortical locus of the disturbance. Usually the movements spread from central muscle groups to others and may involve one whole side of the body. This spreading of the seizure is termed *Jacksonian march*.

epilepsy, Jacksonian sensory A form of focal epilepsy analogous to JACKSONIAN MOTOR *EPILEPSY, except that the primary symptoms are specific and localized sensory disturbances.

epilepsy, major Epilepsy characterized by gross convulsive tonic-clonic seizures, loss of consciousness and loss of control over various autonomic functions (e.g. bladder and bowel control). Also called *grand mal epilepsy*, and the seizures *grand mal seizures*. The term *tonic-clonic epilepsy* is also found denoting that the seizures are marked by both TONUS and CLONUS.

epilepsy, minor A general label for any epilepsy characterized by nonconvulsive seizures (or their epileptic equivalent). Often there is only a momentary lapse of consciousness and/or minor sensorimotor dysfunction. Also called *petit mal epilepsy*.

epilepsy, photogenic Epileptic seizures brought on by a visual stimulus, most commonly a flickering light.

epilepsy, psychomotor A form of epilepsy characterized by periodic behaviour disturbances manifested typically as repetitive and often highly organized movements that are carried out unconsciously and semi-automatically.

epilepsy, symptomatic A general term for any epilepsy for which there is a known organic cause.

epilepsy, temporal (lobe) Epilepsy in which the focus of the dysfunction is the temporal lobe of the cortex.

epilepsy, tonic-clonic See MAJOR *EPILEPSY.

epileptic equivalent A general term for any episodic sensory or motor symptom which an epileptic may experience instead of convulsive seizures.

epileptogenic Characterizing factors that cause epilepsy or circumstances that produce seizures in individuals with epilepsy.

epinephrine One of the CATECHOLAMINES that is synthesized from NOREPINEPHRINE. It is

classified as a HORMONE when carried in the blood and a NEUROTRANSMITTER when released in a synapse. Large amounts are secreted from the adrenal glands when stimulated by anger, fear or alarm and help prepare the body for emergencies. When released into the blood stream, it increases oxygen and glucose levels in the brain, boosts heart rate and the strength of contractions, produces vasodilation in skeletal muscle and vasoconstriction in the gut and the skin. It also suppresses digestive system functions and the immune system. The term itself comes from the Greek and translates as *on the kidney*. It is the preferred synonym of ADRENALIN: see that entry for reasons why. Note, however, that the adjectival form in general use is still ADRENERGIC; *epinephrinergic* has just never taken hold even in the technical literature.

epinosic gain SECONDARY GAIN.

epiphenomenalism A term used primarily within a metaphysical context to refer to the doctrine that 'mental life', 'mind', 'consciousness' and other similar constructs are but the manifestations or by-products of a complex neurological system and are without causal influence. In short, to the epiphenomenalist, the mental is real but causally inert. O. H. Mowrer put it most succinctly: '…epiphenomenalism posits that the physical world is the only true reality and that psychic events are inconsequential excrescences'.

epiphenomenon Any event that occurs in the presence of or incidentally accompanies some other process or event but in fact plays no part in that process or event. For example, a good case can be made for the notion that dreams are epiphenomena that merely accompany biochemical and neurological events during sleep. This point of view contrasts strongly with the Freudian view that dreams have strong causal roles in symbolically disguising unwanted thoughts and images.

epiphysis 1 In the developing infant and child, a bone forming (ossification) centre attached to another bone by cartilage. The degree of ossification can be used as a measure of growth. **2** A shortened form of *epiphysis cerebri*, the PINEAL GLAND.

episcotister A piece of lab equipment used in experimental psychology's early days for presenting visual displays.

episode Any relatively well-defined event or coordinated sequence of events that is perceived as a unit, as a whole. Episodes are generally marked as occurring in particular times and places. See e.g. EPISODIC *MEMORY, PSYCHOTIC EPISODE.

episode marker MARKER, EPISODE.

episode theory INSTANCE THEORY.

episodic amnesia AMNESIA, EPISODIC.

episodic buffer In Baddeley's updated model of WORKING *MEMORY, a component that stores multimodal information about complex episodes. The buffer's store is assumed to be much larger than the other components (PHONOLOGICAL LOOP and VISUO-SPATIAL SKETCHPAD) and to have links with long-term memory.

episodic memory MEMORY, EPISODIC.

epistemic Of or relating to knowledge. See EPISTEMOLOGY.

epistemic value The extent to which something increases knowledge. Theories with explanatory power, cognitive processes that increase understanding and beliefs systems that have positive social impact are all considered to have high epistemic value.

epistemology The branch of philosophy that is concerned with the origins, nature, methods and limits of human knowledge.

epistemophilia Love of knowledge, derivation of pleasure from the acquisition of knowledge.

epithelium Any thin layer of tissue that covers the surface or lines the cavity of an organ. Generally performs a secreting or protective function.

epoch A period of time. In psychological usage, the periods are usually short. For example, in physiological work a period of a few hundred milliseconds during which a neuron responds will be called an epoch.

EPP END-PLATE POTENTIAL.

epsilon motion MOTION, EPSILON.

EPSP Abbrev. for *excitatory postsynaptic potential;* see POSTSYNAPTIC POTENTIAL.

EQ EDUCATIONAL QUOTIENT.

equal and unequal cases method A variation on the *method of constant stimuli;* see MEASUREMENT OF *THRESHOLD.

equal-appearing-intervals method A method of scaling in which the subject is asked to sort stimuli into groups separated by equal steps. The technique is used in psychophysical work, where the stimuli may be lights, weights, tones, etc., and in social psychology, where the stimuli may be statements of opinions, attitudes, preferences, etc. See also METHODS OF *SCALING, THURSTONE-TYPE SCALES.

equal-interval scale SCALES.

equality, judgement of Quite literally, the judgement that two (or more) stimuli are equal. However, the term must be applied loosely since two compared stimuli rarely if ever give the impression of true equality; a judgement of equality is really a judgement of doubt concerning the confidence of a person that he or she has in fact detected a real difference between the stimuli. See also SIGNAL-DETECTION THEORY.

equality, law of A Gestalt principle of perceptual organization stating that, as the several components of a perceptual field become more similar, they will tend to be perceived as a unit.

equal-sense differences method Another term for EQUAL-APPEARING-INTERVALS METHOD.

equated score(s) Any two sets of scores from different tests or from different parts of the same test (assuming that the same variable is being measured) that have been reduced to a common scale (i.e. equated) to facilitate comparisons. *Percentile scores* and STANDARD *SCORES are both examples.

equation, empirical Any mathematical equation that is used to fit observed data. An empirical equation is essentially an after-the-fact attempt to characterize quantitatively a set of observations, and the value of such an equation is given by the closeness of the 'fit' between it and the data; theory is not an important issue here. Fechner's psychophysical law is a classic example. Compare with RATIONAL *EQUATION.

equation method MEASUREMENT OF *THRESHOLD.

equation, rational A logical or mathematical expression based on (rational) assumptions about processes. Such equations differ from EMPIRICAL *EQUATIONS in that their parameters are derived by deduction from theoretical assumptions and not simply from attempts to fit data. See STIMULUS SAMPLING THEORY for an example.

equi- Word element meaning *equal* or *equally*.

equifinal Descriptive of a situation in which two different antecedent conditions result in the same outcome.

equilibration 1 Generally, achieving a balance between opposing forces. **2** In Piagetian theory, the process by which a balance between ASSIMILATION and ACCOMMODATION is maintained and whereby conflicting *schemas* can be integrated into new structures. In a sense it is a cognitive analogue of the physiological notion of *homeostasis*, with the added element that as a child centres on new aspects of the environment, the process of maintaining equilibrium becomes the mechanism that ultimately produces the transition to a higher cognitive state.

equilibrium Basically the term is used as a synonym of *balance*, with several special usages: **1** In physiology, the point at which opposing biochemical reactions are stable; *homeostasis*. **2** In perception, the sense through which the body maintains a stable upright posture with respect to its centre of gravity. Sometimes called the *equilibrium sense* or *static sense*. **3** The point at which the body is in an upright, stabile position. **4** In social psychology, the theoretical tendency for a social system to bring about corrective changes to maintain itself as a functionally integrated unit. Note that this usage carries the notion of a *process*; the others represent equilibrium as a point of balance, with the process that we know must be there left implicit. **5** In Piaget's theory, a cognitive state whereby the information available to a child is in balance with the existing cognitive schemas held. Such states may be quite temporary, especially during the early sensorimotor, preoperational and concrete operational stages; or they may be rather stable and permanent, as at the formal operational stage.

equipotentiality Lit., of the same potential. There are several specialized usages: **1** In embryology, a generalization which states that any section of the embryonic tissue can develop into any part of the fully developed organism. In its extreme form this generalization is incorrect, but within limits (i.e. during the germinal phase prior to production of specific enzymes) the phenomenon may be observed. **2** In neurophysiology, the hypothesis, first articulated by Karl Lashley, that all the neurons which mediate a given sensory modality have a common competing function in addition to their specific functions. That is, each has 'equal potential' for participating in a sensory event within that modality. **3** By extension, the notion that within certain limits one portion of the cerebral cortex can take on the functions of another part.

equity theory A general label for a class of broad social-psychological theories that seek to explain behaviour by reference to the concept of equity, i.e. those conditions in which the rewards for individuals in a group are in proportion to their efforts on behalf of the group. The chief argument of its proponents is that such diverse phenomena as *altruism, power, aggression* and *cooperation* can be subsumed under an analysis of equity/inequity.

equivalence In general, any relationship between two things such that one may be substituted for the other in a particular setting and not significantly alter the situation. The term is often modified so that the particular form of equivalence is specified; e.g. *stimulus equivalence* refers to two or more stimuli that are sufficiently similar that they evoke the same or nearly the same response, while *response equivalence* refers to similar responses made to similar stimuli.

equivalence belief A term coined by E. C. Tolman for the hypothesized internal state of an organism such that it responds to a subgoal as it would to the goal. Hence it was used as roughly synonymous with *secondary reinforcement*.

equivalence class Collectively, all the

stimuli or events in a group that display EQUIVALENCE.

equivalence, coefficient of A correlation coefficient used to evaluate the consistency or reliability of a particular test. Generally carried out by comparing scores on two separate but equivalent forms of the test. See COEFFICIENT OF *RELIABILITY and ALTERNATE FORMS *RELIABILITY.

equivalence of cues, acquired ACQUIRED DISCRIMINATION OF CUES.

equivalent forms ALTERNATE FORMS *RELIABILITY.

equivalent groups procedure MATCHED GROUPS PROCEDURE.

erectile disorder MALE ERECTILE DISORDER.

erethism An unusually high sensitivity to sensory stimulation.

ERG ELECTRORETINOGRAM.

erg 1 In physics, the work done by a force of 1 dyne acting through a displacement of 1 cm (0.4 in.) in the direction of the force. **2** In psychology the term is used in a variety of combinations that are metaphoric and relate to energy, force, purpose or dynamic qualities.

ergic Purposive. In the work of R. B. Cattell, pertaining to innate drives or predispositions.

-ergic Suffix denoting *work, function, purpose*. It is used in physiology to characterize a neuron or a neural pathway in terms of the operative neurotransmitter; e.g. *dopaminergic* refers to a neural structure in which dopamine is the substance that 'does the work'.

erg(o)- Combining form meaning *work*.

ergodic In probability theory, characteristic of any stochastic process in which every sequence of events is statistically the same and therefore may be taken as representative of the whole.

ergograph Any device for measuring the amount of work accomplished by a muscle or muscle group.

ergonomics The science of the 'fit' between jobs and persons, the study of the relationship between an individual's anatomy, physiology and psychology and the demands of particular forms of work. See also HUMAN FACTORS.

ergot A cover term for a group of toxic alkaloids derived from a fungus that grows on grains. Among their many effects are uterine contractions and derivatives have been used since the middle ages to induce labour or abortion. Biologically similar to LSD, episodes of 'ergotism' marked by hallucinations, irrational thinking and a 'burning' skin (caused by severe peripheral vasoconstriction) have occurred throughout history when contaminated grains are eaten. Because of its complex neurological and circulatory functions, the less toxic ergot derivatives are under study as possible psychopharmacologic agents. Currently one, *ergotamine*, is used in the treatment of migraine.

ergotropic Descriptive of processes that mobilize bodily functions and ready an organism for environmental challenges. Contrast with TROPHOTROPIC.

ERN ERROR-RELATED NEGATIVITY.

erogenous zones Areas of the body the stimulation of which gives rise to erotic or sexual sensations. Occasionally called *erotogenic zones*.

Eros The Greek god of love. In Freudian theory, *Eros* refers to the whole complex of life-preservative instincts. Included among these, of course, are the sexual instincts. Compare with Freud's use of THANATOS, the totality of death instincts.

erotic Generally, sexual or libidinal. Used broadly, the term may pertain to: **1** Feelings arising specifically from the genitals. **2** A more general sense of sexual arousal. **3** The stimuli that give rise to sexual arousal. **4** Any motive or need that has sexual components. **5** Love in any of its manifestations.

erotic apathy SEXUAL APATHY.

erotic delusion DELUSIONAL DISORDER, EROTIC.

eroticism 1 Sexual arousal. **2** A greater than average disposition for the sexual, a tendency to be easily aroused sexually. **3** Sexual excitement arising from areas other than those specifically sexual, i.e. other than the genitals. Usually the area is specified, e.g. *anal eroticism*. var., *erotism*.

erotization A psychoanalytic term for the process by which a body part or bodily function becomes a source of erotic pleasure.

eroto- Combining form meaning pertaining to *sex, sexuality, love*.

erotogenic zones EROGENOUS ZONES.

erotomania General term for any exaggerated sexual drive.

ERP EVENT-RELATED POTENTIAL.

error There are several *general* senses in which this term is used: **1** A departure from correctness. **2** A mistaken belief. **3** The state of holding a mistaken belief, as in the common expression, to be 'in error'. **4** In statistics, a departure from a true score, a DEVIATION. **5** In an experiment, any variation in the dependent variable caused by factors other than variation in the independent variable. **6** An inappropriate or incorrect response that results in a delay in the learning of the correct response.

There are also scores of specialized usages of this inherently appealing term, as in the following entries. Note that qualifiers are often used to locate the source of or characterize the nature of error.

error, absolute The absolute value (i.e. without regard to sign) of the difference between an observed value and the true value of a measure. For example, *over*estimating someone's height by 2 in. (5 cm) produces the same absolute error as *under*estimating by 2 in.

error, A not B See A NOT B ERROR.

error, anticipation Any error characterized by the making of a response before it should properly be made.

error, average Lit., the average error in a series of observations or judgements.

error, chance Simply, an error that arises from chance factors. Since such errors are in principle random and unbiased they tend to cancel each other out, and the sum of chance errors, when a sufficiently large number of cases is considered, approaches zero. Also called *variable error, accidental error, random error*. Compare with CONSTANT *ERROR.

error, compensating Any error that cancels out a previously made error. It may be introduced deliberately to correct for another source of error.

error, constant An error produced by some factor that affects all observations similarly so that the errors are always in one direction and do not cancel each other out. Usually a constant error can be detected and corrected for during statistical analysis. Also called *systematic error*.

error, experimental This term covers a large class of possible errors the origins of which lie in the inadequacy of an experimental design or procedure. The history of psychology is well salted with legendary experimental errors due to improper control of some important factor. The most common are failures to control for practice effects, temporal factors, time errors, observer differences, experimenter biases, physiological and species differences and the ubiquitous sampling errors.

error, grouping Any error introduced by the manner in which data are combined or grouped. In general when data are grouped into classes the statistical operations carried out on those classes are based on the assumption that the combined scores are symmetrically distributed around the midpoint of each class. As a quick look at SAMPLING *ERROR will show, this assumption is often not met and hence some measure of grouping error will emerge during such procedures.

error, instrumental A constant error due to a bias in the apparatus.

error, measurement Any constant error due to a bias in the process of measurement. It may be due to the apparatus, the observer, the subject or the experimenter.

error, perseverative Generally, any tendency for a subject to persevere inappropriately with a particular response.

error, probable Occasionally used as a measure of the error of estimate or of the sampling error. The probable error is exactly 0.6745 of the STANDARD ERROR.

error-related negativity (ERN) An EVENT-RELATED POTENTIAL that occurs roughly 100 msec after an error was made. The ERN arises in the *anterior cingulate* and is markedly larger when accuracy is stressed over speed. It is not clear to what extent the ERN is caused by the commission of the error or the belief that one has made one. Also known, jokingly, as the *blunder blip*.

error, sampling A general term used for any difference between the true value of a statistic within a population and the estimated value of that statistic derived from a sample of that population. Since nearly all work in psychology is based on samples, not complete populations, there will almost always be some sampling error. Naturally, one tries to keep this kind of error to a minimum by selecting samples which are representative of the true population and by using as large a sample as is conveniently possible. Note, however, that sampling errors may emerge in two fashions. The first, the one which is inescapable and hence regarded as a legitimate form of error, results from inexorable laws of probability and sampling. The second, the kind which is in principle preventable, results from nonrepresentative, sloppy, incomplete or biased sampling. See SAMPLING et seq.

error, stimulus To commit the stimulus error, according to E. B. Titchener's brand of structuralism, was to lapse during introspection from the 'psychological' point of view to some other perspective. A stimulus error would result when the subject allowed mediated experience to interfere with the introspection of immediate experience. A butcher who, because of experience with estimating weights, reports that a 2 lb (0.9 kg) object is 'twice as heavy' as a 1 lb (0.45 kg) object commits the stimulus error because the response is based on mediated experience with weights rather than on the basis of immediate experience with the weights as they feel at the time of the experiment.

error, subjective A systematic error introduced into observation or interpretation due to an individual's biases or prejudices.

error, time An error in judgement concerning comparisons between two or more events or stimuli based on their temporal order of presentation. By convention, if the first of two objectively equal stimuli is erroneously judged the greater it is termed a *positive* time error; should the second be so judged it is termed a *negative* time error.

error, (Type I and **Type II)** In testing the significance of an experimental result one is, in essence, determining whether to accept or reject the null hypothesis. Under such conditions one is laid open to one of two types of error: (a) the erroneous rejection of a true hypothesis; or (b) the failure to reject a hypothesis that is, in fact, false. The first of these is called a *Type I error* (or, on occasion, an *alpha error*); the second is known as a *Type II error* (or *beta error*). Note that Type I and Type II errors are inextricably linked. If one sets a particularly stringent level of *significance* (or *alpha level*), a Type I error becomes very unlikely but the possibility of a Type II error is raised accordingly; a lenient alpha level lowers the chance of a Type II error but markedly raises the possibility of making a Type I error.

error variance That proportion of the VARIANCE that cannot be attributed to controlled factors. Error variance will be inflated by sampling errors, measurement errors, experimental errors, etc.

erythr(o)- From the Greek, a prefix meaning *red*.

erythropia Vision in which objects are tinged red. It can result from overexposure to intense light, as in snow blindness. var., *erythropsia*.

ESB ELECTRICAL BRAIN STIMULATION.

E scale MEASUREMENT OF *AUTHORITARIANISM.

escape from reality FLIGHT FROM *REALITY.

escape learning (or **conditioning**) A form of learning in which an organism acquires an instrumental or operant response that permits it to escape a noxious or painful stimulus. Escape learning is often discussed in conjunction with AVOIDANCE LEARNING.

escape mechanism A loose synonym for DEFENCE MECHANISM.

escape training Generally, any experimental procedure in which the subject must learn an escape response.

esotropia A form of STRABISMUS in which one eye turns inward when the other fixates on an object.

ESP EXTRASENSORY PERCEPTION.

essentialism A philosophical position that

maintains that for every kind of entity there will be a particular set of 'essential' features that characterize the category to which it belongs. In psychology, essentialism is of interest to those concerned with questions such as how to define a particular category and how children learn them (see CATEGORY et seq.). It is also an element of folk psychology since most people assume that natural objects have such hidden essential properties (e.g. all tigers have an essential 'tigerness' that is captured by stripes, aggression, cat-like, whiskers, etc.).

EST 1 Abbreviation for *electroshock therapy*. 2 An acronym for *Erhard Seminar Training*. A form of psychotherapy based on the 'theor-ies' of Werner Erhard (né Jack Rosenberg, a one-time sales manager). Once popular, it is now thankfully losing its cachet.

estimate 1 n. Loosely, a reasonable guess concerning the value of some factor. 2 n. In statistics, somewhat more precisely, a 'best guess' of the value of some variable or statis-tic based on refined computational proced-ures which provide both the estimated value as well as a measure of the likelihood that that value falls within ascertainable limits of the true value. An estimate in this sense is an inference about a population based on measurements made on a sample.

eta 1 A correlation coefficient for curvilinear relationships. Compare with PRODUCT MOMENT *CORRELATION, which expresses linear relationships between two variables. 2 A measure of EFFECT SIZE interpretable as the pro-portion of total variance that is attributable to group membership or treatment group in a FACTORIAL *DESIGN when there is more than one *degree of freedom* in the factor of interest. Various formulas exist for measuring eta and most are known to overestimate the propor-tion of variance attributable to the factor of interest. Also denoted as η.

eta squared The square of the value of ETA (1). It is an estimate of the proportion of the variance in the data in a curvilinear relation-ship that can be attributed to the relation-ship.

ethics A branch of philosophy concerned with that which is deemed acceptable in human behaviour, with what is good or bad, right or wrong in human conduct in pursuit of goals and aims. There is a tendency to use the term in consideration of theor-etical treatises, or examinations of the ideal; when actual human behaviour in social and cultural settings is under consid-eration (particularly with regard to develop-mental issues and the acquisition of codes of ethics) many authors use *morality* and related terms. For more discussion see MORAL et seq.

ethinamate A nonbarbiturate sedative used primarily as a sleeping pill. Its effects are similar to those of *chloral hydrate*.

ethnic group Originally this term was used to refer to groups of people who were bio-logically related. The usage has been inten-tionally expanded and an ethnic group is now seen as any group with common cul-tural traditions and a sense of identity. Thus, ethnic groups may be bound together by a sense of history and tradition (Jews), language (the Dakota Indians), geography (Scandinavians), a sociological definition of race (American Blacks), religion (Muslims), etc. Usually the term is reserved for minority groups, although not always; some social psychologists call the dominant group in a society an ethnic group. Although ethnic groups are often racial groups, these two terms are no longer used synonymously.

ethnic psychosis CULTURE-SPECIFIC SYNDROME.

ethnocentrism 1 The tendency to view one's own ethnic group and its social stand-ards as the basis for evaluative judgement concerning the practices of others, with the implication that one views one's own stand-ards as superior. Hence, ethnocentrism con-notes a habitual disposition to look with disfavour on the practices of alien groups. The term is the ethnic analogue of egocentr-ism. 2 In some instances, a synonym of SOCIOCENTRISM, but see that entry for more detail.

ethnography A division of anthropology devoted to the comparative study of individ-ual cultures. var., *ethnology*.

ethnomethodology A term originally coined by the sociologist H. Garfinkel to describe the study of the 'resources' available to participants in social interactions and how these resources are utilized by them. The term, which Garfinkel later came to regard as a shibboleth, is generally used to refer to a body of sociological and psychological research on conversational rules, negotiation of property rights and other socially motivated interactions. Such research is generally carried out using naturalistic observation techniques.

ethogram As total a record as is possible of the behaviour of an animal in a naturalistic setting. The term carries a theoretical assumption in the notion that within the behavioural repertoire of a species there is only a finite number of fixed, repeatable behaviour patterns that can enter into an ethogram. See ETHOLOGY (4).

ethology The term derives originally from the Greek *ethos* meaning *character* or *essential nature* and *-ology* meaning *study of*. Hence, it has been applied to: **1** The study of ethics, especially comparative examination of ethical systems. **2** The empirical investigation of human character. **3** The study of cultural customs. All three of these meanings are, however, rarely intended today. The term is now, in contemporary psychology, applied almost exclusively to: **4** An interdisciplinary science, combining zoology, biology and comparative psychology, concerned with precise observation of the behaviour of animals in their natural environment and the development of theoretical characterizations of that behaviour with regard to the subtle interplay of genetic and environmental factors. The science has its origins in the work of the European naturalists Lorenz, Tinbergen, Thorpe, von Frisch and others. The primary focus of ethological research is the complete, exhaustive analysis of behaviour using techniques of NATURALISTIC OBSERVATION. In this respect it is usually distinguished from COMPARATIVE PSYCHOLOGY, in which experimental-manipulative techniques and controlled laboratory techniques are the rule.

etiology AETIOLOGY.

etymology The study of the historical origins and development of linguistic forms.

eu- Combining form meaning *healthy, well, normal, advantageous*.

Euclidean space SPACE (1).

eufunction A term occasionally used as the antonym of DYSFUNCTION. Since *function* is, strictly speaking, a value-neutral term,

eufunction is sometimes used to specify positive, healthy function.

eugenics The study of human heredity patterns with the goal of improving the species through selective breeding. *Positive* eugenics emphasizes encouraging individuals with 'desirable' traits to procreate, and *negative* eugenics focuses on discouraging those with 'undesirable' traits from procreating (often by unethical procedures such as forced sterilization). Unfortunately (or should we say fortunately?), agreement about which characteristics it is desirable to perpetuate has not been reached. Since the founding of the discipline by Francis Galton in the 19th century, eugenicists have been unable to extricate themselves from their own ethnocentrism.

eunuch A prepubertally castrated male. The term is also used to describe the physical characteristics of a eunuch – poor muscle tone, lack of bodily hair, undeveloped genitalia. Occasionally the term is used to refer to a prepubertally ovarectomized female.

euphoria 1 A sense of extreme elation generally accompanied by optimism and a deep sense of well-being and heightened activity. In pathological cases it may be totally unrealistic, contain delusions of grandeur and invulnerability and include manic levels of activity. ant., *dysphoria*. **2** H. S. Sullivan also used the term to refer to a feeling of deep satisfaction, well-being and comfort. However, compared with meaning 1, the emotion in this sense is rather constrained and relaxed.

eupsychia A. Maslow's term for the humanistic utopia which would be reached when all persons were psychologically healthy – at least psychologically healthy in the sense characterized by Maslow's particular brand of optimistic humanism. See, in this regard, HUMANISTIC PSYCHOLOGY and NEED HIERARCHY.

eurymorph BODY-BUILD INDEX.

Eustachian tube Small tube of bone and cartilage that connects the middle ear with the pharynx, serving to equalize air pressure on either side of the tympanic membrane.

euthanasia Easy and painless death, or the means for bringing this about. Advocated by many for those suffering from the intractable pain that accompanies the terminal stages of many incurable diseases. A distinction worth noting (in respect of matters legal and ethical) is that drawn between *passive* euthanasia, when one simply ceases to supply requisite extraordinary support measures needed to keep an individual alive, and *active* euthanasia, when specific means are taken to terminate life.

euthenics The discipline that seeks to improve the lot of the human being by regulating the environment. The insurmountable ethical problems of EUGENICS have contributed to the development of this field.

euthymia From the Greek for *good mood, serenity*. While it is often used as an antonym of DYSTHYMIA, this is not quite right. *Dysthymia* is a distinctly negative emotional state, one of depression and sadness; *euthymia* is properly used for a state of calmness and serenity, not necessarily one marked by happiness. Compare with EUPHORIA.

euthymic mood A mood characterized by EUTHYMIA.

evaluation 1 Generally, the determining of the value or worth of something. **2** More specifically, the determination of how successful a programme, a curriculum, a series of experiments, a drug, etc. has been in achieving the goals laid out for it at the outset. See OUTCOMES ASSESSMENT. **3** One of the three hypothesized universal dimensions of *semantic space* in Osgood's theory of word meaning. See SEMANTIC DIFFERENTIAL.

evaluation research An area of applied psychology concerned with development of procedures for testing the effectiveness of social, educational, therapeutic or other applied programmes. See EVALUATION (2), OUTCOMES ASSESSMENT.

evaluative semantic priming method See PIPELINE TECHNIQUES.

event An occurrence, a phenomenon, a slice of reality, indeed anything that happens that has a beginning and an end and can be specified in terms of change. Thus, one speaks of stimuli, responses, reinforcements, outcomes of trials and so on as events. The word is ubiquitous in psychology and everyone uses it in whatever fashion makes them comfortable.

event-related potential (ERP) EVOKED POTENTIAL.

evidence-based approaches 1 Generally, therapeutic approaches that have strong empirical evidence of effectiveness. Also called *empirically supported treatments, evidence-based practices,* or *evidence-based treatments*. **2** Assessments that measure a disorder or problem as accurately, efficiently, comprehensively and directly as possible. Of course, the empirical evidence for the former rests on the latter.

eviration 1 Castration. **2** Loss of masculine characteristics. **3** A delusion in a man that he has become a woman.

evocative therapy A general term used primarily by behavioural therapists for any form of psychotherapy that focuses on underlying causes of psychological disorders, i.e. the psychoanalytic and psychodynamic. The term was coined by J. D. Frank to emphasize that these approaches functioned by attempting to evoke changes in internal conditions and thereby produce socially acceptable behaviours.

evo-devo See EVOLUTIONARY DEVELOPMENTAL BIOLOGY.

evoke To elicit, call forth. Generally used to refer to responses that are elicited from an organism or from a part of an organism by stimulation.

evoked potential A regular pattern of electrical activity recorded from neural tissue evoked by a controlled stimulus. The term usually applies to potentials from large masses of central-nervous-system tissue, specifically the brain. Also called *event-related potential*. Qualifiers are often used to specify a type of potential, e.g. *visual evoked potential* for neural responses to visual stimuli.

evolution 1 Generally and loosely, orderly development. Here one finds reference to evolution of thought, of theory, of style and the like. **2** More specifically, the process by which plant and animal forms have developed by descent, with modification, from earlier forms. See here EVOLUTIONARY THEORY.

evolutionary developmental biology A subfield of biology that focuses on: (a) the study of how patterns of developmental processes inform our understanding of *evolution* and vice versa; and (b) the comparison of the developmental paths of different species to derive information about their probable evolutionary and biological relationships. It integrates ONTOGENY and PHYLOGENY and blends them with ecological perspectives (ECOLOGY (1)) and modern genetics. A related approach, *evolutionary developmental psychology* studies similar issues but emphasizes behaviour rather than biological mechanisms. The informal expression 'evo-devo' is found referring to either or both.

evolutionary psychology A broad approach to the study of psychology that seeks to understand behaviours in their evolutionary contexts. Although the approach shares with SOCIOBIOLOGY a focus on genetic and biological constraints, it places more emphasis on the role of social and cognitive factors, which tend to be neglected by sociobiologists.

evolutionary theory Frequently one sees the terms *evolution, evolutionary theory, theory of evolution* and others used as though they were synonyms and all denoting the particular position put forward by Charles Darwin. This pattern of usage tends to be misleading. Evolution is not theory, it is fact; the 'gradualist' position of the origin of species by natural selection put forward by Darwin (see DARWINISM) is one attempt to explain that fact. Defenders of creationism frequently mistake disputes over the best characterization of the process of evolution as indications that biologists themselves regard evolution as merely a theoretical notion.

Evolutionary theory has been the stage for many vigorous disputes, ranging from early (indeed, pre-Darwinian) arguments over the role of Lamarckian processes (see INHERITANCE OF *ACQUIRED CHARACTERISTICS) to the current debate between the gradualists, who, with Darwin, argue that new species develop slowly (relatively speaking) and in an orderly way, and the saltationists, who defend the position of punctuated equilibrium that argues that new species appear suddenly (relatively speaking) and abruptly, to the seemingly endless argument over whether principles of organic evolution can be applied to the social and cultural milieu (see SOCIOBIOLOGY). These disputes notwithstanding, the impact that evolutionary theory has had upon scientific thought, philosophy and theology is incalculable.

In psychology, evolutionary doctrine produced a genuine revolution. It ushered in the study of individual differences with its emphasis on mental testing; it provided the rationale for the field of comparative psychology and made legitimate the inference from animal work to human; it stressed the concepts of adaptation, function and purpose which became dominant in American and European psychology during the 20th century; it focused attention on the role of genetic material, eventually culminating in the discipline of behaviour genetics; and finally, by stressing inheritance, it profoundly influenced the field of developmental psychology. Indeed, there is probably no area of contemporary psychological thinking that has remained immune from its influence.

ex- Prefix indicating *out, out of, away from*.

exafference REAFFERENCE.

exaptation In evolutionary biology, the process whereby forms or structures that evolved to serve one function are co-opted to serve other functions. The human use of the tongue for speech is a good example. The possibility of traits and functions developing through such a process was first proposed by S. J. Gould. See SPANDREL for a related phenomenon.

exceptional child As used in child psychology the term refers to extremely talented and gifted children as well as to those with low intelligence or other learning disabilities. The application of the term to the latter group was well motivated, to remove the stigma of being classified as 'retarded' or 'minimally functional'. Unfortunately, the effect seems to have been one of altering and contaminating the meaning of the term *exceptional* rather than changing the characterization of the methods of dealing with children so designated.

exchange theory SOCIAL EXCHANGE THEORY.

excitable Generally, capable of being aroused or excited. The term is widely used as descriptive of: (a) living tissue, specifically neural tissue, that is in a state such that it will respond to a stimulus; (b) a person who is in a state such that he or she is easily aroused to emotional reactions; (c) a person who is characteristically easily aroused, etc.

excitant Rare synonym of STIMULUS.

excitation 1 In physiology, a process whereby some stimulus energy pattern sets up a change or pattern of changes in a receptor. The energy here may be either physical or other neural activity; see STIMULATION. 2 In the study of learning, a general high level of activity in the whole nervous system; a reasonable synonym here is *drive state*. 3 In social psychology, an increase in psychological tension; this meaning is intuitively close to conventional usage.

excitatory conditioning CONDITIONING, EXCITATORY.

excitatory irradiation IRRADIATION.

excitatory postsynaptic potential (EPSP) POSTSYNAPTIC POTENTIAL.

excitatory potential ($_sE_R$) In Hull's theory, a hypothesized state assumed to reflect an organism's tendency to make a response.

excitatory threshold THRESHOLD (3).

excitement–calm (or excitement–quiescence) One of the dimensions of Wundt's three-dimensional theory of emotion. The others are: *pleasantness–unpleasantness* and *tension–relaxation*.

excitotoxin Any agent that overstimulates nerve cells to the point of destroying them.

executive Used primarily in models of cognition, particularly those represented as computer models, this term refers to a hypothesized 'master programme' that controls and directs small, more limited subprogrammes. In some ways the executive programme is the modern version of the HOMUNCULUS.

executive area In neurophysiology, a term used loosely to refer to any cortical area that serves integrative, organizing functions.

executive control See EXECUTIVE FUNCTIONS.

executive functions Collectively, those functions that comprise volitional activities such as planning, organizing, self-awareness, self-regulation and initiation of action. The term tends to be used in a distinctly loose fashion simply because there is no simple list of identifiable functions here. Rather, it refers to a variety of interlocking networked processes involving self-regulation, planning and maintaining goal-directed efforts, the capacity to make inferences, to appreciate the ramifications of choices and to control action and thought. Some authorities also include logical reasoning, the capacity for symbolic representation and abstract thought although there are reasons for keeping these functions separate since clinical syndromes exist where such 'rational' capabilities are lost but the other functions remain intact. There is also evidence that short-term memory functions play a role and various emotional states are known to be integrated with executive function. It is unclear exactly what cortical structures are involved although the frontal lobes are certainly implicated. Also called *executive control*, and *central executive*.

exemplar theory INSTANCE THEORY.

exercise, law (or principle) of The generalization, first formulated by E. L. Thorndike, that 'other things being equal', repeated performance of any act makes the behaviour easier to perform, more fluid and less prone to error.

exhaustion 1 Physiologically, a state in which the metabolic process has been depleted, producing fatigue, weariness and a general lack of responsiveness. 2 In ethology, the draining of action-specific energy for a particular instinctive act by constant repetition. When used in this sense metabolic depletion is not entailed since the muscles used in the act are not themselves necessarily fatigued. This meaning is also found vaguely represented in the way some psychoanalysts characterize the draining off of libido. 3 Shortened form of EXHAUSTION STAGE.

exhaustion delirium An acute delirium occasionally observed under conditions of extreme exhaustion brought about by intense extended physical effort or by other debilitating conditions such as high fever.

exhaustion stage The third stage in the GENERAL ADAPTATION SYNDROME.

exhaustive search SEARCH, EXHAUSTIVE.

exhibitionism 1 Generally, a strong tendency to make oneself the constant centre of attention. **2** A PARAPHILIA characterized by a compulsion to expose one's genitals under socially inappropriate circumstances.

existential analysis The generally accepted translation of *Daseinanalyse*. See the discussions under EXISTENTIALISM and EXISTENTIAL THERAPY.

existential anxiety A profound experience of apprehension, alienation and ANGST (1) that is regarded within EXISTENTIALISM as a critical element of life.

existential crisis A critical moment in an individual's life, a point where, as per the classical model of EXISTENTIALISM, a person confronts the need to find meaning in life, purpose in their existence and to take responsibility for choices and decisions. Outside of existentialism the term is used loosely for moments where hard choices need to be made.

existentialism An important 20th-century philosophical movement which carved out a domain for itself between rationalistic idealism and totally objective materialism. The emphasis is upon personal decisions to be made in a world without reason and without purpose. Existentialism emphasizes subjectivity, free will and individuality and has acted as a philosophical counterbalance to theories that stress the role of society and social groups. It has also spawned a form of psychotherapy (see EXISTENTIAL THERAPY) that focuses on free will and the necessity for individual choice, action and judgement.

existential psychology This label was once used for the point of view espoused by E. B. Titchener (see STRUCTURALISM). However, when found today it almost invariably refers to one or another version of the psychological positions that have emerged from EXISTENTIALISM.

existential therapy A form of psychotherapy based upon the philosophical doctrine of EXISTENTIALISM. In practice the existentialist approach is highly subjective and focuses on the immediate situation (see BEING-IN-THE-WORLD and DASEIN). It differs from most other therapies in that there is a strict avoidance of intellectual explanation and interpretation; the focus is on the immediate reality shared by client and therapist. Exist-

entialism, by design, resists easy codification, and its therapeutic practice runs from the pessimism of the Europeans, especially the followers of Ludwig Binswanger, to the smiling optimism of the American HUMAN POTENTIAL MOVEMENT.

exo- Prefix designating *out, outside of, external to.*

exocrine Used of glands that secrete hormones through a duct. Contrast with ENDOCRINE and see the discussion under GLAND.

exocytosis The process by which a cell secretes its products. The secreted material is held in a container which migrates to and fuses with the cell's outer membrane and then bursts, dumping its contents into the extracellular fluid.

exogamy Marriage outside of one's social or cultural group. Contrast with ENDOGAMY.

exogenous (or **exogenic**) Lit., originating from without. Used to refer to phenomena the origins of which are external or outside the body. Contrast with ENDOGENOUS.

exogenous depression REACTIVE *DEPRESSION.

exogenous opiates Literally, any OPIATE introduced into the body. Compare with ENDOGENOUS OPIATES.

exophthalmia Abnormal protrusion of the eyeball.

exopsychic Characterizing mental activity that has effects outside a person.

exosomatic method A method of evaluating the GALVANIC SKIN RESPONSE.

exotropia Divergent STRABISMUS.

expansive delusion A delusion of grandeur accompanied by feelings of wealth, power, influence, etc.

expansiveness 1 Generally, outgoingness, friendliness, reactiveness, loquaciousness, etc. However: **2** In K. Horney's writings, a neurotic condition resulting from the mistaken sense that one has actually achieved IDEALIZED *SELF (2). Here the characteristic behaviours are arrogance, narcissism, vindictiveness, etc.

expectancy 1 Occasional synonym of EXPECTED VALUE. **2** An internal state, an attitude or set of an organism that leads it to anticipate (or expect) a particular event. Note that in this sense the term is used by both behaviourists and cognitive psychologists: for the former, expectancy must be inferred from objective behaviour and is characterized by attentiveness, muscle tension, etc.; for the latter, it is treated as a mental set with a good deal of conscious cognitive processing involved and is assessed phenomenologically.

expectancy effect EXPERIMENTER EXPECTANCY EFFECT.

expectancy theory One of several names used for E. C. Tolman's purposive psychology. The basic assumption here is that what is learned is a disposition to behave toward stimulus objects as though they were signs for other objects or events the occurrence of which is contingent on the appropriate behaviour. Thus, in this conceptualization, reinforcement becomes confirmation.

expectancy-value theory Not so much a theory as a way of looking at motivation and behaviour. The essential notion here is that any organism (human or otherwise, although the theory is generally used to characterize human motivation) behaves in accordance with the expected outcomes of various courses of action and the values associated with each of those outcomes. See EXPECTATION, EXPECTED VALUE.

expectation 1 The anticipated outcome of a probabilistic situation, the EXPECTED VALUE. **2** The TRUE *MEAN. **3** An emotional state of anticipation.

expected value Most generally, this is the anticipated outcome, in the long run, of a particular strategy. For example, suppose you are invited to play a game in which a head on a coin flip wins you 6 units while a tail loses 5 units. The expected value of this game is + 0.50 units on each toss. The calculation is simple: multiply the value of each outcome by its probability of occurrence and combine them. Expected values can be calculated for any situation in which the probabilities of the several events are known. In statistical analyses, expected values become extremely important because they reveal critical characteristics of distributions. In

particular, the mean is the expected value of a distribution. In the theory of decision-making, the expected value of a decision is one of the more important determinants of people's behaviour. See also in this context GAME, SUBJECTIVE PROBABILITY, UTILITY.

experience Generally, the term is used in ways commensurate with lay language; hence: **1** Any event through which one has lived. **2** The knowledge gained from participation in an event. **3** The sum total of knowledge accumulated. However, recent reintroduction of some classic philosophical problems of epistemology into the study of cognition has produced a fresh nuance; namely, some now use the term with reference specifically to the real world, meaning experience is characterized in terms of what is 'out there', while others use it to refer only to personal, subjective phenomena, meaning experience is characterized in terms of what is 'in the head'. To appreciate this distinction consider whether or not the 'pink elephants' seen by an alcoholic count as *experiences*.

experiential avoidance The efforts of a person to avoid contact with unpleasant thoughts, situations and emotions. The term is used in the cognitive-behaviour therapy field to express a concept similar to that captured by the psychoanalytic construct of SUPPRESSION (3), although experiential avoidance does not require the avoided emotion or situation to be unacceptable – merely unpleasant.

experiment Modern scientific psychology prides itself (perhaps a bit self-consciously) on being *experimental*. The intent here is to let it be known that psychological principles are founded on well-controlled and repeatable experiments. In essence, any experiment is an arrangement of conditions or procedures for the purpose of testing some hypothesis. The design of an experiment focuses on: (a) the antecedent conditions themselves, usually referred to as the INDEPENDENT *VARIABLES (or *treatments* or *experimental variables*), and (b) the outcome or results of the experiment, usually called the DEPENDENT *VARIABLES. The critical aspect of any experiment is that there be *control* over the independent variables such that cause-and-effect relationships can be discovered without ambiguity.

There is a tendency to use the adjectival form *experimental* in a broader and looser sense to cover casual observations or simple trial procedures that are not always well controlled. This usage is not wrong in any etymological sense, although it should be avoided for it detracts from the rigorous meaning. See also CONTROL (1), EXPERIMENTAL *DESIGN, SCIENTIFIC *METHOD.

experimental artifact ARTIFACT, EXPERIMENTAL.

experimental control CONTROL (2).

experimental design DESIGN, EXPERIMENTAL.

experimental error ERROR, EXPERIMENTAL.

experimental extinction EXTINCTION.

experimental group (or condition) A group (or condition) in an experiment that is exposed to the independent variable(s) under investigation. Usually the experimental group is matched with a control group (or condition) that receives similar treatment except for the critical independent variable(s).

experimental method EXPERIMENT and SCIENTIFIC *METHOD.

experimental neurosis A condition originally described by Pavlov. It is a 'neurosis' that results from an attempt to classically condition an impossible discrimination. For example, the positive stimulus may be a circle and the negative one an ellipse. Over several trials the ellipse is gradually formed into a circle so that the discrimination becomes impossible to make. Dogs treated in this manner behaved 'neurotically'. They attempted to avoid entering the laboratory, barked violently during the study, tore and bit at the apparatus, etc. A similar phenomenon may be established by punishing behaviour necessary for existence such as shocking a rat every time it tries to eat or drink. The use of the term *experimental neurosis* has been deplored by some as it adds to the already confused state of the meaning of *neurosis*, but it has been applauded by others because it provides a possibility for operationalizing the term. The issue, however, has been rendered lexicographically moot (at least in North Amer-

ica) since the *DSM* (DIAGNOSTIC AND STATISTICAL MANUAL) no longer uses the term *neurosis*.

experimental psychology A very general term that can be applied to any approach to the study of psychological issues that uses experimental procedures. Once the term was limited to 'laboratory' psychology but now it is used ubiquitously.

experimental variable INDEPENDENT *VARIABLE.

experiment, controlled In a sense this term is redundant since the assumption is that all experiments are adequately controlled. Nevertheless, one often finds it used to refer to experiments which employ both experimental and control groups.

experimenter bias EXPERIMENTER EXPECTANCY EFFECT.

experimenter expectancy effect A bias introduced into an investigation by the experimenter. Such biases can enter most insidiously into many experiments, even those with lower organisms. The common denominator is that if an investigator has certain expectations about the outcome of an experiment these can contaminate the entire scientific process. The experimenter can subtly (unconsciously?) alter his or her behaviour in carrying out the experiment in any of a number of ways and so produce biased results. For details on a few of these biases see DEMAND CHARACTERISTICS, SELF-FULFILLING PROPHECY and CLEVER HANS. Also known by a variety of other names, including *expectancy effect*, *experimenter bias* and, after the researcher who did much of the early work, *Rosenthal effect*.

experiment, mental A kind of speculative nonexperiment in which the investigator considers the possible results *if* certain manipulations were carried out. Generally, such *thought experiments* (as they are often called) are useful heuristics for exploring the implications of particular theoretical models or for musing about the implications of accumulated facts. Also called *Gedanken experiments*, from the German for *thought*.

experimentum crucis CRUCIAL EXPERIMENT.

expert witness An individual deemed by a court to be acceptable as a witness in legal settings based on his or her qualifications, experience, training, licensure and so forth. Opinions of expert witnesses in psychiatry and psychology are often sought in cases ranging from those in which the INSANITY DEFENCE is claimed to those involving perceptual and cognitive functions, e.g. cases depending upon EYEWITNESS TESTIMONY.

expiatory punishment PUNISHMENT, EXPIATORY.

explanation An account of a phenomenon or an event or the characterization of a object. Many a scientist's and many a philosopher's lifetime's work has been invested in explication of just what form of account of a thing can be regarded as a true explanation of that thing. Explanations come in various guises, to wit: (a) *causal* – which lays out the necessary and sufficient antecedent conditions for the phenomenon; (b) *historical* (or *ontogenetic*) – which focuses on articulating the previously occurring events that led to the event of which an explanation is sought; (c) *reductive* – which recasts the phenomenon under scrutiny in simpler or more fundamental terms; (d) *constructive* (or *generalized*) – which is concerned with the elaboration of more general principles or laws that lay out the relationship between the event to be explained and others. Generally, one distinguishes between an explanatory effort and a descriptive one, on the grounds that the latter is restricted to reports of observations while the former extends to articulation of relationships between those things observed. In practice, of course, this distinction is not always so easily made. See CAUSATION, DEFINITION, DESCRIPTION.

explicit 1 Generally, characterizing that which is direct and clearly specified. 2 By extension, characterizing that which is *overt* and open for observation. 3 By further extension, characterizing that which is consciously known; explicit cognitive processes are those a person is aware of using. Compare here with IMPLICIT.

explicit learning LEARNING, EXPLICIT.

explicit memory MEMORY, EXPLICIT.

exploitive character E. Fromm's term for one who derives satisfaction from exploiting others, who uses others to satisfy his or her own needs without concern for the needs of those others. var., *exploitative*.

exploratory behaviour Generally, any series of movements or acts the apparent purpose of which is to bring an organism into contact with the various portions or aspects of its surroundings. Such exploratory behaviour was something of a problem for early learning theories (particularly Hull's) since there did not appear to be any clear drive state motivating it. The solution to the conundrum was to hypothesize an exploratory drive. Today, with the development of ethological approaches to behaviour, such behaviour is regarded as 'natural' and common to locomoting species (including *H. sapiens*) that require information about the nature of novel situations so as to be able to make appropriate responses. The term is also occasionally used to refer to some cognitive processes, such as the tendency for people to shift thought patterns from one aspect to another of a novel situation, or to consider a variety of possible strategies for action in a particular situation.

exploratory drive EXPLORATORY BEHAVIOUR.

exploratory study Any preliminary study designed to provide some feeling for or general understanding of the phenomena to be studied. A good exploratory study will yield cues as to how to proceed with the major investigation. Also called *pilot study*.

explosive disorder INTERMITTENT EXPLOSIVE DISORDER.

exposition need H. Murray's term for the need to explain, demonstrate to and (alas) lecture others.

ex post facto From the Latin, meaning *by subsequent action*. An *ex post facto* experimental design is one in which the groups are matched after the independent variables have already been administered or after the occurrence of the event to be studied. A common example is the examining of census data collected for other reasons. An *ex post facto* explanation is one that explains the findings after the research has been completed. Although *ex post facto* experiments and explanations are less desirable than predictive experiments and explanations, they are often unavoidable.

exposure therapy See ANXIETY-INDUCTION THERAPY.

expression Generally, any outward display. Somewhat more restrictively, an outward display that is taken as implying a particular internal state; see here EMOTIONAL EXPRESSION.

expressive 1 adj. Characterizing an expression; a term typically used with regard to facial and/or vocal displays but occasionally extended to cover bodily gestures. **2** n. A class of SPEECH ACT which is generally used without any specific function other than to keep social interactions going smoothly. Included here are expressions like *please, thank you* and *excuse me*. Unlike most other speech acts, these appear to be learned by children purely by rote.

expressive amusia AMUSIA.

expressive aphasia BROCA'S *APHASIA.

expressive dysphasia DEVELOPMENTAL *LANGUAGE DISORDER.

expressive functions Loosely, those functions involved in the manifestation of underlying mental activity. Generally included are speaking, writing, drawing, manipulating, gesturing, and specific facial and bodily expressions and movements.

expressive language disorder DEVELOPMENTAL *LANGUAGE DISORDER.

expressive methods A general label for a variety of diagnostic and therapeutic techniques all of which require that the individual freely act out (or express) some particular role, part or fantasy. Included here are *psychodrama, play techniques* and *role-playing*. Expressive methods are generally regarded as forms of PROJECTIVE TECHNIQUES.

expressive writing disorder, developmental A disorder marked by impairment in the development of expressive writing skills. Written texts are marked by spelling and grammatical errors, poor punctuation and poor organization. The term is not used in cases in which the disability is the result of mental retardation, inadequate schooling or a neurological disorder.

extension 1 The spatial property of an object. **2** The movement by which the ends of something are pulled apart; hence, any muscle movement that straightens a limb. Contrast here with FLEXION. **3** In logic, the domain of a term or concept made up of all

those things which fall within it. In less formal terms, *extension* is roughly equivalent to DENOTATIVE *MEANING. See and compare with INTENSION.

extensor A muscle the action of which straightens a limb. Contrast with FLEXOR. Extensor and flexor muscles generally act to form a pair of ANTAGONISTIC MUSCLES.

external aim AIM (3).

external auditory meatus The canal from the external ear to the tympanic membrane.

external inhibition INHIBITION, EXTERNAL.

externalization A term with a number of usages in a number of disparate areas in psychology. All, however, share the underlying notion that some 'thing' initially internal or 'inside' gets represented, projected or manifested in the external world. Thus: **1** In learning, the process through which a drive becomes activated through external stimulation; e.g. hunger aroused by the smell of food, sexual desire by erotic literature. **2** In developmental psychology, the process through which a child gradually comes to differentiate between self and the external world, or not-self. **3** In social psychology and personality theory, the attribution of cause of behaviour to external factors, to chance events or to other fortuitous happenings over which one has (or feels one has) little control. See here INTERNALIZATION (1) and LOCUS OF CONTROL. **4** By extension, some use the term as approximately synonymous with PROJECTION (especially 1–6). This meaning derives from K. Horney's terms *active* and *passive externalization*, of which the former refers to the process whereby feelings about oneself are experienced as feelings about others, and the latter to the process whereby feelings toward others are experienced as their feelings about oneself. **5** In studies of *expressive function*, reacting to an event with an overt behavioural reaction, but little or nothing in the way of covert physiological responses.

externalizing behaviours In the study of children's problem behaviours, their reactions to stressors are commonly divided into *internalizing* and *externalizing* behaviours. In the former, stress is dealt with by focusing on the self, sometimes resulting in problems like depression or shyness. In the

latter, stress is dealt with by active behaviours directed toward the outside world,
sometimes resulting in displays of aggression, defiance and hyperactivity. Note that
while the original distinction rested on a particular model of psychopathology, the terms
are often used in a more descriptive, atheoretical manner.

external rectus One of the muscles controlling the eye.

external validity CRITERION-RELATED *VALID-
ITY.

exteroceptor A sensory receptor that is
stimulated by changes in the exterior
world. Compare with INTEROCEPTOR and PRO-
PRIOCEPTOR.

extinction Outside of evolutionary biology, in which it refers to the disappearance
of species, this term is used in two ways
which are often not kept separate. **1** An
experimental procedure in which the stimulus event that maintains the behaviour is
removed. In classical conditioning this
means presentation of the CS (conditional
stimulus) without the US (unconditional
stimulus); in operant or instrumental conditioning this amounts to withholding the
reinforcer even though the response occurs.
The term *experimental extinction* is occasionally used here. **2** Somewhat more loosely, the
actual decrease in the learned response
which results from this extinction procedure, i.e. the product of the procedure, not
the procedure itself.

extinction burst A sudden burst of rapid
and often vigorous responding that frequently occurs when an organism is shifted
from reinforced responding to extinction.

extinction, latent In the ordinary extinction procedure using operant or instrumental behaviour, an organism makes responses
that go unrewarded. If, prior to running
standard extinction trials, the organism is
placed in the usual setting but without the
opportunity to respond, a subsequent sharp
decrease in responsiveness is observed when
the extinction procedure is later introduced.
This effect of extinction without responding
is called latent extinction because of the conceptual parallel with LATENT *LEARNING.

extinction, secondary The weakening of

one response when a similar response undergoes experimental extinction.

extinction trial TRIAL, EXTINCTION.

extinguish Following the two meanings of
the term EXTINCTION: **1** To carry out the procedure of experimental extinction. **2** To
diminish the responsiveness of an organism
by running experimental extinction.

extinguished Generally, characterizing a
response that has been subjected to extinction procedures. There is also a curious tendency to speak of the organism itself as
having been extinguished when the
response no longer occurs. This sense of
the term is somewhat misleading but fairly
common.

extirpation Removal, usually surgical, of
an organ or bodily structure. When only
part of an organ or structure is removed the
term ABLATION is generally used.

extra- Prefix meaning: **1** *Outside of, beyond,
beside*, e.g. *extrasensory*. **2** By extension, *more*
of a thing; usually hyphenated, e.g. *extra-
strong*. var., *extro-*.

extracellular thirst VOLUMETRIC *THIRST.

extraception H. Murray's term for an outlook on life that is objective, concerned with
facts, sceptical. Contrast with INTRACEPTION.

extradimensional shift REVERSAL *LEARNING.

extrafusal fibres Muscle fibres that mediate the force extended by contraction.

extrajection An occasional synonym of
PROJECTION (especially 1–3).

extraocular muscles EYE MUSCLES.

extrapolate To estimate, from a series of
known values, the values of a variable that
are higher or lower than the known range.
The estimation is made on the assumption
that the trends already observed in the data
will continue. Extrapolations are useful but
subject to error because of unpredictable factors that may only reveal their effects at the
higher and lower ends of a continuum. Contrast with INTERPOLATE.

extrapunitive Characterizing the tendency
to react to frustration by showing anger
toward, and investing blame in, others. Con-

trast with INTROPUNITIVE and compare with IMPUNITIVE.

extrapyramidal motor system A set of complex, diffuse neural structures, both cortical and subcortical, including the basal ganglia, cerebellum, parts of the reticular formation and their connections with the motor neurons of the spinal cord and nuclei of the cranial nerves.

extrapyramidal syndrome A neurological disorder with a variety of signs and symptoms, including tremors, muscular rigidity, a shuffling gait, restlessness and difficulty in initiating movements. It results from dysfunctions of the extrapyramidal motor system and may occur as a side effect of some psychotropic drugs, especially the phenothiazine derivatives, which are used as antipsychotics. See also TARDIVE DYSKINESIA.

extrasensory perception (ESP) Lit., perception which occurs outside any known sensory system. An umbrella term for a number of hypothesized paranormal phenomena, including *clairvoyance*, *precognition* and *telepathy*. See PARAPSYCHOLOGY for a general discussion of these and related terms.

extraspectral hue Any hue that cannot be characterized by a single wavelength. Purple, which requires a mixture of long wavelengths (red) and short wavelengths (blue), is a good example.

extrastriate cortex Visual association cortex that surrounds the primary visual cortex (STRIATE CORTEX). It receives fibres from both the primary visual cortex and the superior colliculi (COLLICULUS). Also called *circumstriate cortex* and *prestriate cortex*.

extraversion Lit., turning outwards. Used primarily in personality theory to refer to the tendency to direct one's energies outwards, to be concerned with and derive gratification from the physical and social environment. var., *extroversion*. Contrast with INTROVERSION and EXTRAVERSION–INTROVERSION.

extraversion–introversion A hypothesized dimension of personality with two theoretical poles, EXTRAVERSION and INTROVERSION. Originally the dimension was considered to reflect two unitary personality types which were presumed opposites of each other. Today most theorists doubt that either exists

as a singular type and instead regard both as collections of a number of different patterns of behaviour. Moreover, it also seems unlikely that the two poles can be validly regarded as opposites since many persons exhibit aspects of both and may increase their display of behaviours reflective of one pole without necessarily diminishing display of behaviours reflective of the other.

extravert A label applied to an individual who displays the behaviours discussed under EXTRAVERSION. Jung also used the term for one of his personality types.

extrinsic 1 Characterizing a property of something that derives its essential nature from relationships with outside factors. Contrast with INTRINSIC. 2 Characterizing a property of something that lies wholly external to the subject. Contrast here with INHERENT.

extrinsic eye muscles EYE MUSCLES.

extrinsic interest Interest in an object or an activity that derives from its relationship to other, outside factors; e.g. learning to paint because of the prestige or income that might accrue from the skill. Compare with INTRINSIC INTEREST.

extrinsic motivation Lit., motivation that originates in factors outside the individual. Behaviour that is motivated by rewards and/ or punishments administered by outside forces is extrinsically determined. Usually the question of inner satisfaction or dissatisfaction is considered secondary. Thus, for example, many students strive mightily in school for the extrinsic reward of good grades with little concern for any knowledge or understanding that may be acquired along the way – their behaviour is said to be extrinsically motivated. Contrast with INTRINSIC MOTIVATION and see the extended discussion under the base term MOTIVATION.

extro- Variation of EXTRA-. Generally (but not always) used in contrast with INTRO-.

extroversion EXTRAVERSION.

extrovert EXTRAVERT.

eye The visual organ. Anatomically the term covers the eyeball (and related structures) and that portion of the optic nerve lying within the eye socket. Moving from the inside of the eye out, there are three coats that make up the eye itself. The innermost is the *retina*, which contains the RODS and CONES, the specific visual receptors, and a number of other neural structures that mediate the initial processing of visual input; see RETINA for details. Next is the *uvea*, which is collectively composed of the choroid, the ciliary body and the iris and is primarily nutritional in function. The outermost layer is made up of the *sclera* and *cornea*. Two cavities are enclosed between these layers: the anterior is the space lying in front of the lens and is filled with a watery *aqueous humour*; the cavity behind the lens is much larger and is filled with the gelatinous *vitreous body*.

eye-balling Laboratory slang for taking a quick look at one's data to see if any obvious trends can be perceived prior to (although one hopes not instead of) performing careful statistical analyses.

eyeblink conditioning EYELID CONDITIONING.

eyebrow flash A rapid raising of the eyebrows lasting about 1/6 second. It is a virtually universal sign of either greeting or flirtation.

eyelid conditioning A classical conditioning procedure used commonly with humans. The response is the BLINK REFLEX, usually evoked in response to a puff of air directed at the eye–cheek area.

eye movement desensitization and reprocessing therapy (EMDR) An INNOVATIVE THERAPY in which the person being treated focuses on an external perceptual stimulus such as the therapist's moving finger while holding in mind clinically relevant images and thoughts suggested by the therapist. Although there is some evidence that the procedure can ameliorate anxieties, this might be due to *general factors* or specific *cognitive-behavioural therapy* principles. Also called *rapid eye movement therapy*.

eye movements Obviously, movements of the eye. There are, however, several kinds of such movements; see e.g. CONVERGENCE, DIVERGENCE, FIXATION, NYSTAGMUS, OCULAR *PURSUIT, RAPID EYE MOVEMENT, SACCADE.

eye muscles The term covers two categories of muscles. The *extrinsic* or *extraocular* muscles are a set of six muscles attached to the tough outer coat of the eyeball (the *sclera*) that control the movements of the eyes. The *intrinsic* muscles are those of the iris and ciliary body and are typically not called, collectively, eye muscles but referred to by the structures they control.

eye regression REGRESSION (4).

eye span READING SPAN.

eye–voice span A measure of how far the eye is ahead of the voice in oral reading. Specifically, the number of words that a person can read out loud after the lights are turned off and the room becomes dark. It is often used as a measure of reading skill and as a procedure for investigating reading processes.

eyewitness testimony Basically a legal term for the use of an eyewitness to a crime to provide testimony in court about the identity of the perpetrator. The term, however, is common in FORENSIC PSYCHOLOGY, which has a large literature dealing with the reliability of eyewitnesses and the validity of their testimony.

Eysenck Personality Inventory A self-report personality inventory developed by the German-born British psychologist H. J. Eysenck. The inventory is based on Eysenck's factor theory of personality, which assumes three basic dimensions: *extraversion–introversion, neuroticism* and *psychoticism*.

F

F **1** Fahrenheit. **2** *F* RATIO. **3** *F* TEST. **4** FORMANT.

F$_0$ FUNDAMENTAL TONE.

F$_1$, F$_2$ **1** In genetics, the first and second filial generations. F$_1$ represents the offspring of two unlike individuals; F$_2$ represents the offspring of two individuals of the F$_1$ generation. **2** See FORMANT.

f **1** Frequency. **2** Fluency. **3** Function.

fables test A test in which the subject is required to provide interpretations of fables. Such tests have been used (not terribly successfully) as tests of intelligence and as projective devices (using ambiguous fables).

face blindness A deficit in the ability to identify faces. Unlike PROSOPAGNOSISA, which is caused by damage to brain areas that are involved in the identification of faces (e.g. the FUSIFORM GYRUS), this dysfunction appears to occur spontaneously in the population and to be familial, suggesting that there is a genetic basis for it. There is a suggestion that it might be a component in some cases of AUTISTIC SPECTRUM DISORDER.

face-en-face French for 'face-to-face'. This version of the phrase is found in the developmental literature for the face-to-face social interaction of parents, caretakers and young infants.

face-inversion effect The finding that inverting a human face impairs recognition to a greater degree than inverting a non-face figure does.

face saving In social psychology this term is used with essentially the same meaning as in common parlance: the protection of one's public image.

face-to-face group GROUP, FACE-TO-FACE.

face validity VALIDITY, FACE.

facial action coding system A system for classifying the emotional expressions of faces. Developed by Paul Ekman and collaborators, it is based on the analysis of specific muscles and the impact they have on facial features.

facial nerve The VIIth *cranial nerve*. A mixed nerve with efferent fibres to the facial muscles, the platysmal muscle of the neck and the sublingual glands and afferent fibres from the taste buds of the front two-thirds of the tongue.

facial paresis A disorder characterized by a partial paralysis of the facial muscles. In the *volitional* variety, which is caused by damage to the facial region of the primary motor cortex, the patient loses the ability to express an emotion voluntarily. However, when they experience the emotion their face reflects it appropriately. In the *emotional* form, in which the damage can be anywhere from the thalamus, through the white matter of the frontal lobe, to the insular region, the reverse pattern is seen. Both forms are usually lateralized and affect only one side.

facial vision Not vision at all; rather, the term refers to the ability to detect the presence of an object specifically without vision. Often found in the blind, the cues are provided primarily by echoes and, to a lesser extent, by air currents. Compare with OBSTACLE SENSE.

facies Loosely, the appearance of a thing. More specifically, characteristic of a face, particularly with regard to its appearance in a medical condition. Commonly used of the flat, muted expression seen in Parkinson's disease.

facilitated communication An approach to working with autistic children in which a facilitator holds the child's hand steady so he or she can type out messages on a keyboard. There are reasons for suspecting that the procedure may be of value in the case of children with neurological disorders that compromise physical functioning; there is no evidence whatsoever that it is of value for autism, despite the lavish claims of its supporters.

facilitation Generally, the act of making something easier, removing impediments or difficulties. The term is found in many combined forms, some of which follow; others may be found under the listing of the modifying term.

facilitation, neural Lowering the threshold for nerve conduction along a neural pathway. It may occur in a number of ways; e.g. by SUMMATION of several neural processes, by repeated excitation of the pathways or by inhibiting inhibitory fibres that converge on the synapse.

facilitation, retroactive Strengthening of the association between a stimulus and a response by the formation of new associations.

facilitator A term used for a therapist who serves as the 'leader' in particular kinds of group therapy settings. The notion is that the leader's role is not to direct so much as to help and guide the group members in their search for their own personal insights.

fact A proposition that has been, in S. J. Gould's words, 'confirmed to so high a degree that it would be perverse to withhold provisional assent'.

factitious **1** Characteristic of an artifact, made by humans. **2** Not real, not genuine.

factitious disorder An umbrella term for any psychological or psychiatric disorder the symptoms of which are voluntarily produced; factitious disorders are feigned and the disabilities displayed are simulated. Usually, however, this classification does not include MALINGERING, in which the illness is claimed for a particular purpose; in a factitious disorder there seems to be no obvious aim other than to play the 'patient role'. These disorders are often classified by patterns of symptoms and referred to accordingly; e.g. *factitious disorder with psychological symptoms* (also called *pseudopsychosis*), *factitious disorder with physical symptoms* (also called *Münchausen's syndrome*). Distinguish from SOMATOFORM DISORDER, the symptoms of which are not produced voluntarily and are not under the control of the individual.

factitious disorder by proxy A FACTITIOUS DISORDER in which one individual produces symptoms in another for the purpose of indirectly assuming the role of a sick individual. It is most commonly seen in a parent artificially creating physical symptoms in a child. When the second individual plays no active role in the creation of the symptoms, they are called *induced factitious symptoms*. Also called *Münchausen's by proxy*.

factitious disorder with physical symptoms The most common factitious disorder, characterized by the plausible presentation of physical symptoms that are apparently under the individual's control. A wide range of symptoms may emerge including back pain, nausea, vomiting, dizziness, rashes, abscesses, fevers of undetermined origin and secondary bleeding stemming from ingestion of anticoagulants. The patient's medical knowledge and imagination are the only limits. The patient with a true *Münchausen's syndrome* (as it is also called – after Baron Karl von Münchhausen, a notorious teller of tall tales) has typically had multiple hospitalizations and often multiple surgical procedures performed during them. Note that in the naming of the syndrome, the Baron lost an 'h'.

factitious disorder with psychological symptoms A factitious disorder characterized by the production of various symptoms of psychological disorders seemingly under the voluntary control of the patient. The condition is virtually always superimposed on a severe personality disorder, although the particular symptoms displayed are not explained by that disorder. A typical pattern is for the patient to complain of memory loss, hallucinations, and dissociative and conversion symptoms, and, often, to be discovered to have been secretly taking various drugs to produce symptoms that support the diagnosis of a nonorganic mental disorder. Also called *pseudopsychosis*.

fact memory MEMORY, FACT.

factor 1 Generally, anything that has some causal influence, some effect on a phenomenon. In this sense a factor is an antecedent condition, a cause. **2** By extension, an independent variable. This usage is common in statistical procedures based on analysis of variance; see FIXED *FACTOR, RANDOM *FACTOR. **3** In mathematics, any of the numbers which when multiplied together yield a specified product. **4** By extension of 3, one of the products of a factor analysis. Note that the factors in this sense are strictly no more than numbers in a factor matrix that function as in meaning 3, even though they are typically presented as though they represent some underlying trait (e.g. a *number factor* or a *verbal factor*). See FACTOR ANALYSIS for clarification of this usage.

factor analysis This term does not really represent a unitary concept, rather it serves as a cover term for a number of statistical procedures all of which function so as to locate a smaller number of dimensions, clusters or FACTORS (4) in a larger set of independent variables or items. The primary, distinctive element of a factor analysis is data reduction. Beginning with an array of correlation coefficients between all of the initial variables in the database (the number of which may be very large, especially if they are items from a personality inventory or an intelligence test), the factor-analytic techniques extract a small number of basic components that may be viewed as source variables that account for the interrelations observed in the data. Variables that correlate highly with each other become identified as representing a single factor; variables that do not correlate with each other are identified as representing orthogonal (or independent) factors. The ideal factor analysis would identify a small number of factors which were orthogonal to each other; that is, in spatial terms, they would lie at right angles to each other when graphed.

Note that the procedures are all strictly statistical; the factors that emerge from an analysis still have to be subjectively examined to determine whether they represent salient psychological dimensions. For example, in an IQ test the scores on a number of items may be found to correlate highly with each other and emerge as a statistical factor. Later examination of these items may reveal that all contain mathematical elements and thus may lead one to hypothesize the existence of a mathematical factor.

There is a tendency, particularly when factor-analytic techniques are applied to personality inventories, to identify the factors that emerge as *traits*. Strictly speaking, a factor is not a trait: a trait is inferred from a factor. A factor represents an underlying regularity in the data base, and the two terms should not be treated as synonymous. The establishment of a valid trait requires additional inferences; see TRAIT for discussion of usage and associated problems of meaning.

Factor analysis is an important tool in areas of psychology in which underlying components are suspected but difficult to discern, such as intelligence testing, personality assessment and semantics. The procedures themselves are quite complex, and some degree of mathematical sophistication is needed to understand and utilize them. In many of the entries that follow the conceptual basis of factor analytical terms is given; for the mathematical foundations and methods of application the reader should consult a text on factor analysis. vb., *factor analyse* (not *factor*, which is to find the multipliers of a product); adj., *factor analytical* (not *factorial*, which derives from FACTOR (1, 2)).

factor analysis, confirmatory Any factor analysis in which the number and content of factors is specified in advance in order to test whether a theoretical model is borne out by the data. Other parameters of the factors may also be specified in advance.

factor analysis, exploratory Any factor analysis in which the content of factors is not specified in advance, but determined by the statistical structure of the data themselves. The number of factors may or may not be specified in advance.

factor analysis, inverse A factor analysis applied to a correlation matrix of 'units' (e.g. individual persons, groups, objects) rather than to the individual items that each unit 'responds' to, which is the more usual technique. Often called the Q *technique* or Q *factor analysis*.

factor axes The set of coordinates that represent the relationships of the various factors to each other and to the full correlation matrix. The particular set that best represents a given database is determined by a process of FACTOR *ROTATION.

factor coefficient FACTOR LOADING.

factor configuration In factor analysis, the position of the system of lines or vectors that represents the several tests in the full correlation matrix. In spatial terms, the angles of the vectors to each other specify the correlations between them; right angles reflect orthogonal (or uncorrelated) vectors, acute angles reflect correlations with the degree of acuteness reflecting the degree of correlation. Note that the exact configuration of the factor structure is not unique and one solution may be transformed into another. There are many statistically equivalent ways to represent the underlying dimensions.

factor, first-order A factor that emerges from the matrix of test scores, from the original set of intercorrelations. Compare with a *second-order factor*, which is one that is derived from the intercorrelations among the first-order factors.

factor, fixed Any independent variable in an experiment in which the values that the variable may take are set (or fixed) by natural circumstances. For example, suppose there exist only 7 different brands of aspirin; an experiment evaluating and comparing them would have the 'brand' variable as a fixed factor. The results that emerge from the study are called *fixed effects*, and the data-analysis technique used to evaluate them is termed the *fixed effects model*. Compare with RANDOM *FACTOR.

factor, general (g or G) 1 Generally, a factor that is found in all of the tests subjected to a factor analysis. 2 Specifically, a factor hypothesized to be basic to all tests of ability. The notion of a general factor (or *g-factor* or, more simply, *g*) was first put forward in 1904 by the British psychometrician Charles Spearman as representing a single ability that could be taken to represent intelligence. It must be appreciated that *g* has not (and probably cannot) be shown to exist as a separate measurable entity. Spearman identified it on the basis of factor analysis of the various components of an intelligence test. The logical argument is that since the several component skills assessed tended to be positively correlated with each other (i.e. high scores on verbal subtests are accompanied by high scores on numerical subtests, etc.), then they can all be thought of as reflective of a general ability that underlies them. However, it must be recognized that, since *g* is identified in this manner, it is an outcome of a particular form of factor analysis – not all factor analytic procedures will yield such a characterization even when applied to the same database. This point was made by L. L. Thurstone when he showed that other procedures lead to the uncovering of a number of PRIMARY *FACTORS rather than a single core factor. With Thurstone's methods, *g*, if it exists at all, is found only as a *second-order factor* and accounts for very little of the data from intelligence tests; with Spearman's methods it accounts for most of the data. Hence, *g* must be viewed not as a 'real' ability but as a hypothetical ability the existence of which is dependent on methodological procedures.

factor, group A factor that emerges from high intercorrelations between two or more tests in the set of tests analysed but does not correlate with all tests. Most of the factors that have emerged from factor-analysing intelligence tests (e.g. verbal, arithmetic, analytical) are group factors.

factor, hereditary Simply, a gene. By extension, any transfer of information via the genetic material.

factorial design DESIGN, FACTORIAL.

factorial invariance The extent to which the results of a factor analysis remain unaltered when new tests are introduced and the full analysis is repeated, or when a new set of subjects is run and the full set of data is reanalysed.

factoring Generally, finding FACTORS. However, *factoring* is usually reserved for finding FACTORS (3); for finding FACTORS (4) the preferred term is *factor analysing*.

factor loading A value that expresses the degree to which any given factor accounts for the total variability of the full set of correlations on which a factor analysis has been carried out. That is, the extent to which it correlates with the test itself or the full set of items analysed. The higher the factor loading, the more salient the factor. Also called *factor weight* or *weighting*.

factor matrix In most general terms, a table (i.e. matrix) that gives the factor loadings that emerge from a factor analysis. Actually, a variety of specific kinds of factor matrices may be found depending on the kind(s) of transformations one makes on the data. In such cases qualifiers are used to indicate the kind of matrix under consideration.

factor, primary Any of the factors that emerge in the final stages of factor analysis; i.e. the point at which further mathematical manipulations fail to account for substantially more of the variance and the factors have been located (by ROTATION) so that the number of factors needed to account for the intercorrelations is minimized. Also called *terminal factor*.

factor, random Any independent variable in an experiment in which the values that the variable may take are very large (or infinite) and the actual values of the factor used in the study are selected at random. Results from a study using such variables are termed *random effects* and the data-analysis technique used to evaluate them is called the *random effects model*. Compare with FIXED *FACTOR.

factor reflection REFLECTION (4).

factor resolution R. B. Cattell's term for the finally accepted interpretation of a factor analysis; that is, the particular position of the factor axes after rotation in relation to the test vectors. Thurstone originally used the term FACTOR STRUCTURE here and many still do.

factor rotation ROTATION (2).

factor space The region within which a set of factors may be represented. The factor space is defined by the set of intercorrelations in the analysis and is not necessarily two-or three-dimensional and not necessarily Euclidean.

factor, specific A factor that is found in only one test or one unique group of items all of which reflect the same variable. Compare with GENERAL *FACTOR and GROUP *FACTOR. Also called *unique factor*.

factor structure FACTOR RESOLUTION.

factor theory A general label applied to any theory of psychological phenomena that characterizes things in terms of various FACTORS. The term is typically used for theories of personality and of intelligence that have extracted their hypothesized factors from factor-analysing batteries of tests or personality inventories. However, there is also a tendency to use it for any theory that hypothesizes two (or more) distinguishable processes or components for a psychological process; e.g. the so-called two-factor theory of learning, which maintains that both classical and operant conditioning processes are needed to explain complex behaviour, or the *two-factor theories of memory*, which assumes both episodic and semantic memory systems. The key to distinguishing these two patterns of usage is to note that the base term *factor theory* generally uses FACTOR in sense 4, while terms that begin *n-factor theory* generally use it in sense 1.

factor weight FACTOR LOADING.

factual knowledge DECLARATIVE *KNOWLEDGE.

faculty psychology Historically, a faculty was defined as a general power of the mind, a cognitive ability such as intellect, will, memory or understanding. Faculty psychology approached the study of the human mind by attempting to account for mental processes in terms of a fixed number of such powers or abilities. The *phrenologists* presented the ultimate in this kind of theorizing. Although regarded as a discredited historical curiosity for decades, faculty psychology has recently been revived under the name of *modularity*, coined owing to the practice of hypothesizing cognitive and perceptual modules (e.g. a language module, a numerical module). See MODULARITY HYPOTHESIS.

fading A technique in behaviourally oriented training in which a new stimulus is presented along with an old one to which a response has already been learned. The old stimulus is then gradually diminished in size or intensity or clarity (i.e. faded) and the new one gains control over the response.

failure to thrive Inadequate weight gain and generally overall poor physical, motor and cognitive development in infants under the age of two. It may be due to low levels of GROWTH HORMONE or REACTIVE ATTACHMENT DISORDER. The former has a good prognosis with appropriate treatment; the latter, less so.

faith healing Healing presumably accomplished through faith or belief in the power of the healer, the therapist, the therapeutic procedure or something else. See PLACEBO and PLACEBO EFFECT for more insight into how such 'healing' occurs.

fallacy An argument involving logically invalid or improper reasoning, and, by extension, a conclusion reached by such unsound reasoning. Note that the meaning of the term depends on the reasoning and not on what is reasoned. Although fallacies usually lead to false conclusions they do not do so by definition; it is quite possible to reach a valid conclusion by faulty means.

fallacy of personal validation See BARNUM EFFECT.

fallacy, planning The common underestimation of the amount of time it will take to complete a task. It appears to be due to a tendency to focus only on some of the steps that need to be completed.

fall chronometer A rather clever device from experimental psychology's early days for measuring short time intervals by assessing the distance a weight fell.

fallectomy Surgical severing of the Fallopian tubes. See SALPINGECTOMY.

false That which is not TRUE (1 and 2).

false alarm In SIGNAL-DETECTION THEORY, the statement by a subject that a stimulus was present when in fact no stimulus occurred. Contrast with HIT.

false-belief task A task used with young children to assess their understanding of reality and how other people perceive it. Children are asked to predict how some deceptive object will appear to another person. For example, after children are shown a candy box that turns out to hold pencils, they are asked what someone else will expect to see when they open the box. Children around the age of 3 consistently believe the other person will expect to see pencils, older children correctly believe that others will

expect candy. The task is often used to determine whether a child has a THEORY OF MIND. See also APPEARANCE-REALITY TASK.

false-consensus effect (or **bias**) The tendency to overestimate the degree to which one's opinions and beliefs are shared by others. It derives from the AVAILABILITY HEURISTIC, in that people tend to spend more time with others who think and believe as they do.

false hope syndrome A cognitive-behavioural cycle of attempts at self-change characterized by: (a) setting a goal which is probably unattainable (e.g. losing one-quarter of body weight in 3 months); (b) failure to attain this unrealistic goal (e.g. losing only one-tenth of body weight); (c) attribution of failure to factors that are unstable or modifiable (e.g. wrong diet); and (d) re-attempting to reach the goal rather than acknowledging that the goal is unrealistic and should be modified. It is easy to understand how the syndrome got its name.

false memory MEMORY, FALSE.

false memory syndrome See FALSE *MEMORY and RECOVERED *MEMORY.

false negative A case of improper exclusion. Since all tests (e.g. civil service exams, college entrance exams) are less than perfect, some individuals who score below the cut-off and are thus excluded would actually perform successfully; they are the *false negatives*. Similarly, there are those who score above the cut-off and are included but later fail to perform successfully; these are the *false positives*. The concepts underlying this example are quite general and the terms are found widely in medical science, in decision-making, in psychophysical investigations, etc.

false positive FALSE NEGATIVE.

false pregnancy PSEUDOCYESIS.

false transmitter A substance that binds with postsynaptic receptors but does not activate them. Such substances act as antagonists in that by occupying the receptor sites they prevent the normal NEUROTRANSMITTER from exerting its effects.

false vocal cords VENTRICULAR FOLDS.

falsificationism The philosophical point of view, associated with the philosopher of science Sir Karl R. Popper, that holds that scientific theories cannot be proven to be true but only subjected to attempts at refutation. From this point of view, a scientific theory is accepted not because it is demonstrably a correct codification of a class of phenomena but because it has not yet been shown to be false. This position is usually contrasted with the older position of *verificationism*, which argues that scientific work consists of the attempt to substantiate (i.e. verify) the correctness of a theory by logical and empirical means.

familial Lit., pertaining to the FAMILY. Generally used with the notion of *common to* members of a family, and in this sense may refer either to factors that are hereditary and genetic or to factors that make up a family's social or cultural heritage.

familial Alzheimer's disease ALZHEIMER'S DISEASE.

family 1 Most strictly, the fundamental unit of kinship. In its minimal or nuclear form the family consists of mother, father and offspring. In broader usage the term may refer to the *extended* family, which may include grandparents, cousins, adopted children, etc., all operating as a recognized social unit. Sociologists and anthropologists have literally dozens of other special classifications for various kinds of family units as they are represented in different cultures and societies. **2** By extension, a group of people with close social or personal ties, even though there may be no blood relationships between them. **3** By further extension, any collection of closely or formally related items or events; hence, in mathematics one refers to a family of curves, in social psychology to a family of traits or attitudes, in linguistics to a language family, etc. **4** In biology, a taxonomic classification of related genera (or sometimes a single genus) within an order.

family constellation The complex set of relationships within a family, dictated in large part by the number of family members, their ages and the pattern of functional interactions between them.

family therapy An umbrella term for a number of therapeutic approaches all of which treat a family as a whole rather than singling out specific individuals for inde-

pendent treatment. The term is neutral theoretically; one can practise family therapy within many different frameworks.

fan effect The phenomenon whereby it takes longer to retrieve any particular fact about a concept as one learns more about it. The term refers to the fanning out of the information base. One explanation is that, as the information base fans out, the individual associations connecting facts to the concept are weakened.

fantasy Generally, the mental process of imagining objects, symbols or events not immediately present. However, it is also used to refer to a symbol or image itself. In general, fantasy is assumed to be normal, even indicative of psychological stability and health. It is usually pleasant, often whimsical and frequently creative. The pathological aspects that are often cited are restricted to those cases in which a fantasy becomes delusionary or when it dominates a person's mental life and serves as a retreat from reality rather than an adjunct to it. var., *phantasy*.

FAP (or fap) FIXED ACTION PATTERN.

far point The most remote point distinctly visible under conditions of relaxed accommodation. Contrast with NEAR POINT.

farsightedness Any visual condition where objects at a distance are seen relatively clearly but near objects are out of focus. See PRESBYOPIA and HYPEROPIA for specific forms.

FAS FOETAL ALCOHOL SYNDROME.

fasciculus Any bundle of nerve fibres; an occasional synonym of TRACT.

fashioning effect The fact that the social role adopted by a person influences both that person's behaviour and their self-perceptions.

fastigial nucleus A deep cerebellar nucleus; it receives information from the *vermis* and sends its outputs to the *vestibular nucleus* and the motor nuclei in the *reticular formation*.

fasting phase A metabolic phase during which the digestive system does not supply nutrients. The body's needs during this period are derived from other sources, specifically from glycogen, proteins and adipose tissue.

fast mapping MAPPING.

fast (twitch) muscle MUSCLE TWITCH (1).

fatal familial insomnia INSOMNIA, FATAL FAMILIAL.

fatalism The philosophical view that all events are predetermined and subject to fate, a deity, the stars, etc. Free will or any act of volition is assumed to be futile. Differentiate fatalism from DETERMINISM; the latter stresses that all events have antecedent causes but does not assume that they are metaphysically *pre*determined.

father complex OEDIPUS COMPLEX.

father figure One who takes the place and hence the role of a real father. The term may be used with either of two connotations: **1** The sense that the person has taken over the full complement of functions of the real father he has replaced; i.e. a stepfather or foster-father. **2** The sense that the person fulfils psychologically important functions, in particular that of becoming the male adult with whom a child identifies. As the word *figure* suggests, meaning 2 is the dominant one and indeed may be what is intended even when the father figure has taken on the role described in 1. Some authors use *father surrogate* for 1 to prevent confusion. Also occasionally called *father imago*.

father fixation An excessive focusing of emotional attachment on the male parent. The term implies a rigid focusing, so that there is difficulty in shifting affective attention away from the father to other more socially accepted persons. The equivalent process centred on the female parent is called, not surprisingly, *mother fixation*.

father imago FATHER FIGURE.

father surrogate One who stands in place of the real father. See FATHER FIGURE and SURROGATE for details.

fatigue 1 n. The diminution in ability to do work that results from previous efforts. **2** n. The internal state or condition experienced as a feeling of weariness or tiredness that results from extended effort and underlies the diminished capacity to perform. These meanings are very general; a number of more specific senses are often intended and are usually marked by a qualifier that identifies the source of or the basis for the fatigue. Thus, *sensory fatigue* refers to the reduced responsiveness of a sense organ following prolonged exposure to stimulation (see ADAPTATION (1)); *neuronal* or *neural fatigue* is a heightened threshold of nerve fibres caused by previous neural activity (see REFRACTORY PERIOD et seq.); *muscle fatigue* refers to the reduced capacity of muscle tissue to contract owing to a build-up of metabolic waste products such as lactic acid; *emotional fatigue* is the general debilitated state resulting from excessive conflicts, frustrations, anxieties, etc.; *mental fatigue* refers to a cognitive weariness stemming from either extended mental concentration or boredom; and so forth. Note that these specialized terms are employed to identify the source of the fatigue, some by specifying the external conditions that produce it (e.g. *emotional, mental*), and some by specifying the underlying neurological and/or physiological effects that are responsible for it (e.g. *neural, muscle*). Note that some authors take a behaviouristic stance here and treat fatigue purely in terms of performance decrements; others take a sharp physiological line and view it in terms of biological (dys)function; still others treat it more phenomenologically as an experienced internal state; most, alas, confound all of these meanings. vb., *to fatigue*. See also EXHAUSTION.

fatty acid Any of three substances (stearic acid, oleic acid and palmitic acid) that, along with GLYCEROL, make up the adipose (fatty) tissue found beneath the skin and in various locations in the abdomen.

F distribution DISTRIBUTION, *F*.

fear An emotional state in the presence or anticipation of a dangerous or noxious stimulus. Fear is usually characterized by an internal, subjective experience of extreme agitation, a desire to flee or to attack, and a variety of sympathetic reactions (see AUTONOMIC NERVOUS SYSTEM). Fear is often differentiated from ANXIETY on one (or both) of two grounds: (a) fear is treated as involving specific objects or events while anxiety is regarded as a more general emotional state; (b) fear is considered a reaction to a present danger, anxiety to an anticipated or imagined one. See also PHOBIA, a specific, persistent, irrational fear.

fearful style ATTACHMENT STYLES.

fear-induced aggression AGGRESSION, FEAR-INDUCED.

fear module A hypothesized MODULE that underlies the emotion of fear. The modularity notion is based on the fact that fear has a fairly specific neural locus (the *amygdala*), operates independently of conscious control and has a reasonably well-understood evolutionary history.

fear of success SUCCESS, FEAR OF.

feature Shorthand for DISTINCTIVE FEATURE.

feature detector A general term used for any built-in perceptual mechanism hypothesized to detect single distinctive features in complex displays. Usually the feature detected is specified; e.g. *line detector* or *edge detector* in vision, *voice-onset time detector* in speech perception.

feature model A class of models of human memory based on the assumption that information is stored in the form of a set of distinctive (semantic) features that uniquely identify each concept. See SEMANTIC FEATURE for more detail and compare with SEMANTIC NETWORK MODEL.

febrile Feverish.

Fechner's colours Subjective colour sensations that appear when black and white sectors are rotated moderately rapidly on a colour wheel. If the rotation is slowed, the sensation is of a series of black radii on a white background called *Charpentier's bands*.

Fechner's law A psychophysical generalization which states that the intensity of subjective sensation increases as the logarithm of the stimulus intensifies. That is, when physical stimuli increase geometrically the psychological experience increases arithmetically. Formally, $\psi = k$ logS, where ψ = sensation, S = stimulus and k is a constant. Named after its discoverer, the great 19th-century psychophysicist Gustav Theodor Fechner (1801–87), the law is based on early work by E. H. Weber. See also WEBER'S LAW and WEBER–FECHNER LAW.

Fechner's paradox The surprising finding that an object viewed monocularly increases in brightness after being viewed binocularly.

fecundity The capacity to produce offspring, often used with the connotation of being highly fruitful, bountiful. adj., *fecund*, vb., *fecundate*. Compare with FERTILITY.

feeble-minded MENTAL DEFICIENCY.

feedback **1** Originally, in engineering, information that signals an ongoing operation in a system or the state of a system at a point in time. A speedometer provides feedback to a driver about distance travelled per unit of time. **2** In *cybernetics* the meaning was expanded to include such information as is utilized by a system to make adjustments and modifications in its operations. A thermostat uses feedback about room temperature to turn the heating system on or off. See SERVOMECHANISM. Meaning 2 has been enthusiastically borrowed by psychology and applied to a variety of situations. Hence: **3** In studies of sensorimotor processes, the information provided by kinaesthetic report from receptors in muscles and points to guide directed movement. See e.g. FITT'S LAW. **4** In learning, any information about the correctness or appropriateness of a response. The early cognitive theorists adopted this meaning as a replacement for the behaviourist notion of reinforcement. For example, a light that signalled whether a choice was correct or not in a problem-solving task was *feedback* to a cognitivist – somehow it hardly seemed to qualify as a *reinforcer* in the sense that that term was also applied to food for a rat at the end of a maze. **5** In social psychology, any reaction from the environment (including other people) that serves as a basis for future action. A return smile is termed *social feedback*. As a generalization, it seems safe to conclude that the term may be applied to any information about the functioning of one or more components of a system that leads to modification of functioning. Occasionally it is used to refer to the process or the system itself rather than the information that is 'fed back'. To prevent confusion some authors use *feedback loop* or *feedback circuit* for the process.

feedback loop FEEDBACK.

feedforward networks In connectionist systems (see CONNECTIONISM (2)), networks in which the information from the input units is fed upwards (i.e. forward) through successive hidden layers to the final output units.

feeding behaviour An umbrella term for all the behavioural components involved in normal eating, including preparatory behaviours, such as foraging for food, actual consumption of food, and the large number of physiological processes involved in the utilization of what has been eaten.

feeding centre A term occasionally used to refer to the lateral hypothalamus, which, when stimulated, causes an animal to begin eating. See HYPOTHALAMUS for more detail.

feeding disorder EATING DISORDERS.

feeding disorder of infancy or early childhood A general term for any feeding disorder characterized by an infant's or child's persistent failure to eat adequately so that he or she either loses weight or fails to gain it at a normal rate. Examples are RUMINATION DISORDER OF INFANCY and PICA.

feeding problem A loose term for any difficulty in getting a child to eat properly. It is not applied to serious EATING DISORDERS.

feeling It is particularly difficult to isolate precise usages of this term since even the most technical are contaminated by popular connotations. **1** Most generally, experiencing, sensing or having a conscious process. More specifically: **2** A *sensory impression*, meaning a sensation such as warmth or pain. **3** An *affective state*, as in a sense of well-being, depression, desire, etc. **4** One of the dimensions of emotion, particularly in reference to the hypothesized elementary emotional continua, such as in Wundt's three dimensions of feeling. **5** *Belief*, as in a vague opinion or notion about something not supported by any real evidence.

The difficulty with the term is that its use is nearly always metaphoric and somehow we all seem quite convinced that we know what we mean when we use it. See also EMOTION et seq., especially THEORIES OF *EMOTION, for more on the terminology of this area of psychology.

feeling of knowing A general, vague sense that we know the answer to a question or have seen or experienced a particular stimulus. The underlying mechanisms that pro-duce this experience are thought to be ones that mediate IMPLICIT *MEMORY and IMPLICIT *LEARNING. Often abbreviated FOK, although be careful when pronouncing this acronym.

feeling type One of Jung's hypothesized personality types. See FUNCTION TYPES.

female impersonator TRANSVESTISM.

femaleness The condition of possessing the physiological and anatomical characteristics of a female as they relate to reproductive capacity. Distinguish from FEMININITY.

female orgasmic disorder ORGASM DISORDERS.

female sexual arousal disorder A SEXUAL AROUSAL DISORDER marked by a woman's persistent or recurrent inability to attain or maintain an adequate lubrication–swelling response to sexual excitement.

feminicula From the Latin, the female form of HOMUNCULUS.

femininity Lit., the state of an organism reflecting or displaying the appearances, traits and behaviour patterns characteristic of the female of the species. Distinguish from FEMALENESS. See also MASCULINITY.

fenestra Latin for *window*. See OVAL WINDOW (*fenestra ovalis* or *vestibuli*) and ROUND WINDOW (*fenestra rotunda*).

fenfluramine A serotonin *agonist* that is used to suppress appetite in obese patients. It has been linked with heart valve problems and has been withdrawn from most markets.

feral child *Feral* means wild or existing in a state of nature. A feral child, then, is one reared in social isolation either by animals or with only indirect contact with humans. The large number of myths about 'wolf children' and the like have great popular and literary appeal, although carefully documented cases are rare. See WILD BOY OF AVEYRON for one excellent case.

Féré phenomenon (or method) GALVANIC SKIN RESPONSE.

Ferry–Porter law The generalization that critical flicker frequency increases with the log of the brightness of the stimulus. The relationship is independent of the wavelength of the stimulus. Also known as *Porter's law*.

fertility 1 Reproductive capability. 2 Figuratively, mental productivity or creativity, the having of many novel ideas. adj., *fertile*. Compare with FECUNDITY.

fertility, differential 1 Generally, differences in the fertility rate in various segments or classes of a society. 2 More specifically, the difference in the fertility rate of the upper and lower socioeconomic classes of a society. Typically the former is low relative to the latter – a fact which predictably bothers some and not others. 3 Most specifically, the number of offspring of any one couple compared with others.

fertility rate An index of the fertility of a large population. It is typically taken as the number of offspring born per 1,000 women of childbearing age. Note that various upper and lower limits are used to define this age; the broadest range commonly used is 15–49.

fertilization The impregnation of an ovum by a spermatozoon.

festinating gait An abnormal gait seen in PARKINSON'S DISEASE. It is marked by difficulty in initiating walking with a stuttering start followed by slowly speeding up to normal and an upper body lean for balance.

fetal FOETAL.

fetal programming FOETAL PROGRAMMING.

fetish 1 Generally, any object of blind devotion or reverence. 2 The object of a FETISHISM. 3 Popularly, a fetishism itself.

fetishism 1 This term connotes a kind of religious activity that emphasizes the worship of inanimate objects believed to have magical or transcendent powers. Often found in connection with ANIMISM. 2 A PARA-PHILIA characterized by obtaining sexual arousal and satisfaction with some object or some part of the body not generally considered erogenous. Fetishes are usually articles (e.g. shoes, gloves, handkerchiefs) used by others, often but not always of the opposite sex, or parts of the body (e.g. hair, feet).

fetus FOETUS.

FFF Abbreviation for *flicker fusion frequency*. See CRITICAL FLICKER FREQUENCY.

FI Abbreviation for *fixed interval*. See SCHEDULES OF *REINFORCEMENT.

fibre Any thread-like strand of living material; several fibres running together make up tissue. *Fibre* is also occasionally used synonymously with *nerve fibre* or *neuron*. var., *fiber*.

fibril Any small, fine filament which runs through the cell body passing out into axons and dendrites and to peripheral processes.

fibrillation 1 The process of formation of fibrils or other minute fibres. 2 Rapid quivering contraction of muscle fibres.

fibromyalgia syndrome A chronic disorder with a variety of poorly defined symptoms, including muscle aches, fatigue, sleep disturbances, bowel problems and anxiety. Problems in identifying and diagnosing the syndrome are similar to those encountered in cases of CHRONIC FATIGUE SYNDROME.

fiction Generally in psychology, and especially in psychoanalytic approaches, any hypothetical entity, internal state or theoretical process that is treated as if it actually existed; see here the discussion under 'AS IF'. The term is particularly common in Adler's approach to personality; see here FICTIONAL FINALISM, GUIDING *FICTION.

fictional finalism A term coined by Alfred Adler to encapsulate his beliefs that (a) one is motivated more by one's expectation for the future than by one's experiences in the past, and (b) such projected expectations are often fictional in that they may be unrealizable or unattainable. In Adler's positivistic outlook fictional finalism may function to motivate great accomplishments. A classic Adlerian neurosis emerges, however, when one cannot step outside the fiction and confront reality.

fiction, guiding In Adler's approach to personality, a persistent but largely unconscious train of thought or principle by which a person directs, coordinates and categorizes experiences. In the well balanced, guiding fictions are assumed to approximate reality and to be quite flexible and adaptive. In the neurotic they are assumed to be somewhat divorced from reality and tend to become rigid and nonadaptive. Note that *fiction* is used here to denote an abstraction or schema which is not necessarily fictitious and tends to function as if it were true. Hence, many Adlerians prefer to use the phrase *guiding idea*, which is less ambiguous.

fiducial limits CONFIDENCE LIMITS.

field 1 Generally, a bounded area. In the most straightforward physical sense areas are defined by boundaries. The notion of an area without bounds is nonsensical: a field of green is defined by the points at which the green ceases. However, in psychological parlance usage tends toward the metaphoric. Generally this presents no problems since the term is rarely used without some qualifier that specifies the boundaries of the field and hence defines it. Examples include *visual field*, meaning all those points in space that can be seen at a point in time and from a particular location, and *attentional field*, meaning those objects, thoughts and concepts within one's consciousness. **2** In discussions of FIELD THEORY the term takes on a more dynamic and extended meaning. Here it becomes a generalized kind of psychological space that includes an organism and its environment. The various forms of field theory all emphasize the interactions between an organism and the configuration of the organism's perceptions.

field dependence (and **independence**) Simply, these two terms refer to a continuum along which an individual may be placed to characterize the extent to which his or her perceptions are dependent on (or independent of) cues in the environment (or field). In the first and simplest test used to study this factor a subject had to align a stimulus (such as a rod) so that it was truly vertical when a second stimulus (such as a frame around the rod) was varied with respect to the true vertical. Persons who can set the rod relatively accurately independently of the orientation of the frame are called field independent, because they rely on bodily sensation cues rather than on cues in the field. The more the tilt in the field influences the setting of the rod, the more field dependent a person is. More elaborate studies were carried out later using chairs and whole rooms that could be tilted. The study of the trait of field dependence/independence began as an investigation of perception, but the large individual differences that were found gradually moved

the research into the areas of personality, cognitive style and even psychopathology.

field force FIELD THEORY.

field investigation FIELD RESEARCH.

field of regard REGARD.

field research Research carried out in a natural setting ('in the field'). Included here is almost all the work in ethology using naturalistic observation techniques, a good deal of the work in developmental psychology, and in applied areas such as market research and industrial psychology.

field theory Loosely, any theory that focuses on the total psychological environment (i.e. the 'field') and attempts to explain behaviour as resulting from the dynamic interaction between forces in it. Field theory developed from Gestalt psychology primarily through the work of Wolfgang Köhler and Kurt Lewin. Köhler drew the parallel between psychological field processes and electromagnetic fields of force. His argument was that any psychological process is dependent upon the interactions in the field and cannot be viewed except from this dynamic point of view. The position is sharply holistic and critical of elementaristic approaches. Köhler extrapolated the general theory into the areas of physiological psychology, particularly the physiological basis of perception, and argued for the existence of electrical brain fields that corresponded to phenomenological experience. See ISOMORPHISM (2).

Lewin's theorizing focused more on social psychology and personality theory. The field represented the total environment, including the individual and all significant other people, and came to be known as the LIFE SPACE. Behaviour was represented as movement through the regions of the life space, some of which are attractive (i.e. those with positive valence) and others unattractive (those with negative valence). Like Köhler's position this perspective is holistic and dynamic.

figural aftereffects Distortions of perception that occur after long exposure to certain stimulus conditions. For example, if a slightly curved line is fixated on for several minutes and then replaced by a straight line, the straight line will appear to curve in the opposite direction. The process underlying such effects is quite complex and not well understood. They can occur in any sensory modality that can yield the experience of form – for example, holding a curved block in the hand will produce a figural aftereffect in *haptic* perception; they are not receptor-specific – expose the left eye and the after-effect is produced in the right eye; and they can last for days.

figural cohesion The tendency for all parts of a figure to 'hang together' even though they may be but disjointed lines.

figural fluency tests A general label for a group of related tests in which the subject is required to produce a variety of figures. In some tests the figures are copied, in some they are drawn following instructions, in others dots must be connected. They are useful in diagnosis of various neurological disorders.

figural synthesis U. Neisser's term for the notion that form perception is based on a process of active construction of meaning from a stimulus.

figurative language LANGUAGE, FIGURATIVE.

figure Of the multitude of meanings found in standard dictionaries two figure importantly in psychology: **1** A kind of unitary, cohesive, perceptual experience. Figures in this sense are characterized by contour, structure, coherence and solidity; see FIGURE–GROUND. **2** A person who represents the essential attributes of a stereotyped role, e.g. a *father figure*.

figure, ambiguous An umbrella term for any visual stimulus that permits of more than one interpretation. Although a good case can be made that ambiguity is an inherent feature of *all* displays, the term is typically reserved for a class of stimuli that readily lend themselves to two (or more) interpretations which look different from each other and in which contextual constraints affect what one perceives. The classic example here is Boring's old woman/young woman drawing, reproduced above.

Note also that some authors treat REVERSIBLE *FIGURES and EMBEDDED FIGURES as belonging in this category. While this inclusion is defensible in that such figures are indeed ambiguous, other authorities argue that they should be kept separate. The arguments here are: (a)

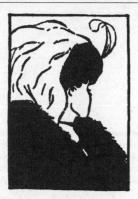

embedded figures are not really available for multiple interpretations but merely difficult to detect owing to the context within which they are embedded; and (b) reversible figures have the property that they shift back and forth spontaneously and are relatively immune to any imposed interpretative bias. There is, however, precious little consistency in terminology here.

figure–ground A term used to describe the perceptual relationship between an object of focus (the figure) and the rest of the perceptual field (the ground). The figure generally has form or structure and appears to be in front of the ground. The ground is seen as relatively homogeneous and as extending behind the figure. The relationship, in many instances, can be reversed by focusing on or attending to the ground rather than the figure.

The best way to conceptualize the notion of a figure–ground relationship is to appreciate that the CONTOUR or boundary that 'separates' the figure from the background *physically* belongs to both of them but *perceptually* belongs to the figure. Hence, the figure is given form and shape and the background is left unshaped and lacking in form.

figure, hidden Synonym of *embedded figure*.

figure, impossible Any of a class of figures in which the several components produce conflicting interpretations. In the example given here the right side has cues for a two-pronged object but the left for a three-

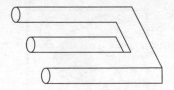

pronged object. Resolution of the whole figure is thus rendered impossible.

figure, reversible Any of a class of figures that undergo spontaneous reversal of perspective when steadily fixated on. The orientation of the Necker cube given here shifts when stared at.

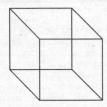

file drawer problem A problem that emerges in attempts to determine, through published research, whether a particular effect is real. The difficulty emerges when the effect is small (or perhaps nonexistent) and so is only obtained occasionally. Those researchers who find it report it; those who fail to find it tend not to publish their work, leaving it instead in their file drawers. A noneffect can be made to appear real when large numbers of nonfindings are stuck in file drawers while the few anomalous positive findings are published, misleading all concerned. PARAPSYCHOLOGY is an area seriously contaminated by this problem.

filial Pertaining to offspring and descendants.

filial generation F_1, F_2.

filial piety The set of moral obligations between children and parents. There are large cultural differences in how strict these obligations are and in their importance in the development of social roles.

filial regression, law of A principle of genetics characterized by a regression toward the mean of traits between the members of filial generations. That is, offspring of two very tall parents will tend to be taller than the average of the whole population but less than the average of their parents' heights. Naturally, the principle is a generalization that holds only when large populations are considered.

filiform papilla LINGUAL PAPILLA.

filled pause PAUSE, FILLED.

filler (material) Material unrelated to the specific experimental manipulations of a study. Such material is often used in studies on language, in questionnaires, on attitude scales, etc., where the filler items help to disguise the true nature of the investigation. Also called *filler items, buffer items* or *buffer material*.

film colour COLOUR, FILM.

filter Any device that screens out (i.e. filters) particular stimuli or specific components of a complex stimulus, permitting other stimuli or parts thereof to pass through. The term is used broadly: it may be a lens that only transmits certain wavelengths (a light filter), an electronic device that allows only particular sound frequencies to pass (an acoustic filter), a highly restrictive acoustic filter that only passes a narrow band of frequencies (a band pass filter), etc. Note that the term is also used metaphorically in reference to hypothesized perceptual and cognitive processes; see FILTER THEORY.

filter, Gabor Named for the Hungarian physicist Dennis Gabor, a filter defined by complex mathematical relations between harmonic and Gaussian functions. Gabor filters have been proposed as a mechanism for how cells in the primary visual cortex function since they can, in principle, account for how cells filter specific stimuli and allow for detection of edges, orientations and stimulus intensities. A *Gabor pattern, stimulus* or *patch* is a graphic representation of the operating characteristics of a Gabor filter.

filter theory In research on PATTERN RECOGNITION, any theory that proposes a neural mechanism tuned to either detect or block certain patterns of perceptual input. Early theories like the TEMPLATE MATCHING MODEL specified cell groups that would block all except certain inputs so that an 'A'-filter would block any visual input other than an 'A' from proceeding to be processed by appropriate brain centres. More recent theories posit neural cells and/or cell assemblies that are maximally sensitive to particular patterns in the neural stimulation they receive. That is, they fire most rapidly when the input matches their tuning characteristics – much as a tuning fork or guitar string will vibrate in response to a particular sound – thus 'signalling' that a particular pattern has occurred. Most contemporary theorists treat the process as one that results from a series of such filters applied to input (e.g. GABOR *FILTER). They also allow for the fact that some cells display their 'filtering' functions by decreasing their rate of firing if the input matches their tuning characteristics.

fimbria 1 A complex fibre bundle that runs from the lateral surface of the HIPPOCAMPAL FORMATION to various other regions of the forebrain. The section that runs rostrally from the *hippocampus* forms the *fornix*, which, in turn, is divided into the *precommissural fornix*, the axons of which run from the *medial septum* to the *hippocampus* and from there to the *lateral septum*, and the *fornix columns*, which convey axons from the *subiculum* to the *anterior thalamic nuclei* and to the *mammillary bodies* of the *hypothalamus*. **2** The long fringe-like extremities of the *Fallopian tubes*.

final common path C. S. Sherrington's term for the lower motor neurons of the spinal cord and cranial nerve nuclei in their role within any decision-making process involving motor action. Sherrington's point was, simply, that all processes that are to influence movement, be they monosynaptic spinal reflexes or 'purposive' higher brain functions, must do so by ultimately acting on the motor neurons – hence they are the final common path.

finalism A synonym of TELEOLOGY.

fine motor movement Simply, fine movements which require subtle muscular coordination in cases where delicate control is needed. Compare with GROSS MOTOR MOVEMENT.

finger agnosia TACTILE *AGNOSIA.

finger spelling A mode of manual communication in which 26 discrete arrangements of the fingers correspond to the letters of the alphabet, allowing words to be spelled out manually. It is an important adjunct to SIGN LANGUAGE.

first-line treatment The standard treatment for a disorder or disease. It is usually the procedure most likely to be effective in the presenting condition. For example, in current psychiatry the first-line drug for depression is one of the SELECTIVE SEROTONIN REUPTAKE INHIBITORS.

first moment The *mean* of a distribution. MOMENT (2).

first-order correlation CORRELATION, FIRST-ORDER.

first-order factor FACTOR, FIRST-ORDER.

first-signal system SECOND-SIGNAL SYSTEM.

Fisher's exact probability test A nonparametric statistical test useful in cases in which the data are from two relatively small samples and fall into two mutually exclusive categories.

Fisher's test A statistical test for determining the significance of a correlation coefficient.

Fisher's Z-transformation Z-TRANSFORMATION.

fishing expedition DATA SNOOPING.

fission 1 Cell reproduction by division. Each part grows into a normal cell identical to the original. **2** The term is also used analogously in social psychology, and the terms *social fission* and *group fission* relate to the splitting of a coherent social group into two separate groups each of which adds members and functions in a manner either similar to or derivative of the original.

fissure Any deep groove in the surface of an organ, specifically the brain, e.g the CENTRAL and LATERAL FISSURES. Compare with SULCUS, which is used for the shallow ones.

fistula A narrow opening or passageway in an area of tissue produced either artificially by surgery or by abnormal development or incomplete healing. Note that the term is used in two ways: (a) when the opening is an aspect of the tissue of the organism itself, and (b) by extension, when the opening is a surgically implanted tube that functions to keep a passageway in the tissue open. Strictly speaking, in the latter case the tube is not the fistula, but usage here tends to be loose.

fit 1 n. Medically, a sudden attack or convulsion. See EPILEPSY et seq. **2** n. Statistically, a degree of conformity between observed data and expected data. See GOODNESS OF *FIT. **3** vb. To adjust data to bring them into conformity with some standard. This process is only defensible when there is a set of strongly motivated principles to guide one, otherwise one ends up 'fudging' the data, not fitting them. Distinguish from CURVE FITTING, which does not involve any modification of the data themselves.

fit, goodness of 1 An expression of how well any set of observed data conforms to some expected distribution. There are several tests for evaluating goodness of fit based on the sum of the squared deviations between the observed and the expected values. See e.g. CHI-SQUARE and LEAST-SQUARES PRINCIPLE.

fitness 1 Generally, the extent to which an organism is prepared to succeed in some endeavour. **2** In evolutionary theory, the degree to which an organism is successful in production of viable offspring. Distinguish from ADAPTATION (3): an individual may have an extremely adaptive phenotype but if it is sterile its fitness is zero. *Darwinian fitness* also carries meaning 2. See also INCLUSIVE FITNESS.

Fitt's law A generalization about sensorimotor processes relating movement time (MT) to the precision of the movement and to the distance of the movement. Specifically, $MT = a + (b \log_2 2D/W)$, where a and b are constants, D is distance moved and W is the width of the target moved toward (the measure of precision). The generalization derives from feedback principles: the longer or the more precise a movement must be the more corrections are needed to perform it and these 'in course' corrections take time.

five factor theory A theoretical model of human personality (and, indeed, the personality of some nonhuman animals) that maintains that the various complex aspects of personality can be understood in terms of five fundamental dimensions: NEUROTICISM, EXTRAVERSION, OPENNESS to new experiences, AGREEABLENESS and CONSCIENTIOUSNESS. See each entry for details. The model is grounded in over a century of empirical personality research. Also called the *big five model*, occasionally the name will be capitalized.

5-HT SEROTONIN.

fixated response A response that continues to be emitted despite attempts to extinguish or alter it.

fixation 1 Generally, the process whereby something becomes rigid, set, inflexible; the operation of holding something in a fixed position. This meaning is broadly applied in many areas in psychology: learning, perception, cognition, personality, social psychology, etc. Frequently, a qualifier designates a specific variety of fixation, as the entries that follow reveal. **2** Within psychoanalytic theory, an extremely common shortened form of AFFECTIVE *FIXATION.

fixation, abnormal Persistent, compulsive behaviour seemingly without rational motivation. Within psychoanalytic theory it is usually assumed to result from AFFECTIVE *FIXATION.

fixation, affective In classical psychoanalytic theory, the process whereby a person becomes excessively attached to (or affectively fixated on) an object or person appropriate to an earlier stage of development. The person is thus said to have become affectively fixated at an immature stage. This condition is assumed to produce a variety of neurotic behaviours, such as excessive or irrational attachments to people or objects and an inability to form normal, mature relationships. Sometimes the attachment object itself is called a *fixation*, and the point in the developmental sequence at which the individual is arrested is called the *fixation point*. The full term is often (indeed, usually) shortened to *fixation*. Context-specific modifiers are often added, e.g. *father fixation*, *oral fixation*, etc.

fixation, law of In learning theory one speaks of overlearned behaviour that is seemingly permanent as being *fixed* or *fixated*. *Law* here simply means a generalization that states that such fixing of behaviour will occur if there is sufficient reinforced practice.

fixation line VISUAL *FIXATION.

fixation of affect AFFECTIVE *FIXATION.

fixation pause A brief moment when the eyeball is at rest. It is during fixation pauses that visual discrimination is possible. For example, the visual input for reading takes place during these pauses. See also READING SPAN, SACCADE.

fixation point 1 AFFECTIVE *FIXATION. 2 FIXATION PAUSE, VISUAL *FIXATION.

fixation, visual The orienting of the eyeball so that the projection of the viewed object falls on the fovea and is in focus. The object or location in space is called the *fixation point* and lies along the *fixation line*, which can be 'drawn' from the fovea through the pupil to the object.

fixed action pattern (fap) An ethological term applied to any behavioural sequence that typically occurs in a fixed, stereotyped fashion when evoked or released by a specific stimulus (see RELEASER). Within classical ethological theory, a fap was assumed to be evoked or released in a relatively autonomous fashion when the appropriate species-specific stimulus was encountered. The stereotypy of the fap turns out not to be as dramatic as once thought, hence the term has been largely replaced by *species-specific* or *species-typical behaviour*.

fixed alternative FORCED CHOICE (TECHNIQUE).

fixed-effects fallacy The results of an experiment run with FIXED *FACTORS do not avail themselves of generalizations beyond the fixed values used. The aptly named fallacy is committed when the experimenter supposes that the experiment was run with RANDOM *FACTORS when in fact the variable used was actually a fixed one. The classic example is selecting a subset of the large (infinite) set of possible English sentences for a psycholinguistic experiment and treating it as representing a random factor. On the surface this seems right, since the stimuli were taken at random from an infinite population. However, in practice the particular set of sentences selected may (indeed, usually will) have rather specific idiosyncratic properties which produce results that do not generalize to the rest of the language. This fallacy can be circumvented most easily by using a different subset of materials for each subject run.

fixed effects model FIXED *FACTOR.

fixed factor FACTOR, FIXED.

fixed idea IDÉE FIXE.

fixed image STABILIZED IMAGE.

fixed interval (FI) SCHEDULES OF *REINFORCEMENT.

fixed ratio (FR) SCHEDULES OF *REINFORCEMENT.

fixed time (FT) SCHEDULES OF *REINFORCEMENT.

flaccid Flabby, low in muscle tone.

flaccid paralysis PARALYSIS.

flagellation The practice of whipping. The term *flagellant* was originally applied to members of a 12th-century sect of religious fanatics who did religious penance by whipping. Flagellation also has strong sexual-arousal properties for some people, and the term is commonly used with this connotation. See MASOCHISM, PARAPHILIA, SADISM.

flanker A visual distracter that occurs 'next to' a TARGET (2) where 'next to' may mean on one side, on both flanks or totally surrounding. See FLANKER EFFECTS.

flanker effects Any of several visual effects produced by a FLANKER. For example, a subject is told 'press the left button if ← appears and the right button if → appears' in the midst of a group of flanking arrows. If the flankers are congruent (face the same way as the target) reaction times here tend to be faster than if they are incongruent. The term *flanker effect* refers specifically to the difference in reaction times.

flashback The spontaneous recurrence of the imagery and hallucinations of a drug-induced experience without further doses of the drug being taken. Most commonly associated with the hallucinogens (e.g. LSD), such flashbacks may occur as long as 1 or 2 years after the last ingestion of the drug.

flashbulb memory MEMORY, FLASHBULB.

flattening of affect The absence of appropriate, outward emotional responses.

flavour A general term used to describe the combined effects of olfactory (smell), gustatory (taste) and touch and temperature sensations of objects in the mouth. var., *flavor*.

flehmen A lip curl: a common facial expression of mammals, usually associated with sniffing, that probably functions to convey substances to the VOMERONASAL ORGAN.

Flesch index (or **formula**) A formula for evaluating the reading difficulty of a passage of English prose.

flexibilitas cerea Latin for *waxy flexibility*. See CATATONIC WAXY FLEXIBILITY.

flexion Bending inward, particularly of a limb at a joint. Contrast with EXTENSION (2).

flexor A muscle the action of which bends (or flexes) a limb. Contrast with EXTENSOR. Flexor and extensor muscles generally act to form a pair of ANTAGONISTIC MUSCLES.

flicker Generally, any rapid alternation in a stimulus, typically a visual stimulus. The point at which the periodic aspect of the stimulus ceases and the flickering effect 'fuses' into a continuous one is called the CRITICAL FLICKER FREQUENCY.

flicker, auditory Periodic sound alternation. *Flicker* is really the wrong word here, particularly because of its association with visual stimuli; *flutter* is better and found with increasing frequency. *Jitter* is also used.

flicker fusion point CRITICAL FLICKER FREQUENCY.

flight from reality REALITY, FLIGHT FROM.

flight into health A phrase used to characterize the sudden 'recovery' of some emotionally distressed people when they suddenly come face to face with psychotherapy. The usual interpretation is that this retreat (or flight) is a defence mechanism set up to avoid the self-examination required in therapy.

flight into illness A phrase occasionally used to characterize a sudden emergence of psychiatric symptoms. Within psychoanalysis it is viewed as a defence mechanism that is used to mask a deeper conflict, the examination of which is deferred while the new syndrome is made the focus of analysis.

flight of colours A succession of coloured images seen as an afterimage following an intense, short-duration stimulus viewed against a dark background.

flight of ideas A continuous, fragmentary stream of ideas, thoughts and images without any coherent pattern or focus, as expressed in speech. Often observed in the manic phase of bipolar disorders.

floaters Tiny substances in the humours of the eye which, although always present, generally go unnoticed. Occasionally they are seen as floating specks in the visual field. In some disorders, such as detached vitreous, they can become quite numerous and rather annoying. Also called by the French term *mouches volantes* (flying flies).

floating affect A psychoanalytic term used to refer to emotional states that are not associated with any specific object or event. The term FREE-FLOATING *ANXIETY is often used in this fashion to refer to generalized feelings of distress which have been 'set free' from the particular circumstances that caused them.

floccillation Random purposeless plucking of clothing or bedding. A common symptom of dementia and also seen in febrile states and cases of delirium.

floccinaucinihilipilification A word assembled from a set of Latin words which mean 'worthless' or 'of little value'. In psychology, it is used to refer to the act of judging oneself and/or something else as worthless. When chronic, it is thought to contribute to a *depressive* world view. The increased use of technical terms like this can induce the dysfunction so referenced.

flocculonodular lobe A lobe located at the caudal end of the cerebellum that is involved in postural reflexes. It receives inputs from the *vestibular system* and projects its axons to the *vestibular nucleus*.

flooding An ANXIETY-INDUCTION THERAPY in which the client is exposed to highly anxiety-provoking stimuli. The exposure may take place in a real world setting (in what is known as the *in vivo* approach) or through the use of imagery (the *imaginal* approach).

floor effect CEILING EFFECT.

flow M. Csikszentmihalyi's term for an ongoing perceptual, cognitive process characterized by unimpeded concentration on a goal, thorough enjoyment of the activities that lead to the goal, and such complete absorption in the activity that the sense of self is completely enveloped by the activity.

flow chart *Flow* here refers to a sequence of events, hence a flow chart is a graphic or pictorial representation of such a sequence. Originally used in computer programming, the term has been borrowed by psychology along with the general technique, which is used as a means of displaying schematically the sequence of events hypothesized to take place in information processing.

fluctuation 1 A generic term characterizing any oscillation or any cyclic change. 2 In biology, a slight variation in form and structure within a species. Contrast here with MUTATION. 3 In statistics, a variation in the values of a statistic calculated from successive samples. 4 In perception, a shift in the perceived object when there has been no objective change in the physical stimulus. This meaning is also expressed by the term *fluctuation of attention*, although such perceptual shifts are not necessarily the result of shifts in attention but may be caused by more basic physiological processes, e.g. adaptation effects.

fluctuation of attention FLUCTUATION (4).

fluency The ease, facility or efficiency in any processing system that results from repeated exposure and practice. *Perceptual fluency* is used for an increase in the ability to process incoming stimuli rapidly and efficiently; *cognitive fluency* for facile decision-making, problem-solving or game playing; *linguistic fluency* for effective speaking of a language.

fluent aphasia WERNICKE'S *APHASIA.

fluoxetine An ANTIDEPRESSANT DRUG in the SELECTIVE SEROTONIN REUPTAKE INHIBITOR (SSRI) group. It was among the first of the SSRIs to be put on the market and, although there are others that are more effective and with fewer side effects, is still widely prescribed. Trade name Prozac.

fluphenazine An antipsychotic drug of the phenothiazine group.

flutter AUDITORY *FLICKER.

fluvoxamine A SELECTIVE SEROTONIN REUPTAKE

INHIBITOR used as an ANTIDEPRESSANT DRUG and for treatment of obsessive-compulsive disorder. Trade name Luvox.

Flynn effect The tendency, first documented by James Flynn, for IQ RAW *SCORES to rise, over time. The relationship between scores and time since standardization is often, but not always, monotonic. The reasons for the effect are unclear.

fMRI FUNCTIONAL MAGNETIC RESONANCE IMAGING.

focal 1 Descriptive of the point at which light rays are in focus. 2 By extension, characterizing any integral point that lies at the core of some effect or phenomenon.

focal attention ATTENTION, FOCAL.

focal epilepsy EPILEPSY, FOCAL.

focalism The common tendency to focus on only some aspects of a task or event. The WEAPON-FOCUS EFFECT is a simple example. Other examples are AFFECTIVE *FORECASTING and the PLANNING *FALLACY.

focal length As descriptive of a particular lens, it is the distance from the lens to the point at which parallel rays of light are brought into focus.

focal lesion Any LESION that is localized and limited in the area affected.

focal stress The primary vocal stress in a spoken sentence. Such stress plays an important role in the interpretation of an utterance, as can be appreciated by repeating the simple sentence 'What are you doing?' four times with focal stress on a different word each time.

focal therapy A restricted form of psychotherapy in which one particular problem is singled out and made the focus of the therapy.

focus 1 n. The point at which the light rays passing through a lens converge. 2 n. The object upon which one's attention or thinking is centred. 3 vb. To adjust an optical system (including the eye) so that the light rays converge at a point. 4 vb. To centre one's attention on a particular thing.

focus group A small COHORT (2), usually between 8 and 12 people, brought together to discuss some topic of common interest.

Originally designed for use in marketing where the group focused on consumer reactions to products, they are now used widely in a variety of domains including, perhaps not surprisingly, politics.

focus of attention The object, event, idea, problem, thought, etc. upon which one is concentrating.

foetal Pertaining to the FOETUS. var., *fetal*.

foetal alcohol effects A syndrome characterized by some of the features of FOETAL ALCOHOL SYNDROME (FAS), such as hyperactivity, memory disorders, language learning problems and motoric deficits, but typically not as severe as FAS.

foetal alcohol syndrome (FAS) A cluster of abnormal developmental features in a foetus resulting from alcohol consumption by the mother during pregnancy. The high level of alcohol in the blood combined with a generally reduced level of normal nutrients can produce all (or all) of a number of anatomical and psychological deficits, including microcephaly, growth deficiencies, mental retardation, hyperactivity, heart murmurs and skeletal malformations. See also TERATOGEN.

foetal antigen hypothesis See MATERNAL IMMUNIZATION HYPOTHESIS.

feotal familial insomnia INSOMNIA, FEOTAL FAMILIAL.

foetal programming In biology and medicine, the concept that antenatal events programme or condition the foetus in a way that affects postnatal development. The term is moving into psychology with efforts to identify which, if any, antenatal events influence later psychological development.

foetus An organism in the latter stages of prenatal development. In humans, from the third month of pregnancy to birth is called the foetal stage. Prior to that time the developing child is called an EMBRYO. var., *fetus*.

FOK FEELING OF KNOWING.

foliate papilla LINGUAL PAPILLA.

folie à deux French for *insanity in pairs*. Descriptive of instances in which two closely related people (e.g. siblings, husband and wife) display the same mental disorder at

the same time. If the number of individuals displaying symptoms is higher *folie à trois*, *folie à quatre*, etc. are used. See also INDUCED PSYCHOTIC DISORDER.

folium A convolution or fold on the cerebellum. pl., *folia*.

folklore The complex of songs, legends, stories, etc. that make up the unwritten traditional oral literature of a culture.

folk mind GROUP MIND.

folk psychology 1 Everyday, common-sense psychology. The kinds of psychological notions, principles, understandings (and misunderstandings) that are held by most lay people. The term has neutral connotations in most contexts. However, some, particularly defenders of MATERIALISM (2), use it in a critical manner for such perspectives on the grounds that the 'folk' usually put too much emphasis on beliefs, free will and other 'mentalist' notions. 2 An inappropriately literal translation of Wilhelm Wundt's approach of *Völkerpsychologie* which was actually much closer to *social* or *cultural* psychology.

folkways Social norms or traditional patterns of behaviour in a culture. Folkways are implicit and learned by successive generations through socialization and hence are distinguished from MORES, which are explicitly presented and obligatory standards.

follicle Generally, any small secreting cavity.

follicle, hair A cylindrical invagination in the epidermis with associated sebaceous glands and small muscles through which a hair grows.

follicle-stimulating hormone (FSH) MENSTRUAL CYCLE.

following reaction The species-specific tendency for young to follow their mother after IMPRINTING has taken place.

fontanel The area in the cranium of an infant that has not yet become ossified. The so-called soft spot. var., *fontanelle*.

food aversion (or avoidance) CONDITIONED *AVOIDANCE.

foot anaesthesia GLOVE *ANAESTHESIA.

foot candle An obsolete term for a unit of

ILLUMINANCE defined as the illumination on a surface by a standard candle at a distance of 1 ft (0.3 m). The preferred measure is the LUX. See also CANDELA and CANDLE.

foot fetish A FETISHISM (2) for feet, shoes, boots and occasionally, stockings. The foot and associated coverings are probably the most common objects of fetishes. Also called *retifism* to 'honour' the 18th-century French writer, Nicolas-Edem Rétif, an early devotee.

foot-in-the-door technique A way of obtaining compliance whereby an individual first makes a small, even trivial, request and once this is granted escalates to larger and more important requests. Compare with DOOR-IN-THE-FACE TECHNIQUE.

foot lambert An obsolete term for a unit of LUMINANCE defined as the *luminous flux* produced by a perfectly reflecting and diffusing surface the brightness of which is uniformly 1 foot candle. The LUMEN is now the preferred measure.

foraging In studies of feeding behaviour in natural environments the various activities involved in obtaining foodstuffs, e.g. search, identification, procurement, handling and storage.

foramen magnum A foramen is any opening or passageway; the foramen magnum is the opening in the occipital bone of the skull through which the spinal cord passes to become the medulla. Also called the *intervertebral foramen*.

forced-choice (technique) A general label for any procedure in which the subject is required to select one item or answer from a fixed set of two or more alternatives. There are several variations on the technique and they are used in such diverse areas as personality assessment, determination of personal preferences, studies of memory and examinations of decision-making. The basic technique is an extremely important one for it allows one to control for a number of extraneous factors that could easily contaminate the results of an experiment. For example, in the commonly used self-rating personality inventories, social desirability can often disrupt one's findings because in a free-choice setting people tend to put down answers that reflect what society prizes rather than what is appropriate for them. The forced-choice technique demands of the testee the selection of one alternative from a given set even if he or she feels that all (or none) of those provided really fit. By carefully counterbalancing items the social-desirability factor is controlled for. Similarly, in recognition-memory studies individual biases to respond 'yes' or 'no' when in doubt as to an item's status can be eliminated by always giving two or more stimulus items only one of which is correct. Also called, particularly in personality assessment, *fixed-alternative technique*.

force field In physics this term can be given precise meaning; in psychology it is used almost entirely metaphorically and typically refers to any or all of the influences on behaviour. It tends to be used rather holistically – the force field encompasses all significant factors. Such usage unfortunately tends to be so broad that it robs the term of any real descriptive value.

fore- Prefix meaning *in front of, before*.

forebrain During embryonic development the brain evolves three separate portions: the hindbrain, midbrain and forebrain. The last of these subdivides into the telencephalon and diencephalon. The telencephalon then develops into the cerebral cortex, the basal ganglia and the limbic system. The diencephalon becomes the thalamus and the hypothalamus.

forecasting, affective The act of predicting how one will feel in the future. Typically, people's predictions are more extreme than they actually turn out to be. The negative component, where people overestimate the degree of negative affect that they will experience, is stronger than the positive.

forecasting efficiency, index of A measure of the extent to which one can use knowledge of one variable to make predictions about another variable given that the correlation between the two is known. Usually symbolized as E, the index is given as $1 - \sqrt{(1 - r^2)}$, where r is the correlation coefficient.

foreconscious Synonym for PRECONSCIOUS.

foregrounding A general term for any action taken by a person designed to draw another person's attention to a particular aspect of a stimulus environment. A spoken sentence like 'Look at this book' is a good example; it places the book in the person's perceptual/conceptual foreground. Foregrounding is very common in parent–child interactions.

foreign hull In K. Lewin's field theory, all those nonpsychological aspects of the environment that lie outside but adjacent to the LIFE SPACE. It is composed of the physical environment and the social and cultural environments that may invade or penetrate the life space.

forensic From the Latin, meaning *of the forum*. Hence: **1** Argumentative, suited for argumentation. **2** Pertaining to the courts of law and judicial procedure. See following entries for specifics.

forensic medicine The application of medical knowledge and medical practice as it pertains to legal issues.

forensic psychiatry A branch of psychiatry dealing with legal questions such as determination of SANITY (see that term for clarification of usage), issues of mental responsibility for acts committed, and committability of an individual (to an institution). Generally distinguished from FORENSIC PSYCHOLOGY, although on occasions a forensic psychiatrist may be called to testify on issues that fall within the range of issues discussed under that term.

forensic psychology The field of psychology concerned with the application of psychological knowledge and principles to legal issues. Generally distinguished from FORENSIC PSYCHIATRY, it is concerned with an array of problems of a psychological nature including the reliability of various kinds of evidence, the reliability of such as eyewitness testimony, the role of human memory, the psychology of decision-making (particularly group decision-making – as in juries) and questions of the general credibility of witnesses. For a referential subtlety, see LEGAL PSYCHOLOGY.

foreperiod Generally, the first part of an experiment; specifically, in experiments on reaction time, the period between the 'ready' signal and the presentation of the stimulus.

fore-pleasure In the classical psychoanalytic approach erotic pleasures are divided into those associated with increasing erotic tension (the *fore*-pleasures) and those associated with release of the tension (*end*-pleasures). Thus, *fore-pleasure* will be found denoting any activity that functions to increase the desire for end-pleasure.

foreshortening The decrease in apparent length of a line, looked at in an alignment parallel to the line of regard, as compared with its apparent length when seen so that it is at an oblique angle relative to the viewer.

forgetting 1 Broadly, the loss of the ability to recall, recognize or reproduce that which was previously learned. This definition is fairly straightforward and reflects the term's general meaning. However, usage within psychology tends to be tinged with various nuances, nuances that stem from particular theoretical characterizations of the nature of the processes underlying forgetting. In particular: **2** In the traditional approaches to learning, forgetting is the weakening of an associative bond. This is presumed to be brought about either by non-reinforcement or by the action of various inhibitory or interfering processes. See here e.g. INHIBITION, PROACTIVE *INTERFERENCE, RETRO-ACTIVE *INTERFERENCE. **3** In psychoanalytic theory forgetting is treated as the result of REPRESSION; that is, memories are assumed not to be totally lost but rather rendered non-retrievable by the action of defence mechanisms. **4** In Gestalt theory, since perception and learning were assumed to be predicated on the organization of coherent wholes, forgetting was viewed as the result of the disruption of or interference with the structured memory. Material was either 'lost' because the coded structure was not retrieved, or 'modified' by reorganization so thoroughly that it was no longer recognizable as the original. While the Gestalt movement is dormant these days, the notion that access to memories may be compromised by disturbances in the underlying structure of the representations is very much a viable hypothesis. **5** The contemporary cognitive-information-processing approach postulates three types of memory each with a hypothesized forgetting mechanism: (a) the SENSORY-INFORMATION STORE is very short-lived and information is lost through a rapid process of neural decay; (b) SHORT-TERM *MEMORY is a limited-capacity system that retains material through rehearsal and loses it through decay if rehearsal is interfered with. In both (a) and (b) material that is forgotten is assumed to be irrevocably gone; (c) LONG-TERM *MEMORY is a theoretically unlimited memorial system containing all relatively well-coded and organized knowledge. When information is 'lost' from this store the mechanism of interference is generally implicated; forgetting from long-term memory is treated as failure to retrieve. See also MEMORY and related entries.

form Generally, this term refers to the outline, shape or overall structure of an object or figure. The critical psychological aspect of any form is that the pattern of the whole figure is usually perceived as more important or significant than the several elements that make it up. The notion of form and form perception is critical in psychology. It was first made into an important issue by the Gestalt psychologists, who argued convincingly that form takes precedence over superficial aspects of any display; both o and O are seen as circles, and a melody is recognizable whether sung by a baritone or a soprano. See GESTALT PSYCHOLOGY and related entries.

formal 1 Pertaining to FORM. **2** Pertaining to an emphasis on general rules or overall patterns and principles rather than on content.

formal discipline The approach to education which advocates that some subjects ought to be studied independently of any content that they might have because they acquaint the student with basic principles (or *forms*) that will ultimately prove of value in other ways and generally serve to 'train the mind'. The enthusiasm for this approach has waxed and waned over the years.

formalism A general orientation to the gathering of knowledge that places primary emphasis on organization, consistency and the development of formal principles. Within psychology there have been relatively few theoretical approaches that qualify as formalisms; the most recent reasonably successful ones are Anderson's ACT theory and the new CONNECTIONISM (2). The formalist approach is generally balanced against the ECLECTIC; see that term for further discussion.

formal operations A set of cognitive operations cited by Piaget as characteristic of the thought of a child in the FORMAL OPERATORY STAGE. Such thought involves abstract thinking that is no longer tied to physical objects and events. It is propositional in nature and is concerned with the hypothetical and the possible rather than the real and the perceived. Compare with CONCRETE OPERATIONS.

formal operatory stage (or **level** or **period**) In Piagetian theory, the stage of cognitive functioning following the CONCRETE OPERATORY STAGE and assumed to begin around age 12 with the development of abstract thinking. According to Piaget it is regarded as the culmination of 'intellectual' development, although this particular point is vigorously debated by other theorists.

formal operatory thought A term used by Piaget to characterize the 'formal', logical, cognitive processes manifested by a person in the FORMAL OPERATORY STAGE.

formal organization ORGANIZATION (2).

formal thought disorder THOUGHT DISORDER.

formal universals LINGUISTIC *UNIVERSALS.

formant A spectrographic representation of a speech sound reveals that energy is concentrated in bands at particular frequencies. The concentrations of energy show up as dark areas which are called formants. Each speech sound can be described by the location in the frequency spectrum of four separate formants. The first two (counting up from the lower frequencies) appear to be the critical ones for processing human speech. The formants are labelled numerically in increasing order of their frequencies such that F1 is the lowest frequency formant, and F2 is the next highest frequency formant. See SPECTROGRAPH, FUNDAMENTAL TONE.

formatting SCAFFOLDING.

formboard test A class of performance tests in which the task is to fit a set of blocks of varying shapes into slots of varying shapes.

form constancy OBJECT CONSTANCY.

form from motion effect Induction of form in a moving visual display by mentally organizing all the points that move together into an object. For example, one is unlikely to see a snake lying on the ground, but the form of the snake pops out visually as soon as it moves. Also called *structure from motion effect*.

form–function relation (or **distinction**) In general, this term refers to the role of a thing (its *function*) compared with or distinguished from its physical characteristics (its *form*). The classic distinctions here occur in the study of the psychology of language, in which it is often necessary to distinguish between the formal properties of an utterance and its function in a particular setting. For example, the sentence 'Can you close the door?' is formally a question about one's capabilities but it functions as a request for action.

formication From the Latin *formica*, meaning *ant*. A hallucinated sensation that insects, or in some cases snakes, are crawling on or under the skin. It is a form of PARAESTHESIA and a common side effect of long-term abuse of cocaine and amphetamines.

forms, comparable Two or more comparable or correlated forms of a test. Also called *alternate* or *alternative forms*.

fornication Noncoerced sexual intercourse between persons not married to each other.

fornix See the description of the neural pathways of the FIMBRIA (1).

fornix columns FIMBRIA (1).

45,X TURNER'S SYNDROME, in which there are only 45 chromosomes, with only a single sex chromosome (X), present in the genotype.

47,XXX TRIPLE-X SYNDROME.

47,XXY KLINEFELTER'S SYNDROME, in which there are 47 chromosomes, including 3 sex chromosomes (XXY), present in the genotype.

47,XYY XYY SYNDROME.

foster-child fantasy The childhood delusion that one's parents are not one's real parents but adoptive or foster parents.

founder cells Cells in the VENTRICULAR ZONE that, during early development, give rise to the cells that make up the central nervous system.

founder effect In genetics, differences between two (or more) populations brought about as a result of one population having been founded in a new locale by a small group of individuals who happened to be carrying a subset of genes from the general population. Some unusual patterns of incidence, such as the high rate of schizophrenia among the residents of the area of Sweden above the Arctic Circle, are thought to be *founder effects*.

four-card problem WASON TASK.

fourfold-point correlation PHI COEFFICIENT.

Fourier's law The mathematically demonstrable generalization that any complex periodic pattern, such as sound waves, may be described as a particular sum of a number of sine waves. The sine waves so used are called a *Fourier series* and the description itself is a *Fourier analysis*.

four plus or minus one (4±1) Early research on the limits on unprocessed information suggested that SEVEN PLUS OR MINUS TWO discrete elements was the upper bound of short-term memory. More recent work suggests that this estimate was a bit too high and that working memory really can only hold some four or so unencoded or unchunked pieces of information.

fourth moment The KURTOSIS of a distribution. See also MOMENT (2).

four-walls technique A technique for obtaining compliance by presenting a person with a set of questions, the answers to which are designed to produce *cognitive dissonance* should the person fail to comply with the ultimate request. The classic case is the encyclopedia salesperson who begins by asking the customer questions like 'Do you feel that education is important for your children?' and 'Do you believe that having good reference materials will help your child's education?'

fovea (**centralis**) A small pit or depression in the retina. When light enters the eye along the visual axis it falls on the portion of the retina called the macula lutea (or yellow spot), in the middle of which is the fovea, a rather small area covering only about 2° of visual angle. The fovea is densely packed with cones (it is rod-free) and is the area of clearest vision. When you focus or look at an object you are turning the eye so that the image of the object is projected on the fovea.

foveal vision FOVEA and PHOTOPIC VISION.

FOXP2 Short for *forkhead box P2*, a gene on chromosome 7 that has been implicated in language function. It was discovered during the study of a family, several members of which have mutant FOXP2 genes and marked language and speech dysfunctions. Some researchers have argued that the existence of the gene supports claims for a specific *language acquisition device* (see LAD). Others have noted that individuals with the mutant gene also have a variety of difficulties not specific to language such as facial and oral motor problems, difficulty in processing words, generally low IQ and neurological abnormalities in the caudate nucleus. The gene itself is evolutionarily quite old. It underwent a single mutation from mouse to chimpanzee and two more since the *Homo* line diverged. The specific mutation appears to cause difficulties during embryonic development that produce abnormalities in brain pathways with a variety of symptoms, some of which involve human speech. It should not be thought of as a 'grammar gene'.

FR Abbreviation for *fixed ratio*. See SCHEDULES OF *REINFORCEMENT.

fractional antedating goal response (r_G) A hypothetical reaction assumed to occur in a long response chain. In successive trials it is assumed to move progressively earlier in the chain and provide additional cues which become conditioned to successive responses leading to the goal. Also called *functional anticipatory goal response*.

fractional goal stimulus (s_G) A proprioceptive stimulus which is assumed to occur as a result of a *fractional antedating goal response*.

fragile X syndrome A genetic disorder caused by a mutation on the X chromosome. Symptoms include mental retardation, low muscle tone and elongated face often with large ears. Males have large testicles. Females often are subclinical, primarily because of the protection provided by the other, unaffected X chromosome. The syndrome often has a variety of behavioural characteristics including stereotyped actions, shyness

and poor social development to the point where they may reach the diagnostic criteria for autism (see AUTISTIC SPECTRUM DISORDER).

frame **1** In ARTIFICIAL INTELLIGENCE, a set of fixed elements that define (i.e. frame) a situation. For example, the elements in a *room frame* are walls, a ceiling, a floor, doorways, etc. This usage is associated with the work of the American theorist Marvin Minsky. **2** In social psychology the term is used in similar fashion but much more loosely. Any social situation can be defined in terms of basic principles that affect and control the ways in which people involve themselves with and experience it. These definitions are frames. Note that the term is used here specifically to refer to the *perceived* and *experienced* organization, the agreed-upon frame within which people function. It is not used to express any necessary statements about objective social reality. This meaning was first introduced by G. Bateson but is primarily associated with the work of the sociologist Erving Goffman.

frame analysis An approach to the study of the experiencing of social situations by analysing them in terms of FRAMES.

frame of reference The overall context within which a particular event takes place and, hence, is interpreted or judged. See FRAME (2).

frame problem In philosophical psychology, the problem confronted by a person (or other device, see ARTIFICIAL INTELLIGENCE (AI)) when some action causes changes in some aspects of the general FRAME (1) within which one is working. For example, if an AI is programmed to turn the TV on when it enters a room, how does it 'know' that this act has an impact on some other parts of the frame (e.g. the light and sound levels) but not others (the location of the furniture)? It seems like a trivial issue but careful thought will show that it is not simple at all.

framework theory In developmental psychology, a theory of how conceptual change takes place in young children. Infants and young children are proposed to hold INTUITIVE (3) theories that are specific to each domain. With age and experience, the child begins to integrate these theories and organize them into more abstract, regular laws, rules and categories. Thus, the child constructs 'frameworks' that bridge different knowledge systems with general principles such as hierarchical relationships, theories of animacy and agency, and so on. The term is used to refer both to the general developmental theory and to the newly organized theories themselves.

framing A COGNITIVE *HEURISTIC in which people tend to reach conclusions based on the 'framework' within which a situation is presented; e.g. people are more likely to recommend the use of a new procedure if it is described as having a '50% success rate' than a '50% failure rate'.

fraternal twins DIZYGOTIC *TWINS.

F ratio In statistics, the ratio of the variances (σ^2) of two samples. The ratio was named in honour of the statistician Ronald A. Fisher and is given by $F = \sigma_1^2/\sigma_2^2$, where σ_2^2 is always the smaller of the two variances. The size of an F ratio may be used to determine whether there is homogeneity of variance between the two samples from which the two values of σ^2 were estimated.

free association ASSOCIATION, FREE.

freedom A term with two distinct uses in psychology: **1** The sense that one has personal control over one's choices, decisions, actions, etc.; the feeling that external factors play little or no role in one's personal behaviour. This meaning is conveyed by the expression 'freedom to...' **2** The state in which one is (relatively) unburdened by painful situations, noxious stimuli, hunger, pain, disease, etc. This sense is usually intended by the expression 'freedom from...'
To be sure, in the pragmatics of everyday life these two kinds of freedom are intimately intertwined, but failure to keep them conceptually distinct leads to philosophical and political muddle. The former is close in conceptualization to the doctrine of FREE WILL; the latter relates to issues of CONTROL (2). SOCIAL *POWER and the behaviourist position on the role of REINFORCEMENT and PUNISHMENT.

free-feeding AD LIB.

free-floating anxiety FREE-FLOATING *ANXIETY and FLOATING AFFECT.

free fusion The act of focusing visually behind or in front of a STEREOGRAM so that its features fuse and a three-dimensional object or scene emerges. Successful free fusion is not instantaneous implying that this type of BINOCULAR *PERCEPTION is cortical rather than occurring in brain centres that produce more basic percepts. vb., *free fuse*.

freeloading Not doing one's share in social settings. It is used in the technical literature as in normal language; a freeloader is someone who benefits from the actions of a group while deliberately putting in less effort or fewer resources than is expected of members of the group. Also called *free-riding*.

free morpheme MORPHEME.

free nerve endings The microscopic, branched endings of afferent neurons that innervate all body tissues unconnected to any specific sensory receptor. They function as pain receptors, and are also believed to contribute to the perception of mechanical touch and possibly temperature. The thin, slow *C fibres* mediate the slow, diffuse, dull sense of pain; the thicker, myelinated, faster *A-delta fibres* mediate the sharp, localized sense of pain.

free operant A response that may be emitted at any time in a particular situation. In most operant-conditioning experiments the organism is free to respond, and measures of behaviour are based on response rate or the number of free responses made per unit of time. The key concept here is *emitted*; see EMIT and also the discussion under OPERANT CONDITIONING.

free recall An experimental procedure used in memory research in which the subject is free to recall, in any order, the items given for memorization. Compare with SERIAL RECALL.

free responding FREE OPERANT.

free running In the study of CIRCADIAN RHYTHMS, maintaining an organism in either constant darkness or light so that the normal day/night cycle that constrains the circadian rhythms is no longer present and biological rhythms 'run free'.

free will 1 A most general term used to refer to a broad class of philosophical positions all of which have in common the assumption that to some degree or another behaviour is under control of the volition of an individual. Contrast with DETERMINISM. **2** A hypothesized (and often reified) internal agency that functions independently of externally imposed forces, as meant in the often-asked question 'Don't you think people have free will?'

freezing 1 Assuming a position of tonic immobility. The ethological term DEATH FEIGNING is used when the response is a natural one for a member of the species, while *freezing* is used by some for the response when it develops as a learned reaction. **2** A temporary inability to move seen in patients with Parkinson's disease. It often occurs when a patient encounters a change in the pattern on the floor or when he or she is in a doorway or exiting a room.

Fregoli syndrome A DELUSIONAL MISIDENTIFICATION DISORDER that two or more people are in fact a single person who constantly changes appearance or disguises. There is a distinct paranoid element in that the patient believes they are being stalked or persecuted by the person. The name comes from the Italian actor, Leopold Fregoli, a renowned quick-change artist.

frequency 1 The number of occurrences of the several values of some variable. **2** Cycles per second in periodic vibration, e.g. in sound waves or electric current. **3** By extension, the number of times a visual pattern repeats within one degree of VISUAL ANGLE. The latter is often termed *spatial frequency* to distinguish it from the other meanings.

frequency distribution DISTRIBUTION, FREQUENCY.

frequency, law of The generalization that the more often a response is made the more robust and resistant to extinction it becomes. Also known as the *law of repetition*.

frequency method MEASUREMENT OF *THRESHOLD.

frequency polygon A way of pictorially presenting a frequency distribution. The frequency of each class interval (see GROUPED FREQUENCY *DISTRIBUTION) is plotted and a line is drawn connecting the points. See also HISTOGRAM.

frequency theory THEORIES OF *HEARING.

Freudian Of or pertaining to the points of view associated with the brilliant Viennese neurologist Sigmund Freud (1856–1939). Many of the details of specific terms, concepts and principles that emerged from this orientation are dealt with elsewhere in this volume; this eponymous adjective itself is used freely in conjunction with them all. However, there are particular core concepts that characterize the pure term *Freudian*: (a) a focus upon the unconscious, specifically the role of unconscious processes as motivators of behaviour; (b) an abiding concern with the cognitive and the symbolic; (c) an affiliation with the basic biological progenitors of human behaviour, especially the sexual and the aggressive; (d) a strong presumption that early experiences are the causes of later behaviours; (e) a penchant for deep interpretation, for rummaging down through the layers of the psyche to seek understanding and explanation; (f) the elaboration of the methods of psychoanalytic therapy as a means of producing changes in behaviour, thought and feeling.

The many terms that spring to the minds of most educated lay people like *id, ego, superego, cathexis, displacement, psychosexual stage,* etc. are not really viewed as pure representations of Freudianism any longer. They have become so much a part of the various analytical or depth psychologies that Freudians no longer hold a special claim to them. What truly represents the appellation is: (g) an overarching concern with the most profound conflict of human existence, the agony of recognition of our 'creatureliness' with all of its evolutionarily dictated baseness balanced against our rich cognitive capacity for transcendent thought with its extensions to symbolism, religion and aesthetics – and the knowledge derived from this mental capacity that the base creature must eventually die.

Freudian slip PARAPRAXIS.

fricative A speech sound produced by nearly closing the oral cavity so that there is a turbulent air flow, e.g. the *f* in *fat*, the *th* in *thin*, both of which are voiceless fricatives, and the *v* in *vat* and the *th* in *this*, both of which are voiced.

frigidity 1 Generally, a lack of sexual desire. **2** More specifically, an inability to enjoy or complete sexual intercourse. **3** Most specifically, an inability to achieve orgasm. The term is used almost exclusively with respect to women; IMPOTENCE is used for men. The term is no longer used in the technical literature. Its demise in the nontechnical would not be mourned. See HYPOACTIVE SEXUAL DESIRE DISORDER and ORGASM DISORDERS.

fringe consciousness As first used by William James, a vague halo of experience, the edge of consciousness where mental events and processes can occur. The basic idea is also carried by the term FRINGE OF CONSCIOUSNESS although here the sense is that something is not in this 'fringy' state but on the 'fringe' of normal consciousness. See also MARGIN OF *ATTENTION.

fringe of consciousness An occasional synonym for MARGIN OF *ATTENTION.

frontal Pertaining to the anterior part of a body or organ.

frontal abulia An ORGANIC *PERSONALITY DISORDER resulting from injury to the left prefrontal area of the brain. The syndrome is marked by cognitive and motivational impairments including emotional blunting, difficulty initiating behaviour and loss of curiosity.

frontal lobe Approximately, that portion of the cerebral cortex that lies in front of the precentral gyrus.

frontal-lobe syndrome Loosely, any disorder due to neurological damage to the frontal lobes. Characteristic symptoms include disruptions of EXECUTIVE FUNCTION manifested by emotional lability, problems with impulse control, general apathy, a marked tendency to perseverate and impaired social judgement. Similar patterns of behaviour are often, although not always correctly, classified under several other headings including FRONTO-TEMPORAL *DEMENTIA, ORGANIC *PERSONALITY SYNDROME and DYSEXECUTIVE SYNDROME.

frontal lobotomy LOBOTOMY et seq.

frontal section SECTION (2).

frontopolar cortex See ANTERIOR PREFRONTAL CORTEX.

fronto-temporal dementia DEMENTIA, FRONTO-TEMPORAL.

frottage The act of rubbing one's genitals

against another person for the purpose of sexual pleasure.

frotteurism A SEXUAL DISORDER characterized by intense sexual urges involving touching and rubbing against another, nonconsenting, person. The act itself (*frottage*) is usually carried out in crowded places such as buses or subways. See also PARAPHILIA.

frozen noise NOISE, FROZEN.

frustration Technical usage of this term in psychology is generally limited to two meanings: **1** The act of blocking, interfering with or disrupting behaviour that is directed toward some goal. This is the operational definition; the behaviour may be almost anything from overt, physical movement to covert, cognitive process. **2** The emotional state assumed to result from the act in 1. It is typically assumed that this emotional state has motivational properties that produce behaviour designed to bypass or surmount the block.

frustration–aggression hypothesis A 'double-barrelled' proposition which assumes that frustration always leads to aggression (whether covert or overt) and that aggressive behaviour is always an indication of frustration. Stated this way the hypothesis is circular and an unsatisfying account of behaviour. However, the link between frustration and aggression is an intuitively compelling one; what is needed to rescue the hypothesis is independent evaluations of frustration and aggression.

frustrative nonreward (hypothesis) A generalization that assumes that the withholding of a reinforcer is an actively punishing and aversive (i.e. frustrating) event. The hypothesis predicts that behaviour following frustrative nonreward will show greater vigour.

F scale MEASUREMENT OF *AUTHORITARIANISM.

FSH Abbreviation for *follicle-stimulating hormone.* See MENSTRUAL CYCLE.

FT Abbreviation for *fixed time.* See SCHEDULES OF *REINFORCEMENT.

F test A parametric statistical test that uses the *F* RATIO to determine whether the variances of two samples are significantly different. This simple test forms the basis for the most utilized of all statistical techniques, the *analysis of variance*. The extension was first worked out by Sir Ronald A. Fisher (the *F* honours him), who showed that more than two conditions can be evaluated by setting up an *F* ratio between a variance estimate based on variability *among* several means and one based on variability among scores *within* each condition.

fugue From the Latin for *flight*, a psychiatric disability the defining feature of which is a sudden and unexpected leaving of home and the assumption of a new identity elsewhere. During the fugue there is no recollection of the earlier life and after recovery there is amnesia for events during it. Often called *dissociative psychogenic fugue* to distinguish it from other syndromes that have similar symptoms but are caused by known organic dysfunctions.

Fullerton–Cattell law A psychophysical generalization that the error of observation increases with the square root of the stimulus intensity. Proposed as a substitute for WEBER'S LAW on the grounds that errors of observation are more psychologically germane than the classic procedures that use introspection to determine a 'real' *just noticeable difference*.

full-scale intelligence quotient The composite IQ score derived from all the subtests of an intelligence test. When one sees a reference to an IQ score in a technical manual or journal it is almost invariably to this measure. Early in testing, IQ used to be a measure of the ratio of mental age to chronological age. With the development of sophisticated developmental norms, IQ is now given in numbers that reflect the score on each subtest (usually verbal and performance scales) and the *full-scale* quotient.

function 1 In mathematics, a quantity that varies systematically with variation in some other quantity. In the expression $y = f(x)$, variations in y are given as a function of variations in x. The changes are not necessarily proportional, but are expressed by the nature of f. When used psychologically, x is the INDEPENDENT *VARIABLE and y the DEPENDENT *VARIABLE. Graphic representation can be made of such functional relations by plotting values of x on one axis and values of y on the other. **2** Often the term is used in something like this mathematical fashion but without

the quantification that the above usage reflects. Thus, one will encounter expressions like 'persuasion is a function of the credibility of the source', in which the mathematical meaning is implied with the connotation of one thing being dependent on something else but the quantification of the variables is either missing altogether or represented on a scale of less power (see the discussion under SCALE and related entries for clarification of usage here). **3** The proper activity or appropriate behaviour of a person, an organ, a structure, a machine or even a socially defined role. Thus one sees references to the function of a teacher, a computer, the liver, a group leader, etc. Compare here with STRUCTURE (especially 1) and see also FUNCTIONALISM and STRUCTURALISM. **4** A variation on 3 is also found in which some purpose or goal is specified along with the behaviour or activity, e.g. 'a function of the adrenal glands is the production of epinepherine'.

There are other subtle distinctions in the use of the term, but most of them can be subsumed under these general meanings. When variations of meaning are intended they are usually signalled by the use of qualifiers.

functional 1 Referring to the useful features of a mechanism, object, process, etc. **2** See FUNCTIONAL DISORDER.

functional amnesia AMNESIA, FUNCTIONAL.

functional analysis 1 Generally, an analysis of a complex system with an eye to the functions of the various aspects of the system and the manner of integrated operation. Such an analysis usually soft-pedals the actual form or structure. The system analysed can be essentially anything; the term is used in this fashion very broadly. **2** Somewhat more specifically, the term is associated with the strong behaviourist point of view of B. F. Skinner. Here the full term is *functional analysis of behaviour* and the stress is on examining behaviour *per se* while eschewing appeals to internal cognitive or physiological components.

functional antagonism DRUG *ANTAGONISM.

functional autonomy AUTONOMY, FUNCTIONAL.

functional disorder An umbrella term for any disorder for which there is no known organic pathology. In actual practice the term is used for (a) those disorders in which there is *no known* organic pathology (e.g. psychogenic FUGUE) as well as for (b) those disorders in which there is *known to be no* specific organic pathology that could be directly responsible for the symptoms (e.g. GLOVE *ANAESTHESIA). In older texts reference to HYSTERICAL (2) disorders reflects this meaning. See HYSTERIA for reasons why that term has been dropped from the 'official' lexicon.

functional fixedness A conceptual set whereby objects that have been used for one function tend to be viewed as serving only that function even though the situation may call for their use in a different context. For example, a hammer just used for pounding nails may not be perceived as appropriate for use as a pendulum weight. Also called *functional fixity*.

functional fixity FUNCTIONAL FIXEDNESS.

functional integration INTEGRATION, FUNCTIONAL.

functionalism Within psychology: **1** A general and broadly presented point of view that stresses the analysis of mind and behaviour in terms of their functions or utilities rather than in terms of their contents. **2** A school of thought formally established at the University of Chicago under J. R. Angell and H. Carr during the 1910s and 1920s.

While the school of thought in 2 reflected many of the characteristics of the approach in 1 it is important to distinguish between them. The school (which is often capitalized: the *Functionalist* school) represented a particular programmatic approach to the study of consciousness. It had a set of basic tenets put forth by Angell and was designed as a replacement paradigm for the then dominant Structuralist school (see STRUCTURALISM (1)). Functionalism in sense 1, which is rarely if ever capitalized, represents a particular perspective that emerged from several influences, namely Darwin's evolutionary theory, with its emphasis on adaptation, James's and Peirce's pragmatism, with its open-mindedness and liberal attitudes and its focus on the practical utility of action, and Dewey's holism, with its bias toward

examination of the intact, functioning organism interacting with its environment.

While the school of thought of the Chicagoans has expired, the functionalist perspective is still very much alive. It is manifested in modern empiricism, and common terms such as *purpose, adaptation, function, utility, role* and many others are its legacy.

3 In philosophy, an approach to the study of mind that views mental states as functional states. Functionalism in this sense is distinguished metaphysically from physicalism in that rather than arguing that two identical mental states are physically identical it argues that they should (can) only be viewed as functionally equivalent. This point of view is represented in work in such fields as artificial intelligence, where a theory of an automaton would be represented in terms of functions rather than of real internal (i.e. physical) structures.

functional knowledge PROCEDURAL *KNOWLEDGE.

functional magnetic resonance imaging (fMRI) A form of MAGNETIC RESONANCE IMAGING in which the brain activity is scanned while it is actually taking place. The use of fMRI techniques has been a major advance in the cognitive neurosciences, since ongoing neural processes can be examined whereas older techniques were limited to 'snapshot' views of a static brain.

functional psychology FUNCTIONALISM (1, 2).

functional reasoning A kind of deductive reasoning whereby one's knowledge of the world allows the reaching of a valid conclusion about things not previously known. In the classic example, we probably don't *know* that bananas are not grown in Greenland but by virtue of what we know about geography, climate and growing bananas we can surmise this simple fact.

functional relation A relation between two variables such that change in one results in change in the other. Philosophically, a functional relation can be characterized as a causal relation.

functional stimulus STIMULUS, FUNCTIONAL.

function engram Jung's hypothesized genetic neurological 'imprint' that serves as the underlying representation of archetypes and endows symbols with their meanings.

function types Jung's classification of personality types was based on four functions: feeling, thinking, sensing and intuiting. Feeling and thinking were considered *rational*, sensing and intuiting *irrational*. All persons were assumed to possess all four of these functions, and the typing was a reflection of which style dominated in an individual's overall make-up.

function word Any word that has a grammatical (syntactic) role in a sentence as opposed to a lexical (semantic) meaning. Prepositions, auxiliary verbs, conjunctions, interjections, articles, etc. are function words. Also called *functor*. Compare with CONTENT WORD.

functor FUNCTION WORD.

fundamental attribution error ATTRIBUTION ERROR, FUNDAMENTAL.

fundamental colour(s) Colours (or, strictly speaking, *hues*) that are assumed to correspond with the fundamental colour-vision responses of any particular theory of colour vision. Thus, in the Young–Helmholtz theory there are three fundamental colours (red, green and blue) which when mixed in proper proportions yield all possible hues with a saturation greater than that possible with any other three wavelengths. See also THEORIES OF *COLOUR VISION.

fundamental needs The most basic of the BASIC NEEDS in Maslow's theory of human motivation. They include those generally related to physiological deficits such as hunger, thirst, etc.

fundamental skill Any skill that is a prerequisite for further progress.

fundamental tone The lowest-pitched tone in any compound sound. Practically every sounding or vibrating body vibrates in parts, each part putting out a pure tone dependent on the overall physical structure of the body. The perceived pitch of the resulting compound tone corresponds to the frequency of the *fundamental*. All higher-pitched tones are called *harmonics*, *partial tones* or simply *partials*.

fungiform papilla LINGUAL PAPILLA.

funnel technique A technique used in interviewing and in the construction of questionnaires or inventories whereby broad, general questions are used at the beginning and then the scope is gradually narrowed to specifics.

fusiform face area An area on the *fusiform gyrus* on the underside of the brain. It is part of the extrastriate cortex of the occipital lobe and is on both sides of the brain – although the right hemisphere area appears to be more important. While it is intimately involved in the perception of faces it should not be thought of as a pure 'face recognition' area since it is also known to be involved in recognition of items in other domains, provided that the person has had extensive experience. For example, it is activated when expert dog fanciers view pictures of dogs. There are suggestions that it functions abnormally in some cases of autism and damage to it can cause PROSOPAGNOSIA.

fusiform gyrus FUSIFORM FACE AREA.

fusion 1 A generic term used to refer to any process in which the several elements of a complex stimulus are blended or fused together in a whole so that the component parts cannot be perceptually distinguished. The term is very broadly used in this sense, and the stimulus may be almost anything from a straightforward physical one in a study on perception to a complex social one in a study of personal interaction. **2** In classical psychoanalytic theory, the balanced coordinated functioning of the life instincts and the death instincts. Fusion is regarded as 'normal', although different behavioural patterns are assumed to result depending on which instincts dominate. *Defusion* is assumed to lead to various neuroses, especially obsessions.

fusional language SYNTHETIC LANGUAGE.

fusion, binaural The combining of the sounds presented to each ear into a unitary auditory experience.

fusion, binocular The combining of the images presented to each eye into a single visual experience. Also called *retinal fusion*. See BINOCULAR RIVALRY for more discussion.

fusion frequency CRITICAL FLICKER FREQUENCY.

future shock A term coined by A. Toffler as a way of expressing the view that people in Western society are becoming overloaded in terms of what they can process. The 'shock' produced by rapid changes in social structures, social values and consumer products is so great that, Toffler argued, many persons simply cannot cope or adapt. It was a clever idea but there doesn't seem to be much evidence to support it.

fuzzy set (or **restriction**) The calculus of fuzzy sets is a relatively recent innovation in mathematics dealing with domains and concepts the boundaries of which are not sharply defined. Since much of human cognition seems to operate with such fuzzy concepts (e.g. 'hot', 'young', 'approximately equal'), there are many who foresee important applications of this novel calculus to the psychology of thinking, concept formation, judgement, decision-making, etc.

fuzzy trace A loose, gist-like memory or representation of a stimulus. Fuzzy memory traces lie at the opposite pole from *verbatim traces*, which are quite concrete and capture the full set of encoded features that characterized the stimulus.

fuzzy trace theory The generalization, due largely to C. Brainerd and V. Reyna, that memory needs to be viewed as ranging from highly inexact and intuitive representations (the FUZZY TRACES) to exact, verbatim representations. The theory assumes that, while everyone prefers fuzzy to verbatim representations, development can be seen, in part, as a movement from a reliance on the fuzzy, characteristic of the young, to a greater reliance on the encoded, logical forms of knowledge.

G

G 1 Abbreviation for GOAL, especially in Hullian theory. **2** Abbreviation for GENERAL FACTOR, also denoted as *g*. **3** A statistic expressing the degree of CONTINGENCY (2) or ASSOCIATION (4).

g 1 In Hull's theory, a fractional part of a goal reaction. See here FRACTIONAL ANTEDATING GOAL RESPONSE. **2** Abbreviation for GENERAL •FACTOR, also denoted as *G*.

GABA GAMMA-AMINOBUTYRIC ACID.

GABAergic Denoting neurons and neural pathways where GAMMA-AMINOBUTYRIC ACID is the neurotransmitter.

gabapentin A medication originally developed as an ANTIEPILEPTIC DRUG, but now also used to treat pain, particularly neuropathic pain, because of its minimal side effects. Named after its mimicry of GAMMA-AMINOBUTYRIC ACID. Trade name Neurontin.

Gabor filter FILTER, GABOR.

GAD GLUTAMIC ACID DECARBOXYLASE.

GAF GLOBAL ASSESSMENT OF FUNCTIONING.

Gage, Phineas One of neuropsychology's most famous patients. In 1848, Gage survived an explosion that propelled a large iron bar through his left cheek, up through his brain and out just to the left of the midline of the frontal lobes. Before the accident, Gage was a temperate, relaxed and highly competent man. Afterwards, his personality was dramatically changed. He became irascible and impulsive and showed exceedingly poor judgement – patterns of behaviour now associated with a variety of ORGANIC •PERSONALITY SYNDROMES caused by damage to the frontal lobes.

Gaia A theory developed initially by James Lovelock that views the sum of all life on earth, along with the planet itself, as a singular living, self-correcting system. The theory is certainly radical enough and has received both blistering criticism and enthusiastic support. The jury is still out.

gain by illness ADVANTAGE BY ILLNESS.

galact(o)- Combining form meaning *pertaining to milk* and occasionally, by extension, to *the breast, milk ducts, lactation*, etc.

galactosemia A genetic metabolic disorder characterized by an absence of the enzyme required for conversion of galactose (the sugar in milk) to glucose. If untreated it can lead to irreversible mental retardation. Treatment consists primarily of adjustment of diet to eliminate galactose milk sugar.

galanin A neurotransmitter found in the hypothalamus (interestingly, in the same terminal buttons as *norepinephrine*). Release of galanin alters the secretion of insulin and corticosterone and stimulates the intake of fats.

galantamine An ACETYLCHOLINESTERASE inhibitor that appears to have some ability to slow the progression of ALZHEIMER'S DISEASE and other dementias.

Galton bar A device for determining the *just noticeable difference* for visual distance.

Galton whistle A primitive device emitting very high-pitched tones once used extensively to determine upper-pitch thresholds. It is not very accurate.

galvanic Pertaining to direct current.

galvanic skin response (GSR) A measure of the electrical response of the skin as measured by a galvanometer. Two techniques are used: the Féré measure, which records changes in the resistance of the skin to the passage of a weak electric current, and the Tarchanoff measure, which records weak current actually produced by the body. Since the Féré measure increases with increasing perspiration it has often been assumed to be an indicator of emotional tension or anxiety. This assumption has proven difficult to substantiate, however, and it is probably best to consider the measure as merely an indicator of physiological arousal; see LIE DETECTOR, POLYGRAPH. The GSR has a seemingly endless array of alternative names, including *skin conductance response* (SCR), *skin resistance response* (SRR), *skin potential response* (SPR), *psychogalvanic response* (PGR), *electrodermal response* (EDR), *electrical skin response* (ESR), *Féré phenomenon* and *Tarchanoff phenomenon*.

galvanometer An instrument which measures electric current.

galvanotropism An orienting response to electric current. Also called *galvano-taxis*. See TAXIS and TROPISM for a distinction in terminology.

gambler's fallacy This is explained most easily with an example. Suppose you have just flipped a fair, unbiased coin seven times in a row and got seven heads. If you think that the chance of getting a tail on the next flip is very high (at least over 0.5) because 'a tail is due', then you have committed the gambler's fallacy: the probability of a tail is still only 0.5. Events such as coin flips are independent of each other and the probabilities of their occurrence are not altered by past outcomes. However, you are not alone: in most experiments on choice behaviour, people's intuitions about the probabilities of independent events do not coincide with a rational implementation of simple probability theory.

gambling The risking of something of value with the possibility of ultimate gain. Not a great deal is known about gambling behaviour apart from what has been derived from studies of risk-taking and game theory and through clinical evaluations of pathological gamblers. The term tends to be used in a restricted fashion to refer to the risking of money in organized settings such as casinos or race-tracks. Actually, the deeper meaning – the notion of risking something of value for potential gain – is a much broader notion, and in this larger sense gambling is a fundamental feature of human behaviour. Ironically, this general sense tends to be found more in nontechnical writings than in the psychological literature. It is probably worth pointing out that professionals who play games like poker often do not call themselves gamblers, on the simple grounds that they do not gamble in the above sense of the term: rather than wagering on the *possibility* of ultimate gain they do so on the virtual *assuredness* of it in the long run.

gambling, pathological An IMPULSE CONTROL DISORDER characterized by chronic inability to resist impulses to gamble. The term is generally not used unless the pattern of behaviour disrupts and damages personal, familial and vocational life. Like most impulse control disorders, pathological gambling rarely occurs in isolation. Pathological gamblers typically have a variety of other difficulties, commonly alcohol and drug abuse.

game A generic term for any pattern of social interaction or organized play with well-defined rules.

gamete A general term for a reproductive cell, either a sperm or an egg cell, in its mature state.

game theory A branch of mathematics concerned with providing a formal analysis of decision-making, specifically the decision-making process that takes account of the actions and options for action of another party whose decisions present a conflict (which, after all, is what a game is). In principle, the analyses carried out within this often abstruse realm of mathematics apply to more than simple games. Variations on the basic theory have been directed at studies of interpersonal interactions, economics, labour-management negotiations and international diplomacy. For not too abstruse an example often studied in the laboratory, see PRISONER'S *DILEMMA.

game, zero-sum Any game of which the expected value of playing it is zero for all participants, i.e. a game in which in the long run, one expects (probabilistically speaking) to lose exactly as much as one wins. Note that games and the strategies players adopt in playing them can usually be evaluated in terms of this notion of expected gain or loss. Naturally, many games and/or playing strategies yield positive expected values (so-called *plus-sum games*) and others result in negative expectations (*minus-sum games*). See also EXPECTED VALUE.

gamma (γ) In psychophysics, the distance of any stimulus from threshold.

gamma afferent GAMMA *MOTOR NEURON.

gamma-aminobutyric acid (GABA) An amino acid that functions as an important inhibitory neurotransmitter in many central-nervous-system locations. It is found throughout the grey matter, in the cells of the basal ganglia that project to the substantia nigra, in the Purkinje cells of the cerebellum and in the dorsal horn of the spinal cord. GABA has been implicated in the neurological disorder *Huntington's disease*, and imbalances are thought to play a role in severe anxiety disorders. Note that there are three known GABA receptors, usually denoted $GABA_A$, $GABA_B$ and $GABA_C$. All three are complex, $GABA_A$ having at least five distinct receptor sites. These sites bind a variety of substances, including the BENZO-DIAZEPINES, the BARBITURATES and various steroids.

gamma motion MOTION, GAMMA.

gamma motor neuron MOTOR NEURON, GAMMA.

gamma rhythm (or **wave**) A pattern of electrical activity in the brain characterized by a cycle of approximately 40 Hz. It is present during awakening and during REM sleep, and so thought to be associated with changes of consciousness. Some researchers classify this pattern along with the slightly slower BETA RHYTHM because both indicate consciousness. Also called *gamma cycle*.

gam(o)- Combining form used to indicate a marital relationship or a sexual union. Used as a prefix, although the suffix forms *-(o)gamous* and *-(o)gamy* are also used, for adjectives and nouns respectively.

ganglion A collection of cell bodies or nerve cells usually outside the central nervous system. The term is also used on occasion for collections of grey matter in the central nervous system, e.g. the *basal ganglia*. Specific ganglia are listed under the modifying term.

ganglion cells Cells in the retina that receive information from the bipolar cells. Their axons give rise, at the optic disc, to the optic nerve.

Ganser syndrome A FACTITIOUS DISORDER (or pseudopsychosis) in which there is voluntary production of (often severe) psychological symptoms. Typically these are worse when the patient is cognizant of being observed. The displayed symptoms are almost always a reflection of the patient's own concept of some disorder and rarely conform to recognized diagnostic categories. The syndrome is often seen among prisoners and army draftees who seek, consciously or otherwise, to receive special treatment by virtue of their 'disorder'. Also spelled *Ganzer*.

Ganzfeld From the German for *complete* or *homogeneous field*, a Ganzfeld is a visual field produced by a set-up in which the entire retina is stimulated by homogeneous light. It has no contours or forms and is totally undifferentiated. In effect, such stimulation is equivalent to no stimulation at all. For example, a coloured Ganzfeld becomes an undifferentiated grey after a few minutes and the distance of the field becomes unstable. The easiest way to approximate one outside the laboratory is to cut a ping-pong ball along the seam and place the halves over the eyes.

Garcia effect CONDITIONED *AVERSION, TOXICOSIS.

garden-path sentences A rather clever name given by psycholinguists to sentences in which the initial few words suggest an interpretation that the later words prove to have been inappropriate. For example, 'The horse raced past the barn fell.'

gargoylism HURLER'S SYNDROME.

GAS GENERAL ADAPTATION SYNDROME.

gaster(o)-, gastric(-), gastro- Combining forms meaning *stomach* or the *stomach region*.

gate-control theory A theory of pain perception that, building on the principle of GATING, assumes that pain is only experienced when input from peripheral neurons passes through 'gates' at the points where they enter the spinal cord and lower brainstem. Support for the theory comes from the fact that neurons in the PERIAQUEDUCTAL GREY in the midbrain have descending axons that terminate on inhibitory neurons in these gates, which in turn inhibit transmission of the messages from the peripheral neurons.

gating Essentially, selective damping or inhibiting of sensory input. The 'gate' metaphor is apt: the essence of the effect is that only certain afferent messages get through to be processed consciously. For example, while intently watching a football game one is simply unaware of other aspects of the environment such as itches, cold feet, pickpockets, etc. Also called *sensory gating*.

Gaussian distribution (or **curve**) The normal distribution or curve is often called Gaussian or, simply, Gauss's distribution or curve, in honour of C. F. Gauss (1777–1855), the great German mathematician and astronomer.

gay A sobriquet for *homosexual*. It has gradually worked its way from the common language into the scientific and is now used regularly in journals and textbooks. Note that some authors only use this term for males; those that do so will typically use *lesbian* for homosexual women. See HOMOSEXUALITY et seq. for more detail on usage.

Gedanken experiment MENTAL •EXPERIMENT.

gemellology The study of twins, particularly the use of twins as the primary data source for evaluating the contributions of heredity and environment to behaviour.

gender Strictly speaking, a grammatical term used for classifying nouns. However, because of the many denotative and connotative difficulties with the term SEX, it has gradually emerged as the term of choice in discussion of male/female differences, identity, societal roles and the like. The following entries give examples of contemporary usage; see also SEX et seq. for other conceptually related terms.

gender assignment Classification of the sex of an infant with ambiguous external genitalia. At one time the assignment was made primarily on the basis of the physical features and determination of the success of various surgical procedures. Today it is done

primarily with regard to the genetic sex of the child since biological factors are now know to play a dominate role in GENDER IDENTITY.

gender differences SEX DIFFERENCES.

gender dysphoria Distress or discomfort with one's gender.

gender identity One's IDENTITY (1) as it is experienced with regard to one's individuality as male or female. This sense of self-awareness is generally treated as the internal, private experience of the overt expression of GENDER ROLE. See also SEX IDENTITY.

gender identity disorder A class of disorders characterized by a strong and persistent sense of inappropriateness concerning one's gender. See, e.g. GENDER IDENTITY DISORDER IN CHILDHOOD, TRANSGENDER, TRANSSEXUALISM.

gender identity disorder in childhood A GENDER IDENTITY DISORDER characterized by a compelling sense that one is the wrong sex. As the name implies, it is usually first noted in childhood primarily by the child displaying preferences for clothing, games and pastimes typical of the other sex and a tendency for cross-gender role-playing. In adolescence and adulthood there is a marked desire to be the other sex, frequent 'passing' for the other sex, a wish to be treated by others as a member of the other sex and a tendency to feel discomfort with one's genitals and secondary sex characteristics, such as hair and muscles in men and breasts and menstruation in women. There is often depression and considerable psychological distress although these symptoms typically do not manifest themselves until adolescence or adulthood. They are rarely seen in childhood and, indeed, in some cases are totally absent. Some authors use *gender-role disorder in childhood* interchangeably on the grounds that IDENTITY (1) is the private experience of the outward expression of ROLE. Both terms should be reserved for extreme cases and not used in instances of GENDER NONCONFORMITY.

genderlect D. Tannen's term for the particular communication styles or dialects that are exhibited by men and women. Her argument is that cultural factors have a marked impact on the manner and style of speaking and communicating and that one of the most compelling of these factors is gender.

gender nonconformity Quite literally, failure to conform to society's characterization of appropriate sex-role behaviour. The term is typically used in reference to children who display preferences for toys and activities generally associated with the opposite sex and who do not show the more common signs of appropriate sex-role identification, i.e. boys who say they just don't 'feel' very masculine, or girls who don't 'feel' feminine. Distinguish from GENDER IDENTITY DISORDER IN CHILDHOOD.

gender role The overt expression of behaviours and attitudes that indicates to others the degree of one's affiliation to maleness or femaleness. It is generally assumed that gender role is the public expression of GENDER IDENTITY. See also ROLE and SEX ROLE.

gender-role disorder in childhood GENDER IDENTITY DISORDER IN CHILDHOOD.

gender schema Quite literally, a SCHEMA about gender; that is, a set of beliefs and expectations that guide the way people process information about gender and sex.

gender script A temporally organized GENDER SCHEMA, a sequence of actions typically associated with a particular sex in a particular culture.

gene Any of the functional units of the chromosomes. Genes manifest themselves in heredity by directing the synthesis of proteins. See DEOXYRIBONUCLEIC ACID.

gene expression The degree to which particular genes or inherited traits are displayed phenotypically. The term is not used for a 'pure' gene process; there are many well-documented phenomena in which environmental effects dictate gene expression.

gene pair Two genes, one from each parent, that combine to determine a particular inherited trait. The pair is called *homozygous* if both determine the trait in the same way and *heterozygous* if they have different effects. See also ALLELE.

general ability The hypothetical broad-based cognitive ability that some presume to be basic to all the special or *specific abilities* displayed in particular situations. In short, a synonym for INTELLIGENCE. See also GENERAL *FACTOR.

general adaptation syndrome (GAS) Hans Selye's three-stage characterization of an organism's biological reactions to severe stress. The first stage, the *alarm reaction*, is characterized by two substages: a *shock phase* and a *countershock phase*. During the shock phase body temperature drops, blood pressure falls, there is a loss of fluid from the tissues, muscle tone decreases, etc. During the countershock phase there is an increase in adrenocortical hormones and a general biological defensive reaction against the stress begins. The second stage is a *resistance stage*, which continues the recuperative processes begun during countershock. Bodily functions, blood pressure, temperature, etc. gradually return to normal or near normal. However, if the stress is too severe or prolonged, the third stage, *exhaustion*, ensues. Here the general pattern of the initial shock phase reappears and ultimately death results.

general aptitude (test) See discussion under APTITUDE TEST.

general factor FACTOR, GENERAL

general factors In clinical psychology, a cluster of factors that all effective therapies share. Included are a good relationship between therapist and client, the genuineness of the therapist, and the client's motivation to change. Distinguish from GENERAL FACTOR.

generalizability The degree to which findings can be taken to apply to other situations, groups, and so on. See GENERALIZATION for a related discussion and GENERALIZABILTY THEORY for a particular application of the term.

generalizability theory In psychological testing and assessment, the theory that test scores are a result of multiple identifiable factors, and not just the result of a TRUE *SCORE plus ERROR (4, 5). From this perspective, work in test construction, reliability and validation should allow one to isolate precisely which aspects of test score variance are due to which factors. The theory maintains that only when all sources of variance are understood will we be able to specify the degree to which scores and findings can be generalized to real-life performance, other groups, and so on. Also called *G-Theory*.

generalization **1** A process of forming a judgement or making a decision that is applicable to an entire class or category of objects, events or phenomena. There are several features of this meaning that deserve mention. First, generalization in this sense nearly always involves a process of induction; it is derived from a limited number of observations of members of a class and extended (i.e. *generalized*) to the other members. Second, generalization here is the other side of the coin from DISCRIMINATION (1). That is, when one generalizes a judgement or a response over all members of a category one is, in effect, not discriminating between the individual tokens within that category. See GENERALIZATION GRADIENT for more on this issue. **2** The process of extending a principle or conceptualization to new objects, events or domains. Note, this process may be similar to 1, in that one discovers that the new objects can be classified in a known group and thus included in a previously made generalization, or it may deal with a wholly new set of objects that are still distinguishable from other events but have been shown to lend themselves to explication by some known principle. **3** In science, any broad principle that can encompass a number of observations. That is, the process of a generalization in sense 2 may yield one in sense 3. **4** In studies of expressive functions, reacting to an event with both an overt behavioural response and a covert autonomic nervous system response.

Because these meanings are themselves so general, the term is often qualified by various modifiers that delineate the kind of generalization under consideration. See the following entries for some common examples.

generalization, acoustic A form of STIMULUS *GENERALIZATION along an acoustic dimension. One rather compelling example of this kind of generalization is the startled response that invariably accompanies hearing someone loudly exclaim, 'Oh, sit!' in public. This stimulus evokes an emotional reaction because it is acoustically similar to a taboo word. Distinguish from SEMANTIC *GENERALIZATION.

generalization gradient In both RESPONSE *GENERALIZATION and STIMULUS *GENERALIZATION there is a gradient such that: **1** in response generalization, the more alike the several responses are to the original, the more likely they are to occur in response to the stimulus; and **2** in stimulus generalization, the more similar the several stimuli are to the original, the more likely they are to produce the response. See GRADIENT.

generalization, mediated Any STIMULUS *GENERALIZATION that is mediated through some other process. The most common form is SEMANTIC *GENERALIZATION, in which the generalization occurs through the semantic content or meaning of a word.

generalization, response The tendency for responses similar to the original reinforced or conditioned response to be made in the conditioning situation. The response is said to be *generalized* to the situation.

generalization, semantic A form of STIMULUS *GENERALIZATION in which the generalization process operates through the semantic properties of the stimuli. For example, a response originally established to the word *style* may be elicited by the word *fashion*. For more on this general notion, see PRIMING (3).

generalization, stimulus The tendency for stimuli similar to the original stimulus in a learning situation to produce the response originally acquired. Generalization gradients are typically found when the stimuli are systematically varied: the more dissimilar a stimulus is from the original, the less likely the response.

generalization, verbal Simply, GENERALIZATION with verbal materials, e.g. ACOUSTIC *GENERALIZATION, SEMANTIC *GENERALIZATION.

generalized anxiety disorder A subclass of ANXIETY DISORDERS characterized by persistent *free-floating anxiety* and a host of unspecific reactions such as trembling, jitteriness, tension, sweating, light-headedness, feelings of apprehension and irritability. The term is applied only to functional disorders, not to organic disabilities, which can produce similar symptoms. Also called, simply, *anxiety reaction*.

generalized inhibitory potential ($_sI_R$) In

Hull's learning theory, inhibition conditioned as a result of stimulus generalization.

generalized other A term introduced by the sociologist George Herbert Mead to refer to a person's inculcated notions of some abstract social class or group. An individual develops a generalized other by a process of social interaction through which the attitudes, values, expectations, points of view, etc. of the members of the group gradually become one's own. Although the initial phases may be quite specific, with particular aspects of the group's values being adopted, over time the full complex of factors becomes interrelated and generalized and it no longer reflects specific attitudes of specific persons. It is through this generalized other that a person comes to interact successfully within the group and reflect its values. Moreover, according to Mead, the generalized other also serves as the basis for abstract thought and problem-solving. See also SIGNIFICANT OTHER and SOCIALIZATION.

generalizing assimilation ASSIMILATION, GENERALIZING.

general paresis (general paralysis) PARESIS.

General Problem Solver (GPS) One of the first computer programs to do a respectable job of simulating some limited aspects of human cognitive processes. GPS, developed in 1959 by A. Newell and co-workers, used heuristically guided trial-and-error processes to solve some simple problems and to do so in ways that approximated those used by adults.

general psychology 1 An antiquated term once used for an approach to psychology that sought broad general explanatory principles. **2** Loosely, psychology as it is presented in the typical introductory text.

generation 1 The process of procreation, the forming of a new organism. **2** By extension, any process of creation. Here the meaning extends beyond the organic; see e.g. GENERATIVE *GRAMMAR. **3** The offspring of an ancestor the same distance removed; e.g. *filial generation* – see here F_1, F_2. **4** The average period of time between the birth of parents and the birth of their children. This period differs from culture to culture.

generative grammar GRAMMAR, GENERATIVE.

generative semantics SEMANTICS, GENERATIVE.

generator potential Any graded change in electrical potential that occurs in a receptor organ or receptor cell. Generator potentials are related to the initiation of the action potential in the associated afferent neurons; they function much like POSTSYNAPTIC POTENTIALS in that they raise or lower the likelihood of a neuron firing. Differentiate from RECEPTOR POTENTIAL and ACTION POTENTIAL.

generic 1 General, having wide application – at least within the class of objects or events under consideration. **2** Pertaining to a GENUS.

generic knowledge KNOWLEDGE, GENERIC.

generic name The general chemical name for a drug, the nonproprietary name.

genetic 1 Pertaining to the origins and development of any single organism or to an entire species. One uses the term *ontogenetic* when referring to the development of a single organism and *phylogenetic* when referring to the evolutionary development of a species. **2** Pertaining to GENETICS. **3** Pertaining to GENES; see GENIC.

genetic algorithm A computational procedure for discovering optimum solutions in complex domains using a technique analogous to natural selection. The procedure has applications in a wide variety of settings including code breaking, game theory, linguistics and even aesthetics. For example, it is possible using this technique to find an aesthetically pleasing bottle. People are given an array of bottles of various shapes, sizes and colours and asked to pick the ones they like best. The array is then systematically shifted, keeping the objects liked best (i.e. selected) and adding others. The process continues iteratively until the ideal or optimum bottle is revealed.

genetic counselling A general term for any health service that tests, advises and counsels prospective parents on any genetic disorder that they may pass to their offspring.

genetic drift Changes in the genetic composition of a population, or, more precisely, of the gene pool of a population, from generation to generation. The meaning here is not synonymous with NATURAL SELECTION as the changes in the gene pool are not given direction by selection.

genetic epistemology An approach to psychology that focuses on the study of the development of knowledge. The label itself is usually associated with the orientation to development of the Swiss psychologist Jean Piaget. This point of view stresses: (a) that knowledge develops in the sense of becoming increasingly organized and adaptive to one's surroundings; (b) that this process of development is not based on innately given ideas nor any simple automatic maturation but rather as active construction on the part of the individual; and (c) that this construction of knowledge is initiated and carried through by the need to overcome contradictions produced by functioning in a complex, changing environment. See also PIAGETIAN.

geneticism One of several terms used for the view that behaviour is largely a result of innate characteristics. Note that one could stress either species-specific characteristics shared by all members of the species or the individually inherited traits of single organisms. The distinction is usually marked by appending *phylogenetic* or *ontogenetic* to the base term for these two meanings.

genetic memory MEMORY, GENETIC.

genetic psychology A rough synonym of the more common term DEVELOPMENTAL PSYCHOLOGY. Note, however, that genetic psychology also includes COMPARATIVE PSYCHOLOGY and tends to focus on developmental processes that underlie phenomena studied in the mature organism.

genetics A branch of biology that deals with heredity in any of its manifestations.

Genevan school The school of psychology founded by Jean Piaget. For details see GENETIC EPISTEMOLOGY and PIAGETIAN.

genic Relating to genes or to that which is caused by genes. A preferred synonym of GENETIC (3).

-genic Combining form used with a variety of prefixes to characterize: **1** The locus or point of origin of something, e.g. *endogenic* = originating from within. **2** The agent origin of something, e.g. *mutagenic* = mutation-causing.

geniculate bodies Two sets of paired oval tissue masses lying under and to the rear of the thalamus. The LATERAL GENICULATE BODIES are important synaptic stations for vision, the MEDIAL GENICULATE BODIES for audition; see each for details.

genital Pertaining to the genitals.

genital anomaly SEX ANOMALY.

genital character In psychoanalytic theory, the mature synthesis of the previous stages of psychosexual development culminating in the GENITAL STAGE.

genital eroticism Sensual or sexual pleasure derived from the genitals. var., *genital erotism.*

genitalia GENITALS.

genitals (or **genitalia**) The reproductive organs.

genital stage (or **level**) In psychoanalytic theory, the culminating level of psychosexual development characterized by the development of relationships with persons of the opposite sex.

genital zones The external genitals and adjacent areas, one of the *erogenous zones.*

genius Loosely used, the term refers to the highest level of intellectual or creative functioning, or to a person endowed with such. Although there have been several efforts at formulating an explicit definition (e.g. at one time an IQ of 140 or over was considered to indicate genius), such attempts only provide illusory objectivity. Unfortunately (or fortunately) there doesn't appear to be any clear set of attributes that defines genius; all behaviours, including the intellectual and creative, are subject to a variety of noncognitive factors such as motivation, temperament, emotion and the demand characteristics of the environment, and people who display genius in one setting do not necessarily display it in others. Furthermore, the common language has played such havoc with the term that its usefulness is now suspect even in the most technical context.

genome The full collection of genes of an organism.

genotype 1 The genetic constitution of an

individual organism, the particular set of genes it carries. The genotype includes hereditary factors that may be passed on to future generations even though they are not manifested in the organism's PHENOTYPE. Usage here, particularly in the study of developmental psychology, typically focuses on the notion of the genotype as a collection of hereditary factors that influences the development of an individual. Rather than referring directly to inherited traits *per se*, the term relates to inherited influences that help the development of particular traits. Meaning here reflects the complexities of the interaction between heredity and environment and the recognition that a given genotype can be expressed in a variety of phenotypes. **2** In Lewin's theory of personality, the full compilation of causes responsible for any behavioural phenomenon. This usage is much more inclusive than 1 and is rarely intended any more.

-genous Combining form meaning: **1** *Producing*. **2** *Produced by*. Often used as a variation of -GENIC.

gens SIB (2).

genus **1** In biology, a classification encompassing related SPECIES (1). **2** In Aristotelian logic, a broad category containing subclasses of SPECIES (2). pl., *genera*.

-geny Combining form denoting: **1** *Origin* or *cause*. **2** *Generation*.

geometric illusion Any of a large class of visual illusions produced by perceptual distortions of straight lines, curves, etc.

geometric mean MEAN, GEOMETRIC.

geometric series A series that increases or decreases by a constant proportion or ratio, e.g. 2, 4, 8, 16, 32. A geometric series is logarithmic. Contrast with ARITHMETIC SERIES.

geon Any of the simple three-dimensional forms that, according to Biederman's theory, make up the perceptual components of more complex forms. Examples of geons are cubes, cylinders, wedges and slices.

geotropism An orienting response to gravitational forces. Also called *geotaxis*; see TAXIS and TROPISM for a distinction often ignored.

geriatrics The medical speciality dealing with treatment of the aged.

geriopsychosis SENILE *DEMENTIA.

germ cell A general term for a reproductive cell in any stage of development. Distinguish from GAMETE, a mature germ cell.

germinal stage (or **period**) The earliest stage of gestation. In humans, it is the period of approximately two weeks from the moment of conception. See EMBRYO.

gerontology The study of the aged and the aging process. The field is extremely broad and encompasses essentially all aspects of life – physiological, social, psychological, medical, economic, etc. – as they are relevant to the understanding of aging.

Gerstmann's syndrome A syndrome characterized by a cluster of specific dysfunctions including *acalculia, agraphia,* a left–right spatial disorientation and a *finger agnosia*. These various dysfunctions tend to occur together when there is damage in the left parietal-occipital region.

Gesell Developmental Schedules (or **Scales**) The first of the DEVELOPMENTAL SCALES to be constructed and standardized. The schedules were developed by Arnold Gesell and his colleagues to assess four major areas of behaviour in the young child: motor, adaptive, language and personal–social. Unlike some later scales (e.g. BAYLEY SCALES), they are weighted toward physical development and are largely based on simple observation of the behaviour of the infant and preschooler, and when they are used it is as a supplement to medical, neurological examinations. Two scales are available, an *Infant Schedule* and a *Preschool Schedule*.

gestagen Any of the group of hormones that function to promote and support pregnancy.

Gestalt (or **gestalt**) A German term which unfortunately has no exact English equivalent. Several terms have been proposed, such as *form, configuration* and *shape*; however, *essence* and *manner* are also acceptable translations. By and large, the term itself, rather than any inadequate translation, has moved over into English and is now often spelled without the initial capital.

The primary focus of the term is that it is used to refer to unified wholes, complete structures, totalities, the nature of which is not revealed by simply analysing the several parts that make them up. An aphorism spawned by this idea is 'The whole [i.e. the Gestalt] is different from the sum of its parts.' This principle forms the core of the Gestalt psychology movement. See the following entries for more details on terminology. pl., *Gestalten* or *Gestalts*.

Gestalt factor Any stimulus situation which tends to produce a perceptual experience of wholeness or unity, a GESTALT. All of the Gestalt laws (or principles) of organization utilize Gestalt factors.

Gestalt laws of organization A cover term for all of those principles of organization that identify the factors that lead to particular forms of perceptual organization. A few of them, with examples, are:

continuation: the tendency to perceive a line as maintaining its established direction, e.g. this figure tends to be seen as two uprights and a diamond rather than a W on top of an M.

closure: the tendency to perceive incomplete objects as complete, e.g. a square is seen as such despite a gap.

proximity: events or stimuli that are close to one another spatially or temporally are perceived as belonging together, e.g. three groups of two lines.

similarity: parts of a stimulus field that are physically similar tend to be perceived as belonging together, e.g. alternating columns of light and dark dots.

good shape or form: the tendency to perceive figures in their symmetric, uniform and stable way, e.g. seeing an irregular form as a circle.

Gestalt psychology A school of psychology founded in Germany in the 1910s. Arguing originally against the structuralists, the Gestaltists maintained that psychological phenomena could only be understood if they were viewed as organized, structured wholes (or Gestalten). The structuralist position that phenomena could be introspectively broken down into primitive perceptual elements was directly challenged

by the Gestalt point of view that such an analysis left out the notion of the whole, unitary essence of phenomena (e.g. is an apple *really* a particular combination of primitive elements such as redness, shape, contour, hardness, etc., or does this analysis miss some fundamental 'appleness' that is only apprehensible when the whole is viewed as a whole?).

The early Gestaltists were masters of the elegant counterexample and presented sufficiently convincing arguments and demonstrations to damage seriously the orthodox structuralist view. For example, a particular melody is easily recognized even when its component parts are dramatically altered: it may be sung (in any voice range), played (by any combination of musical instruments), changed in key, embedded in multiple variations, etc., without destroying its recognizable Gestalt. Further, each of the several notes in any particular melody has a different phenomenological sense if played alone or if introduced into a new melody. In all cases, they argued, the whole dominates the perception and it is experienced as different from simply the sum of its several parts.

Learning was regarded by the Gestaltists not as associations between stimuli and responses (as the behaviourists maintained), but as a restructuring or reorganizing of the whole situation, often involving INSIGHT as a critical feature. The physiology of the brain was viewed in like fashion. Rather than accepting the then conventional view that the cortex was a static, well-differentiated system, they argued for a coordinated physiology in which the cortex was conceptualized as the place in which incoming stimuli interacted in a field of forces. See here ISOMORPHISM (2). In social psychology their work led to FIELD THEORY, and in education the stress was on productive thinking and creativity.

In general, Gestalt psychology is antithetical to atomistic psychology in all of its varieties (see here ATOMISM, ELEMENTARISM) and equal hostility was directed toward the behaviourists and the structuralists. Although as a separate theory Gestalt psychology hardly exists today, many of its discoveries and insights have been incorporated into the contemporary body of knowledge, particularly in the field of perception. The main exponents of the school were Max

Wertheimer, Kurt Koffka, Wolfgang Köhler and, by philosophical allegiance, Kurt Lewin.

Gestaltqualität A German term roughly translated as *form quality*. Originally introduced by C. von Ehrenfels, a precursor of the Gestalt movement, it refers to the quality or property of a whole that emerges out of a pattern of stimulation. See also GESTALT PSYCHOLOGY, the proponents of which disputed von Ehrenfels's suggestions that a *Gestaltqualität* is merely another perceptual element.

Gestalt therapy A form of psychotherapy associated with the work of Frederick (Fritz) Perls. It is based loosely on the Gestalt concepts of unity and wholeness. Treatment, which is usually conducted in groups, focuses on attempts to broaden a person's awareness of self by using past experiences, memories, emotional states, bodily sensations, etc. In short, everything that could contribute to the person forming a meaningful configuration of awareness is an acceptable part of the therapy process.

gestation 1 The carrying of the embryo in the womb. **2** The period of intrauterine development from conception to birth. **3** By extension, a period of 'incubation' for the development of an idea, a work of art, a scientific theory, etc.

gestational age CONCEPTION *AGE.

gestural language A broad term for any communication system based primarily on gestural operations. See NONVERBAL COMMUNICATION and SIGN LANGUAGE.

gesture Any bodily or facial movement used for communication. Gestures may accompany speech or may be used independently, as in sign language.

geusis The process or act of tasting.

g factor GENERAL *FACTOR.

ghrelin A hormone that increases eating. High blood levels are found during fasting and are reduced after a meal. It is released in both the brain and the stomach.

Gibsonian Pertaining to and characterizing the theoretical position of James J. Gibson (1904–80). Gibson's work was focused on that oldest of questions, 'How do we learn about the world?' His answer was simple yet radical: by direct pick-up of information

about the invariant properties of the environment. It was simple because it dispensed with the need to take raw sensations into account and because it eliminated the need to hypothesize about internal organizing and inferencing systems that structure and code sensations. It was 'radical' for these very same reasons. See also AFFORDANCE, DIRECT PERCEPTION, ECOLOGICAL OPTICS and ECOLOGICAL VALIDITY for more on Gibson's system.

gifted Characterizing a person with a special talent. The talent may be a general intellectual one or quite specific such as for music or chess. The word *gift* implies that the talent is inherited, a shaky hypothesis at best and one that probably cannot be applied uniformly to all gifted individuals. The term also suffers from the same kind of definitional fogginess that surrounds other similar terms, such as GENIUS. See GIFTED CHILD.

gifted child 1 A label for any child whose intellectual aptitude and performance dramatically exceeds the norms for her or his age. **2** More broadly, a child who displays special talents in any area of human behaviour that society values. This meaning is based on the notion that giftedness may extend beyond those characteristics and talents assessed through standardized testing instruments. Contrast with SPECIAL CHILD.

gigantism Abnormal overdevelopment of the skeleton caused by malfunctioning of the anterior pituitary gland before adulthood. See GROWTH HORMONE.

gigantocellular tegmental field A group of cells in the pons. Activity here is hypothesized to be an important component in the control of REM sleep.

GIGO An acronym for 'garbage in garbage out'. The term is used in computer sciences for the notion that if unreliable data form the input only unreliable outcomes are possible. The acronym has, not surprisingly, achieved wide usage in a variety of psychological contexts.

Gilles de la Tourette's syndrome TOURETTE'S SYNDROME.

given-new distinction A label for those aspects of communication whereby the speaker assumes that the listener knows something (see here PRESUPPOSITION) and then elaborates upon it by adding new information.

glabrous Smooth, without hair. Usually used of skin.

gland Very generally, any organ or structure that forms a bodily substance or secretes it can be called a gland. There are various subdivisions and classification systems for the glands, to wit: (a) glands of *external secretion* (e.g. sweat glands, kidneys) vs. glands of *internal secretion* (e.g. thyroid, pituitary); (b) *endocrine* glands, which are ductless and produce hormones (e.g. pituitary, adrenals) vs. *exocrine* glands, which have ducts (e.g. salivary); (c) *cytogenic* glands, which produce new cells (e.g. lymph nodes, bone marrow, spleen) vs. all others. Moreover, the classifications overlap since some glands (e.g. testes, ovaries, liver) produce a hormone as well as a secretion which flows from a duct.

glans The bulbous end of the clitoris or penis.

glaucoma A pathological condition of the eye caused by increasing intraocular pressure resulting in atrophy of the optic nerve, gradually increasing visual dysfunction and, ultimately, blindness.

glia Collectively, the supportive cells in the central nervous system. Four primary classes of glia cells have been identified: (a) *astroglia* (or *astrocytes* – so called because of their star-like shape), which play a physical and nutritional supporting role and are involved in 'house-cleaning' (the clearing of dead cells) and the formation of scar tissue following injury (recent evidence suggests they may also exchange information with neurons); (b) *micro-glia* (so named owing to their small size), which serve as phagocytes (see here PHAGOCYTOSIS); (c) *oligodendroglia*, which function to produce the *myelin sheath* found on many (but not all) of the axons in the central nervous system; and (d) *radial glia*, which function during feotal development to guide nerve cells to their final location. See also SCHWANN CELLS. Also called *neuroglia*. Recent evidence suggests that glia may also play a role in the formation of synapses in the neurons with which they interact. There are also suggestions that glia play a role in behavioural and cognitive processes,

functions generally thought to be restricted to nerve cells.

glial Pertaining to GLIA.

gliosis The replacement of dead neurons with glia cells.

glissades Small adjustments of the position of the eyes following a SACCADE. The typical saccade does not 'land' at a point for optimal viewing of an object; these small eye movements correct for these errors.

global amnesia AMNESIA, GLOBAL.

global aphasia APHASIA, GLOBAL.

global assessment of functioning Any procedure that assesses the overall level at which a person functions in social, personal and employment domains. Some measures break down functioning across the different areas of a person's life: their social lives, work setting, home, etc.

global processing Processing the overall form or gestalt of a complex stimulus. The processing in these cases appears to be predominately a right hemisphere function most likely in the temporal lobe.

globus hystericus A feeling of a lump in the throat. The term is reserved for a psychogenic syndrome often associated with conversion disorder in which the illusory lump can actually interfere with swallowing.

globus pallidus One of the subcortical nuclei that make up the BASAL GANGLIA. It functions as an excitatory structure of the extrapyramidal motor system. Also called *pallidum* and *paleostriatum*.

glossal Pertaining to the tongue.

glossiness The degree to which a perceived surface reflects light.

glosso- A combining form from the Latin for *tongue*.

glossolalia Artificial, fabricated speech devoid of real, linguistic content. It is observed in persons during religious ecstasy ('speaking in tongues'), under hypnosis and in some psychopathological cases.

glossopharyngeal nerve The IXth CRANIAL NERVE. It contains afferent components from the rear third of the tongue and the soft palate which mediate taste and efferent components to muscles in the throat.

glossosynthesis   In reference to pathological states, the invention of nonsense words. Were it not for the (presumed non-pathological) glossosynthetic predilections of scientists this volume would be about 40% shorter. See also NEOLOGISM.

glottal   **1** Pertaining to the glottis. **2** A speech sound produced by constriction of the glottis, e.g. the *h* in *hot*.

glottal stop (or **catch**)   A speech sound produced by a stopping of the air flow by closing the glottis.

glottis   The opening between the vocal folds or cords.

glove anaesthesia   ANAESTHESIA, GLOVE.

glucagon   A hormone of the pancreas that functions as part of the process that converts glycogen into glucose.

glucocorticoids   A group of hormones of the adrenal cortices that play an important role in the metabolism of proteins and carbohydrates, particularly when the body is subjected to conditions of stress. Included are CORTISOL and CORTICOSTERONE.

glucoprivation   A drop in the level of fatty acids available for cells. Whether brought about by a drop in blood levels of glucose or by drugs that inhibit its metabolism, it causes what is known as *glucoprivic hunger*, which stimulates eating. See also LIPOPRIVATION.

glucoprivic hunger   GLUCOPRIVATION.

glucoreceptors   Cells that are sensitive to glucose. They are found in the lateral hypothalamus and the liver. Also called *glucose receptors*.

glucose   A simple sugar that plays a critical role in metabolism. Along with the *ketones*, glucose constitutes the major source of energy for cerebral tissues.

glucostatic theory   A generalization that satiety and hunger are determined by the level or availability of glucose in the blood.

glutamate   An amino acid that functions as an excitatory neurotransmitter. It is the most common of neurotransmitters and is found in virtually half of all neural tissue. See GLUTAMATE RECEPTORS for more detail. Also called GLUTAMIC ACID.

glutamate receptors   A class of receptor sites on neurons that bind with glutamate. There are two primary types, IONOTROPIC and METABOTROPIC. The ionotropic has three subtypes, NMDA, AMPA and KAINATE; the metabotropic one, MGLUR. See each for details.

glutamic acid   GLUTAMATE.

glutamic acid decarboxylase (GAD)   An enzyme that converts glutamate into GAMMA-AMINOBUTYRIC ACID (GABA).

glycerine   GLYCEROL.

glycerol   A soluble carbohydrate that, along with the FATTY ACIDS, makes up the TRIGLYCERIDES found in adipose (fatty) tissue. Glycerol is converted into glucose by the liver. Also called *glycerine*.

glycine   An AMINO ACID suspected of functioning as an inhibitory neurotransmitter in the spinal cord and lower portions of the brain.

glycogen   A polysaccharide (often called animal starch), glycogen is one form in which carbohydrates are stored. It is converted into glucose for use.

glycogenolysis   The process of conversion of glycogen into glucose.

-gnosia, -gnosis   Combining forms from the Greek for *knowledge* and used widely to denote *knowing, cognition, recognition*, etc.

goal   In psychology the basic meaning is little different from that found in a standard dictionary in that in most usages some end result or object is implied. There are, however, a few subtleties that are worth mentioning: (a) Often the physical location of an object is called a goal (such as the goal box in a maze) rather than the object itself (food, water, etc.). (b) Occasionally there is a loss of clarity in the distinction between the actual, objective goal and some internal, subjective motivational state. This confusion is most often found when *purpose* is used as if it were a synonym of *goal*. While it is probably true that there can be no goal unless there is some motivational state, purpose is still internal and goal, strictly speaking, external and operational. (c) In some approaches (e.g.

Adler's) a goal may be treated as a rather abstract entity, such as *superiority*, which one strives toward.

goal-directed behaviour A neobehaviourist term intended to serve the same semantic function as the more mentalistic term *purpose*. To wit: goal-directed behaviour is a response, or a set of responses, which can only be interpreted in terms of attainment of a known goal. E. C. Tolman once remarked, 'Behaviour reeks of purpose.' He was certainly right, but orthodox behaviourists would have been much more comfortable had he said, 'Behaviour reeks of goal-directedness.' So much for poetry.

goal gradient A phrase used to describe the general finding that the closer an organism gets to a goal the more efficient its behaviour becomes; that is, its speed may increase, its error rate go down, etc. This generalization clearly has limits: when high emotional tone accompanies the approach it often interferes with performance.

goal object Not quite synonymous with GOAL, this term is reserved for cases in which there may be a series of subgoals in a complex task and is used to characterize the final, ultimate goal in the sequence.

goal orientation A general tendency to turn toward or position oneself in the direction of a goal. It applies to cases in which the turning is physical as well as to more metaphoric orientations of thinking and attention.

goal response Any overt response made to or toward a goal. See GOAL-DIRECTED BEHAVIOUR.

goal stimulus Any proprioceptive stimulus arising from behaviour toward a goal.

Goldstein–Scheerer tests A series of tests of concept formation and abstraction used in the diagnosis of brain injuries.

Golgi apparatus A complex of irregular structures of parallel membranes in the cytoplasm of a cell. Basically it is a cell's 'packaging plant'. Secretory cells wrap their products in a membrane produced by the Golgi apparatus, and this membrane bursts and releases the products after migrating to the outer cell membrane.

Golgi–Mazzoni corpuscles Bulbous encapsulated nerve endings found in the dermis. Once thought to be thermoreceptors, they are currently suspected of mediating pressure sensations.

Golgi neurons (Type I and **Type II)** Multipolar neurons in the cerebral cortex and the posterior horns of the spinal cord. Type I have long axons, Type II short axons.

Golgi tendon organ Nerve ending located at the juncture of tendon and muscle. It consists of stretch receptors, i.e. receptors that detect stretch exerted by the muscles (via the tendons) on the bones to which they are attached. Also called *spindle tendon* and *neurotendinal spindle*.

gonad 1 The embryonic sex gland prior to anatomical differentiation into a definitive testis or ovary. **2** The generic term for a sex gland, either testis or ovary.

gonadotrophic hormone Any hormone produced by the anterior pituitary gland which stimulates activity in the gonads. For example, FOLLICLE-STIMULATING HORMONE and LUTEINIZING HORMONE. Also called *gonadotrophin*. Also spelled *gonadotropic*.

gonadotrophin-releasing hormones Hormones that stimulate the gonads, which in turn release their hormones. The onset of puberty occurs when cells in the hypothalamus begin secreting these hormones. Also spelled *gonadotropin*.

gon(o)- Combining form meaning *genitals, seed, generation, offspring*.

gonococcus The organism that causes gonorrhoea.

go/no go task Generally, any task in which the subject must make some response to certain stimuli and refrain from responding to others. Popular in perceptual and cognitive studies, such tasks are also useful in neurological evaluations of patients with frontal lobe damage who often have difficulty withholding responses to the 'no go' stimuli.

gonorrhoea A venereal disease caused by the gonococcus bacterium. In males the primary symptoms are discharge from the penis, pain and burning sensation during urination. Infected females may be asymptomatic initially but more commonly there is urethral or vaginal discharge, pain during urination and occasionally lower abdominal pain; severe cases can lead to pelvic inflammatory disease, which is quite painful. var., *gonorrhea*.

good In psychodynamic and psychoanalytic approaches, the appealing, attractive and nurturing elements of objects.

good continuation GESTALT LAWS OF ORGANIZATION. Also known simply as *continuation*.

Goodenough Draw-a-Person Test An intelligence test used with young children (usually under 12) in which the subject is asked to draw the best picture of a person he or she can. The test is scored according to the amount of detail present and an assessment of qualitative features. Previously known as the *Goodenough Draw-a-Man Test*.

good Gestalt Any basic, stable configuration. See PRÄGNANZ.

goodness of fit FIT, GOODNESS OF.

good shape, law of GESTALT LAWS OF ORGANIZATION.

Gottschaldt figures A set of simple figures embedded in more complex ones. They are used as tests for form perception. See EMBEDDED *FIGURE.

government and binding A class of models of language that are derived from TRANSFORMATIONAL GRAMMAR. Government and binding theory soon becomes quite complex but is based on a rather simple assumption, specifically that all grammatical operations are captured by a single transformation 'move X', X being some abstract aspect of the language such as a noun phrase. The argument is that specifying the parameters for each particular structure X will uncover the universal aspects of all natural languages.

GPS GENERAL PROBLEM SOLVER.

gradation methods A general term for any of the psychophysical methods that use stimuli that change gradually in small, discrete steps, e.g. the *method of limits* (see MEASUREMENT OF *THRESHOLD).

graded potential Any slow, gradual electrical potential in a receptor cell or neuron, including GENERATOR POTENTIAL, POSTSYNAPTIC POTENTIAL and RECEPTOR POTENTIAL. Compare with ACTION POTENTIAL.

grade equivalent A score in a test that represents a level of achievement or performance in that test according to the norms for the population in each school grade.

grade norm The score – or, more commonly, a range of scores – that is representative of the typical level of achievement in the school population for any given grade. If a single score is used it is almost always the 50th percentile; when a range is used it is usually a fairly narrow one around the 50th percentile.

grade score GRADE EQUIVALENT.

gradient Any standard dictionary will provide several meanings for this term. All of them are variations on the basic connotation: a progressive, continual change in some quantity or variable. In this sense the term is used in both adjective and noun forms in many psychological contexts. For some examples see APPROACH GRADIENT, AVOIDANCE GRADIENT and GENERALIZATION GRADIENT.

gradient of effect If, in a sequence of S–R connections, one response is reinforced or punished, those responses preceding and following it show the effects of the procedure. The effect is revealed as a gradient in that responses temporally close to the rewarded or punished response show a larger effect than those more remote. See also SPREAD OF *EFFECT.

gradient of texture One of the monocular cues for depth perception. The fineness of detail or texture that can be seen decreases systematically with increasing distance between observer and stimulus.

graduated and reciprocated initiatives in tension reduction (GRIT) A strategy developed to reduce tensions between two hostile parties. Basically, the idea is to get one side to make a small step toward peace, hopefully followed by the other side making a small step, and so on, each step encouraging the next.

Graduate Record Examination (GRE) An examination widely used in the USA as a means of selecting from among applicants for graduate training. The exam has three general sections and one specialized section.

The general sections test verbal, mathematical and analytic skills; the specialized section tests a student's specific area of concentration.

grain A term descriptive of the record from a CUMULATIVE RECORDER. If the record consists of relatively evenly spaced responses it is said to have a *smooth* grain; if there are bursts of responding with pauses in between it is said to have a *rough* grain.

-gram Suffix denoting *written*, *drawn*, *sketched*. See also -GRAPH.

grammar The structure of a language; the system of rules that dictates the permissible sequences of language elements that form sentences in a language. It is generally assumed in linguistics and psycholinguistics that a mature speaker-hearer of a language knows, in some implicit fashion, the grammar of the language. That is, she or he knows a set of rules – rules of phonology, morphology, reference, semantics and syntax – that enable the production, or *generation*, of an indefinitely large number of grammatical utterances. It is this knowledge, and as yet unanswered questions about how something so complex is acquired, that make grammar an important topic in psychology.

Note that this usage of the term differs from that in the early school grades. The best way to understand this distinction is to appreciate that the grammar taught in the early grades is *prescriptive* – it consists of rules which dictate usage patterns – while the contemporary grammars of linguistics are *generative* – they specify formal rules for the production of sentences (see GENERATIVE *GRAMMAR). For more on usage patterns see the following entries.

grammar, artificial Any arbitrary set of rules that can be used to determine the order in which stimulus items can appear. They are called 'grammars' because, like the grammars of natural languages, they determine which sequences of stimuli are acceptable ('grammatical') or not ('nongrammatical'). These synthetic systems are used mainly in the study of IMPLICIT *LEARNING.

grammar, descriptive A description of the structure of a language. Distinguish from PRESCRIPTIVE *GRAMMAR.

grammar, generative 1 A field of study in linguistics and psycholinguistics that focuses on the development of a set of formal rules that can provide an explanation of language. **2** The set of formal rules itself. The point is that rather than treating grammar as simply a set of *prescriptive* rules about acceptability of sentences, or a set of *descriptive* rules that characterizes a particular corpus from a language, it is viewed as an abstract set of rules that is, in principle, capable of *generating* all, and only, the grammatical sentences of a language. The development of an acceptable generative grammar is one goal of linguistic science. The interest psychologists have in the topic comes from the simple observation that people *generate* sentences: we continually create novel utterances, we are not merely parroters of previously encountered sentences. Thus, the hope is that a linguistically sound generative grammar will express, in some fashion, the knowledge that normal speaker-hearers of a language possess.

grammar, phrase-structure A class of GENERATIVE *GRAMMARS that characterizes a language as a set of rules for arranging the elements of that language. The formal base of a phrase-structure grammar is quite simple and is similar to the old 'parsing' systems for analysing the structure of a sentence; i.e. assigning labels to parts of a sentence and determining the grammatically relevant subparts of phrases. See REWRITE RULE and TREE (2) for examples of the operations involved.

grammar, prescriptive A characterization of the structure of a language in terms of what is regarded as 'proper'. Prescriptive grammarians see themselves as the 'guardians' of their language, ruling on what they consider 'good' grammar and 'proper' speech. They rail against the use of words like *ain't*, they critique double negatives and hate split infinitives. They are also fighting a losing battle, as linguistic historians know. Distinguish from DESCRIPTIVE *GRAMMAR.

grammar, transformational (generative) A class of GENERATIVE *GRAMMARS originally developed by Noam Chomsky. They are attempts to develop formal characterizations of the basic components of natural languages and are based on several distinct components of language, specifically: a *semantics* component, which contains rules for meaning and feeds into a *deep structure* component, where the underlying meaning is represented; a *transformational derivation* component, which is a set of rules for rewriting or mapping deep structures on a *surface* form; and a *phonological* component, which consists of a set of rules for providing the appropriate sound patterns of the language. For more details on these terms see DEEP STRUCTURE, LANGUAGE, PHONOLOGY, PSYCHOLINGUISTICS, SEMANTICS, SURFACE STRUCTURE, TRANSFORMATION (5). Recently, linguists have begun to downplay transformational grammars in favour of those based on principles of GOVERNMENT AND BINDING.

grammar, universal A hypothesized set of basic grammatical principles assumed to be fundamental to all NATURAL LANGUAGES. It is argued by some, notably Chomsky, that a universal grammar, formally presented, would also be a theory of the human faculty for language.

grandiose delusions DELUSIONAL DISORDER, GRANDIOSE TYPE.

grand mal EPILEPSY et seq., especially MAJOR *EPILEPSY.

grandmother cell A hypothesized neural cell (or, better, group of cells) that are specifically tuned to a single mental representation; in this case, your grandmother. Such specificity is unlikely, cortical representations tend toward more diffuse, coordinated processing but the notion of a cell group that *is* the memory is engaging. See ENGRAM.

granular layer 1 Usually, the fourth layer of the cerebral cortex, characterized by many small bipolar cells with short axons. **2** Occasionally, the fifth and seventh layers of the retina, which have a similar granular structure.

granuloma inquinale A venereal disease characterized by the appearance of a small, painless lesion on the skin in the genital area followed by a spreading ulceration of surrounding tissue. Treatment is usually with the antibiotic tetracycline.

graph A representation in *n*-dimensional space of the relationship between *n* variables (in psychology generally *n* = 2). The graph is the actual representation of the data, be they statistical, clinical or experimental, in terms

of lines, curves or figures that reflect the relationship(s) between the variables.

-graph A combining form from the Greek, meaning *written*, and used to denote: **1** Something written or drawn. **2** The instrument or device that writes or records. In this latter sense (e.g. *electrocardiograph*) the written output should, for clarity, be referred to with *-gram* (e.g. *electrocardiogram*). This convention is not always followed.

graphic analysis Simply, the use of a graph to analyse results. Since a graph can present an enormous amount of information in simple visual form, significant relationships between variables may often be detected and appreciated much more easily than when the data are presented in tabular or numerical form.

graphic individuality Pertaining to the fact that each of us has an idiosyncratic and unique handwriting. See GRAPHOLOGY.

graphic language Broadly, a means of communicating via written symbols. See ORTHOGRAPHY (the preferred term) for details.

graphic rating scale RATING SCALE, GRAPHIC.

grapho- Combining form meaning *writing, drawing*.

graphodyne A device for measuring handwriting pressure.

graphology 1 The investigation and study of handwriting. Forensic graphology has some scientific and legal base: a specialist can detect forgeries or identify certain changes in psychological states by analysing changes in a person's handwriting. Unfortunately, this limited foundation has spawned a host of charlatans and frauds who make unsubstantiated claims about the value of graphology in assessing personality, diagnosing illness, etc. **2** Any writing system, e.g. the Roman alphabet or Cyrillic script.

graphometry A projective technique in which a blindfolded person draws a picture and then describes it, first while still blindfolded and then again while looking at it.

graphorrhoea Uncontrollable urge to write, generally resulting in extended nonsense. var., *graphorrhea*.

grasp reflex An automatic grasping of an

object when it is used to stimulate the palm. It is a normal response in infants and is also found in the foot when the sole is stimulated. Also called *grasping reflex*.

Grassmann's laws Those relationships implied by the COLOUR EQUATION that have been found to follow the rules of algebra.

gratification The state of satisfaction following the recognition that one has achieved a desired goal.

gray GREY.

GRE GRADUATE RECORD EXAMINATION.

great commissure CORPUS CALLOSUM.

great-man theory A point of view in historical investigations which contends that accomplishments in a field are due primarily to the efforts of *great men*. This personalistic approach is usually contrasted with the naturalistic approach (often called the *Zeitgeist theory*, from the German for *spirit of the times*), which stresses the role of the social, cultural and intellectual climate within which the investigator works and lives. For example, the former would argue that John Watson was responsible for the rise of behaviourism in the early 20th century; the latter that he was merely a historical puppet and that had he not presented this particular theory someone else would have. Doubtless both of these orientations are incorrect in the extreme, although, equally without doubt, both have elements of truth in that both the individual and the *Zeitgeist* interact in important ways. As an editorial note, perhaps the first reasonable thing to do would be to change the name of this theory to the great-*person* theory. That reflects our *Zeitgeist*.

Greco-Latin square ORTHOGONAL *LATIN SQUARES.

green The PRIMARY *COLOUR experienced when the normal eye is stimulated by light in the vicinity of 515 nm.

Greenhouse-Geisser correction A statistical adjustment to the number of degrees of freedom in a repeated measures FACTORIAL *DESIGN thereby yielding a more conservative statistic. Also called *Greenhouse-Geisser conservative test*.

Greenspoon effect An experimental effect found in some studies on verbal conditioning in which a speaker's use of certain classes of words (e.g. plural nouns) may be made to increase in frequency when reinforced by the listener making appropriately timed gestures of assent, like saying 'Mm-mmm' or 'Uh-huh'.

gregariousness 1 With respect to animals, the tendency found in many species to live in herds or flocks. **2** With respect to humans, the tendency to want to belong to groups or to derive satisfaction from group activity or group work. Because meaning 1 strongly suggests an innate disposition there has been a tendency to assume that meaning 2 is also reflective of an instinctive propensity; it is probably wise to resist this extrapolation.

grey An achromatic visual experience encompassing the brightness dimension from black to white. The greys have neither hue nor saturation. var., *gray*.

grey matter A general term for those parts of the spinal cord and the brain that contain a predominance of cell bodies (which are grey in colour) over myelinated nerve fibres (which are whitish).

grief An intense emotional state associated with the loss of someone (or something) with whom (or which) one has had a deep emotional bond. Not used as a synonym of DEPRESSION.

GRIT GRADUATED AND RECIPROCATED INITIATIVES IN TENSION REDUCTION.

grooming In animals, the removal of dirt and parasites from, and the smoothing of, the fur. Grooming is performed in pairs, when two animals groom each other (as in many species of primate), and singly (as in rats and cats). Interestingly, grooming frequently appears as a DISPLACEMENT (2) activity when animals are under stress or placed in a position of conflict.

groove In neurophysiology, a narrow channel or depression. See SULCUS.

gross motor movement Generally, any large muscular coordination in which strength is primary. Contrast with FINE MOTOR MOVEMENT.

gross score SCORE, GROSS.

ground 1 The background. See FIGURE-

GROUND. **2** The basis for action; a justification for a belief.

group **1** n. A collection or assemblage of things, where 'things' may be taken to cover almost any definable category or class of people, animals, events, objects, data, etc. Buried under this notion are a number of several important issues; see the discussions under the related terms CATEGORY, CLASS and CONCEPT. **2** A social group; i.e. a group in sense 1 but in which the members are all persons who are classified together on the basis of some social/psychological factor(s). Here the implication is that there is some degree of interrelatedness or interdependence among group members. In many combined terms in sociology and social psychology *group* (as adj.) and *social* are used interchangeably; for such terms not found below see those following SOCIAL. **3** vb. To place in classes, to categorize.

group atmosphere SOCIAL CLIMATE.

group autonomy AUTONOMY, GROUP.

group behaviour Actions of a group that are a result of the subtle interworking of the group as a whole, a kind of emergent property of a group and not simply the summation of the separate behaviours of the individuals in the group. Presumably the activities of the members of a group could not occur were they acting independently. Occasionally the term is used as a rough synonym of *teamwork*, but this usage is rather superficial.

group climate SOCIAL CLIMATE.

group, coacting A group of persons engaged in a task at which they work side by side but without interacting.

group cohesion SOCIAL COHESION.

group consciousness SOCIAL CONSCIOUSNESS.

group contagion The rapid spread of an emotional reaction across all of the members of a group.

group decision A decision made by a group. It may be reached by the group acting as a whole, a sort of consensus, or by each member acting individually, in which case the decision usually represents the majority opinion.

group differences Generally, any reliable differences between two or more groups each taken as a whole.

group dynamics **1** Generally, any of the collective interactions that take place within a group. **2** The study of group processes focusing on issues such as power, power shifts, leadership, group formation, how one group reacts to other groups, cohesiveness and decision-making. Note that some restrict this use of the term to small groups and small-group analyses on the grounds that these dynamic components only emerge when the social unit is small enough for meaningful interactions between members.

grouped frequency distribution DISTRIBUTION, GROUPED FREQUENCY.

group experiment Generally, any experiment in which a (large) number of subjects are run together in a group.

group, face-to-face A loose term for any small group in which the physical proximity of the members to each other is such that face-to-face interactions are possible.

group factor FACTOR, GROUP.

group, horizontal A group resulting from selection of individuals from a single social class or level in a hierarchy.

group hysteria MASS HYSTERIA.

group identification IDENTIFICATION.

grouping **1** Generally, the process of classification. Specifically: **2** In statistics, the organizing of data into classes or groups. **3** In education, the classification of students into similar groups, grades, classes, etc.

grouping error ERROR, GROUPING.

group integration INTEGRATION, GROUP.

group intelligence test Any of a number of paper-and-pencil intelligence tests designed to be administered in groups.

group locomotion Movement and shifting of a group toward a goal or decision.

group, marginal A group on the edge or margin of a culture, one only partially assimilated into the dominant cultural patterns.

group marriage CENOGAMY.

group mind A hypothesized, collective, transcendent spirit or consciousness which has been assumed by some to characterize a group or a society. The idea appears in many places, from the theoretical writings of some usually sane philosophers, such as Kant, and the social theories of William McDougall, who often enthusiastically embraced the outlandish, to the work of some contemporary ethologists who maintain that some social species (e.g. termites, honey-bees) function so that some, at least metaphoric, sense of an emergent collective mind can be inferred. This *collective consciousness*, as it was sometimes called, was presumed to exist independently of any single, individual member of a group but to emerge as a synthesized creation when the size of a cohesive group reached some critical mass and organization. Recent theories based on the notion of a TRANSACTIONAL MEMORY SYSTEM have begun to provide a more coherent picture of how something akin to a group mind might emerge and operate. Also called *folk mind*.

group norm NORM (2). For a distinction in usage, see SOCIAL NORM.

group polarization The tendency for the individuals in a group to exaggerate their initial points of view so that the group as a whole takes a more polarized position than the members themselves initially held. Put a group of moderately liberal politicians together and they become more liberal; put together a group of moderately conservative politicians and they become more conservative. See also the related RISKY SHIFT.

group, primary A group consisting of persons with common values, goals and standards of behaviour, and in which there is close personal contact. The adjective *primary* was originally used to emphasize that these groups (of which the *family* is the prime example) have the earliest impact on the development of an individual's socialization. Compare with SECONDARY *GROUP.

groups, comparable Two groups selected from the same population. The notion of comparability here is not strict but based on principles of unbiased sampling; that is, the groups are not expected to be identical in all respects, merely to reflect the same char-

acteristics of the population from which they are taken.

group, secondary A group consisting of persons who share some values and have some common standards of behaviour but only with respect to limited segments of their lives. Professional organizations, fraternities, clubs, etc. are regarded as examples. Compare with PRIMARY *GROUP.

group, selected Generally, any group or sample which results from the application of some rule such that the members are specially selected from a larger population. Note that a selected group may be chosen so as to be either (a) deliberately nonrepresentative of the population, e.g. a group composed of Nobel prize-winners or a group of psychologists who have authored lexicons, or (b) deliberately more representative of the population than a similarly sized random sample could reasonably be expected to be, e.g. a stratified sample, as is often used in modern polling techniques. See SAMPLE et seq.

group selection SELECTION, GROUP.

group, sensitivity SENSITIVITY TRAINING.

group solidarity SOCIAL COHESION.

group structure Quite literally, the structure of a group. Analysis of group structure typically involves examination of such factors as power and power relationships, subgroups (their formation and their roles with respect to the rest of the group), the various roles that individual members play in the group (i.e. leader, follower, cooperative, competitive, etc.), and so forth. Note that the term is eclectic enough to be employed by sociologists, social psychologists, ethologists, zoologists, clinicians, etc.

group superego COORDINATE MORALITY.

group test TEST, GROUP.

group therapy Any psychotherapeutic process in which a group of individuals meets with a therapist/leader. The interactions among the members of the group are assumed to be therapeutic and in many cases to be more effective than the traditional client–therapist diad.

groupthink Within group decision-making procedures, the tendency for the various members of a group to try to achieve consensus. The need for agreement takes priority over the motivation to try to obtain accurate knowledge to make appropriate decisions. This tendency has been suggested as one of the prime reasons why politicians operating in closed groups so often make disastrous decisions.

group, vertical A group composed of persons from more than one social class or level in a hierarchy.

growth Generally, gradual progressive increase. The term is widely applied and may refer to: **1** Increases in size of an individual organism or its parts. **2** Increases in effectiveness or competence of a function, e.g. growth of cognitive capacity in a child. **3** Differentiation and refinement of parts and/or functions. This meaning differs from the above in that sheer increases in magnitude, as in 1, or performance, as in 2, are not entailed; e.g. growth of understanding in a young adult, where the implication is of increasing maturity. **4** In mathematics, the increases in a function or a curve.

growth curve A graphic presentation of the growth over time of some measure or variable.

growth, differential Characterizing those circumstances in which the rate of growth within a complex system does not occur at the same rate in all parts of the system. *System* here is taken very generally, and the term is applied in economics, anatomy, mental and intellectual assessment, etc.

growth hormone A pituitary hormone necessary for normal bodily growth prior to adulthood. It also plays a role in regulation of food intake in that it causes the conversion of glycogen to glucose. Also called *somatotrophic hormone*.

growth needs METANEEDS.

growth principle A principle in Carl Rogers's *humanistic psychology* which maintains that emotional and intellectual growth will take place normally in all persons when they are freed from coercion, arbitrary social pressures, punishment or the fear of it, censure and other common components of our daily lives.

grue 1 In philosophy, a cover term for the following interesting riddle introduced by Nelson Goodman. Suppose that every emerald you have seen is green and you are quite certain that emeralds are, indeed, green. However, it is also true that each of these emeralds is 'grue', where 'grue' is an object that is green up till some time, *t*, when it suddenly becomes blue. How, Goodman asked, can you tell whether emeralds are really green or grue? If this seems totally odd, it is not. After all, these kinds of state changes take place all the time. Usually, of course, we know when *t* has or will occur. For example, a new acquaintance is 'a nice person' (so far…). **2** A colour term for that part of the spectrum that includes 'blue' and 'green'. In both meanings *bleen* is used synonymously.

GSR GALVANIC SKIN RESPONSE.

G-theory GENERALIZABILITY THEORY.

guanine One of the four nucleotide bases that make up DEOXYRIBONUCLEIC ACID and RIBONUCLEIC ACID.

guessing bias Any tendency on the part of a subject to display a bias when guessing among possible responses. Such biases are often observed in experiments on learning, decision-making, psychophysics, etc. when the subject does not know the correct response; e.g. a tendency to guess the first alternative presented or to guess the item on the left, etc. Such biases are a source of CONSTANT *ERROR.

guidance Counselling, leading, directing, advising, assisting, influencing, etc. The term has three broad uses: **1** *Educational guidance*, in which the focus is on providing assistance and advice in school work using instruction, testing and counselling. **2** *Vocational guidance*, in which the aim is to assist a person in finding a suitable vocation. A vast battery of tests – intelligence, vocational, interest, aptitude, achievement, etc. – is used. **3** *Child guidance*, which is concerned with the vast array of potential educational, emotional and behavioural problems that children may display. The focus here is generally interdisciplinary and based on coordination between medical, psychological and educational aspects in attempts to assist the child toward the development of a more satisfying life.

guided participation Generally, all of the

patterns of child–adult interactions during mundane daily activities that function to slowly shape a child's cognitive system. The process generally takes place through shared communication and coordinated participation in ordinary tasks, with the adult guiding the child. It has been proposed as an extension to Vygotsky's notion of the ZONE OF PROXIMAL DEVELOPMENT.

guiding fiction FICTION, GUIDING.

guiding idea GUIDING *FICTION.

guilt An emotional state produced by the knowledge that one has violated moral standards. Most authorities recognize an emotional state as guilt only when the individual concerned has internalized the moral standards of his or her society; thus it is distinguished from simple fear of punishment from external sources – guilt is, in a sense, a self-administered punishment. Distinguish from SHAME, where others' knowledge of the transgression is part of the concept.

gust A psychophysical unit of taste defined as the subjective sense of sweetness produced by a 1% sucrose solution.

gustation The sense of taste. adj., *gustatory*.

gut A term, in surprisingly common use, for the entire digestive system including the oesophagus, stomach, intestines and bowel.

Guttman scaling A method developed by N. Guttman for the measurement of attitudes. Items in a cumulative attitude scale are ranked so that a positive response to any given item is assumed to reflect positive responding to all items of lower rank.

gyn- Combining form from the Greek, meaning *female*, *woman*. vars., *gyne-*, *gyno-* and the suffixes *-gyny* (for nouns) and *-gynous* (for adjectives).

gynandry ANDROGYNY.

gynecomastia The development of breasts on a male. The condition may occur spontaneously, through hormone malfunction, or as a direct result of hormone treatments.

gyrus A convolution or fold on the surface of the cerebral cortex. *Gyri* are bounded by FISSURES (or sulci).

H

H 1 HERITABILITY although the lower case 'h' is more frequently used. **2** HARMONIC •MEAN. **3** ENTROPY. **4** The amount of INFORMATION contained in an array, measured in *bits*. **5** HABIT STRENGTH. In the case of 4, *H* is the base abbreviation for an array of theoretical terms, all within the now obsolete behaviourist framework of C. L. Hull. A few of them are: $_sH_R$ = habit strength, $_s\bar{H}_R$ = effective habit strength, $_s'H_R$ = generalized habit strength.

h, h^2 Abbreviations for HERITABILITY. Some authors reserve the h^2 notation for the *heritability coefficient*. See HERITABILITY for discussion.

Haab's pupillary reflex A contraction of both pupils on turning toward a bright stimulus in an otherwise dark environment.

habit 1 Generally, a learned act. Originally the reference was to motor patterns, physical responses; this limitation is no longer recognized and perceptual, cognitive, affective habits are commonly cited. **2** A pattern of activity that has, through repetition, become automatized and fixed and is easily and effortlessly carried out. This meaning, when found in cognitive psychology, connotes behaviour that is carried out in a kind of 'bottom-up', implicit fashion without much in the way of conscious thought or deliberation. When found in studies of personality, the meaning is very close to that of TRAIT (see that entry for some problems in usage that pertain here as well). **3** An addiction to a drug. The preferred term here is DRUG •DEPENDENCE. **4** A pattern of action that is characteristic of a particular species of animal, e.g. 'the habits of baboons'. Note that this last meaning differs sharply from the preceding in that it usually connotes an innate, species-specific pattern of behaviour, while the other usages all clearly entail the notion of the behaviour as learned.

habitat The geographical area within which conditions are well suited to the life of a particular species.

habit family hierarchy A concept introduced into psychology by Hull to characterize the fact that there are generally several possible paths to a given goal. As the word HIERARCHY (1) implies, there is preference ordering among the habits, so that if one is blocked the next most preferred is most likely to be adopted.

habit formation Obviously, forming a habit: but there have been problems with this term. First, the tendency to use it as a synonym of *learning* should be resisted: such usage implies that all learning is the formation of habits, a theoretical position few would choose to defend any longer. Second, the very word *formation* invites confusion over whether to apply the term to the actual acquisition of a new habit or to the novel use of a previously acquired habit. For example, rats can certainly run down runways, thus the formation of the habit of straight-alley running relates mainly to the novel use of old behaviour. However, in the case of a rat bar-pressing there really is the formation of a new habit. Application of the term is generally restricted to behaviourist approaches to psychology. See CONCEPT FORMATION and CONCEPT LEARNING for a related terminological muddle within the cognitive approach.

habit-forming A nontechnical term used loosely to characterize substances that produce either *psychological* or *physiological* *dependence*. See DRUG •DEPENDENCE and related terms.

habit hierarchy 1 In Hull's theory, an ordering of all of the responses that gain in habit strength by virtue of reinforcement of one of them, organized according to amount of gain. 2 More generally, the organization of simple actions or patterns of behaviour (i.e. HABITS (1, 2)) into more complex, hierarchical systems, each level of which is subsumed into the level above. A variety of complex behavioural systems are representable in this fashion, e.g. typing, language. Note, however, that when the behaviouristic realm of overt acts is left behind (as in the case of language), *habit* is often dropped and the behaviour is described simply as *hierarchical* or *hierarchically organized*.

habit interference A circumstance that occurs when two or more incompatible responses are acquired to the same stimulus. Either both responses are inhibited and weakened or one becomes dominant.

habit strength In Hullian theory, this term refers to the bond between a stimulus and a response and was used synonymously with *learning*. Symbol: $_S\bar{H}_R$.

habituation 1 In keeping with the meaning of HABIT (1, 2), the gradual elimination of superfluous activity in learning. 2 A form of non-associative learning whereby each repetition of a stimulus results in a progressively diminished response. The effect is easily demonstrated in infancy which has led to the development of the HABITUATION TECHNIQUE. See also ADAPTATION (1). 3 See PSYCHO-LOGICAL *DEPENDENCE.

habituation, drug An occasional synonym of PSYCHOLOGICAL *DEPENDENCE.

habituation technique A procedure that uses HABITUATION (2) to assess what a preverbal infant is processing. For example, show an 8-month-old infant a scene where a puppet moves across a table, disappears behind a screen and reappears on the other side. The typical infant will initially show considerable interest but, after several repetitions, will habituate and pay little attention. Now show the same puppet disappearing but *two* puppets suddenly appearing on the other side. If the infant now looks intently at this 'impossible' scene, it suggests that he or she is sensitive to the change in number.

haem(a)- HAEMO-.

haemat(o)- HAEMO-.

haematocyte 1 A red blood cell. 2 Any blood cell. var., *hematocyte*.

haem(o)- Combining form from the Greek for *blood*. vars., *haem(a)-*, *haemat(o)-*, *hem(o)-*, *hem(a)-*, *hemat(o)-*.

haemocyte HAEMATOCYTE.

hair cell A type of cell with hair-like projections (or cilia). They are found in several places, e.g. in the inner ear and in the ampullae at the ends of the semicircular canals, where they function as receptors. The manner of action is similar in both locales: physical force causes a stretching of the membrane to which the hair cells are attached, resulting in a stretching or shearing of the cilia, which produces the receptor potential.

halazepam A BENZODIAZEPINE used in the treatment of anxiety and in some cases of insomnia. It has a conveniently long half-life so it only needs to be taken once a day.

half-life In pharmacology, the length of time it takes for the measured concentration of a drug in the blood to be reduced by 50% from its peak. Half-life is affected by a large number of factors including metabolic action, age and potential interactions with other drugs.

halfway house Originally, a facility for persons released from mental or penal institutions designed to ease their transition back into the community. Many such facilities function more broadly, however. Rather than being only 'halfway out' houses they may also serve as semi-protective environments for those 'halfway in' persons who can still function productively in the community but need a supportive, caring shelter.

hallucination A perceptual experience with all the compelling subjective properties of a real sensory impression but without the normal physical stimulus for that sensory modality. Hallucinations that are not drug-induced are taken as classic indicators of a psychotic disturbance and are a hallmark of various disorders like schizophrenia. Hence, the term is not usually applied to a variety of other false perceptions that occur normally, such as the images that often accompany the transition from waking to sleeping (*hypnago-*

gic), or those that occur when first awakening (*hypnopompic*), or those that occasionally accompany vivid religious experiences. In actual usage the term is generally modified so that the particular modality involved is specified, e.g. *auditory hallucination, tactile hallucination*. Distinguish from both ILLUSION and DELUSION.

hallucinogen Loosely, any of a large group of psychoactive chemical compounds capable of producing hallucinations. See PSYCHEDELIC.

hallucinogen dependence A DRUG *DEPENDENCE in which the drug is a *hallucinogen*.

hallucinogen intoxication Intoxication brought about by use of a *hallucinogen*. It is typically marked by maladaptive behavioural changes, marked anxiety or depression, impaired judgement, paranoid thoughts, perceptual changes and a host of physiological affects including palpitations, tachycardia and tremors.

hallucinosis A general term for a condition of extreme susceptibility to hallucinations. It is reserved for conditions in which there is a substance-induced or organic basis for the hallucinations, e.g. ALCOHOL HALLUCINOSIS.

halo effect A tendency to allow an overall impression of a person, or one particular outstanding trait, to influence the total rating of that person. It often emerges as a bias on personal-rating scales.

haloperidol An ANTIPSYCHOTIC DRUG of the BUTYROPHENONES group. Once commonly prescribed, it has largely been replaced by the ATYPICAL *ANTIPSYCHOTICS.

Halstead-Reitan battery A neuropsychological battery including tests for a variety of functions including language, memory, abstract thought, sensorimotor integration and dexterity. Designed to assess cortical function, the tests are more reliable for acute disorders than chronic ones. Once highly popular, its use has diminished in recent years.

halving method A variation of the *method of equal-appearing intervals* whereby a second stimulus is adjusted so that it appears to be half of a given standard (i.e. half as loud, half as bright, etc.). See METHODS OF *SCALING.

hammer MALLEUS, AUDITORY *OSSICLES.

Hampton Court maze The famous English garden maze that was used as a model for many early maze-learning studies.

handedness Generally, a preference for the use of one hand over the other. In actual practice it can be surprisingly difficult to determine such a preference unambiguously. In literate persons the hand used for writing is usually taken as the criterion for determining handedness, although even in these relatively clear cases the other hand may occasionally be used preferentially for other tasks, such as throwing an object.

handicapped Having an encumbrance or disadvantage that produces a less-than-normal ability to perform. Usually the term refers to the physically impaired but may on occasion be used of the mentally retarded. See also CHALLENGED and DISABLED.

haphalgesia Pain sensation when a usually innocuous stimulus touches the skin.

hapl(o)- Combining form meaning *single* or *simple*.

haploid number The normal number of chromosomes in each *gamete* (or sex cell, i.e. ovum or sperm) of a particular species. The haploid number (which is 23 in *Homo sapiens*) is half of the *diploid number*, the number of chromosomes in each *somatic cell*.

happy puppet An expression often used of children with ANGELMAN SYNDROME.

haptic Relating to the cutaneous senses. Haptics, in the broadest sense, is the study of touch. Note, however, that some will reserve the term for experiences that come from *active* touch, touching initiated by an individual. The more inclusive term is TACTILE; combined terms may be found there.

hard data Laboratory jargon for objective, concrete data. Compare with SOFT DATA.

hard drug Nontechnical term for any drug that can produce a PHYSIOLOGICAL *DEPENDENCE. Most frequently used of opium-based narcotics.

hardiness The dispositional ability to withstand stress. It is characterized by, among other factors, viewing stresses as opportunities for growth and mastery. Compare with RESILIENCE.

hardness A perceptual quality. **1** In tactile perception it characterizes objects which are relatively unyielding to the touch. **2** In vision, it characterizes colour high in saturation and brightness. **3** In audition, it characterizes high-intensity and/or high-pitch tones.

hard palate PALATE.

hard problem, the A term coined by David Chalmers to refer to the (admittedly) monstrously difficult problem of figuring out how consciousness and phenomenal experience are produced by mere matter, by the physical neurological entity that is the human brain.

hard psychology A colloquial expression used to refer to those psychological endeavours that are patterned after the natural sciences, e.g. learning, sensory and physiological psychology, psychophysics, etc. The term derives from the notion that the data in these areas tend to be objective and more concrete than in other areas such as clinical psychology or the study of personality; see SOFT PSYCHOLOGY. Note that this terminology is generally not appreciated by 'soft' psychologists, who prefer to call their areas *complex* and the 'hard' areas *simple*.

hard-to-get effect In social psychology, the tendency for people who are selective in their social choices to be more desirable than those who are more readily available. The effect is a subtle one because many who act hard-to-get do so in an insensitive manner that simply turns other people off and decreases their social desirability.

hardware In computer terminology, the physical apparatus itself as opposed to the programs or SOFTWARE.

hard wired Genetically preprogrammed. Behaviours that are assumed to be based strongly on genetic factors are spoken of as being 'hard wired'.

harmonic 1 n. An overtone or partial, the frequency of which is a multiple of the fundamental tone. **2** adj. Pertaining to harmony.

harmonic analysis The analysis of a complex wave into its sine and cosine components in accordance with FOURIER'S LAW.

harmonic mean MEAN, HARMONIC.

harp theory THEORIES OF *HEARING.

hashish A gummy substance made from the resins of the hemp plant. When smoked or ingested it has psychoactive properties. See CANNABIS (SATIVA) for further discussion.

hassles Stressors that are not major but which nonetheless add up to cause STRESS (2).

hatred A deep, enduring, intense emotion expressing animosity, anger and hostility toward a person, group or object. Hatred is usually assumed to be characterized by (a) the desire to harm or cause pain to the object of the emotion and (b) feelings of pleasure at the object's misfortunes.

Hawthorne effect Named after the industrial plant where the effect was first observed, a generalization that states that anything new works – new programmes, methods, curricula, organization, working conditions, etc. – at least for a while. The innovations produce positive results independently of the nature of the modification; in the original study even control conditions designed to lower worker productivity resulted in increases. Presumably the phenomenon results from the enthusiasm that participants feel toward any innovation and from the sense that the changes being introduced show that people are interested in them. The existence of this effect makes a true evaluation of any new programme a difficult affair. Note, by implication there is also an opposite *negative* Hawthorne effect that is produced when workers are unenthusiastic about an innovation, in which case possible legitimate improvements are stillborn.

H cells HORIZONTAL (H) CELLS.

headstart A general label for a number of educational and social programmes designed to enhance the performance of children from impoverished backgrounds.

heal To become healthy again; to make whole, to free from impairment. Note that some use *heal* as a synonym of CURE while others distinguish between the two. The distinction is based on the argument that *heal* should be reserved for relatively less severe cases of injury or trauma and *cure* for more serious diseases and disabilities. Also, some use *heal* in the context of providing assistance in the restorative process and *cure* in more dramatic cases of intervention to alter or modify ongoing processes to restore health.

health psychology A field of applied psychology that seeks to use psychological theory and knowledge to promote personal and public health. Specific focuses include problems as diverse as identifying the aetiology of illness, understanding the conditions and correlates of well-being, developing techniques for prevention and treatment of illness and improving health-care delivery systems.

hearing The perception of sound primarily through the ear. Some authorities prefer to reserve the term for the *process*, using AUDITION for the *sense* of hearing.

hearing impaired Characterizing a person with a relatively serious hearing loss. The term is preferred by many over *deaf* and its various qualified forms.

hearing loss A measure of hearing impairment usually presented as either (a) the percentage of normal hearing acuity present for different frequency tones, or (b) the absolute threshold in decibels for different frequency tones. See AUDIOGRAM.

hearing, theories of Explaining hearing adequately has proven a singularly difficult task. There are a number of candidates, two major and several minor. The two most viable are *place* theory and *periodicity* theory. Place theory (also known variously as *resonance, harp* and *piano* theory) originated with the great Helmholtz in the 1860s. It assumes that the perceived pitch of a tone is determined by the place of maximum vibration of the basilar membrane, the portion near the oval window being tuned for high-frequency tones, the far end, near the apex of the cochlea, for low-frequency tones. Loudness and tonal discrimination are assumed to be determined by the number of neurons activated by the incoming stimulus. Periodicity (or *rate*) theory, on the other hand, emphasizes synchronized firing of neurons. It depends heavily on the *volley principle*, which proposes that groups of fibres on the basilar membrane work as squads and fire in synchronized volleys. The volley principle is necessary because the auditory nerve only follows signals with frequencies up to 3,000–4,000 Hz.

The current view seems to favour a kind of amalgamation of these two theories. For stimuli below say 3,000 Hz, place and periodicity combine; for higher-frequency stimuli, place on the basilar membrane is probably the critical factor. Loudness would seem to be mediated by the overall number of impulses arriving at the brain.

There are other earlier, less well-supported points of view. The classical *frequency* (or *telephone*) theory of Rutherford assumed that the basilar membrane responds as a whole much like a telephone diaphragm. Meyer's *hydraulic* theory stressed the amount of the basilar membrane involved in different tonal patterns. The *sound-pattern* theory of Ewald assumed that different patterns of vibrations were imposed on the basilar membrane by stimuli of different complexities or pitches.

heat 1 Intuitively and subjectively, a sensory experience toward one end of the warmth continuum. While it is certainly true that heat is experienced when the skin is exposed to temperatures considerably higher than itself, it is also the case that it is experienced by the separate stimulation of receptors for cold and warm. Grasping a pair of intertwined pipes, one containing cold water and one warm, produces a sensation of burning. The assumption is that heat is mediated through a set of neural processes different from those for warm and cold. **2** A sexually receptive state in a female animal.

Hebb rule Put simply, 'Neurons that fire together wire together.' That is, the generalization first suggested by Donald Hebb that circuits might be formed in the brain by the simple process of the coordinated firing of neurons. This simple principle, while initially presented as a generalization about neural functions, has turned out to have wide impact. For example, it underlies the operation of a class of rather powerful theoretical models known as PARALLEL DISTRIBUTED PROCESSING (PDP) MODELS. Note that the learning that occurs in Hebbian systems is treated as *unsupervised* and involves only BOTTOM-UP PROCESSING. See DELTA RULE for an example of a *supervised* learning rule with TOP-DOWN features, and NETWORK MODELS for further discussion of usage.

hebephrenia DISORGANIZED (TYPE) *SCHIZOPHRENIA.

hebetic Relating to youth generally or to occurrences at the time of puberty specifically.

hebetude Emotional dullness, listlessness, a withdrawn lethargy.

hedge Any verbal device that functions to let the listener know that the speaker is not quite as sure as he or she may appear to be, e.g. 'I suspect…' or 'I have heard that…'. A hedge functions to free the speaker from full responsibility for the veracity of an utterance.

hedonic Pertaining to or descriptive of the hypothesized affective dimension of pleasure–unpleasure.

hedonic relevance A term used in social psychology to describe the fact that one's personal involvement in another's behaviour affects the view one has of the other. If your behaviour hurts me personally, I am more likely to have a low opinion of you than if your behaviour hurts others but does not affect me. See PERSON PERCEPTION.

hedonic tone The subjective quality of an experience in terms of the hypothesized pleasure–unpleasure dimension.

hedonism 1 In psychology proper, the theory that behaviour is motivated by approach toward pleasure and avoidance of pain. **2** In ethics, the doctrine that the goal of human conduct ought to be the striving for pleasure and the avoidance of pain. The first usage is descriptive, the second prescriptive.

Heller's syndrome CHILDHOOD DISINTEGRATIVE DISORDER.

heliocotrema The small opening at the apex of the cochlea where the scala tympani and scala vestibuli connect.

heliotropism PHOTOTAXIS.

helping behaviour The providing of assistance to someone in need. The term is applied in situations in which the behaviour involves no sacrifices, real or potential, on the part of the helper. Distinguish from ALTRUISM, the giving of assistance at the risk of personal privation. See also BYSTANDER EFFECT.

helping professions Collectively, all those professions of which the theories, research and practice focus on the assistance of others, the identification and resolution of their problems and the extension of knowledge of the human condition to further those aims. Included are medicine, psychiatry and clinical psychology, as well as various specialized fields such as educational and school psychology, social work, and speech and hearing sciences.

helplessness, learned A term coined by M. Seligman to characterize the generalization that helplessness is a learned state produced by exposure to noxious, unpleasant situations in which there is no possibility of escape or avoidance.

This sense of helplessness has a significant impact on how people react to events, particularly those that have a noxious element to them. It is also possible to countermand it, provided the proper circumstances are present. Individuals who have been given an opportunity to avoid or escape the noxious events tend to become 'immunized' against the feelings of helplessness. Individuals who are provided with options that can help them diminish the aversiveness of the experience also show lessened impact of punishment. The notion has played an important role in approaches to depression (see here HOPELESSNESS THEORY) and cognitive-behavioural approaches to psychotherapy.

hemeralopia A condition in which vision is normal under dim illumination but poor under normal or high light levels. It is seen in those with *achromatopsia*, or total colour blindness, and *albinism*. Also called *day blindness* and in some older writings, incorrectly, *night blindness*, the proper term for which is NYCTALOPIA. var., *hemeralopsia*.

hemi- Prefix meaning *half* or, when used with respect to organs or organisms that display bilateral symmetry, *on one side*. Most of the combined terms using this prefix are easily understood from their etymological roots (e.g. *hemianalgesia* is lack of sensitivity to pain on one side of the body, *hemiplegia* is paralysis of one side of the body); those that are obscure or used in special ways are given below.

hemianopia Blindness in one half of the visual field. It results from a variety of lesions in the optic pathways and can take a variety of forms. Often used with qualifiers to specify the particular form; e.g. *bitemporal* = affecting only the temporal half of the visual field of each eye, *unilateral* = affecting only one eye. vars., *hemiopia, hemianopsia*.

hemiballism BALLISM.

hemi-inattention NEGLECT (2).

hemilateral Synonym of UNILATERAL.

hemineglect NEGLECT (2).

hemiopia HEMIANOPIA.

hemiplegia Paralysis to one side of the body; usually the result of damage to the PRIMARY MOTOR CORTEX accompanied by lesions in the BASAL GANGLIA.

hemispatial neglect See NELGECT (2).

hemisphere Either half of the cerebrum or cerebellum.

hemispheric specialization LATERALITY.

hem(o)- HAEMO-.

Henning's prism A classification system for smell based on human judgements in which six (theoretically) pure odour qualities (flowery, fruity, spicy, resinous, burnt, putrid) form the corners of a prism with the intermediate qualities lying along the surfaces. See also STEROCHEMICAL THEORY for a contemporary model based on seven odours.

Henning's tetrahedron A classification system for taste in which the four primary tastes (sweet, sour, bitter, salty) are arranged at the corners of a four-sided pyramid with all other tastes arranged at various locations to represent how they are combinations of two or more of the primaries. See TASTE (2) for a more up-to-date framework.

Herbartianism An early system of psychological thought developed in the 1820s by J. F. Herbart (1776–1841). It stressed the notion that ideas compete and struggle for recognition. A central concept was *apperceptive mass* (see APPERCEPTION (2)), the previously acquired set of ideas to which any new idea must be related. Since these assumptions imply a level of mind of which we are not conscious,

Herbart is seen as a precursor of psychoanalytic thought. Herbart's system was also highly mathematical; he was the innovator of mathematical descriptions of the formulation and interaction of ideas. Moreover, he was highly influential with educators and is regarded by many as the initiator of modern educational theory.

herding GREGARIOUSNESS (esp. 1). Also called *herd instinct*.

here and now A term popularized by advocates of the HUMAN POTENTIAL MOVEMENT. It refers, quite literally, to the here and now, the present. It is argued that many maladaptive, neurotic behaviours derive from continuous focusing on past problems and injustices and that it is therapeutic to concentrate on what is happening now, to savour the moment.

hereditarianism A label used for any position stressing the role of heredity in the determination of behaviour. Contrast with ENVIRONMENTALISM; differentiate subtly from NATIVISM and HEREDITY–ENVIRONMENT CONTROVERSY.

hereditary factor A gene.

hereditary predisposition An inherited predisposition toward a particular trait. The term is generally reserved for pathological conditions; one speaks, for example, of a hereditary predisposition toward schizophrenia or epilepsy. Whether or not the pathology develops depends on environmental circumstances. Compare with BIOLOGICAL PREDISPOSITION.

heredity Most broadly, the biological transmission of genetic characteristics from parent to offspring. The study of heredity is predicated on several fundamental considerations: (a) the biological principles of genetics and genetic transmission; (b) the impact of the environment, the conditions under which an organism is raised and lives; and (c) the complex manner in which these two broad factors interact with each other. That is, the actual set of physical, behavioural traits manifested (the *phenotype*) is a complex product of the cumulative interactions between the genetic material available at fertilization (the *genotype*) and the various environmental factors that impinge on the developing organism.

Hereditary is the most common adjectival form, although many others are used more or less interchangeably, e.g. *genetic, biological, inborn, inherited, innate* and *natural*. When used to modify a characteristic or trait they carry the connotation that that characteristic or trait is due, *in some measure*, to genetic factors. However, all these terms must be used with caution since none of them carries any lexical component that denotes the *relative* contribution of the hereditary component to the characteristic under consideration – to describe eye colour as hereditary is to suggest one thing, to describe intelligence as hereditary is to suggest quite another. For more on this point see HEREDITY–ENVIRON-MENT CONTROVERSY. Distinguish all adjectival forms from CONGENITAL, which means simply *present at birth*.

heredity–environment controversy Also referred to as the *nature–nurture debate* or, in philosophical writings, the *nativism–empiricism controversy*, this is a debate of long standing over the relative contributions of experience (nurture, environment, learning) and inheritance (nature, heredity, genetic predisposition) to the make-up of an organism, especially a human organism.

In its earliest incarnation the dispute turned on questions of innate qualities of mind that were assumed to be universal and found in all nonpathological instances. A case in point is vision, where everyone perceives a three-dimensional, Euclidean world: is this because, as the Cartesians argued, we are born with this particular spatial knowledge or, as the empiricists following Locke and Hume maintained, because we learn to see spatial relationships through experience? (See MOLYNEUX'S QUESTION.) This particular form of controversy is recognizable today in the analogous dispute between modern nativists, who follow linguist Noam Chomsky in arguing that we are born with the underlying representation of universal grammar that guides language acquisition, and the more empiricist-oriented theorists, who maintain that there are very general learning principles that can account for how a natural language is acquired without assuming such a rich inherited system.

However, the nature–nurture dispute has been most explosive when attention has focused not on consideration of those capacities that are *universal*, like vision and language, but on consideration of the roots of the *differences* between individuals, as displayed for example in their scores on intelligence tests. To wit: to what extent does an individual's genetic endowment determine his or her anatomical and behavioural phenotype as it is manifested in ways that are important in terms of society's evaluations? This issue hinges on the notion of HERITABILITY, the proportion of the variance in a population of some measurable trait that can be attributed to genetic factors. See also ENVIRONMENTALISM and HEREDITARIANISM and, for a characterization of a recent genetically based theoretical approach to these issues, SOCIOBIOLOGY. Finally, see EVOLUTIONARY PSYCHOLOGY, which extends these issues into such areas as mate selection and group identity, where social and cognitive factors play a strong role in moderating the genetic foundations.

Finally, it should be appreciated that this tendency to call it a 'controversy' is waning. This label came about because early approaches tended to see it as an 'either/or' issue, which it is not. Virtually all forms, functions, traits and behaviours are products of complex interactions between hereditary factors and the environments within which organisms live. Genes don't do anything on their own; they need environments to express themselves – differences in parental nurturance can produce different reactions to stress in genetically identical offspring. In addition, genetic predispositions can also influence behaviour – monozygotic twins raised in separate households often exhibit particular behaviours that cause adjustments in child-rearing patterns so that the two families end up with similar parenting behaviours. Indeed, the question of nature vs. nurture is now viewed as a complex interacting web of interdependent and coacting genetic and environmental factors.

Hering afterimage The first POSITIVE *AFTERIMAGE following a brief, bright, visual stimulus.

Hering greys A series of 50 neutral grey papers graded in subjectively equal steps along the achromatic dimension from extreme white to extreme black.

Hering illusion As shown; the two vertical lines are straight.

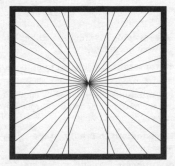

Hering theory of colour vision THEORIES OF *COLOUR VISION.

heritability That proportion of the variance of a particular trait in a population that can be traced to inherited factors. The *heritability coefficient* (or *ratio*) represents this notion as $h^2 = V_G/V_T$, where h^2 is the heritability coefficient, V_G is the variance in the population due to genetic (inherited) factors and V_T is the total variance, that is, the sum of the variance due to genetic factors and that due to environmental. There are three critical implications of this idea that must be recognized: (a) Even if the value of h^2 approaches 1.0, it does not necessarily mean that there are *large* genetic differences between individuals. In this case, it is true that if the environment were perfectly controlled and identical for all individuals (i.e. if the variance due to experience = 0), then any observed differences would be due to genetic factors (since $V_G = V_T$). However, such a state of affairs would have no bearing on the size of those observed differences. Another way to consider this is to appreciate that a century ago blindness would have been scored as low in heritability while today it would be scored as considerably higher. There has not been any change in the occurrence of genetically caused blindness; rather, the overall variability (V_T) has been reduced by the development of safety measures and advances in medicine, which are environmental factors, leaving the heritability ratio to increase. Completely removing all environmental causes of blindness might leave a value of V_T equal to that of V_G and an h^2 of 1.0. (b)

The value of h^2 is only interpretable given a population of individuals: it has no implications for individual cases. One cannot argue that so many centimetres of a person's height are determined by heredity and so many by the environment. That is, h^2 cannot be read as a statement of the amount of a characteristic attributable to genes, but only as a statement about the parcelling out of the variability due to genetic or environmental factors within a given population. (c) No observed group differences on objective measures, no matter how large or small they may be, can be taken as reflective of genetic causes independently of the value of h^2 because h^2 is based on *within*-group variance, not *between*-group variance. For example, one half of a batch of genetically diverse seeds can yield a set of rather tall plants (on average) and the other half yield a set of rather short ones (on average) simply by adjusting the richness of the soil. Or, put another way, the fact that one racial or ethnic group scores consistently lower on an IQ test than another group does not mean that the differences between them are genetic in origin even though the value of h^2 for IQ is above 0 as assessed by within-group designs and twin studies. Interestingly, the concept emerged from the work of agricultural breeders who wished to know if it was worth attempting to select for a particular trait. See also ENVIRONMENTALITY.

heritability coefficient (or **ratio**) (**h^2**) Whereas *heritability* is a general notion that refers to the degree to which inherited factors contribute to specific traits or behaviours, 'coefficient' is added when the reference is specifically to the calculation of this value from a given data set. See HERITABILITY for details on usage.

heritability ratio HERITABILITY COEFFICIENT.

heritage A generic term for transmission from generation to generation. It may refer to either biological heredity or to social transmission of customs and traditions.

hermaphrodite 1 In humans, an individual in whom the structures of the reproductive system are so nondifferentiated that an unambiguous assignment of male or female cannot be made. The term derives from Hermaphroditos, the son of Hermes and Aphrodite, who combined with his consort to become a single body possessing both male and female characteristics. Contrast with ANDROGYNY and PSEUDOHERMAPHRODITE. **2** Characteristic of a species (e.g. many plants) in which both male and female reproductive parts are found in all members.

hermeneutics Interpretative procedures, or the science of such. Originally the term was used to refer to interpretation of scripture but it is used today rather more broadly to encompass any interpretative operations.

hermetic Airtight. Occasionally used metaphorically for a pure, uncontaminated process.

heroin An opiate derived from MORPHINE with analgesic, euphoric and sedative effects. As with all the opiates, repeated dosages lead to development of tolerance and a marked DRUG •DEPENDENCE. The effectiveness of heroin to alter mood, relieve tension, fears and anxieties and produce a gentle drowsy euphoria has made it the most abused of the narcotics.

Hertz (Hz) One cycle per second. The term honours the German physicist Heinrich R. Hertz.

Heschl's gyrus A prominent GYRUS in the primary auditory cortex. Bilateral damage causes cortical deafness, i.e. deafness independent of any peripheral damage.

hesitation pause PAUSE, HESITATION.

Hess image A third POSITIVE •AFTERIMAGE that appears after the first two (known respectively as the Hering and Purkinje afterimages). It is exceedingly faint and there is some uncertainty concerning its description.

hetero- Combining form from the Greek, translated variously as *different, other, unlike,* etc. Contrast with HOMO-.

heterodox Any belief that is different from what is generally accepted, or the person holding such a belief. The treatment given a heterodox varies widely: in theological realms he or she may be seen as a heretic, in scientific work as creative and progressive.

heteroerotic Characterizing sexual attraction toward another person. The term is the antonym of AUTOEROTIC and is neutral as to hetero- or homosexuality.

heterogeneity Generally, dissimilarity.

Used of groups, data, variables, etc. that show marked differences among instances.

heterogeneity of variance See HOMOGENEITY OF VARIANCE.

heterographia Writing something other than what one intended.

heteromorphous Differing from the normal or usual form.

heteronomous Originating or controlled from the outside, externally controlled, the antonym of AUTONOMOUS.

heteronomous morality stage MORAL REALISM STAGE.

heterophemy Saying something other than what one intended.

heterophily The tendency of people to form social ties with people with distinctly different characteristics and lifestyles from oneself. Contrast with HOMOPHILY. adj., *heterophilous*.

heterophoria A general term used for any lack of muscular coordination or balance between the two eyes.

heteroscedasticity SCEDASTICITY.

heterosexism A cultural point of view that identifies heterosexual attraction and conduct as appropriate and proper and denigrates homosexuality, usually regarding same-sex attraction and sexual behaviour as abnormal, even depraved. Unlike HOMOPHOBIA, it refers to a wide set of social values without the sense that homosexual individuals or activity is feared. The term is an odd one and one needs to resist the temptation to assume that it denotes an anti-heterosexual bias.

heterosexual 1 n. An individual whose sexual orientation is for persons of the opposite sex. **2** adj. Characterizing HETEROSEXUALITY.

heterosexuality 1 Sexual contact between persons of opposite sexes. **2** An attraction to persons of the opposite sex, the condition in which one's sexual orientations are for the opposite sex. Compare with HOMOSEXUALITY.

heterosis Increased strength, size, vigour and growth rate resulting from cross-breeding of genetically dissimilar members of the same species. Also called *hybrid vigour*.

heterotropia STRABISMUS.

heterozygote A heterozygous organism.

heterozygous Descriptive of any organism possessing two unlike ALLELES for a particular trait. Contrast with HOMOZYGOUS.

heuristic A method for discovery, a procedure for solving a problem, a technique that operates as a vehicle for creative formulation. Essentially, any sophisticated, directed procedure that functions by reducing the range of possible solutions to a problem or the number of possible answers to a question.

Heuristics operate in the actual doing of science in fundamental ways; they are provisional characterizations that allow for testing, evaluation and refinement of ideas and theories. They emerge, moreover, in a good deal of complex human behaviour, particularly in problem-solving, decision-making, concept-learning, memory and the like. See COGNITIVE *HEURISTIC. Compare with ALGORITHM, which is a procedure that guarantees the finding of a solution, which heuristics do not. adj., *heuristic* or *heuristical*.

heuristic, cognitive A term generally reserved for any of the various HEURISTICS that people use when making decisions, solving problems and forming beliefs. For some examples, see ANCHORING, AVAILABILITY, FRAMING, REPRESENTATIVENESS.

hex(a)- Prefix meaning *six*.

5-HIAA HYDROXYINDOLEACETIC ACID.

Hick–Hyman law A generalization that reflects the fact that reaction time (RT) increases as a function of the amount of information transmitted in making a response. That is, $RT = a + bH$, where a and b are constants and H is the amount of information measured in bits. Thus, as the number of choices available to the subject is increased, RT increases; as the number of errors made increases, RT decreases; as the probability of individual choices goes down, RT goes up; and so forth. See INFORMATION and BIT for details of the patterns of usage of these terms.

hidden figure EMBEDDED FIGURE.

hidden observer In Ernest Hilgard's conceptualization of hypnosis, a hypothesized concealed consciousness that is inferred to experience events differently from (although in parallel with) the hypnotized consciousness.

hierarchical linear model A type of LINEAR *REGRESSION used when data can be viewed as hierarchically organized, as when the individuals in a study can be grouped into higher order units such as classes, schools, school districts, and so on. Also called *multilevel analysis* and *multilevel linear model*.

hierarchy 1 Any system of things, events, persons, concepts, etc. in rank order. A very general term, it is found in many cases where the writer wishes to convey the notion of things ranked from 'high' to 'low'. See following entries for some examples. **2** A system of organization that places elements into superordinate categories, e.g. my pet Phideaux is a collie, which is a dog, which is a mammal, which is… ˙

hierarchy, dominance 1 A HIERARCHY (1) of potential responses ranked in terms of the relative likelihood of occurrence under particular stimulus conditions. See HABIT HIERARCHY. **2** In ethology and comparative psychology, the ranking of members of a group according to relative importance or dominance. The term corresponds to the layman's expression *pecking order*, which comes, not surprisingly, from the fact that chickens typically establish such dominance hierarchies within a group.

high Colloquial term for the psychological state produced by psychotropic drugs, especially the hallucinogens and psychedelics.

higher brain centres (or structures) An early term used loosely for cortical areas suspected of being critical for carrying out the so-called *higher mental processes*. Efforts to identify exactly which these were proved futile. If the term is found in modern texts, it usually refers to the frontal lobes, specifically the prefrontal cortex and the *executive functions* supported.

higher mental processes A generic label used to refer collectively to thought, imagery, memory, ideation, language, abstraction, symbolization, judgement, etc. Rare these days in technical writing.

higher-order conditioning Classical conditioning in which a conditioned stimulus

(CS) from an original conditioning series is used as the unconditioned stimulus (US) in a new experimental setting. Also called *secondary* or *second-order conditioning*.

higher response unit Loosely, any complex, integrated response composed of simple responses.

high-grade defective See DEFECTIVE (2).

hillock AXON HILLOCK.

hindbrain During embryonic development the brain evolves three separate portions: the hindbrain, midbrain and forebrain. The first of these is evolutionarily the oldest; it differentiates into the metencephalon and the myelencephalon. The metencephalon gives rise to the cerebellum and the pons, the myelencephalon to the medulla.

hindsight bias The tendency, after an event has occurred, to think that we knew what was going to happen beforehand.

hippocampal formation A neurologically complex region of the limbic cortex in the temporal lobes which includes the *entorhinal cortex*, the *subicular complex*, the *dentate gyrus*, and the HIPPOCAMPUS itself. It extends from the narrow dorsal part that runs along the corpus callosum to the broad ventral part that forms the floor of the inferior horn of the lateral ventricle. In humans the hippocampal formation plays an important role in the formation of long-term memories; damage to this region or to its inputs and outputs causes ANTEROGRADE *AMNESIA for episodic and declarative memories. It has also been implicated in the encoding and representation of spatial knowledge (see PLACE CELLS). Note that the term *hippocampus*, although strictly the name of only one part of the formation, is often loosely used for the whole hippocampal region.

hippocampus A part of the HIPPOCAMPAL FORMATION. Cells in the hippocampus itself connect with cortical regions in the brain through the ENTORHINAL CORTEX and subcortical regions through the fimbria/fornix. Also called *Ammon's horn* and *cornu ammonis*.

histamine A *biogenic amine* that functions as a *neurotransmitter* in several cerebral pathways playing a significant role in wakefulness and arousal. It is also present in nearly all bodily tissue and is released whenever tissues are injured and in allergic reactions. Histamine causes a local red spot, which turns bluish in a minute or two, followed by a spreading redness and a localized swelling which typically itches.

histo- Prefix indicating *relating to tissue*.

histogram A type of BAR GRAPH of a frequency distribution in which the number of cases per class is presented as a vertical bar.

histology The discipline that studies the microscopic structure of bodily tissue. Basically, it is a branch of biology but histological analyses are an integral part of physiological psychology.

historical method A general term for any form of therapy, analysis or counselling that deals with the individual by focusing on life history.

histrionic personality disorder A personality disorder usually characterized by immaturity, self-centredness, attention-getting, manipulativeness and, quite often, a vague seductiveness. Such persons are overly dramatic, reactive and intense in their interpersonal relationships and frequently play out classic roles like 'princess' or 'victim'. Also called, especially in older texts, *hysterical personality*.

hit The accurate statement by a subject that an objectively present stimulus was, in fact, present and perceived. Compare with FALSE ALARM and see discussion under SIGNAL-DETECTION THEORY.

HM The sobriquet of one of neuropsychology's most important early cases. Operated on for intractable epilepsy, HM underwent a bilateral midtemporal lobe resection of the amygdala, the anterior two-thirds of the hippocampus, and surrounding cortical tissue. The procedure made the epilepsy manageable but resulted in a severe anterograde amnesia. It was largely through this case that the importance of the midtemporal lobe, especially the HIPPOCAMPAL FORMATION, in explicit memory was first appreciated.

hoarding, compulsive A COMPULSIVE CONDUCT DISORDER in which a person excessively and uncontrollably acquires and hoards items. The disorder is extremely difficult to treat. Also called *pack-rat syndrome*.

hobbits and orcs A puzzle used in studies of problem-solving. Three hobbits and three orcs must cross a river in a boat that can only hold two people. If the hobbits are ever outnumbered on the river bank they will be eaten and the canoe must have at least one passenger on each crossing. Try it. Also called, somewhat insensitively, *missionaries and cannibals*.

Hobson's choice From the Elizabethan Thomas Hobson, described by the early 18th-century essayist Richard Steele; a choice that is not a choice at all. Hobson, a stableowner, would only lend out the one horse nearest the stable door no matter how many other of his horses were free. Hence, being presented with Hobson's choice is to be confronted with a situation in which there are nominally many alternatives from which to choose but the constraints of the situation are such that one's actual choice is forced upon one. The situation presented to the chooser is of considerable interest in social psychological theories of choice behaviour. See, for example, REACTANCE THEORY, REACTIVE (2, 3).

hodological space Hodology is a branch of geometry that characterizes geometric relationships in terms of vectors and their paths. K. Lewin's topological theory of personality is based (somewhat informally) on the mathematics of such spaces. See FIELD THEORY, TOPOLOGY.

Höffding step In the terminology of Gestalt psychology, the mental step through which the perception of an image makes contact with a memory trace. If you see a table and think 'chair', the sight of the table does not trigger the associated memory of 'chair' directly. There is an additional step necessary, the step whereby the stimulus 'table' contacts the memory trace of 'table' which then contacts the memory 'chair'. Although the need for the Höffding step has been recognized for nearly a century it has only become regarded as important for theories of pattern perception and pattern recognition in recent years.

hold index In neuropsychology, a measure of a patient's performance on cognitive ability tasks that are thought to be relatively resistant to the effects of brain damage (e.g. vocabulary) relative to performance on other tasks thought to be sensitive to neurological problems (e.g. memory). The index was originally developed to represent an individual's relative preservation of ability in the face of aging and neurological problems. Unfortunately, it has not stood up well to empirical tests. Also called *hold–don't hold index*. The converse is often called the *deterioration index*.

holergasia Obsolescent term for any psychiatric disorder that affects the entire emotional, cognitive and behavioural repertoire of an individual.

holism A general label applied to any philosophical approach that focuses on the whole living organism. The basic axiom of a holistic position is that a complex phenomenon cannot be understood by an analysis of the constituent parts alone. Contrast with ELEMENTARISM and ATOMISM. Gestalt and Freudian theories are classic examples of holistic approaches in psychology.

holistic Pertaining to the whole rather than the components of an object or situation. The term is used in a number of specialized ways, e.g. *holistic perception* or *holistic processing* where it reflects the core connotation that the material is handled in a global, Gestalt-like fashion.

Holland codes A set of six career types (artistic, conventional, enterprising, investigative, realistic and social) identified by John Holland and used as part of an occupational coding scheme. Holland argued that each individual is typically dominated by two or three types. The Holland codes are used for scoring the STRONG–CAMPBELL INTEREST INVENTORY.

Hollingshead scales Formulas that allow one to convert the occupation and education level of adults into ordinal scales of socioeconomic status (SES). Intriguingly, even though the Hollingshead is among the most used scales for determining SES, the latest version never appeared 'officially', that is, in a peer-reviewed journal or book. Everyone simply uses the unpublished manuscript Hollingshead left behind when he died. The UK equivalent is called the *Registrar General's scale/categories*. See also OCCUPATIONAL HIERARCHY.

Holmgren test An early (19th-century) test

for colour blindness using skeins of yarn of various colours that had to be classified into three groups determined by a set of three standard-coloured skeins. The test has also been used to evaluate abstracting ability, particularly in patients with brain damage.

hol(o)- Combining form meaning *complete, whole, homogeneous.*

holographic memory MEMORY, HOLO-GRAPHIC.

holophrase A single-word utterance that may function as a whole phrase or even a sentence. See HOLOPHRASTIC STAGE.

holophrastic stage An early stage in the development of language in a child in which single-word utterances dominate. Some theorists argue that such single words (or holophrases) are reduced or telegraphic sentences (e.g. 'Milk' represents 'I want milk'), and suggest that memory and motor-control limitations of the young child force their use. Other theorists argue that the holophrastic stage is presyntactic and that one should not infer that the child in any way knows sentence formation rules, merely that the holophrases are used to indicate primitive concepts like desire, possession, location, etc.

homeo- Combining form denoting *sameness* or *resemblance.*

homeostasis From the Greek for *same-state.* The American physiologist W. B. Cannon introduced the term for any process that modifies an existing condition or a set of circumstances and thereby initiates other processes that function in a regulatory manner to re-establish the initial condition. A thermostat is a mechanical homeostat. The term is used in physiological psychology to encompass a number of complex biological mechanisms that operate via the autonomic nervous system to regulate such factors as body temperature, bodily fluids and their physical and chemical properties, blood pressure, water balance and metabolism. For example, a drop in body temperature initiates a variety of processes, such as shivering, piloerection and an increase in metabolism, that produce and conserve heat until a normal temperature is achieved.

home sign Fant's term for the informal, invented manual gestures often seen in communication between deaf children who have been trained through the use of the ORAL METHOD. See also MANUAL METHOD.

hominid From the name for the primate family Hominidae, this term refers to any of the species so classified. *Homo sapiens* is the only surviving member.

Homo From the Latin for *man.* Usually, but not always, capitalized.

homo- Combining form from the Greek, meaning *same, similar, alike.*

homoerotism 1 Broadly, any erotic feelings toward members of one's own sex. **2** Specifically, HOMOSEXUALITY.

homogamy The tendency for people to select mates who are similar to themselves. It is not clear whether this well-documented tendency is due to a genuine selection of like by like or an artifact of the patterns of social interaction in which people typically spend most of their time with those from similar racial, ethnic and socioeconomic backgrounds. See also PROPINQUITY and HOMOPHILY.

homogeneity Broadly, similarity, sameness. Applied in various settings to refer to groups, subjects, data, variables, etc. when the items under consideration are not appreciably or meaningfully different from each other.

homogeneity of variance Similarity in VARIANCE. Many parametrical statistical tests (e.g. t test, F test) are based on the assumption that the population variances underlying the samples are the same (in order for the test to provide a valid estimate of any statistical effects). In practice homogeneity of variance means *nonsignificant heterogeneity.* That is, one does not expect variances to be identical, merely not significantly different from each other so that one may operate on the assumption that the samples actually came from the same underlying population. The F RATIO is the most convenient test for this.

homograph Any pair or set of words with identical spellings but different etymologies and hence different meanings. One of our favourites is the two verbs *cleave* – each is the antonym of the other.

homolateral IPSILATERAL.

homologous 1 Of biological structures that correspond in type of structure and origin but not necessarily in function. The foreleg of a horse and a bird's wing are homologous structures. Contrast with the biologist's use of ANALOGUE (2), in which the function is similar but the structure and origin are not, e.g. the wings of bees and birds. **2** By extension, of behaviours that show such a relationship; e.g. territoriality in baboons is often considered to be homologous to territoriality in *Homo sapiens*.

homonym One of two or more words with identical pronunciations and spellings but different etymologies and hence different meanings, e.g. *pool* (the game) and *pool* (the place to swim). Compare with HOMOPHONE.

homonymous hemianopia Blindness in the same half of the visual field in both eyes.

homonym symptom A form of speech behaviour observed at times in schizophrenics when a polysemous word sends the patient off in what seems like a bizarre narrative. For example, he may begin by telling what he did with his savings and say, '...I took it all to deposit it in the bank...and there we sat down to fish for a while...'

homophile 1 A lover of mankind. **2** A homosexual.

homophily The tendency of people to form social ties with people who share the same characteristics and lifestyle as oneself. Contrast with HETEROPHILY. adj., *homophilous*.

homophone One of two or more words with identical pronunciations but, owing to different etymologies, different meanings and written forms, e.g. *bare* and *bear* or *to*, *two* and *too*.

homoscedasticity SCEDASTICITY.

homosexual 1 One who is sexually attracted to members of the same sex. **2** One who engages in sexual contact with members of the same sex. **3** One who identifies as having HOMOSEXUALITY as a facet of their sense of self. Note that the first definition is based on attraction, the second on behaviour and the third on identity. All three will be found in the literature and failure to keep them referentially distinct can

lead to all sorts of confusion both in technical writings and the popular press. For example, estimates of the population rate of HOMOSEXUALITY will vary tremendously from relatively rare to quite common depending on which definition or combination of definitions one adopts. Note, in the popular press and increasingly the technical literature, the term *gay* is used for males and *lesbian* for females.

homosexuality A term used rather generally to refer to sexual contact between persons of the same gender. That is, the individuals would be classified as HOMOSEXUAL in sense (2) of that term, with the emphasis on behaviour, not identity or attraction. This contact may be fleeting, non-orgasmic and occasional or it may represent an individual's dominant (if not exclusive) mode of sexual expression. In a very real sense, then, the term may be found in the psychological literature covering persons ranging from those who have had but one or two half-hearted experiences to those for whom heterosexual contacts have been non-existent. Contemporary scientific perspectives treat homosexuality as a simple variation on human sexual expression with no implications of pathology or immorality – a position not necessarily shared by members of the lay public.

homosexuality, ego-dystonic Homosexuality in which the individual has a persistent concern with changing his or her sexual orientation. In the *DSM-IV* this is no longer listed as a psychiatric disturbance. Note that the critical feature is not the sexual orientation *per se*, but the distress and anxiety over it and the persistent desire to be heterosexual. Compare with EGO-SYNTONIC *HOMOSEXUALITY.

homosexuality, ego-syntonic Homosexuality in which the individual is comfortable with and accepts his or her behaviour as a simple manifestation of natural sexual orientation. Compare with EGO-DYSTONIC *HOMOSEXUALITY.

homosexuality, situational Homosexuality that occurs in particular situations, most commonly in same-sex environments like prisons and boarding schools. The term is typically used of heterosexual individuals who return to their usual mode of sexual expression when they leave the setting.

homozygote A HOMOZYGOUS organism.

homozygous Descriptive of any organism possessing two like ALLELES for a particular trait. Contrast with HETEROZYGOUS.

homunculus Lit., a *miniature man*. **1** Through the ages the homunculus has served as a half-serious (and occasionally totally serious) physiological and psychological metaphor. At times he has been viewed as inhabiting the reproductive cells and acting as the agent for genetic transmission, as a kind of gremlin in the body regulating morality, or as a little 'green man' in the brain governing decision-making. The main problem with the metaphor is that it leaves open the question of what kind of beast inhabits the homunculus and governs its acts, *reductio ad infinitum cum absurdum*. **2** In neurophysiology, a schematic representation of the cortical projections for sensory and motor functions. The body is drawn in proportion to the amount of cortical tissue that subsumes each part. Thus, the human motor homunculus has an extremely large mouth, lips, tongue, eyes and hands and a rather diminutive skull, torso, buttocks and legs. The sensory version has a prominent tongue, lips, face, hands, feet, intra-abdominal region and genitals and a small torso, buttocks, skull, arms and legs. Not surprisingly, these proportions correspond to sensory discrimination and motor control of these regions. **3** An obsolete term for a dwarf with normal anatomical proportions.

honestly significant difference test TUKEY HONESTLY SIGNIFICANT DIFFERENCE TEST.

Honi phenomenon Failure of the well-known perceptual distortion effects of the AMES ROOM to occur when a very familiar person such as a parent or spouse is placed in the room. The effect is not named for its discoverer. 'Honi' was the nickname of the family of the subject who first experienced it. Recent research also suggests that the phenomenon may not be as pronounced as first thought.

hopelessness theory A theory of depression that extends Martin Seligman's earlier theory of LEARNED *HELPLESSNESS by focusing on the fact that people differ in their ATTRIBUTIONAL STYLE. Individuals who are prone to

interpreting the negative events in life as stable (not likely to change), global (widespread) and internal (caused by the individual) are viewed as displaying a pessimistic attributional style. These DEPRESSOGENIC attributions, in turn, increase the likelihood that such individuals will encounter situations where they experience helplessness and hopelessness. The spiral of attributions is assumed to be a leading cause of depression.

horizon **1** In perception, the limit of the range of what can be perceived. **2** By extension, the limit of knowledge.

horizontal **1** Pertaining to the horizon. **2** At right angles to the vertical.

horizontal (H) cells Cells in the retinas of vertebrates with colour vision. They have dendrites that hook up with a large number of cones and have been shown to respond in opposite fashion to stimulation of different wavelengths (e.g. red and green). This feature has led to the hypothesis that H cells form part of the neurological mechanism assumed by the *opponent process theory*; for more detail SEE THEORIES OF *COLOUR VISION.

horizontal décalage DÉCALAGE.

horizontal group GROUP, HORIZONTAL.

horizontal mobility Mobility within the same social or occupational class. Also called *horizontal social mobility*.

horizontal sampling SAMPLING, HORIZONTAL.

horizontal section SECTION (2).

hormic psychology A school of psychology associated with the work of English-born social psychologist William McDougall. The system is based on a loose collection of basic 'goal-oriented' or 'purposeful' behaviours that were assumed to be motivated by innate propensities or instincts. The term *hormic* derives from the Greek for *animal impulse*.

McDougall, one of the more vigorous critics of Watsonian behaviourism, initially attracted numerous adherents particularly among social psychologists, sociologists and anthropologists, many of whom considered Watson's position simplistic and sterile. The hormic position, however, suffered from major liabilities, the primary being the lack of precision in the definition and use of the concept of instinct. As this, the central pillar of the theory, came under severe attack from the more sophisticated behaviourists the school lost popularity and influence. Today it is mainly of historical interest.

hormone From the Greek, meaning *urging, striving*. A general term covering a large number of bodily substances that originate in a gland or an organ, are conveyed to other organic sites and have any of a number of effects on these target cells. Individual hormones are listed separately. Note that many substances that are listed as hormones by virtue of their production by glands also function as NEUROTRANSMITTERS (e.g. *norepinephrine* and the *endorphins*).

Horn-Cattell theory (of intelligence) A theory of intelligence developed by R. B. Cattell and expanded by J. L. Horn that proposes that intelligence comprises processes of flexible learning, reasoning and problem-solving (see FLUID *INTELLIGENCE) and the products of those processes (or CRYSTALLIZED *INTELLIGENCE). The theory was later elaborated to include several broad factors such as visualization and auditory abilities.

Horner's law The genetic principle that the most common form of colour blindness (red–green) is transmitted from male to male through unaffected females.

horopter When both eyes are fixated on a particular point in the visual field there exists a collection of points in the field the images of which fall on CONGRUENT RETINAL POINTS; collectively this locus is called the horopter.

hospice A specialized nursing home for terminally ill patients. Hospices are designed to be caring, peaceful, supportive environments where patients can live out their final days in dignity. Note that so-called 'hospice care' is now offered through some hospitals and regular nursing homes.

hospital hopper syndrome A nicely descriptive term occasionally used as a synonym of FACTITIOUS DISORDER.

hospitalism REACTIVE ATTACHMENT DISORDER.

hostile media phenomenon The tendency for people on opposite sides of an issue to view the same balanced coverage as hostile to their side. This phenomenon is a prime example of how SCHEMAS can influence our interpretation of information.

hostility A long-lasting emotional state characterized by enmity toward others and manifested by a desire to harm or inflict pain upon those at whom it is directed. Often distinguished from ANGER on the grounds that anger is a more intense and momentary reaction. See also ANIMUS (1), ANIMOSITY and HATRED.

hot Loosely, characterizing actions, processes and functions that are active, vigorous and intense. Hence, common references are found to 'hot' emotions (e.g. anger, rage), 'hot' cognition (e.g. intense efforts at problem-solving) and even 'hot' colours (e.g. reds and oranges).

hot-chair technique A procedure used in Gestalt therapy where the client sits in a chair next to the therapist who prompts and encourages the dialogue, leading the client to work through feelings and beliefs. A group therapy variation is also used.

hot hands A colloquialism that has found its way into serious scientific work, it refers to the notion that an athlete like a basketball player can get on a shooting streak where they are making shots at a rate far above their normal, base rate. That is, they have 'hot hands'. Virtually everyone who plays games like basketball or bowling or golf will attest to the subjective sense that the effect is real. However, the psychologically interesting question is whether these streaks really occur at rates higher than statistical models predict or whether they are subjective illusions. The issues are complex and the jury is still out.

House–Tree–Person Test A projective test in which the subject is requested to draw a house, a tree and a person. The drawings made are interpreted according to a more or less standardized set of criteria involving amount of detail, speed of execution and any comments made by the subject.

5-HT *5-hydroxytryptamine* SEROTONIN.

hue That dimension of visual sensation corresponding chiefly to the wavelength of the light. The term is roughly synonymous with the common term *colour* and, indeed, hues are specified by names like red, green, yellow and blue. Note that hues are also secondarily related to the amplitude of the light waves since a perceived hue will change somewhat with light intensity. See also entries under COLOUR and SPECTRUM.

hue, pure A hue of which the stimulus is a light source with but a single wavelength. Lasers produce pure hues; they are never seen in the 'real world'.

hues, unique PRIMARY *COLOURS (esp. 2).

Hullian Pertaining to the theoretical and empirical point of view of the American psychologist Clark Leonard Hull (1884–1952), specifically the behaviourist perspective he espoused. Although Hull's work spanned several diverse areas, including tests and measurements, hypnosis, concept formation, motivation and learning, the term is generally applied only to his work in these last two. Hull developed in the final two decades of his life a rich, elaborate behaviourist theory of learning and motivation. The Hullian approach was wedded to the use of the HYPOTHETICO-DEDUCTIVE METHOD, in which one deduces hypotheses from postulates and tests them empirically. Those found wanting are taken as guides to the adjustment of one's postulates so as to deduce new hypotheses, and so forth. Thus, the system was designed to be self-correcting.

The basic principle was that HABIT STRENGTH is increased by reinforcement. A variety of secondary principles articulated the manner in which it could also be modified by drive level, various forms of inhibition and excitation, stimulus and response generalization, etc. The full-blown Hullian system eventually expired of its own hypothetico-deductive excesses. So many variables needed to be introduced as part of the postulate system that by the late 1940s a research paper in the tradition, with all the elaborate notation used as shorthand for the variables, looked as if someone had spilled alphabet soup on the page. The power of the Hullian approach that gave it its several decades of influence in experimental psychology derived from a number of factors: (a) the inclusion of motivational elements in the theory of learning; (b) the strong adherence to a sophisticated positivist philosophy; and (c) the novel manner in which Hull attempted to account for the action of a reinforcer; see DRIVE REDUCTION HYPOTHESIS.

There are no true Hullians left today but many who were profoundly influenced by his thinking.

human engineering 1 An applied discipline allied with industrial and organizational psychology that focuses on the problems of the design of equipment, machinery, work places, working conditions and the like. **2** The art of managing humans as engineers manage machines.

human factors A generic term used most often as the name of the professional speciality that studies the so-called man (or person)–machine INTERFACE (2). The focus is generally on problems of perception, psychophysics, decision-making and other aspects of information processing. The term, however, is also used on occasion to refer to those elements (or factors) that are important within this speciality, including the equipment, the physical environment, the tasks and the individuals who do the work. See also INDUSTRIAL/ORGANIZATIONAL PSYCHOLOGY, which is generally regarded as the broader field within which human factors is a subdiscipline.

humanistic psychology An approach to psychology developed largely by theorists such as Abraham Maslow, Carl Rogers, Erich Fromm and Rollo May. They proposed it as 'a third force' after psychoanalysis, which was, in their view, too concerned with the neurotic, and behaviourism, which they saw as excessively focused on that which was explainable with mechanistic theory. Humanism in Maslow's sense was supposed to produce a psychological science concerned with higher human motives, self-development, knowledge, understanding and aesthetics. It never fully succeeded.

human nature An absolutely undefinable term. Usage typically connotes innateness but precisely what the characteristics are presumed to be genetically given tends to depend entirely on the prejudices of the writer. The term's most common use seems to be as an apology for inhuman behaviour.

human potential movement A general label covering the vast array of presumably therapeutic techniques such as encounter groups, sensitivity training and assertiveness training. While these and other techniques are widely used, critics view them as largely irresponsible commercial enterprises which prey upon people's vulnerabilities and fears.

There have been enough positive results from the use of some of the techniques for a number of them (particularly sensitivity training) to have actually been introduced into schools and businesses. However, many authorities are highly critical of the movement as a whole because of its tendency to follow the intuitions of practitioners who tend to accept uncritically the claimed virtues of such disparate approaches as Zen Buddhism, psychodrama, art, dance, poetry, mysticism, yoga, meditation, fasting, acupuncture, rolfing, astrology or just plain 'letting it all hang out', independent of any coherent theoretical analysis, controlled experimentation or systematic follow-up on the efficacy of these techniques. In recent years it has blended in with the New Age movement without, alas, gaining anything in reliability, validity or coherence.

humour 1 Any bodily fluid such as the aqueous humour in the eye. Archaic physiological theories assumed that temperament depended on the relative proportions of four cardinal humours in the body. Note that the vestiges of this point of view are still with us in that in common parlance *humour* can be used synonymously with *mood*. **2** The quality of being pleasant, sympathetic, amusing or funny. var., *humor*.

Humpty-Dumpty rule A rule or principle which has been, perhaps more than any other, the driving force behind the idiosyncratic and often baffling manner of usage of terms in science. It derives, of course, from Lewis Carroll when he had Humpty speak the words closest to his heart: ' "When I use a word," Humpty Dumpty said in a rather scornful tone, "it means just what I choose it to mean – neither more nor less." ' So it is with the neologistic scientist.

hunger 1 Physiologically, an internal state of an organism that results from particular imbalances in nutrients in the body and the severity of which is determined by the degree of these imbalances. See also GLUCO-STATIC THEORY. **2** An internal state that results from food deprivation and the severity of

which is measured by the duration of the deprivation. This meaning is essentially an attempt to provide an operational definition of the term. **3** The phenomenologically experienced state that results from either of the circumstances specified in 1 and 2. **4** A drive state resulting from either of the circumstances specified in 1 and 2 that motivates food-seeking behaviour. Note that 4 extends 3 by implying that the experienced state is linked with motivational components. **5** By extension, any craving for something that one has been deprived of, e.g. a hunger for affection, a sexual hunger. Usage here pulls the term out of its alliance with food but any or all of the specific definitional restrictions exhibited in meanings 1–4 may be found here as well.

hunger, specific A need for specific dietary substances. The term, however, is somewhat misleading in that it connotes, quite literally, that there are specific hungers for specific substances; e.g. that an organism deprived of, say, the vitamin thiamine will have a 'hunger' for it and select out foodstuffs containing it over other foodstuffs lacking it. There is, with the possible exception of salt, precious little evidence for such a phenomenon. What there is evidence for is *learned preference* and *learned avoidance*; that is, an organism will eventually learn to prefer a diet containing thiamine over ones that do not because the ones that do not produce metabolic deficiencies. For more on the model that lies behind this conception, see CONDITIONED *AVERSION.

Huntington's disease An inherited neurological disease characterized by progressive cognitive and muscular deterioration and in the later stages by severe alterations in personality. Patients show deficits in such cognitive areas as attention, memory retrieval, problem-solving and visuoperceptual functions. Interestingly, memory dysfunctions are limited largely to recall of material, recognition ability being often unaffected. The disease is caused by a dominant gene, and anyone carrying it will eventually develop the disease. Also called *Huntington's chorea*.

Hurler's syndrome A genetic disorder characterized by severe mental retardation and a variety of physical abnormalities including pronounced spinal curvature and coarse facial features marked by a broad, flat nose, wide-set eyes, low-set ears and a large protruding tongue.

hwa-byung A CULTURE-SPECIFIC SYNDROME in Korea. Attributed to suppression of anger, symptoms include insomnia, fatigue, panic, indigestion and anorexia, generalized aches and pains, and a feeling of a mass in the pit of the stomach.

hyalophagia Eating of glass, a form of PICA.

H-Y antigen A protein that plays an important role in sexual differentiation. Production of the protein is controlled by a gene on the Y chromosome. When present it stimulates receptors on the surface of the primordial gonads and causes them to develop as testes; when not present they develop as ovaries.

hybrid 1 An offspring resulting from the union of gametes of differing genotypes. Generally used with respect to animals or plants when the parents are of different species or well-marked varieties. **2** By extension, one who is heterogeneous in make-up. Here the meaning extends to social, cultural and linguistic forms. adj., *hybrid*.

hybrid vigour HETEROSIS.

hydraulic theory In general, any theory that models the phenomena under consideration in a fashion based on the assumption that things behave like fluids under pressure, ready to break through any weak spots should the pressure exceed some critical level. Meyer's theory of hearing is termed hydraulic, as are Freud's personality theory and the Tinbergen–Lorenz ethological theory (although in the last case the label was applied derisively by critics, not proponents).

hydraulic theory of hearing THEORIES OF *HEARING.

hydro- Combining form meaning *water* and, by extension, *fluid* or *liquid*.

hydrocephalus Lit., water or fluid in the head. An abnormal accumulation of cerebrospinal fluid within the VENTRICLES (3). The pressure on the brain, if not alleviated, can result in permanent damage to cerebral tissue. adj., *hydrocephalic*.

hydrotherapy A cover term for any use of water in a therapeutic manner.

5-hydroxyindoleacetic acid (5-HIAA) A metabolite of SEROTONIN. Low levels of 5-HIAA have been associated with suicidal depression.

5-hydroxytryptamine SEROTONIN.

5-hydroxytryptophan A SEROTONIN precursor currently being explored for possible therapeutic value in motoric disorders, depression and related syndromes. There are problems with potentially serious side effects.

hyp- HYPO-.

hypacusia Impaired hearing.

hypaesthesia Lowered sensitivity. var., *hypesthesia*.

hypalgesia Relative insensitivity to pain. var., *hypalgia*.

hyper- Combining form meaning *above, beyond, in high degree, excessive*. Most of the combinatory forms using this prefix are self-explanatory (e.g. *hypercritical*); less obvious forms are given below.

hyperactive child Strictly speaking this is a nontechnical term, although it is sometimes found in the technical literature. It is used loosely of a child who displays any of the various disorders of childhood that have hyperactivity as a feature; for example, ATTENTION-DEFICIT HYPERACTIVITY DISORDER.

hyperactive child syndrome ATTENTION-DEFICIT HYPERACTIVITY DISORDER.

hyperactivity Vigorous, inappropriate motor activity. See ATTENTION-DEFICIT HYPERACTIVITY DISORDER.

hyperacusia Excellent hearing, although usually accompanied by intolerance of loud sounds.

hyperaesthesia Extreme sensitivity to touch. On occasion the term is used more generally to refer to any sensory hypersensitivity, in which case it is usually qualified, e.g. *acoustic hyperaesthesia*. var., *hyperaesthesia*.

hyperalgesia Extreme sensitivity to pain. var., *hyperalgia*.

hypercalcemia WILLIAMS SYNDROME.

hypercathexis Investing psychic energy (cathexis) in one process for the (unconscious) purposes of furthering or facilitating another. Generally regarded in psychoanalytic writings as a DEFENCE MECHANISM.

hypercomplex cell See SIMPLE CELL.

hypergasia Overactivity characteristic of the manic phase of BIPOLAR DISORDER.

hypergenitalism Excessive early development of the genitals; premature puberty. The condition may be caused by abnormal endocrine secretions of the adrenal cortices or the gonads or by some hypothalamic disorders.

hypergeometric distribution DISTRIBUTION, HYPERGEOMETRIC.

hypergeusia Extreme taste sensitivity.

hyperglycemia Excess of blood sugar.

hyperkinaesthesia Extreme sensitivity to kinaesthetic sensations. var., *hyperkinesthesia*.

hyperkinesis Excessive and inappropriate motor activity, extreme restlessness; usually accompanied by poor attention span and impulsivity. See ATTENTION-DEFICIT HYPERACTIVITY DISORDER. var., *hyperkinesia*. Hyperkinesias are also seen in various neurological disorders such as HUNTINGTON'S DISEASE.

hyperkinetic dysarthria DYSARTHRIA, HYPERKINETIC.

hyperkinetic syndrome ATTENTION-DEFICIT HYPERACTIVITY DISORDER.

hyperlexia 1 Generally, early acquisition of reading. Used specifically of children who learn to read prior to formal reading instruction. **2** A condition characterized by very early and effortless acquisition of oral reading in a child who otherwise shows no special abilities and, in fact, is slow in reaching standard developmental milestones. Used in this sense it refers to what some feel is a form of minimal brain damage.

hypermania Condition exhibiting extreme activity, rapid and erratic behaviour and speech.

hypermenorrhoea 1 Excessive menstrual flow in amount and/or duration. **2** Abnor-

mally frequent menstruation. Each is a form of DYSMENORRHOEA. var., *hypermenorrhea*.

hypermetropia HYPEROPIA.

hypermnesia Lit., excessive memory. Hence: **1** A characteristic of some SAVANTS who have an extraordinary ability to recall names, dates, places, etc. **2** An extremely detailed recollection of a particular past experience. It is observed occasionally in the manic phase of bipolar disorders, during hypnosis and during certain neurosurgical procedures, particularly when the temporal lobe is stimulated. There are questions as to whether these experiences ought to be classified as true memorial phenomena, in that the conditions under which they occur make it nearly impossible to determine whether they are real hypermnesic effects or merely elaborations and/or confabulations of events. **3** An increase in the ability to recall material over time. This meaning appears in experimental studies of memory and is usually contrasted with 'typical' forgetting, in which the tendency is for material, once learned, to be increasingly unlikely to be recalled over time. It is also found in some psychoanalytic writings since the techniques of classical psychoanalysis are predicated on a hypermnesic effect, in that during analysis the individual is able to retrieve memories of past events that were not recallable prior to the psychic probing of analysis.

hypermotility An occasional synonym of HYPERKINESIS.

hyperopia Farsightedness, the inability to focus clearly on near objects. The shape of the lens of the eye is such that the focal point for light entering the eye is behind the retina rather than directly on it. Contrast with MYOPIA.

hyperorexia Excessive appetite. Contrast with ANOREXIA; differentiate from HYPERPHAGIA.

hyperosmia Extreme sensitivity to odours.

hyperphagia Lit., overeating. The term is most often used to refer to a syndrome, experimentally induced by a lesion in the ventromedial area of the hypothalamus, in which the normal feeding regime is disturbed, resulting in excessive intake of foodstuffs, increased accumulation of adipose tissue and obesity. See HYPOTHALAMUS and VEN-

TROMEDIAL HYPOTHALAMIC SYNDROME for more details.

hyperphasia HYPERPHRASIA.

hyperphoria Abnormal tendency for one eye to turn upward.

hyperphrasia Pathologically excessive talking. var., *hyperphasia*.

hyperphrenia 1 Excessive mental activity. Not necessarily effective mental activity though; the term is used to characterize the manic phase of *bipolar disorder*. 2 Unusually high intellectual ability. This meaning is rare owing to the former.

hyperplasia Increase in the size of an organ caused by an abnormal increase in the number of cells. Compare with HYPERTROPHY.

hyperpnoea Increased breathing either in frequency of respirations or in depth. var., *hyperpnea*.

hyperpolarization An increase in polarization; in neurophysiology, the increase in the membrane potential of a neuron. See discussion under DEPOLARIZATION.

hyperprosexia An exaggerated fixating on some idea to the exclusion of others; seen in compulsive disorders.

hypersomnia A sleep disorder characterized by excessive sleeping, uncontrollable sleepiness.

hypertension 1 Excessive tension or tonus in a muscle or organ. 2 A condition marked by abnormally high blood pressure.

hyperthymestic syndrome From the Greek for 'superior memory'. The term is restricted to cases of extraordinary memory with strong autobiographical features such as that displayed by the famous subject, AJ.

hyperthymia Excessive emotionality, excitability.

hyperthyroidism Excessive secretion of the thyroid gland, producing accelerated metabolic rate, extreme excitability and apprehension.

hypertonic 1 Descriptive of a solution in which the osmotic pressures between the liquid and the cells suspended in it are such that there is fluid transmission from the cells into the surrounding medium.

2 Characteristic of a state of greater-than-normal (muscular) tension. Contrast with HYPOTONIC.

hypertrophy Enlargement or excessive growth of an organ or organ part. Application of the term is restricted to increases not caused by tumour or excessive proliferation of cells (see HYPERPLASIA). Opposite of ATROPHY.

hypertropia Upward STRABISMUS.

hyphen psychologist Historically, a sobriquet used by early behaviourists for those with a cognitive orientation, that is, those who theorized about the hyphen in STIMULUS–RESPONSE.

hypnagogic image(s) Hallucination-like images experienced while first falling asleep. They tend to occur when EEG patterns indicate Stage 1 sleep but in the absence of the rapid eye movements (REM) typically seen during dreaming. Compare with HYPNOPOMPIC IMAGES. var., *hypnogogic*.

hypnoanalysis Psychoanalysis carried out with the patient under hypnosis. Although still used by some analysts it was dissatisfaction with hypnosis that originally led Freud to develop other techniques, such as free association and dream analysis. See HYPNOTHERAPY.

hypnogenic 1 Sleep-producing. 2 Causing or aiding hypnosis.

hypnogogic image(s) HYPNAGOGIC IMAGES.

hypnopaedia Sleep learning. Unfortunately for us all there is absolutely no evidence for this phenomenon.

hypnopompic images(s) Fleeting hallucination-like images that often accompany the first few semi-conscious moments during waking. Compare with HYPNAGOGIC IMAGES.

hypnosedatives A class of drugs which have both sedative (quietening, tranquillizing) and hypnotic (sleep-producing) effects. Included are drugs like the barbiturates, which in small doses function as sedatives and in larger doses as hypnotics. See HYPNOTICS and SEDATIVES for more detail.

hypnosis Few terms in the psychological lexicon are so thoroughly wrapped in mysticism and confusion. The problems arise from the tendency, which dates back to the discoverer, Franz Anton Mesmer, to regard the process of hypnotism as one which transports the subject into a separate 'state of mind'. Additional problems emerged because it has attracted a coterie of nightclub entertainers, charlatans and faith healers who make unsubstantiated claims and have shown a singular reluctance to use scientific controls.

The present view is that a hypnotic 'state' does exist. It is somewhat less dramatic than often portrayed but does, in general, display the following characteristics: (a) although it superficially resembles a sleep-like state (which is how it got its name), the EEG pattern does not resemble that of any of the stages of sleep; (b) normal planning functions are reduced – a hypnotized person tends to wait passively for instructions from the hypnotist; (c) attention becomes highly selective – the subject may hear only one person to the exclusion of others; (d) role-playing is readily accomplished, the hypnotized person frequently becoming quite thoroughly immersed in a suggested role; and (e) posthypnotic suggestion is often observed, frequently a specific amnesia that prevents the subject from recalling things he or she has been told to forget.

It should be noted that all of these effects are of a kind, in that they are also characteristic of an unhypnotized person who has voluntarily given up conscious control, a person who evidences extreme suggestibility. Not surprisingly, then, there is a school of thought that argues that there is nothing at all special about the hypnotic state, and that it merely represents an extreme pole on the scale of normal suggestibility.

hypnotherapy A general term for any psychotherapy that makes use of hypnosis. Hypnotherapy is generally classified as a *directive* therapy since hypnosis tends to produce a passivity during which the client accepts direction from others. See HYPNOANALYSIS.

hypnotic 1 Sleep-producing. **2** Pertaining to HYPNOSIS. **3** Pertaining to one of the HYPNOTICS.

hypnotic amnestic disorder SEDATIVE, HYPNOTIC OR ANXIOLYTIC AMNESTIC DISORDER.

hypnotic regression REGRESSION, HYPNOTIC.

hypnotics A group of drugs that produce sleep by a general (i.e. nonselective) depression of the central nervous system. Some of these drugs are also classified as SEDATIVES or HYPNOSEDATIVES in that their effects are dose-dependent – sedative in small doses, hypnotic in larger.

hypnotic withdrawal SEDATIVE, HYPNOTIC OR ANXIOLYTIC WITHDRAWAL.

hypnotic withdrawal delirium SEDATIVE, HYPNOTIC OR ANXIOLYTIC WITHDRAWAL DELIRIUM.

hypnotism The practice or study of hypnosis.

hypnotize 1 To induce a hypnotic state. **2** By extension, to influence another by subtle charm and guile.

hyp(o)- Combining form meaning *lesser, diminished, below, under.*

hypo Popular slang for a hypodermic syringe or the injection itself.

hypoactive sexual desire disorder A SEXUAL DESIRE DISORDER marked by persistent deficient (or absent) sexual fantasies and desire for sexual activity. It is only regarded as a disorder when this lack of libido (to use an older term) causes distress or interpersonal difficulty. Also called *inhibited sexual desire.*

hypochondriac One with HYPOCHONDRIASIS.

hypochondriasis A SOMATOFORM DISORDER characterized by imagined sufferings of physical illness or, more generally, an exaggerated concern with one's physical health. The hypochondriac typically displays a preoccupation with bodily functions such as heart rate, sweating, and bowel and bladder functions, and occasional minor problems like pimples, headaches, a simple cough, etc. All such trivialities are interpreted as signs or symptoms of more serious diseases. 'Doctor shopping' is common; assurances of health are futile. Also called *hypochondria.* adj., *hypochondriacal.*

hypodermic Under the skin.

hypoendocrinism A general term for any abnormal decrease in secretion from an endocrine gland.

hypoergastia Underactivity characteristic of a depressive state.

hypofrontality Reduced blood flow to the

frontal and prefrontal regions of the cortex relative to other brain regions. It is seen as a chronic condition in older, mentally deteriorated schizophrenics and in younger ones who are in an acute state brought about by attempts to solve complex problems. Note that when normals are engaged in such cognitive activity these cortical areas typically show an *increase* in blood supply.

hypogenitalism Underdevelopment of the genitals.

hypogeusia Abnormally diminished taste sensitivity.

hypoglossal nerve The XIIth CRANIAL NERVE, an efferent nerve arising in the medulla oblongata and supplying the muscles of the tongue.

hypoglycemia Deficiency of blood sugar.

hypogonadal syndrome A condition in males characterized by a failure of the testes to produce adequate amounts of testosterone and marked by obesity, infertility, bone fractures and slightly diminished sexual interest.

hypokinesis Abnormally low motor activity.

hypokinetic dysarthria See discussion under DYSARTHRIA, HYPERKINETIC.

hypolexia Retarded reading ability. See DYSLEXIA, which is the more commonly used term.

hypologia Abnormally poor speaking ability. The term is generally reserved for cases due to either mental retardation or motor dysfunction; if due to a cerebral disorder APHASIA is the proper term.

hypomania Literally, 'under mania'. Used for individuals who display unusually high levels of energy, exuberance and enthusiasm. Hypomanics are talkative, need relatively little sleep, are usually upbeat and optimistic and frequently productive and successful. Compare with MANIA (2) and see BIPOLAR DISORDER.

hypomanic disorder An atypical BIPOLAR DISORDER. The label is applied to persons who have had a depressive episode and now display a mild form of mania.

hypomanic episode A mood disorder marked by a period of HYPOMANIA.

hypomenorrhoea A form of DYSMENORRHOEA characterized by low volume of menstrual flow but with normally spaced periods. var., *hypomenorrhea*.

hypometropia MYOPIA.

hypomnesia A general term for any impaired memory ability.

hypophoria Abnormal tendency for one eye to turn downward.

hypophrenia Mental deficiency, rarely used.

hypophysis PITUITARY GLAND.

hypoplasia Defective development of tissue generally producing a structurally diminished organ or organ part. adj., *hypoplastic*.

hypopolarization DEPOLARIZATION.

hyposmia Diminished smell sensitivity.

hyposthenia Subnormal strength, weakness.

hypotension **1** Diminished tension or tonus in a muscle or organ. **2** A condition marked by abnormally low blood pressure.

hypothalamic hormone Any of a number of hormones released by the neurosecretory cells of the hypothalamus. They are transported to the pituitary, where they regulate the synthesis and release of the pituitary hormones.

hypothalamic-hypophyseal portal system A system of blood vessels that joins the capillaries of the hypothalamus with those of the anterior pituitary.

hypothalamic syndromes A general term for any behavioural syndrome that is hypothesized to result from damage to or dysfunction of a part of the hypothalamus, e.g. LATERAL HYPOTHALAMIC SYNDROME and VENTROMEDIAL HYPOTHALAMIC SYNDROME.

hypothalamus A relatively small (peanut-sized) but extremely complex structure at the base of the brain (below the thalamus) that is intimately involved in control of the autonomic nervous system and a variety of functions that are crucially related to survival, including temperature regulation, heart rate, blood pressure, feeding behaviour, water intake, emotional behaviour and sexual behaviour.

Anatomically the hypothalamus is divided into three subdivisions: (a) the *periventricular* region, containing many neurosecretory cells that serve as part of the control that the hypothalamus exerts over the pituitary gland; (b) the *medial* region, containing a number of hypothalamic nuclei, including the supraoptic, paraventricular, dorsomedial and the important ventromedial (see VENTRO-MEDIAL HYPOTHALAMIC SYNDROME); and (c) the *lateral* region, containing a complex system of neural pathways (those of the medial forebrain bundle) and a collection of axons and cell bodies (see LATERAL HYPOTHALAMIC SYNDROME for discussion of function).

hypothermia Lowering of the body temperature.

hypothesis 1 In scientific work, any statement, proposition or assumption that serves as a tentative explanation of certain facts. A hypothesis is always presented so as to be amenable to empirical test and then either supported or rejected by the evidence. **2** By extension, a strategy adopted in order to solve some problem. In most complex learning experiments such as those on problem-solving, concept-formation, decision-making and the like, subjects typically display consistency from trial to trial, operating as it were on the basis of some hypothesis like, 'If conditions x and y are present, I'll make response A; if not, then I'll try B.' Strictly speaking, the hypothesis itself is an internal, covert event the existence of which must be inferred from the subject's behaviour. If the subject is a human being the inference is typically made on the basis of a verbal report from the subject to the effect that he or she *was*, in fact, using such and such a hypothesis – provided that the data from the experiment are in agreement with the verbal statement. If the subject is an animal (or inarticulate human, e.g. an infant) the inference becomes problematical. adj., *hypothetical*; vb., *hypothesize*.

hypothesis, null A HYPOTHESIS (1) of no difference, no relationship. In the standard hypothesis-testing approach to science one attempts to demonstrate the falsity of the null hypothesis, leaving one with the implication that the alternative, mutually exclusive, hypothesis is the acceptable one.

hypothetical construct As the term suggests, a CONSTRUCT that is hypothetical, i.e. some mechanism the existence of which is inferred but for which unambiguous, objective evidence is not (at least yet) available. An interesting example from history is Harvey's hypothesization of the existence of capillaries from his model of blood circulation. Their hypothetical status was only removed when the microscope verified their existence.

hypothetical syllogism SYLLOGISM.

hypothetico-deductive method A scientific method that focuses on, as the name implies, the deduction of hypotheses. Formally, the process begins with a set of undefined primitive terms or 'givens', a set of newly defined terms and a set of postulates. It then proceeds, using logical deduction, to theorems and corollaries. Hypothetico-deductive systems are basically self-correcting: when new facts are found or new principles discovered that the hypothetical component cannot account for, the superstructure is revised by the modification of the postulate system. Newton's theory of classical mechanics is perhaps the best known and most formalized of such systems. In psychology, Clark L. Hull's herculean efforts to develop a systematic behaviour theory (see here HULLIAN) were structured in terms of a hypothetico-deductive model.

hypothymia Lowered emotionality and depression.

hypothyroidism A deficit in secretions of the thyroid gland resulting in a subnormal metabolic rate. In adults the condition is characterized by weight gain, sluggishness and a tendency to tire easily. In infants, if untreated, it leads to cretinism.

hypotonia–obesity syndrome PRADER-WILLI SYNDROME.

hypotonic 1 Descriptive of a solution in which the osmotic pressures between the liquid and the cells suspended in it are such that there is fluid transmission from the surrounding medium into the cells. **2** Characteristic of a state of (muscular) relaxation. Contrast with HYPERTONIC. n., *hypotonia*.

hypotrophy ATROPHY.

hypotropia Downward STRABISMUS.

hypovolemia A reduction in the volume of extracellular fluid.

hypoxia Insufficient oxygen. Hypoxic episodes can produce neurological disorders. For example, hypoxia can damage cells in the hippocampus resulting in anterograde amnesia.

hypoxyphilia The deriving of sexual arousal through oxygen deprivation. Typically a noose or ligature is used to cut off oxygen as orgasm nears, although inhaling of volatile nitrates is also used since they diminish blood supply to the brain by peripheral vasodilation. Needless to say this is a rather dangerous PARAPHILIA in which bad timing or equipment failure can lead to death.

hysteresis 1 Loosely, the lagging of an effect behind its cause. Used in this sense in biophysics and neurology to refer to apparently delayed effects, see BISTABILITY for an example. **2** More specifically, an effect observed in psychophysics and perception where a finding is biased because of an inherent directionality in the methods used. For example, a difference THRESHOLD (3) established by increasing the intensity of a comparison stimulus relative to a standard produces a different result than one that lessens the intensity of the comparison stimulus.

hysteria Of all psychiatric disorders hysteria has the longest and most chequered history. The name derives from ancient Greek, and the condition was, until relatively recently, assumed to be solely a dysfunction of women and caused by a 'wandering' uterus (*hysteron* = uterus). Psychoanalytic theory helped in providing a more reasonable aetiology, but the link between gender and the disorder was not completely severed: males were rarely diagnosed as hysterical. The symptoms that have been cited most often are: hallucinations, somnambulism, functional anaesthesia, functional paralysis and dissociation, symptoms which don't fit with each other particularly well.

The problems with a general classification like this with such an array of symptoms are enormous. The lack of understanding of the disorder may, quite possibly, be due to the fact that there is no single disorder here at all. The contemporary view is that there is no real syndrome and, indeed, in the most recent edition of the DIAGNOSTIC AND STATISTICAL MANUAL there is no specific listing for hysteria. Instead, three, in principle distinguishable, categories of disorder are identified: CONVERSION DISORDER, DISSOCIATIVE DISORDER and FACTITIOUS DISORDER. Between them these encompass all of the classical symptoms. The oft-hypothesized personality type is now called HISTRIONIC PERSONALITY (the Greek roots are still in evidence) and the acute psychotic form is identified as a BRIEF REACTIVE PSYCHOSIS. See these terms for details on contemporary usage.

hysterical 1 Pertaining to or characterizing the symptoms of *hysteria*. **2** Characterizing or pertaining to functional disorders, e.g. hysterical blindness.

hysterical ataxia ATAXIA, HYSTERICAL.

hysterical blindness FUNCTIONAL *BLINDNESS.

hysterical personality HISTRIONIC PERSONALITY DISORDER.

hysteriform Resembling hysteria.

Hz Abbreviation for HERTZ.

I^1 Abbreviation for: **1** *Inhibition*. The symbol has had quite a thorough work-out in HULLIAN theory. Some of the specialized forms that Hull hypothesized are: I_R = reactive inhibition, $s\bar{I}_R$ = inhibitory potential, $s\bar{I}_R$ = effective inhibitory potential. **2** Intensity.

I^2 That aspect of self which represents the knower of oneself, the component that, in William James's terms, 'is aware of the "me"'. See discussion under SELF (esp. 2).

-ia Suffix connoting *abnormal* or *diseased*.

-iasis Suffix meaning *state* or *condition*, used with the connotation of pathology. var., *-osis*.

IAT IMPLICIT ASSOCIATION TEST.

iatric Pertaining to a physician or to medicine.

-iatric Suffix meaning *healing, medical*.

iatro- Combining form meaning *healing* or *medical*.

iatrogenic disorder A disorder produced by a physician or, by extension, any health-care provider or therapist. The term is used generally to refer to any abnormal condition, physical or mental, caused by the effects of attempts at treatment. The connotation is that such problems can be avoided, although such implications are not always fair. Classic examples are functional disorders produced by suggestion or by the anxiety associated with treatment, and drug-related disorders (e.g. DRUG-INDUCED *PARKINSONISM).

iatrogenic schizophrenia SCHIZOPHRENIA, IATROGENIC.

iatrotropic stimulus The event or symptom that causes a person to seek medical attention. The term covers real symptoms and complaints as well as basically nonmedical stimuli, e.g. a medical exam for employment.

-iatry Suffix meaning *medical* or *physical care*.

Icarus complex H. A. Murray's term for a syndrome characterized by fascination with fire, a history of bedwetting, a desire to be immortal, narcissism and lofty but fragile ambition. The complex is named after the figure in Greek mythology who flew with his father on artificial wings and, against fatherly advice, ventured too close to the sun. The wax in the wings melted and he plunged to his death.

ICD INTERNATIONAL CLASSIFICATION OF DISEASES.

icon ICONIC.

iconic 1 Characterizing an image, a pictorial representation of something, an idol. **2** Characterizing a brief visual experience that lasts for a time (perhaps 2 seconds at most) after the termination of a bright stimulus. Often called *iconic memory*, this effect is considered by many to be one of a class of phenomena within the SENSORY INFORMATION STORE. vars., *ikonic, eikonic*. n., *icon*. The auditory analogue is *echoic*.

iconic memory (or **store**) ICONIC (2), MEMORY, ICONIC.

iconic mode ENACTIVE REPRESENTATION.

iconic representation 1 Generally, any form of mental representation based on relatively simple perceptual, ICONIC (1) encoding systems. **2** A particular form of such representation in J. Bruner's theory of development. See ENACTIVE REPRESENTATION for details.

ICS Abbreviation for *intracranial stimulation*. See ELECTRICAL BRAIN STIMULATION.

ICSH *Interstitial cell-stimulating hormone*. See LUTEINIZING HORMONE.

ictal Sudden, abrupt; ictal emotions are transitory, fleeting emotions. Also used to refer to epilepsy.

ictus 1 In medicine, an epileptic seizure or a stroke. **2** In speech, the accentuation of a syllable.

ICV INTRACEREBROVENTRICULAR.

id In the Freudian tripartite model of mind, the primitive, animalistic, instinctual element, the pit of roiling, libidinous energy demanding immediate satisfaction. It is regarded as the deepest component of the psyche, the true unconscious. Entirely self-contained and isolated from the world about it, it is bent on achieving its own aims. The sole governing device here is the pleasure principle, the id being represented as the ultimate hedonist. The task of restraining this single-minded entity is a major part of the ego's function.

All three components of the psychoanalytic psyche are, of course, metapsychological constructs. The id is a kind of biological metaphor, a descriptive device. The language of many psychoanalytic writers, however, has led to a kind of personalization, a reification that is unwarranted, unfortunate and misleading. Freud himself was quite clear on this point: the concept of the id should be used only as a descriptive characterization of a system of actions and behaviours. See also EGO, SUPEREGO.

idea 1 Plato's intellectual equivalent of form. An idea in this sense is what is seen, mentally, via one's intellectual vision. In the pure Platonic sense, only ideas are real and they are often given an initial capital letter to emphasize this. For example, there is no genuine triangle presented to one's senses; the true, the real, triangle is the idea Triangle in the mind. **2** Descartes drops the notion of the true idea in favour of the concept of that which is *perceived directly* in the mind. This point of view carries over into the work of Locke and was developed richly by various of the British empiricists. **3** In contemporary cognitive psychology the term is still used in roughly this fashion. That is, an idea is a mental event, a brain state underlies it, and it is derived in some fashion from experience. In this sense it is treated as being related to the real world with the presumption that the idea itself is the result of some as yet unknown processing of information that yields the phenomenal experience. **4** In layperson's terms, a plan, a scheme, an opinion, an insight, etc.

ideal 1 An abstract representation of the fundamental characteristics of something. **2** A strived-for goal, one that is highly desirable. The term is often used with the connotation that the goal may not be attainable. This meaning is often carried into theories of personality; see e.g. IDEALIZED *SELF.

idealism 1 A philosophical doctrine that holds that the ultimate reality is mental and that this mental representation forms the basis of all experience and knowledge. From this point of view it is meaningless to speak of the existence of things independent of their perception and experiencing by a conscious observer. Contrast with REALISM (2). **2** An attitude characterized by high personal and societal goals and the general attempt to attain them. Contrast with REALISM (3).

idealization 1 In psychoanalytic theory, a defence mechanism in which an object about which one is ambivalent is split into two conceptual representations, one wholly bad and one completely, ideally good. **2** More generally, the process of dealing with conflict or stress by attributing exaggerated positive qualities to others.

idealized image IMAGE, IDEALIZED.

idealized self SELF, IDEALIZED.

ideal observer A theoretical, perfect observer whose sensory and perceptual systems operate without error and devoid of bias. This notion is used in discussion of sensory and perceptual systems as an abstraction against which to compare an actual observer.

ideas of reference A sense that events and incidents occurring about one have a particular meaning that is special to the individual. Distinguish from DELUSIONS OF REFERENCE.

ideational Pertaining to ideas, to cognitive processes.

ideational agnosia AGNOSIA, IDEATIONAL.

ideational apraxia APRAXIA, IDEATIONAL.

ideational learning LEARNING, IDEATIONAL.

idée fixe French for *fixed idea*. A firmly held idea that is maintained without rational reflection and despite the manifest existence of sufficient contrary evidence to persuade a reasonable person of its untenability. Janet used the term to represent an aspect of a neurosis that interfered with the normal flow of information by restricting an individual's attentional capacities.

id-ego **1** Within orthodox psychoanalytic theory, the primitive unit from which the separate id and ego functions become differentiated. However: **2** In various other psychoanalytic approaches, a *single* entity the opposing functions of which are those of the id and ego, at least as those functions are represented in the classical model. It is difficult to see how one of these two positions could provide greater explanatory power than the other.

identical-elements theory The generalization originally proposed by Thorndike that the degree of transfer of learning that occurs between two tasks is a function of the number of common elements they share.

identical retinal points Any two points, one on each retina, that receive stimulation from the same objective point at infinite distance. Distinguish from CONGRUENT RETINAL POINTS.

identical twins MONOZYGOTIC *TWINS.

identification **1** A mental operation whereby one attributes to oneself, either consciously or unconsciously, the characteristics of another person or group. The notion of TRANSFERENCE is central here. **2** A process of establishing a link between oneself and another person or group. Although similar to 1, the connotation of this usage is closer to that of AFFILIATION. **3** An act of recognizing similarity or identity between events, objects or persons. Here the notions of *labelling* and *classifying* are roughly synonymous. There are variations on all of these definitions and in many instances a single use illustrates more than one of them, e.g. the common expression 'identification with the aggressor'.

identification disorders DELUSIONAL MIS-IDENTIFICATION DISORDER.

identified patient SYMPTOM WEARER (or BEARER).

identity **1** In the study of personality, a person's essential, continuous self, the internal, subjective concept of oneself as an individual. Usage here is often qualified, e.g. *sex-role identity*, *racial* or *group identity*. **2** In logic, a relation between two or more elements such that either may be substituted for the other in a syllogism without altering its truth value. **3** Somewhat more loosely, a deep relationship between elements that is assumed to exist despite surface dissimilarities. This meaning is typically qualified to express the level at which the identity is found, e.g. *functional identity*. **4** Within Piagetian theory, a state of awareness that the relationship described in 3 holds. The classic example here is the case of the child who is aware that a liquid maintains its deep identity even though it undergoes various transformations, such as being poured from one container to another of different shape. See CONSERVATION.

identity crisis An acute loss of the sense of one's identity, a lack of the normal feeling that one has historical continuity, that the person here today is phenomenologically the same as the one here yesterday.

identity formation Quite literally, the forming of one's own IDENTITY (1). Most theorists hold to the point of view that mature identity formation emerges when various early, more primitive identifications and influences are rejected.

identity theory In the philosophy of mind, a variation of the more general position of PHYSICALISM. The strong form of identity theory (more properly called *type*-identity theory) argues that every mental event or mental state is identical with a particular brain state, an in-principle specifiable physiological (i.e. physical) event. Moreover, the theory defends the extension that when two persons share something mental (e.g. both believe that water is wet or both image a dog or both desire to understand psychology) they also have in common in-principle specifiable equivalent physical (brain) states. Note that it is this logical extension that has earned the label *type* theory, for here *types* of mental events are assumed to correspond to *types* of physical events. Without this extension one has (merely) a *token* identity theory, which is a considerably weaker position, in which only specific, individual (*token*) mental states are assumed to reflect these equivalences.

ideo- Combining form from the Greek, meaning *idea* or *mental image*. Distinguish from IDIO-.

ideogram LOGOGRAPHY.

ideokinetic apraxia APRAXIA, IDEOKINETIC.

ideomotor act An overt act initiated by an idea.

ideomotor apraxia APRAXIA, IDEOMOTOR.

idio- Combining form from the Greek *idios*. The general connotation is something *personal*, *private*, *self-produced* and, by extension, *unique* or *distinct*. Distinguish from IDEO-.

idiocentrism An approach to social situations and personal relationships characterized by thought and action that emphasizes one's own particular interests over the larger interests of a group. Contrast with ALLOCENTRISM and see INDIVIDUALISM.

idiocy Severe mental deficiency. The term IDIOT, from which it derives, is obsolescent (see MENTAL DEFICIENCY and MENTAL RETARDATION for discussions of nomenclature) but *idiocy* itself survives in a number of combined forms, chiefly of a medical or psychiatric nature, identifying syndromes named years ago, e.g. *amaurotic (familial) idiocy*.

idioglossia CRYPTOPHASIA.

idiographic Relating to or dealing with the concrete, the individual, the unique. A psychological system or theory with this orientation is labelled an idiographic approach. The opposite of NOMOTHETIC.

idiolect Literally, a DIALECT spoken by a single person. Obviously, there are as many idiolects as there are people. Hence, the term is restricted to particularly idiosyncratic manners of speech or patterns of pronunciation. Some people develop these as affectations, others as poetic signatures.

idiom Any expression with a special meaning that cannot be determined from the meanings of its component parts.

idiopathic **1** In medicine, any primary pathological condition; that is, one arising within the affected organ and not as a result of external dysfunctions. **2** Of any disorder of unknown aetiology.

idiopathic epilepsy EPILEPSY, IDIOPATHIC.

idioretinal light A vague grey perceived in conditions of total darkness with the eyes completely dark-adapted. The term is generally used by those who argue that this percept is the result of metabolic processes within the retina; *cortical grey* is the term of choice of those who maintain that cortical action is responsible. The shortened form, *retinal light*, is also found.

idiosyncracy credits In social psychology, a term for the goodwill a group member can build up by adhering to group norms and working toward group goals. It derives from the notion that some amount of subsequent deviant behaviour will be tolerated by the group; i.e. the group member has built up credits that can be spent on being deviant from the group, or idiosyncratic.

idiosyncratic alcohol intoxication ALCOHOL INTOXICATION, IDIOSYNCRATIC.

idiot From the Greek *idiotes*, which translates roughly as a *person in a totally private state*; by extension, then, an ignorant person. The term is little used today: PROFOUND *MENTAL RETARDATION is preferred. See MENTAL DEFICIENCY for a discussion of this and related terms.

idiotropic Lit., turning inward. *Introspective* is an acceptable synonym, *introverted* is not, as it tends to have negative connotations.

idiot savant SAVANT.

I/E ratio The ratio of the rate of inspiration to the rate of expiration. Low numbers usually indicate high arousal.

I.E. scale **1** A scale of *introversion–extraversion* derived from the MMPI. **2** See INTERNAL–EXTERNAL SCALE and LOCUS OF CONTROL. The abbreviation *I–E* is preferred to differentiate it from 1.

ikonic IKONIC REPRESENTATION, ICONIC.

ikonic representation ENACTIVE REPRESENTATION.

il- Prefix used synonymously in some contexts with IN-, e.g. *illicit*.

illegitimate 1 Generally, of things that violate accepted standards, especially sexual standards. **2** Specifically, of children born out of wedlock. Somehow this latter use seems rather unfair: because the parents chose not to conform to societal mores hardly seems grounds for stigmatizing their offspring.

illicit Generally, not authorized, not permitted. Hence: **1** Not accepted by a culture or not sanctioned by a group. **2** In law, contrary to established legal principle, illegal.

Illinois Test of Psycholinguistic Abilities (ITPA) A test designed to assess psycholinguistic disabilities in children aged 5 to 12 years. Originally constructed to reflect Charles Osgood's theory of communication, the current edition (ITPA-3) attempts to remain somewhat faithful to its history while incorporating more recent thinking about language functions. It comprises 12 subtests assessing language abilities across different levels of organization, psycholinguistic functions, channels of input and output, as well as providing a global estimate of language functioning.

illiteracy Generally (and loosely), the inability to read and write when such inability is not the result of either organic dysfunction or mental retardation. Tightening up this loose definition is, however, difficult. Various criteria have been proposed over the years: (a) inability to read at all; (b) inability to read at a particular average school-year level (US school years from 2 through 6 have been suggested); (c) inability to read and follow the directions on a typical government form. Depending on which is selected the sociopolitical hot potato of the national illiteracy rate can be made to mean many different things. See also READING.

illocutionary act SPEECH ACT.

illuminance The light actually falling on a surface. When the source is perpendicular to the surface, illuminance varies with the power of the source and inversely with the square of the distance of the surface from the source. When the source is at an angle with the surface a correction given by *Lambert's cosine law* is made.

illusion Basically, any stimulus situation in which that which is perceived cannot be predicted, prima facie, by a simple analysis of the physical stimulus. Often one sees illusions characterized as 'mistaken perceptions', a designation that is not really correct and misses the point. *Mach bands*, for example, are illusions but they are not mistaken perceptions. Rather, they are perceptions that result from certain retinal and/or cortical processes that cannot be predicted simply from the stimulus itself. If there is a mistake involved it is on the part of psychologists who don't as yet understand the mechanisms that produce the illusions. For a better understanding of the problems here see the separate entries for some of the more common illusions: HERING, MACH BANDS, MOON, MÜLLER–LYER, POGGENDORFF, etc.

Note that the concept of illusion is distinct from the concepts of HALLUCINATION and DELUSION. Illusions are normal, relatively consistent phenomena found across observers and are subject to regular rules. Hallucinations are quite idiosyncratic and despite their compelling sense of reality do not follow interpersonal patterns. Delusions are best thought of as mistaken beliefs. adj., *illusory*.

illusion of control The belief that one has more control over events than one actually does.

illusory conjunction In perception, a phenomenon in which particular features are seen as belonging to the wrong objects. It occurs when stimuli with several features are flashed rapidly, such as a red curved line and a green straight line. In this instance the subject occasionally sees a green curved line or a red straight line.

illusory contour SUBJECTIVE *CONTOUR.

illusory correlation A perceived strong association between variables that is either not there or considerably smaller than one believes it is. Some theorists argue that the tendency for people to form such illusory correlations helps to explain the development and persistence of stereotypes and the prejudice that results from them.

iloperidone An ATYPICAL *ANITPSYCHOTIC that

acts as an antagonist of serotonin, dopamine and possibly norepinepherine. This broad spectrum of action makes it effective against both positive and negative symptoms of schizophrenia. It has fewer side effects than most other antipsychotics and has potential for treating other disorders such as extreme restlessness (see AKATHESIA) and BIPOLAR DISORDER.

im- Prefix connoting *not*.

image The term derives from the Latin for *imitation*, and most usages in psychology, both obsolete and contemporary, revolve around this notion. Hence, common synonyms are *likeness*, *copy*, *reproduction*, *duplicate*, etc. Several important variations on this theme are found: **1** *Optical image* is the most concrete use and refers specifically to the reflection of an object by a mirror, lens or other optical device. **2** By extension, the *retinal image* is the (approximate) point-by-point picture of an object cast on the retina when light is refracted by the eye's optical system. **3** Within structuralism, *images* was one of the three subclasses of consciousness – the others being *sensations* and *affections*. The thrust of this use was to treat the image as a mental representation of an earlier sensory experience, a copy of it. The copy was considered to be less vivid than the sensory experience but still consciously recognizable as a memory of it. This particular sense of the term has been carried forward into contemporary cognitive psychology, in which an image is viewed, putting it somewhat crudely, as **4** a picture in the head. This rather commonsensical notion actually captures fairly well the essence of the term in most contemporary usage but some caveats must be made: (a) The picture is not a literal one – there is no slide-projector/screen arrangement – rather a kind of *as if* picture. That is, imagery is a cognitive process that operates as if one had a mental picture that was an analogue of a real-world scene. (b) The image is not necessarily treated as a reproduction of an earlier event but as a construction, a synthesis. In this sense an image is no longer viewed as a copy; for example, one can picture a unicorn driving a motorcycle, which is rather unlikely to be a copy of any previously seen stimulus. (c) The image seems to be mentally adjustable; one can picture, for example, the unicorn driving toward you,

away from you, around in circles, etc. (d) The image is not necessarily restricted to visual representation – although this is surely the most common forum in which the term is used. For example, one can elaborate an auditory image (try forming an image of some well-known tune), or a tactile image (image a design of, say, a triangle pressed on your back). Some people even claim to have gustatory and olfactory images. Because of these extensions the term is frequently qualified to indicate the form of image under discussion. Finally, (e) this pattern of usage encroaches on the meaning of an etymologically related term, IMAGINATION.

While these are the dominant uses there are others: **5** A general attitude toward some institution, e.g. as in 'the image of China to Westerners'. **6** An element of a dream. **7** As a verb, *to image* means to create an image. Although used as a synonym of *to imagine*, the latter can also connote flights of fancy, which are generally precluded in the case of the former. That is, despite the subtle overlap between image and imagination, to image something is not, strictly speaking, the same mental act as to imagine something.

image, auditory An image in the auditory system. See IMAGE (esp. 4(d)).

image, fixed STABILIZED IMAGE.

image, hypnopompic HYPNOPOMPIC IMAGE.

image, idealized 1 Generally, an inappropriate sense of one's positive aspects. In classical psychoanalysis it is assumed to develop as a defence against the demands of the *ego ideal*. **2** In K. Horney's theory, a neurotic, unconsciously held image of oneself. Identification with this idealized image results, in her theory, in the development of an IDEALIZED *SELF.

imageless thought The reference here is to a theoretical and empirical debate between the Würzburg school (see ACT PSYCHOLOGY) and orthodox STRUCTURALISM (1) over whether or not all thought processes were based upon images. Although the issue was never fully resolved, the fact that under the same stimulus conditions the Würzburgers found no evidence of images and the structuralists found traces of sensory images did not augur well for the method of introspection.

imagery In the most inclusive sense this

term refers to the whole imaging process. Often it refers only to the actual images themselves (especially IMAGE (4)). The whole question of exactly what is being connoted by terms like *image* and *imagery* is most complex; see the discussion under IMAGE.

image, visual An image in the visual system. Because so much imagery seems to involve vision, this term is often taken as equivalent to IMAGE. However, see that term, especially 4(d).

imaginal Pertaining to IMAGE or to IMAGINATION, although usually the former is intended, *imaginary* being the preferred adjectival form from *imagination*.

imaginary companion A fictional friend, an invisible playmate, created by a young child and treated as real. The mythical friend may be very vivid, have a name, a stable personality, characteristics and mannerisms of action, and play an important role in the child's life.

imagination The process of recombining memories of past experiences and previously formed images into novel constructions. See here IMAGE (4(b)). This term is used in the technical literature very much as it is in the common language. That is, imagination is treated as creative and constructive, it may be primarily wishful or largely reality-bound, and it may involve future plans and projections or mental reviews of the past. Often qualifiers are appended for clarity, e.g. *anticipatory* for the future, *reproductive* for the past, *creative* for the novel.

imagine 1 To engage in the mental process of imagination. **2** An approximate synonym of the verb *to image*, although see IMAGE (7).

imaging (technique) Collectively, any of a number of noninvasive techniques used to image internal functions, most commonly those of the brain. For details, see COMPUTERIZED AXIAL TOMOGRAPHY (CAT), FUNCTIONAL MAGNETIC RESONANCE IMAGING (FMRI), MAGNETIC RESONANCE IMAGING (MRI), POSITRON EMISSION TOMOGRAPHY (PET) and SINGLE PHOTON EMISSION COMPUTER TOMOGRAPHY (SPECT).

imago 1 In biology, an adult, sexually mature insect or the mature stage of insect life. The term is used particularly of those forms which undergo a metamorphosis. **2** A term used by Freud to refer to unconscious representations of other persons, typically a parent with whom one identifies closely. Psychoanalytic theory conceptualizes the imago as being formed very early in life and, hence, it is usually an idealized representation and not necessarily reflective of the true person.

imbecile From the Latin *imbecillus*, meaning *weak* or *weak-minded*. It is little used today; see MENTAL DEFICIENCY and MENTAL RETARDATION.

imipramine A TRICYCLIC COMPOUND used as an ANTIDEPRESSANT. It is a noradrenergic and serotonergic antagonist and functions by retarding the reuptake of norepinephrine and serotonin. Like others in this group of drugs, its potentially serious side effects limit its use.

imitation The process of copying the behaviour of others. The term tends to carry a sense of intentionality: the one imitating wants to, and is trying to, model his or her actions on those of another. Distinguish this connotation from that of the related term MIMICRY. *Imitation* also tends to be used so as to imply that the imitative actions are mechanical and performed by rote, a characterization that somehow seems somewhat misleading. A child who imitates his/her mother's way of walking or who adopts his/her peer group's social-interactive manners at play is not 'just' imitating. Such learned behaviours are most complex, and mechanical processes are clearly inadequate as explanations or even descriptions. Imitation of this kind involves the notion that the child must know, in some implicit fashion, the underlying rules that govern the social patterns of his/her peer group. See MODELLING, which is the term preferred by many because of the simplistic connotations associated with imitation. Distinguish from EMULATION, in which the notion of achieving the same *goal* as the model is an element.

immature 1 Not mature, not fully developed. This meaning is basically descriptive and evaluatively neutral. **2** Displaying less-well-developed traits and characteristics than the norm for one's age. This meaning carries clear negative connotations. The term is found with both meanings in a variety of contexts, including the biological and physiological and the emotional, cognitive and social.

immediate 1 Without delay. **2** Without intervening (i.e. MEDIATE (1)) processes.

immediate association ASSOCIATION, IMMEDIATE.

immediate constituent In linguistics a *constituent* is any word or sentential construction that is part of a larger linguistic unit. An *immediate constituent* is any constituent out of which a construction on the next level is directly formed. Lest this sound too obtuse, consider the following example. In the sentence 'The tiger who grew old ate the zookeeper', each word is a constituent, as is 'who grew old', but not 'old ate' (which bridges two phrases). Similarly, 'The tiger' and 'who grew old' are immediate constituents, since they are part of the higher-level unit 'The tiger who grew old'.

immediate experience Early structuralists distinguished between *mediate* and *immediate experience*. Immediate experience was made up of the pure, momentary elements of a perception; mediate experience was an inference or coordinated perception derived from previous learning. If, for example, you look at a table and perceive a pattern of granularity, roughly trapezoidal in shape, with regular shadows around the edge, etc., you are introspecting on immediate experience; if, however, you perceive a *table* you are introspecting on mediate experience. Within orthodox STRUCTURALISM (1), immediate experience was regarded as the proper focus of an experimental psychology, a point of view hotly disputed by, among others, the GESTALT PSYCHOLOGY proponents.

immediate memory MEMORY, IMMEDIATE.

immobility 1 Generally, a state in which there is no visible motion. **2** In ethology, a shortened form of TONIC IMMOBILITY.

immune reactions, nonspecific Immune reactions that are general and do not involve specific antibodies. The INFLAMMATORY REACTION is a good example.

immune reactions, specific Immune reactions that target specific invader cells.

immune system A complex system that functions to protect the body from infection.

The system learns to recognize the proteins that mark invader organisms and produces antibodies (*immunoglobulins*) that attack and kill them. There are two separate systems, one based on antibodies released by the B-lymphocytes developed in bone marrow; the other on ones released by the T-lymphocytes in the thymus gland. See PSYCHONEUROIMMUNOLOGY.

impairment Generally, any loss of or decrement in function. More specifically, such loss or decrement due to injury or disease.

imperative A SPEECH ACT in which the speaker directly commands or orders the listener to do something.

imperceptible Of a stimulus that is too low in intensity to be perceived; of a stimulus below THRESHOLD.

impersistence A neurological condition, often observed in cases of NEGLECT, in which the patient displays an inability to maintain posture or continue motor movements.

impersonal Characterizing: **1** An objective attitude, a point of view not concerned with personal feelings. **2** A lack of concern with persons.

impersonation Conscious and deliberate assumption of the identity of another.

implantation 1 In placental mammals, the attaching of the embryo to the uterine wall. **2** In physiological psychology, the placement of an electrode in the brain or other tissue of an experimental animal.

implicature In SPEECH ACT theory, a proposition that is implied by a statement although its literal truth is not expressed. If one responds to the question 'What did you think of the soprano's performance?' with 'Her dress was stunning,' one says a great deal that is not in the literal utterance. See also PRAGMATICS (2) and CONVERSATIONAL MAXIMS.

implicit 1 Not explicit, hence not directly observable. Watson used the term in this sense to refer to the subtle muscular and glandular responses that he argued underlay conscious processes such as thinking (which he assumed to be subvocal speech). **2** Unconscious, covert, tacit, hence of a process that takes place largely outside of the awareness of the individual. The term is used in this sense to characterize cognitive processes that operate independently of consciousness. See IMPLICIT *LEARNING and IMPLICIT *MEMORY.

Implicit Association Test (IAT) A procedure developed by Anthony Greenwald designed to assess an individual's attitudes. In the original version subjects grouped a series of insect names (cockroach, ant) and flower names (rose, lilac) along with a list of pleasant and unpleasant words. Most individuals find this easy, particularly when the insect names are grouped with the unpleasant words and the flowers with the pleasant. But when the groups are switched so that they were asked to group the insect names with the pleasant words and the flowers with unpleasant, the task was surprisingly difficult and reaction times (RTs) are dramatically slower. The implicit emotional elements of the objects held in mind either speed up or slow down the RTs to specific objects based on whether the attitudes held are concordant or discordant (see PRIMING, esp. 3). By replacing insects and flowers with groups that have social relevance, attitudes toward issues such as race, gender, homosexuality and other sensitive topics can be assessed whether or not the subjects are aware of holding these attitudes. See PIPELINE TECHNIQUES, where similar issues are dealt with.

implicit egotism EGOTISM, IMPLICIT.

implicit learning LEARNING, IMPLICIT.

implicit memory MEMORY, IMPLICIT.

implicit personality theory Not a theory in the scientific sense, but the unconsciously held set of beliefs that most laypeople have about the personalities of others. Basically they establish a complex web of assumptions about the traits and behaviours of others and assume that they will act in accordance with those assumptions. Because people hold such views, they can be shocked to discover that some well-loved, gentle neighbour has committed a violent crime – such an act does not fit with their implicit personality profile of that person.

implicit speech SUBVOCALIZATION.

implosion 1 Generally, a collapsing inward. **2** Laing extended the application of the term to cover the fear of having one's identity destroyed. This fear is assumed to result from a sense of emptiness and vacuousness and the feeling that whatever reality might occupy this void will annihilate one's fragile sense of identity and reality.

implosion therapy A behaviour therapy in which the client is exposed to prolonged, intense experience of a problematic behaviour or reaction until it is extinguished. There are two ways in which implosion therapy is used. In the most common, ANXIETY-INDUCTION version, a *phobia* is treated by directly exposing the client to the anxiety-provoking object. In the second, obsessions and compulsions are treated by having the client repeatedly engage in the problem behaviour without breaks or limits. The therapy is thought to be effective because: (a) the client learns that the problematic behaviour or reaction is not adaptive, (b) the problematic behaviour or reaction itself becomes aversive when experienced so intensely and/or, (c) the client becomes numb to the stimulus or behaviour.

implosive therapy IMPLOSION THERAPY.

Impotence 1 Most generally, lack of potency, weakness, powerlessness. **2** Specifically, male failure to copulate. See PRIMARY *IMPOTENCE and SECONDARY *IMPOTENCE. Currently the term MALE ERECTILE DISORDER is recommended as the general label for 2; however, even in the technical literature *impotence* is still widely used.

impotence, orgasmic ORGASM DISORDERS.

impotence, primary Total coital dysfunction in the sense that there is an inability to achieve or maintain an erection sufficient for coitus on the first and all subsequent attempts. Compare with SECONDARY *IMPOTENCE.

impotence, psychogenic IMPOTENCE (2) in the absence of any organic dysfunction.

impotence, secondary A form of PSYCHOGENIC *IMPOTENCE. Unlike PRIMARY *IMPOTENCE, it is difficult to define, because one wishes to differentiate between a male who experiences occasional coital failure and one for whom failure is common enough to pose a problem. The criterion usually accepted is failure to maintain erection sufficient for coitus in 25% (or more) of attempts. Note, however, that imposing this simple criterion fails to capture important aspects of the syndrome since for many males impotence is specific to certain individual sex objects or particular situations.

impoverished 1 Of stimuli that have been degraded or occluded so that they are difficult to detect or recognize. See MASKING. **2** Characterizing any stimulus display or stimulus environment that fails to present all of the variations that it could properly display. For example, the language that adults direct toward an infant is argued to be impoverished in that not all of the rules of grammar that the child ultimately comes to be able to use are displayed in it.

impression 1 The presumed neural effects of stimulation. This use of the term is a kind of physiological metaphor for whatever it is that occurs in the brain when a stimulus input is processed. **2** A loosely held belief or judgement; see IMPRESSION FORMATION.

impression formation The coordinating of various bits and pieces of information into a general integrated IMPRESSION (2). The term is most often used in social psychology with regard to the various bits and pieces of interpersonal perception that give rise to the impression formed of other persons but, strictly speaking, the meaning applies to other psychological domains as well.

impression management Generally and loosely, the full array of devices that people use both consciously and unconsciously in an effort to influence the impression that others have of them.

impression-management theory In social psychology the theory that many of our actions are motivated not by a motive to *be* consistent but by a desire to *appear to be* consistent.

imprinting An ethological term used to characterize a kind of RESTRICTED *LEARNING that takes place rapidly within a relatively compressed time span, is exceedingly resistant to extinction or reversal and has a profound and lasting effect on later social behaviour with respect to the stimulus objects for the behaviour. The classic example is the following response in a newly hatched duckling, which imprints

on and follows an object (usually the mother) to which it is exposed during the critical period.

imprinting, negative IMPRINTING that produces an avoidance of an animal or object rather than an approach or following reaction. See INBREEDING AVOIDANCE.

impulse 1 Any act or event triggered by a stimulus and occurring with short latency and with little or no conscious control or direction. **2** Any sudden incitement to act; i.e. the internal state that initiates the action in 1, as in 'an impulse to flee'. **3** In psychoanalytic theory, an instinctual act of the id. **4** In physiology, a self-propagating excitatory state transmitted along a neural fibre. ACTION POTENTIAL. **5** (Rare) An awareness of an IMPULSION.

impulse-control disorders A class of disorders all marked by failure to resist an impulse or temptation to engage in some act that ultimately proves harmful to oneself, e.g. PATHOLOGICAL *GAMBLING, KLEPTOMANIA, PYROMANIA and EXPLOSIVE DISORDERS. Typically the affected individual feels a highly increased sense of tension prior to the act and a pleasurable, gratifying feeling afterwards. Guilt may or may not be experienced following the act.

impulsion A state of great urgency in which one is highly susceptible to performing an impulsive act. Differentiate from COMPULSION.

impulsive A general term used of acts carried out without reflection or of a person prone to such acts. See IMPULSE and IMPULSE-CONTROL DISORDERS.

impulsivity REFLECTIVITY–IMPULSIVITY.

impunitive Characterizing the tendency to react to frustration by assessing the events that led to it without necessarily focusing anger or blame either internally (see INTROPUNITIVE) or externally (see EXTRAPUNITIVE).

in- (ir- before words beginning with *r*) Prefix connoting *not* or *lack of*. The usages of terms like *inattention* and *incomprehensible* are straightforward; terms with specialized meanings are given below.

inaccessibility A state of psychological remoteness in which one is unresponsive to ordinary social stimuli. Seen in cases of autism, severe depression and some forms of schizophrenia.

inaccessible memory MEMORY, INACCESSIBLE.

inadequacy Most broadly, any inferiority, incompetence or the feeling of such. The term is typically qualified to specify the type, e.g. *sexual*, *intellectual*, etc.

inadequate personality Loosely, a person who displays a broad range of inadequacies and has a long history of failure.

inadequate stimulus STIMULUS, INADEQUATE.

inanition 1 General physical weakness due to lack of proper nutrition. 2 Emptiness.

inappropriateness of affect APPROPRIATENESS OF *AFFECT.

inattentional blindness The failure to perceive a presented stimulus when one's attention is focused on a different stimulus. The effect, first discovered by Irvin Rock, occurs even when the unattended stimulus is presented in the same location as the attended. Note that the term refers only to consciously perceived stimuli. It is well known that people implicitly pick up information about stimuli although they are not aware of doing so; see BLINDSIGHT, CHANGE BLINDNESS and CHOICE BLINDNESS.

inborn Innate, inherited; of characteristics that result from genetic factors.

inbreeding 1 In genetics, the mating or interbreeding of those closely related. Often used in animals to develop a strain with particular hereditary characteristics; most laboratory animals are the result of many generations of careful inbreeding. 2 More metaphorically, a confinement of intellectual or social resources resulting from interactions limited to those individuals with a particular orientation.

inbreeding avoidance The tendency to avoid mating with close relatives. Various mechanisms have been proposed to explain the phenomenon, from cultural systems such as the incest taboo (see INCEST, WESTERMARCK EFFECT) to precultural, genetically determined systems found in many animals such as *dispersion*, by which the young leave the home or nest and hence do not have the opportunity to mate with close relatives, and

negative imprinting, by which the young learn to avoid mating with those they have been raised with. See also OUTBREEDING.

incentive Several variations on this term are found, all reflecting the underlying notion that an incentive is a *motivator* of behaviour. Indeed, some use the hybrid phrase *incentive motivation* to ensure that this connotation is not missed. Hence: **1** An inducement to respond. In this sense incentives are conditions or objects that are perceived as satisfiers of some need. Water has incentive value for a thirsty organism. **2** A supplemental reward that functions by maintaining behaviour prior to reaching the primary goal. Weight watchers' clubs use incentives in this way. **3** A synonym of *value*; the greater the value of an object, the greater is its perceived incentive. Note that here there is a close tie between incentive and the notions of DRIVE and NEED. That is, the level of the drive state determines the incentive; food has little or no incentive for a satiated organism.

incest Sexual relations between close relatives. *Close* is defined differently in different cultures although almost all appear to have some form of prohibition against incest, the so-called *incest taboo*. Several theories have been proposed to account for this near universality. Some focus on genetic factors, pointing out that the taboo helps to prevent maladaptive, recessive genes from appearing in the population. Others focus on social factors, arguing that the taboo arose because having more than one close sexual relationship in a family is a fragile and potentially explosive arrangement. However, many nonhuman species have also developed strategies that help accomplish the same end as our incest taboos; see INBREEDING AVOIDANCE. adj., *incestuous*.

incest avoidance INBREEDING AVOIDANCE.

incest barrier A psychoanalytic term for the psychosocial prohibitions that operate within a family to free libido from its Oedipal attachment to the opposite-sexed parent and permit the child to become gradually freed from familial ties.

incest taboo INCEST.

incidence Frequency of occurrence of an event or a condition in relation to the population under examination. Distinguish from

PREVALENCE, which covers a much shorter period of time and which provides a snapshot view of the frequency of occurrence.

incidental learning LEARNING, INCIDENTAL.

incidental tests POST HOC TESTS.

inclusive fitness In evolutionary biology, the total measure of the various strategies that an organism may use to ensure genetic success. Inclusive fitness is made up of one's OWN PERSONAL FITNESS (getting one's own genes into the pool, one's personal reproductive success) plus the KIN SELECTION strategy (elevating the reproductive success of a close biological relative).

incommensurable Of two variables having no common measure or standard of comparison.

incompatible The general dictionary meaning – incapable of existing together in harmony – applies in the psychological uses. Thus, one speaks of *incompatible responses* as those which cannot occur at the same time, e.g. anxiety and relaxation; of *incompatible persons* as those whose values or styles conflict so sharply that they cannot associate freely with each other; of *incompatible judgements* as those that cannot both be true.

incompetent 1 Generally, lacking in qualifications, capacities or abilities. **2** More specifically, a designation for an individual judged to be incapable of making rational judgements and choices and hence not legally responsible. Compare with COMPETENT.

incomplete-pictures test A test in which the subject is shown a series of incomplete pictures of an object, each picture revealing more of the object than the one before. The task is to identify the object as early in the series as possible. It is assumed to measure visual organization and/or set and is occasionally used as a diagnostic tool.

incomplete-sentences test A projective test in which the subject is required to complete sentences like 'When I am depressed I—' or 'When angry I—.' The responses may be used as a vehicle for leading the subject into discussing a topic that his or her answers suggest is psychologically important, or they may be analysed for the projection of unconscious themes.

incongruent CONGRUENT.

incontinence Lack of restraint, of ability to hold back. Although the term may be applied broadly (e.g. on occasion one will see it applied to excessive speaking) it usually refers to an inability to hold back bodily functions, typically urination and defecation but occasionally sexual impulses.

incorporation The roots reveal the general sense of the term: *in-* = *into*, *corpora* = *body*; thus, an act of taking something into the body and, by extension, into the psyche or the self. Hence: **1** The ingestion of foodstuffs. **2** The inculcation of a belief or an attitude. **3** In psychoanalysis, a primitive defence mechanism operating as fantasy in which a person or part is ingested (figuratively, of course). Distinguish this last meaning from INTERNALIZATION and INTROJECTION.

increment Generally, any increase in anything can safely be called an increment.

incremental theory ENTITY THEORY.

incremental validity VALIDITY, INCREMENTAL.

incubation 1 A period of brooding required to bring something to a point where it has form and substance. This is the root meaning. **2** In biology, the period required to bring an egg to hatching. **3** In cognitive psychology, a period of time during which no active effort is made to solve a problem but which terminates with the solution.

incubus A demon supposed to descend upon one during sleep; hence, by extension, a nightmare.

incus One of the AUDITORY *OSSICLES.

indecency Obviously, characterizing that which is not decent. Decency, however, is culturally defined and the standards within one society may differ rather dramatically from those in another. Generally, the term is used so that the acceptable degree of exposure of the body is the primary concern.

independence 1 Most generally, a state existing between variables such that there is no significant, relevant correlational or causal relationship between them. In statistical terms this is expressed by stating that changes in one variable are not systematically accompanied by changes in another. **2** In probability theory, a property of two events x and y such that the probability of the occurrence of x is unaffected by the occurrence of y and vice versa. For example, in a random number table each entry is independent of all other entries in just this fashion. **3** In logic, the characteristic of a proposition the truth of which is not contingent on the truth of other particular propositions. **4** An autonomous attitude in which one is (relatively) free of the influence of the judgements, opinions or beliefs of others.

independent variable   VARIABLE, INDEPENDENT.

indeterminate 1 In mathematics, of values that are not or cannot be determined (i.e. fixed). **2** Occasionally, UNDERDETERMINED.

indeterminism   A cover term for any doctrine antithetical to DETERMINISM. FREE WILL (1) is the most oft-proposed of these.

index 1 Most generally, something used to note, identify, guide or direct; an indication, sign or token. **2** A formula or number, often expressed as a ratio, that notes some relationship between measures or dimensions or one between a measure and a fixed standard. **3** In mathematics, an exponent or an integer in a radical indicating the root. **4** In statistics, a *variable*. Note, however, that the two terms are not really interchangeable: *index* is used for cases in which precision and unambiguous quantification are lacking; e.g. in *stage theories* the various levels of development are taken as indices of some theoretical variable (perhaps cognitive sophistication) but are not properly called variables. **5** By extension of 1 and 4, any measurable or observable value that can be assessed fairly directly and rigorously and used as an indicator of some other value that cannot be so determined. For example, occupation and income are taken as indices of social status. Note that there is an interesting terminological wrinkle here: in sociology and social psychology some authors use *indicator* for a single value in this manner and reserve *index* for a complex set of such indicators. pls., *indices*, *indexes*; adjs., *index*, *indexical*.

index case   PROBAND.

index of independence   In statistics, any index that assesses the degree to which one variable is independent of the other variables in the analysis.

index of variability   Lit., any measure of DISPERSION. Usually the STANDARD DEVIATION.

indicant   Any event used as a token or sign of some other event. Rapid pulse and high GSR (galvanic skin response), for example, are indicants of high arousal. In testing, a score on a psychological test is treated as an indicant of the thing the test is supposed to be measuring. Also called INDICATOR (1).

indicator 1 INDICANT. **2** INDEX (esp. 5).

indices   Plural of INDEX.

indifference   A rough synonym of *neutrality*. An *indifferent stimulus* is one that does not elicit a response. A *state of indifference* is when one has no preferences between alternative choices or courses of action. An *indifference point* is the value on some continuum or dimension that represents neutrality.

indifference reaction   A loose label for any of a number of disorders in which normal emotional reactions are not displayed. Some cases result from specific neurological damage to cortical areas where emotions are processed, others are regarded as secondary in that they may be manifestations of other difficulties such as those involving communication and language.

indigenous   Native to a particular geographical area.

indirect 1 Circuitous, not in a straight line, not direct. **2** Mediated, linked by intermediary steps or transformations.

indirect correlation   NEGATIVE *CORRELATION.

indirect directive   A SPEECH ACT in which the order or directive is syntactically of another form. For example, 'Do you know what time it is?' is usually taken as a request for the time (and a request not easily denied in most social situations) even though syntactically the utterance has the form of a simple yes–no question. 'It's hot in here' can be an indirect directive to another person to open a window, although here the form of the utterance is that of a simple statement concerning temperature. Unlike DIRECTIVES, this class of speech acts exerts effects in strictly indirect ways and follows fairly complex social and interpersonal rules.

indirect perception   TOP-DOWN PROCESSING.

indirect scaling SCALING, INDIRECT.

indirect speech act Any SPEECH ACT expressed by a construction superficially designed for a function other than the one actually intended. See INDIRECT DIRECTIVE for an example of a common form.

indissociation In Piaget's theory, a very early stage of development in which cognitive and perceptual systems are relatively undifferentiated.

individual differences 1 A label for an approach to psychological phenomena that focuses on characteristics or traits in respect of which individual organisms may be shown to differ. Also called DIFFERENTIAL PSYCHOLOGY. 2 The differences themselves.

individualism 1 Personality traits, attitudes or behaviours that reflect personal independence; freedom from the attitudes and opinions of others. Note, this meaning can reflect either a positive connotation, in that one who displays it stands above (or at least outside) social and peer pressure, or a negative connotation, in that the set of characteristics may describe one who is uncooperative and uncaring. 2 A social philosophy emphasizing the initiative of the individual over collectivist or governmental social action. See COLLECTIVISM.

individuality Collectively, those characteristics that distinguish an individual from all others.

individual psychology 1 Historically, a synonym for DIFFERENTIAL PSYCHOLOGY. 2 The personality theory of Alfred Adler, see ADLERIAN.

individual selection SELECTION (2).

individual symbol SYMBOL, INDIVIDUAL.

individual test TEST, INDIVIDUAL.

individuation 1 Generally, any process in which the various elements or parts of a complex whole become differentiated from each other, progressively more distinct and individual. The term implies development from the general to the specific. 2 In perception, DIFFERENTIATION (5). 3 In social psychology, the breakdown of social ties and the emergence of individuals lacking in group loyalty. 4 In psychoanalytic theory, the process of

becoming an individual who is aware of his or her individuality.

indoleamines A group of BIOGENIC AMINES including SEROTONIN and TRYPTOPHAN.

indolones A group of ANTIPSYCHOTIC DRUGS that have biochemical structures that are similar to drugs like IMIPRAMINE and are used as ANTIDEPRESSANTS.

induced aggression AGGRESSION, INDUCED.

induced association ASSOCIATION, INDUCED.

induced colour A perceived colour or colour change that is determined by (i.e. induced by) stimulation in other parts of the visual field. See also COLOUR CONTRAST.

induced factitious symptoms FACTITIOUS DISORDER BY PROXY.

induced goal Any goal the attainment of which is induced by outside sources.

induced motion MOTION, INDUCED.

induced psychotic disorder A delusional disorder that develops as a result of close contact with an individual who already manifests prominent delusions. The delusions are usually derived from the common experiences of the individuals who, in the typical case, have been together for a long time relatively isolated from others. Also called *shared paranoid disorder* since the delusions are usually of the paranoid variety. See also FOLIE À DEUX. In the latest edition of the *DSM* this disorder has been renamed *shared psychotic disorder*.

induction 1 A process of reasoning in which general principles are inferred from specific cases. A logical operation which proceeds from the individual to the general: what is assumed true of elements from a class is assumed true of the whole class. The experimental method is basically inductive in nature in that conclusions about populations are drawn from observations of individuals and small samples. Contrast here with DEDUCTION. 2 A process by which effects are transferred from one thing to another. *Thing* here is meant most broadly. Emotions are said to be transferred from person to person through *sympathetic induction*, electrical fields through *induction-coils*, neural excitation or inhibition may be induced in one area by the spread of activity from other areas, response rates through the negative effects of *behavioural contrast*, and so forth. **3** A form of parental discipline whereby parents use verbal reasoning to induce a child to think about his or her actions and the consequences of them.

induction test A general term for any test in which the subject is required to induce a coherent general principle on the basis of a fixed set of exemplars. Such tests are sometimes included as part of more general intelligence-testing batteries.

inductive statistics INFERENTIAL *STATISTICS.

industrial/organizational psychology A branch of applied psychology covering organizational, military, economic and personnel psychology and including such areas as tests and measurements, the study of organizations and organizational behaviour, personnel practices, human engineering, human factors, the effects of work, fatigue, pay and efficiency, consumer surveys and market research. In recent years, as this applied field has grown, there has been a tendency to alter the name by which it is known. Specifically, many contemporary researchers prefer the shortened form *organizational psychology*, on the grounds that the study of organizational behaviour is broader than that implied by the qualifier *industrial* since it deals with social structures far removed from industry, such as hospitals, prisons, universities and public-service agencies. Often abbrev. *I/O psychology*.

industrial psychiatry OCCUPATIONAL PSYCHIATRY.

industrial psychology INDUSTRIAL/ORGANIZATIONAL PSYCHOLOGY.

ineffective stimulus STIMULUS, INEFFECTIVE.

infancy From the Latin *infantia*, which translates as *inability to speak*. This criterion, however, is seldom used and the definition of the stage of infancy depends on who is doing the defining. In law, infancy is often considered to last 18 or 21 years; in developmental psychology, the first year of life is the typically cited period; in layperson's terms, it may be up to 2 or 3 years.

infant Most generally, an organism within the period of INFANCY. Although primarily used to refer to young members of our own species there is a tendency among some to apply the term to the young of other species during the period of development when they are relatively helpless and dependent on their parents.

infantile Characterizing: **1** INFANCY. **2** The behavioural and emotional patterns typical of infancy, particularly with regard to such behaviours when they are exhibited by an older child or an adult.

infantile amaurotic (familial) idiocy TAY-SACHS DISEASE.

infantile amnesia AMNESIA, INFANTILE.

infantile autism AUTISM, INFANTILE.

infantile-birth theories Beliefs of children concerning the actual manner of birth. Since most parents are loath to deal with these issues in a straightforward and anatomically accurate fashion, children tend to fill in the gaps in what they can discern in rather creative ways. The most common of these 'theories' are emergence through the navel and the anus and some surgical removal techniques. The term is used for child-generated theories, not for cultural myths concerning storks, cabbage patches, mushrooms and the like.

infantile hypercalcemia WILLIAMS SYNDROME.

infantile sexuality Within the classical Freudian psychoanalytic theory, the capacity for sexual desire and experience in the infant specifically as manifested by passage through a series of stages beginning with the oral and moving through the anal and early genital.

Since this concept was (is?) so controversial, a comment on terminology is not out of place here. While there are clearly behaviours exhibited by every infant that indicate a focus on the mouth, the anus and the genitals, it is probably the case that the orthodox Freudians were being vaguely anthropomorphic (adultomorphic?) in assigning *sexuality* as the motivator. *Sensuality*, meaning derived from the senses, is probably more accurate and allows us to put the sensuality–sexuality question into a cultural frame where it belongs. Freud, of course, was excoriated by many for assigning a sexual base to all sensuality and all pleasure. This issue, as much as any, caused many analysts (such as Jung, Adler and Horney) to abandon the orthodox position.

infantilism 1 A condition of an older child or adult who, for whatever reasons, still displays cognitive and emotional behaviours characteristic of infancy. **2** Any specific regressive behaviour characteristic of infants observed in those more mature.

infant test (or **scale**) Any test or scale for measuring development during infancy. Despite long years of work to develop reliable and valid scales measuring everything from sensorimotor ability to IQ, it is generally acknowledged that such measures do not correlate with measures taken at a later age. The main value of such tests is not as predictors of future success but as diagnostic instruments, for extremely low scores on them are indicative of genuine dysfunctions or disorders. See BAYLEY SCALES OF INFANT DEVELOPMENT.

infecundity Sterility in women, barrenness.

inference 1 A logical judgement made on the basis of a sample of evidence, previous judgements, prior conclusions, etc. rather than on direct observation. **2** The cognitive process by which such a judgement is made.

inferential statistics STATISTICS, INFERENTIAL.

inferior 1 Generally, below, lower, worse, in a subsidiary position. **2** In anatomical descriptions, of a lower part of an organ or a body.

inferior colliculus COLLICULUS.

inferiority complex As originally coined by A. Adler, this term described a collection of repressed fears stemming from organ or bodily inferiority that gave rise to feelings, attitudes and ideas of a more general inferiority. Popular usage has badly mangled the original sense by using the term to refer to any sense of inadequacy or feelings of inferiority; see INFERIORITY FEELINGS.

inferiority feelings Loosely, any attitudes toward oneself that are critical and generally negative. Strictly speaking, this is the term that should be used in popular discourse when, for example, someone claims to have an *inferiority complex*. The problem is that the term *complex*, when used in this fashion, carries the connotation of some unconscious roots – hence, claimants can know that they have feelings of inferiority but not that they have an INFERIORITY COMPLEX.

inferior temporal cortex An area of visual association cortex located on the ventral part of the temporal lobe. It is important in the analysis of information about form and colour and plays a critical role in the perception of three-dimensional objects and the ability to differentiate them from their backgrounds.

infertility 1 An inability to produce offspring. **2** A diminished capacity or a less than normal ability to produce offspring. This meaning is usually indicated by the qualified term *relative infertility*. **3** The condition of having no offspring. This meaning is rarely the intended one. Note, *infertility* is typically used of conditions which are temporary or reversible; STERILITY is preferred for those diagnosed as permanent or difficult to reverse. See also FECUNDITY, FERTILITY.

infertility, primary Of females, infertility when there has been no prior pregnancy.

infertility, secondary Of females, infertility when one or more pregnancies have occurred prior to development of the condition.

inflammatory reaction A complex NONSPECIFIC *IMMUNE REACTION in which the cells damaged by an invading organism secrete substances that cause the area to become inflamed and which attract white blood cells that destroy the invaders.

inflection Lit., a bend or change in the course or direction of something. Hence: **1** The point in a curve where it changes from concave to convex, or vice versa. **2** In speech, modulation of the voice by changing pitch. **3** In linguistics, the suffixing of bound morphemes to a base of a word to express grammatical form and function. In the so-called *synthetic languages* (e.g. Latin) inflection is the primary mode of expression; in *analytic languages* (e.g. English) it is relatively rare. var., *inflexion*.

informal organization ORGANIZATION, INFORMAL.

informant In the psychological assessment of an individual, a person who is familiar enough with the individual to serve as a source of information, e.g. a caregiver, teacher, spouse, partner.

information 1 Within INFORMATION THEORY the term is used in a formal manner to quantify an array of items in terms of the number of choices one has in dealing with them. By definition, the amount of information, measured in *bits* and abbreviated as H, contained in an array of equally likely choices is given by $\log_2 N$, where N is the number of choices. Thus, the answer to the question 'Is it raining?' will provide exactly 1 bit of information since there are only two choices (yes or no) and $\log_2 2 = 1$. (Note, it does not matter whether or not the answer is true.) If one is selecting from 16 equally likely alternatives, 4 bits of information will be provided as there are four choices ($\log_2 16 = 4$). In general, the less likely an event is, the more information is conveyed by its occurrence.

Intriguingly, this use of *information* parallels what physicists know as ENTROPY or randomness. When an ensemble is highly structured and not characterized by randomness, both entropy and information are low. This meaning of the term is, therefore, concerned not with what is communicated but with what could be communicated; hence, it must be kept conceptually distinct from: **2** Loosely, any material with content. This sense of the term is close to the standard meaning in nontechnical usage. Information here is basically any knowledge that is received, processed and understood. When INFORMATION PROCESSING models were first introduced in cognitive psychology, the term *information* was used in sense 1. However, the difficulty of specifying just how much information was contained in, and hence processed by someone who dealt with, a relatively straightforward but complex message (e.g. this sentence) quickly led to a shift to sense 2.

informational influence In an ambiguous or unfamiliar situation, we often look to others – whom we assume are more familiar with the situation than ourselves – to gain clues about proper behaviour. This form of influence others have on us is called *informational* because it arises from the belief that they have information we do not. Compare with NORMATIVE INFLUENCE.

information processing In cognitive psychology, the processing of INFORMATION. Some clarification is called for here, since *information* may, depending on when the writer was writing, reflect either meaning 1 or meaning 2. As discussed under that term, nearly all contemporary usage reflects meaning 2 – any attended input, any idea, image, fact, knowledge, etc. counts as information. Now, *to process* means, basically, to move toward some goal by going through a series of stages or a sequence of acts. Putting these two together yields the notion of organizing, interpreting and responding to (i.e. processing) incoming stimulation (i.e. information). Hence, when one says that information is processed one means that knowledge of some kind is dealt with in some cognitive fashion.

In general, information-processing models of thought and action view cognitive and perceptual operations as taking place in stages or steps, e.g. input, coding, storage, retrieval, decoding, output, and are schematically represented as FLOW CHARTS. In recent years, however, this approach to cognition has been largely replaced by models based on PRODUCTION SYSTEMS and CONNECTIONISM (2).

information theory More an approach to the study of communications than a theory, it is concerned with the issues of transmission of signals and messages. Strongly interdisciplinary, it draws upon work in engineering, physics, communications, linguistics, psychology, cybernetics, etc. See INFORMATION (1) for details.

informed consent Permission given by a person to participate in a research or medical procedure when the consenting individual is provided with complete information about the procedure including: (a) the nature of the procedure; (b) the potential known risks and benefits; (c) any alternative procedures that are available; and (d) acknowledgement that such consent is voluntary.

infra- Combining form meaning *low, under, inferior, after*.

infradian rhythms Biological rhythms with cycles of considerable duration, e.g. the menstrual cycle.

infrared Pertaining to electromagnetic

radiation the wavelength of which is longer than that to which the normal human eye responds, above roughly 700 nm.

infundibulum 1 Generally, any funnel-shaped passage or structure. 2 Specifically, the stalk attaching the pituitary body to the forebrain.

ingestive behaviour FEEDING BEHAVIOUR.

ingratiation Essentially, the act of trying to make someone like you. In E. E. Jones's taxonomy of common strategies used in SELF-PRESENTATION, ingratiation is a strategy whereby you induce others to do your bidding by making them like you. Prototypical ingratiating actions include flattery, agreement with another's opinions and currying favours.

in-group A select group in which all members feel a strong sense of identity with the group, foster a sense of elitism about the group and tend to act so as to exclude others (the *out-group*). Note that the term connotes strong positive feelings toward the group as an abstraction and not necessarily any such affection toward the individual members of the group, who, in fact, may heartily dislike each other. Also occasionally called the *we-group*.

inhalant use disorder A group of disorders brought about by inhaling the aliphatic and aromatic hydrocarbons found in such substances as glue, paint thinners and gasoline. Also abused are the halogenated hydrocarbons in volatile compounds containing esters, ketones and glycols. Use produces a psychoactive *inhalant intoxication*; abuse leads to *inhalant dependence* and *inhalant abuse* with serious side effects including neurological, renal and hepatic complications.

inherent From the Latin, meaning *sticking to* or *in*; characterizing a property or attribute of something or someone that is inseparable and permanent. The term is a close synonym of INTRINSIC and contrasts with EXTRINSIC (2). It should be kept distinct from INHERIT and related terms, which have a different etymology that typically denotes genetic origins. vb., *inhere*.

inherit To receive from one's predecessors. In biology, the reference is to the process of

genetic transmission; in social, political terms, to a transfer of property and perhaps certain rights and privileges.

inheritance HEREDITY.

inherited trait TRAIT, INHERITED.

inhibited (female or male) orgasm ORGASM DISORDERS.

inhibited sexual desire HYPOACTIVE SEXUAL DESIRE DISORDER.

inhibition From the Latin for *restraint*. Hence, very generally: 1 The restraining, preventing, repressing, decreasing or prohibiting of any process, or the process that brings about such restraining. Somewhat more specifically: 2 In physiology, the restraining of an ongoing organic process or the prevention of its initiation by neurological or physiological means. There are many specialized forms of inhibition here – see the following entries for details. 3 In the study of learning, any reduction in or prevention of a response owing to the operation of some other process. Again, specialized terms abound and the more common are given below. 4 In cognitive psychology, particularly the study of memory, the reduction in performance resulting from the presence of other information that 'gets in the way'. Note that in the case of 3 and 4 there is a tendency for some authors to use *inhibition* as though it were a synonym of *interference*. For meaning 3, the resulting distortion is not serious since the theoretical characterization of such an inhibitory process is that other ongoing processes are interfering with the process under consideration (see e.g. RECIPROCAL INHIBITION). For 4, however, such presumed semantic equivalence is, given contemporary theories of memory, misleading and not recommended. See INTERFERENCE (5) for clarification of this point. 5 In psychoanalysis, the control of instinctual id impulses by the action of the superego. Although some analysts use the term interchangeably with SUPPRESSION (and occasionally even with REPRESSION), this practice is not recommended. In the classical theory *inhibition* is used as equivalent to *prevention*; the instinctual processes may get repressed or suppressed but only if inhibition should fail. 6 By extension (and dilution) of 5, any restraining of a momentary impulse or desire.

Not surprisingly, the base term appears in a vast array of specialized contexts and in many agglutinized forms. vb., *inhibit*; adj., *inhibitory*. Combined terms not given below may be found under the modifying term.

inhibition, central This term is used whenever the assumed inhibitory action is taking place within the central nervous system; e.g. *reciprocal inhibition* as exhibited by antagonistic muscles when the neural message to one muscle to contract is accompanied by a relaxation of the other resulting from an inhibition of its motor nerve cells. When action is in the cerebral cortex the term *cortical inhibition* is used.

inhibition, cortical CENTRAL *INHIBITION.

inhibition, external The inhibition of a conditioned response produced when a novel, irrelevant stimulus is presented along with the conditioned stimulus. First discovered by Pavlov, who assumed that it resulted from simultaneous excitations in the central nervous system. Contrast with INTERNAL *INHIBITION.

inhibition, internal Inhibition that depends on a conditioning process, e.g. that produced by *extinction*, *inhibition of delay* or *conditioned inhibition*. Contrast with EXTERNAL *INHIBITION.

inhibition, latent Inhibition established by nonreinforced exposure to a stimulus. An animal learns not to attend to that stimulus so that when it is presented in a reinforcing situation learning is inhibited. Also called the *stimulus pre-exposure effect*.

inhibition of delay A form of internal inhibition that theoretically produces the characteristic delay of responding during long trace conditioning. The fragile inhibitory nature of the process is demonstrated by the ease with which the response may be *disinhibited* by an extraneous stimulus during the trace or delay period.

inhibition of inhibition The original Pavlovian term for DISINHIBITION.

inhibition of (or **with**) **reinforcement** The lessening of a conditioned response when massed, reinforced trials are presented.

It is presumably a fatigue factor and responsiveness recovers with rest.

inhibition of return 1 A perceptual phenomenon in which individuals show a slower reaction to an object that reappears in a specific location. In the classic case, if a stimulus initially occurs just to the right of a fixation point it will be responded to more slowly if it reoccurs in that spot than if its next appearance is in a different spot, say on the left of the fixation point. **2** In ethology, the tendency of an animal to avoid returning to a spot where they have previously looked for food. This pattern is highly adaptive in foraging species. That spot likely either contains no food or it has already been eaten or gathered.

inhibition, proactive PROACTIVE *INTERFERENCE; see also INTERFERENCE (esp. 4) for why *inhibition* is not the preferred term here.

inhibition, reactive (I_R) Hull's term for the hypothesized inhibitory tendency that builds up as a result of effortful responding.

inhibitory conditioning CONDITIONING, INHIBITORY.

inhibitory postsynaptic potential (IPSP) POSTSYNAPTIC POTENTIAL.

inhibitory potential ($_sI_R$) In Hullian theory, the hypothesized state that results from the making of a response and assumed to reflect an organism's tendency to inhibit the making of that response.

inhibitory reflex REFLEX INHIBITION.

initial insomnia INSOMNIA, INITIAL.

initial teaching alphabet An alphabet that expresses English so that the written form is coordinate with the pronunciation (e.g. 'cough' is spelled 'kawf'). Championed by such luminaries as G. B. Shaw as an adjunct to teaching reading, it has fallen out of favour and been pretty much abandoned.

initiation deficit A neurological disorder characterized by an inability to initiate an action even though the patient knows what is expected of him or her and can carry out the action when it is part of another ongoing series of behaviours. It is associated with frontal lobe damage.

injury Broadly, any damage to bodily tissue.

injury feigning A response to a threatening situation whereby an animal feigns an injury in order to attract the attention of a predator and lead it away. The classic case here is the ground-nesting female plover, who feigns a broken wing to lure an intruder away from her young. See DEATH FEIGNING.

inkblot test A generic term used for any of the several projective tests that use inkblots. The most widely used is, of course, the RORSCHACH TEST.

innate Pertaining to or characterizing that which is natural or native to an organism, that which exists or is potential at birth by virtue of genetic factors. In this vein some more or less acceptable synonyms are *inborn, hereditary, inherited, native, nativistic*. That which is innate is demarcated from that which is acquired, learned or derived from experience. The term is used in two ways: (a) With respect to those properties that are hypothesized to be part of the genetic endowment of each member of a particular species and hence to be observed in the anatomy and behaviour of each member. The focus here is universality, those things that are common to all. This sense of the term, long of interest in philosophy (see INNATE IDEAS), is also represented by work in ethology and in some approaches to developmental psychology. (b) To characterize differences between individual members of a species that are not due to environmental factors. Here the focus is on the attribution of genetic cause to observed differences in phenotype among members of a given species. To appreciate these two senses of the term note that walking is innate in the former sense and individual differences in the ability to walk may be innate in the latter sense. Try thinking about an at least partially innate characteristic, such as body weight, in this manner to appreciate the point. See also the extended discussions on usage under HERITABILITY and HEREDITY–ENVIRONMENT CONTROVERSY.

innate ideas A hoary philosophical doctrine dating back to the Stoics that holds that certain ideas are innate, existing a priori in all human beings. Descartes was probably the most vigorous defender of the doctrine, suggesting that knowledge of time, causality, perfection and even the (Euclidean) axioms of geometry were innately given. Locke and other British empiricists attacked the Cartesian position, stressing the role of experience over native endowment. The doctrine has, however, proven rather robust, reappearing in different forms in the writings of Leibniz and Kant and more recently in the theories of the contemporary American linguist and philosopher Noam Chomsky.

innate releasing mechanism In the Lorenz–Tinbergen ethological theory, a postulated mechanism whereby instinctive acts are assumed to be inhibited until the appropriate stimulus (the SIGN STIMULUS) occurs. See ACTION-SPECIFIC ENERGY, FIXED ACTION PATTERN and VACUUM ACTIVITY for details of how this model attempted to account for various behaviours.

inner-directed Coined by D. Riesman to characterize a tendency to react according to an internalized set of goals or values, this term is used to refer to persons exhibiting such internal characteristics as well as the society that fosters them. Contrast with OUTER-DIRECTED and TRADITION-DIRECTED.

inner ear The innermost component of the ear containing the cochlea and the organs of balance. Also called the *labyrinth*.

innervation 1 The neural distribution of and supply to an organ, gland or muscle. This is the usual meaning. On occasion: 2 The neural excitation of an organ, gland or muscle.

innervation, reciprocal Innervation of a pair of antagonistic muscles through which neural impulses induce flexion in one and extension in the other.

innovative therapies Over the years almost every conceivable form of doing, believing, acting, reacting, hoping, touching, fighting, loving, moving, emoting, provoking, etc. ad nauseam has been turned into some form of psychotherapy. This term acts as an umbrella for them all. A few have shown their worth in controlled settings and with proper evaluation and follow-up of cases (e.g. sex therapy, art therapy), others serve mainly as sources of income for therapists and as something new to try for people who drift about psychically looking for someone somewhere to inject some meaning into their lives. Some of the more exotic extant forms (at the time of writing, anyway – most are short-lived) are: poetry therapy, facilitated communication, rebirthing therapy, herbal therapy, therapeutic touch and a whole range of New Age therapies involving aromas, crystals, psychic energies, channelling and reincarnation. One hardly knows what to make of these. Typically, little attempt is made to validate the techniques used, there is no basis for determining success or lack of it and, most damning, there is no reasonable theoretical basis for assuming that some of them ought to work – short of plain old common sense. A few innovative therapies have indeed been validated; WRITING THERAPY is one. For others, such as EYE MOVEMENT DESENSITIZATION AND REPROCESSING THERAPY, the jury is still out. For the remainder, researchers are urged to apply themselves to the task of validation; for the consumer the best advice is *caveat emptor*.

innumeracy A difficulty with numbers and below-normal abilities with basic mathematic operations like addition, subtraction and multiplication. The term is only used when there is no evidence of organic dysfunction or mental retardation. Basically, it is the arithmetic analogue of ILLITERACY, and like that term, it is singularly difficult to assess objectively because of a lack of consensus on just how poor performance needs be before it is appropriate to apply the term.

inoculate 1 To introduce a microorganism or other substance into the body usually by means of an injection. 2 The substance itself. 3 Metaphorically, to introduce new ideas to someone. 4 By extension, to strengthen. 5 To protect from future negative effects. Although the use of the term in this sense is not entirely consistent with the technical usages, it is a reasonable extension of them in that inoculation provides protection from potentially harmful events. It is used broadly in this sense; e.g. for educational techniques that make one less prone to manipulation or to child-rearing styles that promote a robust, hardy personality.

inoculation hypothesis In the study of attitudes, the hypothesis that one's belief in some point of view can be strengthened by presenting weak and refutable counterarguments to it.

input Obviously, something that is put into a system. Broadly, any stimulus may be represented as input in that it is some form of energy that enters some system (an organism). More specifically, the term characterizes a signal fed to an electrical circuit, a message that acts on a receiver, the information entered into a computer, etc. In general one is counselled to ignore the esoterica; all uses are intuitively obvious.

input/output A hybrid term used in various cognitive theories (e.g. *information processing*) to represent the information to a person (input), the behaviour of the person (output) and the relationships between them.

insanity In popular terminology, *not sane*. The term has regrettably been so brutalized by irresponsible writers over the years that its only remaining technical meaning is a forensic one, in its use as a legal designation for the state of an individual judged to be legally irresponsible or incompetent. See INSANITY DEFENCE.

insanity defence The legal concept that a person cannot be convicted of a crime if it can be shown that he or she lacked 'criminal responsibility', that he or she was (legally) insane, at the time of the crime. Several principles have been accepted by various courts on this issue; see e.g. DURHAM RULE, IRRESISTIBLE-IMPULSE TEST, MCNAGHTEN RULE and ALI DEFENCE RULING.

insect societies SOCIAL INSECTS.

insecurity A lack of assurance; uncertainty, unprotectedness. Some theorists argue, not without foundation, that essentially all neurotic, destructive behaviours stem from feelings of insecurity and the attendant sense of anxiety. It is difficult to say much else about this term and the manner of its use in psychology. The feelings are ubiquitous in humankind and if there is one who cannot sense its meaning from personal experience little can be done to explicate further.

insensible Lit., without sensibility. Hence: 1 Of stimuli that are below threshold or outside the range of the sensory modality under consideration. 2 Characteristic of an organism in a state of unresponsiveness, e.g. one unconscious or in a coma. 3 Descriptive of individuals who are lacking in feelings or sensitivities. This last usage is generally equivalent to the nontechnical term *insensitive*.

insight 1 Most generally, an act of apprehending or sensing intuitively the inner nature of something. There are several more specialized meanings. Two relate to *personal* insight: **2** In standard parlance, any self-awareness, self-knowledge or self-understanding. **3** In psychotherapy, the illumination or comprehension of one's mental condition, which has previously escaped awareness. Note that a distinction is made here between *intellectual* insight, which is a kind of theoretical understanding of one's condition or of the underlying psychodynamics of one's actions but still leaves one alienated from the self, and *emotional* insight, which is regarded as the true, deep understanding. Classical psychoanalysis, for example, regards the intellectual form as a defence mechanism and the emotional form as the critical element of successful therapy.

Two additional meanings relate to situational or environmentally stimulated insights: **4** A novel, clear, compelling apprehension of the truth of something occurring without overt recourse to memories of past experiences. **5** Within GESTALT PSYCHOLOGY, the process by which problems are solved. In this sense, insight characterizes a sudden reorganization or restructuring of the pattern or significance of events allowing one to grasp relationships relevant to the solution. Here, insight represents a kind of learning and is characterized in an all-or-none fashion. See also INTUITION.

insomnia A general term for chronic inability to sleep normally, as evidenced by difficulty in falling asleep, frequent waking during the night, and/or early-morning waking with attendant difficulty in falling back to sleep. Insomnia is most often caused by either anxiety or pain. Over the years a large number of synonyms have been used, including *agrypnia, ahypnia, ahyposia, anhypnia, anhypnosis* and other variations. The current view is that insomnia is not a single disorder but a complex group of related disorders, which has led to the suggestion that the term *disorders of initiating and maintaining sleep (DIMS)* be used in place of *insomnia*. For additional details see SLEEP DISORDER and related terms.

insomnia, delayed sleep-onset SLEEP–WAKE SCHEDULE DISORDER.

insomnia, drug dependency REBOUND *INSOMNIA.

insomnia, fatal familial An inherited neurological disorder characterized by progressive deficits in attention and memory, loss of control over the autonomic nervous system and insomnia. Whether or not the insomnia is a direct contributor to the patient's death or a side effect of the neurological damage is not known.

insomnia, initial Difficulty in falling asleep.

insomnia, middle Frequent awakening from sleep accompanied by difficulty falling back to sleep.

insomnia, primary The most common SLEEP DISORDER, characterized by difficulty falling and/or staying asleep to the point where the individual suffers daytime fatigue and impaired daytime functioning. When the shortened term *insomnia* is used it is typically meant to refer to this disorder.

insomnia, rebound Insomnia that occurs following withdrawal from drugs taken to relieve insomnia. On occasion it is worse than the original insomnia the drug was intended to alleviate. Also called *drug dependency insomnia*.

insomnia, terminal Awakening before one's planned or typical time accompanied by difficulty in falling back to sleep.

inspiration 1 Breathing in, inhaling. **2** A sudden apprehension of the essential nature of a thing. This latter use is derived from the former, owing to the ancient belief that such insights came on the breath of spirits.

inspiration/expiration ratio I/E RATIO.

instability UNSTABLE.

instance theory An umbrella term for a number of theories in cognitive psychology that argue that memory and knowledge systems are built up on the basis of specific instances or episodes. Theorists argue, for example, that if a hairy, four-legged creature should walk into the room, the reason you

instinct

know it is a dog is because it reminds you of an earlier instance in which a similar-looking creature was called a dog. Contrast with ABSTRACTION THEORY. Also called *episode theory* and *exemplar theory*. See MULTIPLE CODE THEORY for a more general position.

instant A 'spot' of time; psychologically, a duration so brief that two or more (perhaps) sequential events are perceived as simultaneous. See SPECIOUS PRESENT.

instantiated memory MEMORY, INSTAN-TIATED.

instigation Arousal, stimulation.

instigation therapy A form of behaviourally oriented, directive therapy in which the therapist sets up positive models for the client and actively reinforces progress toward them.

instinct A term with a tortured history indeed. The root is Latin, *instinctus* meaning *instigated* or *impelled*, with the implication that such impulses are natural or innate. There are four general, distinguishable meanings of the term: **1** An unlearned response characteristic of the members of a given species. **2** A tendency or disposition to respond in a particular manner that is characteristic of a particular species. This disposition (2) is the presumed underpinning of the observed behaviour (1). **3** A complex, coordinated set of acts found universally, or nearly so, within a given species that emerges under specific stimulus conditions, specific drive conditions and specific developmental conditions. This meaning was introduced by ethologists; see e.g. INNATE RELEASING MECHANISM, FIXED ACTION PATTERN and related entries. **4** Any of a number of unlearned, inherited tendencies that are hypothesized to function as the motivational forces behind complex human behaviours. This sense is that expressed by classical psychoanalysis.

In actual use, the manner of application of the term has differed dramatically from theory to theory. The first school of psychology to make instinct a central concept was the FREUDIAN. In his early writings, Freud outlined two classes of instincts: *ego*, or self-preserving, instincts, and *sexual*, or reproductive instincts. In his later works he restricted the term to THANATOS (the death instincts)

and EROS (the life instincts). However, in both schemes Freud was clear that instincts were fundamentally motivators of behaviour but were not presumed to specify particular behavioural manifestations. The emphasis was on that which is *instinctual* rather than on the instincts themselves; that is, meanings 1, 2 and 3 did not apply.

McDougall's HORMIC PSYCHOLOGY used instinct (in senses 1, 2 and 4) as the central theoretical concept. All behaviour was treated as purposive or goal-seeking and motivated by underlying species-specific propensities, the instincts. Unlike Freud, McDougall applied the term broadly to all motivational constructs and the resultant proliferation of hypothesized instincts undermined the scientific basis of the theory.

The use of the term by the early ethologists (primarily in sense 3 but incorporating 1 and 2) has stressed the species-specific and biological aspects. Lorenz's definition made this clear: 'Behaviour which is to a large extent determined by nervous mechanisms evolved in the phylogeny of the species.' Note that this use specifically includes behaviour, as opposed to the psychoanalytic focus on motivation.

Much of the confusion has resulted from several unresolved issues: (a) *The heredity problem:* To what extent are instincts biologically preprogrammed or the result of environmental factors? See here HEREDITY–ENVIRONMENT CONTROVERSY. (b) *Species specificity:* Are instincts general motivators or can they only be explicated within individual species? (c) *Behavioural specificity:* To what degree are specific behaviours to be incorporated into the concept? While it is clear that some behavioural manifestations are always implied (how else to know the existence of the instinct?), this last problem is a serious one. The more specific the presumed behaviours, the greater the chance that the term will take on an unacceptable nebulousness, as it did with McDougall.

Obviously these points are interconnected and, of course, they are not the only ones of import. The problem is that the general concept is too vital to permit banishment of the term from the psychologist's lexicon, as some have suggested. A less robust concept would long ago have succumbed to its own excesses. Handle with care.

instinct, closed An innate species-specific behaviour pattern (i.e. INSTINCT (3)) that is rigid and inflexible. It appears if and only if the proper stimulus is provided and is closed to any environmentally guided modification. Much insect behaviour falls into this category.

instinct, delayed Any instinct the characteristic behaviour of which does not appear until some time after birth or hatching. See here CRITICAL PERIOD.

instinctive Pertaining to instinct. Note that there is a common misuse of this term in nontechnical writings, as in 'the goal tender made a sudden instinctive kick to block the shot'. Here the act is clearly the result of much skilled practice and not in any way truly instinctive; highly practised automatized acts are not instincts in the technical sense. Compare with INTUITIVE.

instinct, life EROS, LIBIDO.

instinct, open An innate species-specific behaviour pattern (i.e. INSTINCT (3)) that displays flexibility so that the behaviour 'drifts' over time and with experience. For example, feedback about the appropriateness of certain materials for nest-building will produce changes in the nest-building behaviour of many species of bird. The use of the term *instinct* here is questioned by some, who would prefer to call such modification by experience RESTRICTED *LEARNING.

instinctual Pertaining to INSTINCT.

instinctual aggression AGGRESSION.

instinctual anxiety A psychoanalytic term for anxiety provoked by fear of one's basic, primal instincts. Used roughly synonymously with NEUROTIC *ANXIETY.

instinctual fusion FUSION (2).

institution 1 In the argot of the sociologist, an organized system of social roles which is a persistent and significant element in a society and which focuses on basic human needs and functions. The term is used broadly and one will find references to economic institutions, institutions of higher learning, marriage as an institution, military institutions, religious orders as institutions, etc. **2** More specifically, and less technically, the term is also used for local clubs, prisons, hospitals,

etc. **3** Most specifically, the buildings occupied or used by such organizations. See ORGANIZATION (2).

institutionalization 1 The process of development of the stable and formal patterns of behaviour that make up an institution. The usage here is quite broad and derives from sociology. **2** The habituation of a person to the patterns within an institution, often to the extent that the person may not be capable of normal functioning outside. **3** The process of having someone placed in an institution.

institutionalize A transitive verb that refers to the process of INSTITUTIONALIZATION (2, 3) of a person by either (a) indoctrination into a system of social roles or (b) physical placement in an institution such as a prison or a mental hospital. Note that in practice, although not necessarily in theory, the former connotation is subtly implied in the latter; individuals placed in institutions (theoretically for rehabilitative or therapeutic reasons) are expected to conform to the 'appropriate' modes of behaviour of the place of confinement and hence to become institutionalized.

institutional review board In North America, a board of persons responsible for reviewing research proposals and ongoing research in order to protect the rights of research subjects. Commonly called *IRB*.

institution, total A specialized use of INSTITUTION denoting a place of confinement (total or partial) where lifestyle is sharply restricted, formalized and under the control of special staff. Traditionally, prisons, army camps, convents, mental hospitals, boarding schools, etc. are so classified.

instruction(s) 1 In the singular, directing, teaching, imparting knowledge. **2** In the plural, directions for carrying out some procedure. Used commonly in this sense to mean a set of directions to a participant in an experiment.

instrument 1 Characterizing instruments and tools. **2** Characterizing behaviours that are goal-directed.

instrumental Obvious meanings about instruments and tools aside, the psychologist generally uses this term to characterize beha-

viours that are goal-directed. See e.g. INSTRU-
MENTAL BEHAVIOUR, INSTRUMENTAL CONDITIONING.

instrumental aggression   AGGRESSION,
INSTRUMENTAL.

instrumental behaviour (or **act**)   Very
generally, any behaviour or act that is goal-
directed, a means to some end. See INSTRU-
MENTAL CONDITIONING.

instrumental conditioning   An experimental procedure in which reinforcement
occurs only after a subject has made the
proper response. Mazes, straight alleys, puzzle boxes and the like are all examples of
experimental apparatuses used to study
instrumental conditioning. There are several
things of note about this term: (a) The name
derives from the fact that the occurrence of
the proper response is *instrumental* in producing the reinforcement. Contrast with CLAS-
SICAL CONDITIONING, in which the US
(unconditioned stimulus) appears regardless
of whether or not the CR (conditioned
response) occurs. (b) Many authors prefer
to use the term *operant conditioning* rather
than instrumental conditioning. It is, however, not simply a matter of replacing one
term with another. Instrumental conditioning traditionally covered discrete-trial situations in which the subject had to perform
some act within a structured environment.
Operant conditioning covers 'free' behaviour as well as discrete-trial behaviour and
includes behaviour in which the subject
responds in some way which changes (or
operates on) the environment. Hence,
instrumental conditioning is really a special
case of operant conditioning. (c) In general,
the term is used to refer both to the actual
learning that takes place and to the experimental procedure itself. See also CONDITION-
ING and OPERANT CONDITIONING.

instrumentalism   A term introduced by
John Dewey to characterize his moderate
variation on the philosophy of pragmatism.
This approach shares with *operationalism* and
other forms of *empiricism* an emphasis on the
need to verify concepts through empirical
testing, but it is somewhat looser in that it
does not insist on operational definitions
and allows for more conceptual and theoretical analysis.

insufficient justification   One of the classic means of inducing *cognitive dissonance*; a
technique whereby participants are induced
to behave in a way that is inconsistent with
their beliefs or self-perception but are not
given sufficient reason to justify such behaviour to themselves. The original example, in
work by Festinger and colleagues, involved
getting participants to lie about the intrinsic
interest of a task and paying them just one
dollar to do so.

insufflation   The delivery of a drug by sniffing it so that it makes contact with the nasal
mucosa.

insula   A part of the cortex buried deeply
inside the Sylvian fissure of the brain behind
the rostral part of the temporal lobe. Largely
because of its inaccessibility, there is no clear
understanding of the role of the insular cortex. It has been implicated in the processing
of somatosensory stimuli, particularly those
relating to feeding (e.g. odour, taste) as well
as various motor functions from those
involved in feeding (e.g. swallowing) to
those that play a role in the articulation of
speech. Other research suggests it plays a role
in emotion, particularly negative emotions
(disgust, guilt) and in the processing of aversive stimuli. Also called the *island of reil*.

insulin   A hormone secreted by the beta cells
of the islets of Langerhans in the pancreas.
Insulin is an essential component of proper
metabolism; it facilitates entry of glucose
and amino acids into cells, provides for
proper metabolism of glucose by aiding in
its conversion into glycogen and facilitates
production of fats in adipose (fatty) tissue.
Diminished secretion leads to inadequate
metabolism of carbohydrates and fats and
the hyperglycaemia of diabetes. Secretion
of insulin is determined by (a) blood-glucose
concentrations, with high levels triggering
secretion and low levels inhibiting it, (b) a
rise in the level of amino acids, and (c) direct
efferent nerve impulses from the brain to the
pancreas.

insulin resistance syndrome   METABOLIC
SYNDROME.

insulin shock (or **coma**)   A hypoglycaemic
state produced by excess insulin, resulting in
a lowering of blood sugar and a comatose
state.

insulin-shock therapy   A form of therapy

for certain psychological disorders utilizing a dose of insulin large enough to induce shock and coma. It is a procedure with very real dangers and insufficient evidence for any therapeutic effects; as a result, it is virtually never used anymore.

insult Occasional synonym for *injury*.

integrate 1 Generally, to bring into a harmonious or coordinated whole by rearranging, organizing and occasionally adding or deleting elements or parts. **2** Specifically, to carry out such an operation when the elements are persons who are distinguished by characteristics that play important socioeconomic roles in a culture, e.g. race, sex, religion, social class.

integration Very generally, the process of coordinating and unifying disparate elements into a whole; see INTEGRATE. A variety of special usages is found, typically with qualifiers appended, as in the following entries.

integration, behavioural The blending, chaining or combining of several separate behaviours into a coordinated whole.

integration, cultural The blending of cultural traits, which were originally conflicting, to form a modified, integrated system.

integration, functional A general term used to denote the functional, operative aspects of any integration.

integration, group Any FUNCTIONAL *INTEGRATION in which the system under examination is a group and the several parts are people. The term is used roughly synonymously with SOCIAL *INTEGRATION.

integration, social There are two slightly different uses here: **1** The process of uniting disparate elements or groups into one unified group. **2** The adoption of existing group standards by an individual so that he or she is accepted into an existing group. In the first, the new group may be totally different after this process; in the second, the group standards remain unchanged.

intellect Originally this term referred specifically to the *rational* thought functions of the human mind; today it is a generic term covering the cognitive processes as a whole.

intellectual 1 adj. Pertaining to the intellect or to intelligence. **2** adj. Pertaining to one with abiding interests in ideas, thinking, creativity. **3** n. A person devoted to matters of the mind. A strange term in many ways, its affective connotations have varied greatly over the years. With skill it can be used as either a high compliment (connotations of intelligence) or a dashing insult (connotations of being narrow, otherworldly, neglectful of emotions, affections, sensations, etc.).

intellectualism A general term for any doctrine that focuses exclusively on intellectual functioning. Used occasionally as a rough synonym of IDEALISM or RATIONALISM, depending on whether the author takes the point of view that the intellectual represents the ultimate reality (idealism) or that it represents the basic process by which knowledge is acquired (rationalism).

intellectualization A defence mechanism whereby problems are analysed in remote, intellectual terms while emotion, affect and feeling are ignored.

intelligence Few concepts in psychology have received more devoted attention and few have resisted clarification so thoroughly. Despite many efforts over the years to develop some independent definition of the term, its connotations have remained intimately intertwined with the techniques developed for its measurement. Binet, the inventor of the individual intelligence test, felt that intelligent behaviour would be manifested in such abilities as reasoning, imagination, insight, judgement and adaptability, so he designed his tests (see BINET TESTS) to evaluate just these functions. Still others have argued that all such abilities are only manifestations of a single underlying factor (the so-called GENERAL *FACTOR) which is presumed to be at the root of all intellectual functioning. In 1927 the frustrations of dealing with the concept were already being felt. Spearman, the great psychometrician, despaired of the whole notion and called intelligence 'a mere vocal sound, a word with so many meanings that finally it had none'.

Such pessimism, however deeply felt, has not dimmed psychology's need for such a concept. Before the tests and measurement movement, the term meant 'the ability to profit from experience', which implies the ability to behave adaptively, to function successfully within particular environments. Hence, any intelligence test that proves to be valid will be one that accurately predicts adaptive and successful functioning within specified environments. Since its inception, the dominant use of the intelligence test has been as a predictor of scholastic success and so, of course, there should be little surprise that the behaviours deemed adaptive and successful have been precisely those of reasoning, judging, learning, dealing with novelty, abstracting, etc. All such intelligence tests are, by their very existence, socioculturally determined. They reflect the ideals and values of the culture of the test designers, and 'adaptive and successful functioning' always means 'adaptive and successful functioning within that culture'.

There is nothing fundamentally wrong with this. The fact that this set of circumstances invites abuse does not deny a society the right to attempt to discern which of its citizens is most likely to profit from what it has to offer them. Ultimately intelligence is, conceptually, what it has always been – the ability to profit from experience – and, pragmatically, what it has become – that which the intelligence tests measure.

intelligence, abstract See ABSTRACT and INTELLIGENCE. The term is used similarly to FLUID *INTELLIGENCE.

intelligence, adult **1** Psychometrically speaking, the level of intelligence reached at which there is a marked decrease in the growth of measured intelligence, or, more formally, of which the year-to-year average increase in measured mental age becomes small relative to the standard deviation in the scores in the whole population. The age at which this point is reached differs from intelligence test to intelligence test but there is vague agreement that it is somewhere during adolescence (roughly 13–18 years of age). **2** The average level of intelligence of the adults in a given population. Meanings 1 and 2 are, in many respects, contradictory. On the one hand, if *adult* covers everyone past adolescence, then the average *measured* IQ in 2 may very well be lower than in 1 since there is some evidence that IQ scores drop off after middle age. But, on the other hand, if maturity, wisdom, insight, understanding and all those other qualities of the mature adult are to count toward a

pragmatic conceptualization of intelligence, then 2 is certainly going to be higher than 1. However, since we haven't the foggiest notion how to evaluate quantitatively such a thing as wisdom but think we know how to measure intelligence, most authorities have placed themselves in the embarrassing position of defining *adult* intelligence as that possessed by the average *adolescent*.

intelligence, analytical In the TRIARCHIC THEORY OF INTELLIGENCE, the ability to analyse situations, make comparisons, evaluate and judge settings, in short, the skills measured by standard INTELLIGENCE TESTS.

intelligence, coefficient of Generally, any index of intelligence derived by forming the ratio of the score obtained by an individual on an intelligence test to the norms for that person's age (usually multiplied by some constant); see INTELLIGENCE QUOTIENT.

intelligence, concrete Generally, the ability to function effectively with CONCRETE problems. The term is used similarly to CRYS-TALLIZED *INTELLIGENCE. See also the general discussion under INTELLIGENCE.

intelligence, creative In the TRIARCHIC THEORY OF INTELLIGENCE, that component of cognitive function linked with creativity, specifically the ability to invent, explore, expand, imagine and uncover.

intelligence, crystallized Intelligence as assessed by those components of an intelligence test that are based on facts and previously acquired skills. The term is used similarly to CONCRETE *INTELLIGENCE.

intelligence, emotional Literally, the capacity to react in emotionally arousing situations, to be able to decode, encode, understand and/or manage emotions in an adaptive manner.

intelligence, fluid Intelligence as assessed by those components of a test that are based on the ability to solve novel problems creatively.

intelligence, practical In the TRIARCHIC THEORY OF INTELLIGENCE, the set of flexible skills that allow one to adapt, shape and adjust to new environments; to apply knowledge in everyday settings.

intelligence quotient A measure of intelligence level. Originally defined as 100 times the mental age (MA, determined by a standardized test) divided by the chronological age (CA), it now represents a person's performance relative to peers. Both procedures establish the average as 100. Nearly always abbrev., *IQ*.

intelligence, successful In the TRIARCHIC THEORY OF INTELLIGENCE, the set of flexible skills that allow one to succeed in life – with the understanding that 'success' is a personal thing and one establishes one's own criteria. It is assumed to emerge from the effective use of ANALYTIC, CREATIVE and PRACTICAL *INTELLIGENCE.

intelligence test Any test that purports to measure intelligence. Generally such tests consist of a series of cognitive tasks each of which has been standardized with a large, representative population of individuals. See INTELLIGENCE for a discussion of issues and problems.

intension In logic, the domain of a general term or concept made up of all those terms or concepts that are necessarily true of it. In less formal terms, intension is roughly equivalent to CONNOTATIVE *MEANING. Compare with EXTENSION (3). Distinguish from INTENTION.

intensity 1 As borrowed from physics, a measure of a quantity of energy. Hence, physical stimuli are characterized in terms of intensity, e.g. the intensity of a light, a tone, an electric current. **2** The degree of experienced sensation as related to some physical stimulus. Here subjective experience is so characterized, e.g. the intensity of a pain or an auditory sensation. Sense 1 is quantitative, thanks to the successes of the physical sciences; sense 2 is usually qualitative, owing to the complexities of the psychological processes involved, but see SCALING and METHODS OF *SCALING for attempts to quantify experienced intensity. **3** The vigour or strength of an emitted behaviour. This sense is common in behaviourist studies of learning and conditioning. **4** By extension of 3, the degree to which an emotion is experienced, a belief held, an attitude adopted, etc.

In all cases *intensity* refers to or implies the existence of a whole dimension along which the variable can be expressed; hence *intense* is taken to mean, simply, *of high intensity*, and

intensive becomes the modifier used to pertain to the full dimension.

intention 1 Generally, any desire, plan, purpose, aim or belief that is oriented toward some goal, some end state. The term is used by most with the connotation that such striving is *conscious*, although it occasionally creeps into psychoanalytic writings without this implication. **2** In the philosophy of mind and the older school of ACT PSYCHOLOGY, the essential feature of all conscious processes in that they involve outward references to objects. See here INTENTIONALITY. Distinguish from INTENSION.

intentional 1 Deliberate, purposeful, goal-oriented. A term generally used to characterize acts undertaken consciously, e.g. INTENTIONAL *LEARNING as opposed to IMPLICIT *LEARNING, or INTENTIONAL *FORGETTING versus 'ordinary' FORGETTING. **2** Pertaining to INTENTION (2); see also INTENTIONALITY.

intentional forgetting 1 FORGETTING due to REPRESSION. Here the notion of *intentional* is compromised somewhat in that it usually carries the connotation of awareness, whereas *repression* denotes an unconscious process. See INTENTION (1). **2** Directed forgetting, forgetting of material following instructions to do so. This is a touchy issue; it evokes images of the old joke about instructing someone *not* to think about pigmy elephants…(see PARADOXICAL INJUNCTION). The argument put forward by some is that such intentional forgetting may result because the person so directed refrains from deep coding or processing of the material and so tends not to be able to recall it later. See here DEPTH OF PROCESSING.

intentionality As borrowed from philosophy, a feature of some (but not all) internal mental or cognitive states in that they are focused outward at objects, events and states of affairs in the real world. The mental state instantiated by saying 'I believe it is raining' would have intentionality. In general, beliefs, intentions, desires, purposes, etc. are *intentional states*. Other mental states characterized by undifferentiated or undirected affect, e.g. depression or anxiety, are not so classified.

intentional learning LEARNING, INTENTIONAL.

intentional state INTENTIONALITY.

intention tremor ACTION TREMOR.

inter- Combining term indicating *between*, *among* or *mutual*. Compare with INTRA-.

interaction Reciprocal effect or influence. In *social interaction* the behaviour of one acts as a stimulus for the behaviour of another, and vice versa. In *statistical interaction* the effects of two (or more) variables are interdependent; e.g. task difficulty and arousal often interact so that increased arousal increases performance on easy tasks but decreases it on difficult tasks.

interactionism DUALISM.

interaction variance In statistics, the proportion of the total variance that is not related to the action of single variables but due to the interaction between variables.

Interactive dualism DUALISM.

interaural differences Differences in the sound arriving at the two ears. There are two kinds of interaural differences: *time* and *intensity*. Together they make up the set of cues for localizing a sound source in the environment. See also BINAURAL TIME DIFFERENCES.

Interbrain DIENCEPHALON.

intercalation **1** Insertion in between the elements of an ordered series. A term generally used with the connotation of extraneous, unnecessary. **2** A speech disorder in which irrelevant, inappropriate sounds or words are inserted.

intercorrelations The correlations of each variable in a set with every other variable in the analysis. A full set of intercorrelations, usually displayed in matrix form, is the basis for a factor analysis.

intercourse **1** Generally, dealings, interactions or communications between persons and/or groups. **2** More specifically, an interchange of affect, of emotion. **3** Most specifically, SEXUAL INTERCOURSE.

interdependence Generally, a pattern of action and thought that focuses on the relationships between self and other(s) and emphasizes the importance of positive interpersonal behaviours such as cooperation. A common example is found in the behaviour of people who think of themselves as being 'good neighbours'. In the study of SELF-CONSTRUAL, it is generally contrasted with INDEPENDENCE (4).

interest One of those terms that slipped unnoticed into the technical vocabulary of psychology, especially educational psychology. Its meaning is loose at best and at one time or another has been used to imply all of the following: attention, curiosity, motivation, focus, concern, goal-directedness, awareness, worthiness and desire. Most authors merely follow their intuitions in its use; it's hard to go wrong.

interest inventory (or **test**) An instrument designed to evaluate a person's interests in or preferences for a variety of activities, e.g. KUDER PREFERENCE RECORD and STRONG INTEREST INVENTORY.

interface **1** In computer terminology, the circuitry that connects the central processing core of a computer and its peripheral parts. **2** By extension, the connection between any two functioning units, including organisms. A common phrase in engineering psychology is *man–machine (or person–machine) interface*.

interfemale aggression AGGRESSION, INTERFEMALE.

interference From the Old French, meaning *to strike each other*. Surprisingly, this original sense can still be felt in contemporary use. Hence: **1** Very generally, any process in which there is some conflict between operations or acts such that a diminution or decrement in performance results. In layperson's terms, things getting in the way of other things. **2** In acoustics and optics, the decrease in amplitude of a complex wave form when two or more wave patterns of different phases come together. **3** In social psychology, a conflict between competing emotions, motives, values, etc. **4** In learning and conditioning, a conflict among associations formed between stimuli and responses. Commonly used here for circumstances in which there are two mutually incompatible responses and a single stimulus. Often INHIBITION (esp. 3) is an acceptable synonym of this meaning; see e.g. RECIPROCAL INHIBITION. **5** In learning and memory, a conflict between information in memory such that either (a) new information becomes difficult to learn because of previous experiences (see here PROACTIVE *INTERFERENCE), or (b) old information becomes difficult to recall because of current information (see here RETROACTIVE *INTERFERENCE). Occasionally one sees INHIBITION (4) used as a synonym here. Unlike 4 above, this usage is misleading, particularly in that the theoretical characterization of these memory phenomena is that they are caused by 'things getting in the way of other things' and not by 'things restraining other things', as connoted by the term *inhibition*. **6** A block or barrier that creates difficulties for another person.

interference, proactive (PI) The interference of material previously learned with material currently being learned. It is proactive in the sense that the effects of information acquired in the past are felt 'forward' in time. Proactive interference builds up surprisingly fast, particularly when a person undertakes several highly similar tasks in a short period of time, and performance may drop off precipitously. See RELEASE FROM *PI. Compare with RETROACTIVE *INTERFERENCE.

interference, retroactive (RI) The interference of newly learned material with the recall of material learned previously. It is retroactive in the sense that current tasks interfere with the retrieval of memories for learning that took place earlier in time. Compare with PROACTIVE *INTERFERENCE.

intergenerational mobility Vertical social mobility from one generation to the next. Typically assessed by comparing occupations of parents with those of their offspring.

interjectional theory THEORIES OF *LANGUAGE ORIGINS.

interlocking schedule SCHEDULES OF *REINFORCEMENT.

intermale aggression AGGRESSION, INTERMALE.

intermarriage 1 Marriage between persons who are blood relations. **2** Marriage between persons of disparate groups. The groups may be defined by social class, religion, ethnicity or race.

intermediate needs In Maslow's theory, a subclass of DEFICIENCY NEEDS (2). Included here are safety, belongingness, self-esteem, secur-

ity, etc. See NEED HIERARCHY for the relationship between the various classes of needs in the theory.

intermetamorphosis A DELUSIONAL MISIDENTIFICATION DISORDER in which the patient believes that two persons well known to him or her have exchanged identities with each other.

intermission A symptom-free period in a chronic disorder. Distinguish from REMISSION.

intermittence tone INTERRUPTION TONE.

intermittent explosive disorder An IMPULSE-CONTROL DISORDER characterized by episodes of aggressiveness resulting in serious assaults on people or property. The degree of aggression displayed is dramatically out of proportion to any precipitating event or known external cause. The term is only used when other psychiatric disorders that are associated with loss of control of aggressive impulses have been ruled out. Note that a subcategory of this disorder previously referred to as an *isolated* form of explosive disorder, in which there was but a single such episode, is, for simple logical reasons, no longer officially recognized.

intermittent reinforcement REINFORCEMENT, INTERMITTENT.

intermittent schedule INTERMITTENT *REINFORCEMENT.

internal aim AIM (3).

internal capsule A wide band of myelinated axons in the CORPUS STRIATUM. It separates the CAUDATE NUCLEUS and the THALAMUS from the LENTICULAR NUCLEUS. There are several subareas within it, each comprised of efferent pathways from the cerebral cortex and afferent fibres from various sensory systems.

internal consistency 1 The degree to which various parts of a test or other instrument are associated with one another empirically, i.e. the degree to which they cohere. **2** Occasionally, the extent to which an individual's behaviour is consistent from situation to situation. The preferred term here is SELF-CONSISTENCY (esp. 2, 3).

internal consistency, coefficient of COEFFICIENT OF *RELIABILITY, SPLIT-HALF *RELIABILITY.

internal ear Collectively, the middle and inner parts of the ear.

internal environment A general term used to refer to any and all processes and their effects occurring inside the body.

internal–external scale A self-report inventory designed to measure the degree to which a person perceives control of his or her behaviours as arising from internal or from external factors. See LOCUS OF CONTROL for more detail. abbrev., *I–E scale*.

internal inhibition INHIBITION, INTERNAL.

internalization 1 The acceptance or adoption of beliefs, values, attitudes, practices, standards, etc. as one's own. In traditional psychoanalytic theory a person's superego is assumed to develop through the process of internalization of the standards and values of their parents. Within traditional approaches to social psychology and the study of personality an important issue is the degree to which a person attributes his or her behaviour to such internalized motives. See here LOCUS OF CONTROL and compare with EXTERNALIZATION. Also, differentiate from INTROJECTION, in which the values are borrowed rather than adopted, and from SOCIALIZATION, a term also used in cases in which the behaviour may conform to societal values without the commitment or belief. **2** The learning of highly abstract rule systems. Thus a child learning to speak is described as internalizing the rules of the grammar of language. **3** In studies of *expressive functions*, reacting to an event with strong physiological indicators but little or nothing in the way of overt behavioural or emotional responses.

internalizing behaviours EXTERNALIZING BEHAVIOURS.

internal rectus One of the muscles controlling the eye.

internal secretion gland GLAND.

internal senses The senses of INTEROCEPTION and PROPRIOCEPTION.

internal validity VALIDITY, INTERNAL.

International Classification of Diseases (**ICD**) A system of classification of diseases developed under the auspices of the World Health Organization. Over the years many revisions of the *ICD* have been published; at the time of writing, the most recent system is the tenth, known as *ICD-10*, published in 1992. The *ICD* has an extensive section on mental and behavioural disorders, which is in wide use in many countries. The other major system in use in clinical psychology and psychiatry is the one laid out in the DIAGNOSTIC AND STATISTICAL MANUAL (DSM), which was developed by the American Psychiatric Association. Happily, in the most recent editions of the *DSM* and the *ICD* the once disparate terminology has been coordinated. Accordingly, the definitions of the various mental and behavioural disorders in this volume reflect the usage patterns of both the *DSM* and the *ICD* and are therefore appropriate for use virtually anywhere.

International Phonetic Alphabet (IPA) A phonetic alphabet of approximately 95 phones. It is rich and flexible enough for all of the phonemes of the world's languages to be represented.

interneuron A connecting neuron, one that lies between sensory (afferent) and motor (efferent) neurons. Found within the central nervous system. Also called *internuncial neuron* and, in older texts, *association neuron*.

internuncial neuron INTERNEURON.

interoception The sense of internal functioning, the perception of events within the body. An *interoceptor* is any sense organ or receptor that is activated by stimuli arising within the body, including hunger, thirst, nausea, visceral sensations and the like.

interoceptor Any internal sense organ or receptor. Contrast with EXTEROCEPTOR and PROPRIOCEPTOR. var., *enteroceptor*.

interocular distance The distance between the pupils when the eyes are in normal position for distance viewing, i.e. focused on infinity.

interpersonal 1 Generally, characterizing relations between two or more persons, usually with the connotation that the interaction is mutual and reciprocal. **2** Relating to phenomena, properties, effects, etc. that result from such interactions. **3** Broadly, of that which is social.

interpersonal control This term refers to a

set of processes whereby a person regulates interactions with others and with the environment. It is considered a dynamic arrangement that changes with conditions to maintain a desired level of interaction.

interpersonal intelligence See MULTIPLE INTELLIGENCES THEORY.

interpersonal theory A label used to characterize the personality theory of H. S. Sullivan, who theorized that personality dynamics and disorders thereof were due primarily to social forces and interpersonal situations.

interpersonal trust scale A scale developed by J. Rotter that measures a generalized expectation of the believability or trustworthiness of others.

interpolate To estimate, on the basis of two known values of a variable, a value that lies between them. Interpolations are based on the assumption that intermediate points conform to overall trends already observed. They are useful and often necessary but can occasionally lead to errors. Contrast with EXTRAPOLATE.

interpolated reinforcement SCHEDULES OF *REINFORCEMENT.

interposition Partial blocking or obscuring of one object in the visual field by another object. One of the monocular cues for depth perception and one of the more compelling. Also called *occlusion*.

interpretation A process that is usually described as 'explaining a thing in a meaningful way', or words to that effect. While not wrong, such a definition glosses over an important and complex implication: the very act of interpretation implies the existence of a conceptual schema or model on the part of the interpreter such that what is being observed and interpreted is assumed to conform logically to the facts and explanations inherent in the model.

Hence, there are two broad classes of usage: (a) Scientific interpretation, in which the model is a theoretical one and explanation is a characterization of reality. Thus, whether one interprets a response from a laboratory rat, the action of a neuron, the behaviour of a group of people or a dream, the process involves induction and generalization from some accepted scientific schema. Indeed, all such data *must* be interpreted; facts do not stand in isolation, they are always seen in relationship to other facts and models about those facts. The collection of data and the scientific interpretation of those data are, *ipso facto*, part of the same process. (b) Cognitive interpretation, in which the model is assumed to be the mental scheme within which all the incoming stimuli are identified, classified and reacted to. The interpretative act here is equally essential, since all stimuli are indeed data for the observer and are meaningless (some would say phenomenologically nonexistent) without cognitive interpretation.

interpretative therapy Loosely, any form of psychotherapy in which the therapist interprets the significance and underlying symbolic meaning of the client's statements.

interquartile range The range between the first and third quartiles (i.e. between the 25th and 75th percentiles) of a distribution.

interrater reliability RELIABILITY, INTERRATER.

interresponse time (IRT) Simply, the time between responses. It is an important dependent variable in evaluating operant behaviour.

interrogative A SPEECH ACT in which the speaker requests information from the listener.

interruption tone A tone produced by regular interruptions of a constant tone. If the interruptions are slow, beats are heard; if they are rapid, a tone with pitch corresponding to the rate of interruption is heard. Also called *intermittence tone*.

intersexuality The condition of having both male and female characteristics, particularly the secondary sex characteristics. See the discussion under HERMAPHRODITE.

interstice A gap or space in a tissue or in the structure of an organ.

interstimulus interval (ISI) In any procedure that uses two stimuli, the time between the offset of the first stimulus and the onset of the second (compare with STIMULUS ONSET ASYNCHRONY). It is frequently used as an independent variable in experimental work; for example, in classical conditioning as the interval between the conditioned stimulus (CS) and the unconditioned stimulus (US), and in studies of perception and cognition as the time allotted to a subject to process a brief stimulus prior to the presentation of another stimulus. See MASKING.

interstitial cell-stimulating hormone (ICSH) LUTEINIZING HORMONE.

interstitial fluid The fluid that fills the spaces between the cells of the body.

intersubjective Of subjective phenomena that are assumed to be experienced in similar fashion by people other than oneself. The term *intersubjective testability* is used to refer to the essential criterion of any science that no event or effect is to be accepted as a legitimate part of the science unless it is of a type that can be described by more than one person. A *dream* is, from this point of view, not an acceptable datum, but the dreamer's *report* of the dream is.

intersubjectivity Loosely, a mutual exchange of conscious information, knowledge or emotions between individuals. The connotation is that the experience has a distinct empathic element to it (EMPATHY (1, 2)). The exchange need not be explicit and complete, but must involve the individuals understanding each other's motives, assertions, thoughts or emotions to some degree. Some distinguish between *primary intersubjectivity* in which feelings are communicated and exchanged, and *secondary intersubjectivity* in which conventional shared symbolic meanings are negotiated and understood.

intertrial interval (ITI) The time interval between two trials of an experiment. Often used as an independent variable in experiments on learning and memory.

interval of uncertainty (IU) In determining a difference THRESHOLD (3) one may find the *upper threshold* (i.e. the stimulus sufficiently more intense than a standard stimulus so that the subject can just detect the difference) or the *lower threshold* (the stimulus sufficiently less intense for the subject to just detect the difference). The difference invariably produced by these methods is the IU. Also see HYSTERESIS (2).

interval reinforcement   REINFORCEMENT, INTERVAL.

interval scale SCALE, INTERVAL.

intervening variable VARIABLE, INTERVENING.

intervention (technique) A generic term used for any procedure or technique that is designed to interrupt, interfere with and/or modify an ongoing process. It is used in medicine to characterize particular surgical procedures (e.g. cutting an afferent neural pathway to stop intractable pain), in psychotherapy to disrupt ongoing maladaptive behaviour patterns (e.g. removing a child from a home where it is being physically abused), in education to reorient a student's approach to learning (e.g. switching the student to a different school), etc.

intervertebral foramen FORAMEN MAGNUM.

interview A directed conversation. In psychology, interviews usually have either information-gathering or therapeutic purposes. Occasionally qualifiers are appended to denote the specific kind of interview under discussion. For example, in *nondirective* or *unstructured interviews* the interviewer is given discretion in the questions and topics to be covered; in *semi-structured interviews*, questions and topics are specified, but the interviewer is given some flexibility in terms of rewording and pursuit of topics; in *structured interviews* only specified questions and topics are used with little or no flexibility in coverage. In general, the more structured the interview, the more reliable and valid it is found to be.

interview, depth An interview designed to probe beneath the superficial, to allow for exploration of unknown variables and (the hope is) to provide insight into the nature of the factors discussed.

interviewer bias In an interview, the contaminating effect of the interviewer's opinions, expectations or general lack of objectivity. See EXPERIMENTER BIAS for an analogous bias in experimental research.

intimacy disorder A general term for the inability to become intimate with others, to share emotions, trust others or make a commitment to a stable, lasting relationship.

intimacy, principle of The generalization

that the several elements of a Gestalt are intimately related to each other so as to produce, by their mutual interdependence, the perceived whole. Individual elements or parts of a Gestalt may not be removed or replaced without disrupting or changing it; they are not independent from each other nor from the whole percept. See GESTALT PSYCHOLOGY.

intolerance of ambiguity AMBIGUITY, INTOLERANCE OF.

intolerance of uncertainty TOLERANCE OF *UNCERTAINTY.

intonation A general term covering the modulations of the voice, the stress patterns and the rise and fall in pitch while speaking. Such modulations play an important grammatical role in the spoken language. For example, a simple sequence of words like 'Paint the box brown' can be uttered as many different sentences by varying the intonation pattern (well over a dozen can be generated if you make 'Brown' a name). See also INTONATION CONTOUR, STRESS (2).

intonation contour The intonation pattern over a full phrase or sentence. 'Mary slew a tiger' can be either a simple declarative or a question depending on whether the intonation contour falls or rises.

intoxication 1 Generally, from the Greek for *poison*, the state of having been poisoned by some substance. **2** Specifically, such a state produced by excessive alcohol intake. In standard psychiatric terminology, mental disorders that result from substance-induced intoxication are classified as ORGANIC MENTAL DISORDERS and are typically specified by the name of the responsible substance; e.g. alcohol intoxication, caffeine intoxication, amphetamine intoxication.

intra- A prefix from the Latin meaning *within* or *inside*. Compare with INTER- and INTRO- for a subtle distinction.

intracellular fluid The fluid inside the cells.

intraception H. Murray's term for an outlook on life that is subjective, internally motivated, imaginative. Contrast with EXTRACEPTION.

intracerebral Into or within the brain.

intracerebroventricular Into or within any of the cerebral ventricles.

intracranial stimulation (ICS) ELECTRICAL BRAIN STIMULATION.

intradimensional shift REVERSAL *LEARNING.

intrafusal fibres Muscle fibres that function as stretch receptors. They are arranged in parallel with EXTRAFUSAL FIBRES and detect the length of a muscle. Also called *muscle spindles*.

intramural Lit., within the walls; hence, pertaining to events occurring inside the boundaries of an institution.

intramuscular Into or within a muscle.

intransitivity Lit., the state of being incapable of passing over or through. Hence, a characteristic of a relation between elements x, y and z such that x is related to y in some fashion and y is related to z in like fashion but without it necessarily being the case that x is so related to z. Liking is such a relation: the fact that one person, x, likes another, y, and y likes z does not imply that x necessarily likes z. *Intransitivity* implies that the scale being used is multidimensional and the relation multicausal. Contrast with TRANSITIVITY.

intraperitoneal Into or within the peritoneal cavity (the space that houses the abdominal organs).

intrapersonal intelligence MULTIPLE INTELLIGENCES THEORY.

intraocular modification An umbrella term covering any change in the visual signal due to the characteristics of the eye, e.g. refraction by the cornea and lens, light scattering, light absorption.

intrapsychic 1 Of anything assumed to arise or take place within the mind. **2** Of interactions between internal, covert factors; e.g. *intrapsychic conflicts* are conflicts between beliefs, needs, desires, etc.

intrapsychic ataxia MENTAL *ATAXIA.

intraverbal In Skinner's behaviourist analysis of language, a class of verbal operants made up of social responses and incidental conversational utterances.

intraversion A common misspelling of INTROVERSION produced by the failure to

intuition

appreciate the distinction between INTRA- and INTRO-.

intrinsic From the Latin, meaning *inwardly* or *inward*. Used generally to characterize a property of something that reflects the essential nature of the thing. The connotation is that the property derives none of its character from outside sources. Contrast with EXTRINSIC (1).

intrinsic eye muscles EYE MUSCLES.

intrinsic interest Quite literally, interest in an object or an activity that derives from a desire for that object or activity for its own sake, e.g. interest in learning to paint simply for aesthetic pleasure. Contrast with EXTRINSIC INTEREST.

intrinsic motivation A term used to refer to the motivation for any behaviour that is dependent on factors that are internal in origin. Intrinsic motivation usually derives from feelings of satisfaction and fulfilment, not from external rewards. Contrast with EXTRINSIC MOTIVATION and see the discussion under MOTIVATION.

intrinsic validity VALIDITY, INTRINSIC.

intro- Prefix meaning *moving within* or *toward the inside*. Distinguish from INTRA-, from which the notion of movement is absent.

introjection 1 Generally, the process by which aspects of the external world are absorbed into or incorporated within the self, the internal representation then taking over the psychological functions of the external objects. 2 Specifically, in psychoanalysis, that process whereby the parent figures become the external objects and the *introjects* (as they are called) are the values of the parents; the process here is assumed to lead to the formation of the superego. 3 Reversing the directional flow of 1 and 2, a process of projecting one's own characteristics into inanimate objects; see ANIMISM.

intromission Placing or inserting one part inside another.

intropunitive Characterizing the tendency to react to frustration by directing anger and blame toward oneself, the internally focused emotions often being experienced as guilt or shame. Contrast with EXTRAPUNITIVE and compare with IMPUNITIVE.

introspection 1 Generally, the act of looking inward, the examination of one's mental experiences. 2 The report of such an inward glance, specifically the mental contents of one's consciousness. See INTROSPECTIONISM.

introspectionism Roughly synonymous with STRUCTURALISM (1), the early school of psychology founded on the method of careful and systematic introspection. The basic operation was to present trained observers with controlled stimuli and to have them report back their introspections about covert mental processes while perceiving them. As several critics have noted, introspection is not a true examination of the contents of consciousness, as its proponents claimed, but a retrospective glance back at that which has passed through consciousness.

introversion A turning inward. The term is used in personality theory to refer to the tendency to shrink from social contacts and become preoccupied with one's own thoughts. Although presumably a normal characteristic, there are many who feel that extreme forms of introversion border on the pathological. Curiously, in our culture, such suspicions are rarely voiced of those exhibiting extreme EXTRAVERSION.

introversion–extraversion EXTRAVERSION–INTROVERSION.

introvert A label for an individual who displays the behaviours discussed under INTROVERSION. Jung also used it for one of his personality types.

intrusion response (or **error**) In an ordered or serial recall experiment any response that either (a) was not in the original list or (b) occurred in the wrong position in the list.

intuition A mode of understanding or knowing characterized as direct and immediate and occurring without conscious thought or judgement. There are two distinct connotations which often accompany this term: (a) that the process is unmediated and somehow mystical; (b) that it is a response to subtle cues and relationships apprehended implicitly, unconsciously. The former borders on the unscientific and is not recommended, although it is certainly common enough in the nontechnical literature; the latter hints at a number of difficult but fascinating problems in the study of human behaviour in the presence of complex situations. See here IMPLICIT *LEARNING, LEARNING WITHOUT *AWARENESS and INTUITIVE.

intuitive 1 Pertaining to INTUITION. **2** Characterizing belief and knowledge systems held by children and by most laypersons within a culture, e.g. *intuitive physics* is the non-scientist's understanding of the physical world. Intuitive knowledge systems tend to be more than simple, situation-specific rules. They typically have abstract features and general principles but these are not as abstract and formalized as those held by specialists in the field. Note that these systems need not be explicit and conscious and, indeed, most are held implicitly. The terms *naïve* and *folk* are common synonyms. See FOLK PSYCHOLOGY.

intuitive type One of Jung's hypothesized personality types. See FUNCTION TYPES.

in utero Latin for *within the uterus*.

in vacuo Latin for *in a vacuum*. Often used metaphorically to refer to operations or processes carried out without knowledge of related factors.

invalid 1 Failing to fulfil the canons of logic; a term used of any statement, proposition, argument or method that does not follow logically from the premises. **2** By extension, of any test or other evaluative device that fails to measure what it was intended or designed to measure. See VALIDITY et seq.

invalidate 1 In logic, to render an argument or conclusion invalid, to prove it false. **2** By extension, to demonstrate the lack of worth of an experiment and its conclusions either by demonstrating the lack of coherent theoretical analysis of the problem it was designed to explicate or by showing that the procedures used were improper.

invariable (or invariant) hues Hues that do not show the BEZOLD-BRÜCKE EFFECT, those that do not change with changes in illuminance. Three spectral hues – 478 nm (a yellow), 503 nm (a green) and 578 nm (a red) – and one extraspectral hue that is a mixture of short and long wavelengths (a purple) are invariant.

invariance Generally, the quality of not changing. The term is most often used with the qualifier *relative*. That is, few things in this world are truly invariant but some display greater invariance, greater consistency from circumstance to circumstance, than others. In general, in the study of perception and learning, those aspects of the stimulus world that display greater invariance are learned most quickly and easily.

invasive 1 Generally, pertaining to any therapy or procedure that invades the body in some direct manner, particularly surgical. **2** Pertaining to tumours or growths that have a tendency to spread. Contrast with NONINVASIVE.

inventory An ordered listing or cataloguing of items. The term applies broadly; any check-list, instrument, test or questionnaire that assesses traits, opinions, beliefs, aptitudes, behaviours, etc. may be so labelled, e.g. the *Minnesota Multiphasic Personality Inventory*.

inverse correlation An occasional synonym of NEGATIVE *CORRELATION.

inverse factor analysis FACTOR ANALYSIS, INVERSE.

inverse nystagmus ROTATIONAL *NYSTAGMUS.

inversion 1 Generally, any process of turning inside out or upside down, or the result of such a process. **2** In statistics, transposing a series of numbers. **3** In mathematics, a momentary reversal of a function or the curve of a function. **4** In genetics, CHROMOSOMAL ALTERATIONS. **5** Shorthand for the more specific SEXUAL *INVERSION. **6** In older psychoanalytic writings, HOMOSEXUALITY.

inversion effect The generalization that visual displays that are inverted are more difficult to process, recall and recognize than when presented in the usual upright orientation. It is particularly strong for faces.

inversion of affect Sudden switching between two emotions that are at opposite poles on a continuum, usually love and hatred. Typically seen as a sign of a deep ambivalence.

inversion, sexual A more-or-less obsolete

term that has been used at various times to mean: **1** Hermaphroditism. **2** Transvestism. **3** Homosexuality, specifically the taking on of the role of the opposite sex in sexual acts.

inverted factor analysis INVERSE *FACTOR ANALYSIS.

inverted Oedipus (complex) In psychoanalysis, an OEDIPUS COMPLEX in which the parent of one's gender becomes the object of libidinal attachment.

inverted sadism Repressed *sadism*. Note that, as the term is used, it refers to an unconscious state the existence of which is hypothesized on the basis of an extreme withdrawal from any conscious display of aggression, violence, hostility, etc.

inverted-U curve (or **distribution**) Quite literally, any distribution the curve of which is shaped like an inverted letter U, with high frequency for moderate values and low frequency for both very low and very high values. A classic example is performance of a task as a function of arousal level; performance is optimal at moderate levels and drops off with either increases or decreases in arousal.

investment From the Latin, meaning *clothing*. **1** In psychoanalysis, an approximate synonym of *cathexis*; the connotation is of expanding psychic energy, of 'dressing up' an object or figure with one's affect. If one has fear of an authority figure then the fear is said to be *invested in* that figure. **2** In physiology, a covering or sheath.

in vitro Latin for *in glass*. Hence, a term used to refer to biological or physiological tests or experiments carried out in isolation (e.g. in a test tube) rather than in the whole organism. Contrast with IN VIVO.

in vivo Latin for *in the living body*. Compare with IN VITRO.

in vivo desensitization DESENSITIZATION PROCEDURE.

involuntary 1 Characterizing that which is not volitional, that which occurs because of external compulsions. **2** Characterizing those psychological processes or behaviours that are not under voluntary control. Involuntary behaviours and processes are typically: (a) reflex-like and elicited from an organism by a particular stimulus (see here CLASSICAL CONDITIONING); or (b) FIXED-ACTION PATTERNS, which are part of the genetic make-up of a particular species; or (c) extremely well-learned, automatized responses that occur without the sense that one has willed them.

involuntary memory MEMORY, INVOLUNTARY.

involution From the Latin, meaning *roll into*, used in the sense of a degeneration, a retrograde change, a turning inward. An occasional synonym of *menopause*.

involutional depression An obsolete term once applied to depressions that occurred in women following the onset of menopause (see INVOLUTION). Similarly obsolete are the terms *involutional psychotic reaction* and *involutional melancholia*.

involutional melancholia INVOLUTIONAL DEPRESSION.

involutional psychotic reaction INVOLUTIONAL DEPRESSION.

I/O Abbreviation for: **1** The field of INDUSTRIAL/ORGANIZATIONAL PSYCHOLOGY. **2** INPUT/OUTPUT.

ion A charged molecule; *anions* have negative charge, *cations* positive.

ionotropic receptors Receptors that operate by directly opening *ion* channels that allow specific ions to flow in and out of a cell. Compare with METABOTROPIC RECEPTORS.

Iowa gambling task An experimental task used in studies of decision-making. The subject is presented with stacks of cards and told that each card drawn will yield a monetary reward. However, they are also told that a small percentage of cards drawn will incur losses. The amounts of the rewards and losses actually differ across stacks of cards, with two of the stacks ultimately yielding a net gain and the other two a net loss. After some trials, healthy adults will switch to drawing only from the stacks that yield a net gain, but patients with orbitofrontal cortex dysfunction will generally fail to make this behavioural shift even once they realize that they are losing money.

IPA INTERNATIONAL PHONETIC ALPHABET.

iprindole A tricyclic compound used as an ANTIDEPRESSANT DRUG.

iproniazide A monoamine oxidase inhibitor used as an ANTIDEPRESSANT DRUG.

ips(a)- Prefix meaning *of one's own, of the self, the same.* var., *ips(o)-*.

ipsative Reflected or measured against the self. An ipsative personality test, for example, might reveal that an individual has a greater need for achievement than for affiliation, but not reveal whether either need is high or low relative to national norms.

ipseity Selfhood, the sense of having an individual identity

ipsilateral Pertaining to the same side. Also called *homolateral*. Contrast with CONTRALATERAL.

ips(o)- IPSA-.

IPSP Abbreviation for *inhibitory postsynaptic potential*. See POSTSYNAPTIC POTENTIAL.

IQ INTELLIGENCE QUOTIENT. Probably the best-known abbreviation in psychology.

ir- IN-.

iris The pigmented muscular membrane that projects from the ciliary body of the eye. The aperture in the centre is the pupil, which adjusts to control the amount of light entering the eye.

iris reflex PUPILLARY REFLEX.

iritic reflex PUPILLARY REFLEX.

iron deficiency anaemia A condition of impaired cognitive development in childhood caused by a deficiency of iron in the diet.

irradiation The central notion here is diffusion or radiation of something from a central point of origin, and all specialized uses of the term involve this idea of spread. **1** In optics, the spreading of radiant energy from a light source; measured in relation to the radiant flux per unit area. **2** In perception, the phenomenon whereby a bright stimulus appears larger when viewed against a dark background. **3** In physiology, the spread of afferent neural impulses. **4** In Pavlovian conditioning: (a) The elicitation of a conditioned response by stimulation similar but not identical to the original stimulus. This use is essentially synonymous with that of STIMULUS *GENERALIZATION. (b) Spread of cortical activity from a central point. Note that this last meaning was introduced by Pavlov to explain that given in 4(a).

irradiation theory An out-of-date term for a theory of learning that makes essentially the same assumptions as TRIAL-AND-ERROR *LEARNING, which itself is also out of date as a general theory of learning.

irrational In violation of the rules of logic. Typically used of such cognitive acts as thought, judgement and decision-making that do not follow the canons of logic, with the (often implicit) assumption that RATIONAL thought or judgements could reasonably be expected under the conditions. Distinguish subtly from NONRATIONAL, used when reason and logic are seemingly absent but not necessarily violated. A common connotation of *irrational* is that acts so described are assumed to have been carried out under the pressures of emotional factors that have, somehow, overridden the logical, rational faculties – a connotation which is certainly legitimate in many contexts but which should probably not be applied as widely as it is.

irrational type RATIONAL TYPE.

irresistible-impulse test A legal principle set in 1922 in the USA for the establishment of an INSANITY DEFENCE. It states that a person is not to be held responsible for a criminal act if it can be shown that he or she acted through an 'irresistible impulse' which he or she was unable to control because of a mental disorder. It has been rejected by most courts and is rarely used today.

irresponsibility The basis of an INSANITY DEFENCE. In forensic psychiatry and legal parlance, the principle that an individual is not to be adjudged guilty of a crime if it can be determined that the normal conditions under which he or she could be held responsible for his or her actions do not, in fact, pertain. Various legal precedents have been established (and revoked) over the years; see e.g. ALI DEFENCE RULING, DURHAM RULE, IRRESISTIBLE-IMPULSE TEST, MCNAGHTEN RULE.

irritability 1 Generally, excitability. All specialized meanings reflect this sense. **2** Of all living tissue, the property of responding to stimulation. **3** By extension, the property of an organ, muscle or part thereof such that it responds to particular classes of stimulation. **4** Of persons, excessive responsiveness, oversensitivity, impatience.

IRT 1 INTERRESPONSE TIME. **2** ITEM RESPONSE THEORY.

ischaemia Reduced blood flow to a part of the body. var., *ischemia*.

ischemic attack, transient A temporary reduction of blood flow to the brain, often an indicator that a more serious stroke is imminent. The symptoms are similar to those of a stroke, and often include visual blurring and facial numbness.

Ishihari colour plates A series of colour plates printed in various hues such that coherent figures (e.g. letters, numbers) are visible to the normal eye but not to the colour-blind or colour-deficient eye. The plates consist of dots that are carefully selected to control saturation and brightness so that only the hue dimension reflects the figures. See also STILLING TEST.

ISI INTERSTIMULUS INTERVAL.

island of Reil INSULA.

-ism A richly polysemous, noun-forming suffix used to denote *usage, action, practice, condition, principle, characteristic* or *doctrine*. The most common is the last of these and, as some wit put it, if you have enough -ists in agreement you have an -ism.

iso- Combining form meaning *equal* or *the same*.

isochronal 1 Equal in rate, frequency or time of occurrence. **2** Equal in CHRONAXIE. var., *isochronous*.

isocoria The normal condition in which both eyes show equal pupil size even though there may be different amounts of light falling on the two eyes.

isocortex NEOCORTEX.

isolated explosive disorder INTERMITTENT EXPLOSIVE DISORDER.

isolation 1 Generally, separateness, apartness. The meaning here is carried into several specialized usages: **2** In genetics, the condition in which a breeding population is separated from other members of the species. This separation may be brought about by complex social/cultural factors or by simple geographical conditions. Such a group is said to be made up of *breeding isolates*. **3** In psychoanalysis, a defence mechanism that is assumed to function by severing the conscious psychological ties between some unacceptable act or impulse and its original memory source. In this sense, the original experience is not forgotten but it is separated from the affect originally associated with it. The classical theory views this mechanism as a common one in obsessional neuroses. Also called *isolation of affect*. **4** In Jung's terms, a feeling of psychological estrangement from others. Also called *psychic isolation*. Jung argued that it derived from deep secrets, originally from the collective unconscious, which one feels must be kept from others.

isolation amentia An obsolete term for the mental retardation observed in cases of anaclitic depression.

isolation effect VON RESTORFF EFFECT.

isolation of affect ISOLATION (3).

isometric contraction (or **twitch**) Muscle contraction that causes tension but no movement, as when pushing against a wall.

isomorphism 1 In mathematics, a formal point-by-point relationship between two systems. **2** In Gestalt psychology, the hypothesis that there is such a structural similarity between excitatory fields in the cortex and conscious experience. Note that the correspondence here is not presumed to be between the physical stimulus and the brain but between the *perception* of the stimulus and the brain.

isophilia Nonsexual attraction toward and affection for members of one's own sex. Distinguish from HOMOSEXUALITY.

isophonic contour Lit., equal-sound contour. The line or contour representing the set of coincidences between values of separate dimensions of sounds that are perceived as identical. The point about an isophonic contour is that the dimensions of sound co-vary: loudness, for example, is not merely a function of sound pressure but is dependent on the frequency of the tone. To take one case, a tone of 400 Hz at 61 db is heard as equal in loudness to a tone of 600 Hz at 59 db.

isotonic Lit., of equal tension. Hence, an *isotonic contraction* is a muscle contraction in which there is equal tension in a muscle throughout a movement, as in a simple lifting of the hand; and an *isotonic solution* is a solution in which the osmotic pressure between the fluid and a cell suspended in it is such that there is no transmission across the cell membrane. Contrast with HYPERTONIC and HYPOTONIC.

isotropic Drawn equally in all directions. By extension, not fixed, channelled or constrained, therefore influenced by a variety of factors. Most commonly used to describe functions that are not rigid or encapsulated but free to vary.

-ist Suffix used to denote *agent* or *actor*, an advocate of an -ISM.

It **1** Originally a psychosomatic entity, an inner power or psychic force that was assumed to shape both body and mind. **2** Later, in classical psychoanalysis, the ID.

ITA INITIAL TEACHING ALPHABET.

itch Itching is, oddly enough, a source of much interest and confusion. It is, as we all know, a rather attention-demanding condition although little is known about the underlying physiology. Presumably, an itch is produced by a fairly low level of irritation of free nerve endings in the skin. The irritation may be chemical, electrical or mechanical, although itching has also been reported in the phantom limbs of amputees, indicating that a central component is involved as well. The two main unanswered questions are: (a) What is the relationship between itch and pain? (b) Why does scratching relieve an itch?

item analysis Generally, the detailed analysis of the individual items of a test or a questionnaire for the purpose of assessing their reliability and validity. Such analysis can focus on content and form or it can be carried out quantitatively in terms of how effectively each item contributes to the overall reliability and validity of the test. In the broadest sense the term covers any analysis, including that concerned with factors such as item ambiguity, difficulty, time components, etc. In a narrower sense, the term is used specifically to refer to an assessment of how effectively each individual item contributes to the overall validity of a test. See VALIDITY.

item difficulty Quite literally, the difficulty of an item in a test. It is defined in terms of the frequency with which the individuals who attempt the item answer it correctly.

itemized rating scale RATING SCALE, ITEMIZED.

item reliability RELIABILITY, ITEM.

item response theory The theory of testing and test construction that maintains that items on a test should be related to the parameters of a construct. The theory supports the use of ITEM ANALYSIS that focuses on how each item of a test is related to the underlying or latent construct. Also called *latent trait theory*.

item validity The degree to which an individual item in a test assesses what it is designed to assess. See VALIDITY et seq.

-itis A suffix denoting *inflammation*.

ITPA ILLINOIS TEST OF PSYCHOLINGUISTIC ABILITIES.

IU INTERVAL OF UNCERTAINTY.

IV INDEPENDENT *VARIABLE.

J In Hullian theory, an abbreviation for delay of reinforcement.

jabberwocky Laboratory slang for artificially constructed verbal materials that are formed using English function words and morphological forms to represent the structure of a sentence frame but using only nonsense for the content words. The term, of course, comes from Lewis Carroll's famous poem in which extensive use of this technique is made ("Twas brillig, and the slithy toves...'). Jabberwocky, perhaps not surprisingly, is much easier to read than pure nonsense (i.e. without the function words) but more difficult than ordinary prose.

Jacksonian epilepsy (and related terms) See EPILEPSY, JACKSONIAN et seq.

Jacksonian march JACKSONIAN MOTOR *EPILEPSY.

Jacksonian motor epilepsy EPILEPSY, JACKSONIAN MOTOR.

Jacksonian sensory epilepsy EPILEPSY, JACKSONIAN SENSORY.

Jackson's principle (or **law**) The generalization that the degree of resistance of a mental function to disease or natural deterioration is directly related to the evolutionary antiquity of that function; that is, recently evolved cognitive functions are lost first, those of greater evolutionary age are lost later. Analogous principles have been argued to hold for learned behaviours: the earlier in an individual's life something is learned the more robust that knowledge will be in the face of disease or other insult.

Jacobson's organ VOMERONASAL SYSTEM.

jactation A rare term for an extreme restlessness with uncontrollable jerky movements.

jamais vu French for *never seen*. An illusory experience in which the familiar suddenly feels unfamiliar. The experience is not uncommon in the aura phase that often precedes an epileptic seizure. Compare with DÉJÀ VU

Jamesian Characteristic of or pertaining to the work, theories and overall orientation of the American psychologist/philosopher William James (1842–1910). Although there is no broad, structured theory associated with James's work, the adjectival form is used with regard to the particular point of view that formed the empirical and philosophical underpinnings of his intellectual life. Specifically, these are pragmatism and functionalism, a strong affiliation with evolutionary theory and an open-mindedness concerning novel and often unorthodox views. For a glimpse of the Jamesian point of view on a few topics see STREAM OF CONSCIOUSNESS, THEORIES OF *EMOTION, TIP-OF-THE-TONGUE STATE.

James–Lange theory of emotion THEORIES OF *EMOTION.

jargon 1 Speech that is meaningless to others. Thus, the specialized language of a group or profession is jargon to one not trained in it and the nonsensical babble of some aphasics is jargon to all. **2** A type of prelanguage vocalization observed in some infants whereby they babble in extended 'phrases' which have an intonation contour like that of real adult sentences. To a casual listener it sounds at first as though the infant is actually talking. Note that 1 generally implies that there is a meaningful message there somewhere, whereas 2 does not.

jargon aphasia APHASIA, JARGON.

J coefficient A measure of the validity of the several component tests in a vocational test battery. The technique is based on correlations between test scores and job preference (the J is for *job*) with the special feature that each of the specific aspects of a given job is weighted as to its relative importance by both supervisors and workers. The J coefficient is an index of the SYNTHETIC *VALIDITY of a test battery.

J curve Generally, any curve of a frequency distribution that when plotted is shaped approximately like the capital letter J. That is, distributions have very low frequencies at the low values and rapidly increasing frequencies at successively higher values. There is also a *reverse J curve*, in which the low values reflect high frequencies and vice versa.

jealousy Generally, any emotional state classified as a special form of anxiety and assumed to derive from a lack of sense of security in the affections of one who is loved. The jealousy is directed toward a third party, the rival who is perceived as garnering the affections of the object of love. Distinguish from ENVY, where there need be no loved one, merely a desire for things possessed by the rival.

jigsaw classroom Perhaps the earliest and best-known way of organizing a classroom and a lesson plan in order to promote COOPERATIVE *LEARNING (1). It involves giving a diverse group of students a task to complete and making each child responsible for one piece of the puzzle. The essential component in the technique is structuring the classroom so that students succeed by working together rather than by competing. See COOPERATIVE *LEARNING (3).

Jimmy legs RESTLESS LEG SYNDROME.

jitter AUDITORY *FLICKER.

jnd JUST NOTICEABLE DIFFERENCE.

job analysis A loose term for the study of particular aspects of a given job. Those aspects may range from the tasks and duties of the position, to an examination of the desirable qualities of an employee, to the conditions of employment including pay, promotion opportunities, vacations, etc.

Jocasta complex In Greek mythology, Jocasta was both the mother and wife of Oedipus. In psychoanalysis, the term is used for a mother's libidinous fixation on her son. See OEDIPUS COMPLEX.

John Henry effect The tendency, occasionally seen in industrial settings, for people who know they are in a control group to put forth extraordinary efforts in an attempt to outdo those in the experimental group. Its occurrence can negate the purpose of a control group. The effect is named after the mythical steelworker whose name is a symbol of superhuman effort.

joint event In probability theory, any event that is the simultaneous occurrence of any two (or more) other events. For example, a black five dealt from a deck of cards is a joint event, being both a black card and a card with five marks.

joint probability The probability of occurrence of a JOINT EVENT; it is given as the product of the probabilities of each of the specific events that comprise the joint event.

joking relationship A social relationship that permits the telling of jokes, playing tricks, teasing or displaying a privileged familiarity in a socially approved manner that would be regarded as offensive and insulting if engaged in by persons outside the relationship. It is basically what permits Jews to tell anti-Semitic jokes to each other and Blacks to call each other 'nigger' without offence.

Jost's law The generalization that (a) within a given time interval material learned recently is more likely to be forgotten than memories of greater antiquity and (b) practice with material facilitates recall of older memories more than it does more recent memories. The term is largely obsolete, and both of these principles are now captured by the conceptualization of human memory as comprised of a SHORT-TERM *MEMORY and a LONG-TERM *MEMORY. See these terms for clarification.

Joubert syndrome A genetic disorder marked by a failure of the VERMIS to develop normally. Symptoms include discoordinated motor movements (ATAXIA), abnormal breathing and mental retardation. Various physical deformities may present including extra digits, cleft palate and an abnormal tongue.

judgement 1 Generally, the process of forming an opinion or reaching a conclusion based on the available material; the opinion or conclusion so reached. 2 The hypothesized mental faculty that functions so as to carry out such judgement. This meaning is only found in older writings. 3 In logic, a statement of the relation between symbols in sentence form. This sense has now been taken over by the term PROPOSITION. 4 A critical evaluation of some thing, event or person. 5 In psychophysics, the decision concerning the presence or absence of a signal, or estimations of its intensity relative to other stimuli.

Juke The fictitious name of a large extended family allegedly riddled with all manner of unsavoury characters, social misfits, criminals and degenerates, fully half of whom were supposedly 'feeble-minded'. Studies of this family and the equally (in)famous KALLI-KAKS were carried out in the late 19th and early 20th centuries and were taken by many as providing strong evidence for the hereditarian position on intelligence, temperament, socialization, etc. The actual investigations, however, were so badly performed, and the role of the environment was so thoroughly neglected in the analyses, that they are no longer taken seriously. See HERED-ITY–ENVIRONMENT CONTROVERSY.

Julesz's stereogram STEREOGRAM.

jumping stand LASHLEY JUMPING STAND.

juncture In linguistics, a SUPRASEGMENTAL that marks the manner in which speech sounds are joined, specifically the pausing patterns. For example, by changing the pause point 'light housekeeper' becomes 'lighthouse keeper'.

Jungian Pertaining to or representative of the analytical psychology of Carl Gustav Jung (1875–1961). Although Jung wrote broadly on such diverse topics as word association, mythology, religion, telepathy, spiritualism and flying saucers, the adjectival form of his name is primarily associated with an approach to psychoanalysis that placed, relative to Freud's, little emphasis on the role of sex and sexual impulses and focused instead on the hypothesized deep, inherited, *collective unconscious* with its universal ideas or images, the *archetypes*. Jungian

analysis is of the 'deep' variety and concerns itself with rich interpretation of symbols and makes extensive use of dreams.

junk-box classification A sobriquet applied (critically) to any of a number of diagnostic classifications, especially *aphasia*, *autism* and *schizophrenia*. The implications of the label are that the diagnostic category does not really represent a well-defined syndrome (or disease or condition) but rather is a loosely constructed conceptual 'junk box' into which all manner of individual cases are thrown because of superficial similarities (e.g. all aphasics show some form of language loss) and/or because the diagnostician frankly is unclear about how else to classify them.

justification Generally, the rationale for action, choice or belief or the result of such. The term is used widely with varying connotations. In Piagetian theory it is a neutral term for a person's explanation of an answer, particularly one given by a child. In clinical settings the connotation is defensive implying that the client is providing an inappropriate excuse for knowingly indefensible actions or feelings. In moral philosophy it suggests a carefully thought through set of principles for established ethical standards.

justification of effort The tendency for people to report greater liking of an object or a status that they had to work hard to achieve than one which came easily. Apparently, we need to justify expending all that effort, so we glorify the object of our labours. This tendency can be seen as a specific manifestation of COGNITIVE DISSONANCE.

just noticeable difference (jnd) The difference between two stimuli that is, under properly controlled experimental conditions, just noticeable. Given the variability of our sensory systems, a stable value cannot be found for the difference. Rather, the jnd is determined to be that difference between two stimuli that is detected as often as it is undetected. Thus, it is viewed as a statistical estimate of the resolving power of a sensory system. For more detail on usage here see the discussion under THRESHOLD and MEASUREMENT OF *THRESHOLD.

just-world bias The belief that we live in a

just world and that life really is fair. People who hold this bias tend to blame the victims of crimes or disasters on the grounds that those who suffer must, for some reason, deserve to suffer.

juxtaposition 1 Generally, the positioning of two things next to each other. **2** In Piagetian theory, the cognitive tendency of a young child to tie elements to each other in a kind of primitive 'and then' manner rather than see causal or logical links between them. Contrast this process with SYNCRETISM (2).

K

K In Hullian theory, incentive motivation.

K' In Hullian theory, physical incentive.

k 1 The COEFFICIENT OF *ALIENATION. **2** Abbreviation for KILO-.

kainate One of the ionotropic GLUTAMATE RECEPTORS. Less well understood than the others, kainate receptors activate postsynaptic membranes but also have an inhibitory function in modulating release of GABA through a presynaptic mechanism.

kainic acid An excitatory amino acid that stimulates kainate GLUTAMATE RECEPTORS. In large doses it is neurotoxic and can overstimulate neurons and destroy their cell bodies.

kairos Within existential psychology, a critical moment of decision in life, a moment of compelling personal experience when the meanings and values attached to living undergo transformation and when decisive personality changes occur. See also EXISTENTIALISM and EXISTENTIAL THERAPY.

kakosmia CACOSMIA.

Kallikak A pseudonym used of two branches of a family tree both of which ostensibly sprang from the loins of one man. The 'good Kallikaks' (who were all, according to H. H. Goddard's report in 1912, fine, moral, upstanding members of the community) supposedly came from his marriage with a middle-class woman; the 'bad Kallikaks' (who, in Goddard's analysis, were nearly all degenerates, feeble-minded, criminals and/or vagrants) descended from his brief affair with a retarded woman. Goddard's eugenicist analysis was so tainted by his own peculiar prejudices concerning the role of heredity in shaping behaviour that this once-celebrated case is no longer of any scientific value. See also JUKE and the discussion under HEREDITY–ENVIRONMENT CONTROVERSY.

Kanner's syndrome A term occasionally used for INFANTILE *AUTISM.

kappa A statistical index of INTERRATER *RELIABILITY used to determine whether the obtained degree of agreement is expected by chance.

kappa effect An illusion based on the interaction between time and physical space. In the classic case three equally bright lights A, B and C are arranged so that A and B are a bit closer together than B and C. If they are flashed in succession with identical time intervals, the time between A and B will be perceived as shorter than between B and C. There is an analogous 'real world' effect; if one takes two trips of equal duration the one that covered less distance will seem to have taken less time. See also TAU EFFECT.

kary(o)- Combining form meaning *nucleus*.

karyotype A systematic array of the chromosomes of a single cell in graphic form.

kata Variation of CATA-.

katasexuality A rare PARAPHILIA characterized by a sexual preference for deceased persons (also called *necrophilia*) or animals (also called *bestiality*).

K complex A sudden, brief, high-amplitude wave-form in the EEG of a sleeping person. Such wave-forms typically occur at about one-minute intervals during Stage 2 SLEEP but can be triggered by outside noises.

Keller plan A form of personalised instruction developed by the behaviourist Fred Keller. Based on principles like shaping by successive approximations and the careful use of reinforcement, it once enjoyed considerable popularity. It is little used today, largely because of any compelling evidence that it worked any better than traditional educational methods.

Kendall tests Any of several nonparametric measures of correlation useful when data do not satisfy the assumptions of standard correlational analyses. See e.g. COEFFICIENT OF *CONCORDANCE, TAU COEFFICIENT OF CORRELATION.

Kent–Rosanoff List (or Test) A free-association test originally developed for assessing imagery and thought patterns in which an individual's associations to a standardized list of words are compared with a set of norms. Although the test itself is not in common use today, the norms continue to be used in studies of memory.

keratoconus A condition in which the cornea thins and develops weak spots and distortions. It can cause pain and vision loss.

kernel sentence A simple, active, declarative sentence. The term comes from early conceptualizations of TRANSFORMATIONAL *GRAMMAR in which such sentences were seen as linguistically (and perhaps psycholinguistically) significant because they are derived from the base with the fewest transformations.

kernicterus A neurological disorder resulting from excess bilirubin in the blood during infancy. Symptoms include lethargy and lack of appetite.

ketones Organic acids that are broken down into carbon dioxide and water, releasing energy in the process. They result from the breakdown of fats and, along with glucose, are readily metabolized by the brain and serve as an important energy source. Also known as *keto bodies* and *keto acids*.

ketosteroid A steroid produced by the adrenal cortices and the gonads.

key By extension from locksmithery, any device that contains information necessary to 'unlock' a message, to understand something. Hence: **1** The set of rules or principles that allows one to encode and decode messages. **2** The set of correct answers in a test. **3** The legend on a graph, table or chart that reveals the significance of the notation system in use. **4** A signal that sets the context within which a particular event is to be regarded; e.g. an art class is keyed to the acceptance of the nudity of a model in a nonsexual manner. **5** In operant-conditioning studies with pigeons, a small disc that a bird must peck in order to receive reinforcement.

Kiddie Mach Test A test designed to assess MACHIAVELLIANISM in children. See also MACHIAVELLIAN SCALE.

kids' culture A half-joking term with a serious and interesting reference. It refers to the notion that children have their own culture, with social rules, games, specialized language devices, rituals, etc. Each person passes through the culture and is appropriately acculturated but only temporarily. An adult peering back to childhood finds it as difficult to apprehend fully the culture as does an anthropologist studying a culture very different from his or her own.

kilo- Combining form meaning *1,000*, or *multiplied by 1,000*. abbrev., *k*.

kin RELATIVES (4).

kinaesthesis The sensory modality that picks up information from the muscles, joints and tendons. The kinaesthetic sense provides feedback about movements, muscle tension, posture and position using sensors such as stress receptors in muscles and joints. Occasionally it is used as a synonym of PROPRIOCEPTION although, properly, that term is more inclusive and also covers the sense of balance or equilibrium. The area of study is called *kinaesthesia*. var., *kinesthesis*.

kinaesthetic intelligence MULTIPLE INTELLIGENCES THEORY.

kinaesthetics Lit., *feelings of motion*. An umbrella term for the sensations originating in muscles, tendons and joints. Along with PROPRIOCEPTION and EQUILIBRIUM (2), kinaesthetics make up the sensory system that acquires its information from INTEROCEPTORS.

kinase Any *enzyme* that produces movement. The term is used as a combining form in physiology and physiological psychology.

kine- Combining form indicating *motion*, *movement*.

kinematics The study of motion.

kineme KINESICS (1).

kinemorph KINESICS (1).

kinephantom A movement illusion, particularly of shadows. The most common example is the experience of a rotating spoked object like a fan or wheel appearing to move in reverse direction.

kinesia Motion sickness.

-kinesia Combining form meaning *movement*.

kinesics **1** The study of the movements of the body and their communicative functions. The approach, perhaps not surprisingly, shares some interesting parallels with descriptive linguistics. For example, it is possible to identify *kinemes*, which are analogues of *phonemes* in that they are classes of movements which are treated as conceptual categories inasmuch as variations within them are nonmeaningful. Combinations or sequences of kinemes make up *kinemorphs*, which are analogues of *morphemes*. **2** Those facets of movement and muscle perception readily accessible to consciousness.

kinesiology The study of human movement. An interdisciplinary science, it incorporates physiology, psychology, sociology, the neurosciences and biomechanics.

kinetic Pertaining to physical motion.

kinetic depth effect A perceptual effect in which a visual pattern appears to be flat (two-dimensional) when stationary but when moved gives rise to an experience of depth (three dimensional).

kin group A group of persons recognized as being related by blood or marriage.

King's (or Queen's) English The idealized, standard form of 'proper' English of Great Britain. In studies of dialectology it is used as the basis for phonetic, semantic and syntactic distinctions in other regional and social class dialects. See also RECEIVED PRONUNCIATION, STANDARD ENGLISH.

kinocilia In the inner ear, the tallest of the hairs projecting from the surfaces of the cells of the semicircular canals. Compare with STEREOCILIA.

kin selection SELECTION, KIN.

kin selection altruism ALTRUISM.

kinship A general term used to refer to any social relationship based upon family, including consanguinal (blood) relationships and those recognized by cultural convention, e.g. marriage and adoption. The roles, rights and obligations that such related individuals have with respect to each other are determined by their culture and not purely by the closeness of biological relationship.

kinship, ritual A kinship relation based on a societally defined relationship. The most common example is godparent–godchild.

Kleine–Levin syndrome A syndrome characterized by HYPERSOMNIA and BULIMIA. Typically observed in adolescent males.

kleptolagnia Sexual desire and excitement associated with stealing.

kleptomania An IMPULSE-CONTROL DISORDER characterized by recurrent inability to resist impulses to steal. A defining feature of the disorder is that there is no immediate need or use for what is stolen. Typically there is little or no planning involved, merely a sudden, acute impulse which is acted on.

Klinefelter's syndrome A chromosomal anomaly characterized genotypically by an XXY pattern in the sex chromosomes. Phenotypically such persons are male, but the penis may be unusually small and the testicles abnormally small and often undescended, and there are often marked feminine characteristics such as breast development.

klismaphilia A PARAPHILIA characterized by the deriving of sexual stimulation from having an enema administered.

kluge Hans, der CLEVER HANS.

Klüver–Bucy syndrome A collection of bizarre behaviours including visual *agnosia*, compulsive exploration, hypersexuality and profound changes in emotionality. It is not infrequently observed following removal of a brain tumour or injury to the temporal lobe of the brain and has been induced experimentally in monkeys by bilateral temporal lobectomy with partial destruction of amygdaloid nuclei and pyriform cortex. The interesting and puzzling aspect of the syndrome is that it involves behaviours that are quite cognitive (e.g. VISUAL *AGNOSIA) as well as those that are quite clearly emotional.

knee-jerk reflex A reflex of the lower leg produced by a sharp tap on the patellar tendon just below the kneecap. It was this reflex that Twitmeyer studied in the first experimental investigation of classical conditioning (several years before Pavlov). Because of its long history in the study of the psychology of reflexes, the phrase *knee-jerk* has taken on vaguely insulting properties and is often used synonymously with *unthinking*.

knockout In biology and genetics, an organism in which a gene has been artificially deactivated or eliminated. Usually the species is given, e.g. 'knockout mouse'.

knowing how PROCEDURAL *KNOWLEDGE.

knowing self The I. See also SELF (1, 2).

knowing that DECLARATIVE *KNOWLEDGE.

knowledge 1 Collectively, the body of information possessed by a person or, by extension, by a group of persons or a culture. **2** Those mental components that result from any and all processes, be they innately given or experientially acquired. Both senses carry the implication that knowledge is deep, abstract and not simply a compendium of dispositions for action.

Within the philosophical and cognitive psychological approaches to EPISTEMOLOGY and COGNITIVE SCIENCE, various forms of knowledge are typically distinguished; see the following entries for the more commonly cited. Note that *memory* is often used as a virtual synonym of *knowledge*. Combined terms like *episodic knowledge* and *declarative knowledge* are used interchangeably with *episodic memory* and *declarative memory*. See MEMORY et seq. for more detail and for combined terms not given here.

knowledge by acquaintance As distinguished from both PROCEDURAL *KNOWLEDGE and DECLARATIVE *KNOWLEDGE, knowledge of which we are directly aware, knowledge of people, places and things derived from sense data.

knowledge, core Knowledge that is presumed to be innate, or at least emerge very early in infancy, and that continues to struc-

ture thinking throughout the lifespan. The term is used particularly in the study of the acquisition of knowledge about objects and basic physics, where understanding of principles such as the solidity and continuity of objects can be demonstrated as emerging within the first few months of life.

knowledge, declarative Knowledge about the world that can be represented as consciously known, factual knowledge. That is, knowledge about which a person can make a declaration, e.g. 'A rose is a kind of flower.' Gilbert Ryle liked to refer to it by the phrase *knowing that*. Also called *factual knowledge*. Compare with PROCEDURAL *KNOWLEDGE.

knowledge, generic General knowledge about things in the world that is held independent of any specific events or episodes. The term is used interchangeably with *semantic knowledge* and SEMANTIC *MEMORY.

knowledge of results Very general term used for any feedback of information to: (a) a subject in an experiment about the correctness of his or her responses; (b) a student in a learning situation about success or failure in mastering material; (c) a client in psychotherapy about progress made, etc.

knowledge, personal Michael Polanyi's term for the idea captured by TACIT KNOWLEDGE. It emphasizes the notion that this kind of knowledge has a highly personal component to it.

knowledge, procedural Knowledge about how to do something; knowledge that is operational, practical. Unlike DECLARATIVE *KNOWLEDGE, procedural knowledge lies outside an individual's realm of consciousness. Some classic examples are knowing how to ride a bicycle or tie a knot or, interestingly, speak a language. Procedural knowledge lies behind complex actions and typically is rather resistant to attempts to make it conscious; try explaining to someone how to tie a shoelace – it's much easier to show than to tell. Gilbert Ryle called it *knowing how* or *practical knowledge*.

knowledge, tacit Knowledge held independently of awareness, knowledge that is IMPLICIT.

known self The ME. See also SELF (1, 2).

Kolomogorov-Smirnov test A nonparametric statistical test that may be used to test the significance of the difference between one sample of scores and a population or the difference between two samples. The 'vodka test', as it is jokingly called, is one of the more powerful nonparametric tests, invariably more sensitive to differences than *chi-square* and approximating the sensitivity of the *t test*.

kolytic From the Greek for *hinder*, used of processes that are inhibitory.

König bars A set of bars used for measuring visual acuity. The standard for normal vision is a set of bars subtending 3 minutes of visual angle with 1-minute separations between them. Sometimes adapted to measure tactile acuity.

koniocellular system That portion of the pathways of the primate visual system that carries information about the presence of short wavelengths and is thought to be responsible for the ability to distinguish blue and yellow. Compare with MAGNOCELLULAR SYSTEM and PARVOCELLULAR SYSTEM.

koro A culture-specific disorder found among Southeast Asian males. The primary symptom is a fear that the penis will retract into the abdomen and the belief that this will cause death.

Korsakoff's syndrome An AMNESTIC SYNDROME often found in chronic alcoholics and named after its first systematic describer, the Russian physician S. S. Korsakoff. The most significant symptom is the loss of memory of recent events, although memory of the more remote remains intact. That is, patients display ANTEROGRADE *AMNESIA but little in the way of RETROGRADE *AMNESIA. Intriguingly, Korsakoff's patients show much less disturbance of IMPLICIT *MEMORY and IMPLICIT *LEARNING than they do of learning and memory functions that are based on consciousness and awareness. Autopsies have tended to implicate the medial thalamus and the hippocampus as the brain structures involved. Also spelled *Korsakov* and *Korsakow*, and also known as *Wernicke–Korsakoff's syndrome*, *alcohol amnestic disorder* and *alcoholic dementia*.

Korte's laws A series of generalizations concerning the optimum apparent motion (see BETA *MOTION) in the PHI PHENOMENON. In par-

ticular, they express the fact that relationships hold between spatial separation of the successively presented stimuli, the intensity of the stimuli, the exposure times and the interstimulus interval. Specifically: it is more difficult to see apparent motion when the two stimuli are far apart, spatial separation is very wide, illumination is very low and the interstimulus interval is very short, although decrements in one or two variables can be compensated for by increments in the other(s).

Krause end bulb One of the several encapsulated receptors that innervate the skin. It is found typically in mucocutaneous zones, tissue that is transitional between dry, glabrous skin and mucous membranes. Once thought to mediate temperature, it is now suspected of being responsive to mechanical stimulation.

Kretschmer types CONSTITUTIONAL THEORY.

Kruskal–Shepard scaling A type of multidimensional scaling procedure developed relatively independently by the mathematician J. B. Kruskal and the psychologist R. Shepard. The technique requires that subjects make judgements of the similarity of various stimuli; these judgements are then analysed to determine the underlying psychological dimensions that were used to make them.

Kruskal–Wallis test A nonparametric analysis of variance. Although it only handles one-way effects (i.e. it cannot test the effects of more than one variable) its sensitivity to difference is quite high, making it a useful test particularly when the assumptions of the *F-test* are not met.

K scale A specialized scale within the *MMPI* that is presumed to detect defensiveness.

K strategy In evolutionary biology, a type of reproductive breeding utilized by many species in which one (or, on occasions, two or three) offspring is born at one time. The K strategy involves considerable investment of energy and resources in the rearing of each offspring and a relatively long interbirth period. This strategy has been adopted by many mammals, most significantly by the great apes and, of course, by *Homo sapiens*. Compare with R STRATEGY. Also called *K selection* or *K selection strategy*.

Kuder Occupational Interest Survey The current version of the KUDER PREFERENCE RECORD.

Kuder Preference Record The prototype of the so-called *interest inventories*. The respondent is presented with a series of triads comprising three different occupations or activities and asked to mark which of these is the least and most liked options. From these responses, a profile of preferred academic subjects and occupations is generated. The current adult version is known as the *Kuder Occupational Interest Survey* and is referred to by practitioners as simply 'The Kuder'.

Kuder–Richardson formulas Frequently used measures of RELIABILITY of a test. There are several variations for specialized situations although all are based on the correlations between comparable forms of the test.

Often abbreviated as *K-R formulas* or *K-R coefficients of equivalence*.

kurtosis A statistical term used to describe the overall shape of a frequency distribution. The normal curve is *mesokurtic*, a peaked curve is *leptokurtic* and a flat curve is *platykurtic*. Kurtosis is the fourth MOMENT (2) of a distribution.

kymograph A general term for any device that makes a graphic recording of events. It operates by using a moving pen or marker that responds to pressure applied to it to make a trace on paper wrapped round a revolving drum. Rarely used any more, having been replaced by more sophisticated devices like polygraphs and computer output systems.

kypho- Prefix meaning *humped*.

kyto- A variation of CYTO-.

L

L Abbreviation for: **1** LAMBERT. **2** LUMEN. **3** LIMEN.

L₁,₂,... In the study of bi- and multilingualism, L_1 is used to note the first language learned, L_2 the second, etc.

la belle indifférence BELLE INDIFFÉRENCE, LA.

labelling theory An appellation used of contemporary psychiatry by many of its critics who regard most approaches to clinical phenomena as little more than ways of labelling people. Their point, put most simply, is that the traditional diagnostic systems of Western psychiatry are not reflective of any true underlying mental illnesses, rather merely apply labels to behaviour patterns deemed 'abnormal' because they are unacceptable to society. Further, they argue, once a label has been attached, professionals, friends and even the designated individual come to reflect the expectations of the label and behave accordingly, resulting in a classic instance of the SELF-FULFILLING PROPHECY. This point of view is, to be sure, an extreme one and disputed by most mental-health professionals (although in gentler moments they will admit that it has some merit).

labia (sing. **labium** = lip). **1** The lips. This meaning is found commonly in linguistics to refer to speech sounds that use the lips, see LABIAL. **2** The fleshy folds that surround the vagina. The inner, richly vascular folds are called the *labia minora* and the outer, fatty folds the *labia majora*.

labial Adjective form of *labium, labia*. Used of lips in general, but most commonly with reference to the oral lips. In linguistics it is descriptive of phones produced using one or both lips; e.g. *b* and *p* are *bilabials*.

labile Changeable, adaptable and, by extension, not stable. The term is used widely in psychology, most commonly of the changing expression of emotions. Here the connotation is negative, implying a lack of emotional stability.

labile personality CYCLOTHYMIC DISORDER.

labiodental A class of speech sounds produced by using the lower lip and the upper teeth, e.g. *f* and *v* in *five*.

labyrinth **1** From the Greek for *maze*, any structure of intricate pathways. **2** Because of its complex and intricate membranous and bony construction, the inner ear, which contains the sense organs for hearing and balance.

lachrymal Variation of LACRIMAL.

lacrimal Of or relating to tears. var., *lachrymal*.

lacrimal gland The tear gland. It lies beneath the upper eyelid and secretes tears, which moisten the cornea. The tears drain into the nose through the *lacrimal duct*.

lactate **1** vb. To produce milk. **2** n. A salt derived from lactic acid.

lactation The production of milk by mammary glands.

lactogenic hormone PROLACTIN.

lacuna A gap, a blank space, a hole. Most often used metaphorically to refer to gaps in memory or in consciousness, the term is occasionally applied to specific neurological deficits; e.g. *cerebral lacuna* refers to a small area of damaged brain tissue like that resulting from occlusion of a branch of a cerebral artery.

lacunar amnesia EPISODIC *AMNESIA.

LAD (or **LAS**) An acronym for *language acqui-sition device* (or *system* – bad jokes about mas-culine and feminine forms abound). It was originally hypothesized by N. Chomsky to be an innately given mechanism that operated upon the linguistic input to elaborate a rep-resentative grammar, a kind of 'language organ'. In Chomsky's conceptualization, the LAD is preprogrammed with the under-lying rules of universal grammar and will, depending on the language to which a child is exposed, select from the full set of rules those that are appropriate for the one spoken. The status of the LAD is highly equivocal and most psycholinguists and cog-nitive psychologists find the idea fascinating but doubtful. However, others treat it as though its reality were as unchallenged as, say, that of the pituitary gland. Also called the LRCS, for *language-responsible cognitive structure*.

Ladd–Franklin theory An early theory of colour vision, not generally accepted today, that assumed a complex photosensitive mol-ecule that responded differentially to red, green, blue and yellow light by releasing sub-stances that stimulated respective nerve end-ings. The theory was evolutionarily based: dichromatic vision was explained by assum-ing a less highly developed molecule, and achromatic vision by assuming an even more primitive one. See THEORIES OF *COLOUR VISION.

lag 1 Generally, any time delay between events. Usually the term is qualified to iden-tify the nature of the lag, e.g. *response lag*, *culture lag*. **2** A brief period after a stimulus has been removed when it may still be per-ceived. See here ICONIC.

-lagnia Combining form meaning *lust*.

laissez-faire The idea, first promulgated in 18th-century France, that government should not exert control or influence over the economy. By extension, in social psych-ology the term is used to characterize any leadership system that operates with min-imal control. In the true *laissez-faire* system no control is provided by the leader, not even assistance or guidance.

laissez-faire **atmosphere** K. Lewin's term for the general sociopolitical climate estab-lished when the nominal leader of a group maintains a hands-off policy and there is lit-tle or no guidance or direction imposed. Contrast with AUTHORITARIAN ATMOSPHERE and DEMOCRATIC ATMOSPHERE.

-lalia Combining form meaning *speech*, used specifically in reference to disorders of speech.

lallation 1 An unintelligible, infantile bab-bling. **2** The constant use of *l* in place of *r*. Also called *lalling*.

lalo- The prefix form of *-lalia*.

laloplegia Inability to speak owing to par-alysis of all the muscles used for speech except the tongue.

lalorrhoea LOGORRHOEA.

Lamarckianism (or **Lamarckism**) INHERIT-ANCE OF *ACQUIRED CHARACTERISTICS.

Lamaze method A method of psycho-logical preparation for childbirth. named after a Frenchman, F. Lamaze. The procedure is a modification of a technique first intro-duced in the Soviet Union based on Pavlo-vian conditioning principles. The method focuses on proper anatomical and physio-logical knowledge, breathing techniques, conditioned relaxation, cognitive control and a social support system. Also known as the *psychophylatic method*.

lambda (λ) Designation for wavelength of a light.

lambert The luminance of a perfectly dif-fusing surface either reflecting or emitting light at the rate of 1 lumen per cm^2. As this is a rather intense level of light, the millilam-bert (1 mL = $\frac{1}{1000}$ lambert) is the preferred unit.

Lambert cosine law The illumination of a surface varies as the cosine of the angle of incidence of the light and the surface.

Landau–Kleffner syndrome (**LKS**) An aphasia-producing seizure disorder. It occurs in childhood and is marked by acute or pro-gressive loss of language ability characterized by comprehension deficits and verbal audi-tory *agnosia*. Also called *progressive epileptic aphasia, epileptiform aphasia* or *acquired epi-leptic aphasia*.

Land effect First demonstrated by Edwin Land (who also developed the Polaroid cam-era), the effect produces the perception of colour from black and white photographs. In the simplest form, two black and white pictures are taken of a scene, one through a red filter and one through a blue–green filter. The two are projected together on a screen, the former through a red filter, the latter through a green one. The resulting scene is seen as composed of a wide variety of colours, including blues that are not normally produced by a mixture of red and green.

landmark agnosia AGNOSIA, LANDMARK.

Landolt ring(s) A doughnut-shaped figure with an opening in it used for measuring visual acuity. The standard ring has a thickness of 1 minute of visual angle and an opening of 1 minute, other rings have smaller and larger openings.

language All know the meaning of this term: a language is what we speak, the set of arbitrary conventional symbols through which we convey meaning, the culturally determined pattern of vocal gestures we acquire by virtue of being raised in a particular place and time, the medium through which we code our feelings, thoughts, ideas and experiences, the most uniquely human of behaviours and the most ubiquitous behaviour of humans. Yet, as the term is used, it may mean all of these, none of them, or even things very different.

The conviction that we know the meaning of the word *language* lasts only so long as we refrain from attempts at specifying what we know. To appreciate the problems of definition and use here consider the following questions: (a) Is the system of manual signs used by the profoundly deaf a language? (b) Are the synthetic systems developed for the programming of computers true languages? (c) Are the invented coding systems of sociopolitical reformers such as Esperanto to be classified as languages? (d) Should the sequences of motor movements, body positions, gestures and facial expressions that convey meaning be regarded as language? (e) Are there valid reasons for labelling the communication systems of other species languages; for example, those of bees, parrots, dolphins and chimpanzees? (f) At what point in the emerging vocalizations of an infant do we want to conclude that it now has language?

These questions and many more like them cannot easily be answered. They are presented here to illustrate the complexity that the word carries, a complexity that renders any straightforward definition useless. See also LINGUISTICS, PARALINGUISTICS, PSYCHO-LINGUISTICS, SIGN LANGUAGE and related terms.

language acquisition device (or **system**) LAD.

language centres Those cortical areas known to be involved in the production and/or comprehension of spoken and/or written language. BROCA'S AREA and WERNICKE'S AREA are the two most often cited. However, the term needs to be used with caution, for these hypothesized centres cannot be thought of as circumscribed areas of the brain that encapsulate all linguistic functions. Other regions of the cortex are known to play a role in linguistic behaviours and neurological injuries in other sites can result in language deficits.

language-delayed child Loosely, any child whose language development is significantly behind the norms. The term is applied to children who are autistic, retarded, have suffered neurological damage, or have merely been raised in linguistically deprived environments. Those who catch up later on are often called, somewhat informally, *late talkers*.

language disability An umbrella term for any nonnormal language function. Use is nearly always restricted to children: a child displaying it is classified as *language disabled* when the syndrome is general and *specific language disabled* when only fairly precise dysfunctions are identified. There is a tendency to use the term as though it reflects some underlying, subtle, organic dysfunction, and the language-disabled child is often assumed to have some form of minimal brain damage. See also DEVELOPMENTAL *LANGUAGE DISORDER.

language disorder, developmental A general label for a number of disorders evidenced by significant impairment in the development of language skills during childhood. The term is restricted to cases in which there is no known neurological or anatomical defect. Often the disorders are divided into the *expressive* types, in which vocal output is disordered but language comprehension is normal, and a *mixed receptive-expressive* type, in which both are impaired. Note, the term *developmental aphasia* has been used to refer to these disorders, but incorrectly: APHASIA is reserved for language functions that are *lost*, not for those unacquired. The acceptable synonyms for these varieties of disorder are *expressive* and *receptive dysphasia* respectively; see DYSPHASIA. See also LANGUAGE DISABILITY, which tends to be used more often in the educational literature than in the clinical.

language, figurative A cover term for those aspects of language used to express ideas through metaphor, simile, allusions and analogies. Figurative language is nonliteral and often idiomatic.

language, natural To circumvent some of the problems posed by the term LANGUAGE, the adjective *natural* is often appended when the writer wishes to be clear that only the naturally occurring verbal expression systems of *Homo sapiens* are being referenced. That is, a *natural language* is what the layperson generally means when referring to *language*.

language origins, theories of Three general classes of theories were developed during the 19th century. All were highly speculative and dealt only with single words: (a) the *onomatopoetic*, which argued that imitations of sounds of animals and natural events were the beginnings; (b) the *interjectional*, which assumed that emotional exclamations ('Ow!', 'Ah!') were the first words: and (c) the *natural response* theory, which held that automatic vocal reactions to specific environmental stimuli were the initial verbal communications. All three points of view are seriously lacking in explanatory power and are mostly known today by the rather absurd names bestowed by their critics: the 'bow-wow' theory, the 'pooh-pooh' theory, and the 'ding-dong' or 'splish-splash' theory. There is a great deal of enthusiastic research being done by contemporary anthropologists, psychologists, linguists and biologists on the problem of language origins but no well-developed or widely accepted theory is currently about.

lanugo 1 Fine, downy, infant-like hair. **2** Such fine hair that briefly covers the body of the foetus during the later stage of gestation.

lapse 1 Generally, a slip, a mistake, an error of omission. **2** A brief period during which one is unaware of one's surroundings, especially in mild forms of epilepsy.

lapsus Latin for *slip*. Used in several combined phrases: *lapsus calami* = slip of the pen, *lapsus linguae* = slip of the tongue, *lapsus memoriae* = lapse of memory. Within psychoanalysis all such momentary failures are examples of PARAPRAXIS and assumed to be due to unconscious factors.

large numbers, law of In mathematically simplest terms, the larger a sample of data the more likely it is that the mean of the sample lies arbitrarily close to the true mean of the population from which it was drawn. In essence, given that there are no sampling biases, the larger the database the more confident one may be that the sample statistics provide accurate estimates of the population parameters.

larynx A cartilaginous structure that sits atop the windpipe. It contains a 'valve' made up of a double set of muscular folds covered with a layer of mucous membrane. The lower set is the true vocal folds (or 'cords'), which open and close rapidly during vocalization. During quiet breathing the muscles that control the laryngeal cartilages relax and the folds form a V-shaped opening (called the *glottis*) to allow free passage of air.

Lashley jumping stand A device used for experimenting on small animals (usually laboratory rats). An animal is placed on a stand and must jump toward one of two or more stimuli placed in front of it. The device has been widely used in studies of discrimination and choice behaviour.

Lashley-Wade model In CLASSICAL CONDITIONING, the theory that the GENERALIZATION GRADIENT is influenced by prior experience in discriminating the CONDITIONED STIMULUS from other stimuli.

latah syndrome A rare psychiatric syndrome characterized by symptoms of excitement, *echolalia*, *echopraxia*, *coprolalia* and, sometimes, *fugue* and *hallucinations*. var., *lattah*.

late See EARLY.

late luteal phase dysphoric disorder A MOOD DISORDER associated with the late luteal phase of a woman's menstrual cycle. The term is still found in many texts although it has been dropped from the last several editions of the *DSM* and replaced by PREMENSTRUAL DYSPHORIC DISORDER (see for details).

latency Generally, a period of inactivity within a system. The system is generally an organism and the period of inactivity is marked by some stimulus that initiates it and the occurrence of some response that ends it. The term is broadly used and often qualified as to the particular system and/or the kind of effect referred to; see the entries below for examples. adj., *latent*.

latency period In classical psychoanalytic theory, the period of time from the end of the Oedipal period to the beginning of puberty, during which sexual interest is presumed to be sublimated.

latency, response The time between the onset of a stimulus and the occurrence of the overt response to that stimulus. See ASSOCIATION TIME (1), REACTION TIME and VERIFICATION TIME for some specialized types of response latencies.

latent Existing in hidden form, dormant but capable of being evoked or developed. The term is used adjectivally in a variety of contexts, some of which follow as illustration.

latent content LATENT AND MANIFEST *CONTENT.

latent extinction EXTINCTION, LATENT.

latent homosexual Although psychodynamic theories of personality and sexuality go to great lengths to explain this term it seems clear that a latent homosexual is merely a heterosexual.

latent inhibition INHIBITION, LATENT.

latent learning LEARNING, LATENT.

latent process Very generally, and lit., any process that is *latent*. In psychoanalytic theory an infant's ego processes are often said to be latent; in cognitive psychology particular intellectual processes that have not yet manifested themselves are referred to as latent; and so forth.

latent schizophrenia SCHIZOTYPAL PERSONALITY DISORDER.

latent social identity A social role that, although not 'officially' a factor in functioning in a society, nevertheless has significant impact upon an individual's behaviour in a social organization. Gender, race, religion, etc. form part of a person's latent social identity.

latent traits Generally, those genetic traits that do not manifest themselves in the phenotype of an individual but which can be passed on to future generations.

late (onset) paraphrenia Generally, any DELUSIONAL DISORDER that emerges late in life. Sixty years of age is the standard criterion.

lateral Of or relating to the side, away from the median axis. Used to characterize any number of structures, as the following entries show.

lateral-basomedial group A cluster of nuclei in the *amygdala* that receives visual, auditory and somatosensory information and sends it to the *forebrain* and *hypothalamus*.

lateral corticospinal tract CORTICOSPINAL PATHWAYS.

lateral differences A cover term for any behavioural, cognitive or affective differences between the two hemispheres of the brain and/or the associated peripheral processes. See e.g. LATERALITY and HANDEDNESS.

lateral dominance Preferential use of one side of the body. The term is used broadly and covers preferred use of a hand, an eye, an arm or a hemisphere (especially for language). To get a feeling for the range of issues tucked under this term see DOMINANCE (esp. 5, 6) et seq., HANDEDNESS and LATERALITY.

lateral dorsal nucleus DORSOLATERAL NUCLEUS.

lateral fissure The deep groove on the lateral surface of the hemispheres of the brain that marks the border between the frontal and parietal lobes (above the fissure) and the temporal lobe (below it). Also called the *Sylvian fissure* or the *fissure of Sylvius*.

lateral geniculate nucleus Two cell nuclei of the thalamus, located at the termini of each optic tract, from which the visual pathways proceed to the striate area of the occipital cortex. Each lateral geniculate nucleus has a laminar structure such that for the left side the three left layers receive axons from the left side of the left retina and the three right layers receive axons from the left side of the right retina. For the right side the reverse is found. Also called *lateral geniculate bodies*.

lateral hypothalamic syndrome A behavioural syndrome observed in animals following lesions in the lateral area of the hypothalamus (LH). It is characterized by *aphagia* (lack of eating) and *adipsia* (lack of drinking). If left to their own devices, LH-lesioned animals will die. However, careful nursing and forced feeding will keep them alive and a second stage will be observed during which they recover (more or less – they are still abnormal in other ways) and establish a new, lower but stable, body weight. At first the syndrome was assumed to implicate the LH as a feeding centre that operated in reciprocal fashion with the ventromedial hypothalamus (see here VENTROMEDIAL HYPOTHALAMIC SYNDROME). The contemporary viewpoint, however, is that a set of extremely complex neural pathways involving sensory and motor systems – all of which have been shown to play a role in feeding – pass through and around the LH, hence lesions here disrupt the normal pattern of eating and drinking. The LH is thus not a feeding centre but part of a network of structures and pathways all of which are part of the complex sensory, motor and affective components of feeding.

lateral hypothalamus (LH) HYPOTHALAMUS, LATERAL HYPOTHALAMIC SYNDROME.

lateral inhibition A set of conditions established when two or more neural cells are interconnected so that excitation of one produces inhibition in the other. Complex lateral inhibitory systems are responsible for the 'sharpening' of perceptions, particularly in the visual system.

laterality Lit., sideness. In general, the term can refer to any preference for one side of the body over the other, such as having a preferred hand or eye. Recently, however, it has come to be used largely to characterize the asymmetry of the hemispheres of the brain with regard to specific cognitive functions. It is often used to characterize the fact that the brain is organized so that language and speech functions are mediated in the left hemisphere (for most of us, anyway). Although these linguistic capacities are the ones most clearly associated with laterality, there is a growing body of evidence to suggest that a variety of other cognitive, perceptual and affective components of behaviour may also be lateralized: specifically, that the left hemisphere is *analytic* and functions in a sequential, rational fashion, and that the right hemisphere is *synthetic* and functions in a more holistic, arational manner. Being precise here is difficult but, to carry this speculation further, some researchers argue that such analytic skills as problem-solving and hypothesis-formation and testing, even perhaps consciousness itself, are left-hemispheric, whereas other skills, such as art and music, and perhaps even the unconscious, are right-hemispheric. All this is great fun, but if we can learn anything from past researches into brain function, it is that these sharp delineations in hemispheric function for specific capacities are painful oversimplifications. See also DOMINANCE (5, 6).

lateralization The process by which different functions and processes become associated with one or the other side of the brain. For more detail see LATERALITY.

lateral lemniscus LEMNISCAL SYSTEM.

lateral posterior nucleus A thalamic nucleus that interconnects with the parietal cortex.

lateral preoptic area PREOPTIC AREA.

lateral thinking A *heuristic* for solving problems in which the individual attempts to look at a problem from many angles rather than searching for a direct, head-on solution.

latero- Combining form meaning LATERAL.

late-selection model See EARLY-SELECTION MODEL.

late talker LANGUAGE-DELAYED CHILD.

Latin square A balanced two-way classification scheme in which each condition occurs just once in each row and column. For example:

conditions or trails

	a	b	c
subjects	b	c	a
	c	a	b

This balancing is often incorporated into experimental designs so that the order of administration of treatments is perfectly balanced across subjects. Two such Latin squares are orthogonal if, when combined, the same pair of symbols occurs only once in the combined square. This composite square is called a *Greco-Latin square*. For example:

conditions or trails

	ab	bc	ca
subjects	bc	ca	ab
	ca	ab	bc

latitude Freedom from narrow restrictions. The term is used in the study of attitudes to refer to the point of view that attitudes, beliefs, opinions and the like should not be viewed as points along a dimension but rather as ranges with some average point representing the core or dominant position taken. That is, each attitude that a person holds exists with some degree of flexibility or *latitude*.

lattah syndrome LATAH SYNDROME.

law 1 In science, see SCIENTIFIC *LAW and STATISTICAL *LAW. **2** In legal parlance, a governmentally imposed rule of conduct.

law, empirical A principle or generalization relating variables to each other and based on observations or experimental findings. Such laws are basically no more than descriptions of the concordance of events or of facts; WEBER'S LAW is a good example of an empirical law.

law, natural 1 In the natural sciences, a SCIENTIFIC *LAW. **2** In social discourse, any established custom or practice adhered to independently of formal legislation. In 1 the sense is of that which occurs in *nature*, in 2 of that which occurs *naturally*.

law of effect EFFECT, LAW OF.

law of exercise EXERCISE, LAW OF.

law, scientific When a generalization or

principle has been verified sufficiently often (or has resisted frequent and strong attempts at refutation), when the data base is well defined and when those concerned are satisfied that the relationships specified are, under the appropriate conditions, universal, then one may begin to speak of a scientific law. Psychology, despite frequent premature announcements, has shown itself to be a discipline particularly resistant to the establishment of such laws. Indeed, it is good counsel to recommend that for the social sciences in general the terms GENERALIZATION (esp. 3) and PRINCIPLE (1, 2) are the terms of choice, as they tend not to mislead. See also STATISTICAL *LAW.

law, statistical A SCIENTIFIC *LAW, when expressed in terms of the probability that the specified relationships will obtain, is a statistical law – given, of course, that the probability is less than 1.0. In some respects such laws are major advances, particularly when they reveal that the underlying lawful processes are themselves probabilistic in nature; in other respects they are admissions of ignorance about the possibility that other poorly understood effects are operating such that precise predictions cannot be made. Most 'laws' in psychology are of this latter kind – an assessment that is generally construed not as criticism of the scientific stature of the field but rather as an acknowledgement of the complexity of its subject-matter.

lax In phonetics, a DISTINCTIVE FEATURE (2) descriptive of speech sounds produced when the vocal tract is in its normal resting position. Opposite of TENSE (3).

lay Characterizing a nonprofessional, i.e. a layperson.

lay analyst One who has received psychoanalytic training and is qualified to practise but who has not taken a degree in medicine.

lazy eye AMBLYOPIA.

LD Abbreviation for: **1** LEARNING DISABILITY. **2** LANGUAGE DISABILITY. Generally used in reference to a child diagnosed as having one of these disabilities.

L-DOPA Short for *levodopa*, a precursor of DOPAMINE. Because L-DOPA crosses the blood–brain barrier, which dopamine does not, it is used as a standard treatment in PARKINSON'S DISEASE.

leader Anyone who holds a position of dominance, authority or influence in a group. Usually an adjective is affixed to characterize the form of leader or leadership under consideration. See the following entries.

leader, authoritarian A leader with absolute authority, with no requirement to consult with other members of the group in decision-making. Authoritarian leaders are often found in the military, in dictatorships, and in many organizations, youth gangs, families, etc. In fact, the prevalence of this type of leader has generated considerable interest in social scientists and much concern in social reformers. See also AUTHORITARIANISM; contrast with DEMOCRATIC *LEADER.

leader, bureaucratic A leader whose authority stems from the official bureaucratic position he or she holds. No other personal or individual characteristics are implied.

leader, charismatic A leader whose authority stems from the emotional, cognitive and behavioural commitment of the group to the vision formulated and articulated by the leader.

leader, democratic A leader whose authority springs from the consensus of a group and who acts in accordance with the beliefs and desires of the members of the group both individually and collectively.

leader, nominal A leader in name only but with no actual leadership role. The implication is that another is actually providing the leadership.

leadership The only really proper use for this term is to characterize the exercise of authority and influence within a social group; that is, to function as a leader is to manifest leadership. It is often used, however, as if it were a personality trait, as if there were a collection of specific skills that reflect leadership capability. Although there is a certain intuitive truth here, this use leads to hopeless confusion because it neglects the role of a situation itself in determining leadership behaviour.

leading eye EYE *DOMINANCE.

leading hemisphere Occasionally used for either **1** the hemisphere of the brain that is primarily responsible for a particular behaviour or mode of cognition, or **2** the dominant (i.e. linguistic) hemisphere. The term was first used by the English neurologist J. H. Jackson in 1868 in sense 2 on the grounds that language represents the highest mental process and hence the linguistic hemisphere is the one which 'leads' in cognitive functions. See CEREBRAL DOMINANCE.

learned flavour (or **food** or **taste**) **aversion** (or **avoidance**) CONDITIONED *AVERSION

learned helplessness HELPLESSNESS, LEARNED.

learning 1 The process of acquiring knowledge or the actual possession of such; scholarship. This meaning is very loose and is used in like fashion within various disciplines, such as educational psychology and cognitive psychology. The connotations and entailments of this meaning in the technical literature are essentially the same as they are in the nontechnical. However, this looseness is regarded as unsatisfactory within the more behaviourally oriented approaches; hence, here: **2** In G. Kimble's terms, 'a relatively permanent change in response potentiality which occurs as a result of reinforced practice'. This definition captures the features that behaviourist theory was most concerned with, specifically: (a) 'Relatively permanent': the point here is simple – the exclusion of momentary changes in behaviour brought about by fatigue, satiation, habituation and the like. (b) 'Response potentiality': this phrase is included in recognition of the learning–performance distinction. It allows the inclusion of the phenomena of LATENT *LEARNING and INCIDENTAL *LEARNING, in which changes in behaviour are not immediately observable, and reflects the truism that learning is really a hypothetical event recognizable solely through measurable changes in performance. (c) 'Reinforced': regarded as the crux of the issue in the heyday of behaviourism, since, presumably – so far as most behaviourists are concerned – without reinforcement extinction will occur. Today's more cognitively oriented theorists are less concerned with the role of reinforcement, although most acknowledge that it plays a role. See REINFORCEMENT for details. (d) 'Practice': the point here is that, for learning to emerge, sooner or later the behaviour must be emitted, and repeated (reinforced) occurrences will improve learning. This consideration is generally accepted in psychology, although some allowances need to be made for the effects of IMITATION, MODELLING and OBSERVATION *LEARNING. The notion of practice also allows for the exclusion of other behavioural changes of a relatively permanent kind that are generally not considered to be instances of learning, such as native tendencies of particular species (e.g. imprinting) and maturational changes (e.g. flying in birds).

Oddly, the definition and manner of use of the term *learning* have caused relatively little controversy among theorists and it is used with relatively few encumbrances by developmentalists, educators, cognitive psychologists, behaviourists, etc. The tendency is to use it as a 'chapter heading' word and allow the socially accepted meaning to prevail. The difficulties that do emerge in usage show up when theoretical processes and mechanisms for explaining learning are proposed. Several of the more hotly disputed are discussed under LEARNING THEORY.

learning, all-or-none Learning that either takes place completely and successfully 'all at once' (i.e. on a single trial) or not at all (i.e. not on that particular trial).

learning, associative Learning an association, learning that occurs through the process of linking or binding. What becomes linked or associated is a theoretical question that has received many different answers over the years, from the *ideas* of the early empiricists to the *stimuli* and *responses* of the behaviourists and the *propositions* and *images* of more modern cognitivists. That the term has survived such dramatic shifts in the hypothesized elements is perhaps itself of some significance. See CONNECTIONISM.

learning, context specific The general principle that, since learning occurs in particular contexts, material is best accessed or recalled in the context in which it was acquired. Our favourite study here is one that showed that subjects who learned material while under water in scuba diving gear evidenced better recall when tested under water than when sitting by the pool, and vice versa for subjects who learned while sitting by the pool. For a similar phenomenon see STATE-DEPENDENT *LEARNING.

learning, cooperative This term is used in three different but related ways: **1** The act of learning through cooperation. That is, learning where students must work together to accomplish their task. **2** A technique used in the classroom to promote (1). **3** A philosophical approach to education, based on the idea that children learn better when they cooperate in mastering the material. See also JIGSAW CLASSROOM.

learning curve Any graphic representation of the process of learning or, more precisely, the performance assumed to reflect the learning. Generally the independent variable is plotted on the horizontal axis and the dependent on the vertical. Several decades ago there was a flurry of theoretical activity concerning the shape of *the* learning curve presumed to underlie the process. Although there is something of a consensus that the typical shape is negatively accelerated, there is such a large number of variables that can affect the course of learning that no firm generalizations are possible.

learning, declarative Learning that results in knowledge that can be communicated to others. Learning that produces DECLARATIVE *KNOWLEDGE. Often used synonymously with EXPLICIT *LEARNING.

learning disability **1** In Britain, MENTAL RETARDATION. **2** In North America, a syndrome found in children of normal or above-average intelligence characterized by specific difficulties in learning to read (*dyslexia*), to write (*dysgraphia*), to do grade appropriate mathematics (*dyscalculia*), and/or to read nonverbal social cues (*dyssemia*). Since other cognitive functions are normal it is assumed by most authorities that these disabilities stem from some form of MINIMAL BRAIN DYSFUNCTION. Often abbreviated *LD*, with a child so diagnosed referred to as an *LD child*. Note that while the disorder is typically detected and subjected to remediation in childhood, its manifestations are also seen in adults who throughout their lives may have difficulty with particular kinds of verbal and/or quantitative materials.

learning disorder The *DSM-IV* term for any of the various disorders discussed under ACADEMIC SKILLS DISORDERS and/or LEARNING DISABILITY.

learning, explicit Learning that takes place consciously and results in knowledge that is available to consciousness; learning of which one is aware. When most people use the term *learning* with reference to the acquisition of complex knowledge in humans, they tend to use it in this sense; that is, the learning is thought of as a *conscious* process that results in DECLARATIVE *KNOWLEDGE. However, see IMPLICIT *LEARNING.

learning, ideational Loosely, learning based on abstractions, on comprehension. Contrast with ROTE *LEARNING.

learning, implicit A term coined by A. S. Reber for learning that takes place largely independent of awareness of both the process of acquisition and the content of the knowledge so acquired. Material that has been learned in this fashion, often termed PROCEDURAL *KNOWLEDGE, can be used to guide behaviour, make decisions and solve problems, although the individual is typically unaware of the complex knowledge held that enables him or her to act in this fashion. The classic examples are the acquisition of language and the process of socialization: individuals come to speak their natural language and become inculcated with their society's norms and mores but without conscious knowledge of the underlying principles that guide their behaviour. Of course, when implicit learning is examined in the laboratory, artificial systems of considerably less complexity are used. See also IMPLICIT *MEMORY.

learning, incidental Rather literally, learning that takes place in the absence of intent to learn or instructions to that effect. Distinguish from EXPLICIT *LEARNING, in which there is a clear intention to learn.

learning, latent Learning that has taken place but has not yet manifested itself in changes in performance. The term comes from a series of classic studies carried out some decades ago which showed that if fully satiated animals are allowed to explore a maze they will, when hungry, learn to traverse it for food reinforcement more rapidly than controls which have not had the previous, nonreinforced exposure.

learning, motor A generic term covering, very loosely, any learning in which the basic changes in performance are motoric. Although some movement is ultimately involved in essentially all learning, the term is typically used in contrast with cases in which the critical components are perceptual or cognitive.

learning, observation(al) A term coined by A. Bandura to characterize learning that takes place simply by having the learner observe someone else perform the to-be-acquired response. See also MODELLING, SOCIAL LEARNING THEORY.

learning, one-trial A term used to represent the point of view of E. R. Guthrie, that all learning takes place on a single trial. It only *appears*, he argued, that extended practice improves performance, because the behaviours usually under investigation are complex and the gradual improvement reflects a large number of simple components each of which is acquired on a single trial. Contrast with the position expressed by CONTINUITY THEORY. See also ALL-OR-NONE *LEARNING.

learning, paired-associates Essentially an experimental procedure that is used for investigating a variety of phenomena including memory, concept learning, transfer and interference. The subject is required to learn paired (or associated) relations between a set of stimulus items and a set of response items. The usual procedure is to present the stimulus items one at a time and for the subject to reply with the associated response items. Often abbreviated *PA learning* or even *PAL*.

learning, perceptual Learning in which the learner comes to perceive the stimuli differently with exposure and practice. Definitionally not much more can be said, but the simplicity of the term is illusory. Specification of exactly what mental changes occur when a perceptual change takes place, and explaining the mechanisms underlying such changes, are enormous tasks. The major problems surround the issue of *nativism* versus *environmentalism* and the distinction between *enrichment* and *differentiation*.

learning, place Once upon a time there was a very intense theoretical debate over whether an animal learning a maze learned to go to a particular *place* (the goal box) or whether it learned to make a particular set of motor *responses* that led it to the goal box. The issue of contention was that the advocates of place-learning were espousing cognitive mechanisms, the response-learners peripheral processes. The outcome of the dispute was that both were right – it depends on the experimental setting. Simply, if location of the goal box is clearly marked relative to the general surroundings, then place-learning will emerge; if it is not, then the animal will, of necessity, resort to conditioned motor responses.

learning, probability (PL) Learning the probabilities with which events occur. It is typically studied in simple situations where each of two or three events (e.g. flashing lights on a computer screen) occurs with different probabilities and the subject attempts to predict the event that will occur on each trial. In the typical experiment, subjects' prediction frequencies come to approximate the actual probabilities of occurrence of the several events.

learning, procedural Learning that produces knowledge that is highly resistant to being communicated to others; learning that results in PROCEDURAL *KNOWLEDGE. Often used synonymously with IMPLICIT *LEARNING.

learning, relational A generic term covering cases in which the critical components to be learned are the relations or patterns between stimuli. Roughly synonymous with PATTERN LEARNING but see also PATTERN RECOGNITION for details.

learning, response See the discussion under PLACE *LEARNING. Note that the term is also used more generally on occasion to refer to *any* situation in which the subject must learn the response to be made in a particular setting.

learning, restricted An ethological term for a species-specific learning ability whereby the animal possesses the capacity to extract a critical piece of information from the environment that results in precise alterations in the animal's behaviour. Restricted learning is close, if not identical, to OPEN *INSTINCT.

learning, reversal This term covers a variety of learning situations in which, at some point during discrimination-training, the original cues for correct responding are

modified so that they no longer serve as indicators for the original correct response. For example, a child may be trained to press the right-hand button on a panel whenever a triangle appears and the left button for a circle. After learning has reached some criterion the cues are reversed so that now the right button is correct for circles and the left for triangles. Originally this procedure was called the *cue-reversal technique*, and early work focused on simple motor responses and simple physical cues. However, the technique has been adapted so that it lends itself to the examination of symbolic processes as well. The point is that the reversal need not be so simple as replacing triangles with circles. For example, suppose the original stimuli are circles that vary in brightness and size. On initial training trials all large circles are 'correct' independent of brightness. Now, on reversal trials there may be an *intradimensional* (or *reversal*) shift so that all small circles are now deemed 'correct', or there may be an *extradimensional* (or *nonreversal*) shift so that size becomes irrelevant and all white circles are 'correct' and all dark 'wrong'. Developmental level and phylogenetic differences have both been shown to affect learning, implicating symbolic processes underlying the behaviour.

learning, rote Learning (really memorizing) that takes place purely through repetition devoid of meaningfulness of the material or of other operations such as organization, inference or the use of mnemonics.

learning, rule This term is commonly used in roughly the same manner as *concept learning*, with the implicit distinction that the *rule* is the formal statement of the structure or pattern that underlies the *concept*. See CONCEPT FORMATION and LEARNING.

learning, selective A very general term applied to those learning situations in which one or a few specific responses are singled out (by an experimenter or by environmental contingencies), reinforced and hence learned while other similar responses go unreinforced and hence remain unlearned.

learning, serial An experimental procedure whereby stimulus material consisting of a list of items is presented in a fixed order and the subject is required to adhere to that order in attempts at recall. Also called *serial list* *learning*; see also SERIAL RECALL (which is used similarly) and compare with FREE RECALL.

learning set Most broadly, a kind of attentional focus, a determining tendency that functions so that the subject's perceptual or cognitive system is 'primed' or 'set' for a particular stimulus or pattern of stimuli. The meaning here is close to that of the old German term *Einstellung*. The concept has served as a theoretical device for explaining various phenomena such as FUNCTIONAL FIXEDNESS and LEARNING TO LEARN.

learning, single-loop A behaviour pattern in which individuals learn to act so as to minimize emotionality and negative feelings in their relationships. Such learning is frequently seen in business and political organizations where members learn to 'minimize unpleasant messages' (or 'MUM'). Unfortunately, once these patterns become fixed they often prevent decision-makers from receiving critical information. Moreover, because these processes are rarely conscious, the behaviour, once established, can be difficult to modify.

learning, S–R Abbreviation for *stimulus–response learning*; this is one of those relatively rare cases in which the abbreviated form is almost always used. It stands as a kind of cover term; that is, any kind of learning is assumed to be fundamentally governed by the forming of some link or bond between a particular stimulus and a specific response.

learning, S–S Learning based on the association between two stimuli. The term, which is typically used in this abbreviated fashion, is short for *stimulus–stimulus learning*.

learning, state-dependent This term refers to the general principle that recall of a past event is enhanced if one returns to the original setting of the event. One is much more likely to be able to remember the names of one's first-grade classmates if one returns to the original classroom. The inference is that the learning of the material was dependent upon the original state. For a similar effect see CONTEXT SPECIFIC *LEARNING.

learning, statistical Learning based on apprehending and representing the statistical properties of a data set. The term is used frequently in the development of COM-PUTATIONAL MODELS, especially those attempting to model the acquisition of complex materials, e.g. language learning. Distinguish from PROBABILITY *LEARNING, which is a very specific type of statistical learning.

learning theory Any effort to codify and systematize the operations, and to hypothesize about the underlying mechanisms, of that 'relatively permanent change in response potential' (see LEARNING) can qualify as a learning theory. Over the years nearly every conceivable form of theory has been seriously proposed, from the purely peripheral behaviourism of Watson to the strongly centralist positions of modern cognitive science; from those wholly dependent upon reinforcement, such as Thorndike's and Skinner's, to those for which the concept is irrelevant, like Guthrie's; from those that are founded upon physiological function, such as Pavlov's and Köhler's, to those that eschew all efforts to physiologize, like Skinner's behaviourism. Given all this variation it should be clear that there really is no such thing as a single theory of learning. Theorizing about learning is an exercise in generalization and can often be as polemical as it seeks to be empirical.

learning theory, mathematical A general label for a particular kind of approach to theory construction in the area of learning. The focus is far from unitary; rather, it represents an agreement between theorists to try to use mathematics as the vehicle for maximum precision in the statement of the theory. See, for more detail, MATHEMATICAL MODEL, MATHEMATICAL PSYCHOLOGY, STATISTICAL-LEARNING THEORY, STIMULUS-SAMPLING THEORY.

learning to learn The term refers to the fact that with successive presentations of problems of a similar form the subjects become increasingly successful in learning how to solve them: that is, they learn how to learn. According to some theoretical accounts, learning to learn is predicated upon the formation of an appropriate LEARNING SET.

learning trial TRIAL, LEARNING.

learning, trial-and-error Quite literally, learning that is characterized by trial-and-error responding. The course of such learning is typified by the gradual elimination of ineffectual responses and the strengthening of those responses that are satisfactory. Thorndike, in his early theorizing, argued that this process was central to the acquisition of *all* complex acts, a position now all but totally abandoned. Contrast with INSIGHT and OBSERVATIONAL *LEARNING.

learning without awareness AWARENESS, LEARNING WITHOUT.

least-effort principle The *heuristic* that, given various possibilities for action, an organism will select the one requiring the least expenditure of effort. It has been used to theorize about how rats learn mazes, how children develop articulation skills, how adults act in social settings and how economic systems operate, to name just a few.

least-squares principle The statistical principle that the line of best fit for a body of data is the line which minimizes the sum of the squares of the deviations of the data points about it. Most CURVE FITTING (1) procedures are based on this principle. See also GOODNESS OF *FIT.

leaving the field Confronted with insoluble conflict or intensely frustrating circumstances an organism may simply take leave of the field. Escape may be a quite literal physical act or a psychological one, such as diverting attention or changing the subject.

Leboyer method A natural childbirth method developed around the assumption that child-bearing can be made less violent for the infant. Delivery takes place in a darkened room, the infant is bathed in warm water and then placed on the mother's abdomen, and the severing of the umbilical cord is delayed.

Lee-Boot effect The gradual slowing down of the OESTRUS CYCLES of a group of female mice which are housed together. If they are then exposed to the odour of a male (or to his urine), their cycles begin again. This latter effect, which is called the *Whitten effect*, is caused by a PHEROMONE in the male's urine.

left parietal apraxia APRAXIA, LEFT PARIETAL.

left–right effect The greater difficulty preschool children have learning to make left–right than up–down discriminations. Note that the effect is named after the poorer capacity.

left-to-right bias The tendency to SCAN (4) a display from left-to-right. It is most marked in people who are literate in a language that is read left-to-right, but, surprisingly, is also seen in people not literate in such a language. There is also an analogous top-to-bottom bias.

legal authority AUTHORITY, LEGAL.

legal psychology Because the term FORENSIC PSYCHOLOGY is often used in a manner that focuses on the clinical and psychopathological aspects of psychology and the law, this term was introduced to identify the approach that focuses more on empirical research and theory. It hasn't really caught on.

lek (lekking) A form of mating behaviour whereby members of one gender congregate in specific areas and 'set out their wares' for the other gender. Various insect, bird and mammal species use this mating pattern. In most, it is the males that congregate.

lemma In logic, a proposition accepted as true for use in the proof of another proposition. Lemmas are usually distinguished from POSTULATES in being, in principle, provable (or supposedly so).

lemniscal system A polysynaptic pathway that ascends through the reticular formation. Made up of the *lateral lemniscus*, which runs rostrally through the medulla and pons carrying fibres of the auditory system; the *medial lemniscus*, which ascends through the medulla and pons carrying somatosensory fibres; and the *trigeminal lemniscus*, which runs parallel to the medial carrying afferent fibres from the trigeminal (VIIth cranial) nerve to the thalamus.

lens 1 Any transparent refracting medium. **2** In vertebrate eyes, the transparent, crystalline structure lying just behind the pupil which helps to focus light on the retina. See ACCOMMODATION (2).

lenticular nucleus Collectively the *putamen* and *pallidum* of the BASAL GANGLIA (see that entry for details).

-lepsia, -lepsy Combining forms meaning *seizure*.

leptin A protein secreted by adipose tissue (fat cells). It causes an increase in metabolism, a rise in body temperature and decreases in food intake. Because it also appears to be associated with feelings of satiety, there were early hopes that it might function as a weight-loss drug for the obese. Unfortunately these have not been borne out. Most overweight individuals are not lacking in leptin; the difficulty seems to be associated with reduced receptivity to it.

lept(o)- Combining forms meaning *small, thin, fine* or *weak*.

leptokurtosis KURTOSIS.

leptomorph BODY-BUILD INDEX.

lesbian A female homosexual.

Lesch–Nyhan syndrome A genetic metabolic syndrome marked by abnormally high levels of uric acid resulting in severe mental retardation. The main behavioural characteristic of the syndrome is a pattern of severe self-mutilation, including lip-biting and finger-chewing, often to the point of causing serious deformities. The disorder is associated with a recessive X-linked inheritance, and males are primarily affected.

lesion 1 Most generally, any impairment or flaw produced by an injury. **2** More specifically (and commonly), a circumscribed area of impairment to organic tissue caused by injury, disease or surgical intervention. vb., *to lesion*.

lethologica A temporary inability to recall a proper noun or a name.

letter-by-letter dyslexia An acquired learning disability in which a person reads each letter sequentially rather than as a whole word. Hence, 'cat' is read as 'c-a-t' rather than as a single, unified chunk.

letter cancellation test A general term for any of a variety of tests in which participants are asked to cancel out particular letters from a complex array. In the simpler tests, letters are presented in rows on a sheet of paper and the task is to cross out all instances of a particular letter. The task can be made more complex by changing the target letter from row to row, mixing up the rows, etc. Used as a test of attention deficits and such neurological syndromes as *neglect*.

letter-number sequencing A test in which letters and numbers are presented intermixed and the participant is asked to report the numbers in ascending order and the letters in alphabetic. It is used as a measure of working memory and is often part of standard tests of cognitive function (e.g. it is one of the subtests in the WECHSLER MEMORY SCALE).

letter reversal REVERSAL(S).

leuc(o)-, leuk(o)- Combining forms meaning *white, colourless*. As prefixes they are found in a variety of terms pertaining to disorders of white blood cells and cerebral white matter; e.g. *leukoencephalopathy* is a disease of the white matter of the brain.

leucotomy LOBOTOMY.

leukocyte A white blood cell. var., *leucocyte*.

level 1 Position or rank on some continuum, e.g. *intelligence level*. **2** A uniform concentration of a substance in the body, e.g. *glucose level*. **3** The magnitude of a quantity measured according to a specified reference value, e.g. *decibel level*. **4** A measure of performance, e.g. *sixth-grade reading level*. Compare with PHASE and STAGE.

levelling The tendency to smooth over the unusual, irregular or novel aspects of a situation, an event, a story or a drawing such that details are glossed over and what ultimately ends up in memory is a more homogeneous, less incongruous version than what was objectively presented. The reverse tendency is *sharpening*, in which details are (over) emphasized and accentuated. Some have suggested that together these two tendencies represent the poles on a dimension of *cognitive style*; others that essentially everyone displays both tendencies to some extent or other depending on the circumstances and the nature of the material.

level of achievement ACHIEVEMENT, LEVEL OF.

level of aspiration ASPIRATION, LEVEL OF.

level of confidence 1 SIGNIFICANCE LEVEL. **2** CONFIDENCE (2). Note, these two meanings are related but different.

level of significance SIGNIFICANCE LEVEL.

levels of consciousness LEVELS OF *AWARENESS.

levels of processing DEPTH OF PROCESSING.

levodopa See L-DOPA.

Lewinian Of or pertaining to the general point of view of the Prussian-born psychologist Kurt Lewin (1890–1947). Lewin's work was influenced by the Gestalt movement and by the Freudian psychoanalytic school, both of which emphasized the dynamic and the structured elements of human personality. His general position often goes by the name of FIELD THEORY, with the concept of the LIFE SPACE holding a central position. Much of Lewin's theorizing about the life space was highly esoteric and was concerned with his attempts to develop a model of personality based on the topology of HODOLOGICAL SPACE. There has been little lasting impact of this specific work; his influence on modern psychology derives largely from his emphasis on groups and group dynamics and from his intellectual and personal style, which was democratic, generous and accepting.

lexical-decision task An experimental technique for evaluating the manner in which verbal information is stored in memory. The task simply requests the subject to decide as rapidly as possible whether a string of letters presented briefly is a real word or a nonword. The pattern of response latencies that the subject produces is a sensitive measure of LEXICAL *MEMORY. Also called *word–nonword task*.

lexical memory MEMORY, LEXICAL.

lexicon Most generally an alphabetic listing of the words of a language, a dictionary. By extension, in cognitive theories of human memory the term is used loosely for the storehouse of words that a person knows, although the restriction that the ordering be alphabetic is always dropped when talking about a mental lexicon. See LEXICAL *MEMORY.

lexicostatistical method A technique for estimating the historical connection between two languages. By comparing the number of cognates in a standard list of common terms, an evaluation can be made of the duration of separation and evolution from a common parent language.

LH 1 *Luteinizing hormone* (see MENSTRUAL CYCLE). **2** *Lateral hypothalamus* (see HYPOTHALAMUS).

libidinal The adjectival form of *libido*; hence, relating to the sexual energy derived from the id; highly sexual. Distinguish from LIBIDINOUS.

libidinal (infantile) development In classical psychoanalysis, the series of stages of growth through which each individual passes from infancy to the latency period; namely, the *oral, anal* and *genital*.

libidinal object The object (person or thing) in which libido is invested.

libidinous Excessively sexually active. Distinguish from LIBIDINAL, from which the connotation of excess is absent.

libido 1 In psychoanalysis, the hypothesized mental energy which, being derived from the id, is most fundamentally sexual. Freud, who introduced the term, modified his usage of it considerably in his later works so that the purely sexual component became less prominent and it took on a meaning closer to *life* energy. This meaning developed along with his reinterpretation of *instinct* to include only Eros and Thanatos, with libido being the energy of Eros. Within the larger scope of psychoanalysis these later modifications never dominated thinking to the extent that the early theory did and *libido* itself has tended to retain its strongly sexual connotations. Owing, however, to these somewhat conflicting senses of the term it is frequently taken simply to represent: **2** any sexual or erotic desire or pleasure, or **3** any psychic energy independent of sexuality. Between these two the vast majority of contemporary usages is covered. adj., *libidinal*.

library In cognitive psychology, especially in the study of long-term memory, the term serves as a metaphor for the totality of information about the world that a person carries about.

Librium CHLORDIAZEPOXIDE.

lie detector An instrument that measures several physiological processes that may be interpreted as indicators of emotional arousal, e.g. heart rate, blood pressure, breathing rate, galvanic skin response. It is, of course, not a lie detector at all; rather, it detects autonomic reactions that are argued to accompany the telling of deliberate falsehoods. Put simply, it detects physiological arousal, not guilt, and therein lies the problem. Such arousal may indeed accompany guilt but it also accompanies many other emotionally arousing circumstances. Law-enforcement officers typically have more faith in the device than do trained scientists. See also POLYGRAPH.

lie scale A subscale of the MMPI designed to detect attempts on the part of test-takers to present themselves in an unrealistically positive light (i.e. to detect lying).

life 1 The collective total of those properties that differentiate the living from the nonliving. The unsatisfying circularity of this definition will have to suffice for now. It is said with truth that biologists only began making progress when they gave up trying to define this term. **2** The actual state of being alive as manifested by the carrying out of various functions associated with life, e.g. metabolism, growth, reproduction and adaptation to the environment. **3** The time between inception and death. Fixing the two poles here has proved troublesome. The question of whether life (in the sense of an individual, distinct organism) begins at conception, at birth or at some intermediate point during gestation (e.g. the point at which the foetus becomes capable of survival outside the womb) has troubled judges, theologians, philosophers and scientists for a long time with no, as yet, satisfactory resolution. Similar problems arise in defining DEATH.

life chance(s) The likelihood of any person achieving particular goals, e.g. in education, earning power, marriage, prestige, influence. Strong relationships exist in all stratified societies between such factors as one's sex and race, the socioeconomic status of one's family and one's life chances. See also SOCIAL CLASS.

life cycle 1 The sequence of stages that each member of a particular species goes through from inception to death. **2** By extension, the analogous stages of other social units such as groups, societies and institutions. Note that the term *cycle* here implies that all members or social units undergo these stages and that they recur from generation to generation.

life goal In Adler's conceptualization, the fundamental aim of achieving the particular form of superiority that will allow one to compensate for one's primary, felt inferiority.

life instinct Synonym for EROS. See also LIBIDO.

life lie Adler's term for one's primary defensive rationalization(s) about what one cannot do, what one will surely fail at if one attempts it, owing to one's personal feelings and weaknesses.

life plan Adler's term for the full complement of defensive reactions and rationalizations that one uses in attempts to achieve superiority and to justify failure. See also GUIDING FICTION.

life space The central notion in Kurt Lewin's personality theory. Influenced by the Gestalt perspective, he characterized the world of each individual as a dynamic life space composed of regions representing all the states of affairs, persons, goals, objects, desires, behavioural tendencies, etc. germane to the individual. Lewin developed topological models complete with vectors and valences to characterize 'movement', 'direction' and 'force' within the life space and hoped that mathematical models could be developed to formalize the system. For more detail, see FIELD THEORY and LEWINIAN.

lifespan 1 The actual duration of life of an individual organism from inception to death. **2** By extension, the duration of a whole species.

light The stimulus for vision, specifically electromagnetic radiation of wavelengths between approximately 400 and 700 nm. Light may be characterized as either individual particles (quanta) or as waves; the latter is most useful for work in psychology, as this definition reflects.

light adaptation The process of adjustment of the eye to light of relatively high intensity, the shift from the *scotopic* system to the *photopic* system. In the light-adapted eye the pupil is constricted and the cone system is operative, rendering the eye relatively insensitive to lower intensities. Compare with DARK ADAPTATION.

light induction VISUAL INDUCTION.

lightness That attribute of an OBJECT COLOUR

according to which it is positioned on the black–grey–white spectrum.

lightning calculator A person who is capable of performing complex feats of mathematical calculation in his or her head. There are several variations on this general theme. Some such persons can carry out massive multiplication problems, such as squaring seven digit numbers; others are capable of calendar 'look-up' feats, such as figuring out the day of the week on which 11 March 2040 will fall. Little is known about the operations or processes used by these people, who frequently (but not always) display little or no other special intellectual talent. See SAVANT. See also MNEMONIST.

light reflex The pupillary response. Generally it includes both dilation, when light levels drop and constriction when they are raised, although it is occasionally used only for the constriction response.

likelihood 1 Commonly used as a synonym of *subjective probability*; i.e. the estimation by a person of the probability of some event occurring. **2** In statistics, the probability that a sample statistic arose from a particular set of parameters in the population from which the sample was drawn.

likelihood ratio In simplest form, the ratio of the probability that a signal was present and detected by the subject (a *hit*) to the probability that a signal was not actually present but was apparently detected by the subject (a *false alarm*). For elaboration of this usage see SIGNAL-DETECTION THEORY. Naturally, this concept has considerable generality, for *signal* can be variously interpreted to mean scientific hypotheses, beliefs, stories, expectations about events and the like; hence, the mathematical system underlying likelihood ratios can be applied to more subjective realms of psychology, such as choice behaviour, decision-making and statistical testing.

Likert scale A scale developed by Rensis Likert and used primarily in measurement of attitudes. The respondent is given a series of attitude statements and asked to rate them according to his degree of agreement or disagreement. Usually there are five levels, running from 'strongly agree' through 'uncertain' to 'strongly disagree', although scales with three, seven or even more choices

are used and called Likert scales. The importance of the technique is due to the fact that the resulting data are easily amenable to factor analysis, which allows the basic underlying dimensions of the tested attitudes to be evaluated.

liking scale A scale developed to measure interpersonal liking. The scale is based on two primary components assumed to reflect liking: a feeling that the liked person is similar to oneself and an overall favourable evaluation of the liked person. Compare these with the components of the LOVE SCALE.

limb apraxia APRAXIA, LIMB.

limbic system A complex set of evolutionarily old structures of the forebrain lying in an arc below the corpus callosum. The specific structures generally classed as limbic are the *hippocampus, anterior thalamus, amygdala* and *septum*, and parts of the *hypothalamus* and their interconnecting fibre bundles. For more details, see the entries for these separate structures.

limen Latin for THRESHOLD.

liminal Of or pertaining to THRESHOLD. Usually used in combined forms, e.g. *subliminal, supraliminal*.

limit 1 The terminal value of a series. **2** The end(s) of some continuum, especially a sensory continuum. **3** The ASYMPTOTE.

limits, method of MEASUREMENT OF *THRESHOLD.

limulus The horseshoe crab. Important in psychology because of a very large compound eye that lends itself nicely to experimental study. Much of the work on lateral inhibition was performed on limulus.

linear 1 Generally of or relating to a line. **2** Specifically, of or relating to a straight line. **3** Continuous, as opposed to discrete. n., *linearity*.

linear correlation CORRELATION, LINEAR.

linear-operator model An early mathematical theory of learning based on a linear equation that specifies how the probability of a response is hypothesized to increase or decrease as a function of the occurrence of particular events or 'operators', such as reinforcement or punishment.

linear perspective A monocular depth cue based on the geometric fact that as the distance of an object increases, the visual angle that it subtends on the eye of the observer decreases. The familiar railroad tracks receding to a single point in the distance are perhaps the most frequently cited example.

linear regression REGRESSION, LINEAR.

lingual 1 Of or pertaining to the tongue. 2 By extension, pertaining to languages. 3 In articulatory phonetics, characteristic of sounds made with the tip of the tongue.

lingual papilla A visible protuberance on the surface of the tongue associated with the taste buds. Anatomically, there are four kinds of papillae: *circumvallate, folate, fungiform* and *filiform*. All but the last contain taste buds.

linguistic relativity WHORFIAN HYPOTHESIS.

linguistics Broadly, the study of the origins, evolution and structure of language(s). At one time, linguistics and psychology benignly followed their own bents quite independently of each other; but no more. Since the work of Noam Chomsky in the 1960s the two disciplines have become importantly interrelated; in fact, Chomsky has characterized his own discipline of linguistics as a branch of cognitive psychology. See also LANGUAGE, PSYCHOLINGUISTICS.

linguistic universals UNIVERSALS, LINGUISTIC.

linkage In genetics, two or more genes are said to be linked if they tend to be passed from generation to generation as a unit. The mechanism of linkage is chromosomal and the closer the genes are to each other on the chromosome the more closely they are linked. Thus, all the genes on a given chromosome are said to form a *linkage group*. Note, however, that even closely linked genes can become separated as a result of *crossing over*.

lipoprivation A drop in the level of fatty acids available for cells. Whether brought about by a drop in blood levels of lipids or by drugs that inhibit the metabolism of fatty acids, it causes a state called *liproprivic hunger* which is a stimulus for eating. Also see GLU-COPRIVATION.

liproprivic hunger LIPOPRIVATION.

liquid In phonetics, the 'flowing' speech sounds *r* and *l*.

lisp An articulatory speech disorder in which sibilant sounds (*s, z, sh, ch*) are mispronounced, usually by substituting a *th* sound.

Lissajou's figures Revolving abstract designs, produced either by reflections from vibrating mirrors or on an oscilloscope screen. When watched closely for a time the direction of apparent rotation reverses.

lissencephaly Literally, smooth brain. A disorder in which the gyri fail to develop normally, producing a smooth cortical surface. Not surprisingly, the syndrome is associated with severe mental retardation.

literacy The state of being literate, the ability to read and write. Specifying precisely what level of ability in these skills equates to functional literacy has proven to be something of a problem. See ILLITERACY; see also READING.

lithium (salts) Usually classified as *antipsychotic drugs*, lithium compounds are used primarily in the treatment of BIPOLAR DISORDERS, particularly the manic aspect. The lithium salts have rather pervasive effects on the nervous system. The most commonly used form, lithium carbonate, has a significant impact on the action of sodium at neural junctures, interferes with both the synthesis and the reuptake of several neurotransmitters and modifies the concentrations of serotonin and its precursor, tryptophan. Consequently, it has been difficult to discern which of its many actions is responsible for its mood-stabilizing effects. It is also highly toxic and dosage must be carefully controlled. Common side effects include dizziness, slurred speech and ataxia. Note that occasionally the lithium salts are referred to as *antidepressant drugs*. However, they differ from the typical antidepressants in that they are only effective with the depression that accompanies bipolar disorder.

litigious paranoia A form of PARANOIA marked by feelings of persecution, particularly with regard to beliefs that one's rights have been abused. As the name suggests, such individuals often have a history of filing law suits to seek redress for imagined wrongs.

Little Albert The 11-month-old boy used by Watson and Rayner in 1920 to demonstrate that phobias could be produced by simple classical conditioning. They paired a white laboratory rat (which Albert had previously shown a liking for) with a loud clanging noise that scared him. After several pairings of the rat with the aversive sound, Albert displayed a classic CONDITIONED EMOTIONAL RESPONSE to the rat and to other similar objects by pulling back from them and crying. The original study is somewhat infamous owing to questions about the exact procedure used as well as the ethical issues that Watson and Rayner (as well as everyone else in those days) seemed oblivious to.

Little Hans The pseudonym of one of Freud's most famous cases, the psychoanalysis of a young boy with a phobia of horses. It was, and still is today, cited by many as a source of supportive evidence for the Freudian theory of psychosexual development in children and how neuroses emerge from deep psychic conflict. It is also cited by many others as a classic case of flagrant overinterpretation – these persons typically are those with a behaviourist orientation who view phobias as the result of conditioning processes.

LKS LANDAU–KLEFFNER SYNDROME.

Lloyd Morgan's canon Articulated in 1894 by the British physiologist/psychologist Conwy Lloyd Morgan, this cautioned against the explanatory excesses of the new field of comparative psychology by stating that in interpreting the behaviour of an animal it is always preferable to use the psychologically simplest interpretation. Specifically, it is preferable to use the lower or more primitive explanation rather than to assume the action of a higher, more mentalistic process. The canon was very influential in the work of early behaviourists such as Watson and Thorndike. See also OCCAM'S RAZOR and the PRINCIPLE OF *PARSIMONY, with which the canon shares a philosophical basis.

loading FACTOR LOADING.

loafing SOCIAL LOAFING.

lobe Any reasonably well-defined part of an organ.

lobectomy Generally, the surgical removal

of a lobe, or part of a lobe, of the brain. The term is usually used with a qualifier to denote the lobe(s) in question.

lobotomy, prefrontal A surgical procedure severing the white-matter tracts between the frontal lobes and the diencephalon, especially those of the thalamic and hypothalamic areas. The original operation was developed by A. E. Moniz in the 1930s and was so heralded as a psychosurgical procedure for severe psychological disorders that he received a Nobel prize for his work. With the accumulation of data from tens of thousands of lobotomies (including one performed on one of Moniz's own patients, who, ungrateful wretch, shot the good doctor, causing a partial paralysis), the general conclusion is that the procedure does not work. Whatever beneficial results may occasionally be obtained must be balanced against the negative side effects of apathy, insensitivity, impaired judgement and seizures, all of which are irreversible. Recent years have fortunately witnessed its demise. Also called *prefrontal leucotomy*. See PSYCHOSURGERY.

lobotomy, transorbital A procedure for performing a PREFRONTAL *LOBOTOMY in which a surgical knife is inserted above the eyeball and moved to cut brain fibres.

localization 1 Perceptual act of locating the spatial position of a stimulus. The term is used with respect to audition (locating a sound source in the environment), vision (locating a stimulus in the visual field) and tactile sensations (making references to the point of stimulation on the skin). **2** LOCALIZATION OF FUNCTION.

localization of function A general hypothesized principle concerning brain function that, all things considered, specific functions have relatively precise and relatively circumscribed cortical locations. Contrast with the principle of MASS ACTION.

local sign According to the perceptual theory of the 19th-century philosopher Rudolph H. Lotze, every tactile and visual sensation has its particular local sign or 'signature', an experiential intensity that is specific for the point stimulated, either on the skin in the case of the tactile or on the retina in the case of the visual. The perception of space was, according to Lotze, produced by the relationships between the local signs as the stimulation shifted across the receptor system.

location error (or **bias**) SPACE ERROR OR BIAS.

loci, method of A mnemonic device in which the memorizer uses as the basis for learning new material a well-known geographical or architectural structure as a set of locations. For example, the Russian mnemonist S (as he is known in the literature), studied by Luria, used to 'place' objects to be recalled in a mental picture of a well-known street. To recall the list of objects he would merely take a 'mental walk' down the street and 'pick up' the objects where he had placed them.

lock-and-key model A model of synaptic transmission based on the assumption that a neurotransmitter affects only those postsynaptic receptor sites that have the correct shape for that particular molecule, much as a key fits into a lock.

locomotion Aside from the standard meanings, *locomotion* was used by Lewin in a figurative manner to refer to the movement of a person through his or her LIFE SPACE.

locomotor ataxia ATAXIA.

locus Generally, a locale, a spot or a place. Used widely as follows: in perception, a point in space; in genetics, the position of a gene on a chromosome; in physiology, a circumscribed area on or in an organ; etc. pl., *loci*.

locus coeruleus A group of cell bodies located in the dorsal pons. Axons from cells here branch widely and release *norepinephrine* throughout the neocortex, hippocampus, thalamus, the cortex of the cerebellum, medulla, and the rest of the pons. Activity in the locus coeruleus is closely associated with the sleep–waking cycle.

locus of control A general term in social psychology used to refer to the perceived source of control over one's behaviour. It is measured along a dimension running from high *internal* to high *external*, with internal persons being those who tend to take responsibility for their own actions and to view themselves as having control over their own destinies, and externals being those who tend to see control as residing elsewhere and to attribute success or failure to outside

forces. Note that *reality* is not being measured here; the question is not whether true control derives from endogenous or exogenous sources but how the individual *perceives* it. See also ATTRIBUTION THEORY, INTERNAL–EXTERNAL SCALE.

log 1 LOGARITHM. **2** LOG(O)-.

logagnosia A condition in which the patient can see and read words but not identify them in terms of their meanings. Some classify it as a form of AGNOSIA, most regard it as a type of APHASIA.

logamnesia A condition in which the patient is unable to recognize spoken or written words. See APHASIA, of which it is a common symptom.

logaphasia An older term for MOTOR *APHASIA.

logarithm The exponent to which a number (called the *base*) must be raised to equal a given number. Hence, $\log_{10} 1,000 = 3$, since the base (10) must be raised to the 3rd power to yield 1,000. The most common log bases are 2 (see INFORMATION), 10 (most of the arithmetic calculations used in psychology) and *e* (the natural logarithmic system in mathematics in which *logarithmic* is abbreviated *ln*).

logarithmic curve (or **relationship**) Any curve in which the variables are related to one another according to the equation $y = \log x$.

logarithmic mean GEOMETRIC *MEAN.

-logia Suffix meaning *relating to speech* or *speaking*.

logic That normative branch of philosophy that deals with the criteria of validity in thought, the canons of correct predication and the principles of reasoning and demonstration. Logic concerns only the reasoning process, not the end result. Incorrect conclusions can be reached through logical means if the original assumptions are faulty. See also FORMAL *LOGIC, SYMBOLIC *LOGIC.

logic, affective Sequencing of ideas or deductions in which the connecting factors are emotional.

logical 1 Pertaining to LOGIC. **2** Characterizing reasoning that is sound, correct.

logical-mathematical intelligence MULTIPLE INTELLIGENCES THEORY.

logical positivism POSITIVISM, LOGICAL.

logic, formal Logic based on FORMAL (2) propositions as opposed to logic based on meanings.

logic, symbolic Originally *logic* referred only to linguistic manifestations of reasoning – see here LOGO-. Symbolic logic was developed using a logical/symbolic language to formalize logical processes and thus remove them from the ambiguities of natural languages.

logistic regression REGRESSION, LOGISTIC.

log law Term used for FECHNER'S LAW.

log(o)- Combining form from the Greek *logos* meaning *word* and, by extension, *speech* and even, on occasion, *thought*.

logogen John Morton's term for a memory unit that is assumed to represent a 'node' that interlinks all aspects of a word's representations (i.e. its semantic, auditory, visual and pictorial properties). A logogen is viewed as an integration of all the relevant information with regard to any particular word or concept.

logography Any ORTHOGRAPHY based on the use of signs to represent words or morphemes. Mayan, early Egyptian and Chinese are examples.

logomania LOGORRHOEA.

logopathy General label for any speech disorder.

logorrhoea The roots of the word should be familiar enough. The literal meaning is, of course, an excessive flow or stream of words, usually incoherent. It is often accompanied by an *anosognosia*, in that the patient is unaware of the disorder and may become angry when people fail to understand what he or she is saying. Also called *logomania*, *lalorrhea* and *verbomania*. var., *logorrhea*.

logotherapy Viktor Frankl's term for his form of psychotherapy based on focusing the client on a recognition and acceptance of himself or herself in a meaningful way as part of a totality, including the real world within which he or she must function. Often characterized as the third Viennese

school (Freudian and Adlerian being the first two), Frankl's approach embodies elements of the dynamic psychologies, *existentialism* and *behaviourism*, the latter particularly with regard to the role of learning in the development of neurotic behaviours. Frankl's orientation is also seen as an important component of the HUMANISTIC PSYCHOLOGY movement.

-logy Combining form meaning *speech* and, by extension, *knowledge* or *science*.

Lombrosian theory A theory of criminality proposed in the late 19th century by Cesare Lombroso. His thesis was that criminality was biological and that 'criminal types' could be identified through physical analysis of head shape. It was without scientific foundation and its main impact was to make life rather unpleasant for some unfortunates with the 'wrong' head shape.

longitudinal 1 Pertaining to length, along the length of something. **2** In anatomy, pertaining to direction or position along the long axis of the body.

longitudinal fissure SAGITTAL FISSURE.

longitudinal method Research carried out by following a number of subjects over an extended period of time. Compare with CROSS-SECTIONAL METHOD.

long-term depression (LTD) 1 A long-term decrease in excitatory postsynaptic potentials. It operates in a fashion opposite to LONG-TERM POTENTIATION. Just as frequent stimulation increases the ease with which neurons are activated, infrequent stimulation decreases it. It allows for the unlearning of associations as the contingencies in the environment change. **2** DEPRESSION (2). Meaning 1 is almost always the one intended, although in the clinical literature one will see references to depressions that last a long time.

long-term memory (or **store**) MEMORY, LONG-TERM.

long-term orientation A social-cultural philosophy emphasizing a focus on the future and on delay of need gratification over more *short-term* goals such as consumption, quick results and enjoyment of leisure activities. The construct is more complex than this simple definition suggests, and encompasses a variety of social and personal values. In general, people in economically stable East and South Asian countries are higher on long-term orientation than are people from European, North American and African countries, leading some to put forward *Confucian values* as a replacement.

long-term potentiation (LTP) A relatively permanent increase in the excitatory POST-SYNAPTIC POTENTIAL (or EPSP) at a synapse. It can be produced by delivering a rapid train of impulses to the presynaptic neuron and is manifested by stronger and more prolonged EPSPs. First observed in the dentate gyrus of the hippocampal formation, LTP has since been found in a variety of pathways throughout the cortex and the cerebellum. LTPs are thought to be the basis for the long-term modification of neural pathways and, thus, represent the neural foundations of learning and memory. Recent work suggests that they are maintained by a protein kinase, PKMζ. There is also an opposing LONG-TERM DEPRESSION (1).

long-term working memory MEMORY, LONG-TERM WORKING.

looking-glass self A term introduced by C. H. Cooley to characterize a person's perception of him- or herself as a reflection of how he or she appears to others. A person's self-image is formed as a consequence of the attitudes others have about him or her.

look–say method WHOLE-WORD METHOD.

looming A term used to describe the complex of gradient transformations produced as one rapidly approaches some object, or vice versa. Essentially, looming is the cue for an impending collision.

loosening of associations A thought disturbance in which ideas shift in a helter-skelter manner from subject to subject, producing an incoherent stream.

LOP abb. for *levels of processing*. See DEPTH OF PROCESSING for details.

lorazepam An ANTIANXIETY DRUG of the BENZODIAZEPINE group. It has few side effects and, unlike other benzodiazepines, puts no extra demands on liver function making it a useful compound in treating alcoholism.

lordosis 1 A severe concavity of the spine and back. **2** A concave arching of the back in response to specific stimulation. It is a common sexual response in many species.

lose–shift strategy WIN–STAY LOSE–SHIFT STRATEGY.

lost-letter technique A procedure for evaluating HELPING BEHAVIOUR. A number of addressed, stamped letters are 'planted' in various places such as street corners, hallways and buses. The data consist of the number of letters picked up and mailed by passers-by.

loudness The psychological attribute of an auditory stimulus corresponding to the physical dimension of intensity.

love Psychologists would probably have been wise to have abdicated responsibility for analysis of this term and left it to poets. The confusing litter left behind by lack of wisdom and excess of boldness can, however, be codified by the following classification scheme. First, the two most general uses of the term: **1** An intense feeling of strong liking or affection for some specific thing or person. **2** An enduring sentiment toward a person producing a desire to be with that person and a concern for the happiness and satisfactions of that person. Note that both of these meanings may or may not carry sexual connotations. Certainly 1 is often used in reference to cats, tennis, teachers or academic disciplines, and 2 to refer to parents or children – all without sexual or erotic connotations. However, 1 may apply equally well to paramours and 2 to wives and husbands and lovers. The primary role played by love in either of these senses is that it is an affective state that is assumed to colour all interactions with and perceptions of the person or thing loved. It is this component, of course, that makes love so attractive to psychologists.

In psychoanalytic theory, where one might hope to turn for clarification, one finds, in the British analyst C. Rycroft's words, 'as much difficulty defining this protean concept as elsewhere'. The term is used variously to mean: **3** Any affective state defined as the opposite of *hatred*. **4** An emotion liable to sublimation or inhibition. **5** An equivalent of Eros, an instinctive force close either to the life instincts or to the sexual instincts – depending on whether one is affiliated with the early or late Freudian point of view (see LIBIDO for clarification).

Meaning 3 seems to be of little value to psychologists: it merely defers the definitional obligation. Meanings 4 and 5 are close to the classic psychoanalytic meaning, particularly in that here all manifestations of love – love of self, of children, of humanity, of country or even of abstract ideas – are viewed as manifestations of a basic instinctual force and, hence, subject to the action of defence mechanisms. However, complications do arise, particularly since some theorists append the notion of *object* love, and reinterpret the ideas contained in 4 and 5 as a manifestation of a need to relate to objects – which may include, of course, people.

Using love as a scientific term produces several types of conflict which we specify here with no attempt at resolution. First, there is the issue of sex and sexual expression: is this an essential component or can love exist totally divorced from it? Second, there is the instinct issue: is love innate or is it an acquired emotional response? Third, there is the problem of the manner or manifestation of the emotions: can the feeling be dissociated from the behaviour or does the emotion always contaminate the behaviour? Fourth, and probably most troubling to many, is love merely an emotive state that results from particular neurochemical actions and, by implication, crassly manipulable?

love, agape Selfless, unconditional love. Rarely observed in real world relationships, it is a central component of many religions.

love, companionate Love that is based on a secure and trusting relationship.

love, romantic According to Rubin, that kind of love hypothesized to exist between opposite-sexed peers. See LOVE SCALE.

love scale A scale devised by Z. Rubin to measure ROMANTIC *LOVE. The scale is constructed to evaluate three components: affiliative/dependent needs; predispositions to help; and exclusiveness. Differentiate these components from those used in the LIKING SCALE. Note that this effort to specify the underlying dimensions of romantic love is accomplished by dramatically circumscribing the domain discussed under the more general term LOVE.

love withdrawal A form of discipline in which parents control a child's behaviour by expressing disapproval. Although the technique consists of making disapproving statements to the child like 'That was a stupid thing to do', the implication is that the parent has, by making such a statement, withdrawn his or her love.

low-balling A two-step device for obtaining compliance in which the individual first secures agreement by requesting something simple and then steps up the request by revealing hidden costs. Compare with THAT'S-NOT-ALL TECHNIQUE; contrast with FOOT-IN-THE-DOOR TECHNIQUE and DOOR-IN-THE-FACE TECHNIQUE, in which the second step involves a new request, not a change in the original deal.

low-grade defective DEFECTIVE (2).

loxapine An ANTIPSYCHOTIC DRUG used primarily in the treatment of schizophrenia. Because it blocks the reuptake of both serotonin and dopamine and is chemically related to CLOZAPINE, some have argued that it should be classified as an ATYPICAL *ANTIPSYCHOTIC.

LRCS Abbreviation for *language-responsible cognitive structure*. See LAD.

LSD LYSERGIC ACID DIETHYLAMIDE.

LTD LONG-TERM DEPRESSION.

LTM LONG-TERM *MEMORY.

LTP LONG TERM POTENTIATION.

LTS Abbreviation for *long-term store*. See discussion under LONG-TERM *MEMORY.

Luchins water-jar problem(s) WATER-JAR PROBLEM(S).

lucid dream DREAM, LUCID.

lucid interval A period of relatively normal mental functioning between bouts of a psychotic disorder.

lucidity Clarity, especially of mind.

ludic From the Latin *ludere*, meaning *to play*. **1** Pertaining to behaviours that are seemingly primary, in that all members of a species display them, yet have no obvious biological basis. Generally included as ludic activities are exploration, curiosity, intellectual games, humour and the like. **2** In Piagetian terminology, characterizing that which is make-believe.

lumen In light measurement, the amount of light within a unit solid angle coming from a 1 candlepower source. abbrev., *L*.

luminance The *luminous flux* emitted, reflected or transmitted by a surface and measured in candles/m². Luminance is directly related to the ILLUMINANCE at the surface times the reflectance of the surface. Thus luminance is equal to RC/d^2, where R is the reflectance of the surface, C is the candle-power of the source and d is the distance of the source from the surface.

luminosity A term with an often confusing array of uses. Once used rather indefinitely for *brightness*, in the contemporary visual sciences it now refers to the property of a stimulus such that the physical characteristics of the energy radiating or reflecting from it are adequate for exciting sufficient numbers of visual receptors for the experiencing of a visual sensation. In older texts this concept was rendered by the term VISIBILITY. Some authors use SPECTRAL SENSITIVITY as a synonym of *luminosity*. This is not wrong, although spectral sensitivity when unqualified is a rather more general term and applicable to any spectrum, not just the visual (e.g. the auditory spectrum).

luminosity coefficient(s) Any of the coefficients expressing the relative luminosity of the visual system to the various wavelengths of the visible spectrum. The coefficients are normalized measures of sensitivity of the system given, relative to the wavelength of peak sensitivity. For the SCOTOPIC system the peak is at approximately 510 nm, for the PHOTOPIC it is at approximately 555 nm. In older texts the term *visibility coefficient* is often used.

luminosity curve(s) Spectral sensitivity curve(s) for the visual system showing the sensitivity of the system to all wavelengths within the visible spectrum. There are a number of such curves depending on a variety of factors, such as whether the eye is dark-adapted or not and whether one is evaluating the SCOTOPIC or the PHOTOPIC function.

luminous flux The amount of light radiated or emitted by a source, measured in LUMENS.

luminous intensity Luminous flux emitted per unit angle about a light source, measured in international *candles* or *candelas*.

lunacy An obsolete term for legal INSANITY.

lupus An autoimmune disease marked by a variety of central-nervous-system symptoms including stroke, seizures, dementia, peripheral neural dysfunctions and, occasionally, psychosis. *Systemic lupus erythematosus*, as it is properly known, is almost certainly not a single disease but a heterogenous group of neurological disorders, each with potentially different aetiologies.

lure An item used to attract attention away from a correct answer. Lures are an important technique in the construction of multiple-choice tests and are used in investigations of topics like the NEGATIVE SUGGESTION EFFECT. Often the term *critical lure* is used, particularly when a number of lures are used but only one of which is of theoretical importance.

lurking variable A third, hidden variable that might explain a correlation between two other variables. For example, there is little doubt that there would be a correlation between infant distress and ice-cream sales in a northern urban environment like New York City. The correlation, however, would be driven by a third variable – temperature – 'lurking' behind the data.

luteinizing hormone (LH) A hormone that, in the female, regulates progesterone production during the latter stages of the menstrual cycle and, in the male, regulates the production of androgen. Also called *interstitial-cell-stimulating hormone*. See also MENSTRUAL CYCLE for more detail on its manner of action in females.

luteotropic hormone PROLACTIN.

lux A unit of ILLUMINANCE equal to the amount of light falling on a surface 1 m from a source of 1 international *candle* or *candela*.

Luys, nucleus of SUBTHALAMIC NUCLEUS.

lycanthropy The delusion that one is, or can change into, a wolf.

lymph The alkaline fluid of the lymphatic

vessels. Lymph differs from blood in that red corpuscles are absent and the protein content is lower. It is found in tissue spaces all over the body; it is gathered into small vessels and carried centrally, eventually entering the bloodstream at junctions with the large veins near the heart.

lymphocytes Specialized white blood cells that manufacture dozens of the natural chemicals involved in the body's immune reactions. The T-lymphocytes are produced in the thymus, the B-lymphocytes in the bone marrow.

lysergic acid diethylamide (LSD) An exceedingly powerful psychoactive drug capable of producing extreme alterations in consciousness, hallucinations, dramatic distortions in perception and unpredictable mood swings. It was originally classified as a *psychotomimetic* drug because it appeared to produce a state that mimicked a psychosis (in particular, schizophrenia), although this parallel now seems to have little to recommend it. It is difficult to predict what a person's reactions to LSD (or, for that matter, any psychoactive drug) will be. The effects are dependent on a number of factors other than dosage, such as the expectations of the user, the setting in which the experience takes place and the individual's general psychological state of mind at the time. There was, for a time, hope that it might have some therapeutic role to play, and a few researchers reported some success in treating various disorders from schizophrenia to alcoholism. Follow-up work failed to confirm these early reports and today the drug is regarded as having essentially no clinical value. As a recreational drug it harbours a number of very real psychological dangers.

-lytic Suffix indicating *opposition*, often used of drugs that oppose a form of action; e.g. a *sympatholytic* drug opposes sympathetic-nervous-system effects.

M

M Abbreviation for MEAN. Often set in italics, *M*.

m 1 Matter. **2** MEANINGFULNESS.

MA MENTAL *AGE.

mμ Millimicron (10^{-9} metre).

μ The Greek letter *mu*, a common abbreviation for *micron*.

MacBeth illuminometer A now-obsolete device for measuring the visual effectiveness of light that uses a person's own eye as the basic measuring instrument. It is rarely used any more since much more efficient and precise photometric instruments now exist; see PHOTOMETRY.

Mach bands A phenomenon of brightness contrast produced when a dimly illuminated area is adjacent to a more brightly illuminated one. The perceived change in brightness is considerably sharper than the actual change in light intensity, and two bands of dark and light are seen on either side of the gradation. These two bands are named after the 19th-century scientist Ernst Mach.

Machiavellianism Descriptive of a pattern of behaviours, including manipulation of others through guile, deviousness, deception and opportunism, with the increase of power and control as the central motive. The term 'honours' the 16th-century Italian court adviser Niccolò Machiavelli.

Machiavellian Scale A scale designed by R. Christie to measure Machiavellianism. The subject is asked to agree or disagree with a series of statements, many of which are actually direct quotes from Machiavelli's writings. Also known by the shortened form *Mach Scale*.

Machover Draw-a-Person Test A popular projective test in which the subject is asked to draw a person and tell a story about the drawing. Both drawing and story are then analysed. Designed for use with ages 2 and up. Also known as the *DAP Test*.

Mach Scale MACHIAVELLIAN SCALE.

MacLean's theory of emotion Taking PAPEZ'S THEORY as a base, MacLean's major modifications were that other areas of the limbic system, particularly the hippocampus and the amygdaloid complex, were involved in emotion as well as the hypothalamus and that the more primitive layers of the cortex played a major role in integrating information. MacLean's theory is part of his more general characterization of the TRIUNE BRAIN.

macro- Prefix connoting *large, long* or *thick*. Compare with MICRO- (1). See also MEGALO- et seq. for terms not found here.

macrobiotic Long-lived; characterizing that which functions to prolong life.

macrocephaly A cover term for any of a number of pathological conditions marked by abnormal enlargement of the head.

macroelectrode A large electrode used for recording the activity of a large number of neurons. Compare with MICROELECTRODE.

macromania MEGALOMANIA.

macropsia Abnormal enlargement of perceived size of visual stimuli.

maculae acusticae Collectively, the *macula sacculi* and *macula utriculi*, the two patches of sensory cells in the utricle and saccule in the vestibular apparatus of the inner ear.

macula fibres Neural fibres which leave the

retina from the *macula lutea* and form the central core of the optic nerve.

macula lutea A small yellowish spot in the centre of the retina. It contains a pit or depression known as the FOVEA. Also called the *yellow spot*.

mad hatter's disease A condition marked by mental confusion, emotional disturbances, muscular weakness and, in advanced cases, a full psychosis. It is caused by chronic mercury poisoning; the name came from its high incidence among hatters who worked with furs and felt treated with mercury.

madness A strictly nontechnical term for INSANITY, which itself has only a very specialized technical use.

magazine In operant-conditioning procedures, any mechanical device that delivers food, water, etc. to the experimental subject.

magazine training A part of the process of shaping an operant response. The subject is trained to associate the sound and sight of the MAGAZINE with reinforcement.

magic Sociologists and social psychologists will classify a practice as magic when: (a) the practitioners believe that supernatural powers are the cause of events; and (b) it is not a part of an organized religion, although this latter criterion tends to be applied rather ethnocentrically.

magical number 7±2 SEVEN PLUS OR MINUS TWO.

magical thinking The belief that thinking is equated with doing. Seen in children as a normal stage of development, during which they believe that their thoughts and hopes are the cause of events happening about them. Also observed in adults in a variety of psychiatric disorders. See also OMNIPOTENCE OF THOUGHT.

magico-phenomenalist In Piaget's theory, a description of an infant in terms of his or her presumed quality of perception prior to the development of OBJECT PERMANENCE. Basically the idea is that such infants are thought to perceive the world through unorganized, fleeting, sensory impressions.

magnacide The act of assassinating a famous person for no other reason than the fact that he or she is famous.

magnetic resonance imaging (MRI) A noninvasive procedure that provides a detailed picture of body tissue. An MRI resembles a CAT-scan (see COMPUTERIZED AXIAL TOMOGRAPHY) but uses a strong magnetic field instead of X-rays. Strong magnetic fields cause the nuclei of some molecules in the body to spin. When a radio wave is passed through the body, the nuclei emit energy at various frequencies, which are picked up by the MRI scanner; a computer then interprets the pattern of emissions and assembles a picture of a slice of the tissue. MRI-scans have several advantages over CAT-scans and PET-scans (see POSITRON EMISSION TOMOGRAPHY). They present fine detail more clearly; they do not use potentially damaging X-rays; and they can make scans in the sagittal or frontal planes as well as the horizontal. While MRI techniques are still widely used, particularly in medicine, researchers in the cognitive neurosciences favour the fMRI (FUNCTIONAL MAGNETIC RESONANCE IMAGE), in which the scan is carried out while the cognitive tasks are actually taking place.

magnetoencephalography (MEG) An IMAGING (TECHNIQUE) based on the use of sensitive devices (SQUIDs) to measure the magnetic fields produced by brain activity. Because MEG has extremely high temporal resolution (down to 1 msec), it is a good complement to FMRI, which lacks such. Its main limitation is that it doesn't pick up activity from subcortical structures.

magnetotropism An orienting response to a magnetic force.

magnitude estimation METHODS OF *SCALING.

magnitude production METHODS OF *SCALING.

magnocellular system That portion of the pathways of the visual system that is responsible for the perception of form, movement, depth and small brightness differences. The system is named after the large, rapidly conducting, evolutionarily old cells that make up the magnocellular layers of the lateral geniculate nucleus. Often termed *M channel*. Compare with PARVOCELLULAR SYSTEM and KONIOCELLULAR SYSTEM.

main effect In statistical analysis of data, the basic relationship between a single independent variable and a single dependent variable.

mainstreaming The educational practice of removing children with special problems (physical, mental and/or emotional) from special classes and schools and placing them in regular classroom settings.

maintaining stimulus Generally, any stimulus the mere continued presence of which is sufficient to continue to elicit a particular response.

maintenance functions All those physiological processes and behavioural activities that serve to keep an organism in a relatively stable (i.e. *homeostatic*) condition.

maintenance level The physiological steady state of a mature organism after growth has ceased and diet and environmental conditions serve to keep things relatively constant.

maintenance schedule A schedule of feeding, watering, exercising, etc. that keeps an organism at MAINTENANCE LEVEL.

major affective disorder MOOD DISORDERS.

major depressive episode DEPRESSIVE EPISODE, MAJOR.

major epilepsy EPILEPSY, MAJOR.

major solution K. Horney's term for a form of NEUROTIC SOLUTION in which one engages in vigorous compulsive activity as a way of avoiding anxiety and conflict.

major tranquillizer TRANQUILLIZER, MAJOR.

mal French for *sickness, disorder, evil*. Used in some combined forms, e.g. *mal de mer* = seasickness, *petit mal* = minor epilepsy, *grand mal* = major epilepsy.

mal- Prefix used to express *faulty, ill, imperfect*. Essentially synonymous with DYS-, although the latter is properly reserved for words of Greek origin.

maladaptive Lit., of that which is not adaptive. There are three primary usages here: **1** In biology, characterizing aspects of an organism that limit its chances of developing the behavioural repertoire needed for survival; also descriptive of an organism with such features. **2** By extension, in evolutionary biology, of such characteristics when displayed

by a species. **3** In psychiatry and clinical psychology, of patterns of behaviour likely to produce so much psychic distress or dysfunction that therapy is needed. This usage, which is growing in popularity, was introduced to de-emphasize the medical or disease aspects of much standard psychiatric terminology. The argument put forward by those who favour this term is that many clinical syndromes are fundamentally maladaptive behaviour patterns or maladaptive ways of thinking, not necessarily signs of *mental illness* or *mental disease*. See ADAPTIVE (2).

maladjustment ADJUSTMENT is basically the relationship that any organism establishes with respect to its *environment* (although see that term for nuances). The connotation is that when this relationship is adaptive the state of adjustment exists, and when it is not there is a condition of maladjustment. Generally, the term is used with respect to social or cultural standards and values, although it may legitimately be applied to more basic biological conditions as well. See ADJUSTMENT DISORDER.

malapropism The inappropriate substitution of one word for another similar in sound. See also SPOONERISM.

mal de ojo A CULTURE-SPECIFIC SYNDROME found in the Mediterranean. The term translates as *evil eye*, and the condition is especially found in children. Symptoms include fitful sleep, crying without apparent cause, fever and various digestive problems.

male erectile disorder (or **dysfunction**) A SEXUAL AROUSAL DISORDER in males marked by a persistent or recurrent inability to maintain an adequate erection. While this term is the one recommended in *DSM-IV*, IMPOTENCE and its variations are still very much in use.

maleness The condition of possessing those physiological and anatomical characteristics of a male that relate to his reproductive capacity. Distinguish from MASCULINITY.

male orgasmic disorder ORGASM DISORDERS.

malevolent transformation H. S. Sullivan's term for the development of the (neurotic) sense that one is living in the midst of one's enemies, particularly persons with some measure of control over one's life, e.g. doctors, nurses, teachers, parents.

malformation Generally, any deformity. The term is frequently used with the connotation that a deformity is congenital.

malign **1** adj. Tending to harm, damaging, malignant. **2** vb. To speak about a person in an injurious manner which denigrates or causes harm.

malignant adj. Characteristic of a condition which is growing worse; virulent, harmful, ultimately fatal. Contrast with BENIGN. n., *malignancy*.

malignant narcissism NARCISSISM, MALIGNANT.

malingering Deliberate feigning of illness, disability or incompetence. Contrast with HYPOCHONDRIA, in which the condition is not faked but believed. See also FACTITIOUS DISORDER.

malleus One of the AUDITORY *OSSICLES.

malpractice Incorrect or negligent treatment or other professional action especially by a physician, psychologist or other health practitioner. The term has both ethical and legal implications.

Malthusian theory The rather pessimistic theory of Thomas Malthus (1766–1834) which states that the population of a species tends to increase geometrically while its food supply only increases arithmetically. Hence, some check on the population must occur and Malthus cited war, pestilence, famine, disease and plague as those most likely while counselling birth control and limitations in family size. The implications of Malthus's arguments became an important element in the development of Darwin's theory of evolution through natural selection. See EVOLUTIONARY THEORY.

mammal Any member of the Mammalia class of vertebrates. Mammalian characteristics include, in addition to the obvious mammary glands for milk secretion and suckling, hair, a diaphragm for respiration, a lower jaw consisting of a single pair of bones, and the ossicles of the middle ear.

mammary glands The compound glands of the female breast that secrete milk.

mammillary bodies Two small rounded projections in the medial area of the hypothalamus that have been implicated in emotional behaviour and sexual motivation.

man **1** The genus *Homo* of the primate order, of which the species *Homo sapiens* is the only surviving member. **2** By extension, any member of this species. **3** By de-extension, any male member of this species. Raised consciousnesses everywhere concerning the nonequivalence of these meanings have created no end of linguistic havoc. In this volume we have tried to use gender-neutral language as much as possible, hence *man* is only used when it refers to the species as a whole, as in 1, and to the male of the species, as in 3.

management **1** The carrying out of functions of planning, organizing and directing any enterprise. **2** Collectively, those persons in an organization who perform these functions.

managerial psychology A subarea of industrial/organizational psychology focusing on the role of the manager or supervisor in an organization and the interactive processes between the supervisor and those supervised.

MANCOVA MULTIVARIATE ANALYSIS OF COVARIANCE.

mand A category of verbal behaviour proposed by Skinner in his analysis of language. A mand represents a large class of utterances that make demands upon the hearer and are reinforced by fulfilment of the demand. Classic examples of mands are 'Please pass the salt' and 'Get me my book.' See also AUTOCLITIC and TACT.

mandala A mystic symbol of the cosmos generally of circular form with representations of deities arranged symmetrically around it. Used chiefly in Hinduism and Buddhism as an aid to meditation, it has become popular in the West for similar functions. In Jungian theory it is the symbolic representation of the striving for unity of the self.

mandibulofacial dysosostosis TREACHER COLLINS SYNDROME.

mania **1** Loosely and nontechnically, madness; violent, erratic behaviour. **2** A mood disorder characterized by a variety of symptoms including inappropriate elation, extreme motor activity, impulsiveness and excessively rapid thought and speech. It is a component in several MOOD DISORDERS, particularly the manic aspect of BIPOLAR DISORDER. adj., *maniacal, manic.*

-mania A suffix used to indicate an obsessive preoccupation with a particular activity or pattern of thinking or a compulsive need to act in some deviant fashion; see e.g. KLEPTOMANIA, MEGALOMANIA, PYROMANIA.

maniacal MANIA.

mania, unipolar MANIA (2). The qualifier *unipolar* is used for cases in which there are recurrent episodes of mania without the appearance of the depressive phase observed in the classic BIPOLAR DISORDER.

manic 1 adj. Characteristic of MANIA. **2** n. One diagnosed as having MANIA (2).

manic bipolar disorder BIPOLAR DISORDER, MANIC.

manic-depressive psychosis (or **illness, reaction** or **syndrome**) BIPOLAR DISORDER.

manic episode A distinct period during which the predominant mood is MANIA (2).

manifest anxiety Overt, displayed anxiety; anxiety about which one is conscious. Note, when the term is used in psychoanalytic writings the assumption is that such anxiety is a symptom of a deeper, repressed conflict.

Manifest Anxiety Scale (MAS) A scale for measuring manifest or admitted anxiety. It is distinct from other devices for assessing anxiety, which are classified as *projective techniques* since they are designed to deal with repressed or unconscious aspects. The MAS was derived from the *MMPI* and consists of a set of descriptions of anxiety symptoms which the respondent identifies as characteristic or not characteristic of the self.

manifest content LATENT AND MANIFEST *CONTENT.

manipulandum Basically, any characteristic of an object that can be manipulated. The term is most commonly used to refer to the physical object the movement of which is associated with reinforcement in an operant-conditioning situation.

manipulation check Generally, any procedure that checks to ensure that an experimental manipulation has had its intended effect. For example, suppose an experiment on motor learning uses a preliminary task designed to fatigue participants. Some independent procedure needs to be used to ensure that the manipulation functioned as claimed. It is not enough to point to the fact that performance fell off and therefore the participants must be tired; they may have simply become bored by the manipulation and stopped trying.

manipulative drive A motive to manipulate objects, to handle and explore them. It was hypothesized by neobehaviourists that organisms, including many lower species, have this drive since they are known to perform other behaviours in which the only reward is the opportunity to manipulate a complex novel object.

mannerism A characteristic quirk or habitual oddity in an individual's behaviour or speech.

Mann–Whitney U A nonparametric statistical test based on rank-order data. It compares two samples of scores by evaluating the probabilities of the distribution of rankings. One of the most powerful of the nonparametric tests, it is often used in place of the *t test* when the assumptions of parametric tests are not met. There is also an extension of the test to three samples known as the *Whitney extension*.

MANOVA MULTIVARIATE ANALYSIS OF VARIANCE.

mantra Specifically, a Vedic hymn. More generally, any ritual verbal incantation used devotionally or as an aid in meditation.

manual alphabet FINGER SPELLING.

manual language SIGN LANGUAGE.

manual method A method of teaching communication to the deaf through the use of sign language. For many years a controversy has raged over whether this method is preferable to the so-called *oral method*, in which the teaching is through carefully shaped speaking and lip reading. The manual method has the major drawback that it can only be used with others trained in sign language, which eliminates the vast majority of the hearing; the oral method's primary liability is that only a small percentage of those who undergo training reach the fluency needed for easy communication. Most teachers of the deaf today aim for a combination of the two, teaching signing first so that the deaf can communicate with each other and using the oral method later.

MAO inhibitor MONOAMINE OXIDASE INHIBI-TOR.

mapping In the study of vocabulary acquisition, the procedure whereby words are attached to meanings. Novel word mapping is the procedure by which one learns that a newly encountered word refers to a novel object, concept, attribute or action (see WHOLE-OBJECT ASSUMPTION). By extension, *fast mapping* is the phenomenon of rapid vocabulary growth during the toddler period, when children learn several new words almost every day, often without direct instruction. There is considerable research on the mechanisms that enable children to accomplish this task, whether adults show similar fast mapping, and whether it applies to concepts and general knowledge or only to vocabulary.

marasmus Originally, the deterioration of tissue in the young caused by poor nutrition. The term is also used as roughly synonymous with ANACLITIC DEPRESSION and thus incorporates a sense of emotional deterioration as an outcome and social and sensory deprivations as causes.

marathon group An aptly named group-therapy technique in which a group of individuals, usually with a fairly singular focus or purpose, meets for an extended period of time ranging anywhere from roughly 6 hours up to 48 hours.

Marbe's law The generalization that in word-association tasks the more frequently a response occurs the more rapidly it tends to occur; latency is inversely related to frequency.

Marfan's syndrome A genetic condition consisting of large, bony fingers, hyper-extensible joints and a gaunt, angular face. Often cardiac abnormalities are present, including a weakened aorta.

marginal 1 Generally, on the margin; characteristic of an instance or event of uncertain classification or one on the borderline between two classes or categories. **2** MARGINAL FREQUENCY. **3** In significance testing, an

observed probability that approaches but fails to meet the *a priori* chosen significance level for rejecting the null hypothesis. Most typically, an obtained probability between .10 and .05 is termed marginal.

marginal frequency (or **total**) In any data matrix, the sum of any one of the rows or columns, i.e. the frequencies in the margins. For example, in a tabulation of persons by sex and height one set of marginals (as they are often called for short) would give the number of men and the number of women without regard to height; the other set would give the totals of each height without regard to sex.

marginal group GROUP, MARGINAL.

marginal intelligence An occasional synonym of BORDERLINE INTELLIGENCE.

marginalization In cultural psychology, the process whereby individuals or groups fail to identify with any national or cultural group. Commonly found in immigrants who identify with neither their culture of origin nor their host culture, and those whose idiosyncratic beliefs or practices keep them on the margins of society. Some use *marginal man* or *marginal person* in this manner to refer to both individuals and groups. Also spelled *marginalisation*.

marginal man (or **person**) MARGINALIZA-TION.

margin of attention ATTENTION, MARGIN OF.

margin of consciousness MARGIN OF *ATTEN-TION.

marijuana (or **marihuana**) CANNABIS (SATIVA).

marital therapy Therapy aimed at the resolution of problems of married couples. Typically both parties are in therapy conjointly although on occasion each may be seen individually. The focus is generally broad, embracing psychodynamic elements, sexual issues, economic factors, etc. The term COUPLES THERAPY is preferred by many for it encompasses unmarried unions as well. See also FAMILY THERAPY.

marked–unmarked adjectives In adjectives that represent poles along a dimension often one can be 'neutralized' to represent the whole dimension and is considered to be *unmarked* while the other, which cannot be so neutralized, is called *marked*. For example, in the pair *long–short, long* is unmarked and can represent neutrally the concept of time, as in the question, 'How long was the movie?' If, however, one asks, 'How short was the movie?' the question is not neutral but presupposes that the film was inordinately short.

marker 1 In linguistics, a signal that indicates (i.e. marks) a function or a feature. The easiest way to grasp the use here is to note that markers generally designate the presence or absence of distinctive features. Thus, a full stop is a sentence-boundary marker, voicing marks the phone [b] and distinguishes it from [p], -*ed* marks the past tense of regular verbs in English, etc. **2** In medicine generally and psychiatry specifically, any sign that can be used diagnostically with respect to a specific disorder. Three kinds are identified: EPISODE, RESIDUAL and VULNERABILITY *MARKER.

marker, episode A MARKER (2) or specific symptom that occurs in particular disorders, e.g. fluid in the lungs in pneumonia, auditory hallucinations in schizophrenia. Episode markers allow one to confirm a diagnosis. Compare with RESIDUAL and VULNERABILITY *MARKER.

marker, residual A MARKER (2) which is an aftereffect of a disorder and hence marks a patient as having had that disorder even after it has subsided, e.g. certain antibodies following viral infections, subtle sensorimotor deficits following some psychiatric disorders. Compare with EPISODE and VULNERABILITY *MARKER.

marker, vulnerability A MARKER (2) that exists before, during and after a particular disorder. Vulnerability markers are, generally speaking, risk factors associated with particular disorders and include such things as particular genes that predispose one to a particular syndrome. Compare with EPISODE and RESIDUAL *MARKER.

market research The application of statistical and experimental procedures to the study of buying habits, selling techniques, advertising and other attendant economic components of the marketplace. See also MOTIVATION RESEARCH.

marriage Common parlance tends to miss the point that marriage is an institution, a set of social norms. In all cases it sanctions, according to local customs, a union between two (or on occasion more) persons and, at least theoretically, binds them to a system of obligatory behaviours for the purpose of maintaining a family unit. Although we need not list them here, it should be noted that anthropologists and sociologists distinguish over a score of different kinds of marriage.

marriage counselling MARITAL THERAPY.

masculine protest An Adlerian term which can take two forms. The uninteresting use is to describe a desire on the part of the female to be male. The interesting one is to characterize the drive for power and superiority which can, of course, be displayed by either sex.

masculinity Lit., the state of an organism reflecting or displaying the appearances, traits and behaviour patterns characteristic of the male of the species. As defined, the label does not necessarily implicate gender; it should not be used as a synonym of MALENESS. See also FEMININITY.

masculinity–femininity scale (MF scale) A scale designed to measure the degree of masculinity and femininity in a person. Note that the scale is gender-free; that is, one's sex does not limit one to scoring on either extreme. This type of scale must always be viewed as tightly culture-bound since what characterizes masculinity or femininity differs dramatically from culture to culture.

masking A general term in the study of perception for any process whereby a detectable or recognizable stimulus (called the *target*) is made difficult or impossible to detect or recognize by the presentation of a second stimulus (the *masker*) in close temporal or spatial proximity to it. Masking may occur in any sensory system; e.g. it may be: auditory, when an above-threshold tone is masked by the introduction of a second tone; visual, when a recognizable form is rendered unrecognizable by introducing an overlapping figure; olfactory, when one odour is covered by another. Masking may also be produced by several temporal arrangements of the target and masker. In *simultaneous masking* the two are presented together; in *backward masking* the masker is presented some (usually very short) time after the target; in *forward masking* the order of presentation is reversed. See also METACONTRAST, which refers to visual masking when the target and masker are spatially separated.

masking, lateral MASKING of a visual stimulus by other stimuli on either side of it. Note that in such cases there will always be mutuality; the target stimulus will mask the masker as well as being masked by it, and often the term *mutual lateral masking* is used. See also METACONTRAST.

masking, remote In audition, the masking of low-frequency tones by high-frequency noise stimuli. It is hypothesized that the effect is produced by distortion processes in the inner ear.

masochism The term derives from the name of the Austrian novelist Leopold von Sacher-Masoch, and refers most broadly to any tendency to direct that which is destructive, painful or humiliating against oneself. Special uses abound: *sexual masochism* is used when erotic pleasure is associated with the treatment; *moral masochism* is used when such tendencies dominate to such an extent that they seem to represent a character trait, the presumption here being that the person seeks to alleviate guilt by subjecting him- or herself to continuous punishment; *psychic masochism* is used of any kind of hostility or destructive impulse turned upon oneself, a usage which is very general; *mass masochism* refers to whole populations subjecting themselves to pain and hardship.

masochistic personality disorder SELF-DEFEATING PERSONALITY DISORDER.

masochistic sabotage A psychoanalytic term for blatant, overt, self-destructive acts. Such acts are assumed within the theory to result from unconscious motives to punish oneself.

mass In social psychology, any large number of people both diverse in make-up and without social organization. The interesting aspect of the term is the implication that although the mass is without discernible structure the people involved tend to behave in a relatively uniform fashion. See here MASS BEHAVIOUR. Distinguish from MOB.

mass-action principle A generalization concerning cortical functioning put forward by the American physiological psychologist Karl S. Lashley. In simplest terms he argued that the cortex operates as a coordinated system, that large masses of tissue were involved in all complex functioning. This position contrasts with the oft-proposed theory that specific local areas of the brain mediate specific behaviours. Lashley's theory rests upon the demonstration that the degree of disruption of a learned behaviour is due not simply to the location of brain lesions but to the amount of tissue involved. Note that Lashley was not suggesting that there was no localization of function but that such localization was only part of the story.

massa intermedia Tissue that connects the two lobes of the THALAMUS.

mass behaviour Collective behaviour of a MASS without any obvious direct or personal communication or mutual influencing of the individuals making up the mass. Fads and fashions, dress styles, political movements, etc. are examples. The assumption is that mass-communication systems are the channels through which the societal influences occur. Also called *mass contagion*.

mass contagion MASS BEHAVIOUR.

massed practice PRACTICE, MASSED.

Massformel German for *measuring formula*. It was Fechner's label for his grand achievement; see FECHNER'S LAW.

mass hysteria A form of MASS BEHAVIOUR where pathological or maladaptive behaviour is exhibited by large numbers of people. Such episodes can be deadly (e.g. WERTHER SYNDROME) or merely expensive (e.g. TULIPMANIA). Also called *collective hysteria* and *group hysteria*.

mass movement Spontaneous behaviour of a mass of people with some particular focus or goal. Although there may be a common aim the term does not imply that the movement is controlled or organized. In fact, reflecting the meaning of MASS, the assumption is that there is no overall plan.

mass noun COUNT/MASS NOUN DISTINCTION.

mass reflex Generally, any reflex-like

response involving large numbers of muscles and glands, e.g. the *startle response*.

mastery The achieving of some preset level of functioning on some task.

mastery test TEST, MASTERY.

mastoid From the Greek for 'breast' and 'resembling', the small bony projection just behind the lower part of the outer ear. When a vibrating solid is placed there, the vibrations are translated directly to the inner ear and a sound is heard.

masturbation The accepted meaning of the term is the production of erotic stimulation of the genitals, usually to the point of orgasm, by manual means. Although not explicit, the usual inference is that the stimulation is self-induced. The Latin roots of the term are interesting, particularly in light of so many of the Puritan myths about masturbation: *manus*, meaning *hand*, and *stupare*, meaning *to defile* or *dishonour*.

MAT MILLER ANALOGIES TEST.

matched-groups procedure An experimental procedure in which control is achieved by matching the groups of subjects on those variables not specifically under investigation. In cases in which very fine control is required individual subjects in each group are matched against each other, the so-called *matched-pairs procedure*. Also called *equivalent-groups procedure*. See also YOKED CONTROL, which is a variation on the general procedure.

matched pairs MATCHED-GROUPS PROCEDURE.

matched sample SAMPLE, MATCHED.

matching law The generalization that an organism will select each of several alternatives with a probability that matches the overall probability that each of the alternatives actually occurs. See PROBABILITY MATCHING, a somewhat more neutral term that merely describes rather than claims 'lawful' status for this phenomenon.

matching test MATCHING TO SAMPLE.

matching to sample An experimental procedure, simple in basic form but with many complex variations. Most succinctly, the subject is shown a target stimulus and required to choose from a set of alternative stimuli the one that matches the target. Simple variations allow for exploring a host of psychological processes. For example, memory can be studied by introducing a delay between the target and presentation of the alternatives; category representation can be examined by having the correct alternative be physically distinct from the target (e.g. oak tree as target and maple tree as match) and even abstract concepts can be explored by having the match be on the number of objects or their functions.

materialism 1 In a sociological sense, a preoccupation with the pursuit of things material to the neglect of the mental or the spiritual. **2** As a philosophical position, the doctrine that the only means through which reality comes to be known is through an understanding of physical matter. Contrast here with MENTALISM and VITALISM and compare with MECHANISM.

maternal aggression AGGRESSION, MATERNAL.

maternal behaviour Collectively, all those behaviours related to or associated with being a mother. The term is often used synonymously with *caring for the young*. This usage, understandable given much of the behaviour of specific species, is misleading when applied universally. In many species the father displays nurturant behaviour, and we would do well to use the neutral word CAREGIVER (2) as the general term with *maternal* and *paternal* reserved for specific cases.

maternal-deprivation syndrome A group of symptoms, including stunted physical growth and retarded emotional development, associated with infants who have been deprived of handling and nurturing. Interestingly, the syndrome emerges in species other than humans and has been documented in several mammals, including monkeys and mice. See MATERNAL BEHAVIOUR for some terminological issues regarding gender.

maternal drive (or **instinct**) Generally, the tendency of the female of a species to engage in the so-called maternal behaviours of feeding, sheltering and protecting the young. The term can be misleading: the adjective *maternal* suggests falsely that males do not display these behaviours, and the nouns *drive* and/or *instinct* imply that the behaviours are wholly innate and unitary. The situation is complex. Under a variety of conditions females will fail to display the behaviours, and under other conditions males will actively engage in them. Moreover, when the various aspects of the criterial behaviours are measured and compared, they are found not to correlate. Overall, a term best discarded from the psychologists' lexicon.

maternal immunization hypothesis The hypothesis that the well-documented increase in likelihood of homosexuality in later-born males is due to the development of maternal antibodies to antigens released by earlier male foetuses during prior pregnancies. The assumption is that these antibodies inhibit development of male characteristics in the brain and possibly the hormonal systems. Also called *foetal antigen hypothesis*.

maternal impression, influence of The doctrine that a mother's experiences, feelings and thoughts during pregnancy directly affect the foetus. This thesis is of considerable antiquity and is even represented in the Book of Genesis. While it is certainly true that many experiences of the mother have an impact on the foetus (e.g. drugs, diseases, diet), in the strong form that the doctrine is usually put forward it is utterly false. Listening to Beethoven will not produce musically precocious offspring, nor will a sudden fright produce a birthmark or other deformity.

mate selection Collectively, any and all mechanisms, strategies and processes used to choose an appropriate partner for reproduction. Individual species have evolved an amazing array of strategies for searching out 'desirable' partners. See PARENTAL INVESTMENT for one based on shared resources and responsibilities that plays a significant role in many species.

mathematical learning theory LEARNING THEORY, MATHEMATICAL.

mathematical model Any model or theory expressed in formal mathematical terms, and, hence, one making precise quantitative predictions.

mathematical psychology A cover term for any systematic effort to frame psycho-logical ideas, hypotheses and theories in formal mathematical terms. Mathematical psychology does not represent any one idea or interest, although some issues have been found to be more amenable to mathematical analyses than others. In *psychophysics, decision-making, learning* and *information-processing* some progress has been made; other areas, such as clinical, personality and social psychology, have been virtually untouched.

mathematico-deductive method An occasional synonym of HYPOTHETICO-DEDUCTIVE METHOD.

mating Loosely and collectively, all the behaviours associated with reproduction including selecting one's mate (see MATE SELECTION), courtship behaviour and eventual copulation. The term was first used by ethologists and animal behaviourists and referred primarily to species other than *Homo sapiens*. However, it has developed considerable currency in EVOLUTIONARY PSYCHOLOGY and is now routinely used to refer to human behaviour.

mating, assortative Mating of individuals within a species that are more similar (or more dissimilar) phenotypically than would be expected if only chance mating were to occur. It is termed *positive* when the mating is between phenotypically similar individuals and *negative* when between dissimilar. Compare with INBREEDING.

mating, random Mating that occurs essentially by chance, where there are no particular biases that encourage selection of a mate with any particular phenotypic characteristics. Compare with ASSORTATIVE *MATING.

mating system Any structured pattern for mating based on the number of males and females involved. Most species have a particular strategy that developed over evolutionary time. See, for example, MONOGAMY, POLYANDRY, POLYGAMY, POLYGYNANDRY and POLYGYNY.

matriarchy A social organization using the female (or, more literally, the *mother*) as the base. Sociologists and anthropologists distinguish between various forms of matriarchies depending on which societal aspects are involved. Thus, a *matriarchal family* is a family group organized around the mother as the head and dominant person, and a *matriarchal society* is a larger social and/or governmental system in which political and administrative power is invested predominantly in females. Note that in this latter case the sense of *mother* is no longer strictly present.

matrilineal descent The passing on of the family name or inheritance through the female line. Also called *uterine descent*.

matrix 1 Any arrangement of data (or numbers or symbols) into a table of rows and columns. **2** A frame or structure that provides form or meaning, a context. Used figuratively, especially for a cognitive or perceptual context that helps to set or determine the meaning of a situation. pl., *matrices*.

matrix, correlation A matrix giving the coefficient of correlation between each variable in a data set with every other variable.

matrix, simplex A CORRELATION *MATRIX in which the component correlations display a simple, orderly linear relationship.

maturation The core meaning of this is relatively straightforward and parallels that in common language: the developmental process leading toward the state of MATURITY. The manner in which the term is used by various writers, however, introduces connotative subtleties that reflect the theoretical complexities that underlie it. Nearly all the varieties of usage revolve around one prime issue: the relative contributions of heredity and environment to the maturation process. Consider three 'definitions' found in the literature: **1** Maturation as a pure biological unfolding. In its simplest form the implication here is that the process is biologically 'prewired' and that all behavioural and morphological changes are inevitable. Practically no one holds this position any longer since even the most primitive of maturational processes require some environmental input in order to emerge in normal fashion. **2** Maturation as a process occurring within inherited boundary conditions. The notion here is that environmental input is needed for normal developmental changes to occur but that its role is circumscribed by biologically imposed limits. Some who take this position like to think of the environment as acting first as a trigger that initiates the process (this idea is, of course, also captured in the above use) and second as a dictator of the manner in which the biological processes

are manifested. **3** Maturation as that proportion of the variance in developmental change that is attributable to hereditary factors. The technical term for this meaning is *heritability*, and the position is one that reflects the commonly accepted view that heredity and environment interact with each other to control developmental/maturational processes. The various subtleties of usage here are the same as those raised under the more general term HEREDITY-ENVIRONMENT CONTROVERSY. Note also that in all of these usages the notion of *species specificity* is implicit. All maturational changes must be viewed within the framework of the individual species under consideration.

maturity From the Latin, meaning *ripeness*; the state of adulthood, of completed growth, of full functioning; the end of the process of MATURATION. The term is widely used, generally with an adjective prefixed to specify the kind of growth achieved, e.g. sexual maturity, intellectual maturity, emotional maturity, etc. Note that while some of these can be reasonably well defined, such as sexual maturity, most cannot. They generally entail value judgements made of persons to reflect how successfully they correspond to socially and culturally accepted norms. What is considered emotionally childish in one society may very well be an aspect of emotional maturity in another.

maxim A type of HEURISTIC; a general principle usually regarded as somewhat less compelling than a CANON.

maximal 1 Pertaining to or characteristic of a MAXIMUM (1, 2). **2** MAXIMUM (3).

maximal age AGE, MAXIMAL.

maximize Generally, to engage in any decision-making strategy that optimizes gain. The gain can be objective, as in studies of economic behaviour where the focus might be on heuristic and algorithmic strategies that maximize financial gain or it can be more subjective, as in social psychology where decision-making strategies aim at the best possible outcome, given that a variety of typically subjective factors are in play, e.g. maximizing happiness. Compare with SATISFICE.

maximum 1 n. The highest value of a variable, a series or a continuum. **2** n. In a curve, a value that is higher than those immediately preceding and following it. In this sense there can be several maxima in a given function. pls., *maxima, maximums*. **3** adj. Characteristic or descriptive of such values in either of the above senses. In most psychological contexts the maximum value is given by the functional capacity of the organism; e.g. the maximum intensity of a stimulus is the one beyond which further increases in the physical produce no increments in sensation. vb., *maximize*.

maximum-likelihood estimator According to the PRINCIPLE OF *MAXIMUM LIKELIHOOD, the best estimators of true population values are those which, when substituted for the population value, maximize the likelihood of the sample result. To be a good estimator a statistic should be unbiased, consistent, efficient and sufficient.

maximum likelihood, principle of A statistical principle that reflects the very spirit of empirical science and either implicitly or explicitly underlies all statistical inference. To appreciate the sense of the term, note that there are two broad classes of inference that one may want to make: (a) the inference that the obtained values in a sample are truly representative of the population; and (b) the inference that the observed results are in keeping with theoretical expectations (or, better, the inference that one's theoretical predictions accurately reflect the empirical findings). The principle of maximum likelihood states, essentially, that when faced with two or more possible values any one of which may be the true population (or true theoretical) value, then the best guess (i.e. the one with the maximum likelihood) is that value which would have made the actual empirical sample have the highest probability.

Maxwell discs Slotted coloured discs that can be mounted on a rapidly rotating spindle. By controlling the amount of overlapping of discs of various hues the basic principles of colour mixture can be represented.

maze Any experimental apparatus consisting of pathways and culs-de-sac (blind alleys) leading from a start box to an outlet or goal box. Mazes were, along with puzzle boxes, essential pieces of laboratory equipment in the early studies of instrumental behaviour. The variety available is rather impressive, from the simplest *T-maze* to the complex *Hampton Court maze*. The most common form is the multiple *T-maze* (and its progeny, the *Y-mazes*). There are also water mazes that must be swum through, elevated mazes that consist of narrow ramps, paper-and-pencil mazes, temporal mazes, straight-alley mazes (which are hardly mazes at all), verbal mazes, etc.

MBD Abbreviation for MINIMAL BRAIN DYSFUNCTION or DAMAGE (the former is preferred).

McCarthy Scales of Children's Abilities A set of developmental scales for assessing the abilities of preschoolers between the ages of 2 and 8. Since the scales were last revised in 1972, their use has diminished.

McClintock effect The synchronization of menstrual cycles in women who live together. It is taken by some to suggest that humans are affected by PHEROMONES.

McCollough effect (or **afterimage**) A persistent afterimage produced by saturating the eye (or, more precisely, the brain) with red and green patterns of different angularity. In the typical experiment a pattern of bright red and black horizontal lines is alternated with a pattern of bright green and black vertical lines every five seconds for several minutes. Following these exposures a pattern of black and white lines at various angles is presented, and when the afterimage appears the horizontal white lines are seen as tinged with green and the vertical with red. If the head is tilted 90° the colours change, taking on the appropriate coloration. The effect may last up to four or five days, or in some cases even longer.

McGurk effect See CROSS-MODAL.

MCI MILD COGNITIVE IMPAIRMENT.

McNaghten (or **M'Naghten**) **rule** A legal precedent for the establishment of an INSANITY DEFENCE set in the British House of Lords in 1843. It states that a person is not to be held responsible for a crime if he 'was labouring under such a deficit of reason from disease of the mind as not to know the nature and quality of the act; or if he did know it, that he did not know that what he was doing was wrong'. Compare with DURHAM RULE.

McNemar test A nonparametric test that evaluates whether changes in the variable under consideration are, for a given set of subjects, significant. Since the test is a test of changes, it is particularly useful in experiments in which each subject is used as its own control and scores before and after a particular treatment make up the data.

MDA Short for methylenedioxyamphetamine. It is a metabolite of MDMA which many suspect is the compound responsible for that drug's actions. Like MDMA, it has mild hallucinogenic properties.

MDMA Short for methylenedioxymethamphetamine. A hallucinogen with catecholamine properties and an amphetamine-like reaction that produces a mild euphoria along with feelings of togetherness and closeness that some have referred to as almost 'spiritual'. Onset is rapid and the experience can last for hours with residual effects occasionally felt for days. MDMA is one of the most frequently used 'party' or 'club' drugs. Because it disrupts serotonin functions, a variety of unpleasant side effects frequently accompany the high including depression, memory dysfunctions and disturbed decision-making and self-control. The street name for the drug is *Ecstasy*.

md, mdn Abbreviations for *median*.

me That aspect of SELF (esp. 1, 2) that represents those components of one's total self that derive from the environment, including material possessions, internalized social values, indeed the full collection of one's states of consciousness. William James called this me the *empirical* or *known self* and differentiated it from the I, the KNOWING SELF. George Herbert Mead also used the term in a similar fashion but with, predictably, a stronger focus upon the social aspects. Also called the *psychological self*.

mean 1 n. In statistics, any of several measures of central tendency. Properly, the particular measure used is noted (e.g. *arithmetic mean, geometric mean*); when unqualified the term invariably refers to the ARITHMETIC *MEAN. **2** vb. To form an INTENSION. **3** vb. To express a reference, to convey a meaning, to denote or connote something, to imply.

mean, arithmetic The sum of a set of values (or scores) divided by the number of values (or scores). It is the most commonly used and most useful measure of central tendency since, unlike the *median* and *mode*, it uses all of the data in the distribution and it serves as the basis for the measures of variability or dispersion. When the shorthand form *mean* is used without the qualifier it can safely be taken as a reference to the arithmetic mean. Symbol: M or $\bar{X}$.

mean, assumed Quite literally, a value assumed as a first guess to be the mean of a set of scores.

mean deviation AVERAGE *DEVIATION.

mean, geometric A measure of central tendency for a set of n values given by the nth root of the product of the n scores. Less often used than the arithmetic mean, it finds its greatest use in the study of average rates of change. Also called *logarithmic mean*.

mean, harmonic A measure of central tendency of a set of values given by the reciprocal of the arithmetic mean of the reciprocals of the set of values. Of limited use, it is found mostly in averaging rates.

meaning Let us begin with a simple truism: communication consists of three components – a transmitter, a medium and a receiver. Therefore, the *meaning* of a message as communicated, or any element thereof (e.g. a word, a phrase or a gesture), may be defined from any of three perspectives: **1** That which the speaker or writer intended to convey. As Lewis Carroll put it, speaking through Humpty-Dumpty, 'When I use a word, it means just what I choose it to mean – neither more nor less.' **2** The representation associated with the physical symbol used, the thing that it designates: 'X marks the spot', '♀ means female', 'ψ stands for psychology.' **3** The apprehended representations of the hearer or reader, the significance of the message as received.

Several cautionary notes are needed here: (a) Specification of senses 1 and 3 is no mean task. There are philosophers and linguists who will tell you that it is the single most difficult task confronting them – and there are others who will tell you it is a hopeless one. No matter what one's view is here, attempts to come to grips with the problem have spawned a large number of specialized forms of meaning; those significant in psychology are given below. (b) Sense 2, taken by itself, is something of an absurdity. The point here is that no symbol 'carries' or 'has' meaning; the meaning is in the mind of the speaker/hearer. The symbol functions as a device for achieving denotative and connotative mutuality. (c) Although meaning (broadly) is often dealt with as though it were codifiable, representable and, at least in principle, explicable, it almost assuredly is a concept that can only be made to make sense when couched in a contextual frame. For example, the standard meaning of *bachelor* is *unmarried male*, but somehow sentences like 'Oscar Wilde was a bachelor' or 'The Pope is a bachelor' or 'My ten-year-old son is a bachelor' miss the mark; they provide contextual frames that do violence to the standard dictionary meaning. Put another way, meaning is in the mind of the beholder. The ludicrous implication of this point is that dictionary-writing is a bad joke, for if words only have meaning (senses 1 and 3, of course) in particular contexts, then giving them explicit definitions is an exercise in futility. Recognizing this problem we have attempted to present the terms in this volume as expressing manner of usage; see DEFINITION for more on this problem. (d) Much of the conveyance of meaning is dependent on the degree of coordination between the intentions of the speaker/writer and the suppositions of the hearer/reader about those intentions. For example, 'She has a lovely voice' can be uttered as a compliment about a singer or a sarcastic remark about a dreadful dramatic performance, and if meaning 1 is to be coordinate with meaning 3, intentions and suppositions must be equivalent.

meaning, affective Basically, if one lists the words that can be used to characterize the sense of another word, that list will capture the affective meaning of the original word. Note that this sense of MEANING is quite close to that presented under CONNOTATIVE *MEANING. Osgood's SEMANTIC DIFFERENTIAL was designed to measure such meaning.

meaning, associative Loosely, all the things that a person thinks of upon hearing a word represent the associative meaning of that word. Note that these may well include connotative meanings (one thinks of *safety* in relation to *home*), denotative meanings

(*flare* in relation to *danger*), referential meanings (*Fido* in relation to *dog*), and many other links. See also MEANINGFULNESS.

meaning, connotative Logicians use *connote* as equivalent to *imply*. Taking off here, then, connotative meaning is that which is suggested or implied or signified by a word, symbol, gesture or event. Connotative meanings usually define abstract qualities, common properties or classes of objects, or emotional components. Contrast with DENOTATIVE *MEANING.

meaning, denotative Meaning conveyed by the objects or instances to which a word refers, or, by extension, by the generic idea or concept that is represented by a word.

meaningfulness (m) A measure developed in an effort to arrive at an objective characterization of how meaningful a particular word is. It is given as the average number of associations to a word that are produced in one minute. Meaningfulness, not surprisingly, correlates highly with other dimensions, such as imageability, familiarity and frequency of use of the word in the language, and, as a result, is rarely used in contemporary work.

meaning, referential The particular object or event (i.e. the referent) designated by a word. Usually referential meaning is highly context-dependent and quite specific.

mean length of utterance (MLU) As it says, the mean length, measured in morphemes or words, of the utterances in a sample of speech. It is one of the more frequently used measures of the linguistic sophistication of a child. Although it is a relatively gross measure and does not reflect a child's use of particular syntactic or semantic forms, it gives an excellent first approximation of the stage of linguistic development and allows for quantitative comparisons between children.

mean, sample The mean of a sample of scores. When the scores are a REPRESENTATIVE *SAMPLE, it will be the best estimator of the TRUE *MEAN.

means–ends analysis A *heuristic* or rule of thumb incorporated into several models of human problem-solving. In a means–ends analysis the solver moves toward a final solution by setting up subgoals, each of which is a means toward the final end. The term was first introduced formally in the context of a computer-based model of problem-solving: A. Newell's GENERAL PROBLEM SOLVER.

means–ends readiness In E. C. Tolman's theory of purposive behaviour, an organism's state of selective readiness such that it would acquire certain expectancies. Note how this concept enabled Tolman to sneak a subjective unobservable element like *belief* and weave it into his supposedly objective behaviourism.

means object (or situation) In Tolman's theory, any object (or situation) that brought an organism closer to a goal. He used the term as roughly equivalent to *cue*, on the assumption that a means object functioned by arousing an expectation concerning a goal.

mean square The average of a set of squared deviations from the mean, i.e. the VARIANCE. The root mean square is the square root of the mean square or the STANDARD DEVIATION.

mean, trimmed The mean calculated after the effects of extreme scores (see OUTLIERS) have been dropped.

mean, true (or population) The theoretical value representing the mean of the full compilation of all the possible scores under consideration. The sample mean is always the best estimate of this, the true mean.

measure 1 vb. To evaluate quantity or magnitude; to make a measurement. **2** n. A value obtained by an act of measurement. **3** A statistic.

measurement There is little difficulty with definition here. The one most generally agreed on comes from S. S. Stevens: 'The assignment of numerals to objects or events according to rules.' The difficulty with using the term in a scientifically legitimate fashion comes with the problems involved in constructing SCALES OF MEASUREMENT and understanding the properties that can be ascribed to them.

measurement scales SCALES OF MEASUREMENT and related terms.

meatus A passageway or an opening.

mechanical ability (or aptitude) Quite simply, ability or aptitude for the mechanical. Generally regarded as a relatively low-level intellectual ability and hence often contrasted with ability or aptitude for the abstract, for ideas.

mechanical causality 1 A class of explanations whereby the occurrence of events is represented in terms of physical (mechanical) contacts. **2** In Piagetian theory, a stage in a child's development of an understanding of causality at which he or she can analyse the various components of a causal chain of events; i.e. the child appreciates that when one ball hits another it causes the second one to move.

mechanism 1 A philosophical doctrine that maintains that all events or phenomena, no matter what their complexity, can be ultimately understood in a mechanistic framework. The position is strongly deterministic and opposed to a host of other positions, including DUALISM. See also IDEALISM and VITALISM. Moreover, it implicitly assumes the possibility of REDUCTIONISM to basic principles of physics and physiology. **2** A theoretical process through which events can be understood and explained. Note that a hypothesized mechanism in this sense can be quite concrete and 'mechanical' (e.g. classical conditioning as understood through the existing mechanism of the reflex arc), or it can be quite abstract (e.g. operant control of autonomic activity as understood through the mechanism of biofeedback). In the approach to science that characterizes most of Western psychological thought, a mechanism of this kind is considered essential for the establishment and acceptance of a phenomenon, and the failure to provide one leads invariably to scepticism and often outright rejection of purported findings. For a case study here see the discussion under PARAPSYCHOLOGY. **3** A habitual adaptive response; for example, the DEFENCE MECHANISMS of psychoanalytic theories. **4** A purely mechanical device or machine the actions of which are clearly specifiable in terms of physical cause-and-effect systems.

mechanistic organization ORGANIZATION, MECHANISTIC.

mechanistic theory MECHANISM (1).

medial **1** Pertaining to or situated in the middle. **2** Toward or near the middle of the body. See MEDIAN.

medial dorsal nucleus DORSOMEDIAL NUCLEUS.

medial forebrain bundle A pathway in the limbic system leading from the precommissural fornix and the olfactory bulb through the basal forebrain and lateral hypothalamus. It contains axons that connect with structures in the midbrain and forebrain and has been found to produce highly reinforcing self-stimulation.

medial geniculate nucleus Either of two cell nuclei lying near the rear of the thalamus which are important synaptic way stations in the ascending auditory pathways. Afferent pathways connect the inferior colliculi with the medial geniculate nuclei, and these, in turn, project onto the auditory cortex.

medial lemniscus LEMNISCAL SYSTEM.

medial phoneme Any phoneme pronounced in the middle of the oral cavity, e.g. /r/.

medial plane The sagittal or midline plane that divides the body into right and left halves. Also called *median plane*.

medial preoptic area PREOPTIC AREA.

medial syllable Any syllable in the middle of a word.

medial temporal area See VS.

medial temporal lobe (MTL) The area of the TEMPORAL LOBE containing, among other structures, the AMYGDALA and the HIPPOCAMPAL FORMATION. Damage to cells in the MTL can cause a variety of disorders including dysfunctions in emotions, abnormalities in spatial representations and TEMPORAL LOBE *AMNESIA.

median The middlemost score in a distribution of scores ordered according to magnitude. As a measure of central tendency it is used less often than MEAN; its primary value is in dealing with distributions that are dramatically skewed. Although the term is used mostly in statistics, it is also an occasional synonym of MEDIAL. abbrev., *md* or *mdn*.

median plane MEDIAL PLANE.

median test A nonparametric statistical test that evaluates the significance of the difference between the medians of two samples. The test is useful when the data consist only of ranked scores and one cannot be sure that they lie on an interval scale.

mediate **1** adj. Descriptive of stimuli, responses, items or events that are in between other stimuli, responses, items or events. **2** adj. Descriptive of behaviour or action that is dependent on an intervening process. **3** vb. To arbitrate between two or more disputants. **4** To act as a MEDIATING *VARIABLE.

mediate association IMMEDIATE *ASSOCIATION.

mediated generalization MEDIATED *GENERALIZATION and SEMANTIC *GENERALIZATION.

mediate experience IMMEDIATE EXPERIENCE.

mediating variable VARIABLE, MEDIATING.

mediation theory A descriptive label for those neobehaviourist approaches to the study of learning that assumed some event(s) intervened between the stimulus and the response and that explanations of behaviour required explication of this process. This approach and the term itself are closely tied to the S–R behaviourist orientation. Contemporary theorists take it for granted that most of what is interesting about psychological processes takes place internally and don't even bother with a term here.

medical model A general label for any approach to psychiatry and clinical psychology based on the assumption that abnormalities and disorders are produced by specific causes and that cure is only possible by removing the root cause. The analogy with the medical approach to somatic diseases is obvious. The term is used relatively neutrally; those who are critical of this particular approach will often call it the DISEASE MODEL, a term always used with clearly negative connotations.

medication-induced movement disorders Movement disorders produced by the taking of medication designed to cure or alleviate some other condition. The most common are the NEUROLEPTIC-INDUCED disorders. See also IATROGENIC DISORDER.

mediola The bony part of the division between the scala media and the scala tympani of the cochlea.

meditation A state of extended reflection or contemplation. Although the term and the characterization of the mental state itself have suffered from considerable abuse – administered mainly in response to those who make unsubstantiated claims about its therapeutic value – a few aspects of the meditational state have been documented: the EEG pattern generally shows alpha waves, oxygen consumption drops, energy expenditure is lowered and subjective reports are consistent in describing the experience as relaxing and salutary.

medium **1** Any intervening substance through which forces act or events are produced. **2** More generally, the environment. **3** More specifically, and of doubtful validity, a person through whom paranormal phenomena occur.

medroxyprogesterone acetate An ANDROGEN antagonist used in the treatment of repeated sex offenders. It is the drug used most often in HORMONAL *CASTRATION.

medulla **1** Generally, the central or inner core of a structure or an organ. **2** The MEDULLA OBLONGATA.

medulla oblongata The lowest or hindmost part of the brain, continuous with the spinal cord and containing nuclei which control vital bodily functions such as breathing, circulation, etc.

medullary sheath MYELIN SHEATH.

MEG MAGNETOENCEPHALOGRAPHY.

mega-, megalo- Prefixes from the Greek, meaning *bigness, greatness, power*, often with the implication that the characterization is exaggerated. See also MACRO- et seq. for combined terms not found here.

megalomania An exaggerated self-evaluation or sense of self-worth. A common component in narcissistic personality disorder. Also called *macromania*.

megalopsia MACROPSIA.

megavitamin therapy ORTHOMOLECULAR THERAPY.

megrim MIGRAINE.

meio- Combining form meaning *decrease in size* or *in number*.

meiosis The cell-division process in the formation of gametes. The products of meiosis (sperms and ova) are haploid cells containing half the full complement of chromosomes found in diploid cells. Meiosis consists of two successive cell divisions which superficially resemble MITOSIS, but the chromosomes are duplicated only once, with each daughter cell ending up with the haploid number.

Meissner's corpuscles Specialized encapsulated nerve endings found in the papillae of hairless skin. It is thought that they are one of the sets of receptors for the sensing of pressure and, on occasion, are referred to as tactile receptors.

mel By definition, the pitch of a 1,000 Hz tone 40 db above threshold is equal to 1,000 mels. Thus, the mel becomes the psychological unit for a scale of pitch.

melancholia From the classic Greek for *black bile*. The archaic theory of temperament was tied to the hypothesized humours or bodily fluids and their balances in the body. Today the term refers to a pronounced depression with feelings of foreboding, sleeplessness and loss of appetite.

melatonin An INDOLEAMINE produced by the PINEAL GLAND. It has a wide variety of effects including regulating seasonal physiological changes, playing a role in puberty as secretions inhibit the development of sexual maturation and modulating the sleep–wake cycle. It is sold as an over-the-counter sleep aid and appears to help in hastening sleep onset.

member **1** In Gestalt theory, the preferred synonym of *part*. The purpose is to communicate the idea that, in accordance with Gestalt principles, a given component of a larger whole is not a separate entity but rather an integrated constituent (i.e. member) of the functioning system or whole. The whole here may be anything from a simple perception to a society, and the member an aspect of a physical stimulus or a person. **2** In organizational psychology, an individual within a group. Note the semantic implications are the same as in meaning 1. Other uses of the term are in keeping with the general dictionary meaning.

membership character Extending the Gestalt use of the term MEMBER (1), the notion is that each member of a group is, to some extent, dependent on the structure of the whole group and each will be affected to a greater or lesser degree by changes in the group. Although the changes, or *characters* as they are called, are presumed to characterize any whole (or Gestalt), the term was rarely used outside the LEWINIAN approach to social psychology. See also FIELD THEORY.

membrane Any thin, flexible layer of tissue.

membrane potential The −70 mV electrical charge inside a neuron. The message that is conducted down an axon (see ACTION POTENTIAL) is nothing more than a momentary charge in the membrane potential.

meme Richard Dawkins's term for the minimal unit or component of transmission within a culture. Memes (and, yes, the term was chosen so that it rhymed with *gene*) are theorized to function as the bases of evolution of culture. Virtually any complex idea or notion can be a meme. Religious beliefs, foods, recipes for preparing foods, the wheel, wearing clothing, technologies and war all qualify. As engaging as this notion is, it should be clear that its universality of application is a serious weakness in that there are no clear boundaries to the use of the term. Recent efforts have focused on attempting to define the term using underlying neurological mechanisms but a satisfactory referential resolution is still outstanding.

memorial Of or pertaining to memory or to that which is in memory.

memorist Occasional synonym of MNEMONIST.

memorize To commit to memory. Generally the term carries the implication that the memory process used is rote memory by repeated practice.

memory Since the demise of behaviourism nearly everything about the way in which psychologists characterize memory has changed save the working definition(s) of the generic term. *Memory* refers to one of the following: **1** The mental function of retaining information about stimuli, events, images, ideas, etc. after the original stimuli are no longer present. **2** The hypothesized storage system in the mind/brain that holds this information. **3** The information so retained.

Within these definitions there are numerous and varied meanings to be found in the psychological literature. Most of the specialized uses derive from the simple fact that memorial processes are extremely complex and different memory tasks recruit different ones. For example, the rat that 'remembers' to turn left to a bright light and right to a dim one is most assuredly using a different memorial process from the one employed by the medical student who can recall the twelve cranial nerves, and this latter case is just as profoundly different from that of the person who can recall the meaning of a Socratic dialogue. As a result, *memory* is used almost invariably in psychology with some adjective preceding it to set limits on the kind of memory processes under discussion. The following entries are those in most common use. Note that in nearly every case the type of memory being specified is intimately tied in with the task of the person trying to store away the material and with the type of material being so stored. The exceptions to this pattern are those memorial systems that have theoretical pretensions.

Note also that the following virtual blizzard of specialized terms, all of which can be found in the contemporary literature, suggests that these various memory systems and functions can actually be distinguished and that terminology corresponds with an agreed-upon reality. Caution is advised here. For example, some will use *immediate memory* and *primary memory* to refer to distinct mechanisms, others will use them as synonyms; some authorities regard *implicit memory* as equivalent to *procedural memory*, others draw distinctions; *working memory* will be found as a convenient semantic replacement for *short-term memory* in some cases but not in others. Worse, the terms *memory* and *knowledge* are often used interchangeably. See KNOWLEDGE et seq. for more details and for any combined terms not found here. *Caveat lector.*

memory afterimage An obsolescent term for the kind of memory experience now captured by the term SENSORY INFORMATION STORE. The older term has been largely abandoned because the word *afterimage* is misleading.

memory, associative This term is used as a label for any memory system that is hypothesized to rest on the notion of an association. Thus the British empiricist assumption of association between ideas, the behaviourist S–R bond, the cognitivist propositionally based associationism and connectionist notions are all classifiable as associative-memory theories.

memory, autobiographical Memory for events that have occurred in one's life. It is a kind of EPISODIC *MEMORY.

memory, biological Used synonymously with **1** Jung's RACIAL *MEMORY and **2** GENETIC *MEMORY.

memory, body An odd term used by some to refer to an assumed capacity for the body to store away information, particularly about experiences of abuse or trauma. Memories, however, are stored in neural tissue. Peripheral systems involving muscle and connective tissue are modified by experience but these are not regarded as memories in the standard sense. The real difficulty with this term, however, comes from its use by those who maintain that one's body 'recalls' or 'knows' about 'forgotten' childhood abuse and that techniques like hypnosis or suggestion can be used to extract this information. See FALSE *MEMORY and RECOVERED *MEMORY for more detail.

memory, colour Memory for colours which, perhaps surprisingly, is notoriously poor. It appears that we do not store colours in an accurate form but rather organize our memory for them around prototypes such as primary colours.

memory, declarative Conscious memory, memory that one can communicate (or declare) to others. Often contrasted with PROCEDURAL *MEMORY. A rough synonym of EXPLICIT *MEMORY.

memory drum An early piece of laboratory equipment that presents a series of stimuli to a subject for memory experiments. The stimuli are printed on a rotating drum that stops at controlled intervals so that only one stimulus item is visible at a time. It has been largely replaced by computers.

memory, echoic A residual sensory memory that lasts for a short time (perhaps 2–3 seconds) after a brief auditory stimulus. See the discussion under ICONIC (2) and SENSORY INFORMATION STORE.

memory, episodic A form of memory in which information is stored with 'mental tags' about where, when and how it was picked up; i.e. the material in memory concerns fairly sharply circumscribed episodes. Compare with SEMANTIC *MEMORY.

memory, expert Memory for material within a domain that one is an expert in. It is typically fast, efficient and accurate and highly organized, particularly when compared with that of a non-expert. Chess masters, for example, can look briefly at a game in progress and accurately store the configuration of all of the pieces on the board. Such memorial feats utilize various cognitive devices such as CHUNKING, and the information so stored plays a role in LONG-TERM WORKING *MEMORY.

memory, explicit Conscious memory, memory for material of which one is aware. Explicit memory for previously presented material is tapped by tasks like *recall* and *recognition* when the individual is consciously aware of the knowledge held and can recall it or recognize it among several alternatives. When most people use the term *memory* they tend to use it in this sense; that is, memory for material is virtually always thought of as *conscious* memory. However, see IMPLICIT *MEMORY to appreciate that not all knowledge held in the mind is available to consciousness.

memory, fact Memory for specific facts events, or other information carried in a message. Often compared with SOURCE *MEMORY.

memory, false Quite literally, memory for some event that in fact did not happen. False memories are quite common and surprisingly easy to create; e.g. see RECOVERED *MEMORY.

memory, flashbulb Roger Brown's term for the memory that surrounds a particular, significant event in one's life. Such memories are typically very clear and poignant, consisting of where one was, what one was doing, who was there, etc. when the event occurred. In order for such sharp memories to be formed both a high level of surprise and a high level of emotional arousal must be present.

memory, genetic A hypothesized 'memory' for biological events that have occurred during the aeons of evolution of a species. *Memory* here is used in a metaphorical fashion to refer to a genetically coded propensity for particular behaviours and patterns of action which are vestiges of evolutionarily important modifications of the species. The fear of falling and the reflex reactions to a possible plummet have been put forward as an example reflecting an evolutionary adaptive reaction which any successful brachiating primate with a high body-mass-to-surface-area ratio must have. Also called *biological memory*.

memory, holographic A hypothesized memory system suggested by the neuropsychologist Karl Pribram. It is a neurophysiological model of memory based on the assumption that the principles of holography serve as an analogue of the neurological processes of memory.

memory, iconic A residual sensory memory that lasts for a short time (perhaps up to 2 seconds) after a brief visual stimulus. See ICONIC (2) and SENSORY INFORMATION STORE.

memory, immediate Most often, a synonym of SHORT-TERM *MEMORY. However, some use it as equivalent to *iconic memory*; see ICONIC. To complicate matters, others use it for the first, early stages of short-term memory.

memory, implicit Unconscious memory, memory for material of which one is unaware. Implicit memory for previously presented material can be tapped by a variety of tasks, most commonly PRIMING (3). The existence of implicit memory is compellingly displayed in cases of AMNESIA, in which, despite the patient's inability to explicitly recall previously presented material, performance on tasks like priming is virtually normal. See also IMPLICIT *LEARNING.

memory, inaccessible A general term for any memory that, while not actually lost,

cannot, for any number of reasons, be retrieved. See IMPLICIT *MEMORY.

memory, instantiated Memory based on instances, items or events that have occurred. Instantiated memories tend to be concrete and based on the properties of the original stimuli. As a result they show less flexibility than memories based on abstractions or reconstructions. See INSTANCE THEORY.

memory, involuntary A memory that emerges unanticipated, unplanned and unintended. Unlike IMPLICIT *MEMORY, where the individual is unaware of memorial content, involuntary memories are conscious. It is the process of calling them up that takes place outside of consciousness. Also called *spontaneous memory* and *unintended memory*.

memory, lexical Loosely, memory for the words that one knows – not their meanings but the words themselves, with their graphological and phonological features. When used in this manner, the meanings of these lexical items are assumed to be stored in SEMANTIC *MEMORY.

memory, long-term (LTM) Memory for information that has been well processed and integrated into one's general knowledge store. Once input information has been processed or interpreted in a reasonably deep fashion the underlying abstraction is stored away in this so-called *long-term* system. Thus, LTM is presumed, unlike either SENSORY INFORMATION STORE or SHORT-TERM *MEMORY, to be without limit either in capacity to store information or in duration of that which is stored. Most of the research on LTM is highly specialized. The search is for the organizational principles and the form(s) of memorial representation that will explicate memory generally, but the work itself tends to focus on specific types of information storage. To appreciate this and get a feeling for the terminological distinctions that are often made, see SEMANTIC *MEMORY, EPISODIC *MEMORY, LEXICAL *MEMORY, ASSOCIATIVE *MEMORY and IMAGE, all of which are presumed to be special cases of the long-term memory processing system. Also called *long-term store (LTS)*, *secondary memory* and *permanent memory*.

memory, long-term working Memory for complex, interrelated material that is held in long-term store and used for problem-solving or task completion. For example, an architect might hold in memory an immense amount of interlocking pieces of information about materials, size, stress factors, design, aesthetics and more while making decisions about the design of a building.

memory, mood-congruent A form of STATE-DEPENDENT *MEMORY where an individual's current emotional state affects what is recalled. Happy people tend to recall happy previous episodes; depressed individuals, depressive ones. Because one cannot make assumptions about the emotional state when the original memories were formed, mood-congruency is distinct from MOOD-DEPENDENT *MEMORY.

memory, mood-dependent A form of STATE-DEPENDENT *MEMORY where the emotional state an individual is in during the encoding of input is a factor in retrieval of that information. Material learned when sad is recalled better when one is sad than when one is happy. The effect is best assessed using RECALL, not RECOGNITION PROCEDURES. Distinguish from MOOD-CONGRUENT *MEMORY.

memory, motor As it says, memory for motor actions and motoric skills. Often regarded as a subcategory of PROCEDURAL *MEMORY.

memory, noetic Endel Tulving's term for memory of general facts, knowledge that one has and knows that one has. In Tulving's model noetic memory is distinguished from both anoetic memory, which is knowledge held and retrieved independent of consciousness, and autonoetic memory, which is personal memory of events in one's life. All three of these are used in ways that overlap with a host of other hypothesized memory systems. Anoetic is an approximate synonym of IMPLICIT *MEMORY, noetic is used similarly to SEMANTIC *MEMORY and autonoetic to EPISODIC *MEMORY.

Memory-Operating Characteristic (MOC) curve A statistical procedure for analysing the data from a memory experiment. The technique is the same as that used in analysis of the data from a sensory-detection experiment except instead of plotting detection rates one plots correct recognition responses. For details see RECEIVER-OPERATING CHARACTERISTIC (ROC) CURVE.

memory, primary A troublesome term. Some use it as a synonym of SHORT-TERM *MEMORY. Those who do so will also use *secondary memory* as referentially equivalent to LONG-TERM *MEMORY. Those who do not tend to treat it as a subcategory of short-term memory in a manner close to SENSORY *MEMORY.

memory, procedural Memory for procedures or complex activities that have become highly automatized and are acted out without conscious thought about their processes, such as driving a car or riding a bicycle. Compare with DECLARATIVE *MEMORY. The term is used by some as a rough synonym of IMPLICIT *MEMORY.

memory, prospective Remembering to perform an intended action such as checking one's calendar before buying concert tickets. It is not regarded as a distinct memory system but a function served by WORKING *MEMORY, CUED *RECALL, and METAMEMORY.

memory, Proustian In honour of Marcel Proust's *Remembrance of Things Past*, a memory experience in which a simple cue triggers a vivid sequence of recollections of a previous event.

memory, racial A hypothesized storehouse of memories, feelings, ideas, etc. which, according to Carl Jung, we have inherited from our ancestral past. Racial memory in Jung's theory is a part of the COLLECTIVE UNCONSCIOUS. See also GENETIC *MEMORY, a concept to which it is related but which is free of some of the mystical connotations of Jung's characterizations.

memory, recent and **remote** Terms often used in the neuroclinical literature to refer to memories formed at different times in life. *Recent* denotes memories formed within the last few hours, days, weeks or even months; *remote* denotes those formed long ago, specifically in childhood.

memory, recognition RECOGNITION.

memory, reconstructive Descriptive of the type of memory hypothesized to operate according to principles of reconstruction rather than reproduction. Theories of reconstructive memory assume that abstract principles about the input material are stored away and that the memory is actually reconstructed according to these principles during recall of the material. W. James's theory, outlined in 1890, was the first of this kind and, after a period of many decades during which theories based on REPRODUCTIVE *MEMORY dominated, it is viewed with favour today.

memory, recovered Material that has supposedly been brought back into conscious memory by the use of various techniques such as hypnosis and suggestion. This is a very touchy issue, particularly in legal settings, where such memories have been used in evidence in cases of abuse and assault. Alas, there is absolutely no evidence that hypnosis or suggestion can function to recover lost memories; worse, they tend to encourage confabulation and elaboration. Recovered memories are rarely true memories; they tend rather to be constructed at the prompting of the hypnotist or therapist. See FALSE *MEMORY.

memory, redintegrative From the word *redintegrate*, memory of events that is a re-establishment of the original information based on only partial recall of the original material. It is the ability to recall, by piecemeal reconstruction, a past experience by recollecting events, the circumstances surrounding the events, etc. Try, for example, to recall your high-school graduation ceremony, your wedding, your first date or some other such event to appreciate the processes involved.

memory, remote RECENT and REMOTE *MEMORY.

memory, reproductive The type of memory hypothesized to operate by reproducing the original stimulus input. Reproductive-memory theories imply that images or other forms of mental representations of the original material are stored away and reproduced during recall. Contrast this characterization of memory with that of RECONSTRUCTIVE *MEMORY.

memory, screen A psychoanalytic term for the memory for events dating from early childhood, fleeting, elusive memories that have managed to filter through the ego's defensive efforts at repression. The usual interpretation is that such memories function as 'covers' for other emotionally dangerous information, which they in fact help to repress. Hence, a common synonym is *cover memory*.

memory, secondary PRIMARY *MEMORY.

memory, semantic Put simply, memory for meanings. Some theorists consider the study of semantic memory to be equivalent to the study of LONG-TERM *MEMORY on the grounds that all long-term, relatively permanent memories are those that are coded and stored on the basis of their meaning. However, see EPISODIC *MEMORY for another theoretically valid possibility. Compare with LEXICAL *MEMORY. Also known as *reference memory*.

memory, sensorimotor Literally, memory for sensorimotor actions. Used roughly synonymously with PROCEDURAL *MEMORY and MOTOR *MEMORY.

memory, sensory Memory for a specific stimulus input, the material as it was sensed. Some authorities don't like referring to this function as 'memory' because the representations are so fleeting. For details see SENSORY INFORMATION STORE.

memory, short-term (STM) Memory for information that has received minimal processing or interpretation. According to contemporary theories of memory, STM is a relatively limited-capacity store capable of holding only about seven or so 'items' (although, if the interpretation of the material is rich enough, these items can contain a good deal of information; see 7±2). Material is assumed to be held in STM by the operation of rehearsal, and should such rehearsal be interrupted the material has a half-life of probably no more than 10 or 15 seconds. Compare with LONG-TERM *MEMORY and SENSORY INFORMATION STORE. Also known as *short-term store (STS)*, *primary memory* and *working memory*.

memory, source Memory for the source of a message, e.g. *who* said something rather than *what* was said. Often compared with FACT *MEMORY. See also SOURCE MONITORING.

memory span The number of items immediately reproducible after presentation. True tests of memory span require that the materials used be unrelated sets of symbols, otherwise complex coding systems artificially inflate the estimate of the span.

memory, spatial Memory for the locations of objects in environments including arrangements, direction, orientation and the spatial relationships among all these factors. The HIPPOCAMPAL FORMATION is a key neural structure in these functions; see also PLACE CELLS. Also called *topographic memory*.

memory, state-dependent Memories that are dependent on the emotional or physiological states of acquisition and recall. Memory is best when the states are congruent and diminished when there is a mismatch. See MOOD-CONGRUENT *MEMORY and MOOD-DEPENDENT *MEMORY. Note that the effect occurs even when the state is induced by substances that normally compromise memorial functions (e.g. alcohol). See CONTEXT SPECIFIC *LEARNING.

memory trace The presumed neurological event(s) responsible for any relatively permanent memory. See ENGRAM.

memory, tunnel Not a form of memory so much as a narrowing of focus in EPISODIC *MEMORY that results from negative emotions that emerged during the initial exposure. Seen compellingly in the WEAPON-FOCUS EFFECT.

memory, unconscious 1 Generally, IMPLICIT *MEMORY. **2** Specifically within psychoanalysis, nonretrievable memory for events, feelings and acts that have been repressed.

memory, voluntary Generally, a memory that results from conscious attempts at recall. Compare with INVOLUNTARY *MEMORY.

memory, working (WM) A hypothesized memory system that holds the input while an interpretation of it is worked out. The notion of a working memory is sometimes restricted to theoretical discussions of memory for materials presented in sentence form in which the assumption is that a sentence is held verbatim while its meaning is extracted. Other theorists, however, use the term as equivalent to SHORT-TERM *MEMORY. While this meaning has now become the dominant one, expanding the sense of the term in this way has yielded a subtle confusion that often goes unacknowledged. Specifically, some use WM so that it implies that the process of

'working with' these short-term memories is carried out consciously, with explicit control over how the material is encoded, processed and linked with other knowledge. Others use the term so that it also covers the processing of implicitly held memories, material that is 'worked with' outside of conscious control. *Caveat lector*. See VISUO-SPATIAL SKETCHPAD and PHONOLOGICAL LOOP for examples of some WM functions.

menarche (*menar'kee*) The first menstrual period.

Mendelian Of the genetic principles developed by the Austrian scientist/priest Gregor J. Mendel (1822–84). His three principles were: (a) that separate characteristics are inherited independently of each other via hypothesized elements called genes; (b) that each reproductive cell possesses only one gene from each gene pair; and (c) that some factors are dominant over others.

Ménière's disease A disorder of the inner ear, named for Prosper Ménière who first described it. Classic symptoms are vertigo, ringing in the ears (tinnitus), a feeling of pressure in the ear, and variable hearing loss. Episodes usually last two to four hours.

meninges Collectively, the three membranes (dura, pia and arachnoid) covering the spinal cord and the brain. sing., *meninx*.

menopause That period that marks the permanent cessation of menstrual activity, the period during which menstruation gradually ceases. Also known as the *climacteric* and, popularly, *change of life*, both terms which can be applied to the analogous period of hormonal change in males, although there is no relatively simple criterion to use with them.

mens rea Latin for *a guilty mind*. A legal term, used in forensic psychology and psychiatry in cases in which insanity is raised as a defence and questions of intention and motivation are deemed important in adjudging legal guilt.

menses MENSTRUATION.

menstrual cycle The full cycle of changes in the uterus and associated sex organs connected with menstruation and the intermenstrual periods. It begins with growth of ovarian follicles stimulated by the pituitary gland's release of follicle-stimulating hormone (FSH). The follicles produce oestrogens, which stimulate the hypothalamus, which, in turn, causes the pituitary to produce luteinizing hormone (LH). LH causes the follicle to rupture, releasing the ovum; the follicle becomes a *corpus luteum* that produces progesterone, which stimulates the uterus to prepare its lining for implantation. If the ovum goes unfertilized or is fertilized too late, or if implantation is prevented (e.g. by an IUD), the walls of the uterus slough off and menstruation begins.

menstrual synchrony MCCLINTOCK EFFECT.

menstruation The periodic discharge of blood and uterine material in mature women. This term and *menses* are often treated as synonyms, although occasionally the latter is restricted in meaning to the actual flow or discharge. See MENSTRUAL CYCLE for details.

mental In the most general sense: **1** Pertaining to MIND. Unfortunately, there has been so much bitter dispute as to the very nature of mind that it has never been entirely clear what this adjectival form pertains to. For example, from psychology's earlier days: **2** Within STRUCTURALISM (1), pertaining to the *contents* of an introspectible consciousness. **3** In ACT PSYCHOLOGY, characterizing the *acts* or *processes* of mind. **4** In FUNCTIONALISM (1, 2), pertaining to the *functional, adaptive aspects* of consciousness.

Now, except within the strict confines of each of these theoretical frameworks, it is difficult to appreciate the distinctions among these last three senses of the term. In fact, so much agonizing hair-splitting went on over these issues that the Watsonian radical behaviourists could argue persuasively that the concept was useless and that unobservable mental events (be they contents, acts or functions) had no role to play in a scientific psychology. The difficulty with the radical behaviourist position, however, was that one simply cannot bully a term out of existence because of confusion over its lexical domain. If anything, the fury of the disputation over what the referent of *mental* was should have been a cue that there was something of considerable significance here for psychology. Put simply, the term would not die, rather it shifted in its

connotations to reflect emerging theory. That is: **5** Pertaining to mediational processes, those covert events that were interposed between the overt physical stimulus and the observable response of a subject. This meaning was, and to some extent still is, favoured by those with liberal, neobehaviourist leanings. **6** Pertaining to those functions that are identified as reflective of intelligence. The sense here is to be distinguished from that concerning other internal processes that are regarded as *affective* or *conative*. This meaning, which is rarely intended specifically any more, survives in combined terms like MENTAL TEST and MENTAL RETARDATION. **7** Pertaining to that which is causally located in mind. This sense is carried in terms like MENTAL ILLNESS and MENTAL DISEASE. Note the distinction here between 6, which superficially suggests the intellectual, and 7, which, while it may include such processes as thought and rationality, also clearly embodies the emotional and motivational. Perhaps a better term for 7 would be *psychogenic*, but it has little currency in these contexts in the literature. **8** Pertaining (broadly) to all those operations subsumed under the label COGNITIVE. This is, in contemporary psychology, the dominant meaning; a mental process is a cognitive process and the term connotes all that is normally subsumed under the approaches of COGNITIVE PSYCHOLOGY and COGNITIVE SCIENCE.

mental aberration ABERRATION, MENTAL.

mental age AGE, MENTAL.

mental ataxia ATAXIA, MENTAL.

mental chemistry A label for a point of view which argues that, in principle, an analogy can be drawn between the fundamental combinatorial principles of chemistry and those of mind. That is, if chemical elements can be combined to produce compounds with emergent properties (SEE EMERGENTISM), then, so the reasoning goes, separate mental elements can be combined to yield the complex components of mind. The doctrine was first proposed by John Stuart Mill, who viewed the association as the bond that linked ideas to form synthesized mental compounds. Compare with MENTAL MECHANICS.

mental chronometrics CHRONOMETRICS, MENTAL.

mental content CONTENT (2).

mental defective This term has been so overworked (as an effective insult) that it no longer has any real scientific meaning. See MENTAL DEFICIENCY, which served as a replacement for a time, and DEFECTIVE (2) for more on usage. MENTAL RETARDATION, is the now accepted cover term for all forms of less-than-normal intellectual functioning.

mental deficiency As the term suggests, a deficiency in mental functioning. There have been a number of attempts at developing a systematic nomenclature to classify and grade various forms of such deficiencies according to intellectual, behavioural and forensic yardsticks. One breakdown, now largely obsolete, used IQ range as follows: *borderline deficiency* (70–80), *moron* (50–69), *imbecile* (20–49), *idiot* (below 20). In addition to these, numerous other terms have put in appearances in the literature: *feeble-minded* (*ness*) was used for a time of people with an IQ below 70 (North American usage) or in the 50–69 range (British usage); *subnormal* has been loosely used of anyone with an IQ under roughly 75 or 80; *amentia* is a sometime synonym of *mental deficiency*, although etymologically it should really only be applied in cases of damage to a once-normal intelligence. In any event, given the lack of consistency in usage of these several terms, not to mention the distinctly unfavourable connotations that they all have in the common language, most authorities have ceased to use them and the generic label itself is dropping out of the technical literature. The favoured cover term now is MENTAL RETARDATION; consult that entry for currently accepted classifications.

mental deterioration DETERIORATION.

mental development Broadly, all those progressive changes in cognitive development that occur in an individual with the passage of time. Some restrict application of the term to the period from birth to adulthood, others use it to refer to the full life cycle.

mental discipline FORMAL DISCIPLINE.

mental disease The concept of a mental disease derives from the so-called *medical model* of abnormal behaviour, which operates on the basis of analogy with diseases of the somatic kind. Hence, any disabling psychological maladjustment or behavioural disorder may be so classified. Once the dominant term, but now the synonymous MENTAL ILLNESS is more common. See that term and the separate entry on DISEASE for a discussion of problems of usage of these and related terms.

mental disorder A more neutral term than either MENTAL DISEASE or MENTAL ILLNESS, this is preferred by many because it does not convey the assumptions of the *medical model* of clinical phenomena, although it still suffers from the suggestion that the mental sphere is at once an analogue of the somatic and yet separate from it. See DISORDER for more on terminological issues here.

mental element ELEMENT (1).

mentalese Some psycholinguists, desperate to characterize the hypothesized internal computing language with which the mind represents its contents, came up with this term. With luck it will expire through lack of use.

mental experiment EXPERIMENT, MENTAL.

mental faculty FACULTY PSYCHOLOGY.

mental function Any cognitive process or act; distinguish from mental CONTENT (2). See also FUNCTIONALISM (1, 2).

mental healing An occasional synonym of FAITH HEALING.

mental health Although the focus of this term is somewhat more sanguine than that of its opposite, MENTAL ILLNESS, the same medical, logical and empirical problems attend its use. In spite of these issues, the term will probably persist because it is generally used to designate one who is functioning at a high level of behavioural and emotional adjustment and adaptiveness and not for one who is, simply, not mentally ill.

mental hygiene 1 Originally, the art of developing and maintaining mental health. **2** A loose catch-phrase for courses generally taught at a very unsophisticated level in many US high schools.

mental illness The generally accepted connotation of this term (and its close synonym MENTAL DISEASE) is that of a psychological or behavioural abnormality of sufficient severity that psychiatric intervention is warranted – with the implicit assumption that this abnormality is caused by some psychic 'germ' in a fashion analogous to the manner in which a somatic illness is caused by a biological infestation. There are good reasons for questioning the generality of this assumption; see the discussion under DISEASE and DIAGNOSIS for an overview of contemporary terminology.

mental image IMAGE (3, 4).

mentalism The doctrine that maintains that an adequate characterization of human behaviour is not possible without invoking mental phenomena as explanatory devices; or, phrased another way, that any reductionistic exercise which seeks to explain cognitive processes (mind) by limiting itself to the physical and the physiological will not succeed in accounting for all phenomena observed. See DUALISM.

mentality 1 Loosely, mental or intellectual activity. **2** The quality of mind that is taken as characteristic of a particular individual or class of individuals.

mental level 1 In psychological testing, quite literally, the level of mental functioning. It is expressed by a measure of MENTAL *AGE. **2** In Jungian theory, any of the three divisions or levels of the psyche: *consciousness, personal unconsciousness* and *collective unconsciousness*.

mentally handicapped Loosely, descriptive of a person with a slight to moderate degree of MENTAL RETARDATION. See that entry for usage patterns.

mental maturity Loosely, the level of mental functioning of the average adult. See ADULT *INTELLIGENCE for problems in usage of this or any term intended to capture this general notion.

mental measurement A generic term used to cover any application of measurement techniques to quantify a mental function. It is most often used to refer to various scales that have been developed to assess internal operations and capacities, notably intelligence tests but also personality inventories,

developmental scales and projective devices and, on occasion, the techniques of psychophysics.

mental mechanics The point of view that an analogy can be drawn between the mode of action of complex, mechanical devices and the workings of the mind. The essence of this perspective, which was championed by James Mill, is that the operations of mind can be viewed as linear and sequential. Compare with MENTAL CHEMISTRY.

mental mechanism An occasional (and misleading) synonym of DEFENCE MECHANISM.

mental paper-folding test A test of spatial and configurational skills. Subjects are shown a flat pattern which corresponds to an unfolded cube. They are requested to mentally refold the cube and determine whether or not two arrows printed on separate faces of the flat pattern would meet when the cube was assembled.

mental process It is difficult to specify the meaning of this term without being tautological. A *process* is an ongoing systematic series of actions or events; if it takes place in the mind, it is a *mental* process. See e.g. INFORMATION PROCESSING.

mental process, higher An obsolete term for all forms of *thinking*, particularly as contrasted with the more primitive processes of *sensing* and *perceiving*.

mental representation REPRESENTATION.

mental retardation The contemporary term of choice as the umbrella label for all forms of below-average intellectual functioning as assessed by a standard IQ test. The classification system currently in use in the USA specifies four levels: *mild* (approximate IQ range of 50–69), *moderate* (35–49), *severe* (20–34) and *profound* (below 20). Note that this breakdown is predicated on the notion that the term itself should only be applied to persons below −2 standard deviations from the mean. Those within −1 standard deviation (i.e. with an IQ score between 86 and 100) are regarded as *normal* or, on occasion for those near the bottom end of this range, as *dull normal*; those within −1 and −2 standard deviations (i.e. with a score of 70–85) are regarded as possessing BORDERLINE INTELLIGENCE. See EDUCABLE MENTALLY

RETARDED and TRAINABLE MENTALLY RETARDED for more on the distinctions drawn between *mild* and *moderate* forms of retardation.

Note that there is a lingering peculiarity in the core term: what precisely are the connotations of *retardation*? It literally denotes a slowing down and, indeed, there do seem to be at least two aspects of such a retarding of function. First, the developmental rate of cognitive maturation is slowed, so a retarded child reaches the standard milestones at a later age than a normal child. Second, the cognitive processes themselves appear to be slower, so retarded persons typically take longer to carry out cognitive tasks than those of average intelligence. However, the term also connotes more than a simple slowing; it carries the implication of a lowered potential or ceiling: a mentally retarded child is not expected ever to reach normal levels no matter how much time is allowed for development. In other words, mental retardation is really mental *deficiency* – only that label has been so abused that few use it today (see MENTAL DEFICIENCY for a discussion). One lexical rescue attempt has been the use of *mentally handicapped* as the general term, but HANDICAPPED has, not surprisingly, its own connotative difficulties.

mental retardation, cultural-familial Mild mental retardation that has no detectable organic basis. The term reflects the assumption that the cause is some combination of environmental (cultural) and hereditary (familial) factors, which certainly seems reasonable if not particularly illuminating. Also called *sociocultural mental retardation*.

mental retardation, mild Below-average intellectual functioning commensurate with an IQ score in the 50–69 range. Persons in this category can develop reasonably effective social and communicative skills and during their early years (up to roughly 5 or 6 years) are indistinguishable from normals. They can learn school subjects up to about the sixth year of schooling and can be taught various skills. The category constitutes about 80% of the mentally retarded. The term is used roughly equivalently with EDUCABLE MENTALLY RETARDED.

mental retardation, moderate Below-average intellectual functioning commen-

surate with an IQ score in the 35–49 range. During childhood persons in this category display poor awareness of social conventions, although their communicative skills are reasonably good. Schooling is rarely successful past the second-year level, but with proper assistance and supervision useful unskilled or semiskilled work can be performed. Roughly 12% of the mentally retarded are in this category. These persons are often called TRAINABLE MENTALLY RETARDED.

mental retardation, profound Below-average intellectual functioning commensurate with an IQ score below 20. Persons in this category display minimal sensorimotor functioning as children. As adults they develop some speech and motor ability and can, on occasion, be taught limited self-care. Highly structured environments and constant supervision and aid are required. Only about 1% of the mentally retarded are in this category.

mental retardation, severe Below-average intellectual functioning commensurate with an IQ score in the 20–34 range. During early childhood there is poor motor development, minimal speech and poor or no acquisition of social and communicative skills. Persons in this category are generally unable to profit from vocational training, although they may carry out some simple tasks with close supervision. About 7% of the mentally retarded are in this category.

mental rotation Quite literally, the ability to rotate mentally a viewed object through two or three dimensions.

mental scale Any assessment device or test for determining an individual's level of mental functioning (i.e. their intelligence).

mental set SET (2).

mental state Somewhat tautologically, that set of circumstances in which an individual is in a state that has cognitive or mental content. If you believe that roses are red, then you are in a mental state such that you believe that roses are red. If you are hungry, you are not in a mental state – although if you *believe* you are hungry, you are. An argument oft found in the philosophy of mind is whether other species have mental states, and if they do whether they attribute such to their conspecifics. In this regard, see also INTENTIONALITY.

mental-status examination A full clinical work-up of a psychiatric patient including assessment of overall psychiatric condition, diagnosis of existing disorders, prognosis, estimates of suitability for treatment of various kinds, formulation of overall personality, and compilation of historical and developmental data.

mental test 1 Generally, any TEST (1) that is designed to evaluate a particular mental ability or performance. The term, in this encompassing sense, was first used by the American psychologist James McKeen Cattell in 1890 and served as a kind of umbrella term for the mental-testing movement that began soon after. **2** More specifically, an INTELLIGENCE TEST.

mentation Slightly antiquated term for any mental activity.

menticide Lit., the murder of mind; rarely used today although the general sense of the term is captured by the somewhat more colourful term BRAINWASHING.

meprobamate An ANTIANXIETY DRUG with mild tranquillizing and muscle-relaxing effects marketed under the brand names Miltown and Equanil. Once in wide use to combat insomnia and reduce stress-related anxieties, it is rarely prescribed these days because of high addiction rates and ease of administering an overdose.

mere exposure effect Zajonc's term for the phenomenon that one's liking or preference for a stimulus is increased by simply being exposed to it. Interestingly, the effect emerges even when the individual is unaware of having been exposed to the stimulus. A *structural mere exposure effect* also exists where a preference for previously unseen stimuli is found, provided that the new stimuli share underlying structural features or patterns with the originals.

mere-measurement effect The phenomenon whereby asking people if they intend to engage in a behaviour (e.g. vote) increases the likelihood of engaging in this behaviour (or decreases it if the response was negative). The jury is still out on precisely why this effect occurs and under which conditions the effect is enhanced or diminished. However, the overall effect appears to be strong and can last long after the initial inquiry.

Merkel's discs Flattened epithelia cells found in glabrous (smooth) skin in the same areas as Meissner's corpuscles. Presumed to function as touch/pressure receptors although the evidence for this is less than overwhelming.

merycism RUMINATION DISORDER OF INFANCY.

mescaline A hallucinogenic drug obtained from the peyote cactus. The effects are similar to those of LSD but generally of lesser intensity (depending, of course, on the dosage).

mesencephalon MIDBRAIN.

mesial Obsolescent synonym of MEDIAL and/ or MEDIAN.

mesmerism An old term for HYPNOTISM, from its discoverer, Franz Anton Mesmer.

mes(o)- Combining form meaning: **1** generally, *middle, moderate* or *intermediate*: **2** in medicine, *secondary, partial.*

mesocephalic Lit., moderate head. See CEPHALIC INDEX.

mesocortical system A system of dopaminergic neurons with cell bodies in the *ventral tegmentum* and projections to the *prefrontal neocortex, limbic cortex* and *hippocampus.*

mesoderm Middle layer of embryonic cellular structure that develops into the muscles and bones.

mesokurtosis KURTOSIS.

mesolimbic system A system of dopaminergic neurons with cell bodies in the *ventral tegmentum* and projections to the *nucleus accumbens, amygdala, lateral septum* and *hippocampus.*

mesomorphy 1 In Sheldon's CONSTITUTIONAL THEORY, one of the three primary dimensions of body type (along with *ectomorphy* and *endomorphy*). A mesomorph is one whose physique is dominated by the embryonic mesodermal component: muscles, skeleton, circulatory system. Hence, mesodermic persons are strong and well muscled and have moderate skin-surface-to-weight ratios. **2** See BODY-BUILD INDEX.

mesopic vision The vision that occurs in

the vaguely defined region between *scotopic* (or twilight) and *photopic* (or daylight) vision.

message A communication; the information transmitted in a communication. There is a good deal of latitude in the usage of this term that derives from the fact that it is used for any (or all) of the three aspects of a communication: (a) the sent message, which reflects the intended meaning of the sender; (b) the transmitted message, which is specified in terms of the medium used; and (c) the received message, which is characterized by the meaning as perceived by the recipient. Clearly, the message in each of these cases may be very different in form, structure and content, depending on a host of psychological and physical variables. See INFORMATION THEORY and related entries.

messenger RNA RIBONUCLEIC ACID (RNA).

meta- A common prefix of Greek origin with a host of connotations, including *about, beyond, among, after, between, behind* or *change in*. The first of these is probably the most common, particularly in philosophically oriented works: the others are used freely in various contexts.

meta-analysis A statistical technique that allows one to combine the findings from a number of studies and determine whether significant trends emerge. It is a particularly powerful procedure because it assists a researcher in dealing with a large number of studies on a topic carried out by different investigators with not-always consistent findings. Meta-analyses look for patterns and trends across studies and provide statistical estimates of the likelihood of significant effects. While such analyses have become common in the social and biomedical sciences, some question the legitimacy of combining data from disparate studies and caution that the results may be misleading. Also spelled *metanalysis*.

metabolic syndrome More a combination of disorders than a distinct syndrome, it is characterized by upper-body obesity with adipose tissue mainly around the waist, low levels of HDL ('good' cholesterol), elevated triglyceride and uric acid levels, hypertension and a marked increase in the risk of heart attack and diabetes. Also called *insulin resistance syndrome* although it is not clear whether this feature is cause or effect.

metabolism The sum of the processes of ANABOLISM and CATABOLISM; all the energy and material transformations that occur in living cells.

metabotropic glutamate receptor (mGluR) The only GLUTAMATE RECEPTOR that is METABOTROPIC. Such receptors, unlike the IONOTROPIC, do not open ion channels but operate indirectly by activating a host of other biochemical actions. The mGluRs play both excitatory and inhibitory roles and are found in the hippocampus, the cerebellum and throughout the cortex and the peripheral nervous system.

metabotropic receptors Receptors that operate indirectly. When stimulated, they activate an *enzyme* that initiates a series of metabolic processes that opens an ion channel elsewhere in the cell's membrane, allowing ions to pass in and out of the cell. Compare with IONOTROPIC RECEPTORS.

metacognition Knowledge of one's own thoughts and, importantly, of those cognitive factors that underlie one's thinking.

metacontrast A variety of backward MASKING in which the perception of a visual stimulus (the *target*) is altered by a second visual display (the *masker*). The most commonly used procedures entail (a) using a masker that consists of two separate stimuli which flank the location of the target, and (b) using a masker that is an outline which surrounds the location of the target. A variety of factors involving size, location, brightness and timing yield different metacontrast effects. The term PARACONTRAST is generally used to indicate a similar situation but one in which the interest is on forward MASKING, i.e. where the flanking or surrounding stimuli are presented first and their impact on the target is evaluated. Not all authors, however, make this distinction.

metaesthetic range That domain of cutaneous responsiveness to stimuli that are not quite intense enough to produce a clear sensation of pain.

metaknowledge Knowledge about knowledge. Used to refer to information that people have about things that they and others know and do not know.

metalanguage A language for speaking or writing about an object language. Hence, the language of linguistics as it is used to characterize and describe a natural language is a metalanguage. Similarly, if a treatise on Russian is written in English, then English is a metalanguage in this context.

metalinguistics The study of what people use language for, what they talk about, how they use particular linguistic forms, and how language interacts with the rest of culture. See also PARALINGUISTICS.

metamemory Simply, knowledge of one's own memory, what one knows and how likely it is that any requested arbitrary tidbit can be recalled. Just when and how children develop this is a topic of considerable research.

metameric match A perceived match between two colour stimuli that actually differ from each other in their spectral characteristics.

metamers Colour stimuli that produce METAMERIC MATCHES.

metamorphosis 1 An abrupt transition in form and structure as occurs in insects (egg, larva, pupa, adult). **2** A transformation in personality.

metanalysis META-ANALYSIS.

metaneeds In A. Maslow's theory of personality, the higher human needs, including justice, beauty, order, honour and self-actualization. Metaneeds (or *growth needs* as they are also called) cannot be dealt with, according to the theory, until the prepotent BASIC NEEDS are fulfilled. See NEED HIERARCHY.

metaphor A linguistic device whereby an abstract concept is expressed by means of analogy. It is generally concluded that there are no defining features of metaphors, rather that they are, to some extent or another, violations of literalness, and it is from the form of violation that they draw their emotive and cognitive effects. Metaphor and other forms of figurative language (e.g. SIMILE) have long fascinated psychologists because of problems in understanding how they are recognized and understood,

what it is that distinguishes a 'good' metaphor from a 'poor' one, what role they play in communication, how such fanciful devices are learned by children, etc.

metaphysics A branch of philosophy that seeks out first principles and, of necessity, must go beyond what can be learned by mechanical or physical analyses. Often, because of its intellectual heritage, the term is used as a label for any philosophy that is abstruse. Indeed, William James characterized metaphysics as 'nothing more than an unusually obstinate effort to think clearly'.

metapsychics An occasional synonym of PARAPSYCHOLOGY.

metapsychology 1 A general label for any theoretical enterprise that attempts to synthesize fact, theory and speculation in a major comprehensive fashion. *Meta-* here means *beyond*, in that such a metapsychological effort is one that goes beyond what has been empirically demonstrated and known and attempts to outline completely general principles of psychology. Such approaches are also called NOMOTHETIC psychology. **2** Within classical Freudian psychoanalysis, such an approach that aims at what Freud regarded as the highest levels of abstraction. Specifically, the analysis of psychic processes in terms of their *dynamic*, *topographical* and *economic* aspects, where *dynamic* includes analysis of instinct, *topographical* covers location of a process in the psychic apparatus of id, ego and superego, and *economic* is concerned with the distribution of psychic energy within the system. **3** Occasionally, and unhappily, a synonym of PARAPSYCHOLOGY.

metatheory A general term used to cover the theoretical discussions about the construction of scientific theories. For example, the entry FALSIFICATIONISM contains a discussion that is metatheoretical.

metathetic From the Greek, meaning *changed* or *changeable*, this term is used to refer to stimulus dimensions within which simple quantitative changes in the physical values produce complex qualitative changes in the psychological sensations. The classic example is the wavelength of light, in which alterations in the continuum produce hue changes. Metathetic continua are a problem for the generality of laws of psychophysical scaling. Contrast with PROTHETIC.

metempsychosis The doctrine of the transmigration of souls, the view that the soul survives bodily death and will, in due course, be reincarnated in another (human or otherwise) body.

metencephalon One of the major subdivisions of the HINDBRAIN; its principal structures include the cerebellum and the pons.

MET gene A gene known to influence a wide range of biological processes, including immune functions, gastrointestinal repair and metastasis. It has recently been implicated in AUTISM. The exact mechanism is unclear but studies suggest that individuals with a particular MET variant display a particularly serious and regressive form of autism along with gastrointestinal disorders and compromised immune reactions. Distinguish from the *met* variant of the COMT GENE.

methadone A synthetic narcotic that blocks the effects of other narcotics. It is used occasionally for the treatment of heroin addiction in what are called *methadone maintenance* programmes. However, methadone itself produces a drug dependence of the morphine type and withdrawal from it is just as traumatic as withdrawal from any of the opioids.

methamphetamine (hydrochloride) A quick-acting and long-lasting AMPHETAMINE. Also called *methylamphetamine*.

methaqualone A sedative usually prescribed as a sleeping pill and occasionally combined with an antihistamine, which increases its effects. Its primary effect is to make one drowsy, but dizziness, stomach distress and pins-and-needles are frequent side effects. It is marketed under a number of trade names, including Quaalude, Melsed, Revonal and Paxidorm. As a street drug it is known as *quaalude* or *lude*.

method Very generally, a way of doing things, of working with facts and concepts in a systematic fashion. Now, this is a pretty broad notion and, in practice, the term usually has qualifiers hung on it to specify the form and variety of method under discussion. Several of the more commonly used follow. Note, however, that often the *type* of

method receives so much of the focus that the word *method* itself is dropped; e.g. the *inductive method* is usually referred to simply as *induction*. Hence, for those terms not given here see the qualifying-term entry. See and compare with PROCEDURE and TECHNIQUE.

methodological behaviourism BEHAVIOURISM.

methodology 1 Broadly, the formulation of systematic and logically coherent methods for the search for knowledge. It is, strictly speaking, not concerned directly with the accumulation of knowledge or understanding but rather with the methods and procedures by which knowledge and understanding are achieved. Most are prone to use the term as equivalent to *scientific method*, with the implication that the only acceptable methodology is the scientific. The legitimacy of this equivalence depends on just how one characterizes the SCIENTIFIC *METHOD – in the treatment given below, which is representative of the contemporary 'received view', this synonymity is defensible. **2** Specifically, the actual procedures used in a particular investigation.

method, scientific The best way to handle this term from the viewpoint of the psychologist is to attack the central issue first: the question as to whether or not psychology is a science. Many persons, both layman and scientists alike, have protested that psychology is not a science, owing to the lack of precision in its procedures and lack of generalizability of its principles. Actually, what makes a given discipline a science has precious little to do with the definitiveness of its findings or the precision of its laws. It rests upon whether the practitioners adhere to the accepted canons of the scientific method. Without going into unnecessary detail (for the study of the philosophy and methodology of science is a vast and complex field) one can isolate several critical steps that are symptomatic of the scientific approach to any problem.

First, the problem must be defined. This may be no small endeavour; for example, little progress was made in the understanding of human cognition during the several centuries in which the core question was 'What is the nature of mind?' Defining the problem means characterizing it in such a way that it lends itself to careful investigation. Second, the problem must be stated in a manner such that it can be tied in with existing theory and known empirical fact. Without this stage the outcome of a study may be of little or no value; a science is much more than a compilation of raw facts – it is made up of facts that can be blended with, and interpreted in the light of, theory and accumulated knowledge. See here INTERPRETATION. Third, a testable hypothesis must be formulated. In light of the above, the hypothesis needs to be expressed so that it dovetails with the body of accepted principles and it should be expressed unambiguously so that the outcome of the investigation will be interpretable. There are some fairly rich arguments concerning this particular issue; see FALSIFICATIONISM for one of them. Fourth, the procedures of investigation must be determined. There is enormous latitude here; the possibilities are essentially unlimited so long as one is careful to maintain proper experimental CONTROL. Fifth (and sixth), the data are gathered and analysed and, in accordance with the findings, the hypothesis is either rejected or supported. Seventh, the existing body of scientific knowledge is modified to accommodate the new findings.

Basically, this is a pretty good way to do things, a good way to 'make science'. It has worked well for some time now. It does have some liabilities, to be sure. It seems sometimes to be a rather conservative and ponderous procedure and, on occasion, novel findings which appear anomalous in view of the momentary 'state of the science' are cast aside because they do not fit. The classic example here is Mendel's work on genetics, which gathered dust for many years until the field was ready for it. But the exploration of nature, particularly from the point of view of the psychologist, does not suffer unduly from a touch of conservatism. Empiricism is the touchstone of science, experimental control is essential, falsifiable hypotheses are necessary, and it all works well – no matter the domain of investigation. For more on related terms see DEFINITION and THEORY.

methoxyhydroxphenylglycol MHPG.

methylenedioxyamphetamine See MDA.

methylenedioxymethamphetamine See MDMA.

methylphenidate A stimulant with pharmacological action similar to the AMPHETAMINES. It functions primarily by blocking the reuptake of the CATECHOLAMINES and has been used for some time as an adjunct to antidepressants and to increase alertness in patients with traumatic brain injuries, cancer and dementia. In recent years it has been approved for use in children and adults with NARCOLEPSY and ATTENTION-DEFICIT HYPERACTIVITY DISORDER (ADHD). The former use is straightforward and nonproblematical. The latter, apparently paradoxical use came about when the drug was discovered to increase attention and decrease the impulsivity and hyperactivity of ADHD and its increasingly wide use has prompted controversy. It is unclear whether the therapeutic value of the drug continues after it is withdrawn and there are concerns about possible side effects and the potential for drug abuse. Trade names: Ritalin, Metadate and Concerta.

methylxanthines A class of mild stimulants including CAFFEINE and THEOPHYLLINE.

metonymy A linguistic form in which a particular characteristic of the meaning of a word or an aspect of its reference comes to stand for something and is then used as a reference for either the thing as a whole or for some other aspect or part of it. While that definition seems awkward, it can be clarified by a simple example: the original meaning of *sweat* is *perspiration* but the link between perspiration and work leads to the metonymic use of sweat to denote hard work. Similarly, *dish* (*tableware*) becomes a label for the entrée in a meal. Metonymy differs from METAPHOR in that the latter derives its impact by similarity while metonymy uses contiguity. The interest in these and other linguistic forms (see SYNECDOCHE) comes from questions about language processing and efforts to understand how children learn these abstract linkages.

Metrazol A circulatory and respiratory stimulant that, in large doses, produces convulsive seizures. Metrazol shock therapy, common in the 1940s and 1950s, is no longer used today. Known as Cardiazol in Europe.

metric 1 Generally, pertaining to measurement. **2** More specifically, characteristic of measurement in which the elements measured fall on an INTERVAL or a RATIO *SCALE. Compare here with NONMETRIC. **3** Pertaining to measurement based on the *metre* (38.37 in) as the unit of length, the *gram* (0.03527 oz) as the unit of weight and the *second* as the unit of time. Occasionally the *litre* (US: 1.057 qt liquid, 0.908 qt dry measure; UK: 1.76 pt liquid, 35 fluid oz) is included as the unit of volume.

-metric, -metrica, -metrika Combining forms meaning *pertaining to measurement*.

metric, arbitrary A measurement scale that allows one to quantify a nebulous construct (e.g. anxiety). An arbitrary metric, being arbitrary, does not allow one to make any direct, supportable statements about the construct without further research.

metric system METRIC (3).

-metry Combining form meaning *measurement*.

met variant See COMT GENE.

MF scale MASCULINITY–FEMININITY SCALE.

mGluR METABOTROPIC GLUTAMATE RECEPTOR.

MHPG Abbreviation for *methoxyhydroxphenylglycol*. A metabolite of brain *norepinephrine*, MHPG can be measured in urine, low levels correlating with depression and high levels with mania in patients with a diagnosed BIPOLAR DISORDER.

micro- **1** Combining term meaning *very small, minute*. Compare with MACRO-. **2** In metric measurement, *one-millionth*.

microcephalic Lit., small-headed. The term is reserved for cases in which the abnormality is so great that retardation results.

microcephaly The condition of being MICROCEPHALIC.

microelectrode A very small electrode, specifically one with a tip diameter of between 0.5 and 5 microns. Used in neurophysiology for SINGLE-UNIT RECORDING.

microgenetic development MICROGENESIS.

microgenetic method MICROGENESIS.

microgenesis Loosely, those organizational or developmental changes that take place over relatively short periods of time. The key notion is 'relative' as the time frame in question can be as short as a fraction of a second or as long as a few weeks or months. For example, changes that occur during *microgenetic development*, like learning the alphabet, are not marked by specific time frames other than being too short to be called ontogenetic (see ONTOGENY); studies that use a *microgenetic method* are ones that take place over periods of time shorter than those that use a LONGITUDINAL METHOD.

microglia GLIA.

micromillimetre One-millionth of a millimetre; NANOMETER (preferred).

micron (μ) One-millionth of a metre; this term is used by convention rather than the literal term *micrometre*. pls., *microns, micra*.

microphonia Abnormally weak voice.

microphonic COCHLEAR MICROPHONIC.

micropsia Abnormal decrease in the perceived size of visual stimuli. var., *micropia*.

microtome A precision instrument capable of making extremely fine, even sections of tissue for microscopic study.

micturate Urinate.

midazolam A BENZODIAZEPINE that severely compromises hippocampal function and is consequently used in studies of memory.

midbrain During embryonic development the brain evolves three separate portions: the hindbrain, midbrain and forebrain. The midbrain develops into the TECTUM and TEGMENTUM; see those entries for details.

mid-collicular transection The *cerveau isolé*; see ENCÉPHALE ISOLÉ.

middle ear The air-filled space of the ear between the eardrum and the cochlea containing the AUDITORY *OSSICLES.

middle insomnia INSOMNIA, MIDDLE.

midline nucleus A thalamic nucleus that relays information from the reticular formation to other thalamic nuclei.

midparent The mean of the measurements of both parents along some dimension – usually weighted for known sex differences – as, for example, in weight or height. It is used as a rough predictor of expectations for offspring.

midpoint The middlemost point in an interval.

midpontine transection ENCÉPHALE ISOLÉ.

midrange The mean of the highest and lowest scores of a distribution. A 'quick and dirty' estimate of central tendency.

midsagittal plane A plane through the midline dividing the body into symmetrical halves.

midscore The MEDIAN.

Mignon delusion From the French, meaning *darling*; a common childhood fantasy that one's 'real' parents are famous, illustrious persons who will eventually come to the rescue.

migraine A syndrome characterized by extremely severe headaches, usually unilateral and often accompanied by nausea, vomiting and visual disturbances. Migraines show a familial pattern and are often triggered by stress or by particular foodstuffs. Treatment is tricky but some newer drugs that modulate serotonin levels are effective.

mild cognitive impairment (MCI) A general condition, often seen in the elderly, in which there is a small but detectable loss in cognitive function. Some authorities identify an *amnestic* subtype where the primary problems are with memory and a *multiple domains* subtype where other functions, such as language, are also affected. Also called *early Alzheimer's* because, of those diagnosed, approximately 15% show distinct signs of ALZHEIMER'S DISEASE within a year, 50% within 5 years and nearly 90% within 10 years.

milestone DEVELOPMENTAL MILESTONES.

milieu The surroundings, the environment, the medium within which events occur. The term is generally used to refer to the social environment, although it is extremely flexible.

milieu therapy A general term for any therapeutic setting in which some control is exerted over the socioenvironment to accommodate it to the needs of those in therapy. This is (or at least should be) an essential aspect of all inpatient psychiatric institutions.

military psychology A branch of psychology concerned with the application of psychological principles to the special environment that the military life invariably creates. A rather vigorously researched field of applied psychology, it is concerned with principles and methods of recruitment, evaluation and training of personnel as well as counselling and clinical applications.

Miller Analogies Test (MAT) A test of the ability to formulate (or, actually, to recognize) analogies. The MAT is used mainly as a screening device for selecting students for graduate schools in the USA and in various businesses for hiring and promotion decisions.

milli- Prefix meaning *one-thousandth*.

millilambert One-thousandth of a LAMBERT.

millimicron (mμ) One-thousandth of a micron; NANOMETER (preferred).

Miltown MEPROBAMATE.

mimetic Characterized by MIMICRY; imitative. Also used as a combining form, as in *psychotomimetic*.

mimetics The study of MEMES.

mimicry 1 In ethology and evolutionary biology, a process where one species takes on the phenotypic characteristics of another. Mimicry can take a variety of forms. Among the more common are *Batesian mimicry* which functions to dupe predators into avoidance such as the octopus that can take on the shape and coloration of a toxic sea snake, *Peckhamian* or *aggressive mimicry* where seduction of prey is the aim as in the snapping turtle whose tongue looks like a worm when it lies open-mouthed and motionless on a lake bottom and *Müllerian mimicry* where two species that are toxic develop similar coloration and derive protective benefit from the common appearance. **2** In social psychology, a form of learning where a particular behaviour is copied in a mindless manner without any appreciation of the goal or original intentions. Compare with EMULATION and IMITATION.

mind This term, and what it connotes, is the battered offspring of the union of philosophy and psychology. At some deep level we dearly love and cherish it and see behind its surface great potential but, because of our own inadequacies, we continuously abuse it, harshly and abruptly pummelling it for imagined excesses, and occasionally even lock it away in some dark closet where we cannot hear its insistent whines.

The history of the use of the term reveals two conflicting impulses: the tendency to treat mind as a metaphysical explanatory entity separate and apart from mechanistic systems, and the tendency to view it as a convenient biological metaphor representing the manifestation of the still-not-understood neurophysiological processes of the brain. The following are the more important and common uses of the term, and this basic conflict can be seen in all.

1 Mind as the totality of hypothesized mental processes and acts that may serve as explanatory devices for psychological data. In recent years this has become the dominant use of the term. Here, mental components are hypothesized because they have, in the proper theoretical frame, considerable explanatory power. Of interest here is the reluctance, even refusal, of those who adopt this position to speculate about the neurophysiological structures to which it might relate. The focus is typically on the effectiveness of the hypothesized model of mind to explain – not merely describe – the observations of empirical studies. The most frequent users of this meaning are workers in artificial intelligence, some cognitive psychologists and several schools of philosophy, e.g. FUNCTIONALISM (3). **2** Mind as the totality of the conscious and unconscious mental experiences of an individual organism (usually, although not always, a human organism). Actually, this use represents an effort to avoid the above-mentioned metaphysical problem but it produces a second-order difficulty of the same kind because of the confusion over how to characterize *consciousness*. Often even those with a behaviouristic approach will 'back door' themselves into speculating about mind in this fashion but they will invariably replace *consciousness* with *behaviours* and *acts*. **3** Mind as a collection of processes. Probably the next most commonly held view, the argument here is that the several processes generally studied under the rubrics of *perception* and *cognition* collectively constitute mind. Here, there is no real effort to define, only to enumerate

and to seek to understand those processes enumerated. Strip meaning 1 of theory and you get 3. **4** Mind as equivalent to brain. This position, which goes back to William James, must in the final analysis be true. Its major liability, of course, is that despite recent gains we know precious little about brain function. As a result, it is more of an article of faith than a true philosophical position. **5** Mind as an emergent property. The argument here is that of EMERGENTISM, that when a biological system reaches a point of sufficient 'something', be it complexity or organizational structure or computational power, mind (or consciousness) emerges. Meanings 4 and 5 are actually nicely coordinate, with 5 merely amplifying a sense that is implicit in 4. **6** Mind as a list of synonyms. For example, *psyche*, *soul*, *self*. Nothing is gained by this use, and the definitional problems are compounded. **7** Mind as intelligence. Really only a colloquial use of the term, as in phrases like 'She has a good mind.' **8** Mind as a characteristic or trait. Also used nontechnically, as in phrases like 'the mind of an artist', or 'the Northern European mind'. See also MIND–BODY PROBLEM.

mindblind Characterizing individuals who have difficulty 'reading' the minds of others, in the sense that they do not readily pick up on the social cues, voice intonations and facial expressions that reveal things about what others are thinking or feeling. It is, not surprisingly, strongly associated with AUTISM.

mind–body problem One of the classical metaphysical issues concerning the relationship between that which is mental and that which is physical. The issue has its origins in the ancient dualism of Plato, and since then many 'solutions' to the problem have been offered; the major ones, classified according to whether they are dualisms, monisms or compromises, follow:

Dualisms: (a) *Interactionism*, wherein mind and body are assumed to be separate entities, obeying separate laws but interacting with and mutually influencing each other. (b) *Psychophysicalism* (or *parallelism*), wherein mind and body are treated as two distinct, independent, but perfectly correlated elements.

Monisms: (a) *Materialism*, which assumes only the physical has reality. (b) *Subjective idealism*, wherein a single basic spiritual or mental realm has reality. (c) *Phenomenalism*, which assumes that neither mind nor body can be substantiated and only ideas and sense impressions exist.

Compromises: (a) *Double aspectism*, wherein it is assumed that the two realities of the physical and the mental come about because each is a particular point of view (or aspect) of a single underlying reality. (b) *Epiphenomenalism*, which treats the mental as a non-causal 'shadow' of the physical. See also MIND.

mindfulness The state of being calmly, intentionally and actively aware of what one is feeling, thinking and doing; hence the state of being attentive to the moment without becoming entangled in it. Mindfulness is the aim of some meditation techniques in which the person is trained to be attentive to thoughts, feelings and actions without imposing judgements on the latter. In Western traditions, training in mindfulness has been used to reduce stress and is used in DIALECTICAL BEHAVIOUR THERAPY.

mindlessness A term coined by Langer to capture the fact that much of our behaviour is carried out 'mindlessly'; that is, without conscious reflection on what we are doing.

mind, philosophy of A branch of philosophy concerned with issues relating to the nature of mind and consciousness, their links to underlying neurological structures, the manner and form of mental representations and the connections between thought, language, emotions and action. The topics of interest are similar to those of cognitive psychology but the methods differ with philosophers favouring argument and analysis rather than empirical study.

mind reading The alleged paranormal ability to know what is going on in the mind of another, a variety of telepathy (see PARAPSYCHOLOGY). Note that when mind-reading performances are put on, say by mediums or stage magicians, the phenomenon is quite normal; it consists of the reading not of minds but of subtle facial and muscular cues, and interpretation of such factors as tone of voice, manner of speaking and other pieces of information communicated unconsciously by the one whose 'mind' is being 'read'. See CLEVER HANS and BARNUM EFFECT.

mindsight A mode of perception in which one senses change having occurred in the environment in the absence of being able to specify what aspect of the display actually changed.

mind wandering The state wherein one's attention is not directed to the task at hand. At times this state can be a deliberate choice to 'tune out' an unpleasant or boring task. At other times, one can be quite unaware that one is not attending.

mineralocorticoids A class of CORTICOSTEROID HOMONES (e.g. ALDOSTERONE) that control electrolyte levels, primarily by adjusting the retention of sodium in the kidneys.

minimal Pertaining to a MINIMUM, and often used interchangeably with that term (in its adjectival form), as in *minimum/minimal audible field* and many other similar turns of phrase.

minimal brain dysfunction (MBD) A general cover term for a variety of behavioural, cognitive and affective abnormalities observed in children. It is typically reserved for cases in which the patterns of thought and action are such that one would expect to find some organic abnormality but none is apparent. Generally included as indicative of MBD are ATTENTION-DEFICIT DISORDER, HYPERKINESIS, *impulsivity*, various SOFT SIGNS and any of a number of learning and language disabilities, such as DYSLEXIA and DYSCALCULIA.

The term is often used as though there were an identifiable MBD *syndrome*, a collection of fairly specific disorders that could be taken as hallmarks of some underlying neurological causal mechanisms. Although the issue here is far from settled, the evidence to support a single MBD syndrome is largely unconvincing.

minimal cerebral dysfunction (or **damage**) ATTENTION-DEFICIT HYPERACTIVITY DISORDER.

minimal change, method of MEASUREMENT OF *THRESHOLD.

minimal cue A REDUCED CUE that is still sufficient to produce the response first associated with the original, full cue.

minimally counterintuitive Characterizing settings that test one's credibility but not to the breaking point. A horse that understands mathematics (see CLEVER HANS) would qualify; one that shape-shifted into a cat would not. Pascal Boyer, who coined the term, argues that because such events attract our attention and are highly memorable, they play a role in forming religious beliefs.

minimal pair In linguistics, any two words that are pronounced identically except for a single element, e.g. *bill–pill*. The existence of a minimal pair in a language is evidence that the phonetic elements that distinguish the two words are phonemes.

mini-max strategy A general *heuristic* that emerges in economics, problem-solving, decision-making, choice behaviour, gambling and even the design of experiments. The basic principle behind every mini-max strategy is to control the situation so that some effects are minimized (usually one's losses) and others are maximized (usually one's gains).

Mini-Mental State Examination A brief neurologically oriented assessment used as a screener to determine whether someone is cognitively intact.

minimum 1 n. The lowest value of a variable, a series or a continuum. **2** n. In a curve, a value that is lower than those immediately preceding and following it. In this sense there can be several minima in a given function. pls., *minima*, *minimums*. **3** adj. Characteristic or descriptive of such value(s) in either of the above senses; see MINIMAL. vb., *to minimize*.

minimum audible field The minimum pressure, measured at a point corresponding to the middle of the head, that will produce a just-audible sound. See also MINIMUM AUDIBLE PRESSURE and THRESHOLD.

minimum audible pressure The minimum pressure, measured at the eardrum, that will produce a just-audible sound. See also MINIMUM AUDIBLE FIELD and THRESHOLD.

minimum-distance principle A *heuristic* for sensing the appropriateness of two or more interdependent syntactic forms based on the principle that agreement between them is given by the distance (in number of words) separating them. The perfectly grammatical sentence 'A number of things is going wrong' feels wrong to most English speakers because it violates this principle; i.e.

things and *is* are closer together than *number* (the real subject) and *is*. Also called *principle of proximity*.

minimum separable The minimum interspace between two visual contours (i.e. the edges or lines) that can be seen. The typical finding for persons with normal visual acuity is roughly 1 minute of visual angle in the fovea; see here ACUITY GRATING. See also TWO-POINT THRESHOLD for an analogous situation on the skin. Compare this measure of acuity with MINIMUM VISIBLE.

minimum visible The narrowest visual stimulus that can be detected. Projected on the fovea of a person with normal visual acuity, the typical finding is roughly 1 second of visual angle. Compare this measure of acuity with MINIMUM SEPARABLE.

Minnesota Multiphasic Personality Inventory (MMPI) One of the, if not *the*, most widely used self-report inventories for the assessment of personality. Published in 1942, the first version consisted of a basic set of 550 items, each of which was a descriptive statement about characteristic feelings or behaviours with which the subject indicated either agreement or disagreement. It was originally developed as a clinical diagnostic tool and had eight scales built into it, designed to assess most of the (then) commonly accepted clinical syndromes. Although the MMPI did not prove to be the objective clinical assessment device its developers had hoped for, it turned out to be extremely useful in research into social/personality issues. Indeed, there are currently over 200 separate scales measuring such traits and qualities as *anxiety*, *ego strength*, *masculinity/femininity* and *internality/externality* that have been developed from the original MMPI item pool.

In response to criticisms concerning many antiquated items, as well as possible biases in the item pool and measurement scales, the inventory was updated in the late 1980s and the scoring system was revised to reflect the results from a large, representative sample of Americans. The revised version, known as the MMPI-2, contains 567 items, each of which is a statement about oneself which must be answered as *true*, *false* or *cannot say*. There are now 15 content scales that are related to a variety of psychological problems such as anxiety, depression, anger, social discomfort and family problems. In the early 1990s a new version was developed specifically for adolescents between the ages of 14 and 18 (the MMPI-A). It contains items designed to identify social and behavioural problems relating to family matters, eating disorders, drug dependencies, emotional difficulties and other issues common to this age group.

minor depressive disorder DEPRESSIVE DISORDER, MINOR.

minor epilepsy EPILEPSY, MINOR.

minor hemisphere A term unfortunately used by some for the nondominant or non-linguistic hemisphere. There is nothing minor about its functions. For more detail, see DOMINANCE et seq.

minority group Any identifiable cultural, racial, ethnic or religious group that is subjected to disadvantageous patterns of discrimination and prejudice. As such, the term is not used in its literal meaning; a *minority* group need not be in the numerical minority, and being a minority does not necessarily mean classification as a minority *group*. Thus women, though they are neither a minority nor, strictly speaking, a group, are often referred to as a minority group because of discrimination against them by a male-dominated society. At the other extreme are members of certain wealthy, privileged classes who often do form groups and are numerically in the minority but are not classified as such because of the lack of disadvantageous prejudice. These considerations have led some to recommend the term *oppressed group* as a replacement but it hasn't really caught on.

minor tranquillizers TRANQUILLIZERS, MINOR.

minus-sum game ZERO-SUM *GAME.

mirror drawing test A test of sensorimotor skills that requires that the subject trace an object (e.g. a five-pointed star) while viewing it in a mirror.

mirroring 1 Originally, the matched dance or entrainment of physical movements of two partners in an interaction. **2** In self-psychology, an aspect of the process of development of a self-concept whereby a sense of self emerges from the ways in which others react to one. This meaning is common in theories of development where the 'others' are the parents or caretakers.

mirror neurons Neurons that respond similarly whether one merely observes an action or event, or experiences it oneself. Several mirror neuron systems have been identified in a variety of species. In humans there are ones that respond to the actions of others and mirror the intentions, social meaning and emotional tone of the perceived behaviours. Found in a variety of regions of the brain including the posterior parietal lobe, superior temporal sulcus, insula and the premotor cortex, they are argued by some to be the neural correlates that underlie empathy and the capacity for imitation. Others speculate that the emergence of culture was dependent upon the evolution of mirror neural systems. And, perhaps not surprisingly, there are suggestions that they malfunction in autism.

mirror phase J. Lacan's term for a period in an infant's life when he or she can appreciate that he or she is an autonomous individual and can recognize him- or herself in a mirror. Taking place roughly between 6 and 18 months of age, Lacan argued that this MIRRORING (2) process marked the beginning of symbolic abilities.

mirror self LOOKING-GLASS SELF.

mirror writing Writing that, when held up to a mirror, appears in the proper orientation.

mirtazapine A MIXED-FUNCTION *ANTIDEPRESSANT drug used to treat anxiety and depression. It increases the availability of both norepinepherine and serotonin in the brain by stimulating the release of norepinephrine from presynaptic neurons and functioning as a serotonin agonist in postsynaptic neurons.

mis- MIS(O)-.

misandry Hatred of males.

misanthropy Hatred of (literally) males or (more generally) human beings.

misidentification In neuropsychology, a symptom seen in various delusional disorders whereby the patient misidentifies a well-known individual. See DELUSIONAL MISIDENTIFICATION DISORDER.

misidentification syndromes See DELU-
SIONAL MISIDENTIFICATION DISORDER.

mis(o)- **1** From the Greek, *hated, hating.*
2 From the Latin, *incorrect, improper, mistakenly.*

misogyny Hatred of females.

miss An inaccurate judgement by a subject
that there was no signal present on a trial
when one was, in fact, presented. See
SIGNAL-DETECTION THEORY for more details.

missing fundamental VIRTUAL PITCH.

missing-parts test A general label for any
test in which the subject's task is to point out
the parts that are absent in a complex pattern
or picture. Such exercises are often used as
items on intelligence tests and in diagnosing
various neurological disorders.

missionaries and cannibals HOBBITS AND
ORCS.

miswanting Mistakenly believing that
something will make you happy or, more
precisely, happier than it actually will. The
term was introduced by Daniel Gilbert and
Timothy Wilson for the circumstance where
individuals want things (objects, careers,
goals, other people) only to discover that
these things, when actually obtained, do
not have the anticipated positive impact.
Miswanting is ubiquitous in human affairs
and is due primarily to the fact that people
are rather poor at judging how happy particular outcomes will make them.

mitosis The cell-division process in which
somatic cells divide into daughter cells each
with a full complement of chromosomes (the
diploid number). Compare with MEIOSIS.

mitten grasp Grasping an object without
using the thumb. This is common in human
infants and nonhuman primates of all ages,
but a few human adults retain this method of
holding small objects such as pencils.

Mitwelt EIGENWELT.

mixed **1** A combining term used widely to
note circumstances where more than one
factor or principle is operating. **2** In many
psychiatric classification systems this term
is used to mark disorders that do not display
the standard characteristics. In this sense, it
is a close synonym of ATYPICAL (3).

mixed bipolar disorder BIPOLAR DISORDER,
MIXED.

mixed (cerebral) dominance DOMINANCE,
MIXED (CEREBRAL).

mixed effects model A type of analysis of
variance that combines features of the fixed
effects model (see FIXED *FACTOR) and the random effects model (see RANDOM *FACTOR).

mixed episode A mood disorder marked by
a period of time in which both the symptoms
of a MANIC EPISODE and a MAJOR *DEPRESSIVE EPI-
SODE are present.

mixed-function antidepressant ANTIDE-
PRESSANT, MIXED-FUNCTION.

mixed-motive task Any task or situation
in which an individual may have more than
one conflicting motive operating at the same
time. For example, in the PRISONER'S *DILEMMA,
behaviours that can potentially produce the
most favourable outcomes also carry the
greatest risk.

**mixed receptive–expressive language
disorder** DEVELOPMENTAL *LANGUAGE DISORDER.

mixed schedule SCHEDULES OF *REINFORCE-
MENT.

mixed transcortical aphasia APHASIA,
MIXED TRANSCORTICAL.

mixoscopia Sexual arousal obtained
through watching others engaged in sexual
acts. See VOYEURISM.

MLU MEAN LENGTH OF UTTERANCE.

MMPI MINNESOTA MULTIPHASIC PERSONALITY
INVENTORY.

M'Naghten rule MCNAGHTEN RULE.

mneme A memory trace.

mnemonic **1** adj. Of or relating to memory.
2 n. A MNEMONIC DEVICE.

mnemonic device An umbrella term covering any technique for committing material
to memory or for improving one's memory.
Mnemonics (for short) have a long history,
having been developed originally by the
ancient Greek and Roman orators, who
had, by virtue of their profession, enormous
memorial burdens placed on them. For
examples of some of the more commonly

used techniques see PEG-WORD SYSTEM and METHOD OF *LOCI.

mnemonic trace MEMORY TRACE, ENGRAM.

mnemonist One who is expert in the use of various mnemonic devices and capable of feats of memory that seem to most of us to be evidence of extraordinary mental functions. Although most mnemonists (some of whom make a living putting on performances) are quite ordinary mortals who have worked long and hard to develop facility with the mnemonics they use, there are the occasional cases of persons whose capabilities appear to be congenital. See here 'S' for a remarkable instance.

-mnesia A suffix meaning *memory*.

mob As a technical term in social psychology *mob* differs little in meaning from common parlance: a collection of persons with a specific common purpose and intent. The term is used with the connotation that the emotional level of those in the mob is so high that acts of violence or destruction are likely to occur in the pursuance of the common goal.

mobility Essentially, the reference of this term is the concept of *movement* – either literal, physical movement of a stimulus, an object or an organism, or a metaphoric movement through strata which are social, occupational or even cognitive. Because of this wide range of application the term is usually accompanied by a qualifier to clarify the reference, e.g. HORIZONTAL MOBILITY, SOCIAL MOBILITY, VERTICAL MOBILITY.

MOC curve MEMORY-OPERATING CHARACTERISTIC CURVE.

modal Relating to the MODE, to the most common score or occurrence.

modality A sensory system, a SENSE (1, 2). The term is usually qualified to specify the sense intended, e.g. *visual modality, kinaesthetic modality*.

mode 1 In statistics, a measure of central tendency of a distribution of scores given by the score of the midpoint of the class interval of scores with the highest frequency. Graphically, it is the peak of a frequency distribution. Although it is the least important of the measures of central tendency (see here MEAN and MEDIAN) it does have descriptive value, particularly when the distribution is *bi-* or *multimodal*. **2** A sense MODALITY (which is the preferred term). **3** An accepted fashion, a characteristic way of behaving.

model 1 n. A representation that mirrors, duplicates, imitates or in some way illustrates a pattern of relationships observed in data or in nature. The model may be purely mechanical, such as those often constructed to represent the workings of the ear; mathematical, such as those in mathematical psychology; or even a complex blending of these two, as evidenced by research in artificial intelligence where complex programs are instantiated on specialized hardware. When used in this sense, a model becomes a kind of mini-theory, a characterization of a process, and, as such, its value and usefulness derive from the predictions one can make from it and its role in guiding and developing theory and research. **2** n. An ideal, a standard, an example set up as worthy of imitation or copying. In social-learning theory the concept of a model in this sense plays an important role since much of socialization is assumed to take place through the imitation of the behaviour of a role model. See here MODELLING. **3** vb. To construct a model (in sense 1). **4** vb. To serve as a model (in sense 2). **5** vb. To imitate, to copy.

modelling (or modeling) 1 The act of constructing a MODEL (1). **2** A procedure whereby a subject observes a MODEL (2) perform some behaviour and then attempts to imitate that behaviour. There are many who feel that this is the fundamental learning process involved in socialization.

moderate mental retardation MENTAL RETARDATION, MODERATE.

moderator variable VARIABLE, MODERATOR.

modularity (theory) Any theoretical model that assumes that behavioural and cognitive functions are founded on a limited number of MODULES (1). Included are Fodor's modularity of mind theory and Chomsky's model of language acquisition.

modulation transfer function A transfer function is a statement about how a given system passes an input as a function of the frequency of the input, i.e. how it 'transfers' it to an output. When the system is, for example, the lens of the eye and the input is electromagnetic radiation, then the transfer function characterizes the manner in which the light waves are modulated by the lens; hence, one has a modulation transfer function that describes the lens.

modulator Any of several types of retinal ganglion cells that have relatively narrow ranges of responsiveness across the visible spectrum. Depending on the species, up to four such modulators have been found with spectral sensitivity peaks in the blue, green, yellow and red ranges. Compare with DOMINATOR.

modulator curve A graph of the spectral sensitivity of individual retinal ganglion cells. See MODULATOR.

module 1 J. Fodor's term for a hypothesized, relatively circumscribed faculty. Modules, in this sense, are similar to systems put forward by early proponents of FACULTY PSYCHOLOGY, although in the modern version the structures are more specific in nature, e.g. a spatial-perception module, a FEAR MODULE or a language module such as Chomsky's LAD. In Fodor's approach modules operate above the level of input systems but below the level of executive functions. That is, they are 'cognitively impenetrable' and carry out processing independently of conscious control. They are assumed to be encapsulated in that functions are specific to that module's domain and are not affected by other cognitive operations. Although Fodor did not go into detail, others have argued that modules, if they exist, should have identifiable localized brain areas and show evidence of being specific evolutionary adaptations to particular environmental demands. Fodor's position is often called *modularity theory* or the *modularity of mind*. Unfortunately, the term has become something of a 'buzz word' in psychology, biology and philosophy with an ever-increasing scope of usage. It can be found referring to almost any distinct pattern of processing in virtually any functional domain. This unfortunate semantic dilution is, predictably, stripping the term of its usefulness. **2** In J. Bruner's theory of cognitive development, an integrated, learned unit of behaviour observed in the final phase of the discovery of a solution to a problem (or to a class of related problems) in which the behaviour of the problem solver typically becomes well integrated and well organized. Meaning 1 so dominates current work that Bruner's sense of the term is now found only rarely.

modulus A standard stimulus used as the basis of comparison in studies of scaling of sensory magnitudes.

modus ponens Latin for *method of affirming*; a logical inference of the form *If A, then B; A, therefore B.*

modus tollens Latin for *method of denying*; a logical inference of the form *If A, then B; not A, therefore not B.*

mogi- Combining form from the Greek, meaning *with exertion* or *with difficulty*. Used freely to connote any difficulty in performance or function, e.g. mogigraphia = writer's cramp, mogilalia = a speech defect such as stuttering or stammering.

molar The central idea behind the various uses of this term is that it always refers to large units of behaviour or to behaviours with holistic functions. Thus, it is used: **1** To characterize learning situations which are large and complex, such as problem-solving or game-playing. **2** Within Gestalt theory to characterize that which is holistic, in the sense that such a molar phenomenon cannot be analytically broken down into component parts without loss of the intrinsic nature of the whole. **3** In Tolman's theory to describe behaviour that is purposive. Contrast with MOLECULAR.

molding MOULDING.

molecular 1 Characterizing that which is small. **2** Pertaining to that which can be analysed into units or divisions that are small. Hence, reflexive behaviour is often called molecular behaviour. Contrast with MOLAR (1, 2).

Molyneux's question A query posed in (by most accounts) 1688 by William Molyneux to his friend John Locke. Simply, he asked, would a congenitally blind adult upon suddenly acquiring vision be able to distinguish between a globe and a cube without touching them? Molyneux answered his own question with a vigorous negative and Locke, not surprisingly, agreed. The question, simple though it seems, drove straight at the heart of the extended debate over innate ideas and is today still of deep interest in terms of theories of the extent and form of biological preprogramming of the brain, particularly with respect to questions concerning perception, language and social behaviour.

moment Irrespective of seconds and minutes, there are two specialized uses of this term: **1** In the phrase *psychological moment*, it refers to the very short period of time within which successive stimuli are integrated and perceived as a whole, a kind of discrete quantum of psychological time. For more on this general notion see SPECIOUS PRESENT. **2** In statistics, a moment of a distribution is given by $m_T = \Sigma \chi^i/N$, where m_T is the ith moment, χ^i is the deviation of each score from the mean raised to the ith power and N is the number of scores. The first moment of a distribution is the *mean*, the second moment is the *variance*, the third is the *skewness* and the fourth is the *kurtosis*.

monad According to Leibniz's doctrine, monads are indestructible, uncreatable, immutable but quite active entities which constitute the fundamental units of all reality. Through various organizational processes these elemental units can, Leibniz assumed, be combined into complex units each of which, by virtue of its coherent structure, is itself a monad.

monaural Pertaining to one ear or to the use of only one ear. Also called *uniaural*.

mongolism DOWN SYNDROME.

monism **1** Any of several philosophical positions which argue that there is but one kind of ultimate reality. Several varieties are discussed under MIND–BODY PROBLEM; see also DUALISM. **2** In sociology, CULTURAL MONISM.

monitor To scan or watch, or one who does so. Such monitoring may be of a machine to detect malfunction, of persons to oversee their behaviour or of oneself to evaluate personal, internal processes of a cognitive or affective kind. This last sense is similar to that expressed by the more formal term INTROSPECTION, but without some of its theoretical implications.

mon(o)- Prefix from the Greek, meaning *alone, single, only* or *one.*

monoamine hypothesis The generaliza-

tion that DEPRESSION is caused by an insufficiency in the activity of monoaminergic neurons, specifically the serotonergic and the noradrenergic. The hypothesis gains support from the fact that drugs that are monoamine agonists, such as the MONOAMINE OXIDASE INHIBITORS and the TRICYCLIC COMPOUNDS, relieve depression, while those that are monoamine antagonists, such as RESERPINE, cause it. See also BIOGENIC AMINE HYPOTHESIS for a more general theoretical perspective.

monoamine oxidase (MAO) One of the enzymes responsible for the metabolic breakdown of the AMINES.

monoamine oxidase inhibitor Any of a class of drugs that operate by inhibiting the action of the enzyme MONOAMINE OXIDASE, leading to an increase in release of amines such as serotonin and norepinephrine. They are used as ANTIDEPRESSANT DRUGS, although not as often as the TRICYCLIC COMPOUNDS.

monoblepsia A visual condition in which vision is better when only one eye is used.

monochorionic twins MONOZYGOTIC *TWINS.

monochromacy Complete colour blindness. A monochromat can differentiate colours only on the basis of brightness. The term derives from the fact that such an individual can match perceptually all samples using but a single hue. Two forms exist, one in which cones are totally absent (see ACHROMATOPSIA) and one in which only a single type of cone is present. In the former (*rod-monochromacy*) all wavelengths are seen as grey, in the latter (*cone-monochromacy*) they are all presumably seen as one hue. Several synonymous terms have been used over the years, including *monochromatism, monochromia* and *monochromasy*.

monochromasy MONOCHROMACY.

monochromat One with MONOCHROMACY.

monochromatic vision MONOCHROMACY.

monochromatism MONOCHROMACY.

monochromia MONOCHROMACY.

monocular Pertaining or relating to one eye

or to the use of only one eye. Also called UNIOCULAR.

monocular cue Any visual cue for depth or distance perception that requires only one eye to be processed. Compare with BINOCULAR CUE.

monocular suppression SUPPRESSION, MONOCULAR.

monogamy A mating (or, in humans, a marriage) system in which each party has but a single mate. Contrast with POLYGAMY. The usual connotation of the term is that the pair maintain mutual sexual fidelity.

monogamy, social A mating system in which the partners are socially but not sexually (or reproductively) monogamous. It is seen in several bird species and, of course, in our very own.

monogony Asexual reproduction.

monomania Once used as equivalent to *paranoia*, *monomania* is now used to refer, almost colloquially, to any inflexible, irrational fixation.

monomyoplegia Paralysis in a single muscle.

monophasic Lit., having but one phase. The most specialized use of the term is to characterize a biological rhythm that has only one full phase per day, such as the typical human sleep/waking cycle.

monoplegia Paralysis of a single limb or a single muscle group.

monoptic With one eye, *monocular*.

monorchid A male with only one testicle.

monorhinic Pertaining to smelling with only one nostril.

monosynaptic reflex arc The simplest possible reflex arc, consisting of only two neurons, one afferent and one efferent, with a single synapse between them. Such neural circuits are rare in higher organisms, in which even the simplest reflexive systems are polysynaptic.

monotic With or to one ear. Contrast with DIOTIC and DICHOTIC.

monotonic Characterizing a relationship between two variables in which for each

value on one there is a unique value on the other. A monotonic relationship, when graphed, produces either a continuously rising or a continuously falling function with no level spots and no inflection points.

monovular twins MONOZYGOTIC *TWINS.

monozygotic (MZ) Lit., one zygote; see MONOZYGOTIC *TWINS.

Monte Carlo procedure Any procedure that generates pseudo-data according to a specific set of stochastic rules. Named for the locale of the legendary casino, such mathematical procedures are used in both the social and natural sciences to produce estimated solutions to mathematically intractable problems.

Monty Hall problem (paradox) A problem named after the TV game-show host Monty Hall and used in studies of decision-making, logic and risk-taking. The subject is presented with three doors and is told that an attractive prize (e.g. $20) lies behind one door and unattractive prizes (e.g. $1) behind the others. After the subject picks one door, the experimenter opens a different door to reveal one of the unattractive prizes. The subject is asked whether he or she wishes to stay with the original choice or switch to the other unopened door. Most people stick with the original choice believing that it is a 50–50 proposition so there is no logical reason to change (after all, there are only two doors left to choose from). However, mathematically it is easy to show that switching actually increases the probability of success from 0.50 to 0.67, which leads to the problem being called a paradox (hint: two-thirds of the time the unattractive prize was behind the first door chosen and in these cases switching *always* wins). In the original game show prizes were substantial; a new car might be behind one door and goats behind the others.

mood 1 Any relatively short-lived, low-intensity emotional state. Used freely. 2 A relatively pervasive and sustained emotional state. Although this meaning clearly conflicts with the original usage, this is the sense found in the latest edition of the DSM and is reflected in the umbrella diagnostic category MOOD DISORDERS.

mood-congruent memory MEMORY, MOOD-CONGRUENT.

mood-congruent psychotic features Delusions or hallucinations the content of which is consistent with displayed mood. For example, manic states accompanied by delusions of great wealth, inflated power and grandiosity. Mood-incongruent features are also often seen, e.g. manic states accompanied by delusions of persecution without grandiose content.

mood-dependent memory MEMORY, MOOD-DEPENDENT.

mood disorders A category of disorders characterized by disturbances of mood or emotional tone to the point where excessive and inappropriate depression or elation occurs. Included are the BIPOLAR DISORDERS, CYCLOTHYMIC DISORDER, DYSTHYMIC DISORDER, MANIA (2) and DEPRESSION. Also known as *affective disorders*.

mood disorder with seasonal pattern SEASONAL AFFECTIVE DISORDER.

mood-incongruent psychotic features MOOD-CONGRUENT PSYCHOTIC FEATURES.

mood-stabilizing drugs An umbrella term for several classes of drugs that are used in the treatment of major mood disorders. All function to stabilize the patient's affect. Included are the TRICYCLIC COMPOUNDS and the MONOAMINE OXIDASE INHIBITORS, both of which are used for depression, and LITHIUM, which is used for BIPOLAR DISORDERS.

Mooney faces (or **images** or **stimuli**) Black and white renditions of faces where almost all the detail of the face has been removed, leaving only a contrast between dark and light portions of the display. They are used as stimuli in cognitive and perceptual experiments comparing holistic with analytical processing and in assessments of perceptual closure. Interestingly, Mooney faces of known people are virtually unrecognizable when inverted, unlike normal photographs that merely display the FACE-INVERSION EFFECT.

moon illusion The illusion that the moon appears larger when low in the sky than when viewed overhead, despite the fact that the retinal image is the same size in both cases.

moral All of the subtle nuances in the meaning of this term focus on the central notion of pertaining to considerations of right and wrong conduct, of that which is right and that which is wrong within a particular MORAL CODE. See the following entries for usage patterns.

moral anxiety ANXIETY, MORAL.

moral code A code or set of sanctions and rules for classifying that which is regarded as right and proper within a particular group or society. The implication is that the code is applicable to all who regard themselves as members of that group or society.

moral development The development of morality, the process whereby individuals, particularly children, come to adopt and internalize the standards of right and wrong of their society. As such, the term acts as a cover term for a substantial subarea within the study of developmental psychology. Classic issues within the field concern how children come to perceive what their society's moral code is, how they learn to resist temptations to transgress, how they react should transgressions occur, how they respond to the knowledge or observance of others who have violated the code, etc.

Usage of the term is often bound up with theory. The most influential and frequently referred to is the interactionist stage theory of Lawrence Kohlberg, which is an extension and elaboration of the early work of Piaget on the problem. Kohlberg's analysis distinguishes three primary levels of moral thinking, each with two stages, yielding six (at least theoretically) distinguishable stages. Level I is classified as *preconventional*, in that behaviour is evaluated only on the basis of personal outcomes without any concept of right or wrong. Stage 1 here is characterized by avoidance of punishment, Stage 2 by hedonistic motives and mutual favouritism. Level II is considered to be the *conventional* level, in that behaviour here is dominated by external sanctions. Stage 3 within it is dominated by a desire for approval from others, Stage 4 is characterized by adherence to strong, legitimate authority. It is assumed that guilt emerges during Level II as an anticipation of possible punishment. Level III, the *postconventional*, is regarded as the highest level, in which moral judgement is based on personal principle. Stage 5 is characterized by concern for the values of the community, a just moral order and self-respect, Stage 6 by a reflection upon personal conscience and deep personal principle.

Balanced against this point of view are two other major schools of thought, within which terms like *moral* and *moral development* reflect different connotations. Within psychoanalysis the development of morality is assumed to proceed by stages but here the primary mechanism is assumed to be *identification* with the values of the parents and *internalization* of those values into the superego. The stages here are not stages of moral development *per se* as they are in Kohlberg's theory; rather they are linked to the more general progression through the stages of psychosexual development.

The other major theory is the social-learning theory of Albert Bandura, which emphasizes learning principles, in particular observational learning and modelling. Unlike the other approaches to moral development, Bandura's theory makes no pretence of being a stage theory and hence no specific sequence of moral judgements or behaviours is predicted. Development of morality is assumed to take place through the dispensing of rewards and punishments by adults and peers who serve as models for acceptable behaviour.

Recent theoretical developments have taken a new approach as researchers look toward evolutionary psychology. This orientation, like Bandura's, presumes no specific developmental course. The assumption is that much of moral behaviour is guided by biological predispositions to behave in particular ways owing to evolutionary pressures. Here, the focus is on uncovering the kinds of adaptive mechanisms that likely evolved over evolutionary time and predispose people to make particular kinds of moral decisions, judgements and justifications.

The fact that such disparate theories can all coexist and all be considered viable says something important about the enormous complexity of the problem of moral development, the difficulty of collecting definitive data that differentiate between each position and the lack of precision with which each is posed, rendering empirical comparisons among them exceedingly difficult.

moral dilemma DILEMMA, MORAL.

moral independence (stage) In Piaget's characterization of moral development, the later stage during which a child's determination of what is right and proper is modified to fit the particular circumstances. Compare with MORAL REALISM STAGE. Also called *autonomous morality stage*.

morality 1 A doctrine or set of principles for action, a *moral code*. **2** A quality of an act such that, according to a particular moral code, it is deemed to be right and proper or not. Morality, while it derives from a social codification of right and wrong, may be treated as either internal and hence part of an individual's personal code or external and imposed by society. It is worth noting that recent research suggests that our moral principles likely are grounded on evolutionary mechanisms that favoured particular characteristics (e.g. the golden rule, mutual grooming, altruism) over others (e.g. unabated aggression).

moral obligation An expectation that some particular act is required of one owing to a given set of socially accepted moral standards.

moral realism (stage) In Piaget's characterization of moral development, the early stage during which a child accepts as right and proper those rules given by authority. Compare with MORAL INDEPENDENCE (STAGE). Also called *heteronomous morality stage*.

morals Principles, or the behaviours which are the manifestations of such principles, judged with respect to rightness and wrongness. If MORALITY is an abstraction that underlies action, then morals are the concretizations. The relationship with ETHICS is strong; in fact it is so closely related that many treat the terms as synonymous.

morbidity rate The number of cases of a disease or other disorder per unit of population (usually per 100,000) in a given period of time (usually 1 year). Compare with MORTALITY RATE (1).

Morenogram See SOCIOGRAM.

mores (*more-rays*) Social norms and customs that provide the moral standards of behaviour of a group or a society. Mores are important codes of behaviour: conformity is regarded as essential for proper functioning of a society, and nonconformity is severely sanctioned. Application of the term is typically restricted to social customs that have not been formally enacted into law. sing., *mos* (rare).

Morgan's canon LLOYD MORGAN'S CANON.

moron From the Greek, meaning *dull*. The term is little used today, MILD *MENTAL RETARD-ATION being preferred. See also MENTAL DEFI-CIENCY for further discussion of terminology.

Moro reflex A startle reflex observed in newborns characterized by a drawing of the arms across the chest in an embrace-like manner. Also called *embrace reflex*.

morphed stimulus Any stimulus that changes from one shape or object to another by small, gradual steps over time.

morpheme The minimal linguistic unit that carries meaning. It may be either *free*, in that it can stand alone (e.g. *book*, *eat*), or *bound*, in that it cannot be used without being affixed to another morpheme (e.g. *un-*, *-ed*).

morphine Named after the minor Greek deity Morpheus, the god of dreams and the son of the god of sleep, a powerful narcotic derived from the opium poppy. It is the principal alkaloid of opium; its primary action is as a depressant producing euphoria, drowsiness and relief from pain. Its use as an analgesic is limited by the development of increasing tolerance for the drug and the ease with which drug dependency develops.

morphogenesis The meaning of this term is evident from its roots: *morph = form* or *structure, genesis = origin* and *development*.

morphological Generally, the study of the form or structure of something. The term is used very broadly.

morphological index A single figure derived from the relative proportions of ecto-morphic, endomorphic and mesomorphic characteristics that make up a person's physique. See SOMATOTYPE.

morphology 1 In biology, analysis of the form and structure of organisms. **2** In linguistics, analysis of language at the level of the MORPHEME.

morphophonemics In linguistics, the study of the interrelationship between PHON-EMES and MORPHEMES; it is generally conceded that a full characterization of any natural language has to have a morphophonemic component, since the two levels are intimately interdependent.

Morris water maze WATER MAZE.

mortality rate 1 Specifically, the death rate, usually given as number of deaths per unit of population (typically 100,000) in a specific time period (usually 1 year) and often expressed as an age-specific rate. Compare with MORBIDITY RATE. **2** Metaphorically, the failure rate in colleges, medical schools, training programmes, etc.

mortality salience TERROR MANAGEMENT THE-ORY (TMT).

mortido The energy of THANATOS, analogous with libido as the energy of Eros.

mos MORES.

mosaic 1 Generally, a structure or design composed of many diverse pieces. **2** In genetics, a chromosomal anomaly in which some cells have the normal complement of chromosomes and others do not.

mosaicistic Down syndrome A rare form of DOWN SYNDROME.

Moses test A nonparametric test that assesses the difference between two sets of scores by comparing the number of extreme scores from one sample with the number from the other.

mother complex OEDIPUS COMPLEX.

motherese E. Newport's unfortunate term for what is now called CHILD-DIRECTED SPEECH. A terminological change was needed here because, in addition to the obvious 'political' reasons, fathers and even older children use this particular form of speech when talking to young children.

mother figure The female analogue of FATHER FIGURE.

mother fixation FATHER FIXATION.

mother surrogate One who stands in place of the real mother. See SURROGATE.

motile 1 adj. Of biological entities, capable of movement. **2** n. In the study of imagery, a person whose images of movement are particularly vivid.

motion The displacement of a mass. Compare with MOVEMENT, which, strictly speaking, is the proper form when the mass that is displaced is an organism or a part thereof – a lexicographic nicety that is generally ignored in psychology, in which the two terms are often used interchangeably. For ease of reference all combined forms and varieties have been included here under *motion*, although the terms are often found in the literature under *movement* as well.

motion aftereffects A class of apparent motion effects. All are produced by first fixating for a time on a steadily moving stimulus and then shifting one's gaze to a stationary stimulus, which appears to move in the opposite direction. Watching a spiral spin inward will make a stationary object appear to move outward; staring at a waterfall for a time makes the trees on the bank appear to swim upward.

motion agnosia AGNOSIA, MOTION.

motion, alpha Apparent motion of change in size produced by presenting successively larger or smaller copies of a figure. The perception is of an expanding or shrinking single figure.

motion, apparent A cover term for a large number of perceptual phenomena in which objects that are, in fact, stationary appear to move. For some examples see MOTION AFTER-EFFECTS, AUTOKINETIC EFFECT and PHI PHENOMENON. Also called *phenomenal motion*.

motion, beta The optimal apparent motion in the PHI PHENOMENON. Specifically, perceived motion of an object from one place to another produced by successive static presentations of the object spatially separated from each other.

motion, biological Literally, the particular form of motion exhibited by a moving organism. In Gunnar Johansson's compelling demonstration, watching an array of some twelve tiny lights affixed to the head and joints of a organism that is moving in total darkness produces precisely this experience.

motion, bow A form of BETA *MOTION produced when an obstructing stimulus is introduced between the two stimulus objects

causing the apparent motion to curve (i.e. bow) around the obstruction.

motion, delta A form of apparent motion in which the position of an object appears to shift with changes in illumination.

motion, epsilon A form of apparent motion produced when a white line on a black background is abruptly changed into a black line on a white background.

motion, gamma Apparent motion of expansion and contraction of a figure when the luminance is increased and decreased.

motion, induced The perception of motion of a stationary stimulus object produced by real motion of another stimulus object. If, for example, in an otherwise dark room, a moving square perimeter of light is presented with a stationary dot of light inside it, the square will be seen as stationary and the dot as moving.

motion parallax A general term used to cover a class of cues for the perception of relative motion all of which are reflective of the fact that as the observer moves there are systematic movements in the visual field. See MOTION PERSPECTIVE.

motion perspective J. J. Gibson's term for the flow of visual information surrounding a moving observer. The term is used with the focus on the critical point that as one moves about in the environment objects at different distances move at different speeds according to their distance from, and position relative to, the observer. The resulting complex of movements (see MOTION PARALLAX) makes up the overall perspective that provides the cues for the veridical perception of real motion in a complex, three-dimensional world.

motion, pure PHI PHENOMENON.

motion, real Strictly speaking, motion that is perceived when either one (or both) of two conditions occur: (a) the image of a stimulus on the retina remains fixed as the eye tracks the stimulus; or (b) the eye remains stationary and the image travels across the retina. Note, however, that such motion is not perceived during a *saccade*. The cues for the perception of real motion are extremely complex and only partly understood; see here MOTION PERSPECTIVE.

motion sickness The feeling of nausea produced by certain patterns of motion. Oddly, exactly what produces this common and often disabling effect is not known. It seems fairly clear that it involves the semicircular canals but just which patterns of movement are effective and which are not is still an open question. Head movement, vision and anxiety also contribute and, to complicate the issue, there are very large individual differences in susceptibility and adaptability.

motion, stroboscopic Any of a class of apparent motion effects produced by presenting a series of stationary stimuli separated by brief intervals. Motion pictures are the best-known example; there is no real motion on the screen, merely a sequence of still frames presented in succession. The discovery of the PHI PHENOMENON was the major impetus for the study of the more general stroboscopic motion effects.

motivate 1 To impel to action, to induce a state of MOTIVATION. **2** To function as a goal or incentive.

motivated error An error that is (theoretically) caused by some underlying need or desire. In classical psychoanalysis, all errors and mistakes are presumed to be caused by such unconscious motives. See UNCONSCIOUS *MOTIVATION and PARAPRAXIS.

motivation The most typical use of this extremely important but definitionally elusive term is as the name for an intervening process or an internal state of an organism that impels or drives it to action. In this sense motivation is an energizer of behaviour. There are, however, several variations on this theme. Some theorists view the motivational state as one of general arousal without any specific goal or directionality – what is known as a *generalized energizer* or a *generalized drive*. The behaviour that actually occurs, they argue, is the one that is dominant in a particular situation. Most other theorists, on the other hand, argue that motivational states are specific to particular drives and needs and must always be analysed in terms of specific goals and directionality. Indeed, in the study of human psychosocial motivation this aspect is generally taken as axiomatic. Hence, motivation here is often characterized by the notion that a particular behaviour or behavioural tendency is observed *because of* a specific motivational state.

Note, however, that motivation is not a concept that can be used as a singular explanation of behaviour. Motivational states result from the multiple interactions of a large number of other variables, among them being the *need* or *drive* level, the *incentive* value of a goal, an organism's *expectations*, the availability of appropriate responses (i.e. learned behaviours), the possible presence of conflicting or contradictory motives and, of course, unconscious factors.

Most contemporary research on motivation falls into three broad orientations: (a) The *physiological*, which aims at an analysis of neurological and biochemical underpinnings. Most work here is limited to the so-called *primary drives*, such as hunger, thirst, temperature maintenance, pain avoidance, sexual desire, etc., which have clear organic bases. See e.g. DRIVE, HOMEOSTASIS, LIMBIC SYSTEM; (b) The *behavioural*, which is concerned largely with elaborations and refinements of drive theory and learning theory. Note that these two orientations are very strongly complementary See e.g. DRIVE (and related entries), INCENTIVE, NEED; (c) The *psychosocial*, which is oriented toward explanations of complex, learned, human behaviours. Except for a sharing of many similar basic concepts, this latter focus is quite separate from the other two. See here NEED FOR ACHIEVEMENT, NEED FOR AFFILIATION, NEED HIERARCHY, UNCONSCIOUS *MOTIVATION.

Finally, note that the topic of motivation is intimately intertwined with that of EMOTION. Emotional states tend to have motivational properties and the energizing elements of a motivational disposition often have a strong emotional tone to them. Moreover, the physiological structures identified in one context tend to be implicated in the other.

motivational hierarchy NEED HIERARCHY.

motivation research An effort on the part of advertisers and their clients to manipulate the buying patterns of consumers by exploitation of the real and/or imagined motivations of the public. *Research* here relates to systematic and controlled efforts to determine just how to package, label and advertise a product to maximize sales. See also MARKET RESEARCH.

motivation, unconscious By definition, motivation that is not in the conscious awareness of the person. Many agree that herein lies the single most important contribution of one Sigmund Freud: not all motivated behaviour can be seen as the result of the rational, the conscious or the wilful. Much of behaviour is motivated by unconscious factors working through a network of defence mechanisms, symbolic disguises and psychosexual cloaks.

motive 1 A state of arousal that impels an organism to action. **2** A rationalization, justification or excuse that a person gives as the reason for his or her behaviour. Note that this second, largely nontechnical, meaning carries the same essential theoretical component as the first, more technical, one – it provides a characterization of the cause of the behaviour. **3** Occasionally, a general global attitude, as in a phrase like 'his actions reflected altruistic motives'. See MOTIVATION for more details on usage.

moto- Combining form of *motor*.

motoneuron MOTOR NEURON.

motor Very generally, pertaining to or characterizing that which involves muscles, muscular movements and, by extension, glandular secretions. In short, anything that gives rise to or results in stimulation of effector organs. Almost invariably used in combined form, as the following entries show. Contrast with SENSORY.

motor aphasia APHASIA, MOTOR.

motor apraxia APRAXIA, MOTOR.

motor aprosodia APROSODIA.

motor area(s) Most generally, those regions of the central nervous system that have direct descending connections to motor neurons. The area most often cited is the *primary motor area* of the precentral gyrus, which is, in many aspects, a mirror of the sensory area; upon both is found the body representation known as the HOMUNCULUS (2). The innervation here is contralateral, with the exception of the facial area, where there is bilateral control of lower face and jaw muscles. A *secondary motor area* comprised of the *motor association area* (also known as *premotor cortex*) and the *supplementary motor area* is also included. The former lies in the frontal lobes just rostral to the primary motor area; the latter is on the medial wall of the cortex just below the primary area.

Although much smaller, this area seems to have independent output function in that in experimental animals stimulation here produces movement even if the entire primary motor cortex has been destroyed and its accompanying efferent system has degenerated. In the dominant hemisphere in humans this area has been implicated in the planning of the movements and motivation for speech. Lesions here produce TRANSCORTICAL MOTOR *APHASIA. Note that although motor responses can be elicited by stimulation of some *sensory areas* and many of the *association areas*, these are not technically considered motor areas because of the lack of direct connections with spinal and cranial motor neurons.

motor association area MOTOR AREAS.

motor cortex MOTOR AREAS.

motor end plate The terminus of a motor neuron on muscle fibre. See MYONEURAL JUNCTION.

motor equivalence A term used to characterize the fact that many motor responses may be functionally equivalent in that they bring about the same result though they may be very different topologically; a bar press may occur because a rat uses its teeth, its paws or its head, but all will qualify as bar presses that display motor equivalence.

motor homunculus HOMUNCULUS (2).

motor learning LEARNING, MOTOR.

motor memory MEMORY, MOTOR.

motor nerve A bundle of peripheral nerve fibres connecting the central nervous system with an effector.

motor neuron Any single nerve cell that activates an effector.

motor neuron, alpha A motor neuron with cell body in either the ventral horn of the spinal cord or one of the motor nuclei of the cranial nerves. Stimulation produces contraction of extrafusal muscle fibres.

motor neuron, gamma A motor neuron with cell body in either the grey matter of the spinal cord or the motor nuclei of the cranial nerves. They synapse on intrafusal muscle fibres.

motor projection area(s) The motor areas, because they are the parts of the cerebral cortex where the nerve pathways to the striate muscles originate, are often referred to as motor *projection* areas. See MOTOR AREAS for details.

motor reaction type REACTION TYPE (2).

motor response A somewhat redundant phrase used primarily to refer to: **1** An action of an organism that is emitted without significant covert components, a reflex-like response. **2** That portion of a complex series of actions that is motoric; e.g. in a decision-making task a complex sequence of perceptual and cognitive processes may be manifested by the making of a simple *motor response*, such as pressing one of two buttons.

motor sense A more or less nontechnical term for KINAESTHESIA.

motor theory of consciousness The strongly peripheralist theory, originally proposed by the arch-behaviourist John B. Watson, to the effect that consciousness was no more than an epiphenomenon, muscular and glandular action representing the true realities. What one may actually experience is argued to be a mere correlate of action, and what one senses or perceives is presumed to be dependent on how one reacts to it. The theory has precious few adherents these days.

motor theory of speech perception A theory of speech perception due largely to A. M. Liberman. The main point is that speech is assumed to be perceived by an implicit, covert system that 'maps' the acoustic properties of the input against a set of deep motor representations of idealized articulation. The theory was developed to account for the phenomenon of CATEGORICAL PERCEPTION, which indicated that speech was not processed in the same manner as other acoustic inputs. Note that the motor aspect of the theory is at a deep representational level and, hence, the theory should not be confused with the peripheralist MOTOR THEORY OF CONSCIOUSNESS; in Liberman's conceptualization, one does not actually have to *make* a motor response in order to perceive speech properly.

motor unit The basic unit of action of the neuromuscular system; it includes a single efferent neural fibre from a single motor neuron along with the muscle fibre it innervates.

mouches volantes FLOATERS.

moulding A technique used in *behaviour therapy* whereby the therapist shapes or moulds parts of the client's body, such as folding his or her fingers round a pencil or manipulating his or her mouth to make particular sounds more likely. var., *molding*.

mouth feel The tactile perception of a food substance in the mouth. It is not a true TASTE but a cutaneous sense of the texture of food. Many foods such as ice cream are enjoyed as much for their mouth feel as for their taste, and others such as raw fish are rejected because of their mouth feel rather than their taste.

movement **1** Any MOTION. **2** Any change in the position of an organism or of one or more of its parts. Compound forms involving 1 are under MOTION et seq., those involving 2 under MOTOR et seq.

movement afterimage MOTION AFTER-EFFECTS.

movement disorders A class of neurological disorders including TIC DISORDERS and TOURETTE'S SYNDROME.

movement disturbances A cover term for a large array of abnormal patterns of bodily movement, including CHORIFORM MOVEMENT, DYSTONIC MOVEMENT, DYSKINESIA (see in particular TARDIVE DYSKINESIA) and SPASMS.

movement, illusion of Any illusion that a part of one's body or the whole body is moving when it is not.

Mozart effect The finding that exposure to music enhances cognitive and spatial ability (the name was affixed because the original studies used Mozart's compositions). The effect is thought to be attributable to elevation of arousal and mood and is quite short-lived. It is also not specific to Mozart and can be obtained with any upbeat moderately familiar rhythmical activity or music.

MRI MAGNETIC RESONANCE IMAGING.

mRNA Abbreviation for *messenger RNA*, or RIBONUCLEIC ACID.

msec Abbreviation for *millisecond*, i.e. $\frac{1}{1000}$, or 0.001, of a second.

M system A system of serotonergic neurons (see SEROTONIN) that arises in the medial area of the RAPHE NUCLEUS and, unlike the s system, forms synapses with other neurons.

MTL MEDIAL TEMPORAL LOBE.

mucous membrane A general term for any moist epithelium and the underlying connective tissues found in vertebrates.

Müllerian ducts The structures in the embryo that develop into the female internal sex organs.

Müllerian mimicry MIMICRY.

Müllerian system In the developing embryo, the precursors of the internal female sex organs.

Müller–Lyer illusion One of the best known of the visual illusions, in which the perceived length of a line depends upon the shape and position of other lines that enclose it. The simplest form, the so-called arrowhead illusion, is shown here; lines *a* and *b* are exactly the same length.

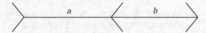

Müller–Urban method In psychophysics, the procedure that sets the threshold as the median value of the ogive fit to the data obtained using a constant-stimulus method. See MEASUREMENT OF *THRESHOLD.

multi- Latin prefix meaning *many*. Properly it should only be used with terms of Latin origin. See POLY-, for those of Greek origin.

multidimensional Of variables and factors that are represented as lying along more than one dimension.

multidimensional analysis A variation on FACTOR ANALYSIS procedures. Rather than searching for basic factors in a complex array of interdependent variables, this type of analysis allows one to identify a small set of dimensions which account for the variability observed in a larger number of scales. See KRUSKAL–SHEPARD SCALING and MULTIDIMENSIONAL SCALING.

multidimensional scaling A statistical procedure for making a multidimensional analysis. All such techniques operate by searching for a small set of dimensions that will provide the best fit for a large number of data points. See e.g. KRUSKAL–SHEPARD SCALING.

multi-infarct dementia DEMENTIA, MULTI-INFARCT.

multimodal Of a distribution with more than one MODE. Compare with BIMODAL, which refers to distributions with exactly two modes.

multimodal theory of intelligence The position that maintains that intelligence is composed of many separate abilities. It is in strong contrast with the theory that holds that all intellectual abilities derive from a single GENERAL FACTOR (2). See also INTELLIGENCE for more on this topic.

multinomial distribution DISTRIBUTION, MULTINOMIAL.

multiparous Pertaining to a female who has borne more than one offspring. Usually the term connotes more than one pregnancy, but it is also applied in cases of multiple births from a single pregnancy.

multiphasic Lit., having many phases. Used to describe (a) testing devices that were designed to measure a variety of facets of personality at the same time, e.g. the MINNESOTA MULTIPHASIC PERSONALITY INVENTORY, and (b) biological rhythms with more than one phase per day. Compare with MONOPHASIC.

multiple-aptitude test APTITUDE TEST.

multiple causation CAUSATION.

multiple-choice experiment Any experiment in which the subject must make a single choice from among several alternatives. Such experiments are most commonly found in the study of perception and cognition.

multiple code theory The theory that experience is coded in a form close to the original experience such that verbal experiences are represented as verbal *representations* or PROPOSITIONS (2, 4), visual experiences as images or other spatial representations, odours as smells, and so on. The theory stands in contrast to theories that maintain a universal type of *memorial* representation for all experiences. See INSTANCE THEORY.

multiple correlation CORRELATION, MULTIPLE.

multiple dissociation procedure DOUBLE DISSOCIATION PROCEDURE.

multiple drafts theory A model of conscious perception put forward by Dennett and Kinsbourne that postulates that there is no single representation of inputs nor a specific cortical location for storage of them. Rather multiple copies (or *drafts*) are distributed widely across sensory cortex. It is an updating of Karl Lashley's MASS-ACTION PRINCIPLE.

multiple intelligences theory Howard Gardner's theory of the ways in which one carries out life's goals. The theory proposes that there are discrete domains of functioning, each of which is mediated by different brain areas, has its own principles and skills and displays individual differences. Gardner identified three original domains of functioning, each of which has several, more specialized functions: (a) a cognitive or thought area which comprises *verbal-linguistic intelligence* (learning and using language) and *logical-mathematical intelligence* (understanding and use of logical, mathematical and abstract symbol systems); (b) a sensate area which comprises *auditory-musical intelligence* (understanding and creating musical and other auditory forms), *visual-spatial intelligence* (understanding and manipulating visual forms), and *kinaesthetic intelligence* (knowing where one's body is and how to manage one's bodily movements); and (c) a communication area consisting of *intrapersonal intelligence* (understanding and managing one's emotions, thoughts and motivations) and *interpersonal intelligence* (understanding and communicating with others). Recently, a domain of *naturalist intelligence* has been proposed to cover the area of sensitivity to one's natural surroundings. Critics of the theory object to the use of the word 'intelligence' – some would prefer that the term 'talent' be used in its place – and to its openness to the addition of new domains of functioning. See also TRIARCHIC THEORY OF INTELLIGENCE.

multiple personality A relatively rare disorder in which the usual integrity of a personality becomes so fractionated that two (or more) relatively independent subpersonalities emerge. The condition of multiple personality is an abnormality of degree, not of kind. Most normal persons show pronounced changes in style, behaviour and reactivity as they move between different social situations and different social roles. The pathological condition is marked by cir-

cumstances in which these varied manifestations of self become so bifurcated that the sense of underlying integrity is lost. There is a suggestion that the disorder is associated with a history of severe abuse during childhood, when fantasy became the only escape from painful reality. The term itself is slowly dropping out of favour, being replaced by DISSOCIATIVE IDENTITY DISORDER (see for more detail). Lay people often confuse multiple personality with schizophrenia, probably because of the persistent and erroneous use of the colloquialism *split personality* for *schizophrenia* (the split is between affect and thought, not between personalities).

multiple regression REGRESSION, MULTIPLE.

multiple-reinforcement schedule SCHEDULES OF *REINFORCEMENT.

multiple suicide CLUSTER SUICIDES.

multipolar cell (or **neuron**) A neuron with more than two neural processes rising from the soma. One of these is the axon, the others are 'trunks' of dendritic 'trees' which undergo multiple branchings. Of the three varieties of neuron (the others are unipolar and bipolar) in the central nervous system, the multipolar is the most common.

multistage theories A generic label applicable to any number of theories that hypothesize the existence of various stages of *processing* or of *development*. The most common of the former kind are *information processing* theories, theories of SEMANTIC *MEMORY and theories of *decision-making*; of the latter kind Piaget's theory of *cognitive development* and Kohlberg's theory of *moral development* are exemplary. In this second category, however, the simpler STAGE THEORY tends to be the term of choice.

multisynaptic reflex arc POLYSYNAPTIC REFLEX ARC.

multi-system atrophies A group of neurodegenerative diseases with early symptoms that can be confused with PARKINSON'S DISEASE. The diagnosis is usually made after the patient fails to show improvement to standard drug therapies or develops atypical dysfunctions. Included are OLIVOPONTOCEREBELLAR ATROPHY and STRIATO-NIGRAL DEGENERATION.

multi-system degenerative diseases See PARKINSON-PLUS SYNDROMES.

multivariate Pertaining to any experimental or statistical situation where more than one variable is assessed simultaneously. See following entries for statistical examples.

multivariate analysis A generic term used to cover any of several statistical techniques for examining multiple variables at the same time, including FACTOR ANALYSIS, MULTIPLE LINEAR *REGRESSION, MULTIVARIATE ANALYSIS OF VARIANCE and MULTIVARIATE ANALYSIS OF COVARIANCE.

multivariate analysis of covariance (MANCOVA) An extension of ANALYSIS OF COVARIANCE to situations in which multiple dependent variables are under analysis.

multivariate analysis of variance (MANOVA) An extension of ANALYSIS OF VARIANCE that permits one to test the effects of an independent variable on more than one dependent variable simultaneously. Unlike a regular analysis of variance, which merely provides significance levels for each dependent variable, a MANOVA also yields an estimate of the proportion of variance in the sample data that can be traced to the dependent variables as a set.

MUM See SINGLE-LOOP *LEARNING.

Münchausen's syndrome FACTITIOUS DISORDER WITH PHYSICAL SYMPTOMS. Also spelled *Münchhausen's*.

Münchausen syndrome by proxy FACTITIOUS DISORDER BY PROXY. Also spelled *Münchhausen*.

Munsell colour system The most widely used of the colour specification systems. In it several hundreds of colour samples are analysed according to their *hue*, *saturation* and *brightness*. The samples in the Munsell Atlas that are used as the basis of comparison for a stimulus were selected to represent psychologically equal steps along the three dimensions, and a notational system was developed that reflects these steps.

Murphy's laws A number of semi-humorous generalizations which, alas, are true entirely too often. Although countless variations on the legendary Murphy and his pronouncements exist, the three original laws are: **1** Anything that can possibly go wrong will go wrong. **2** Anything that goes wrong will do so at the worst possible time. **3** Anything you plan will cost more and take

longer. Anyone with the slightest familiarity with probability theory, or even a touch of fatalism about the outcome of the most carefully planned research, will appreciate the a priori truth of these statements.

muscarinic receptor A type of acetylcholine receptor that is stimulated by muscarine and blocked by atropine. They are found throughout the central nervous system. See also NICOTINIC RECEPTOR.

muscle Any tissue made up of variously modified elongated cells operating together as a contractile unit. Muscles are made up of muscle cells for contraction, connective tissue for binding and vascular tissue for nourishment. Muscles are generally differentiated according to structure of the cells and to function. See e.g. CARDIAC *MUSCLE, SMOOTH *MUSCLE, STRIATE *MUSCLE.

muscle-action potential The sequence of electrical and chemical events that occurs when a muscle cell is stimulated by a motor neuron across the myoneural junction. The polarization reversal that occurs has the same general characteristics as that in a nerve cell when it propagates an impulse. See ACTION POTENTIAL.

muscle, cardiac Specialized muscle tissue found only in the heart. The cells are intermediate in both structure and function between those of smooth and striate muscles and have the automaticity typical of most smooth muscle cells as well as the rapid contraction rate of striate muscle cells.

muscle sensation That aspect of kinaesthesis that provides an awareness of muscle movement and muscle position.

muscle, smooth Specialized muscle tissue found in the viscera, the blood vessels, the sphincters, the iris and the piloerectors. Structurally smooth muscles are the simplest of muscles, functionally they are relatively slow contractors. Innervated by the autonomic nervous system, they are sometimes called *involuntary* muscles, although we can learn voluntary control over some, as in toilet training.

muscle spindles INTRAFUSAL FIBRES.

muscle, striate (or **striped**) Specialized muscle tissue that moves the body about by pulling on the bony levers of the skeleton –

hence, striate muscles are also referred to as *skeletal muscles*. The individual fibres are larger than those in smooth muscle and they have a much faster contraction rate. Often also called *somatic muscle*, it is for the most part under voluntary control.

muscle tone (or **tonus**) The resting, partially contracted state of healthy muscle.

muscle twitch 1 A complex sequence of contraction and relaxation of a muscle following a single momentary stimulus. Muscles are often distinguished on the basis of the speed with which the twitch takes place, i.e. *fast-twitch muscles* have short reaction times and *slow-twitch muscles* long reaction times. 2 Critics of BEHAVIOURISM often referred to that approach as 'muscle-twitch psychology'. This meaning is not found anywhere else.

mutagen Any substance or agent that causes genetic mutations.

mutation A saltatory change in genetic material brought about by factors other than normal Mendelian recombinations. Mutations become part of the genetic material (i.e. they are *genotypic*), although their impact may not be observed in an individual organism's *phenotype*. The majority of mutations involve individual genes, although gross alterations of chromosomes, involving many genes, also occur. A mutation may also take place in a cell body (called *somatic mutation*) and be transmitted by mitosis from that cell. From the perspective of the adaptive value of a mutation for an individual organism, the outcome is strictly random; the role of a mutation in evolution comes about through the process of natural selection. Generally speaking, large (macro) mutations are deleterious to an organism and, hence, do not get passed on; small (micro) mutations, according to the standard viewpoint, are said to be the very stuff of evolution.

mute adj. Descriptive of one who lacks speech. The condition of *mutism* may be due to failure to develop the organs necessary for speech, to congenital or early deafness or to severe emotional factors. n., *mute*.

mutual exclusivity assumption An observed constraint on the learning of the meanings of new words in which the learner assumes that a second novel word for an

object refers not to the object itself but to some part of it. If, on a trip to the zoo, a mother says, 'Look at the ring-tailed lemur', her child, who already knows the word *lemur*, assumes that *ring-tailed* refers to the creature's most distinctive feature. Compare with WHOLE-OBJECT ASSUMPTION.

mutualism An occasional synonym for a true symbiotic relationship; see SYMBIOSIS.

mutual lateral masking LATERAL *MASKING.

mutually exclusive (events) Events that cannot occur simultaneously; the occurrence of one prevents the possibility of the occurrence of the other(s). For example, heads and tails on a coin flip. The concept is extremely important in probability theory and statistics.

mu wave A type of neural activity in the motor cortex that is suppressed during the intention to perform an action and its actual execution. Interestingly, mu waves are also suppressed when an action is observed being performed by another. See MIRROR NEURONS.

myasthenia Muscular disability or weakness.

myasthenia gravis An autoimmune disorder marked by progressive muscular weakness and fatigue, particularly following activity. The disease is caused by antibodies that attack the proteins that make up the acetylcholine receptors. Drugs such as neostigmine or physostigmine that deactivate acetylcholinesterase can relieve the symptoms. Interestingly, these drugs were first used as antidotes for *curare* poisoning.

mydriasis Abnormal dilation of the pupil of the eye. Contrast with MYOSIS.

myelencephalon One of the major subdivisions of the HINDBRAIN. Its principal structure is the *medulla oblongata*.

myelin A white fatty substance that forms a sheath along many nerve axons in vertebrates. The myelin coating usually begins just below the cell body and covers the entire axon except for the very fine terminal end brushes that synapse on other cells. The sheath is interrupted every 2 mm or so by the nodes of Ranvier. Myelinated fibres propagate neural impulses at roughly 20 times the speed of nonmyelinated fibres. In general, small-diameter fibres do not have myelin sheaths, a fact which is apparent from the distinction between *white matter* and *grey matter* in the central nervous system; the former is composed of myelinated fibres, the latter of nonmyelinated fibres.

my(o)- Combining form meaning *muscle*, *muscular*.

myoclonic movement Any sudden arhythmic contraction of a single muscle or a small group of muscles. Although such movements characterize some motor disorders, they are also commonly observed in almost everyone. The most frequent occurrence is the so-called *myoclonic jerk*, which often accompanies the first stages of sleep and can awaken the sleeper.

myogram Any graphic representation of muscular activity; e.g. an *electromyogram*.

myograph Any instrument for measuring muscular strength.

myoneural junction NEUROMUSCULAR JUNCTION.

myopia Near-sightedness, the inability to focus clearly on distant objects. The shape of the lens is such that in normal accommodation the focal point for light entering the eye is in front of the retina rather than directly on it. Contrast with HYPEROPIA. adj., *myopic*; n., *myope* (person).

myosis Abnormal contraction of the pupil of the eye. Contrast with MYDRIASIS.

myotactic reflex STRETCH REFLEX.

myotonia Excessive muscle rigidity.

mysticism 1 A doctrine that knowledge of ultimate reality (theological or otherwise) comes about in nonordinary ways, i.e. through means other than sensory inputs and cognitive processes. **2** The practice of making vague speculations without reasonable foundation. Meaning 1 is not at all derogatory, and the value of establishing such a philosophical position is usually related to current (nonmystical) knowledge and/or lack thereof concerning emotional states, intuition, cognitive processes and other psychological issues. The mystical experiences (or revelations) that have been reported by respected persons reflect an intriguing unanimity, one component of which

is great difficulty in providing verbal descriptions of them except in negative and/or metaphorical terms. Meaning 2, however, is generally a slur applied to those who either eschew the scientific method or apply it badly.

mysticotranscendent therapy An umbrella term used to cover a number of approaches of a therapeutic/religious sort which advocate the achievement of understanding of life and self through mystical and/or transcendental experience. Although most contemporary forms lie outside any well-developed theory of personality or self, the roots of these approaches can be found in the writings of many with an analytic bent, particularly Jung, Fromm and Laing. Frankly, it is not clear that the term *therapy* is really appropriate here; what is generally advocated is a new orientation toward the vagaries of life and a new perspective that transcends the mundane reality – this may or may not prove therapeutic. Indeed, many of the practitioners recommend that one should first be freed of all neurotic tendencies through conventional therapies before one can truly profit from the experience.

myth 1 From the Greek, meaning *tale* or *speech*; a story that is of unknown or unverifiable origin but is part of the traditions of a culture or a group. Usually a myth carries some explanatory component that ostensibly relates historic events, particularly those of importance to the culture. In Jungian theory, the myth became one of the units for analysis of the collective unconscious. **2** A false, unsupportable, but nevertheless widely held, belief.

myxoedema A condition of severe depression of nervous-system activity, the main symptoms of which are lethargy, low basal metabolism rate and general weakness. It occurs in adults with thyroxin deficits. var., *myxedema*.

MZ Abbreviation for MONOZYGOTIC.

MZA (or MZa) Shorthand notation for a pair of MONOZYGOTIC *TWINS reared apart from each other.

MZT (or MZt) Shorthand notation for a pair of MONOZYGOTIC *TWINS reared together in the same home.

N A common abbreviation for *number*, as in the number of scores in a distribution, population, sample or experimental condition, the number of reinforcements, a number factor, etc.

n Abbreviation for: **1** The number of scores or cases in a subclass or subcategory of a larger population. **2** Need, as in *nAch* (*need for achievement*).

N100 The first negative EVOKED POTENTIAL that peaks at roughly 100 msec after onset of a visual stimulus. It is larger for stimuli that are attended to. Also called simply *N1*.

N200 A negative EVOKED POTENTIAL that peaks approximately 200 msec after the presentation of a stimulus. It is thought to reflect correct classification or interpretation of the stimulus and has been observed with a wide variety of stimuli including tones, geometric forms, faces etc. Interestingly, it is reduced or absent in a variety of disorders including ADHD, panic disorder and schizophrenia. Often called simply *N2*.

N400 A negative EVOKED POTENTIAL that peaks at approximately 400 msec poststimulus. It has been extensively studied in language-processing tasks and seems to correspond to violations of semantic expectancies. Often simply referred to as *N4*, particularly in verbal exchanges. See P300 for another potential that appears as a marker of oddity or surprise.

nAch NEED FOR ACHIEVEMENT.

naevus A congenital discoloration of an area of the skin. var., *nevus*. pl., *naevi*.

nAff NEED FOR AFFILIATION.

naïve Lacking sophistication or experience; descriptive of a subject in an experiment who is unaware of the nature and purpose of the experiment. n., *naïveté* (or *naïvety*), *naïveness*. Also written as *naive*.

naïve realism 1 An early philosophical perspective based on the assumption that one's perceptions of the world are accurate reflections of a true reality. Because the position neglects the roles of top-down actions that modulate, interpret and organize inputs, it is no longer regarded as tenable. **2** In social psychology, the belief that one's view of events is unbiased and correct and when others disagree they must be wrong. Found commonly among philosophers and politicians, both of whom should know better.

nalorphine A narcotic antagonist that blocks the primary pharmacological effects of opium-based drugs. When administered alone, however, its effects are of the morphine type.

naloxone An opioid antagonist that reverses the pharmacological action of ENDOGENOUS and EXOGENOUS OPIATES by competing with them for receptor sites in the brain. Used in experimental work as well as in clinical settings to treat opiate overdoses. Unlike other narcotic antagonists, when administered alone it does not have the morphine-type pharmacological effects. Naltrexone, a drug with similar properties but longer lasting, is also in common use.

naltrexone NALOXONE.

Nancy school A 19th-century group of psychiatrists who, under the leadership of Hippolyte M. Bernheim, maintained that the state of consciousness induced by hypnosis was an extension of a normal state of high suggestibility rather than an abnormal state akin to hysteria, as many others argued. SALPÊTRIÈRE SCHOOL.

nano- Prefix meaning *one-billionth*.

nanometer (nm) One-billionth of 1 m. It is the preferred measure for the wavelength of light; 1 nm is equal to 1 mμ (MILLIMICRON).

narcism Variant of NARCISSISM.

narcissism The term comes from the Greek myth about a young man's unfortunate emotional investment in his own reflection. In its most general sense it stands for an exaggerated self-love. However, it may have any of a variety of meanings depending on the particular orientation of the author. For the specific meanings in psychoanalytic theory see PRIMARY *NARCISSISM, SECONDARY *NARCISSISM and NARCISSISTIC NEUROSIS; for the contemporary usage in standard psychiatry see NARCISSISTIC PERSONALITY DISORDER. Note, in some writings narcissism is called *ego erotism*.

narcissism, covert A type of narcissism in which slight negative comments or mild frustration often leads to a sense of *narcissistic injury*. It is assumed to reflect an inflated yet fragile sense of self-esteem, although the person is rarely perceived as grandiose in any way. Contrast with *overt* or *grandiose narcissism*, in which the person appears outgoing and grandiose but tends to ignore or dismiss criticism. In the literature a host of synonyms can be found, including *co-dependent, inverted, sensitive* and *hypersensitive narcissism*.

narcissism, grandiose See COVERT *NARCISSISM.

narcissism, malignant A form of NARCISSISTIC PERSONALITY DISORDER characterized by suspiciousness to the point of paranoia, feelings of grandiosity, and sadistic cruelty accompanied by a complete lack of remorse.

narcissism, overt See COVERT *NARCISSISM.

narcissism, primary In classical psychoanalysis, the early stage of development when libido is overly invested in the self or the ego, or, more simply, in the body. Note that the stage is considered normal in the very young; should it persist into adulthood it is usually classified as a neurosis and is generally characterized by a love of self that precedes, if not precludes, love of others.

narcissism, secondary In classical psychoanalysis, the love of self that results from a withdrawing of libido from objects and persons and the investing of it in oneself.

narcissistic injury A psychological wounding of one's essential self. Such a blow to one's core identity typically lowers one's self-esteem and produces feelings of humiliation, shame and rage.

narcissistic libido EGO LIBIDO.

narcissistic neurosis A neurosis characterized by such excessive self-love that normal love for others is impossible. In the classical theory of psychoanalysis, such a neurosis can prevent the individual from forming a transference. For a nonpsychoanalytic characterization see NARCISSISTIC PERSONALITY DISORDER.

narcissistic object choice As the term suggests, the object that is chosen for narcissistic reasons. The choice is either the self or one very much like oneself.

narcissistic personality disorder A personality disorder characterized by an exaggerated sense of self-importance, a tendency to overvalue one's actual accomplishments, an exhibitionistic need for attention and admiration, a preoccupation with fantasies of success, wealth, power, esteem or ideal love, and inappropriate emotional reactions to the criticisms of others. This symptom-based definition is preferred over that found under the older term NARCISSISTIC NEUROSIS.

narcissistic wound A rather clumsy phrase which simply means any blow to or attack upon one's self-esteem.

narc(o)- A prefix meaning *sleep, numbness* or *stupor*.

narcoanalysis A form of psychoanalysis carried out under the influence of drugs which produces a sleep-like stupor, most commonly one of the barbiturates. The procedure is rarely if ever used today.

narcolepsy An ORGANIC *SLEEP DISORDER characterized by recurrent, uncontrollable, brief episodes of sleep. No more descriptive phrase exists than that in Taber's *Cyclopedic Medical Dictionary* (Philadelphia, 1977): 'Here sleep reasserts itself excessively and under conditions not to the best interests of the patient.'

Narcoleptic sleep is often accompanied by HYPNAGOGIC IMAGES, CATAPLEXY and an immediate onset of REM SLEEP. Although some narcoleptics appear normal except for these transient episodes, many others display related symptoms, including excessive daytime sleepiness, cataplexy and disturbed night-time sleep.

narcomania Obsolescent term for: **1** Extreme desire for narcotic drugs. **2** A psychotic state resulting from long-term abuse of narcotics.

narcosis A state of markedly reduced responsiveness, both in behaviour and in normal physiological functioning, induced by narcotic drugs.

narcotherapy A general term for any therapy that makes use of narcotic drugs. See NARCOANALYSIS, which is sometimes used as an approximate synonym but carries a more restricted set of connotations.

narcotic 1 In psychopharmacology, any drug that has both *sedative* (sleep-inducing) and *analgesic* (pain-relieving) properties. Hence, the classification is restricted essentially to the opiates and opiate-like drugs. **2** In some (ill-advised) legal systems, a drug classification that includes the true narcotics (as in meaning 1) as well as marijuana and cocaine. The problem here is that these other drugs are pharmacologically unrelated to the true narcotics and have different patterns of drug dependence associated with them. Hence the term *narcotic* is rarely if ever used in the technical literature any more. Rather the particular class of drugs under consideration (usually the OPIATES) is specified.

narcotic analgesic NARCOTIC (2).

narcotic blocking agent Any drug that functions as a narcotic *antagonist*. Included are naloxone, naltrexone, methadone and other agents that are structurally similar to the opiates and presumably function by competing with them for the receptor sites in the central nervous system.

nares The nostrils; sing., *naris*.

narratophilia A PARAPHILIA characterized by deriving erotic stimulation from listening to or reading erotic works to the extent that such narratives are necessary for maintaining

sexual arousal and to achieve orgasm. The term is not used for simple enjoyment of erotica or for the use of such literature as an adjunct to sexual activity.

nasal 1 In phonetics, a DISTINCTIVE FEATURE (2) for distinguishing the sounds of a language. A phonetic element is called nasal when the velum is lowered and the sound is permitted to resonate in the nasal cavity (e.g. *m* and *n*); it is marked as nonnasal when the nasal cavity is blocked off (e.g. most of the other phonemes in English). **2** Generally, pertaining to the nose.

nascent Incipient, beginning, just born.

naso- Combining form meaning *nasal, pertaining to the nose.*

nasopharynx Collectively, the nasal passages, the mouth and the upper part of the throat.

native Innate, inherited.

nativism 1 Historically, the doctrine that a variety of human perceptual and cognitive abilities such as the capacity to perceive time and space is inborn. This point of view, in its strongest form, argued for the ability for normal perception independent of experience, a position no longer defensible. See MOLYNEUX'S QUESTION. **2** More contemporarily, and more loosely, any orientation to psychology or philosophy that stresses the genetic, inherited influences on behaviour and thought over the acquired, experiential influences. Modern variations on nativism have focused on issues such as language (see LAD) and social behaviour (see SOCIOBIOLOGY). Compare with EMPIRICISM and see the extended discussion under HEREDITY–ENVIRONMENT CONTROVERSY.

natural category CATEGORY, NATURAL.

natural childbirth A general term covering a number of methods of childbirth in which the focus is on the psychological and social aspects and the meaning of birth rather than on the mechanical, medical and physiological.

natural environment type phobia SIMPLE *PHOBIA.

natural experiment A naturally occurring situation that has many of the trappings of a formal laboratory experiment in that one can identify factors that function as independent variables although they are not controlled in the usual sense. For example, one could study the role of schooling in vocabulary development in children by comparing the number of new words learned during the summer with the number learned during the months just preceding and following.

naturalistic approach ZEITGEIST.

naturalistic observation The collection of data by careful observation of events in their natural setting. The oldest of the various scientific methods, it is used widely in areas such as ethology, ethnomethodology and developmental psychology.

naturalist intelligence See MULTIPLE INTELLIGENCES THEORY.

natural killer cells White blood cells that attack and destroy cells that have been infected by viruses. They are part of the body's immune system.

natural language LANGUAGE, NATURAL.

natural-response theory THEORIES OF *LANGUAGE ORIGINS.

natural selection First proposed by Charles Darwin and Alfred Russel Wallace in 1858, natural selection is now recognized as the primary mechanism of evolution. The principle of natural selection asserts that of the range of inheritable variations of traits in a population, those that contribute to an organism's survival are those most likely to be passed on to the next generation. Hence, the contributions to succeeding generations are not random but are in effect selected by the natural process of the viability of traits. See also DARWINISM, EVOLUTION, EVOLUTIONARY THEORY.

natural sign SIGN (1).

nature Three, more or less distinct, general meanings of this term can be identified: **1** Those traits or characteristics of an organism that are assumed to be innate or inherited. This meaning is reflected in what is often called the nature–nurture or HEREDITY–ENVIRONMENT CONTROVERSY. **2** The complex of events, forces and phenomena that make up the totality of the universe as we know it. Combined with 1 this usage produces a most annoying confrontation of meanings,

since by *nature–nurture* (*nature* in sense 1) we could literally mean 'nature–nature' (nature in sense 2). **3** The intrinsic qualities, attributes or characteristic modes of behaviour of a person. This sense is strictly nontechnical and is found mainly in offhand remarks like 'What do you expect? That's just his nature.'

nature–nurture controversy HEREDITY–ENVIRONMENT CONTROVERSY.

nature, second **1** A nontechnical phrase used to imply that a piece of behaviour is habitual and occurs almost reflexively and without conscious thought. **2** Occasionally, in psychoanalytic writings, the *superego*.

n-back task A task in which the subject is presented with a series of stimuli such as words, and required to report which stimulus occurred a given number (*n*) of instances ago. Often used in investigations of *working memory*.

NDE NEAR DEATH EXPERIENCE.

NE NOREPINEPHRINE.

near death experience (NDE) Subjective experiences reported by individuals who have suffered life-threatening incidents. Among the perceptions and emotions often reported are a cloudy calmness, a sense of separation from the physical and an experience of light. Some regard these as evidence of life after death; others as the manifestation of neurological processes associated with the physiological changes brought about by the episode. The empirical data support the latter.

near point **1** The point closest to the eye at which an object can be clearly seen. Since this point reflects the ability of the lens to focus the image it is often called the *near point of accommodation*. **2** The point closest to the two eyes where an object can be seen with proper binocular fusion. Often called the *near point of convergence*.

nearsightedness MYOPIA.

near vision VISION, NEAR.

necessary condition CONDITION.

Necker cube REVERSIBLE *FIGURE.

necro- Combining form meaning *dead*.

necromania Pathological fascination with death and the dead. Similar in meaning to NECROPHILIA but without the erotic component.

necrophilia A fascination with the dead, specifically an obsessive erotic attraction toward corpses.

necropsy An examination following death to determine its cause, an autopsy.

necrosis Localized tissue death with accompanying degeneration while still in contact with living tissue, e.g. as occurs at the site of a wound.

need 1 Some thing or some state of affairs which, if present, would improve the well-being of an organism. A need, in this sense, may be something basic and biological (e.g. food) or it may involve social and personal factors and derive from complex forms of learning (e.g. achievement, prestige). **2** The internal state of an organism that is in need of such a thing or state of affairs. Note that 1 refers to that which is needed while 2 refers to the hypothetical state of the organism in the deprivation condition.

These two definitions, straightforward though they may be, mask some important subtleties of usage that are reflected in the technical literature. For example, there is a tendency among some, particularly those with behaviourist leanings, to treat *need* as equivalent to DRIVE. This use extends the meanings above in theoretically interesting but occasionally troublesome ways. The equation with drive endows the need state with motivational properties that are not explicitly present in 1, although they are implicit in 2. To appreciate the problem here one must realize that there are needs for which there are no drives, such as the need for oxygen, for the distress felt when you hold your breath is not a drive for oxygen but a drive to reduce carbon dioxide levels.

Attempts have been made to handle the concept of need with a strictly operationalist analysis. That is, a given need is characterized in terms of procedures. An organism's need for food, for example, may be specified by any of several devices such as a statement of its body weight relative to what it would be under normal (ad lib) feeding conditions or a specification of the number of hours since it

has eaten. While this lexicographic device helps to clarify some issues, it doesn't aid in understanding the complex interrelationships between biological needs, social needs and the problem of MOTIVATION.

There are other variations of usage but they are neither as common nor as compelling as these. For example, need is, on occasion, used as a synonym of such terms as *motive, incentive, wish, desire, craving,* etc. The plethora of quasi-synonyms is symptomatic of concepts with the underlying characteristics essential for a theoretically sound psychology but with connotations so diverse that conceptual boundary conditions have not been arrived at. In general, most authors use qualifying phrases to delineate their particular sense of the term, as the following entries show.

need cathexis A more mechanical use of CATHEXIS than that commonly found in psychoanalytic theory. It conveys the same general connotation but physiological needs are assumed in place of *libido*. The need here is assumed to become attached to or invested in some object or person as a means to its gratification or fulfilment.

need–drive–incentive model A model of motivation which assumes that basic, physiological needs are produced by states of deprivation, that such needs produce drives that are the true instigators of action and that the action is directed toward the incentive components of the goal state.

need for achievement As characterized by D. C. McClelland and J. W. Atkinson, the desire to compete with a standard of excellence. It is treated as a socially characterized need with two critical components: a set of internalized standards that represent personal achievement or fulfilment, and a theoretical energizing or motivating condition that impels the person toward attempts to meet these standards. Need for achievement is generally measured with a projective test, using, specifically, several pictures similar to those from Murray's Thematic Apperception Test. Usually written in abbreviated form, *nAch*. See also ACHIEVEMENT et seq.

need for affiliation H. Murray's term for the need to be with other people, to socialize, to form friendships, to cooperate, etc. Often abbreviated *nAff*.

need for cognition A personality variable that reflects the extent to which an individual enjoys effortful cognitive activities. People who are high in need for cognition crave information, like to analyse complex situations and enjoy solving problems, particularly difficult ones.

need hierarchy In A. Maslow's theory all human motives can be viewed as components of a hierarchical need system. Although the hierarchy can be broken up in various ways (see e.g. BASIC NEEDS, INTERMEDIATE NEEDS, METANEEDS and DEFICIENCY NEEDS), the following are the seven main divisions in Maslow's system: 1. Physiological needs – food, water, etc.; 2. Safety needs – freedom from threat, security, etc.; 3. Belongingness and love needs – affiliation, acceptance, etc.; 4. Esteem needs – achievement, prestige, status, etc.; 5. Cognitive needs – knowledge, understanding, curiosity, etc.; 6. Aesthetic needs – order, beauty, structure, art, etc.; 7. Need for self-actualization – self-fulfilment, realization of potential.

Maslow conceptualized the hierarchy as invariant (although this claim is disputed by many theorists) and argued that the lower a need the more prepotent it will become if unfulfilled; e.g. a starving person is unlikely to be much concerned about self-esteem. It is this assumption, of course, that gives Maslow's conceptualization its hierarchical properties; without it all you have is a list.

need-press PRESS.

need, primary Any unlearned need, one determined by innate factors, a *basic need*.

need reduction The result of any event or behaviour that diminishes a need. See also DRIVE REDUCTION.

need state NEED (2).

need, tissue The primary physiological need(s) of tissue for substances necessary for life, such as oxygen, nutrients and water.

neencephalon Lit., new brain; the most recently evolved structures of the brain, the cortex and coordinated structures. All the rest is the *palaeoencephalon* (var., *paleencephalon*) or *old brain*.

negation 1 In logic, the denial of a proposition. **2** Generally, any act of denial or dispute. **3** NEGATIVISM (1).

negative A term with a host of meanings in everyday language although, within psychology, its use is almost always reserved to refer to the downbeat, dispiriting, unhopeful, discouraging aspects of events, situations, syndromes and outcomes. It is also found in an array of phrases where the author wishes to denote these 'negative' elements of whatever is being referenced. The following entries provide definitions where the meaning may not be obvious; for the others we leave it up to the reader. See POSITIVE for a similar state of affairs.

negative acceleration ACCELERATION.

negative adaptation ADAPTATION (1) when there is a gradual diminution in sensitivity.

negative affect reciprocity An unhappy pattern of negatively charged give-and-take behaviours (verbal and nonverbal) between individuals. Because negative feelings presented by one party are often countered with negative messages in return, individuals can easily get caught up in this kind of destructive, reciprocal exchange.

negative afterimage AFTERIMAGE, NEGATIVE.

negative attitude change ATTITUDE CHANGE, NEGATIVE AND POSITIVE.

negative eugenics See EUGENICS.

negative feedback Descriptive of any feedback loop that diminishes or terminates a process. See discussion under FEEDBACK.

negative law of effect See LAW OF *EFFECT.

negative predictive value The proportion of people identified by a test as being 'non-cases' who, in fact, do not have the disorder tested for. If a test for depression identifies 20 people as having no depression, and only one of these actually is depressed, the value is 0.95 (19/20).

negative priming PRIMING, NEGATIVE.

negative punishment PUNISHMENT, NEGATIVE.

negative recency The tendency to predict an event that has not occurred recently. In a simple case like a series of coin flips, the less recently a head has occurred the more likely people are to guess 'heads' on the next flip. Contrast with POSITIVE RECENCY and see the discussion under GAMBLER'S FALLACY.

negative reference group   REFERENCE GROUP, NEGATIVE.

negative reinforcement   REINFORCEMENT, NEGATIVE.

negative schizophrenia   SCHIZOPHRENIA, NEGATIVE.

negative sensation An archaic term for a stimulus the intensity of which is below threshold.

negative suggestion effect The acquisition of false knowledge due to exposure to incorrect information. The deviant input, especially if it is frequently encountered, is later judged as acceptable because it gets stored and competes with or degrades correct knowledge. Politicians discovered this phenomenon long before psychologists.

negative symptoms Symptoms of psychoses characterized by a lack of behaviour or affect that is normally present, e.g. flat affect, thought blocking and social withdrawal. Compare with POSITIVE SYMPTOMS.

negative transfer   TRANSFER, NEGATIVE.

negative transference   TRANSFERENCE.

negativism 1 A general attitude characterized by resistance to suggestions of others (*passive* negativism) and a tendency to act in ways opposite to directions or commands (*active* negativism). The hallmark of such behaviour, particularly when displayed by young children, is the lack of any possible objective reason for the negative stance. **2** A general term for any philosophy based on negative principles, e.g. scepticism, agnosticism.

negativistic personality disorder   PASSIVE-AGGRESSIVE PERSONALITY DISORDER.

neglect 1 Failure to provide appropriate nurturance, emotional support, or to satisfy basic physical needs. See CHILD NEGLECT, ELDER NEGLECT. **2** A neurological disorder in which the patient is simply not cognizant of (i.e. neglects) particular categories of information. In the classic form, the patient is unaware of the left half of the space about him or her (the responsible lesion is virtually always in the parietal lobe of the right hemisphere) and does not consciously see, hear or feel stimuli that originate there. Neglect patients may only see the right half of a painting and typically only eat the food on the right side of their dinner plates. Left-neglect is intriguing for several reasons. For one, patients are typically unaware that there is any problem and will deny that they are not responsive to stimuli in the neglected field. Moreover, while they show no conscious awareness of left-field stimuli, they will make appropriate, automatized responses to stimuli in the neglected field. See BLIND-SIGHT. Neglect is often called *hemineglect, hemispatial neglect, hemi-inattention* and occasionally *unilateral neglect*. A rare form of what is called *altitudinal neglect* is also seen in which the neglected field is vertically oriented. Here, patients neglect the top or bottom half of the field.

neglect dyslexia   DYSLEXIA, NEGLECT.

ne(o)- Prefix used to denote that which is new or recent. Also often used to indicate a theoretical position or a point of view that is derivative of an earlier position.

neoanalyst   NEO-FREUDIAN.

neoassociationism A general term applicable to a number of variations on the classical associationist theory. Neoassociationism tends to be cognitive in character; behaviour is viewed as resulting from links between abstract, mental entities, such as propositions, images and ideas, rather than links between stimuli and responses as in a strict behaviourism. Oddly, these modern theories are hardly *neo* . They are actually quite close in spirit to the associationist ideas of the early British empiricists. For more on usage patterns here see ASSOCIATIONISM.

neobehaviourism A very general label used as descriptive of any theory or approach that, like classical behaviourism, focuses on the behaviours of organisms as the source of one's data but also allows for the use of unobservable and covert processes as explanatory devices.

neocerebellum The evolutionarily newest part of the cerebellum; it is composed of the lateral cortex and the dentate nucleus. Once thought to be concerned solely with rapid skilled movements, there is increasing evidence that its structures may play an important role in cognitive functions such as language and memory. Also called *cerebrocerebellum.*

neocortex The evolutionarily most recent and most complex of neural tissue. The frontal, parietal, temporal and occipital lobes of the brain consist of neocortex.

neo-Freudian A term descriptive of any psychoanalytic approach, theory or individual analyst that departs from or modifies significantly the orthodox FREUDIAN position. Those analysts who emphasized social, cultural and interpersonal factors while still maintaining a basically dynamic point of view, such as Sullivan, Horney or Fromm, are so labelled. Those who made a clean break from Freud and established their own schools of thought, like Jung and Adler, are not so classified.

neologism 1 A new word or phrase or a new meaning attached to an existing word or phrase. 2 The act of coining such; NEOLOGY.

neology The coining of new words or terms or the use of existing words or terms in novel ways. Often considered a creative act of an innovative person, it is also regarded as a symptom characteristic of certain pathological conditions such as schizophrenia and some forms of aphasia.

neonatal abstinence syndrome See NEONATAL DRUG DEPENDENCY SYNDROME.

Neonatal Behavioural Assessment Scale A test of behavioural development constructed by T. B. Brazelton and often simply referred to as 'the Brazelton'. It consists of assessing an infant's reactions to a variety of stimuli, such as a light in the eyes, a rattle or a moving ball. In the latest revision (2000), it contains 26 items designed to assess behavioural characteristics and 14 that focus on neurological factors. It is simple, easily administered, but surprisingly effective at providing an initial assessment of an infant. A variety of abnormalities are easily detected using it.

neonatal drug dependency syndrome A pattern of behaviours observed in the infants of mothers who are dependent on a variety of drugs, usually opiates (see here DRUG DEPENDENCE). The syndrome is characterized by irritability, excessive loud crying, tremors and a voracious appetite unaccompanied by usual weight gain. There is evidence to suggest that the syndrome is associated with decreased attention span and hyperactivity in later childhood. Also called *neonatal abstinence syndrome.*

neonate Lit., a newborn child. Occasionally, however, the term is used metaphorically to characterize anything novel or new, e.g. a neonatal idea.

neopallium All of the tissues of the cerebral cortex except the olfactory area.

neophasia 1 Loosely, any idiosyncratic speech form created by an individual. The connotation is that the language has a coherent semantics and syntax. 2 The peculiar forms of speech occasionally observed in schizophrenia. There is little evidence of regular grammar or vocabulary here.

neophilia 1 Generally, a desire for the new or novel. 2 Specifically, a tendency to try new foods.

NEO-PI-R NEUROTICISM, EXTRAVERSION AND OPENNESS PERSONALITY INVENTORY-REVISED.

neopsychoanalysis NEO-FREUDIAN.

neostigmine An acetylcholinesterase inhibitor, it is used therapeutically for disorders such as *myasthenia gravis* which is marked by diminished supplies of acetylcholine.

neostriatum Collectively, the caudate nucleus and putamen of the BASAL GANGLIA.

neoteny The retention of immature characteristics in adulthood.

nepiophilia A form of PAEDOPHILIA in which infants are the focus of sexual interest.

nerve 1 n. A bundle of independently conducting neural fibres along with accompanying connective tissue. Specific nerves are listed in this volume under the qualifying term. 2 adj. Of or pertaining to such a bundle of neural fibres. There are several adjectival forms freely used with this latter meaning, e.g. *nerve, nervous, neural* and *neuronal.* The standard conventions for usage are as follows:

(a) *Nerve.* Specific reference to anatomical structures, e.g. *nerve tissue, nerve cell, nerve fibre.*

(b) *Nervous.* General reference to pathological conditions, particularly those characterized by instability and excitability. However, also firmly fixed in the physiologist's lexicon as a synonym of *nerve* (above sense), e.g. *central nervous system.*

(c) *Neural.* Originally used to refer to functions and operations of nerve fibres; now often used as a blanket adjective for anything involving nerves and nerve cells – structural or functional.

(d) *Neuronal.* Relating to individual nerve cells; see NEURONS.

While these conventions are followed to a considerable extent, they are hardly adhered to slavishly; all in all these various forms are used with great latitude in the technical literature. If a particular combined form is not found in this volume under one qualifier, see the other three.

nerve block   Temporary inhibition of neural transmission by either chemical or mechanical means.

nerve cell 1 Usually, a NEURON. **2** Occasionally, the CELL BODY of a neuron.

nerve centre 1 Generally, any point in the nervous system that has the function of integrating and coordinating neural information. **2** Specifically, a locus of neural tissue where *afferent* information makes the transition to *efferent* information.

nerve deafness   DEAFNESS, NERVE.

nerve ending   Generally, the terminus of a neuron in a peripheral structure. Usually the term is used in combination with qualifiers that specify structure (e.g. *free nerve ending*) or function (e.g. *efferent nerve ending*). Note, the term is not used of neurons that terminate on other neurons; see SYNAPSE.

nerve fibre 1 An elongated process of a NEURON (usually the axon) that carries neural impulses. This is the preferred reference. **2** Occasionally, a NERVE or a bundle of such nerve fibres. var., *nerve fiber.*

nerve impulse   IMPULSE (4).

nerve-muscle preparation   A procedure used in the study of neural-muscular function. A muscle with its efferent nerve still attached is removed and mounted so that stimulation of the nerve produces muscle contraction.

nerve pathway   The path or route through the nervous system of a particular neural impulse.

nerve process   NEURAL PROCESS.

nerve tissue   Loosely, any and all of the neurons, the cells that comprise the nervous system.

nerve trunk   The main stem of a peripheral nerve.

nervios   ATAQUE DE NERVIOS.

nervous 1 Originally, pertaining to a NERVE. See that entry, especially 2, for various points on usage of the several near-synonyms *nerve*, *neural* and *neuronal.* **2** Loosely and largely nontechnically, descriptive of persons of elevated emotionality, hyperexcitability, tenseness. **3** By extension of these two meanings, referring to a broad class of disorders the origins of which may be either neural or emotional. The looseness of usage apparent in the above has led to a gradual abandonment of this term in the technical literature. Although it still survives in popular parlance (e.g. *nervous breakdown* for a serious acute emotional disorder and *nervous energy* for an elevated level of drive and activity), the technical meanings once associated with it are now for the most part captured by one or another synonym – with the obvious exceptions of phrases like *central nervous system* and *peripheral nervous system*, where usage appears entrenched.

nervous breakdown   A nontechnical term for a severe emotional disorder. See NERVOUS.

nervous habit   Nontechnical term for an oft-repeated set of movements (e.g. nail-biting, finger-tapping, facial and bodily mannerisms) that occur when a person is under tension.

nervous impulse   NEURAL IMPULSE.

nervous system   Collectively, the full system of structures and organs composed of neural tissue. Depending on the focus, various schemes exist for dividing up the nervous system. The most common anatomical division is into the *central nervous system* (brain and spinal cord) and the *peripheral nervous system* (the rest). Other taxonomies focus on function and the division into the *somatic nervous system* and *autonomic nervous* *system*, with the former subserving voluntary, conscious sensory and motor functions and the latter the visceral, automatic and nonvolitional.

nested 1 In experimental design, characterizing factors that are included within other, more inclusive factors. In a study comparing the efficiency of several organizations, the payroll departments would be a 'nested factor' since each is found within the larger organization. **2** In linguistics, descriptive of a phrase contained within another phrase. In the sentence 'James, the fellow who won the contest, was sitting in his new car', 'the fellow who won the contest' is a nested clause.

network Loosely, any system of interactions between elements, where 'elements' can be almost anything. This definition is not particularly helpful but it is accurate. The difficulty is that the term is used promiscuously. A collection of interacting individuals forms a *social network*, coordinated systems of neural pathways form *neural networks*, the various internal factors that characterize an individual's psychological state comprise his or her *mental network*. Use with care.

network models 1 A class of models of SEMANTIC *MEMORY based on the assumption that the representations in memory are stored in a complex network of interrelations and associations. The links between concepts are represented by operations, so that a concept like *apple* would be linked to the concept *round* by a link labelled *is*. Compare with SET-THEORETICAL MODEL. **2** A class of models of learning and memory based on the principles of modern CONNECTIONISM (2). Note that many of the models here are designed to mimic various aspects of the central nervous system and hence are often referred to as *neural network models*.

neural Pertaining to nerves and neurons. See NERVE (2) for comments on the use of this term and its several approximate synonyms.

neural adhesion protein A protein that helps guide the paths of developing neurons during gestation. Its functions are disrupted by alcohol, which is now thought to be a key factor in producing many of the features of FOETAL ALCOHOL SYNDROME.

neural arc Generally, any network or path of afferent, interneural and efferent neurons that forms a functional unit from a receptor through the central nervous system interconnections to an effector.

neural communication Loosely and generally, communication that involves neural mechanisms. It may be within an individual neuron where changes in neural activity take place internally (see ACTION POTENTIAL), or between neurons, where the communication is across a SYNAPSE.

neural conduction The transmission of neural excitation along a nerve fibre (see ACTION POTENTIAL) or between two neurons (see SYNAPTIC TRANSMISSION).

neural crest A band of cells arranged longitudinally along the NEURAL TUBE of a vertebrate embryo that gives rise to the cells that form the cranial, spinal and autonomic ganglia.

neural discharge The firing of an individual neuron, the propagation of a neural impulse down its length and onto either an effector or another neuron. See ACTION POTENTIAL.

neural facilitation FACILITATION, NEURAL.

neural fold One of two longitudinal elevations of the embryonic NEURAL PLATE, which, in vertebrates, unite to form the *neural tube*.

neuralgia Any sharp, relatively severe pain felt along the pathway of a nerve.

neural groove The groove along the *neural plate* in the vertebrate embryo that eventually forms the *neural tube*.

neural imaging A general term used for any IMAGING technique whereby neural tissue is scanned.

neural impulse IMPULSE (4).

neural induction INDUCTION (2).

neural integration The processes by which both excitatory and inhibitory POSTSYNAPTIC POTENTIALS interact to control the firing of neurons.

neural network models NETWORK MODELS (2), CONNECTIONISM (2).

neural plate The thickened layer of ectodermal cells in the vertebrate embryo from which the central nervous system develops.

neural process 1 Anatomically, any filament of a neuron, i.e. an axon, dendrite, terminal branch or collateral fibre. **2** Loosely, any functional change in nerve tissue.

neural pruning PRUNING.

neural quantal hypothesis QUANTAL HYPOTHESIS.

neural reverberation REVERBERATING CIRCUIT.

neural tube The tube formed by the fusing of the NEURAL FOLDS in the vertebrate embryo from which the central nervous system develops.

neural-tube defects A general term for those congenital defects involving a failure of the NEURAL TUBE to close properly during the early stages of gestation. Failure to close at the top results in *anencephaly* (no or at best a rudimentary brain), which is always fatal; failure to close along the spine results in *spina bifida*, which can have either a reasonably hopeful or a very poor prognosis depending on location and other characteristics of the opening.

neurasthenia A psychiatric diagnostic category with a long and confusing history. When in favour it is regarded as a SOMATO-FORM DISORDER characterized by mental and physical fatigue, weakness after performing ordinary chores that normally would not require unusual effort, and a failure to recover with normal periods of rest or relaxation. The exhaustion is often accompanied by headaches, dizziness, sleep disturbances, irritability and intestinal distress.

neuraxis The spinal cord and brain represented as a line of reference along the vertical axis of the body. In anatomy, directions within the nervous system are given relative to the neuraxis.

neurilemma The thin membraneous covering of the MYELIN SHEATH of the axons of peripheral neurons. Neurilemma is made up of SCHWANN CELLS. var., *neurolemma*.

neurin A protein that coats the membrane of presynaptic vesicles.

neuritic plaques Extracellular accumulations found, along with *neurofibrillary tangles*,

in the brains of virtually all Alzheimer's patients and many cases with Down syndrome.

neuritis Inflammation of a nerve, usually associated with a degenerative process.

neur(o)- A combining form meaning *relating to a nerve, neuron, nerve tissue*, etc.

neuroanatomy The study of the structures and functions of the nervous system.

neurobabble PSYCHOBABBLE about things neurological and neurocognitive.

neurobiotaxis The growth of dendrites and the shifts in orientation of nerve cell bodies during development toward the area where their primary impulses are initiated.

neuroblast An embryonic cell from the NEURAL TUBE that gives rise to a neuron.

neuroclinical Referring to approaches to clinical psychology that emphasize the neurological factors that underlie psychopathological disorders. With advances in IMAGING (TECHNIQUE) and the development of sophisticated neuropsychological assessment and diagnostic procedures, this approach is playing an increasingly larger role.

neurocognition See COGNITIVE NEURO-SCIENCE.

neurocyte A nerve cell; see NEURON.

neuroeconomics An interdisciplinary science based on the use of various techniques (e.g. FMRI) to identify the neural structures that underlie economic decision-making and choice.

neuroeffector junction A junction between an efferent neuron and an effector, such as a smooth muscle or a gland.

neuroendocrinology The study of the interactions between the nervous system (considered broadly) and the endocrine system.

neurofibrillary tangles Fine fibrillary material that is found in virtually all cases of ALZHEIMER'S DISEASE.

neurogenesis 1 Growth and development *of* nerve tissue. In this sense, the term can refer to either the processes involved in the first laying down of neural tissue during gestation and the early phases of development as well as to the growth of new neurons in the mature brain. The latter process was, until recently, thought not to occur and in many texts only the first process will be the intended meaning. **2** Growth and development of structures originating *from* nerve tissue.

neuroglia GLIA.

neurogram Synonym of *engram*.

neurohormone Any of several substances that are chemically equivalent to NEUROTRANSMITTERS but classified as HORMONES because they are secreted into the blood rather than onto other neurons.

neurohumour NEUROTRANSMITTER.

neurohypophysis PITUITARY GLAND.

neuroimagery/neuroimaging See SCAN (1, 2, 3) and IMAGING (TECHNIQUE).

neuroleptic induced A cover term for any medication-induced movement disorder that results as a side effect of one of the NEUROLEPTICS. Included are neuroleptically DRUG-INDUCED PARKINSONISM, some forms of *dystonia* and *akathisia*, and TARDIVE DYSKINESIA. See also ANTIPSYCHOTIC DRUGS.

neuroleptics An occasional synonym for the ANTIPSYCHOTIC DRUGS. The term tends to be used only for those dopamine agonist drugs that have their effect through the pathways of the EXTRAPYRAMIDAL SYSTEM.

neurolinguistic programming A technique developed to influence and modify an individual's behaviours and beliefs. It is based on assumed (but largely undocumented) sets of relations between linguistic forms, eye and body position and movement, and memory. It is used primarily as a form of therapy, and its proponents also promote its use in advertising, management and education. There is virtually no reliable evidence of effectiveness.

neurolinguistics A hybrid discipline made up of contributions from psycholinguistics and neurology. The primary focus is on the neurological brain functions and processes that underlie language. It is often included as one of the several disciplines in COGNITIVE SCIENCE. Distinguish from NEUROLINGUISTIC PROGRAMMING.

neurological correlation CORRELATION, NEUROLOGICAL.

neurological soft sign SOFT (NEUROLOGICAL) SIGN.

neuromodulators Chemical substances that function as NEUROTRANSMITTERS but, rather than being restricted to the synaptic cleft, are dispersed widely, modulating the action of many neurons in a particular area.

neuromuscular junction A junction between a somatic motor neuron and a skeletal muscle fibre. Also called MYONEURAL JUNCTION.

neuron A nerve cell, the basic structural and functional unit of the nervous system. Although found in a wide variety of shapes and sizes and subserving a vast array of functions, all neurons consist of a cell body or soma, which contains the nucleus, and its neural processes, an axon and one or more dendrites. var., *neurone*.

neuronal Of or pertaining to a NEURON. See also NERVE (2).

neurontin GABAPENTIN.

neuropathic Variously used in the past as characterizing either organic or functional nervous disabilities. Today the term is generally restricted to the organic, with either *psychogenic* or *neurotic* being the terms used for functional disorders; however, see NEUROSIS for comments on the usage of the latter and related terms.

neuropathology The study of diseases and disorders of the nervous system. Distinguish from NEUROPATHY.

neuropathy Loosely, any disease of the nervous system, most commonly, disorders of the peripheral nerves. Distinguish from NEUROPATHOLOGY.

neuropeptide Any of a large (over a hundred have been identified) group of peptides that function as NEUROTRANSMITTERS.

neuropeptide Y A *peptide* that functions as a *neurotransmitter* and plays a role in feeding. Fasting causes its secretion into the lateral *hypothalamus*; eating diminishes its secretion. If introduced artificially it stimulates ravenous eating. It has also been implicated in control over *circadian rhythms*.

neuroplasticity A general term relating to the capacity of the brain to undergo physical and morphological change. It is used to cover a variety of situations, including cases where functions lost because of brain damage are taken over by other neural tissue and circumstances where the growth of new neurons (NEUROGENESIS) enables new processes to be acquired.

neuropsychiatry A branch of medicine that deals with the relationship between neural processes and psychiatric disorders.

neuropsychological assessment A broad assessment based on evaluations of cognitive, emotional and behavioural functions designed to reveal any neurological problems that may underlie observed compromised abilities.

neuropsychological test A cover term for a wide variety of tests that are designed to explore, evaluate and diagnose disorders due to particular kinds of neurological dysfunctions. There are literally hundreds of such tests; for a few of the more commonly used see WISCONSIN CARD SORTING TEST, COMPLEX FIGURE TESTS and STROOP TEST.

neuropsychology An approach to psychology that examines the interrelationships between neurological functions and the cognitive, emotional and behavioural actions of organisms. It is concerned with both normal, adaptive functioning and the various disorders that can be traced back to neurological dysfunctions. While the term emphasizes the 'neuro' elements, study of the biological and physiological factors that underlie neural mechanisms makes up an important part of the field.

neurosciences Loosely, all those scientific approaches that are founded on neurological studies.

neurosecretory cell A neuron that secretes hormones or similar substances into the extracellular fluid.

neurosis 1 (obs.) A disease of the nerves. **2** A personality or mental disturbance *not* due to any known neurological or organic dysfunction, i.e. a *psychoneurosis*. This meaning, dominant since Freud, has been used: (a) *descriptively*, to denote an identifiable symptom (or group of related symptoms) that, while distressing and painful, is (are) relatively benign in that reality testing is intact and by and large social norms are adhered to, and (b) *aetiologically*, to indicate a causal role played by unconscious conflicts that evoke anxiety and lead to the use of defence mechanisms that ultimately produce the observed symptoms.

Within this conceptual framework a number of specific neuroses have been identified and labelled, beginning with Freud's original four subtypes of *anxiety, phobic, obsessive compulsive* and *hysterical* and expanding to include *depressive, depersonalized, character, narcissistic, organ*, etc. The vagueness of these various syndromes, the failure to find features that reliably characterize each and serve to distinguish it from others, and the inherent ambiguity produced by the use of the core term for both a description and an aetiological process have all conspired to rob the term of any coherent (or even consensual) meaning.

Recent years have seen two terminological adjustments: (a) The use of the phrase *neurotic disorder* as a generic cover term for any enduring mental disorder that is distressing, recognized by the individual as unacceptable and alien, but in which contact with reality is maintained and there is no demonstrable organic disorder. *Neurotic disorder* thus fulfils the *descriptive* role of neurosis but is neutral with regard to aetiological factors. This lexical device is the one adopted in the INTERNATIONAL CLASSIFICATION OF DISEASES.

(b) The elimination of the term as denoting a psychiatrically identifiable diagnosis, accompanied by a reassignment of the various previously recognized neuroses to other diagnostic classifications. This is the resolution of the terminological problem adopted by the DIAGNOSTIC AND STATISTICAL MANUAL of the American Psychiatric Association, in which various specialized terms are introduced for each previously recognized neurotic disorder.

A final note: the term *neurosis* itself is surely not about to expire any time soon. It is deeply entrenched in both the technical literature and the common language. The principle of 'resting semantic inertia' suggests that it will continue to be used technically (especially by those with psychoanalytic training) to mark what many believe to be an aetiological process and popularly to refer to, in Ernst Becker's lovely phrase, 'a miscarriage of clumsy lies about reality'. Specialized forms are listed by defining term. See also NEUROTIC et seq.

neurotendinal spindle GOLGI TENDON ORGAN.

neurotic 1 adj. Pertaining to or characterizing specific behaviours that are actually displayed by a person diagnosed as having a neurosis. **2** adj. Characterizing, loosely, those types of behaviour typical of or resembling those of a neurosis. **3** n. A person displaying such behaviour. See the discussion under NEUROSIS for comments on contemporary usage.

neurotic anxiety ANXIETY, NEUROTIC.

neurotic breakthrough NEUROTIC •DEFENCE.

neurotic character 1 Specifically, in Adler's theory, the collection of qualities and traits that one uses as a defence against feelings of inferiority and which dispose one to develop overt manifestations of neurosis. **2** More generally, an individual with a personality that predisposes him or her to neurosis. **3** Loosely, a label for one diagnosed as having a neurosis.

neurotic claim K. Horney's term for an inappropriate sense of one's superiority such that one feels that others should rightfully fulfil all one's wants and needs.

neurotic compliance COMPLIANT CHARACTER.

neurotic defence DEFENCE, NEUROTIC.

neurotic depression DEPRESSION, NEUROTIC.

neurotic disorder NEUROSIS.

neurotic fiction In Adler's theory, a GUIDING •FICTION that is so inappropriate and divorced from reality that it can never be achieved, leaving the person affected hopelessly in pursuit of selfish, unattainable goals.

neurotic inventory Any questionnaire for examining tendencies toward neuroticism.

neuroticism 1 The state of being neurotic, of having been diagnosed as neurotic. **2** The underlying abstract core that is the aetiological basis for a neurosis. **3** In the FIVE FACTOR THEORY, the broad personality disposition that characterizes the degree to which one is chronically emotionally unstable and

prone to anxiety and psychological distress. See the discussion under NEUROSIS for caveats concerning usage here, especially 2.

Neuroticism, Extraversion and Openness Personality Inventory-Revised (NEO-PI-R) An inventory devised to assess individual personality differences along the dimensions specified by the FIVE FACTOR MODEL. The revision, published in 1992, is based on a total of 240 statements which respondents rate on a LIKERT SCALE from 'strongly agree' to 'strongly disagree'. In addition to the primary factors, the test is designed to assess various subdomains hypothesized to make up each factor. There are two formats, one based on self-report ('Form S') and one in which an adult informant can rate another person ('Form R').

neurotic needs K. Horney's term for irrational solutions to the problems of BASIC ANXIETY. According to her theory, people develop a variety of strategies for dealing with this anxiety, many of which eventually become well-learned characteristics of their personality. They can lead, however, to neuroses because the needs that underlie these strategies are not always rational or appropriate. In the full theory, Horney described ten such needs, including a need for power, a need for prestige, a need for affection, a need to exploit others, etc.

neurotic pride PRIDE, NEUROTIC.

neurotic process In Horney's theory, the core inner conflict between one's idealized self and one's real self.

neurotic solution In Karen Horney's theory, any resolution of a conflict that is based on excluding the conflict from awareness. This may be accomplished by a variety of devices such as distortion, neutralization, minimalization or avoidance, but all are presumed to function by relieving the tension and anxiety produced by the conflict. See also AUXILIARY SOLUTION, COMPREHENSIVE SOLUTION and MAJOR SOLUTION, the three types of these neurotic solutions noted by Horney.

neurotic trend K. Horney's term for a pattern of behavioural tendencies focused primarily on security and the need to decrease basic anxiety. She hypothesized that such a basic trend was almost always acquired in childhood and was manifested as an AGGRESSIVE, a COMPLIANT or a DETACHED CHARACTER.

neurot(o)- Combining form meaning *neurotic*.

neurotoxin Literally *nerve poison*. Any substance that destroys the cell bodies of neurons.

neurotransmitter Any of the many substances that function as the vehicles of communication across the synaptic gap between the terminal buttons of one neuron and the membrane of the receiving cell on the other side. The effect of a neurotransmitter is to produce a brief alteration in the postsynaptic membrane of the receiving cell, either depolarization or hyperpolarization (see here the discussion under POSTSYNAPTIC POTENTIAL). There are many different neurotransmitters of which the actions and locations in the nervous system have been identified, e.g. ACETYLCHOLINE, DOPAMINE, SEROTONIN. Note that some substances that are listed as neurotransmitters by virtue of their production within neurons are chemically identical to substances that also function as HORMONES (e.g. *norepinephrine* and the *endorphins*). See NEUROHORMONES. Also called *neurohumour*, *transmitter substance*.

neurovegetative system Occasional term for the AUTONOMIC NERVOUS SYSTEM, specifically the parasympathetic division.

neutral Indifferent; characterizing values that are not categorized as reflecting properties of specific classes; lying at or arbitrarily close to the zero point on some dimension.

neutral colour Any achromatic colour, one along the black–white continuum.

neutral grey A grey that lies at the midpoint of the continuum of brightness, one that is intermediate between black and white.

neutralization 1 In psychoanalysis, the process by which the sexual and aggressive impulses of infancy are softened (i.e. neutralized) and lose their primitive, infantile quality. **2** More loosely, any psychological defence that lessens the emotional impact of one's actions. It often emerges as a kind of strained rationalization for inappropriate behaviour.

neutral stimulus STIMULUS, NEUTRAL.

Nevo syndrome A genetic disorder marked by curvature of the spine, hypotonia and increased growth that begins in the foetal period. Occasionally misdiagnosed as *Sotos syndrome* because of the rapid early growth typical of both disorders, it is caused by a different genetic mutation.

nevus NAEVUS.

new age therapies See INNOVATIVE THERAPIES.

newborn In humans, by convention, an infant under the age of one month. The term is, however, used loosely, and the upper age limit depends on the species under consideration and the author's preferences.

New Look A label attached to an approach to the study of perception that is today not so new (having been most influential in the 1940s and 1950s). It emphasized the roles of emotion and motivation in perception and produced much interesting work on problems like *perceptual vigilance* and *perceptual defence*.

Newman–Keuls test One of the POST HOC TESTS.

nialamide An ANTIDEPRESSANT DRUG of the monoamine oxidase inhibitor class.

niche picking Selecting a comfortable position within a group or organization. The term was introduced as a pun but, because it identifies nicely an important social behaviour, it quickly became part of the technical literature.

nicotine An alkaloid found in several members of the nightshade family of plants, most notably tobacco. A stimulant, it acts on nicotinic acetylcholine receptors causing an increase in EPINEPHERINE which, in turn, produces increases in respiration, heart rate, blood pressure and glucose levels. In pure form it is highly toxic and causes dizziness, gastric distress and tremors and in large doses death by cardiac arrest and paralysis of respiratory muscles. In low doses such as those from a cigarette, it activates NICOTINIC RECEPTORS producing a wide variety of effects including feelings of calm and an increase in alertness, psychoactive properties that are due largely to increases in DOPAMINE levels in the reward pathways of the brain. It is highly addictive and produces a severe DRUG *DEPENDENCE that is as difficult to break as that on opiates (see NICOTINIC RECEPTORS).

nicotine dependence See NICOTINE, NICOTINE WITHDRAWAL, DRUG *DEPENDENCE.

nicotine withdrawal A syndrome that results from abrupt cessation of use of nicotine-containing substances. It is marked by a craving for nicotine, irritability, feelings of frustration, anxiety, restlessness and increased appetite with occasional weight gain. The symptoms begin within a few hours of cessation and may continue for days, weeks or, in some cases, months. Nicotine withdrawal is regarded by many as an ORGANIC MENTAL DISORDER, and the term *nicotine-induced organic mental disorder* is used synonymously. Also called, in some older texts, *tobacco withdrawal*.

nicotinic receptor A type of acetylcholine receptor that is stimulated by nicotine and blocked by curare. Nicotine receptors are found on skeletal muscles and to some extent in the *central nervous system*. See also MUSCARINIC RECEPTOR.

nictitating membrane A tough, inner eyelid found in many birds, fish and mammals that, when the eye is threatened, moves laterally from the nasal to the temporal side. It is used in studies of the neural basis of conditioning.

night blindness NYCTALOPIA.

night-eating syndrome A syndrome marked by insomnia accompanied by excessive night-time eating during periods of wakefulness. Often disrupted circadian rhythms, erratic daytime eating patterns and high levels of stress are present, although it is not clear what is cause and what is effect. Rare in the general population, up to 20% of obese individuals show some or all of the features.

nightmare Generally, any frightening or anxiety-producing dream. The typical nightmare occurs, like other dreams, during *REM sleep* and is contrasted with SLEEP TERROR DISORDER, which occurs during *NREM sleep*.

nightmare disorder DREAM ANXIETY DISORDER.

night vision SCOTOPIC VISION.

nigro striatal bundle An axon bundle originating in the substantia nigra of the pons and terminating in the caudate nucleus and putamen. It is a dopaminergic pathway and plays an important role in voluntary movement.

nihilistic delusion DELUSION, NIHILISTIC.

nimiety An unpleasant feeling of fullness after eating. It is an unwelcome but common side effect of those who have undergone stomach surgery to lose weight.

nirvana 1 Roughly, the Buddhist notion of liberation from the cycle of death and rebirth. Although there are variations on this theme in the several Buddhist positions, all share the notion that the state is primarily defined as freedom from worldly concerns, particularly concerns of self, self-interest and desire. Such freedom, in principle, allows for the achievement of true wisdom and final liberation. Within some psychoanalytic approaches, total loss of individuality, the so-called *nirvana principle*, is argued to represent the manifestation of Freud's death instinct or Thanatos. **2** In Hinduism, a state of bliss and liberation from individual consciousness. To achieve nirvana in this sense is to have overcome the struggle of birth, death and rebirth and to move beyond the bonds of the real world. **3** In common parlance, any state or place of bliss and peace. Many recent INNOVATIVE THERAPIES promise this state through meditation and work, a goal that cheapens the deeper philosophical meanings carried by the first two.

Nissl bodies Granular bodies found in the cytoplasm of the cell bodies of neurons and glia. Because they are readily stained by various dyes, the Nissl substances make it possible to examine nuclear tissue in the nervous system separately from the fibre bundles, which, made up of axons that do not contain Nissl bodies, are not affected by dyes.

nit A measure of luminance of a surface equal to LUX times 1,000. *Nit* (symbol: nt) is a relatively new term in photometry introduced to replace the *metre-candle* or *foot-candle*. Multiplying it by 0.292 gives *foot-lamberts*.

nitrazepam A long-lasting BENZODIAZEPINE once used as a sleeping drug. Because of its long half-life (nearly 24 hours), it tends to accumulate in the blood stream and is rarely used any more.

nitric oxide A soluble gas that functions as a messenger between neurons. It is found in muscles in the walls of the intestines, in erectile tissue, and in blood vessels in the brain where it is suspected of playing a role in learning. It is produced in many places in a neuron and, unlike other neurotransmitters, is released upon production. Do not confuse with NITROUS OXIDE.

nitrous oxide A gas with mild analgesic properties often used in dental procedures. It also produces a mild sense of elation and giddiness and is colloquially known as *laughing gas*. Distinguish from NITRIC OXIDE.

nm Abbreviation for NANOMETER.

NMDA Short for N-methyl-D-aspartate. See NMDA RECEPTOR.

NMDA receptor A specialized ionotropic GLUTAMATE RECEPTOR with at least six distinct binding sites, four of them on the surface and two within the cell and, consequently, a variety of actions. The NMDA receptor is clearly important although its full functions are not yet understood. One of the sites is, of course, a glutamate receptor. Others allow sodium and calcium ions to enter the cell; one appears to bind with alcohol and another is sensitive to the hallucinogen PCP. Recent research suggests that the NMDA receptor plays a role in working memory and consciousness and some have theorized that dysfunctions may contribute to the development of schizophrenia.

nocebo A 'negative' PLACEBO. Placebo effects were originally assumed to always be positive; they are not. This term was introduced for pharmacologically neutral compounds that participants in a study had aversive or unpleasant reactions to.

nociceptive Pertaining to *pain* or to harmful although not necessarily painful stimuli. Protective reflexes are sometimes referred to as *nociceptive*.

nociceptor Neural fibres that detect noxious stimulation and produce the experience of PAIN. There are at least three known types, a

group of FREE NERVE ENDINGS that are *mechanoreceptors* and respond to extremes of pressure, stretching or pinching, a second group that react to high levels of heat, many acidic compounds and, interestingly, CAPSAICIN and a third type of neuron that responds to diminished blood supply.

noctambulation Lit., walking at night; sleepwalking; SOMNAMBULISM (preferred).

nocturnal emission Ejaculation in males during sleep; usually during a dream.

nocturnal myoclonus A condition characterized by sharp muscular twitches that occur during sleep. It is regarded as an ORGANIC *SLEEP DISORDER, although in mild cases the individual with the disorder is oblivious to it; it only bothers his or her bedmate.

nodal points Two points in an optical system located along the axis of a lens such that a ray of light sent through one produces a parallel emergent ray through the other.

node 1 In anatomy, a knob, a swelling, a protuberance; any small rounded organ or structure. **2** By extension, and metaphorically, a point in a network upon which a number of operations impinge. Set NETWORK MODELS for an example of this usage. **3** The zero amplitude point in a wave.

nodes of Ranvier RANVIER, NODES OF.

noesis 1 In philosophy, a mental event grasped by pure intellect. **2** In psychology, the general functioning of the intellect; cognition. adj., *noetic*.

noetic memory MEMORY, NOETIC.

noetic science *Noetic* has been bandied about for some time as a loose synonym of *consciousness*, although the Greek roots are closer to *intellect, reason* or even *mind*. The appending of *science* was meant to denote a broader approach to the study of consciousness and conscious experience. Unfortunately, 'new age' theorists have commandeered the term and current use carries unhappy mystical connotations involving transcendent or 'cosmic' consciousness.

no-go trial A TRIAL (2) in which the subject is required to inhibit a response to a stimulus. For example, suppose subjects are asked to press a button as soon as a face appears, provided the person does not have red hair – any time a redhead showed up, it would be a no-go trial.

noise 1 Any stimulus that is aperiodic, unstructured and patternless. Although the usual reference here is to auditory stimuli (e.g. WHITE* NOISE), references to *visual noise* are not uncommon. **2** An unwanted, interfering stimulus. The denotations of meaning 2 may be very different from those of meaning 1. For example, a Beethoven symphony could never qualify for 1 but it could very well be noise in sense 2 if it were to interfere with some other ongoing task. On the other hand, real, auditory noise in sense 1 may not be considered noise in sense 2 if, for example, it is used as a background sound that masks other stimuli and assists one's ability to concentrate on some other task. **3** As derived from information theory, any contaminant that clutters up the communication of a message or increases the variability or the error rate in some ongoing process. This general sense has been extended beyond the formal confines of information theory, and one often sees references to 'noisy data' or 'noisy procedures', phrases which imply that various uncontrolled factors have contaminated some process or operation.

noise, frozen A segment of WHITE* NOISE that has been recorded and is repeated over and over. This procedure reduces the variability inherent in standard white noise and ensures that each presentation is equivalent to every other.

noise, pink In acoustics, any NOISE (1) in which the distribution of frequencies is not uniform. Often called *coloured noise*; compare with WHITE* NOISE.

noise, white An auditory stimulus that has all frequencies represented in random fluctuation and sounds like an ongoing 'shhh'. Note that the term derives from the analogy with white light, in which all wavelengths are present. White noise is the most frequently used NOISE (1) in experimental work when a controlled background sound is needed; see here SIGNAL-TO-NOISE RATIO. Compare with PINK *NOISE.

nomadism A tendency to change residences or, by extension, occupations frequently. The term is applied only to pathological cases.

nominal 1 As derived from Latin, pertaining to names or naming; classifying, designating. The connotation here is that of distinguishing one thing from another by their names or designations and not by any factual or empirical properties they may have. **2** By extension, characterizing that which is of limited or only superficial importance.

nominal aphasia ANOMIC APHASIA.

nominal definition DEFINITIONS.

nominalism 1 A philosophical point of view that maintains that abstract ideas or concepts have no objective reality and are therefore not legitimate foci for scientific investigation. Nominalists argue that reality consists solely of objective particulars and that notions like *mind*, *society*, *personality* and so forth are without scientific value. An extreme form of EMPIRICISM. Compare with POSITIVISM and OPERATIONALISM; contrast with REALISM (1). **2** A tendency to accept the naming of something as providing evidence for its reality. Those who espouse 1 eschew 2.

nominal scale SCALE, NOMINAL.

nominal weight WEIGHT (2).

nominating technique A sociometric technique for the exploration of the structure of a group in which each member nominates the person who best satisfies some criterion, e.g. best liked, easiest to work with.

nomological Pertaining to general laws of nature; NOMOTHETIC.

nomothetic From the Greek, meaning relating to or dealing with the *abstract*, the *universal* or the *general*. Any scientific or philosophical system so oriented is called a nomothetic approach. Contrast with IDIO-GRAPHIC. Also called *nomological*.

non- A prefix meaning *not, without*. Generally, the connotation is negative in the sense of the absence of the thing referenced rather than of the opposite or reverse of it. Some specialized terms are given below; the meaning of most others is obvious from the root word.

nonadditive Quite literally, pertaining to objects, variables, scores, etc. that cannot be added together without somehow disrupting the nature of the things so summed. There are at least three important cases of nonadditivity and the reasons for having this property are different in each instance. (a) When variables or objects are measured on a NOMINAL *SCALE they cannot be added because of the lack of quantification in nominal scales; e.g. it makes no sense to add the numbers on football players' uniforms. (b) When objects are reflective of underlying structures that are unrelated they are nonadditive; e.g. one wouldn't add a person's IQ and weight as the resulting number would have no meaning. (c) When a structured configuration, a GESTALT, is under consideration, the elements that comprise it are nonadditive in the sense that each is so intimately related to the whole that they cannot be legitimately distinguished as separate summable entities. Note that case (c) designates the antithesis of (b): in (c) the elements are too closely related to be separately summed, in (b) they are too disparate to be sensibly summed.

nonalcoholic Korsakoff psychosis An AMNESTIC SYNDROME of which alcoholism is not the cause. The term is not recommended since KORSAKOFF'S SYNDROME is specifically associated with long-term alcohol abuse.

nonbarbiturate sedatives SEDATIVES.

non compos mentis Latin for *not of sound mind.*

nonconformity Loosely, a tendency to believe, behave or think in ways that are distinctly different from the standards of one's community or society. The term can be used as a synonym of ANTICONFORMITY (where the decisions are deliberate) or in cases where people are simply ignorant of normative standards. See CONFORMITY for more detail.

nonconscious Not conscious. Used to refer to (a) that which is inanimate and therefore lacking consciousness, and (b) those components of mental functioning in sentient beings that are not part of awareness. In this latter sense the term is properly synonymous with IMPLICIT and COVERT. It is also used as a synonym of UNCONSCIOUS in sense 2a and 2b, but should be distinguished from *unconscious* in senses 3a and 3b.

noncontingent reinforcement REINFORCEMENT, NONCONTINGENT.

nondeclarative memory Occasional synonym of PROCEDURAL MEMORY.

nondecremental conduction A phrase used to characterize the conduction of a neural impulse down an axon which occurs in an all-or-none fashion.

nondetermination, coefficient of COEFFICIENT OF *DETERMINATION.

nondirective therapy A cover term for any therapy in which specific counselling, advice or direction on the part of the therapist is kept to a bare minimum. See CLIENT-CENTRED THERAPY for more discussion. Compare with DIRECTIVE THERAPY.

nondisjunction In genetics, the failure of a pair of chromosomes to separate during meiosis.

nondominant Not dominant; but see the discussion under DOMINANT for specifics on usage.

nonexperimental method An umbrella term for any research method that does not involve the systematic manipulation of independent variables. Naturalistic observation and correlational methods are the most common examples.

nonfalsifiable Characterizing a statement or claim that cannot be subjected to a proper empirical test because no evidence can be presented that would show it to be false. In Karl Popper's FALSIFICATIONISM, such propositions cannot be accepted as scientifically legitimate. Note that the truth or falsity of the statement is not relevant, only the question of whether some outcome from some experiment or observation *could* show it to be false. var., *unfalsifiable.*

nonfluent aphasia BROCA'S *APHASIA.

nonintermittent reinforcement schedule Either *continuous reinforcement* or *extinction.* See SCHEDULES OF *REINFORCEMENT for details.

noninvasive 1 Characterizing devices or procedures that do not invade the body in any direct manner. **2** Pertaining to tumours or other growths that are local and do not spread.

nonlegitimate authority AUTHORITY, NON-LEGITIMATE.

nonlinear Characterizing any curvilinear function, one that cannot be represented by a straight line.

nonlinear correlation CURVILINEAR *CORRELATION.

nonlinear regression CURVILINEAR *REGRESSION.

nonliterate Basically an anthropological term for any culture the spoken language of which does not have a written form. Note, incidentally, that the majority of the world's known languages do not have written forms. Distinguish from ILLITERATE.

nonmatching to sample A variation on the MATCHING TO SAMPLE procedure in which the subject must select the alternative that fails to match the target.

nonmetric 1 Generally, referring to that which is not measured (but not necessarily not measurable) in a quantitative manner. **2** More specifically, characterizing measurement when the elements measured fall on an ORDINAL *SCALE. See METHODS OF *SCALING.

nonmetric scaling METHODS OF *SCALING (esp. 3).

nonnutritive sucking procedures Any of several procedures for assessing an infant's attentional and perceptual processes using a pacifier nipple as the basic apparatus. The infant's rate of sucking is recorded as various stimuli are presented, and inferences about perceptual and cognitive processes are drawn from the observed changes in sucking rate.

nonoperatory thought An occasional synonym of PREOPERATORY THOUGHT.

nonparametric statistics A class of statistical procedures for determining relations between variables which can be used without making assumptions about particular parameters of distributions. Note that although these nonparametric statistical tests are often called *distribution-free* they are not *assumption-free*, for each particular procedure is dependent on certain criteria. Compare with PARAMETRIC STATISTICS and PARAMETER.

nonpreferred Not preferred; see DOMINANT for specifics on usage.

nonprobability sampling SAMPLING, NON-PROBABILITY.

nonrational This term is used quite literally to refer to thinking, believing, decision-making, etc. when the notions of reason and logic are simply not applicable. However, it should be distinguished from IRRATIONAL, which implies that logic and reason are violated and not merely irrelevant. Also called *arational*.

nonregulatory drive DRIVE, NONREGULATORY.

non-REM sleep NREM SLEEP.

nonreversal shift REVERSAL *LEARNING.

nonsense syllable Any pronounceable but nonsensical combination of consonant–vowel–consonant with the restriction that the two consonants be different, e.g. DAX, TUZ. Invented by H. von Ebbinghaus in the 1880s to study memory (relatively) unencumbered by meaningfulness, it has enjoyed over a century of use in experimental psychology. Also called *CVC trigram*.

non sequitur Latin for *it does not follow*. The term is generally reserved for a conclusion that does not even remotely give an appearance of being a valid argument and not for one drawn invalidly simply because of fallacious reasoning. Also used for remarks or comments made that seem to have no semantic or referential relationship to previous features of the conversation.

nonsocial 1 Descriptive of one who remains outside of, or is relatively indifferent to, social groups or gatherings. **2** Pertaining to phenomena that are not social, that do not pertain to groups of individuals or to the effects of such groups. Note that ASOCIAL (1) is an acceptable synonym but ANTISOCIAL is not.

nonsomniac A normal individual who needs little sleep, in some cases as few as one or two hours a night. Differentiate from one who suffers from INSOMNIA, which is a SLEEP DISORDER.

nonspecific 1 Lit., not specific; general. This meaning is straightforward. **2** Characterizing effects or phenomena that cannot be attributed to identifiable causes or factors. This meaning really functions as a gentle euphemism for ignorance; it is used when one simply does not know the origins of some disorder, the causes of some disease, or the basis for the effects that a drug may have on a given individual, etc.

nonspecific immune reactions IMMUNE REACTIONS, NONSPECIFIC.

nonstriate (visual) cortex Loosely, cortical areas that lie outside of the STRIATE CORTEX. The term is used so that it encompasses slightly more cortex than referenced in PRE-STRIATE CORTEX and includes areas in the parietal and temporal lobes that process visuospatial information and play a role in object recognition.

nonverbal This term is almost always used in combined form to express those characteristics of a task, a process or a situation that exclude the specifically linguistic. See the following entries for examples.

nonverbal communication A general term covering any and all aspects of communication that are expressed without the use of the overt, spoken language. Gestures, body positions, facial expressions, contextual factors, presuppositions and the like all fall within the realm of the components of a communication system which transmits information without the use of that which is specifically linguistic. See also KINESIOLOGY, PARALINGUISTICS, PROXEMICS.

nonverbal intelligence Intelligence that is manifested through performance on tasks that require minimal use of verbal materials. Note that the existence of *verbal* and *nonverbal* intelligence tests does not necessarily imply that there are two different kinds of intelligence. The nonverbal (or *performance*) tests were devised to evaluate intelligence in persons who may, for any number of reasons, have problems with verbal materials, e.g. those tested in their second language, those who speak various dialects, the very young, the mentally retarded, those with sensory deficits. See here PERFORMANCE TESTS.

nonverbal learning disorder(s) Any learning disability that is manifested by deficits in nonverbal domains such as social competencies, visual-spatial skills, motor coordination and emotional intelligence.

nonverbal tests PERFORMANCE TESTS.

nonvoluntary INVOLUNTARY.

nonzero-sum game Any game that is not a ZERO-SUM *GAME.

noology Frankl's term for the study of that which is uniquely human. In Frankl's hierarchy, psychology is encompassed by noology (although most of the rest of us psychologists would reverse this inclusionary clause). It's worth noting, just to understand Frankl's perspective, that he has *theology* encompassing *noology*.

nootropic drugs A category of drugs designed to improve cognitive function by increasing neurotransmitter levels, increasing oxygen to the brain or by promoting nerve growth. The term is used broadly. Sometimes it will refer to compounds with actions claimed to be beneficial to normal individuals seeking a boost in memory or intellectual capacity, sometimes to drugs developed specifically for the treatment of the cognitive decline that accompanies various forms of dementia such as ALZHEIMER'S DIS-EASE. There is great promise in the development of effective nootropics but to date the evidence for them is still weak and the risk of misuse is very high.

noradrenalin NOREPINEPHRINE.

noradrenergic Characterizing neurons and neural fibres and pathways which, when stimulated, release NOREPINEPHRINE. Note that although the preferred term for the neurotransmitter itself is *norepinephrine*, this adjectival form, *noradrenergic*, remains in use. See the discussions under ADRENALIN and ADRENERGIC for the reasons for this pattern of usage.

norepinephrine (NE) A CATECHOLEAMINE that functions as a neurotransmitter. In the central nervous system NE-containing cells are found in the locus coeruleus in the brain stem; in the peripheral nervous system NE is the transmitter in the postganglionic neurons of the sympathetic nervous system.

norm 1 Statistically, a number, value or level (or a range of such numbers, values or levels) that is representative of a group and may be used as a basis for comparison of individual cases. In this sense any of the measures of central tendency (or a range of values around the measure, usually 1 or 2 standard deviations) may be taken as a norm. **2** Somewhat less formally, any pattern of behaviour or performance that is typical or representative of a group or a society. See here SOCIAL NORM. **3** An occasional synonym of STANDARD. This usage is not recommended since it deprives *norm* of the quantitative component explicit in 1 and implicit in 2.

normal 1 Generally, as derived from NORM (1, 2), conforming to that which is characteristic and representative of a group; not deviating markedly from the average or the typical. **2** In statistics, characterizing a distribution of scores that does not deviate markedly from the bell-shaped Gaussian curve. See NORMAL *DISTRIBUTION for details. **3** In biology and medicine, regular, natural; not subjected to special consideration or treatment; occurring naturally and not as a result of disease or experimentation. **4** Free from disease, mental disorder, mental retardation or other psychological dysfunction. That is, *not abnormal*.

Meanings 1 and 2 carry statistical, quantitative connotations and so long as this component of the term is intended there are few problems with usage. Meaning 3 also provides sufficiently clear boundaries to defuse confusion. Meaning 4 is, putting it bluntly, a lexicographer's nightmare. The difficulties in usage stem from the original, well-intentioned attempt to have the term reflect the statistical underpinnings of 1 and 2; that *normal behaviour*, for example, should be that behaviour that reflects the typical patterns that are observed in society. Unfortunately, many who use the term allow their theories of behaviour or their own beliefs about the 'quality of life' to determine the boundary that separates normal and abnormal. That is, normal becomes, for them, that which is right and proper, a standard for behaviour and action which may have precious little relationship to the norms that are statistically observed. For more on this definitional problem see ABNORMAL.

One interesting attempt to deal with this problem that has been suggested is the specification of the *norm group*. For example, cannibalism may once have been deemed 'normal' among certain peoples in New Guinea but not in, say, Canada. However, this device does not always work; divorce is still regarded as vaguely abnormal in the United States despite the fact that divorces outnumber marriages in many states. To appreciate the semantic nuances here, compare the sense of the phrases 'divorce is now the norm in America' and 'divorce is now normal in America'. The statistical sense is carried in the former by *norm* but an evaluative element emerges in the latter, and even one who recognizes the truth of the former feels a little uncomfortable accepting the latter. If there is a resolution to this that may work, it lies in the desire of many psychologists to characterize that which is normal in a manner that blends the group-norm idea with the consideration of the individual; i.e. to ask the question: 'Is the behaviour functional and adaptive for that person in that social system?' If so, then it will be considered *normal*, and if not, it will be regarded as *abnormal*. This particular use has much to recommend it, particularly because it helps to remove the subjective opinions of the theoretician and the diagnostician and allows the individual under consideration some rights in making the designation. (See here, for a classic case, the discussion under HOMOSEXUALITY.) Its obvious weakness is that it drastically reduces the strength of the generalizations that one can make concerning what is normal.

normal curve NORMAL *DISTRIBUTION.

normal distribution DISTRIBUTION, NORMAL.

normality The state or condition of being adjudged NORMAL in sense 4 of that term.

normalize 1 To transform a set of scores such that the resulting distribution approximates the NORMAL *DISTRIBUTION. **2** To adjust a set of scores such that the highest score is set equal to 100 and the lowest equal to 0 and, thus, they may be read as percentiles. **3** To adjust something so as to bring it into accordance with an accepted NORM (2).

normative Pertaining to norms or standards. A set of *normative data* is one collected for the purpose of establishing norms and getting a sense of the underlying distribution. See NORM (esp. 1 and 2). Distinguish subtly from the sense of the term borne by the phrase NORMATIVE SCIENCE.

normative influence Any influence on a person's actions or beliefs that comes from what the individual believes others will think of them if they act in particular ways. Compare with INFORMATIONAL INFLUENCE.

normative-re-educative strategy A strategy for social change based on the principle that new attitudes, values and behaviours can only be successfully introduced to a society or group when one takes account of the traditional cultural factors of that society or group and makes allowances for them. Compare with POWER-COERCIVE STRATEGY.

normative research methods A class of nonexperimental research methods based on the collection of observational data from normal subjects of various ages and developmental levels. The purpose is to establish a set of norms that reflect typical behaviour.

normative science Any discipline that seeks to develop correct patterns of behaviour and conduct. Given the standard characterizations of science (see SCIENTIFIC *METHOD), this term is something of a misnomer in that normative science tends to be prescriptive rather than descriptive or explanatory. Ethics and aesthetics are often regarded as normative sciences. See also NORMATIVE

normative survey SURVEY, NORMATIVE.

norm group The group that one uses to establish a standard against which to measure performance or evaluate behaviour. Also called *norming group*.

normless suicide ANOMIC *SUICIDE.

norm of reaction In behavioural genetics, the full range of phenotypic outcomes that can be expressed by a given *genotype*. This notion imposes no practical limits on phenotypic variability and anticipates that, when extreme variations in the environment occur, a larger phenotypic range may be expressed than is generally assumed. See REACTION RANGE.

nortriptyline An ANTIDEPRESSANT DRUG of the tricyclic group.

NOS Abbreviation for NOT OTHERWISE SPECIFIED.

nose The organ of OLFACTION, including the entrance that warms, moistens and filters the air. See also OLFACTORY EPITHELIUM, SMELL and related terms.

nose distance The distance between the noses of two persons in a social interaction. As silly as it sounds, it is actually an important variable in various kinds of personal interactions that occur and in the comfort or discomfort felt by the participants. See DISTANCE ZONE, PERSONAL SPACE.

nos(o)e- Combining form from the Greek, meaning *disease*.

nosology The systematic description and classification of diseases.

nosomania Obsolescent term for the delusion that one is diseased or has a disease.

notochord The embryonic precursor of the spinal cord and brain.

not otherwise specified (NOS) The phrase used in the DSM for disorders with symptoms that do not match the category in precise ways. For example, *amnestic disorder not otherwise specified* would be used to classify a clear case of *amnesia* that failed to meet any of the specified criteria for identified forms of the disorder. The ICD uses the simpler term *unspecified*.

noxious Painful, injurious. The term is commonly applied in the phrase *noxious stimulus*, which is used to characterize (operationally) any stimulus which will function as PUNISHMENT if presented to an organism or as a NEGATIVE *REINFORCER if removed.

NREM sleep Those stages of sleep not characterized by rapid eye movements (REM). Also called *non-REM sleep*; see SLEEP for more details.

nuclear complex (or conflict) Within a number of psychoanalytic or psychodynamic theories, a fundamental conflict that occurs during infancy or early childhood and is assumed to be a root cause of a number of various psychoneurotic disorders that may only emerge later in life. For Freud, the Oedipus complex fulfilled this hypothesized role, for Horney it was a child's feeling of helplessness, for Adler it was feelings of inferiority, etc. A nuclear complex is not the same thing as a UNIVERSAL COMPLEX, although it is true that all nuclear complexes are assumed (within each theory) to be universal. Also called *nuclear problem* or, on occasion, *root conflict*.

nuclear family FAMILY (1).

nuclear problem NUCLEAR COMPLEX.

nuclear schizophrenia See PROCESS *SCHIZOPHRENIA.

nucleic acids A group of complex acids found in the cells of all living things. They are intimately involved in the self-duplication mechanisms that are fundamental to life and form the core of the processes by which hereditary characteristics are transmitted. Those nucleic acids containing ribose are known as RIBONUCLEIC ACIDS (RNA); those containing deoxyribose are the DEOXYR-IBONUCLEIC ACIDS (DNA).

nucleo- Combining form meaning *pertaining to a nucleus*.

nucleolus A spherical organelle contained in the nucleus of a cell that produces ribosomes. pl., *nucleoli*.

nucleus From the Latin, meaning *kernel*. **1** The central portion of an atom. **2** A spherical structure within the cytoplasm of most cells (not, for example, in viruses). It contains the chromosomes and one or more nucleoli and functions as an integral part of the living cell; if it is removed, the cytoplasm dies. **3** A histologically identifiable mass of neural cell bodies in the brain or spinal cord. Specific nuclei are listed in this volume under the modifying term. **4** Any physical core or central point about which elements or factors are gathered, e.g. *governmental nucleus, social-power nucleus*. **5** In factor analysis or multi-dimensional analysis, a cluster of correlations around which many factors or dimensions lie.

nucleus accumbens (septi) A dopaminergic area in the basal forebrain near the septum. Output projections travel through the thalamus to the prefrontal cortex; inputs come from various areas including the prefrontal lobes, the amygdala, hippocampus and ventral tegmental area. The nucleus accumbens is involved in a host of functions involving reinforcement, pleasure and the development of drug dependencies. Eating, drinking, sexual behaviour, the taking of various psychoactive drugs and, interestingly, even contemplating such activities (see MIRROR NEURONS) all produce release of dopamine.

nucleus basalis An acetylcholinergic nucleus in the basal forebrain with neurons that innervate most of the cerebral cortex. It undergoes degeneration in *Alzheimer's disease*.

nucleus of the solitary tract SOLITARY TRACT.

nucleus raphe magnus One of the nuclei of the *raphe*. It receives neural projections from the periaqueductal grey and is involved in producing *analgesia*.

nuisance variable Lab slang for any variable that was not included as one in the original design of an experiment but plays a role and produces an increase in ERROR VARIANCE.

null hypothesis HYPOTHESIS, NULL.

nulliparous Pertaining to a female who has never borne offspring.

null result Any experimental outcome that is not significant. Generally, null results tend not to be reported in the scientific literature – which is occasionally unfortunate since the knowledge that such and such an effect does not obtain is often of considerable importance.

number completion test A test in which the subject is given a series of numbers arranged according to some rule and asked to complete it; e.g. 1, 2, 3, 5, 8, 13…

number factor A factor found in many analyses of performance on intelligence tests and other tests of cognitive ability that emerges as a cluster of skills all of which are seemingly representative of a facility with numerical and quantitative operations.

number form Any conscious spatial mental map of numbers that is used idiosyncratically and habitually by an individual. One person might, for example, think of digits arranged in a circular relationship as on a clock face, while another might think of numbers arranged as seen on a telephone number pad.

numerical value ABSOLUTE *VALUE.

numerosity Quantity, 'manyness'. Young children (and some nonhuman species) can detect fairly subtle distinctions in numerosity in two displays of objects without showing any indication that they have the abstract notion of number. Perhaps the most frequently studied aspect is *relative numerosity*, which involves knowing that fewer items in a display are less in quantity than more items.

nurturance 1 The act of supplying support, food, shelter, protection, etc. to the young, weak or helpless. **2** The tendency to do so.

nurture The collective impact of all environmental factors that affect growth and behaviour. Contrast with NATURE (1, but see also 2).

nutrient Any substance that is part of the normal diet for supporting growth, maintaining bodily health and repairing tissue damage. Included are fatty acids, proteins, carbohydrates and a variety of minerals and vitamins.

nyctalopia Abnormally poor vision under low illumination conditions. It may be due either to a deficiency in vitamin A or to a congenital retinal defect. The former is temporary and correctable; the latter is a permanent condition. Also known popularly as *night blindness*. Beware of incorrect use when HEMERALOPIA is meant.

nyctophilia A preference for darkness or night. Also called SCOTOPHILIA (?)

nymphomania An exaggerated sexual desire in females. The term is used almost unconscionably loosely and is often attached to sexually active women whose erotic desires and behaviours happen to exceed the speaker's own particular preferences about what is right and proper. As a true clinical syndrome it is rare and generally regarded as a manifestation of a deep psychological disorder, and is virtually always accompanied by other symptoms.

nystagmus A set of movements of the eyes made up of small-amplitude, rapid tremors and a large, slower, return sweep. They are normal and, in fact, are critical for proper vision. Their presence and/or absence under various conditions is used in diagnosing a variety of visual and neurological disorders. Compare with SACCADE and STABILIZED (RETINAL) IMAGE for a discussion of the result of neutralizing their function.

nystagmus, caloric Nystagmus produced by introducing either cold or warm water into the canal of the external ear. Warm water produces nystagmus in the direction of the ear stimulated, cold water in the opposite direction.

nystagmus, galvanic Nystagmus produced by a mild electric current passed through the auditory labyrinth.

nystagmus, optokinetic Nystagmus produced by following a moving target with the eyes. The eyes track the target briefly then sweep back to the original position, repeatedly. This appropriately named *optokinetic* response persists for a time after the visual stimulus has been removed.

nystagmus, physiological In the sequence of eye movements described under NYSTAGMUS, the fine, rapid tremors which average roughly 30 Hz with travel no greater than about 20 seconds of arc.

nystagmus, rotational Nystagmus caused by rapid rotating of the body. The slow, large-amplitude phase is in the direction of rotation; when the bodily rotation is stopped, a *secondary* or *postrotational nystagmus* in the opposite direction occurs. See BÁRÁNY TEST.

O

O Abbreviation for: **1** OBSERVER (2), as the subject in studies on perception is often called. **2** ORGANISM. SUBJECT (1) and PARTICIPANT are acceptable synonyms in both cases. **3** OSCILLATION.

ob- Combining form meaning *against, in the way of* or *toward*.

obedience Simply, acting in accordance with rules or orders. In most contemporary work in psychology the term is used as roughly synonymous with COMPLIANCE, i.e. with the connotation that one need not believe in what one in fact does but merely that one feels compelled to obey.

obesity Most definitions of this term are phrased in language that characterizes an individual as being, to some degree or another, overweight. Properly, this is not correct. Obesity is characterized by excess body fat, not excess body weight. While the two are typically correlated, exceptions exist. An athlete, for example, can be 'overweight' when compared with established norms because of extensive muscle development but would not be properly classified as obese. However, since the procedures for determining obesity from a nutritionist's point of view have become quite complex and involve a variety of factors, some general rule of thumb is still needed. Thus, for practical purposes, an individual is regarded as obese if his or her body weight is more than 30% above normal, with normal generally given by standard tables of ranges of optimal weights for age, sex and body type. Obesity can be caused by a large number of factors ranging from the purely physiological to the psychological. Several of the most frequently differentiated types are given in the following entries.

obesity, dietary Obesity which results from simple overeating, particularly when there is an excess of high-fat and high-carbohydrate foods in a person's diet.

obesity, endogenous Obesity the primary cause of which is some organic abnormality, e.g. an endocrine imbalance or faulty metabolism.

obesity, exogenous Obesity the cause of which is external, i.e. it results from excessive food intake and not from some specific organic dysfunction.

obesity, genetic Obesity that is dependent (in part) upon genetic factors. The contemporary point of view is that it results from an overabundance of fat cells which are inherited.

obesity, hypothalamic Obesity resulting from dysfunction of the HYPOTHALAMUS, specifically a lesion in the ventromedial area.

obesity, morbid Obesity in an individual whose weight is in excess of 50% of what is regarded as normal for age, sex and body type.

obesity, ovarian Obesity hypothesized by some to result from imbalances in the sex hormones. This form of obesity is identified with females, who in later life tend more toward obesity than males.

object **1** n. Most broadly, *anything*. **2** n. Within the study of perception and cognition, an aspect of the environment of which one is aware. This sense is expressed in phrases like *stimulus object*, for a physical entity that one detects, senses or recognizes, *object of regard*, for a thing one attends to or looks at, *object of thought*, for something one contemplates or thinks about, and so forth.

3 n. A goal or an end state; here the term is really a shortened form of an *objective*. **4** n. In psychoanalytic theory, a person, a part of a person, or a symbol representative of either, toward which behaviours, thoughts and desires are oriented. In the classical model, an object is required for one to obtain satisfaction of instincts.

Note that these meanings run the gamut from the physical to the perceptual, the conceptual and the symbolic, as well as from the inanimate to the personal. Not surprisingly, the term tends to be used in combined form so that the object or the subject of the object is specified; see the following entries for examples.

object-assembly test A general term for any test in which the subject is required to put together objects which have been disassembled.

object assimilation Modification or alteration of the perceived form or function of an object over time. Jung used the phrase to describe such changes, which he theorized were due to a person's needs. Gestalt psychologists and some contemporary memory theorists use it to refer to modifications in the memorial representation of an object over time, with the stipulation that these modifications bring the memory of the object more in line with that which is typical of the category. See also ASSIMILATION.

object bias The tendency of children to assume that a new word refers to an object as opposed to an action or quality. See WHOLE-OBJECT ASSUMPTION for a similar effect.

object blindness AGNOSIA.

object cathexis In psychoanalysis, investment of energy in an OBJECT (4). See OBJECT CHOICE.

object choice In psychoanalytic theory, an OBJECT (4) as the focus of love, affection or, more generally, libido. When there is identification with an object similar to oneself, it is called *narcissistic object choice*; when identification is based upon differences from oneself, it is called *anaclitic object choice*.

object colour The colour of an object – which is not quite as tautological as it sounds at first, for an object's colour must be either a SURFACE *COLOUR or a VOLUME *COLOUR and

hence differentiated from a FILM *COLOUR. See these terms for details.

object concept In Piagetian theory, a mature object concept is achieved when a child sees an object as a real, physical entity which exists and moves in the same space as him- or herself. See OBJECT PERMANENCE for more on usage.

object constancy 1 A very general term for the tendency for objects to maintain their perceptual characteristics under wide variations of viewing. Full object constancy is produced by several more elemental constancies, namely those of *colour, brightness, size* and *form*. See CONSTANCY. **2** In psychoanalysis, the maintenance of a psychic connection with a specific OBJECT (4). The term is used here with the implication that an object constancy once established functions so that possible replacements for the object tend to be rejected.

object file A term borrowed from computer science used primarily in studies of perception. It refers to an intermediate mental or perceptual representation organized from raw perceptual input. An object file is not viewed as a full category or an abstract, symbolic representation; rather it is assumed to function so that an observer can identify a perceptual input as a particular object, bind the perceptual features into a holistic representation, and track it despite perceptual variations in movement, shading and other changes that might occur in the visual scene.

objectivation A defence mechanism similar to PROJECTION (1) but with a twist. The person upon whom the feelings are projected actually has them.

objective 1 adj. Characterizing an object as a thing that is real, demonstrable or physical (see OBJECT (1, 2 and 3)) and hence the status or function of which is publicly verifiable, externally observable and not dependent on internal, mental or SUBJECTIVE experience. This general sense of the term is reflected in the following, more specific, usages. **2** adj. Characterizing a thing the nature of which is determinable through the use of physical measurement. Weight, wavelength and frequency of a sound wave are *objective* characteristics of things which correspond to the *subjective* dimensions of heaviness, hue and pitch. **3** adj. Free of bias, uncontaminated by the emotional aspects of personal assessment. See CLINICAL *PREDICTION for a classic example of the contrast between *objective* and *subjective*. **4** adj. External to the body or mind. **5** adj. Sensed or experienced as externally localized. **6** adj. Pertaining to an OBJECT, in any of the several meanings of that term. **7** n. A goal; OBJECT (3).

objective anxiety Real anxiety in the sense that there is a clear, objective cause. Note that the meaning here is, in a way, somewhat contradictory to the usual connotations of ANXIETY.

objective examination (or **test**) Any test in which the correct answers are objectively given and no subjective judgements enter into the scoring.

objective psychology A label covering for approach to scientific psychology in which the only data considered legitimate are those based upon measurement in physical, objective terms. Specifically excluded are data based on introspection or interpretation. BEHAVIOURISM is as close to being an objective psychology as one could probably put up with.

objective scoring OBJECTIVE EXAMINATION. Contrast with SUBJECTIVE SCORING.

objective set SET, OBJECTIVE.

objective test OBJECTIVE EXAMINATION.

objective threshold THRESHOLD (1).

objective vertigo VERTIGO.

objectivism In ethics, the point of view that there exist particular moral truths independent of whether or not, in a given society, they are believed in or practised. To take the classic example, one could argue that the stricture 'No one should inflict pain merely to derive pleasure from the suffering of another' is true everywhere, even in a society of sadists, just as 5 + 5 = 10 is true everywhere even in a society in which no one can count. Contrast with SUBJECTIVISM.

objectivity **1** The quality of dealing with objects as external to the mind. **2** An approach to events characterized by freedom from interpretative bias or prejudice. Sense 2 is assumed to be derived from 1 in that the nonsubjective quality results from approach-

ing phenomena on the assumption that they have an external (i.e. *objective*) reality uncontaminated by internal interpretation. See e.g. OBJECTIVE PSYCHOLOGY.

object libido LIBIDINAL OBJECT.

object loss In psychoanalytic theory, the loss of an OBJECT (4) who was perceived as benevolent and loved. The term is used to refer to either the loss of the love or the loss of the object.

object of instinct In psychoanalysis, the OBJECT (4) that is the focus of an instinct.

object, part In psychoanalytic theory, some particular aspect of an OBJECT (4) that plays a role in fulfilling needs, e.g. a breast or a penis.

object permanence A critical aspect of a child's development of what Piaget calls the OBJECT CONCEPT is the notion of its permanence. Specifically, the reference here is to the awareness that a physical object is permanent, that it continues to exist even when the child no longer interacts with it.

object relations **1** Loosely, the full complement of a person's relations with his or her external world. **2** In psychoanalytic theory, relations between SELF (1) and OBJECT (4). The emphasis is more on emotional investment, conceptualization of these relations, and understanding of *the other* than on behavioural or instinctual aspects of relationships the classic Freudians emphasized.

object relations theory A branch of psychoanalysis, due largely to the work of Melanie Klein, that concerns itself with OBJECT RELATIONS (2).

object representation In psychoanalysis, the internal mental representational aspects of an OBJECT (4). The point is that a psychic process, say *object cathexis*, is assumed to take place with respect to one's mental representation of the object and not the real person.

object size Lit., the actual physical size of a thing as opposed to its perceived size. When SIZE CONSTANCY holds, the two measures of size are equivalent.

object, transitional An object used by a child as a comforter. Usually there is considerable emotional attachment invested in the object, which is typically a piece of cloth or a doll. The term derives from psychoanalytic theory, which views the object as a psychological bridge allowing the child to make the transition from primitive narcissism to a more mature emotional attachment to others. It is used by many, however, without the psychoanalytic interpretation.

oblique Characterizing a line or a plane that intersects another line or plane at an angle other than 90°. In graphic representations of factor analysis, two axes (representing factors) that are correlated appear as oblique.

oblique décalage DÉCALAGE.

oblique rotation ROTATION (2).

oblique solution In factor analysis, a solution whereby the axes that represent the underlying factors are situated so that they are not at right angles to each other. In such a solution, the factors themselves are correlated. Compare with ORTHOGONAL SOLUTION. Also called *oblique-axes solution*.

obliviscence An old term for the loss of information from memory. It is currently being resuscitated as a convenient antonym of REMINISCENCE.

oblongata MEDULLA OBLONGATA.

obscenity From the Latin, meaning *of evil omen* and, by extension, *disgusting, offensive*. Modern usage restricts the meaning to those acts, words or pictures that are regarded as indecent and offensive about sexual and excretory matters. The difficulty with the term emerges from the words 'are regarded' in the previous sentence. Typically, appeals are made to 'accepted standards in society' or 'prevailing social morality' or other ill-defined criteria. In the final analysis, obscenity is much like beauty and exists primarily in the eye of the beholder.

observation 1 Most generally, any form of examination of events, behaviours, phenomena, etc. **2** By extension, any individual datum, score, value, etc. that represents an event, behaviour or phenomenon. Note that on occasion observation may be used in contrast with *experiment*. This distinction marks the fact that many regard scientific work based on so-called OBSERVATIONAL METHODS as nonexperimental. In this sense the distinction is justified, although on the other side of the coin lies the argument that such a differ-

entiation is really unnecessary since an experiment is merely one way of making an observation. The terms need to be kept conceptually separate when one wishes to distinguish between research that is controlled by the manipulation of independent variables and research that is carried out using NATURALISTIC OBSERVATION. **3** A casual or informal commentary upon or interpretation of that which has been observed.

observation(al) learning LEARNING, OBSERVATIONAL.

observational methods Generally, any of the procedures and techniques that are used in nonexperimental research to assist in making accurate observations of events. Included is the use of various devices such as audio and video recorders, cameras, stopwatches and check-lists.

observation trial Any trial in an experiment in which the subject is not required to make any response but merely to observe the stimulus presented. See OBSERVATIONAL *LEARNING.

observer 1 One who makes an OBSERVATION. **2** One who is engaged in INTROSPECTION. Note that in sense 1 the observer is the scientist carrying out a study and collecting data, while in 2 the observer is the subject in an experiment who reports on experiences (see INTROSPECTION) or attends to stimuli presented (see OBSERVATIONAL *LEARNING). Symbol (sense 2 only): *O*.

observer bias A BIAS (1, 3, 6) introduced by an OBSERVER (1, 2).

observer drift The tendency for the observers in a study to become inconsistent in the manner in which they make and record their observations. More likely to occur in long-term studies, it is a bias that reduces reliability.

obsession Any idea that haunts, hovers and constantly invades one's consciousness. Obsessions are seemingly beyond one's will, and awareness of their inappropriateness is of little or no avail. Compare with COMPULSION and see also OBSESSIVE-COMPULSIVE DISORDER.

obsessional neurosis Originally, a neurosis characterized by obsessional thoughts, ideas, etc. Because such obsessions tend to occur along with compulsive behaviour, the more inclusive term *obsessive-compulsive neurosis* was introduced. Today, owing to difficulties with the term NEUROSIS itself, the preferred label is OBSESSIVE-COMPULSIVE DISORDER.

obsessive-compulsive disorder (OCD) A subclass of ANXIETY DISORDERS with two essential characteristics: recurrent and persistent thoughts, ideas and feelings; and repetitive, ritualized behaviours. Attempts to resist a compulsion produce mounting tension and anxiety, which are relieved immediately by giving in to it. The term is not properly used of behaviours like excessive drinking, gambling or eating on the grounds that the 'compulsive gambler', for example, actually derives considerable pleasure from gambling (it's the losing that hurts); one burdened with a true obsessive-compulsive disorder derives no pleasure from it other than the release of tension. Recent evidence indicates that the disorder is associated with damage to or dysfunctions of the *basal ganglia, cingulate gyrus* and *prefrontal cortex*. Treatment is with BEHAVIOUR THERAPY, COGNITIVE-BEHAVIOUR THERAPY and ANTIOBSESSIONAL DRUGS.

obstacle sense The ability of many blind persons to avoid obstacles in their path. The sense involved is hearing and the ability is due to ECHOLOCATION. Compare with FACIAL VISION.

obstruction method Any experimental method in which the subject is separated from a goal by some obstruction. Such procedures are useful in exploring motivation, problem-solving and choice behaviour.

obtained mean SAMPLE *MEAN.

obtained score RAW *SCORE.

obtrusive thoughts Loosely, unwanted thoughts or ideas that encroach on one's ongoing mental activity. If frequent and repetitive they can become OBSESSIONS.

Occam's razor The principle *Entia non sunt multiplicanda praeter necessitatem* ('Entities are not to be multiplied beyond necessity'). William of Occam (or Ockham) was a 14th-century Franciscan philosopher and theologian who argued that reality exists only in individual things and events. Often called the *principle of ontological economy*, Occam's razor is similar to the more modern LLOYD

MORGAN'S CANON and to the more general principle of PARSIMONY.

occipital Pertaining to the back part of the head, skull or brain.

occipital lobe The posterior lobe of the cerebral hemispheres, devoted to processing visual information.

occlusion 1 An obstruction, block or closure. The term is used in physiology and medicine to refer to a blockage in or closure of a passageway. **2** INTERPOSITION.

occult From the Latin for *covered* or *concealed*, involving the supernatural. The study of the occult involves magic, spiritualism and other branches of the paranormal, particularly as such 'powers' may be used to control natural events. Modern science is partly occult in its origins, yet oddly most contemporary occultists are vigorously anti-science. See also PARAPSYCHOLOGY.

occupation 1 Specifically, any activity or set of activities carried out for purposes of earning a living. That is, an occupation is a ROLE that has both economic and social elements to it. **2** More generally, any activity that one carries out; whatever keeps one occupied.

occupational analysis JOB ANALYSIS.

occupational family A cluster of occupations or professions all of which share similar training and requisite abilities. Distinguish from OCCUPATIONAL GROUP.

occupational group A group organized and defined by the common occupation of its members. Professional societies, labour unions and the like are examples. Distinguish from OCCUPATIONAL FAMILY.

occupational hierarchy Any ranking or ordering of occupations according to some set of criteria. The most commonly used are: (a) the more or less objective criteria, such as intellectual and/or skill requirements, or the amount of education and/or training needed for success in each occupation; and (b) the social-esteem criteria, such as the prestige and social status associated with each occupation. Although such hierarchies are invariably tinged by social/political biases, they are generally useful in the study of such issues as social mobility, social power and the study of social-class differences. See HOLLINGSHEAD SCALES.

occupational interest inventory INTEREST INVENTORY.

occupational psychiatry Originally classified as a subfield of psychiatry concerned with diagnostic and preventive issues within the workplace. The focus is on problems such as emotional stability in the work environment, absenteeism, accidents and accident proneness, and problems of retirement. It's worth noting that much of the actual practice here is carried out by professionals not trained in psychiatry but in clinical and industrial and organizational psychology. Distinguish from OCCUPATIONAL THERAPY.

occupational therapy Simply, therapy based on giving an individual something purposeful to do. It may be either physical therapy, in which the tasks are designed to exercise and develop certain muscles and sensorimotor coordination, or psychologically oriented therapy, in which the work is designed to improve a person's general sense of self. Distinguish from OCCUPATIONAL PSYCHIATRY.

OCD OBSESSIVE-COMPULSIVE DISORDER.

octa- Combining form meaning *eight*. var., *octo-*.

octave effect A generalization effect observed in classical conditioning in which the CS was a pure tone, tones of varying frequencies are used during generalization testing and at least one of these is an octave of the original. Responses to the octaves are almost always stronger than to other tones, even ones closer in frequency to the original CS.

octo- OCTA-.

ocular Pertaining to the eye. OPHTHALMIC is an acceptable (and the preferred) synonym; OPTIC is not.

ocular apraxia APRAXIA, OCULAR.

ocular dominance 1 An obsolescent term for EYE *DOMINANCE. 2 Descriptive of cells that respond more to stimulation from one eye than from the other. They are common in the STRIATE CORTEX.

ocular dominance columns Vertical columns of neurons in the STRIATE CORTEX that display OCULAR DOMINANCE (2). They lie next to one another and alternate between showing dominance to each eye and are important in binocular vision.

ocular dysmetria Any disability to properly control SACCADES. Also called *saccadic dysmetria*.

ocular pursuit PURSUIT MOVEMENT.

ocular torsional movement TORSION (2).

oculist Obsolete term for *ophthalmologist*.

oculo- Combining form meaning *the eye* or *pertaining to the eye*.

oculogyral illusion The apparent movement of a stationary spot of light when the observer is rotated about rapidly. The illusion of movement is a result of reflexive eye movements caused by the rotation; see here ROTATIONAL *NYSTAGMUS.

oculomotor A cover term used to describe any of the several kinds of eye movements, including the movements of the eyeball as controlled by the extrinsic muscles, the movements of accommodation and the movements of the muscle controlling the iris.

oculomotor nerve The IIIrd CRANIAL NERVE. It originates in the oculomotor nucleus of the superior colliculus and the third ventricle in the midbrain and consists primarily of efferent fibres to all the ocular muscles except the exterior rectus and superior oblique. Although this motor function is primary, the nerve also contains some proprioceptive (afferent) fibres.

oculomotor nucleus OCULOMOTOR NERVE.

OD ORGANIZATIONAL DEVELOPMENT.

oddball task Loosely, any task in which an unexpected stimulus occurs.

odd–even technique SPLIT-HALF *RELIABILITY.

oddity task Any task in which the subject's task is to detect which stimulus is not like the others.

odds In probability calculations, the ratio of success to failure. For example, the odds of drawing a spade at random from a deck of cards is 13 *to* 39 or 1 *to* 3. Note that calculating the odds is not the same as calculating the PROBABILITY (1). The probability of drawing a spade is 0.25 or 1 *in* 4.

odds ratio Quite literally, the ratio between two odds. It is used most often as a statistic that represents the relative risk associated with the presence of a factor. For example, the odds ratio between prenatal exposure to rubella and later development of schizophrenia is approximately 5:1, indicating that foetuses exposed in utero to rubella are 5 times more likely to develop schizophrenia than foetuses not exposed.

odiferous Having an odour.

odor ODOUR.

odorant A substance that has a smell or odour.

odorimetry OLFACTOMETRY.

odor prism HENNING'S PRISM.

odour Either **1** the sensory experience of smelling a gaseous substance, or **2** the substance itself. See OLFACTION, OLFACTORY, SMELL, etc.

oedema EDEMA.

Oedipus complex A group or collection (i.e. a complex) of unconscious wishes, feelings and ideas focusing on the desire to 'possess' the opposite-sexed parent and 'eliminate' the same-sexed parent. In the traditional Freudian view, the complex is seen as emerging during the Oedipal stage, which corresponds roughly to the ages 3 to 5, and is characterized as a universal component of development irrespective of culture. The complex is assumed to become partly resolved, within this classical view, through the child making an appropriate identification with the same-sexed parent, with full resolution theoretically achieved when the opposite-sexed parent is 'rediscovered' in a mature, adult sexual OBJECT (4). Freud viewed the Oedipus complex as the NUCLEAR COMPLEX of all psychoneuroses, and, in his view, a variety of neurotic fixations, sexual aberrations and debilitating guilt feelings were theoretically traceable to an unresolved Oedipus complex.

Interestingly, the theoretical genesis of the complex – which derives its name from the mythical figure Oedipus, the hero of two of Sophocles' tragedies who unknowingly killed his father and married his mother – was Freud's own self-analysis, carried out after his father's death. At first, *Oedipus* referred only to the male complex, *Electra* being used for the female. Today, however, both are subsumed under *Oedipus* largely for convenience, and it should be noted that Electra's sins were different from Oedipus'. Rather than directly murdering her mother, she urged her brother to do it.

Contemporary psychoanalytic theory places somewhat less importance on the complex than did Freud and his immediate followers. There is more emphasis on the earlier relationship between the child and the mother, and the Oedipal behaviours are now viewed as derivative of previous experiences and conflicts. var., *Edipus*.

oestradiol The most biologically potent of the naturally occurring OESTROGENS. It is produced primarily by the ovaries and, in small amounts, by the adrenal cortices. var., *estradiol*.

oestriol An oestrogenic hormone that is regarded as a metabolic product of OESTRADIOL and OESTRONE. var., *estriol*.

oestrogen A generic label for a group of related steroid hormones produced chiefly by the ovaries, but also by the adrenal cortices and, in very small amounts, by the testes. Included are *oestradiol*, *oestrone* and their metabolic product, *oestriol*. Oestrogens are responsible for the morphogenesis of the gonads and the development of most of the female secondary sex characteristics – breast development, maturation of the genitalia, deposition of body fat – but not axillary and pubic hair: growth here is the result of *androstenedione*, an ANDROGEN. They are also responsible for the cyclic changes in the uterus that accompany the MENSTRUAL CYCLE – or, in nonprimate mammals, the OESTRUS CYCLE. See also PROGESTERONE. var., *estrogen*.

oestrone The less potent biologically of the primary OESTROGENS. var., *estrone*.

oestrus OESTRUS CYCLE.

oestrus cycle The ovarian cycle in female subprimate mammals. It has four stages: prooestrus, oestrus, matoestrus and dioestrus. The second stage, *oestrus*, is that associated with ovulation, swelling of the vulva, various uterine processes and receptivity to copulation. The term *oestrus* comes from the Greek, meaning *mad* or *frenetic desire*, and is often used to refer to the periodic sexual desire or *heat* displayed by female animals. var., *estrus*. See also MENSTRUAL CYCLE.

off cell Generally, any cell in the visual system that responds when a stimulus is terminated. Many are found in the retina and others in the visual pathways. Some are GANGLION CELLS, others BIPOLAR. Some are simple; others more complex such as the 'off-centre cells' that are inhibited by light in the centre of a RECEPTIVE FIELD (1) but excited by light on the surround and those in a CENTRE-SURROUND RECEPTIVE FIELD which have a variety of inhibitory and excitatory systems based on the nature of the cells in the field. Analogous neurons with *on* properties respond to the *on*set of stimulation and others with *on–off* characteristics respond to both.

off label A term used to refer to the use of a drug for a treatment other than the one it was originally designed and approved for.

ogive Specifically, an elongated, ∫-shaped curve which results from the transformation of a normal curve into cumulative proportions or frequencies. More generally, although not completely accurately, the term is sometimes used to describe any graph of a cumulative-frequency distribution with this approximate shape.

Ohm's (acoustic) law A principle due to the German physicist G. S. Ohm that says that a complex tone is analysed *by the hearer* into its frequency components. Note that Ohm's law is a theoretical statement about the perceiver and thus must be differentiated from a FOURIER ANALYSIS, which is a theoretical statement about the physical stimulus. Accordingly, it would have been better to have called it Ohm's *auditory* law.

-oid Suffix denoting *resemblance, similarity*.

olanzapine An ATYPICAL *ANTIPSYCHOTIC DRUG used primarily for schizophrenia and acute manic episodes, particularly in cases of bipolar disorder. It is also being used, OFF LABEL, for the treatment of stuttering.

oleic acid FATTY ACID.

olfactie Zwaardemaker's unit for measuring odour intensity. It is established as the number of centimetres exposed on a Zwaarde-

maker olfactometer when the threshold for an odour is reached.

olfaction 1 The sense of smell. 2 The act of smelling. The receptors for olfaction are found in the olfactory epithelium in the upper part of the nose; the stimuli for olfactory experience are chemical substances in gaseous form that can dissolve in the mucus that coats the olfactory epithelium.

olfactometry Measurement of the capacity of a gaseous substance to produce an olfactory experience. Also called *odorimetry*.

olfactory Pertaining to the sense of smell or act of smelling.

olfactory brain RHINENCEPHALON.

olfactory bulbs Two enlargements at the terminus of the olfactory nerve (Ist cranial). They lie at the base of the brain just above the nasal cavity.

olfactory epithelium Two patches of mucous membrane located at the top of the nasal passageways that contain the receptors for the sense of smell.

olfactory nerve The Ist CRANIAL NERVE. An afferent nerve carrying odour information from the receptors in the olfactory epithelium via the mitral cells, the axons of which make up the olfactory bulbs and olfactory tracts, to the cerebrum.

olig(o)- Combining term meaning *little* or *few*.

oligodendroglia GLIA.

oligoencephaly Lit., somewhat like Pooh Bear, 'of little brain'. Specifically, mental deficiency caused by abnormal brain development.

oligologia Lit., of few words. Specifically, having a small vocabulary. Obviously, an affliction uncommon among psychologists.

oligophrenia Generally, any mental deficiency.

olivary body (or nucleus) INFERIOR *OLIVARY NUCLEUS.

olivary nucleus, inferior A rounded, olive-shaped mass of cells in the ventral part of the medulla oblongata that forms part of the reticular system. Also called *olivary body*.

olivary nucleus, superior A small nucleus of cells in the tegmental region of the pons.

olivopontocerebellar atrophy A MULTI-SYSTEM ATROPHY with Parkinson-like symptoms including ataxia, postural instability, rigidity, dysarthria and a flat facial expression. It results from neural damage in the pons and cerebellum and is often misdiagnosed (see PARKINSON-PLUS SYNDROMES).

-ology Suffix denoting *study of, knowledge of* or *science of.*

omega squared A measure of the strength of association between variables. It provides the proportion of the variance in the dependent variable that is associated with the variability in the independent variable. It is somewhat more conservative than other measures of effect size such as r^2.

omission training An occasional synonym of *differential reinforcement of other behaviour*; see SCHEDULES OF *REINFORCEMENT.

omnibus test 1 In statistics, any overall test of statistical significance, such as an ANOVA or MULTIVARIATE ANALYSIS. When omnibus tests yield significance, planned comparisons (see POST HOC TESTS) are run to specify the differences that exist among the groups. **2** In PSYCHOMETRICS, any test that has several subtests distributed throughout it designed to evaluate a number of psychological factors. Most intelligence tests are omnibus tests.

omnipotence of thought 1 Generally, any delusion involving beliefs that one has powers to control events and people simply by thought. **2** In psychoanalytic theory, the belief that one's wishes, hopes or thoughts can affect external reality. Some theorists assume that it is a normal stage of childhood (see MAGICAL THINKING), others regard it as a sign of alienation from, and even denial of, reality. Freud thought that it was a fundamental aspect of the development of animism, magic and religion.

onanism From the practice of the biblical character Onan, *coitus interruptus*. However, the term is often used to refer to sexual self-stimulation, i.e. masturbation.

on cell See OFF CELL.

onco- Combining form meaning *mass, tumour, swelling.*

oneiric Pertaining to dreams or dreaming.

oneiromancy The supposed prediction of the future by the interpretation of dreams. The term is only used in examinations of the paranormal, where it is assumed to refer to one aspect of precognition; it is not used in dream interpretation in psychoanalysis or other depth psychologies.

oneirophrenia A dream-like state with some characteristics of simple schizophrenia but without the dissociation typical of that disorder.

one-tailed test TWO-TAILED TEST.

one-trial learning LEARNING, ONE-TRIAL.

one-way screen (or **mirror**) Any device, commonly a mirror, that permits one to observe events on the other side without being seen.

one-word stage See HOLOPHRASTIC STAGE.

on–off cell See OFF CELL.

onomatomania A disorder in which particular words acquire unnatural, deep significance and are obsessively thought about or repeated.

onomatopoeia The formation of a word by imitation of the thing named; e.g. *cuckoo* as the name of the bird that makes that call. All of the onomatopoeic THEORIES OF *LANGUAGE ORIGINS assume that such mimicking lies at the core of the genesis of human language.

onset 1 In medicine, the point at which a disorder first manifests itself. **2** In experimental psychology, the instant in time when a stimulus is presented. Actually, onset is determined by the point in time when the event is noticed, even though it may have been physically present prior to that time; e.g. the onset of a gradually increasing stimulus is when it is above threshold and the observer first notices it.

onto- Combining form meaning: **1** *existence*; **2** *a living being.*

ontoanalytic model A label occasionally applied to the existential approach; see EXISTENTIALISM et seq. for details.

ontogenic evolution See BALDWIN EFFECT.

ontogeny (ontogenesis) From the roots of the word, the origin and, by extension, the development of an individual organism. By convention, *ontogeny* is used to refer to the abstract and the general, *ontogenesis* to the particular. The term denotes extended time periods, see discussion under MICROGENESIS. Compare with PHYLOGENY and PHYLOGENESIS, the origin and development of species. See also DEVELOPMENT and DEVELOPMENTAL, which are generally preferred in discussions of child psychology.

ontological commitment A social agreement to use words in ways consistent with a particular conception of reality and the existence of particular entities or phenomena. The notion is that the way in which we use words reflects the way we conceptualize the world.

ontology Generally, an aspect of metaphysical inquiry concerned with the question of existence apart from specific objects and events. *Existence* here can be taken broadly to cover cases such as the ontological argument concerning the existence of God, discussions about the conceptual reality of categories, e.g. numbers, trees and languages (see CATEGORY and CONCEPT), and assumptions concerning the underlying conceptual systems of theories of mind.

onychophagia Excessive nail-biting.

oo- Combining form meaning *egg*.

opaque 1 Impenetrable by visible light, not transparent. **2** By extension, not open to conscious awareness.

open adoption Adoption in which, at a minimum, disclosure of adoption and identity of the birth parents is made to the adopted child and family. The openness may range from nominal disclosure through frequent contact with the birth parent(s). In some venues there are legal issues distinguishing this *structural openness* (as it is also called) from *adoption communication openness* where the adoptive parent(s) communicate freely about the adoption with the adopted child in an ongoing fashion. Compare with CLOSED ADOPTION.

open classroom 1 A class(room) made up of children of different ages and achievement levels. **2** A class(room) that the children and teachers can move freely in and out of.

open class words A class of words that permits new items to be introduced. In practice, open class words are the same as CONTENT WORDS. Compare with CLOSED CLASS WORDS and FUNCTION WORDS.

open-ended question Any question that an individual can answer freely, as compared with a CLOSED QUESTION, which has to be answered by selecting one of several specific alternatives. Open-ended questions are often used in political polling, opinion sampling and clinical interviews since they permit a wide range of responses and are not limited by a set of preselected possible answers. They also have a liability in that it is difficult to score and analyse the responses so obtained.

open instinct INSTINCT, OPEN.

openness (to new experiences) The degree to which one seeks and embraces new experiences, knowledge and attitudes. It is one of the factors in the FIVE FACTOR MODEL.

open study (or trial) A preliminary experimental study of a drug or a therapeutic technique in which the experimenter and the subjects know the purpose of the study, what factors are being examined, who is an experimental subject and who a control, etc. Generally used as a pilot study prior to running a fully controlled experiment. Compare with DOUBLE-BLIND.

open system Any system that has flexibility and can be adjusted and modified. **1** In biology, a system which is characterized as not amenable to the standard thermodynamic laws concerning the conservation of energy, entropy, etc., rather is open to new inputs, growth and change. **2** In the study of communication, a system is called *open* if any arbitrary message can be expressed. In this sense, only human languages are truly open. See LANGUAGE and NATURAL *LANGUAGE.

operandum A term preferred by Skinnerians to MANIPULANDUM.

operant 1 n. Any behaviour that is emitted by an organism and can be characterized in terms of its effects upon the environment. Note that the critical feature in this definition is the notion of the changes or effects that the response has on the environment; hence an operant is actually a *class* of responses all of which share the same effect.

For example, a rat in a Skinner box may press the bar with any paw or even with its nose and all will be considered as instances of the same operant – a bar press. To be sure, this issue can be more finely represented so as to include various means of distinguishing between the finer overt aspects of such an operant. See TOPOGRAPHY (2) for a discussion of these. Operants, unlike RESPONDENTS (which are elicited by specific stimuli), occur without specific antecedent stimulus conditions. When an operant has been brought under the control of a discriminative stimulus, OPERANT CONDITIONING has occurred. **2** adj. Pertaining to or characterizing a response that displays these properties. Compare with INSTRUMENTAL.

operant aggression INSTRUMENTAL *AGGRESSION.

operant conditioning A type of CONDITIONING in which an OPERANT response is brought under stimulus control. The operation through which such conditioning occurs is the presentation of reinforcement contingent upon an organism emitting the response. This operational aspect is the critical one in distinguishing the operant conditioning procedure from the CLASSICAL CONDITIONING procedure, in which reinforcement (the *US*) occurs whether or not the organism makes the response. Perhaps the easiest way to view operant conditioning is to regard it as a set of circumstances under which new responses that are within an organism's volitional repertoire come to be strengthened by contingent reinforcement.

Often *operant conditioning* is used synonymously with *instrumental conditioning*, although there are subtle distinctions between these terms that need to be appreciated. See INSTRUMENTAL CONDITIONING for a discussion of these. Finally, note that the phrase operant conditioning itself is used to refer to both the actual procedures as described above as well as to the kind of learning that occurs under such conditions. See also SKINNERIAN.

operant level 1 The rate at which an OPERANT is emitted prior to reinforcement. **2** The response rate after experimental extinction has taken place.

operant reserve The number of operant responses emitted by an organism after the termination of reinforcement. It is used as a measure of resistance to extinction. Occasionally treated as a synonym of REFLEX RESERVE, but see that entry for a distinction.

operant response OPERANT (1).

operating characteristic 1 Generally, a formal statement concerning the likelihood of observing specific effects under specified conditions. This notion appears in various, more circumscribed usages in psychology; to wit: **2** In statistics, the likelihood of failing to reject the null hypothesis, given each statistically defined set of conditions for a particular test of significance. **3** In the study of perception, RECEIVER-OPERATING CHARACTERISTIC (ROC) CURVE. **4** In the study of memory, MEMORY-OPERATING CHARACTERISTIC (MOC) CURVE.

operation Generally, a performing, a carrying-out – or the act so performed or carried out. An operation may be *empirical* if it manipulates aspects of physical reality, *logical* or *mathematical* if it alters the relationships between symbols of a formal system like symbolic logic, or *cognitive* or *mental* if it modifies mental states, ideas, thoughts, images, etc. Note that these usages run the gamut from the objective and physical to the subjective and mental, and various derived terms may reflect one or more of these connotative aspects. For example, OPERATIONALISM stresses the overt, physical and objective, whereas the many combined terms in Piagetian theory (e.g. OPERATORY THOUGHT) deal with processes which are covert and subjective.

operational Generally, pertaining to an OPERATION. However, that term has such a wide range of usages that many writers use the adjectival form only when referring to the overt, objective components of action or to the formal aspects of symbolic systems. The variant *operatory* is then reserved for discussions of the subjective and/or cognitive operations, specifically within the confines of the Piagetian approach. These conventions, needless to say, are not followed by all.

operational definition DEFINITIONS.

operationalism A point of view vigorously expounded (although not originated, as some suppose) by the physicist P. Bridgman. Essentially, it argues that the concepts of science be operationalized – that they be defined by, and their meaning limited to, the concrete operations used in their measurement. Operationalism was embraced in psychology by radical behaviourists, and their theoretical and empirical terminology was derived largely through the use of *operational definitions*. Thus, for example, the strength of a *hunger drive* was defined as a specified number of hours of food deprivation, *classical conditioning* was regarded as a given set of experimental procedures, etc. Even abstract concepts were operationalized: *intelligence* became that which an intelligence test measured – leading to the implication that it would be defined differently according to the test used.

Operationalism, however, was soon discovered to have many problems. While praising its objectivity one needs to recognize its limitations. In the final analysis, many of the critical terms and concepts of psychology carry a 'thingness' or a 'deep' meaning that is simply not captured by even the most thorough operational characterization; the meaning and causal role of *hunger*, for example, is just not represented by the kinds of operational definition given above. Also called *operationism*.

operational research OPERATIONS RESEARCH.

operationism OPERATIONALISM.

operations, cognitive 1 Generally, and loosely, the procedures of thought. 2 Specifically, within the Piagetian approach, the principles involved in OPERATORY THOUGHT as evidenced by CONCRETE OPERATIONS and FORMAL OPERATIONS.

operations research A general term covering any approach to an analysis of a complex system to determine its overall mode of operation and maximize its effectiveness. The system here may be an individual organism, a group of persons, an organization, a machine or any combination of these. Also called *operational research*.

operator 1 In mathematics and statistics, any symbol or number that denotes an operation to be performed on other symbols or numbers. 2 Any individual or part or aspect thereof that carries out some action or process.

operatory Pertaining to an OPERATION. An adjectival form found primarily in the Piagetian approach to cognitive development; see OPERATIONAL for discussion of usage.

operatory stages In Piagetian theory, those stages of cognitive development characterized by OPERATORY THOUGHT.

operatory thought Piaget's general label for the cognitive principles involved in CONCRETE OPERATIONS and FORMAL OPERATIONS. Note that Piagetians restrict the use of the term *operatory* to these two cognitive stages in which a child displays behaviour that reveals thinking that is governed by a logical system. See and compare with PREOPERATORY THOUGHT. Also called, on occasion, *operational thought*; see here the discussion under OPERATIONAL for a note on usage.

ophthalmic Pertaining to the eye. In all terms with the prefix *ophthal-*, the *ph* is pronounced *f*. This is probably the most consistently mispronounced group of words in all of science and medicine. Compare with OCULAR; distinguish from OPTIC.

ophthalmology A medical speciality concerned with treatment of the eye. Ophthalmologists hold the MD degree and their practice includes surgical and pharmaceutical treatment. Compare with OPTOMETRY.

ophthalmometer A device for measuring corneal curvature.

ophthalmoscope An instrument that allows one to see the inside of the eye. Most important, it permits one to make a careful inspection of the retina without any surgical intervention.

-opia (-opy) Suffixes meaning *visual defect*.

opiate receptors Specific, postsynaptic receptors in various parts of the brain (anterior amygdala, central grey regions, hypothalamus) that take up drugs of the opiate group. The opiate receptors function ideally (and naturally) for the ENDORPHINS but will also take up the other OPIATES, the natural as well as the synthetic. At the time of writing three distinct types of receptors have been identified: μ (mu), δ (delta) and κ (kappa).

opiates A broad class of drug compounds including: (a) the naturally occurring opiates, all of which are derived from the opium poppy; morphine is the drug of reference here, codeine the other commonly found alkaloid of opium; (b) the semi-synthetic opiates including heroin and various other preparations such as dihydromorphinone; (c) the synthetic opiates including methadone, meperidine and phenazocine, all of which are wholly synthetic compounds with a morphine-like pharmacological profile; (d) the narcotic antagonists, which when used in conjunction with an opiate block its effects but when used alone have opiate-like properties (note, however, that *naloxone* is an important exception to this pattern, being an opiate antagonist but having no analgesic or narcotic properties by itself); and (e) the ENDOGENOUS OPIATES, which occur naturally and are found in various parts of the brain.

The opiates all have both analgesic and narcotic effects; they also produce (often rapidly) both DRUG *TOLERANCE and DRUG *DEPENDENCE. As research and clinical work involving these compounds focuses less and less on those derived directly from the opium poppy, there is a move to rename the class opioids to indicate that it refers to a variety of chemicals with opium-like effects, with *opiates* being restricted to those compounds that derive from opium. However, this usage has not yet spread to the various compound terms, particularly those involving the endogenous chemicals, which many authorities still refer to as *opiates* on the grounds that they are naturally occurring and have similar biochemical structure to opium and its products.

opinion Generally, a tentatively held and expressible point of view. The term is used with the connotation that an opinion is intellectually held and based on at least some facts or data. This helps differentiate *opinion* from BELIEF, which has an emotional component, and from ATTITUDE (esp. 4), which has a much broader range of semantic implication. To appreciate these distinctions note that we have opinion polls but not belief polls or attitude polls; beliefs and attitudes require more elaborate and intensive devices in order to be properly assessed.

opinion poll Any survey of opinions, most generally through the use of a simple questionnaire.

opinion, private One's internally held opinion on some issue. Depending on various factors, particularly current PUBLIC *OPINION (1) on the issue, a person's private opinion may or may not differ significantly from his or her openly stated opinion – a fact that confounds much work in opinion polling.

opinion, public 1 The general point of view expressed by a group or society, i.e. by the public. The term is used so that it reflects the modal position; there is no implication that the opinion is held universally. **2** An individual's overtly stated opinion on some issue; compare here with PRIVATE *OPINION.

opioids Literally, things resembling opium. Used by many to indicate the class of chemical compounds known originally as OPIATES but see that term for a discussion of usage issues.

opium The substance obtained from the unripe pod of the opium poppy (*Papaver somniferum*). It contains more than 20 distinct alkaloids although virtually all the psychotropic effects are derived from the primary one, MORPHINE. Pharmacologically, it has both narcotic and analgesic properties. adj., *opiate* or *opioid*. See OPIATES for more details.

opponent process Generally, a complex interacting mechanism in which the functioning of one aspect of the system simultaneously inhibits the functioning of the other and vice versa. An opponent-process system operates (roughly) like a balance beam: elevation of one arm depresses the other. This general notion has been incorporated into various theoretical models of psychological processes, e.g. OPPONENT-PROCESS THEORY OF MOTIVATION and THEORIES OF *COLOUR VISION.

opponent-process theory of colour vision THEORIES OF *COLOUR VISION.

opponent-process theory of motivation A theory of motivation, due largely to Richard L. Solomon, which assumes that the functioning of an intact organism is predicated on the maintenance of a moderate position of *motivational normality*. Any swing toward either pole on a motivational dimension produces an opponent process that operates to bring the system back into balance; e.g. terror and fear will produce a tendency toward joy and ecstasy, and vice versa. An axiom of the theory is that excitation of one pole produces a simultaneous inhibition of the other; hence, if the conditions that produced the original state are removed there will be an *overshift* to the opposite side of the balance point owing to the action of disinhibition.

opportunistic sampling SAMPLING, OPPORTUNISTIC.

opposites test A test in which the subject is required to respond to a stimulus word with its opposite, e.g. the ANTONYM TEST.

oppositional defiant disorder A developmental disorder marked by defiant, hostile and negativistic behaviour, but without the serious antisocial characteristics observed in the CONDUCT DISORDERS. Children who have it are argumentative, lose their temper easily, and are resentful, angry and easily annoyed. Typically these patterns of behaviour are only displayed with adults a child knows (such as parents), hence may not be seen during clinical interviews. Often occurs in children with ATTENTION-DEFICIT HYPERACTIVITY DISORDER.

oppressed group MINORITY GROUP.

opsin A protein that occurs in several forms, one of which is one of the metabolic products of the breakdown of RHODOPSIN and is more properly called *rod opsin*.

optic A term originally used to refer to the branch of physics known as *optics*. However, it is also freely used to refer to the eye and to vision and occurs in various combined forms that denote neurological structures, e.g. *optic nerve, optic tract*. var., *optical*.

optic agnosia VISUAL *AGNOSIA.

optic apraxia APRAXIA, OPTIC.

optical axis The line of vision as given by a straight line through the centres of curvature of the lens and the cornea.

optical defect Generally, any impairment of vision that is *optical* in the sense that the light rays are distorted by the eye's optical system (lens and cornea) prior to reaching the retina. Examples include ASTIGMATISM, HYPEROPIA and MYOPIA.

optical illusion Any ILLUSION involving vision.

optical image IMAGE (1).

optical projection PROJECTION, OPTICAL.

optic aphasia APHASIA, OPTIC.

optic ataxia ATAXIA, OPTIC.

optic chiasm The point at the base of the brain where the fibres from the two optic nerves join and diverge. Fibres from the nasal (or inside) areas of each retina cross over at the chiasm; fibres from the temporal (or outside) portions of each retina remain on their original side. Thus the functional distribution of fibres is such that should there be damage to, say, the left *optic nerve* (prior to the chiasm), it would produce blindness in the left eye; damage to the left *optic tract* (after the chiasm) would produce lack of visual functioning in the left half of each retina, which would yield blindness in the right half of the visual field. var., *optic chiasma*.

optic disc The area of the retina where all the nerve fibres collect and leave as a bundle (the OPTIC NERVE). This area is also known as the BLIND SPOT, since there are very few receptors and it is therefore insensitive to light stimulation. Also called the *optic papilla*; var., *optic disk*.

optic flow The VECTORS (1) of an optical display that are produced as one navigates through an environment. The objects directly ahead appear motionless, while the other objects will appear to stream past on all sides. The faster one walks, the faster this stream or flow will appear. If one turns to the left, the visual image flows to the right, and so on. Also called *visual flow*.

optician One who is skilled in grinding lenses and fitting glasses. Distinguish from OPHTHALMOLOGIST and OPTOMETRIST.

optic nerve The IInd CRANIAL NERVE. Composed of two branches, each of which carries visual information from the ganglion cell layer of the retina of each eye to the OPTIC CHIASM, where the decussation (crossing-over) of axons that carry information from the nasal halves of each retina produces two nerve tracts each carrying a representation of half of the visual field to the LATERAL GENICULATE NUCLEI. The portion from the optic chiasm to the lateral geniculate bodies is called the *optic tract*.

optic papilla OPTIC DISC.

optics A branch of physics concerned with the study of light and its relationship to vision.

optic tract That part of the visual pathway from the OPTIC CHIASM to the LATERAL GENICULATE NUCLEI.

optimality theory In evolutionary theory the generalization that the traits that evolve are those that are optimal in the sense that their benefits exceed their costs by a greater amount than all other alternatives. The theory has been applied primarily to analysis of behaviours such as food-gathering and mating, where there are reasonably precise quantitative measures (e.g. calories gained or lost, or number of fertilizations per opportunity).

optimal stopping Ceasing to collect data in a study because the results are so compelling and clear that, from a statistical point of view, it is extremely unlikely that additional data will change the conclusions. Distinguish from OPTIONAL STOPPING FALLACY.

optimum That value from the range of values available that produces the maximum gain for the purpose under consideration. adj., *optimum*, *optimal*; vb., *optimize*.

optional stopping fallacy The unplanned stopping of an experiment at a point other than after the full set of trials that properly should have been run. It occurs in two forms: (a) stopping the experiment when it looks as if one's hypothesis is being supported; and (b) continuing to collect data past the point originally planned because it appears that one's hypothesis has not (yet) been supported. Either procedure leads to the drawing of fallacious conclusions. Distinguish from OPTIMAL STOPPING which is a legitimate procedure.

opto- Prefix denoting *vision* or, on occasion, the *eye*.

optogram The image of an external object on the retina. It results from the bleaching of the photopigments in the receptor cells.

optokinetic Pertaining to eye movements.

optokinetic nystagmus NYSTAGMUS, OPTOKINETIC.

optokinetic reflex The reflex-like movements of the eyes that compensate for head movements so that visual fixation is maintained.

optometrist One trained in OPTOMETRY. Distinguish from OPHTHALMOLOGIST and OPTICIAN.

optometry 1 The actual measurement of the refractive power of the visual apparatus. 2 A label for the profession of correcting vision by exercises and the fitting of corrective lenses. Distinguish from OPHTHALMOLOGY.

-opy OPIA.

oral Pertaining to either 1 the mouth, or 2 its primary product, speech. Most psychological terms embodying the former meaning are psychoanalytic and/or anatomical; most bearing the latter are concerned with language and speech and psycholinguistics. The term is used mainly in conjunction with another word or phrase, as revealed in the following entries. Distinguish from AURAL.

oral-aggressive In psychoanalytic theory, a pattern of aggressive behaviours in an adult which results, at least theoretically, from sublimation of the late oral stage. Behaviours assumed representative are ambition, envy, a pronounced tendency to exploit others and aggressiveness in personal interactions.

oral apraxia BUCCOFACIAL • APRAXIA.

oral cavity The cavity extending from the pharynx to the lips.

oral character In psychoanalytic theory: 1 A personality characteristic displayed by persons with fixations at the ORAL STAGE of development. 2 A personality type characterized by excessive derivation of satisfaction from oral eroticism. In the classic theory such personalities are assumed to be manifested through a tendency to be either (a) optimistic, dependent, generous and elated, or (b) pessimistic, depressed and aggressive. The former cluster of traits is assumed to result from abundant and pleasurable early oral experience, the latter from restrictive and harsh early oral experience.

oral dependence In psychoanalysis, the desire to return to the earliest stage of oral development. This desire is presumed to represent the seeking of the sense of security and safety that characterized this stage. In theory, the specific focus is the comfort of being held to the mother's breast and suckling.

oral drive Broadly, any drive focused on oral satisfaction, most specifically those drives associated with suckling and chewing.

oral dynamism Loosely, the interplay of psychic factors associated with oral characteristics.

oral eroticism Any tendency to obtain pleasure from oral activity. In psychoanalytic theory, oral eroticism normally characterizes the ORAL STAGE of development. When adults display excessive orality it is taken, within the theoretical framework, as evidence of regression to, or fixation at, this stage. Such behaviours as excessive smoking, talking, chewing, etc. are considered to be symptomatic. var., *oral erotism*.

oral-incorporative 1 Generally, in a young child, characterizing the tendency to put nearly everything into the mouth. **2** In psychoanalytic theory the term has the same behavioural reference, but it carries the connotation that this tendency is reflective of the desire on the part of the child to 'incorporate' the mother, particularly through the nipple, into itself. Some analysts argue for a distinct *oral-incorporative stage* of development, others maintain that it should merely be viewed as an aspect of the ORAL STAGE. The classical theory hypothesizes that possessiveness, greed, miserliness and the like are behaviours rooted in this tendency.

oralism See ORAL METHOD.

orality Pertaining to: **1** Specifically, ORAL EROTICISM. **2** More generally, any oral component emerging in a psychoneurosis or other disorder.

oral libido stage ORAL STAGE.

oral method A method of teaching language to the deaf through lip-reading and the shaping of speech. See MANUAL METHOD for a comparison and further discussion. Also called *oralism*.

oral neurosis A term used by some psychoanalysts to refer to various speech impediments such as stammering or stuttering, on the assumption that these result from disorders of the oral libido. There is not much evidence on this point and, frankly, it is far from clear as to what would constitute evidence anyway. See SPEECH DISORDER.

oral-passive RECEPTIVE CHARACTER.

oral personality ORAL CHARACTER.

oral primacy In psychoanalytic theory, the concentration of libido upon the mouth, evidenced by using the tongue and lips to explore things and by deriving pleasure from sucking, biting and chewing. In infancy it is regarded as normal, in adults abnormal.

oral regression A tendency to return to the ORAL STAGE.

oral sadism In psychoanalysis, the desire to inflict pain through oral means. Generally, biting is considered the prime behaviour, although some analysts include verbal attack as symptomatic.

oral stage The first and most primitive of the psychosexual stages of development hypothesized by classical psychoanalytic theory. During this stage the mouth is the focus of the libido and satisfaction is obtained through sucking, biting, chewing, etc. In some analytical frameworks the stage is subdivided into an *early* component characterized by passivity and a *late* component characterized by activity, particularly aggressive activity. Also called *oral libido stage*.

oral test Loosely, any test in which the materials are presented and responded to orally.

oral triad A rather specialized psychoanalytic term applied to three, theoretically coordinated, desires to be suckled by, sleep with and be devoured by the breast.

ora serrata See ORA TERMINALIS.

ora terminalis The very edge of the retina. Also called *ora serrata*.

Orbison figures The figure on page 536 is actually a perfect square, the one on the right a circle.

orbital Pertaining to any orbit but most frequently used in reference to the bony cavity in which the eye is set.

orbitofrontal cortex An area at the base of the frontal lobes just above the orbits. It has an array of complex inputs from various cortical areas, the thalamus, the olfactory bulbs

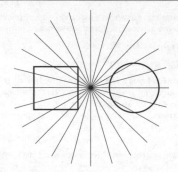

and the amygdala. Its outputs are similarly diverse, going to the hippocampus, areas of the hypothalamus and the amygdala. It plays an important role in emotion and was one of the areas destroyed in the famous case of PHINEAS *GAGE.

orchiectomy Surgical removal of a testicle. See CASTRATION. vars., *orchectomy, orchidectomy*.

orchi(o)- Combining form meaning *testicle*.

order Most of the meanings of this word in psychology derive from standard dictionary definitions. A few, however, rate explication: **1** Any arrangement of facts, data, events, etc. in time (*temporal order*) or space (*spatial order*) or both (*spatio-temporal order*). **2** Any position in an ordered series of events. **3** A category in the phylogenetic classification system just above *family* and below *class*. Meanings 1 and 2 have a verb form, so that *to order* means to arrange facts, events, data etc. in a particular fashion. See the following entries for some special forms. Note, *ordering* is a common synonym of 1 and 2.

order, cyclic An ordering of items that displays a regular cycle, e.g. 112233112233...

order effects Effects that are attributed to the order in which treatments are presented in an experiment. Order effects can confound an experiment and typically COUNTERBALANCING procedures are employed as a control.

order, linear An order in which all items are presented as though they were on a line, e.g. 1st, 2nd, 3rd, 4th. Note that only order is implied here, not magnitude of interval. Thus, for example, the 3rd score is not neces-

sarily larger than the 2nd to the same degree as the 2nd is larger than the 1st. See ORDINAL *SCALE.

order of magnitude 1 An ordering of data or events from the lowest to the highest. This use of the term is essentially synonymous with LINEAR *ORDER. **2** A tenfold increase.

order statistics Statistical tests which can be carried out on data that only reflect ORDINAL *SCALE properties. All order statistics are NONPARAMETRIC STATISTICS, although the reverse is not true.

ordinal (position) A somewhat redundant phrase (in that *ordinal* is a close synonym of *positional*) used to refer to ranked location in an ordered array, i.e. 1st, 2nd, etc.

ordinal scale SCALE, ORDINAL.

ordinate The vertical coordinate of a point in a plane Cartesian coordinate system. Commonly, although strictly speaking not correctly, the *y*-axis is called by this name. In standard notation, values of the DEPENDENT *VARIABLE are plotted on the ordinate. See also AXIS, CARTESIAN COORDINATES.

orectic Pertaining to the appetitive and affective aspects of behaviour. In psychoanalytic writings, the orectic is often contrasted with the cognitive. var., *orexic*. n., *orexis*.

Orestes complex In classical psychoanalytic theory, the (hopefully) repressed desire of a son to commit matricide.

organ Generally, any structural part of an organism that has a specific function (or functions) to perform. Note that the adjectival form ORGANIC has several additional meanings other than, simply, pertaining to an organ.

organelle A specialized part of a cell that performs a specific function.

organ eroticism In psychoanalytic theory, the experiencing of eroticism associated with a particular organ. Also called *organ libido*; var., *organ erotism*.

organic 1 Pertaining to an organ. **2** Essential or vital. **3** Pertaining to the intrinsic organization of a thing, to its existence as a synthesis of elemental parts. **4** Occasionally, pertaining to an organism; ORGANISMIC is preferred here. **5** Pertaining to that which is somatic as opposed to that which is mental. In this last sense, organic is contrasted with FUNCTIONAL. The term, in sense (5), has long been in use in clinical psychology and psychiatry for denoting disorders and syndromes that are due to known biological and neurological conditions, specifically those affecting the brain. The latest edition of the DIAGNOSTIC AND STATISTICAL MANUAL, which is approved for use in the US, has removed many of the clinically relevant diagnostic categories previously marked as *organic*, including *organic affective syndrome, organic brain syndrome, organic delusional disorder, organic dementia, organic hallucinosis, organic mental disorder, organic mood syndrome* and *organic personality syndrome*. However, these terms are still found in many texts and still widely used and definitions of each are included under the appropriate heading.

organic affective syndrome See ORGANIC MOOD SYNDROME.

organic anxiety Anxiety resulting from known organic dysfunction. The term may refer to normal apprehension resulting from the awareness of the very real consequences of a serious disease or to a neurotic overanxious reaction to a disability. See ANGINAPHOBIA for an example of the latter.

organic anxiety syndrome An ORGANIC MENTAL SYNDROME characterized by prominent, recurrent panic attacks or generalized anxiety caused by some specific organic factor such as an endocrine disorder or the abuse of psychoactive substances.

organic approach The position that argues that all disorders, be they psychological, mental, physical, psychiatric (or any other adjective one chooses to use) are, at their core, based on neurophysiological functions. In some very basic way either this is true or some form of dualism is true and most scientists are leery of dualism. However, many are reluctant to embrace this position, feeling that it diminishes the humanity of the client/patient. Also called *organicism*.

organic brain syndrome ORGANIC MENTAL SYNDROME.

organic delusional syndrome DELUSIONAL SYNDROME, ORGANIC.

organic dementia DEMENTIA, ORGANIC.

organic disorder Loosely, any disorder that is caused by a known organic condition. Contrast with FUNCTIONAL DISORDER and, for more details, see ORGANIC MENTAL SYNDROME and ORGANIC MENTAL DISORDER.

organic hallucinosis HALLUCINOSIS.

organicism 1 A sociological theory, first expressed by Herbert Spencer, that treats society as an analogue to an organic, biological system. This 'organic' model draws the parallel between units and elements of society and the biological organ. Sometimes called *social organism model*. 2 See ORGANIC APPROACH.

organic mental disorder An umbrella term in contemporary psychiatry for a large number of disorders all of which are associated with some organic (brain) dysfunction, either transitory or permanent, and of which the aetiologies are either known or can be presumed on the basis of other facts and data. It is this factor regarding aetiology that distinguishes usage of this term from ORGANIC MENTAL SYNDROME. Note, however, that the diagnosis of an organic mental disorder is predicated on an initial diagnosis of an organic mental syndrome; hence a general diagnosis such as *dementia* is regarded as an organic mental syndrome, while specific forms (e.g. *primary degenerative dementia*) are classified as organic mental disorders. Recognize, also, that in contemporary clinical psychology and psychiatry most researchers and practitioners operate on the presumption, taken as an article of faith rather than on any definitive evidence, that ultimately all serious disorders (or psychoses) will be shown to be organic in origin. The existence, however, of distinct classes of organic disorders does not necessarily imply that nonorganic (i.e. functional) disorders are independent of brain processes. Rather, a nonorganic diagnosis tends to be made when either of two criteria pertain: (a) social/behavioural factors provide a cogent characterization of the disorder (e.g. *adjustment disorder*), or (b) the presence of a specific organic factor, although suspected, has not been established (e.g. the *schizophrenias*). Note that the term itself is no longer listed in the *DSM*. See discussion under ORGANIC (5).

organic mental syndrome A cover term for a number of disorders, including AMNESTIC

SYNDROME, DELIRIUM, DEMENTIA, ORGANIC *DELU-
SIONAL SYNDROME, ORGANIC MOOD SYNDROME
and ORGANIC *PERSONALITY SYNDROME. Each of
these disorders is characterized by particular
symptoms, but, unlike the case of the
ORGANIC MENTAL DISORDERS, no reference is
made to their aetiology. Also called *organic
brain syndrome*. This diagnostic category is no
longer listed in the *DSM*. See discussion
under ORGANIC (5).

organic mood syndrome An ORGANIC MEN-
TAL SYNDROME characterized by a prominent
and persistent depressed, elevated or expansive mood resembling the kinds of moods
seen in a MANIC EPISODE or MAJOR *DEPRESSIVE EPI-
SODE. The term is only used when there are
toxic or metabolic factors in the aetiology.
This diagnostic category is no longer listed
in the *DSM*. See discussion under ORGANIC (5).

organic organization ORGANIZATION,
ORGANIC.

organic personality syndrome PERSONAL-
ITY SYNDROME, ORGANIC.

organic psychosis Loosely, any severe
mental disorder due to either known or
strongly suspected brain pathologies. For
more on contemporary terminology, see
ORGANIC MENTAL DISORDER and ORGANIC MENTAL
SYNDROME.

organic repression REPRESSION, ORGANIC.

organic selection See BALDWIN EFFECT.

organic sensations A term now largely
abandoned for the more appropriate VISCERAL
SENSATIONS.

organic variable In post-Watsonian behaviourism, any internal process or state that
was assumed to play a role in determining
the response observed. In the initial behaviourist conceptualization, all behaviours
were viewed simply as S–R processes; that
is, the stimulus (S) was regarded as the sole
causal agent of the response (R) once conditioning was complete. More sober minds
soon recognized that there was a need for
'organic' variables within the behaving
organism upon which the stimuli impinged
and which played a role in the production of
the observed behaviour. abbrev., *O variable*.
See also ORGANISMIC VARIABLE (a descriptively
more accurate term) and INTERVENING *VARI-
ABLE.

organ inferiority As proposed by Adler,
the notion that deficiencies in organ function (real or imagined) can produce a sense
of inferiority.

organism Loosely, any living thing, be it
plant or animal, bacterium or virus. This sort
of definition is only moderately satisfying for
it results in little more than a list of those
entities generally regarded as being organisms. Ideally, we should have a clear definition of what is meant by *living*, and thus
dispense with the list – and also eliminate
arguments over just what things deserved
to be listed; not all would put viruses on it.
The difficulty, however, is that attempts to
define LIFE themselves make for lists; e.g. a
living thing is that which carries out some
(or all) of the basic physiological functions of
ingestion, excretion, reproduction, locomotion, etc. As there is currently no agreed-
upon criterial set of features for determination of that which is living, there is no rigorous definition of that which qualifies as an
organism. Generally speaking, the term is
used in psychology to refer to an animal, particularly one used in an experiment or other
scientific study.

organismic In simplest terms, pertaining to
an organism. However, this straightforward
use is rare. More often, the term is used to
refer to any of several theoretical approaches
that emphasize the need to view a behaving
organism as a biological entity, one which
must be approached as the coordinated functioning of a multitude of interrelated processes. Organismic approaches are
uniformly *monistic*, rejecting mind–body
dualism, and tend to focus on larger, more
molar analyses to the relative neglect of
reductionistic analyses.

organismic determinant DETERMINANT.

organismic psychology ORGANISMIC.

organismic variable Lit., a variable inside
an organism; a process or operation that
occurs internally but is hypothesized to
play a causal role in determining overt
responding. See also ORGANIC VARIABLE.

organization 1 A characteristic of any complex system that reflects the degree to which
its several structurally distinguishable parts
are functionally coordinated and interrelated. **2** The process that operates so as to

bring about such a coordinated system. **3** The system itself as it displays such properties.

This term, particularly in sense 3, represents a very powerful concept in the social (and, for that matter, the physical) sciences. In all cases the central connotation is one of *structure*; diverse parts or elements are coordinated to form an integrated, coherent and systematic whole. This notion of an organization is represented in such areas as: (a) GESTALT PSYCHOLOGY, in which it refers to the processes whereby a perceptual GESTALT is formed (see also GESTALT LAWS OF ORGANIZA-TION); (b) cognitive theory, in which it serves as a vehicle for expressing the notion that thought is more than a simple linear arrangement of primitive processes (see COGNITIVE *ORGANIZATION); (c) social psychology, in which it refers to a GROUP (2) as a structured collection of individuals (see here SOCIAL *ORGANIZATION); and (d) INDUSTRIAL/ORGANIZA-TIONAL PSYCHOLOGY, in which the reference is to a complex social system made up of individuals, their facilities and the products yielded. In this last sense, which is admittedly very general, a small corner shop qualifies as an (albeit relatively simple) organization, as does a multinational corporation, a political party or a university. Because of the great latitude of reference here, several criteria are usually applied so as to limit the meaning. To wit: there must be coordination of effort of the personnel, who must have some set of common goals or purposes, there has to be some division of labour within the larger structure, and there must also be some degree of integrated functioning, including a hierarchy of authority. vb., *organize*; adjs., *organized, organizational*. See the following entries for a number of other specialized usages of the basic term.

organizational assessment Loosely, any process used to assess the functioning of an ORGANIZATION (3), focusing on the basic question, 'Is the organization performing up to expected standards?' See INDUSTRIAL/ORGANIZA-TIONAL PSYCHOLOGY.

organizational development (OD) A subfield within INDUSTRIAL/ORGANIZATIONAL PSYCH-OLOGY that focuses on improving the functioning of organizations. The approach is eclectic and looks at factors such as individual and group dynamics, issues of personal satisfaction and self-esteem and

relations between the various levels in the organizational hierarchy.

organizational dynamics A term used to refer collectively to the various patterns of shifting (i.e. dynamic) elements within an ORGANIZATION (3(d)).

organizational psychology INDUSTRIAL/ ORGANIZATIONAL PSYCHOLOGY.

organization, cognitive An extension of the connotations of the Gestalt PRINCIPLE OF *ORGANIZATION from the study of perception (where it was first introduced) to the subject-matter of cognitive psychology in general. The essential notion remains the same, that it is the coherent, structured whole that dominates what one perceives or knows; however, the force of the qualifier *cognitive* is to drive the meaning of the term organization beyond the perceptual issues and to apply it to the cognitive domain in all manifestations. To wit: the meaning of a sentence is determined by the whole and not by a summation of the meanings of its several words; the meaning of a position in a chess game is given by the entire configuration and not by the individual pieces in isolation; the knowledge that a researcher or practitioner of psychology has of the field is derived from the coordination of many diverse facts, principles and experiences and is not simply a compendium of, say, the terms used in the discipline.

organization, formal A term occasionally used of an ORGANIZATION (3(c) and (d)) to differentiate it from an INFORMAL *ORGANIZATION.

organization, informal A term for the set of integrated and coordinated activities that the individuals in a group have with each other. The adjective *informal* is used to differentiate these patterns of behaviour, which are often spontaneous and function without well-articulated rules or blueprints for interaction, from the more *formal* patterns entailed by the simple term ORGANIZATION (esp. 3(c) and (d)).

organization, mechanistic An ORGANIZA-TION (3(d)) characterized by a rigid overall structure with clearly defined roles for its members and a clearly specified hierarchy of authority. Mechanistic organizations are relatively easy to establish, but have the disadvantage that they do not respond well to change. Compare with ORGANIC *ORGANIZA-TION.

organization, organic An ORGANIZATION (3 (d)) characterized by a loose overall structure without a clear hierarchy of authority and underdefined tasks and responsibilities for its members. Organic organizations are difficult to establish, but once set up have the advantage of responding well to change. Compare with MECHANISTIC *ORGANIZATION.

organization, principle of As proposed by the Gestalt psychologists, the principle that the separate elements of a GESTALT are not all equally important in determining what is perceived. Rather, it is the integration or organized whole that is deemed critical. According to W. Köhler, who championed this view, this structuring of the stimulus information is assumed to occur without consciousness. For an extension of this basic idea, see COGNITIVE *ORGANIZATION.

organization, social **1** The (relatively) stable set of behavioural patterns of individuals and groups within a society, particularly as they are representative of the SOCIAL NORMS, RULES (3) and ROLES of the society. **2** Loosely, a formally established social group; see ORGANIZATION (esp. 3(c) and (d)).

organized play PLAY, ORGANIZED.

organ libido ORGAN EROTICISM.

organ neurosis A term from classical psychoanalysis which has been largely replaced by PSYCHOSOMATIC DISORDER.

organ of Corti The complex structure in the cochlea of the inner ear including the basilar membrane, the hair cells which are attached to it and the tectorial membrane to which they in turn attach. Vibrations produce deflections of the basilar membrane relative to the more rigid tectorial membrane, which stretches the cilia of the hair cells, resulting in the receptor potential. The structure is named after the Italian anatomist Alfonso Corti.

orgasm A complex sequence of processes occurring at the climax of sexual activity involving involuntary movements of the genital organs, voluntary movements of related muscle groups and neurophysiological responses keyed by spinal action that result in strong pleasurable sexual feelings culminating in an abrupt sense of relief of tension and, in the male, the ejaculation of semen. adjs., *orgasmic, orgastic.*

orgasm disorders A category of SEXUAL DISORDERS marked by persistent or recurrent delay in, or absence of, orgasm following a normal phase of sexual excitement. The term is only used when there is no evidence of another condition that can interfere with sexual functioning, such as depression or drug use. It should not be applied unless there is evidence that the condition causes marked distress or interpersonal difficulty. There are many individuals with little or no orgasmic function who are quite content in that state, and applying the term to them is inappropriate. The term is gender neutral. A variety of other terms has been used over the years for these disorders, including *female* (or *male*) *orgasmic disorder, inhibited* (*female* or *male*) *orgasm, orgasmic* (or *orgastic*) *dysfunction* (for females), and *orgasmic impotence* (for males).

orgasmic dysfunction ORGASM DISORDERS.

orgasmic impotence ORGASM DISORDERS.

orgastic dysfunction/impotence ORGASM DISORDERS.

orgone theory A theory due to Wilhelm Reich, a creative and innovative thinker who, in his search for truth, pushed his basically psychoanalytic system into what became, alas, utterly ludicrous and totally dismissible forms. Essentially, it is a theory of being, based on the hypothesization of a specific form of energy (orgone energy) which was assumed to fill all space and account for all life. Such a concept invites all manner of metaphysical problems; not the least is the problem of identifying the orgone, for in order to demonstrate the existence of something one must be able to ascertain where it is not, so as to know where it is. Put simply, if something is uniformly everywhere it might as well be nowhere. Recognition of this problem led Reich to build his 'orgone accumulator', a device which ultimately led to serious legal problems with the US Food and Drug Administration. See also ORGONOMY.

orgone therapy ORGONOMY.

orgonomy The term generally used to refer

to the personality theory and accompanying therapeutic practices developed by Wilhelm Reich. The central theoretical concept is the hypothesized universal energy form, orgone (see ORGONE THEORY), and the therapy (*orgone therapy*) is based on a rather elaborate programme of massage, manipulation, probing and prodding, directing the client toward the ultimate orgastic release that Reich conceived of as the prime evidence of therapeutic breakthrough. See also BIOFUNCTIONAL THERAPY.

orientation   Since originally *the orient* referred to *the East* or *the sunrise*, *orientation* meant turning toward the East. Today the geographical link has been lost but the sense of turning or focusing is still with us. To wit: **1** In ethology, turning or adjusting the body or parts of the body with respect to specific stimulation. See here TAXIS and TROPISM. **2** The specific position of a body or part thereof. Here one sees references to the orientation of a cell, organ, limb, etc. **3** Knowledge or awareness of one's location and position. The term is used in this sense either literally, concerning physical space and time, or, by extension, with regard to one's figurative place in terms of the social, interpersonal and conceptual framework. **4** A cognitive SET (2), a conceptual point of view that yields a characteristic disposition to react to events. **5** A particular world view, a very general perspective on life, science, philosophy, etc. Meaning 5 is distinguished from 4 only in degree of generality. **6** A programme of instruction designed to assist one to orient oneself in any of the above senses. This meaning is, however, typically expressed in a more restrictive fashion and applied to achieving an orientation of types 3, 4 or 5 with a view to carrying out some occupation or task. Indeed, many jobs and occupations have an *orientation programme* for newcomers associated with them. vb., *orient*; adjs., *oriented* (the preferred form), *orientated*.

orientation column   A column of neurons in the VISUAL CORTEX that respond maximally to stimuli in the same orientation. Neighbouring columns display maximal responding to stimuli of slightly displaced orientations.

orienting reflex   ORIENTING RESPONSE.

orienting response   **1** Most generally, any turning of the body with reference to the position of a specific stimulus. In this sense, the term is essentially synonymous with TROPISM. **2** In Pavlovian terms, any attentional response made to a stimulus, e.g. head-turning, ear-raising. **3** Any response of an organism that functions to bring it into a position whereby it is optimally exposed to stimulation. This meaning is an extension of 2, which connotes a rather reflex-like quality (and, indeed, *orienting reflex* is often used for meaning 2), and applies the concept to a more directed kind of behaviour.

orphenadrine   An ANTICHOLINERGIC drug used as a muscle relaxant and as a therapeutic adjunct in treatment of DRUG-INDUCED *PARKINSONISM.

ortho-   Combining form from the Greek, literally meaning *straight* and, by extension, *correct*, *normal*, *proper*.

orthogenesis   Lit., straight from the beginning; hence, a label for any of several doctrines predicated on the notion of development as set at the beginning such that it will proceed in a particular fashion controlled by internal forces unless cata strophically disrupted by outside forces. It has been proposed at various times as a theory of evolution, as a model of ontogeny and as a theory of social and cultural development. adj., *orthogenic*.

orthognathy   An anatomical arrangement in which the jaw does not project far beyond the cranium, i.e. the jaw and the cranium lie approximately along the same vertical plane. Contrast with PROGNATHY.

orthogonal   At right angles. By extension, characteristic of any set of variables in an experiment that are independent of each other.

orthogonal rotation   ROTATION (2).

orthogonal solution   In factor analysis, a solution in which the axes that represent the underlying factors are situated so that they are at right angles to each other. In such a solution, the factors are uncorrelated. Compare with OBLIQUE SOLUTION.

orthogonal trait   In a factor-analysis matrix, any trait that is independent of, and hence shows a zero correlation with, all others.

orthographic dysgraphia   DYSGRAPHIA, ORTHOGRAPHIC.

orthography   A generic term for any writing system. For details on various types see ALPHABET, LOGOGRAPHY, SEMASIOGRAPHY, SYLLABARY.

orthomolecular psychiatry   An approach to psychiatric therapy that focuses on the attainment of appropriate balances and concentrations of normal bodily substances. This approach has as its basic assumption the notion that abnormal behaviours are the result of biochemical imbalances, or, as it is commonly phrased, 'For every twisted mind there must be a twisted molecule.'

orthopractic   From the theological term *'orthodox praxis'*, characterizing religions and belief systems characterized by a rigorous code of conduct.

orthopsychiatry   A discipline dealing primarily with the prevention and early treatment of mental and emotional disorders. Although the term *psychiatry* is included in the name, in practice the discipline extends beyond psychiatric medicine and involves clinical psychology, pediatrics, social work and education.

os   **1** Mouth or opening. pl., *ora*. **2** Bone. pl., *ossa*.

oscillation   A swinging back and forth, a fluctuation between states. Almost all uses in psychology carry this basic notion. Note, however, that often, particularly in usages that derive from physics, the implication is that the oscillation is regular, like a sine wave. This sense is not always carried over into psychological usage, where frequently the notion is that the oscillation is irregular and variable. See e.g. BEHAVIOURAL OSCILLATION. abbrev., *O*.

oscillometer   Any device for measuring oscillations.

oscilloscope   An electronic device for recording and displaying in a visual form the wave form of changing electrical current, voltage or other quantity that can be represented as electrical change.

-osis   A multifunctional suffix. **1** A diseased state, a variation of -IASIS. **2** Development of a form. **3** A process or state.

osm(o)-   Combining form: **1** From the Greek *osme*, meaning *smell* or *odour*. **2** From the Greek *osmos*, meaning an *impulse*, a *thrusting forth*. **3** By extension of 2, pertaining to OSMOSIS.

osmometric thirst   THIRST, OSMOMETRIC.

osmoreceptor   The inferred receptors that respond to changes in osmotic pressure in cells and, hence, serve as the mediators of OSMOMETRIC *THIRST. The available evidence suggests that they are located in the nucleus circularis of the hypothalamus and function by regulating the secretion of antidiuretic hormone.

osmosis   The diffusion of a solvent through a semi-permeable membrane on either side of which are solutions of different concentrations. The solvent passes through from the side of the lower concentration to the side of the higher and tends to equalize the concentrations.

osphresiolagnia   Erotic experience produced by an odour.

osphresis   OLFACTION, the sense of smell.

ossicle   Any small bone.

ossicles, auditory   The set of three small bones (the *malleus* or hammer, the *incus* or anvil and the *stapes* or stirrup) in the middle ear which transmit the vibrations of the eardrum to the cochlea.

ossify   Lit., to become bone-like; figuratively, to harden, to become inflexible.

O technique   R CORRELATION.

Othello syndrome   A serious, morbid jealousy accompanied by delusions that one's spouse is unfaithful.

other behaviour   In operant-conditioning literature any behaviour other than that which is specifically being reinforced or punished.

other conditions that may be a focus of clinical attention   A rather awkward phrase for a group of psychological, emotional or behavioural conditions that call for clinical attention but do not quality for an 'official' diagnosis by criteria outlined in the latest edition of the *diagnostic and statistical manual*.

other-directed OUTER-DIRECTED.

other, the 1 Most generally, everyone and everything but oneself. In essence this meaning encompasses the entire matrix of events, stimuli, persons, etc. that make up the psychological environment. **2** More specifically, a person not oneself. **3** Most specifically, G. H. Mead's term (used in the plural) for referring collectively to the SIGNIFICANT OTHERS in one's life.

otic Pertaining to the ear or, more specifically, to the receptor cells in the inner ear.

otitis Inflammation of the ear; usually marked as *externa, media* or *interna* depending on the location of the inflammation.

ot(o)- Combining form meaning *the ear*.

otogenic tone A tone produced by the mechanisms within the ear and not objectively present in the environment. See e.g. COMBINATION TONE.

otolaryngology A medical specialization dealing with the ear (otology), nose (rhinology) and the throat (laryngology).

otoliths Tiny calcium crystals suspended in the endolymph of the labyrinth of the inner ear. Movements of the head set the endolymph in motion and the otoliths stimulate the receptor cells, thus providing feedback information that assists in the maintenance of body balance.

otology The science concerned with the ear, its anatomy, physiology and pathology.

otosclerosis A condition characterized by chronic, progressive loss of hearing caused by a build-up of bone around the oval window with attendant immobility of the *stapes* or stirrup.

outbreeding The tendency to mate with individuals who are not closely related genetically; the opposite of INBREEDING. The limits on outbreeding are usually established at the species boundary in that matings further removed typically do not produce viable and fertile offspring. See also INBREEDING AVOIDANCE.

outcome Very generally: **1** Any change in the environment that occurs as a result of an organism's behaviour. **2** Any change in an organism as a result of events in the environment.

outcomes assessment A branch of applied psychology that focuses on assessing the outcomes of social or behavioural programmes. In contrast to the similar term *evaluation*, outcomes assessment does not imply the placing of subjective value or worth on the outcomes being measured, and is therefore preferred by many practitioners as seeming less judgemental.

outercourse Loosely, sexual behaviour not involving COITUS. Because SEXUAL INTERCOURSE has loosened its meaning over the years, this term has been introduced for clarity. Clarity it has, we admit, but as a term we hope we will not need to include it in the next edition.

outer-directed Within the sociological framework of D. Riesman, a tendency to conform to societal values and to be overly sensitized to the expectations and preferences of others. According to Riesman, modern urban societies foster such outer-directedness. The term is applied both to the person who displays these characteristics and to the society itself. Also known as *other-directed*. See also INNER-DIRECTED and TRADITION-DIRECTED.

out-group Quite simply, a group comprised of any and all persons not in one's IN-GROUP. Also occasionally called *they-group*.

out-group homogeneity bias The tendency of members of one group to assume that there is greater similarity among the members of out-groups than there actually is.

outlet Loosely, any activity that serves to relieve a state of tension, reduce a drive, satisfy a need, etc.

outlier Any subject or data point that has an extreme value on some variable. Outliers may represent anomalous data points (e.g. a subject who didn't sleep the night before an experiment, a trial during which the subject sneezed) and can distort one's interpretation of the data. Statistical procedures exist that correct for the effects of outliers.

out-of-body experience A compelling sense that one's mind or self has left one's body and is located elsewhere, often experienced as being above the body, looking down on it. Thought by some to be a manifestation of a paranormal effect (see PARA-PSYCHOLOGY), it appears to be the result of inappropriate neural firing in the *angular gyrus*, which is part of a complex multisensory processing system. An out-of-body experience can also be created in normal individuals by a combination of ambiguous inputs created using a virtual reality set-up in which individuals see an illusory image of themselves and are prodded with various physical stimuli.

outpatient Any nonhospitalized patient who regularly visits a hospital or clinic for treatment.

outpatient clinic CLINIC, OUTPATIENT.

output 1 Generally and literally, that which is put out; any response from an organism or any product of a system. **2** In information theory, the signal emitted.

ova Plural of OVUM.

oval window The membrane in the wall of the cochlea to which the *stapes* or stirrup is attached. It is through the vibration of this membrane that sound waves are carried to the inner ear.

ovarian Pertaining to the OVARY.

ovarian follicle MENSTRUAL CYCLE.

ovariectomy Surgical removal of the ovaries. var., *ovariotomy*.

ovary One of a pair of the primary reproductive organs in the female. The ovaries are glandular organs connected via the Fallopian tubes to the uterus. Ovaries produce the *ova* (pl. of *ovum*) and the *oestrogens*.

over- A common prefix meaning *excessive, more than what is required*. In psychoanalytic writing, it often carries the implication of a pathological condition of sheer excess.

overachiever One whose actual performance on a task or in a situation (e.g. school) is higher than one would have predicted. *Predicted* is used rather loosely here; strictly speaking there should be valid test scores from which to make predictions, otherwise labels like *overachiever* and *underachiever* (its opposite) lack real meaning.

There is a curious aspect to these labels:

*over*achiever has a vaguely insulting connotation whereas *under*achiever carries a kind of subtle praise. It is as if we hold higher what we believe people are capable of doing than what they actually do. Or, then again, maybe it is that we think our tests of intelligence and aptitude are better than they actually are.

overanxious disorder A GENERALIZED ANXIETY DISORDER of childhood characterized by excessive and inappropriate anxiety and fearfulness that is not focused on or associated with a specific situation or object and not due to a particular psychosocial stressor. Children with the disorder display an inordinate concern with future events, are overly concerned about their own performance (scholastic, social, athletic) and often have a variety of psychosomatic complaints.

overcompensation A term used with somewhat less precision than the root word, COMPENSATION. The basic idea is that *over*compensatory behaviour is that which is more than what is really required to make up for or offset some liability. Part of the confusion over the term comes from the fact that some writers use it with a distinctly positive connotation (implying that through extraordinary effort a person has achieved great heights in spite of, or perhaps because of, initial deficiencies), while others use it to connote a kind of negative overreaction (implying that the individual is somehow engaging in pathological and harmful excesses).

overconfidence effect The common tendency of people to overestimate the accuracy, appropriateness and effectiveness of their behaviour. Ironically, this tendency is usually strongest in the poorest performers. The effect is exacerbated when the objective standards of performance are not immediately apparent.

overcontrollers See EGO-CONTROL.

overcrowding CROWDING.

overdetermined Generally, having many causes. In psychoanalysis, a dream, an act, an emotion, etc. is considered overdetermined if it appears to have resulted from the expression of more than one drive, conflict or other unconscious determiner.

overeating HYPERPHAGIA.

overexclusion A perceptual/cognitive deficit characterized by a tendency to exclude, rather rigidly, alternative responses or choices. The term tends to be used in cases of genuine deficit, not of simple UNDERGENERALIZATION.

overexpectation In animal conditioning, a learning situation in which two stimuli are conditioned separately and then the combined stimulus is conditioned. Later testing with either of the two original stimuli separately shows lower responding than during initial training. The term is used to suggest the notion that, after the combined training phase, the animal's 'expectations' are raised and the subsequent presentation of either original stimulus alone is something of a 'let-down'.

overextension OVERGENERALIZATION.

overflow activity VACUUM ACTIVITY.

overgeneralization The extension of the use of a word to cover circumstances, events or objects beyond those that it is normally used for. Such *overextensions* (as they are also called) are common among young children, e.g. calling a horse a 'doggie'. Compare with UNDERGENERALIZATION.

overinclusion A perceptual/cognitive deficit characterized by failure to screen out the irrelevant, the inefficient and the inappropriate. The term is generally used only in cases of genuine deficit, not of simple OVERGENERALIZATION.

overjustification The stance adopted by an individual who, having carried out some task for the simple intrinsic pleasure of it, becomes less inclined to perform the task again for no reward after a period in which they have received extrinsic rewards.

overlapping factor In a factor analysis, any factor that is common to (i.e. overlaps with) more than one test.

overlearning Overlearning is said to occur when a response has been overlearned. This painfully tautological definition is not very satisfying; the problem is that one can only classify a response as *overlearned* when one has some established criterion against which to measure it, hence overlearning is always relative. In the typical experimental study of overlearning some defining condition for learning is set, say 10 correct responses in a row. Some subjects are then run to some overlearning point, say 20 consecutive correct responses, and the impact of this additional training is assessed. Thus, the concept itself is necessarily arbitrary and is always definitionally contingent upon some previously set notion of what is to be considered *learning*.

overload Laboratory jargon used primarily in the information-processing approach to cognitive psychology to refer to the condition of having too much information to deal with at a point in time or too much material to commit to memory in the time available.

overpopulation CROWDING.

overprotection A term commonly used to characterize parental behaviour that is indulgent, pampering, solicitous, encapsulating, sheltering, and fostering of dependencies to an excessive degree. The problem with this usage lies in that word *excessive*. Usually, clinicians consider parents to have been overprotective when their child fails to develop normal independence. Hence, the term functions in an entirely *post hoc* fashion.

overreaction Very generally, any response that is greater than one would have expected given the circumstances. The implication is that there is an emotional element to the response, and, indeed, the adjective *emotional* is often prefixed in psychological writings.

overshadowing In animal conditioning, a learning situation in which a compound conditioned stimulus is used but one element of the stimulus (e.g. a rather loud tone) dominates the other (e.g. a dim light). After training, the dominant stimulus *overshadows* the other and only it will produce responding when presented alone. Compare with CONFIGURATIONAL LEARNING.

overshooting In a PROBABILITY LEARNING experiment, predicting the most likely of two (or more) events with a higher probability than actually occurs. Compare with MAXIMIZING and PROBABILITY MATCHING.

overt That which is open, available, detectable by whoever observes it. Overt behaviour is usually what the strict behaviourist argues should be the subject-matter of psychology.

Note that the use of the term has expanded in recent decades as technology has made that which was covert open for observation. See also COVERT.

overtone Any partial tone produced by a vibrating body other than the FUNDAMENTAL TONE.

ovum The female sex cell, the egg. pl., *ova*.

own-control design An experimental design in which each participant serves as his or her own control. It consists of repeatedly alternating procedures with the same individual and assessing the effect(s) that each has. It is used routinely in intensive case studies in psychiatry, particularly in the use of drug-treatment programmes.

own-group conformity pressure The social and behavioural consequences of the expectations of one's social group of origin. For example, someone from a poor or working-class background might be pressured to not be too 'snobbish', or someone from a non-Caucasian group might be pressured to not act 'white'.

own-race bias The tendency of individuals to exhibit better perception and memory for individuals of their own race. It can cause difficulties in the use of EYEWITNESS TESTIMONY in legal proceedings.

oxazepam A BENZODIAZEPINE COMPOUND used to treat drug withdrawal, anxiety and sleep disorders. Sold under a host of trade names: Alepam, Murelax, Serax, Serepax, Seresta.

oxygen deprivation HYPOXIA.

oxytocin A hormone secreted by the posterior lobe of the pituitary gland which acts on blood pressure, strengthens uterine contractions and controls the milk-ejecting function of the mammary glands. Oxytocin levels are also correlated with the formation of mother–infant bonding.

P 1 PROBABILITY RATIO. **2** The symbol for *stability of personality* in Eysenck's theory. **3** SUBSTANCE P. **4** PERCENTILE.

p 1 The *probability* of a specifiable event or outcome. Here the common use is as a statement of STATISTICAL SIGNIFICANCE. **2** The *proportion* of events in a population exhibiting a particular characteristic and distinguishable from a mutually exclusive proportion of events, q, such that $p + q = 1$. **3** A *percentage*.

P300 A positive EVOKED POTENTIAL that peaks at approximately 300 msec after an event, particularly when the event is unexpected or provides useful information for some task. It is easily produced by a novel stimulus (e.g. a circle after a series of triangles) but can also be observed with a non-event (e.g. a moment of silence following a steady series of 'beep' sounds). If the information is complex, the 'P3' (as it is usually called) will be delayed somewhat. It is largest when the stimulus is rare and is only seen when the subject is actively attending to the series of stimulus, all of which has led to the theory that P3 reflects an updating of expectations about ongoing events.

p_rep A statistical derivative of P (1) that represents the likelihood that an effect will be replicated.

PA Abbreviation for *paired-associate* or *paired-association*. See PAIRED-ASSOCIATES *LEARNING.

pacemaker 1 Generally, any physiological structure or system that displays periodicity and has some regulatory output that helps to control another structure or system. The SUPRACHIASMATIC NUCLEUS is often called a pacemaker. **2** More specifically, a region in the heart that functions as an integral part of the system that is rhythmically active and controls the rate of cardiac contraction. The term is also used for an artificial device implanted in the chest to assist in such functions in cases of heart disease.

pacing 1 Controlling the speed (i.e. the pace) of an act. The term is used generally to refer to experimental procedures in which the sequence and timing of trials or behaviours are carefully controlled. **2** Structuring a learning programme or educational curriculum so that materials are introduced gradually over time so as to correspond with the developmental level of the learner.

Pacinian corpuscle Large, specialized nerve endings located in the deep, subcutaneous fatty tissue. The largest of the nerve endings found in the skin, they occur abundantly in the feet and hands, in joints and ligaments, in the genitals and elsewhere. It is likely that these receptors transmit pressure information in response to rapid changes.

pack-rat syndrome HOARDING.

paederosis PAEDOPHILIA.

paedia-, paed(o)- Combining forms meaning *infant* or *child*. vars., *pedia-, ped(o)-*.

paediatric psychology The field of psychology concerned with the healthcare and physical well-being of children. var., *pediatric psychology*.

paediatrics Medical specialization concerned with the diseases of childhood.

paedologia Lit., infantile speech.

paedomorphism Investing adults with child-like characteristics; interpreting adult behaviour using concepts more appropriate to interpreting that of children. Also called *infantilization*. The reverse tendency is called *enelicomorphism*. Distinguish from PAEDOMORPHOSIS.

paedomorphosis The retention of juvenile characteristics into adulthood; used typically when making cross-species comparisons. Distinguish from PAEDOMORPHISM. See also NEOTENY.

paedophilia Lit., attraction to children. However, as the term is used, the attraction is always sexual in connotation and meaning is restricted to the sexual feelings of an adult for a child. Paedophilia is classified as a PARAPHILIA only when it results in actual sexual activity and the child is prepubic.

PAG PERIAQUEDUCTAL GREY.

pain This term comes from the Latin word for *penalty* or *fine* and has an exceedingly wide range of uses, not all of which reflect the original meaning. Here we shall skip the metaphoric, figurative and poetic; in psychology there are three distinguishable primary senses of the term, each with a variety of more specialized forms. To wit: **1** Loosely, the opposite of PLEASURE, that is, UNPLEASURE. **2** Psychological or psychic distress. While now rather common, this admittedly vague meaning emerged within psychoanalysis, where it was often referred to as *unpleasure* or *displeasure* and is assumed to result from an excess of affect caused by tension and/or conflict. It should be noted that Freud used two separate words to differentiate these two forms of pain. One, *Schmerz*, was translated unambiguously into English as *pain*, the physical kind; the other, *Umlust*, is harder to fit in English and although *displeasure* or *aversion* are more or less acceptable, most translators avoided the issue of nuance and simply used *pain* as well, causing no end of confusion. **3** A SOMATOSENSORY experience, evoked by a stimulus that activates any of the NOCICEPTORS. Pain, in this sense, is generally viewed from three perspectives: (a) a sensory component, the actual experiencing of the percept, (b) an immediate emotional experience, the degree to which the experience is unpleasant and (c) the long-term emotional consequences, such as that of chronic pain.

pain, acute Generally, any relatively short-duration pain with known organic cause. Acute pain is contrasted with CHRONIC •PAIN,

both in manner of cause and in the underlying neural pathways that mediate them. By and large, acute pain is externally caused, experienced immediately, and felt as a sharp, sudden sensation that diminishes fairly quickly. Also called *cutaneous pain*, *sharp pain* and *surface pain*. See also PAIN PATHWAYS.

pain, chronic Deep, long-lasting, intractable pain. As contrasted with ACUTE •PAIN, it is caused by internal factors and is experienced as deep, dull and diffuse; it tends to increase in intensity over time. Also known as *deep pain*. See also PAIN PATHWAYS.

pain, clinical Pain resulting from disease, injury, surgery, etc.

pain disorder An umbrella term for a class of SOMATOFORM DISORDERS marked by the existence of pain as part of an individual's overall clinical picture when that pain causes marked distress or significant impairment of social or occupational functioning. The disorder may be subclassified as *psychological type* if psychological factors are judged to be the significant causes, *secondary type* if non-psychological medical conditions account for the condition, or *combined type* if both factors contribute. Also called *psychogenic pain disorder* and *somatoform pain disorder*.

pain endurance Loosely, the ability of a person to endure pain. Many theorists treat it as a personality characteristic, and there is evidence that the ability to tolerate acute pain (see PAIN TOLERANCE), assessed objectively, predicts how well a person will be able to endure chronic pain resulting from natural causes.

pain management Literally, the managing of PAIN. A variety of techniques are used including various analgesic drugs, nerve blocks and a host of more psychologically oriented procedures such as biofeedback, hypnosis, relaxation therapy and imagery.

pain pathways The afferent neural pathways leading from the receptors to the central nervous system that transmit the sensation of pain. The pathways for ACUTE •PAIN are made up of rapidly conducting fibres that travel to the ventrobasal complex of the thalamus and from there to the somatosensory cortex; those for CHRONIC •PAIN are made up of slowly conducting fibres that travel to the midline nuclei of the thalamus and from there to various areas, including the limbic system and the frontal lobes of the cerebral cortex.

pain, pricking A form of ACUTE *PAIN experienced when a sharp momentary stimulus is applied to the skin.

pain principle The striving for death or for nirvana. In Freud's early psychoanalytic formulations this notion is only hinted at; later it was made explicit in the form of Thanatos, the death instinct, which was conceived of as operating along with Eros, the life instinct. There are some terminological confusions to be found in the writings of psychoanalysts with regard to the pain principle. On one hand the form is used as above, but on the other it also finds expression in the compound phrase PLEASURE–PAIN PRINCIPLE, which has rather different connotations.

pain, referred The sensation of bodily pain in a location other than the place stimulated. It is particularly common in the abdominal area and often makes medical diagnosis difficult.

pain threshold The minimal intensity of a stimulus that is perceived as painful. While this threshold appears to be biologically determined, an individual's PAIN TOLERANCE has a large psychological component.

pain tolerance The upper threshold for endurance of painful stimulation. Experimentally, it is assessed by the point at which a subject (a paid volunteer!) terminates the stimulation.

pair-bond In ethology, a lasting male–female union. The term is only applied to nonhuman species.

paired-associates learning LEARNING, PAIRED-ASSOCIATES.

paired-comparisons method 1 A very general procedure for measuring (scaling) objects or stimuli and assessing the dimensions that underlie them. In the standard, complete method of paired comparisons, every object in a set is presented for judgement in a pair-wise fashion with every other object in the set. The method is extremely powerful and general and, in principle, can be used with any collection of objects or stimuli that can be compared with each other in some psychologically real manner. See also SCALING et seq. **2** In industrial/organizational psychology, an extension of the method to individuals who are systematically compared with each other along some measure of performance.

PAL PAIRED-ASSOCIATES *LEARNING.

palaeo- Combining form meaning *ancient, old, prehistoric.* var., *paleo-*.

palaeocerebellum The phylogenetically older parts of the cerebellum including parts of the vermis and the cerebellar pyramids. Inputs come from the dorsal and ventral spinocerebellar tracts (hence, the area is also known as the *spinocerebellum*) and projections go to deeper nuclei in the cerebellum. It is critical in the control of PROPRIOCEPTION in the maintenance of posture. var., *paleocerebellum*.

palaeocortex The phylogenetically older parts of the cerebral cortex. It consists of between three and five distinct cell layers and is primarily given over to processing olfactory information. var., *paleocortex*.

palaeoencephalon NEENCEPHALON.

palaeopsychology An area of psychology that examines psychological processes and functions and theorizes about their emergence in earlier evolutionary eras. Jung first coined this term and used it for his work on the COLLECTIVE UNCONSCIOUS. While Jung's notions, tinged as they were with mysticism, have few adherents today, the term is still used in EVOLUTIONARY PSYCHOLOGY. var., *paleopsychology*.

palaeostriatum GLOBUS PALLIDUS.

palatable Agreeable to the palate, pleasant-tasting. Interestingly, however, the palate is essentially devoid of taste receptors. Nevertheless, the term continues to be used, in even the most formal presentations, to express the acceptability of foodstuff.

palate The roof of the mouth; it is divided into the anterior hard palate and the posterior soft palate.

PA learning PAIRED-ASSOCIATES *LEARNING.

paleencephalon NEENCEPHALON.

paleopsychology PALAEOPSYCHOLOGY.

palilalia Repeating one's own words and phrases. It is a symptom in some TIC DISORDERS. See ECHOLALIA.

palin- Combining form meaning *backwards* or *repetitive*.

palindrome Any word, phrase or sentence that reads the same forwards and backwards. For obvious reasons, two of your authors are rather partial to them.

palingraphia MIRROR WRITING.

palinlexia Reading backwards. There are two forms, one in which a sentence is read with the word order reversed, the other in which each word is read with letter order reversed.

palinphrasia Pathologically frequent repetition of particular words or phrases during speech.

pallaesthesia The sensation of vibration. Also called *palmaesthesia*. vars., *pallesthesia*, *palmesthesia*.

pallesthesia PALLAESTHESIA.

palliative Anything that eases pain.

pallidum GLOBUS PALLIDUS.

pallindotomy A surgical procedure in which the internal division of the globus pallidus is lesioned. It is used in PARKINSON'S DISEASE, particularly in younger patients and those who no longer respond to L-DOPA.

pallium Obsolescent term for the cerebral cortex.

palmaesthesia PALLAESTHESIA.

palmar Pertaining to the palm of the hand or the sole of the foot. syn., especially in older writings, *volar*.

palmar conductance (or **resistance**) Lit., the electrical conductivity or resistance of the skin of the palm. See GALVANIC SKIN RESPONSE.

palmar response The grasping reflex of a newborn when pressure is applied to the palm. It normally disappears at around the fourth or fifth month of life.

palmesthesia PALLAESTHESIA.

palmistry The practice of personality and character assessment based on the interpretation of the lines, wrinkles and other features of the palm. In Ambrose Bierce's terms, the practice often works, for the wrinkles in the palm of a subject invariably spell out 'dupe'. See PSEUDOSCIENCE, of which palmistry is an example.

palmitic acid FATTY ACID.

palpitation(s) Rapid heartbeat. It often accompanies a PANIC ATTACK and can itself be quite frightening.

palsy Generally, paralysis. The term is typically used in combined form to specify the nature, location or type of disability.

palsy, cerebral (CP) A nonprogressive movement disorder caused by perinatal brain injury.

pan- Combining form meaning *all* or *every* (*where*). var., *panto-*.

pandemic In epidemiology, occurring over a wide geographical area; by extension, universal.

Pandemonium An early and influential computer model of pattern perception developed in the 1950s by O. Selfridge.

panic attack A discrete period of intense fear or discomfort accompanied by various symptoms which may include shortness of breath, dizziness, palpitations, trembling, sweating, nausea and often a fear that one is going crazy. The attacks are initially unexpected and typically last no longer than 15 minutes. See PANIC DISORDERS.

panic disorders A class of ANXIETY DISORDERS characterized by recurrent PANIC ATTACKS. The term is not used when a known organic factor is responsible. A panic disorder is typically classified as with or without AGORAPHOBIA.

panpsychism A philosophical position that holds that the ultimate, meaningful (or perhaps *only*) reality is psychic or mental; that all that exists is 'mind-like'. In the final analysis it represents a rather naïve effort to resolve the MIND–BODY PROBLEM, and when taken to its (logical?) extreme emerges as ANIMISM in disguise.

pansexualism A sobriquet thrust often upon the classical Freudian point of view by its critics, who argue that its strong emphasis on sexual determinants is unwarranted.

pantheism The doctrine that God and the cosmic totality are coterminous. It served as a convenient perspective for rescuing SUBJECTIVE IDEALISM from SOLIPSISM.

panto- PAN-.

Panum phenomenon A visual effect obtained using a stereoscope. The viewer is first presented with two parallel lines to one eye and a single line, at the same distance and similarly parallel, to the other eye. Adjusting the single line so that it fuses stereoscopically with either of the two lines from the other eye causes the fused line to appear to be closer to the viewer than the other line. Also called *Panum's limiting case.*

paper-and-pencil test A general label for any test (achievement, aptitude, intelligence, etc.) that uses only pencil and paper as testing instruments.

paper-folding test MENTAL PAPER-FOLDING TEST.

Papez's circuit A complex neural circuit consisting of the mammillary bodies, the anterior thalamus, the cingulate cortex, the hippocampus and the various fibres interconnecting them.

Papez's theory of emotion One of the first theoretical attempts to delineate the specific cortical mechanisms underlying emotion. It was developed by J. W. Papez in the 1930s and proposed three interlocking systems (sensory, hypothalamic, thalamic), all of which were hypothesized to be combined in the cortex, where the 'psychological products' of emotion emerged. The theory has not stood up to careful anatomical study but it was influential in implicating the hypothalamus and by focusing attention on the integrative role of the cortex. See also MACLEAN'S THEORY OF EMOTION, which built on several of Papez's ideas, and the general discussion under THEORIES OF *EMOTION.

papilla Any small nipple-like protuberance. See e.g. LINGUAL PAPILLA.

-para- Combining term with two origins. When from its Greek roots: **1** *Next to* or *along side of.* **2** By extension, *beyond.* **3** By further extension, *unusual, irregular,* even *abnormal.* When from its Latin roots: **4** *To bear, to bring forth.* It is used in this sense to characterize a woman with respect to her viable offspring; e.g. *nullipara* for one who has had none, *multipara* for one who has had two or more. A shorthand expression is also used here, *para-0, para-1, para-n,* for a woman who has had none, one or *n* offspring.

parabiosis 1 Lit., living alongside; hence, of two individuals, the state of being joined together, either congenitally, as in Siamese conjoined twins, or artificially, as in a PARABIOTIC PREPARATION. **2** An obsolete term for a temporary suppression of the conductivity of a nerve.

parabiotic preparation The conjoining of two genetically similar organisms by surgically linking them, usually by suturing their skins together. The animals share circulating blood and the preparation can be used in a variety of research procedures.

parabrachial nucleus A nucleus in the PONS, the lateral branch of which relays information about taste to the gustatory area of the THALAMUS.

paracentral scotoma A SCOTOMA (1) in the area of the visual field that surrounds the region served by the fovea. It can be monocular, in which case the impairment is peripheral, or binocular, where the neural disorders lie further along the visual pathways, after the LATERAL GENICULATE NUCLEUS.

paracentral vision VISION, PARACENTRAL.

parachlorophenylalanine A substance that prevents the synthesis of SEROTONIN by blocking the action of TRYPTOPHAN.

parachromatopsia A general term for colour deficiency; see COLOUR BLINDNESS.

paracontrast METACONTRAST.

paracusia 1 Specifically, selective deafness to low-pitched tones. **2** More loosely, any hearing dysfunction other than simple DEAFNESS.

paradigm 1 Any series of linguistic forms all of which reflect a common underlying element, e.g. *give, gives, gave, giving, given,* etc. This general notion is also found in other levels of linguistic analysis, including the phonemic, morphemic and syntactic. **2** An orientation to or plan for research using a particular focus. Thus one reads, for example, of an attack on a problem using the *psychoanalytic paradigm*. **3** A particular experimental procedure, e.g. the *classical conditioning paradigm*. **4** In T. S. Kuhn's influential analysis of the history of science, the collective set of attitudes, values, procedures, techniques, etc. that form the generally accepted perspective of a particular discipline at a point in time. Note that all of these uses, from the linguistic to the historical/philosophical, reflect the original Greek word *paradeigma*, meaning *pattern*.

paradigmatic association ASSOCIATION, PARADIGMATIC.

paradox A situation wherein, on the basis of a number of premises generally taken to be true, contradictory conclusions are reached without violating logical deductive reasoning. Note that the contradiction here can arise not only from logical deductions, but also from an experimental outcome that contradicts (using that term loosely) the predictions of a generally agreed-upon theoretical analysis. From an empirical standpoint many scientific paradoxes are but momentary states of affairs that are best viewed as symptoms of a lack of understanding; i.e. usually the premises from which one is working should not be so uncritically accepted as true. For a nice example of a still not completely resolved paradox in cognitive psychology see WORD-SUPERIORITY EFFECT.

From a logical point of view there is a large and important class of paradoxes that are significant for philosophy, mathematics and psychology – the *self-referencing paradoxes*. The most famous (and oldest) is the liar paradox, in which Epimenides (who is from Crete) remarks, 'All Cretans are liars.' Attempt to determine whether Epimenides is speaking the truth or not to see the paradox.

paradoxical cold A sensation of coldness when an actually rather warm object of about 45°C (113°F) or above stimulates a COLD SPOT on the skin.

paradoxical intention A psychotherapeutic technique used within Viktor E. Frankl's LOGOTHERAPY, wherein the client is encouraged (with appropriate humour – a point that Frankl strongly emphasizes and which

some others, to their peril, fail to appreciate) to do exactly what he or she is afraid of doing, or to imagine that his or her worst neurotic fears have actually transpired. The technique is used primarily with obsessions; e.g. as in the case of a man who was terrified to leave his house because of an obsession with having a heart seizure and was told, 'Go on out, have a heart attack. Have two, it's still early in the day; might as well use the day well. Have a stroke too.' Clearly, this is a procedure to be used judiciously; it is not recommended for one not trained in Frankl's approach.

paradoxical sleep A term occasionally used for what is now more commonly referred to as REM SLEEP. The phrase paradoxical sleep was introduced because the EEG pattern during REM sleep looks like that of a normally awake person. Also known as *D sleep*.

paradoxical warmth A sensation of warmth when an actually cold object, that is about 30°C (86°F) or below, stimulates a WARM SPOT.

paraesthesia Abnormal skin sensations such as tickling, itching or burning. See e.g. FORMICATION. var., *paresthesia*.

parafovea The area of the retina immediately surrounding the fovea.

parageusia A general term for any gustatory (taste) illusion.

paragraphia Habitual insertion of inappropriate words or letters into writing.

parahippocampal cortex (or **gyrus**) Part of the limbic system adjacent to the HIPPOCAMPAL FORMATION. It and the *perirhinal cortex* relay information between the hippocampus and the rest of the brain.

parakinesis PSYCHOKINESIS (1).

paralalia Habitual substitution of inappropriate sounds during speech.

paralanguage See PARALINGUISTICS.

paraldehyde A quick-acting, nonbarbiturate sedative with anticonvulsive effects. It is normally administered by injection as it is rather foul-tasting and, if taken orally, leaves a distinctly unpleasant odour on the patient's breath and irritates the stomach.

paralexia A form of DYSLEXIA in which words

and/or letters are misread. Often the misreading involves transposition of letters, syllables and even whole words.

paralinguistics The study of those aspects of communication that are not purely linguistic, i.e. not morphophonemic, syntactic or semantic. Specifically, the meanings conveyed by tone of voice, pacing, pausing, emphasis, hems and haws, snorting, etc. qualify as paralinguistic. Note that some use the term so as to include social mannerisms, gestures, facial expressions and the like. A paralinguistic analysis of an utterance or a discourse is one which is concerned primarily with *how* something is said rather than with the actual words used. See also KINESICS, METALINGUISTICS, NONVERBAL COMMUNICATION.

parallax A term borrowed from geometry to refer to the patterns of shifts in apparent motion of objects in the visual field as the observer moves laterally. For more on usage see MOTION PARALLAX and MOTION PERSPECTIVE.

parallel distributed processing (PDP) models A class of theoretical models in cognitive psychology that are based on the assumption that systems operate by having a number of internal nodes or units that function in parallel with each other. For more detail see CONNECTIONISM (2).

parallel forms ALTERNATE FORMS *RELIABILITY.

parallelism, cultural A situation in which a set of similar, if not identical, cultural patterns and conventions are found in widely separated and presumably totally independent cultures.

parallelism, psychoneural A variation on PSYCHOPHYSICAL *PARALLELISM in which it is assumed that for every event in the mental domain there is a corresponding unique event in the neural domain.

parallelism, psychophysical The philosophical doctrine often associated with the empirically oriented psychology of the late 19th and early 20th centuries. It was an attempt to resolve the mind–body problem by assuming that the two domains were merely separate 'tracks' and that for every mental or psychic event there was a corresponding physical event, and vice versa. See MIND–BODY PROBLEM and DUALISM.

parallel play PLAY, PARALLEL.

parallel processing PROCESSING, PARALLEL.

parallel search SEARCH, PARALLEL.

paralogia Literally, *outside logic*. However, the term is used mainly for illogical thinking presumed to lie behind talk.

paralysis Any partial or complete loss of some function. Unless specifically noted, the reference is nearly always to the voluntary musculature. Although there are many special subclassifications of paralyses which we needn't list here, physicians typically group paralyses into the *spastic* and the *flaccid* types. In the former, involving damage to the upper motor neurons, there is loss of control over musculature with tremors or spasms; in the latter, involving the lesions in the lower motor neurons, there is loss of voluntary control and no movement. See -PLEGIA for additional details. Occasionally the term is used figuratively to mean loss of sensory function and even a crippling, or loss of effectiveness, of cognitive processes.

paralysis agitans PARKINSON'S DISEASE.

paralytic dementia PARESIS.

parameter 1 Mathematically, in the simplest of terms, an *unspecified constant*; that is, the value of a constant in a function that satisfies the conditions of the function. **2** In statistics, the value that enters into the mathematical function for a probability distribution. This sense, which is an application of 1, is most clearly realized as a summary measure of a *population* of scores; e.g. the population mean (μ) is a parameter and so is the population standard deviation (σ). Note that the term is not used of *samples*: the mean and standard deviation of a sample of scores are called *statistics*. For more detail on usage here see PARAMETRIC STATISTICS. **3** In various quantitative approaches to psychology the term is found with essentially these same meanings. For example, a PDP model of learning (see CONNECTIONISM (2)) will have a learning parameter that must be specified in order to determine the rate at which the system will set up its representations. **4** In experimental work, any variable that is set for a particular study to one or more values but can be changed to other values for other parametric variations on the original study. For example, one may study one motivational level in one experiment and double or triple that level in a later parametric extension. **5** In psychotherapy, an aspect of a therapeutic programme that can be systematically altered, e.g. the number of therapy sessions, or the length of those sessions. adj., *parametric*.

parametric statistics A general label covering those statistical procedures that require that the sample data under analysis be drawn from a population with a known form, most generally the normal distribution. Moreover, parametric techniques also require: (a) that the samples under analysis are taken independently; (b) that when more than one population is being sampled they have the same variance or a known ratio of variances; and (c) that the data be in a form such that all arithmetic operations (e.g. addition, multiplication) can be carried out on them. As a rule, parametric procedures are to be preferred over NONPARAMETRIC STATISTICS (provided that the conditions hold) because they generally have greater statistical power and are more likely to detect statistically significant effects.

paramimia An APRAXIA where physical gestures and facial expressions are at variance with felt emotions.

paramnesia A distorted or FALSE *MEMORY. See e.g. DÉJÀ VU and CONFABULATION.

paramnesia, reduplicative A DELUSIONAL MISIDENTIFICATION DISORDER marked by a belief that two (or more) persons or places with virtually identical features exist.

paranoia In the standard psychiatric nosology, a functional disorder characterized by delusions of jealousy, and delusions of grandeur and/or persecution, which are not consistent with other disorders such as *schizophrenia*, *organic mental disorder* or *organic mental syndrome*. In the classic form, the delusions develop insidiously and become knit together into a rational and coherent set of beliefs that is internally consistent and, once the initial set of assumptions is accepted, compelling and vigorously defensible. In paranoia, intellectual functioning is unimpaired and the paranoid is quite capable of coherent behaviour within the delusional system. adj., *paranoid* or *paranoiac*; n., *paranoid* or *paranoiac*. In the standard nomenclature, paranoia is considered a DELUSIONAL DISORDER and specialized terms can be found under that heading.

paranoiac (and **paranoid**) Originally *paranoiac* was used to refer to a person suffering from a diagnosed paranoia and *paranoid* to one manifesting some of the suspiciousness and delusional tendencies typical of the disorder. This distinction, which was useful, has pretty well been lost and both terms are often used interchangeably.

paranoid anxiety A psychoanalytic term for anxiety produced by fear of attack from hostile others. Also called *persecutory anxiety*.

paranoid character PARANOID PERSONALITY DISORDER.

paranoid delusions One of the key symptoms of PARANOID (TYPE) *SCHIZOPHRENIA.

paranoid disorders See DELUSIONAL (PARANOID) DISORDER, the currently approved term, and, for more detail, PARANOIA.

paranoid ideation The typical pattern of thinking displayed in cases of paranoia; it is characterized by suspiciousness and the belief that one is being followed, plotted against, persecuted, etc.

paranoid personality disorder A PERSONALITY DISORDER characterized by excessive suspiciousness, hostility and sensitivity to accusations or even hints of accusation. Distinguish from DELUSIONAL PARANOID DISORDER, in that there is no fully developed persecutory system. Called in some old writings *paranoid character*.

paranoid schizophrenia SCHIZOPHRENIA, PARANOID (TYPE).

paranoid state An acute form of DELUSIONAL (PARANOID) DISORDER often brought about by an abrupt shift in occupation or in living conditions. Seen in immigrants, refugees, prisoners of war, young people leaving home for the first time, etc. The condition is almost always temporary.

paranoid trend An older psychiatric term for the pattern of suspiciousness, jealousy and feelings of persecution and/or grandeur often displayed by one with a PARANOID PERSONALITY DISORDER.

paranormal Lit., outside of the normal. Generally used to refer to the phenomena studied in PARAPSYCHOLOGY, and related areas such as the occult, astrology and magic, etc.

paranosic (gain) PRIMARY GAIN.

paraphasia A general term for any habitual inappropriate use of words in speech.

paraphemia The habitual use of the wrong word or the wrong phonetic unit in speech.

paraphilia An umbrella term for any mode of sexual expression in which arousal is dependent upon what are generally considered to be socially unacceptable stimulating conditions. Typically a paraphiliac is not one who simply enjoys an exotic passing fancy for something offbeat but is rather obsessively concerned with and responsive to the particular erotic stimuli of his or her sexual mode. Human sexual expression is extraordinarily varied and a large number of paraphilias have been identified and studied. Those interested in such matters should see COPROPHILIA (2), EXHIBITIONISM (2), FETISHISM (2), FROTTEURISM, KLISMAPHILIA, MASOCHISM, NECROPHILIA, PAEDOPHILIA, PICTOPHILIA, SADISM, SCOPHOPHILIA, SYMPHOROPHILIA, TRANSVESTIC FETISHISM, TROILISM, UROPHILIA, VOYEURISM and ZOOPHILIA. In some classification systems the term will be used synonymously with SEXUAL *PERVERSION.

paraphilia related disorders In some classification systems the term PARAPHILIA is reserved for particularly problematic conditions such as paedophilia, and this term is used for other 'unusual' modes of sexual expression that cause problems because they are socially inappropriate.

paraphobia Any mild form of a phobia.

paraphonia Generally, any weakness or other abnormal change in voice quality.

paraphrase 1 n. The relation that holds between two sentences when they both have the same underlying meaning but differ in their surface forms, such as the active and passive forms of a simple sentence, e.g. 'Max ate the eggs' and 'The eggs were eaten by Max.' **2** n. By extension, shared meanings of larger units of language, paragraphs, essays, stories, etc. The strict relationship between underlying structures in 1 is not implied in this sense; *meaning* is used more loosely here. **3** vb. To produce either form of paraphrase.

paraphrasic error A speech error marked by substitutions of incorrect words or sounds, usually by transposing syllables, words or even whole phrases. Paraphrasic errors are common in the speech of patients with WERNICKE'S *APHASIA.

paraphrenia SCHIZOPHRENIA, PARANOID (TYPE).

paraplegia Paralysis of the lower limbs.

parapraxis Any minor slip-up or error; most typically observed in speech, writing, small accidents, memory lapses, etc. According to Freud, a parapraxis was no mere innocent gesture but a result of the operation of unconscious wishes or conflicts that could often be used to reveal the functioning of the unconscious in the normal healthy individual. Commonly referred to as a *Freudian slip*. pl., *parapraxes*.

paraprofessional Generally, an individual who has received sufficient training in a specialized field to assist and work under the direction of one who has had full professional training.

parapsychology A more-or-less (with the emphasis on *less*) accepted branch of psychology concerned with paranormal phenomena; that is, phenomena that are presumed to be unexplainable using known laws and principles, including extrasensory perception (ESP), telepathy, precognition, telekinesis and clairvoyance. Although there is a great deal of interest in parapsychology, and many actively pursue the scientific basis of the various claims that have been made, the majority of psychologists are deeply sceptical and for good reason.

First, the results of the individual experiments that have reported positive findings have proven notoriously difficult to replicate. Reproducibility is essential in all sciences; it is a touchstone of the scientific method and demand for independent verification is found everywhere. This aspect of science is, moreover, absolutely essential in any branch that makes a frontal assault on accepted laws and principles. Second, the reported phenomena often entail conclusions that violate known laws of science, such as the further away a light source the weaker the light, or the greater the distance between two bodies the weaker the mutual gravitational pull. Yet, *psi* abilities (as they are often called) have been argued to operate equally well at distances of 1,000 km and 3 m. Most scientists are loath to abandon general principles like the inverse square law (which accounts for the behaviour of both light and gravity in the above examples), particularly when the phenomena that 'mandate' their rejection resist replication so thoroughly. It is more reasonable to distrust the data from the nonrepeatable experiment than to jettison laws that function in all other domains. Third, no mechanism has ever been proposed that explains these purported paranormal phenomena in any way that is coherent in view of the rest of scientific knowledge. Precognition, for example, requires time travel, either by one's mind or by some force that moves from the future to have an impact upon someone's mind in the present. Such a mechanism entails reversal of cause and effect (tomorrow affects today), not to mention the fact that it conflicts with the basic principles of relativity theory and the laws of thermodynamics. Fourth – and this reason is perhaps unfortunate – many charlatans and fakes argue strongly for paranormal phenomena, and many of the purported effects have been shown to be the result of outright fraud. If psi effects are real (and scepticism – reasonable scepticism – does not outlaw them nor uniformly reject them), their vigorous espousal by obvious frauds makes objective analysis extremely difficult.

Finally, many of the sceptics wonder why those persons who claim to have these extraordinary capabilities don't simply hie themselves off to the nearest casino or race track and put them to good use. If nothing else, they could use the profits to fund further research in parapsychology.

parasagittal Of a plane parallel to the SAGITTAL (2) plane of an organ or body.

parasexuality Lit., anomalous sexuality or, by extension, perverted sexuality. Unfortunately, since the notion of just what is anomalous and/or perverted in sexual behaviour changes with the passage of time and with the societally regulated attitudes of the persons making the classification, it is simply not clear which behaviours are truly parasexual and which are merely uncommon among clinicians. See PARAPHILIA.

parasomnia A general label for a group of sleep disorders characterized by abnormal episodes that occur during sleep, including REM BEHAVIOUR DISORDER, SOMNAMBULISM, DREAM ANXIETY DISORDER and SLEEP TERROR DISORDER. When these occur in childhood they are usually due to developmental factors; in adults they are primarily psychogenic. Compare with DYSSOMNIA.

parasympathetic nervous system AUTONOMIC NERVOUS SYSTEM.

parataxic distortion H. S. Sullivan's term for a distortion of reality brought about by inferring a causal relationship between events that are actually independent. Contrast with SYNTAXIS.

parataxis From the Greek, meaning *placing side by side*. Hence: **1** In linguistics, characterizing phrases or sentences placed together without a conjunction, as in Caesar's famous remark, 'I came, I saw, I conquered.' **2** By extension, within H. S. Sullivan's theory, a mode of thinking lacking in integration or a personality in which skills, attitudes, personal relationships, etc. are largely separated from each other. See PARATAXIC DISTORTION. **3** By further extension, an emotional disorder in which the various components of emotion (ideas, thoughts, feelings, attitudes) are poorly integrated.

parateresiomania Synonym of VOYEURISM.

parathyroid glands Several small endocrine glands located in the back and lower edge of the thyroid gland. They secrete the hormone *parathormone*, which is essential for calcium–phosphorus metabolism.

paratypic Lit., diverting from a type. Hence, by extension, characterizing influences that are environmental; not inherited.

paraventricular nucleus A nucleus within the hypothalamus. The cell bodies produce antidiuretic hormone and oxytocin and transport these to the posterior pituitary gland. The nucleus has a variety of metabolic effects, including secretion of insulin, breaking down of triglycerides and lowering of body temperature.

paraverbal PARALINGUISTICS.

paravertebral ganglionic chain AUTONOMIC NERVOUS SYSTEM.

paraxial On either side of the axis of the body or of an organ.

pareidolia A phenomenon where unclear, ambiguous stimuli are interpreted as clear and meaningful. Common examples are seeing religious figures in clouds or specific visions in complex, vague stimuli such ~ landscape painting or a still life.

parental behaviour Behaviour characteristic of a parent; behaviour that is specifically focused on the care, protection, feeding, nurturing, etc. of offspring. The term is used to refer to either (a) behaviours that are gender-free, i.e. that can be carried out by either the male or female parent, or (b) all behaviours of both parents. See MATERNAL BEHAVIOUR and PATERNAL BEHAVIOUR for additional comments on usage.

parental investment 1 Loosely, the amount of time, energy and risk to survival that a parent must invest in the production, care, feeding and protection of offspring. 2 The loss of future reproductive capacity to each adult in a mating that results from producing and nurturing each offspring. These two meanings might appear to be semantically equivalent but the latter, by virtue of focusing on future reproductive success, led Robert Trivers to develop PARENTAL INVESTMENT THEORY.

parental investment theory A theoretical generalization due to Robert Trivers that argues that the different amount of PARENTAL INVESTMENT (1, 2) that each parent provides strongly influences the MATE SELECTION strategies that individual species will evolve. The theory has several important entailments. For example, it predicts that species where one parent has greater parental investment than the other will tend to be ones where that sex will be more vigorously competed for by members of the other sex and be more discriminating when choosing a mate. It also outlines how the different degrees of investment tend to produce particular kinds of MATING SYSTEMS.

parent image 1 The image or memory one has of one's parents. Needless to say, this image does not necessarily correspond to reality. 2 A parent SURROGATE (2).

parergasia 1 Meyer offered this term to replace DEMENTIA PRAECOX. It found little support and both were soon replaced by Bleuler's term SCHIZROPHRENIA. 2 A symptom of SCHIZROPHRENIA where the patient performs an inappropriate action to a specific request; e.g. turning around when asked to sit.

paresis 1 Generally, incomplete, partial paralysis of organic origin, e.g. FACIAL PARESIS. 2 Specifically, an ORGANIC MENTAL DISORDER, characterized by progressive mental deterioration and paralysis, that is the result of central-nervous-system damage caused by tertiary syphilis. Also called *dementia paralytica*, *general paresis* and *general paralysis of the insane*.

paresthesia PARAESTHESIA.

Pareto chart Named for Vilfredo Pareto, a bar chart, commonly used in organizational psychology, in which the values (i.e. height of each bar) are arranged in descending order of frequency, cost or other index of interest. For example, a Pareto chart of the reasons for a manufacturing defect would show the various causes as descending bars on the x-axis.

Pareto efficiency A general principle involving the distribution of limited resources in a population. Specifically, any reallocation that benefits an individual without causing harm to another is said to be a *Pareto improvement*. When no further such reallocations are possible, the system is *Pareto optimal*. A *near-Pareto* decision is one that will benefit a large group of people while still imposing minor losses on others. All of the related Pareto proposals are important in economics and organizational psychology.

Pareto principle A generalization that 80% of the consequences will be due to 20% of the causes. It was originally put forward by Vilfredo Pareto based on his observation that 80% of the wealth in Italy was concentrated in 20% of the population. The so-called '80–20 rule' has found application in a wide variety of settings; e.g. 80% of sales volume comes from 20% of the clients; 80% of computation time comes from 20% of the instructions, etc.

parietal bones The parts of the cranium, in the middle of each side, lying between the occipital and the frontal bones.

parietal lobes The areas of the cerebral hemispheres lying below the parietal bones, i.e. between the frontal and occipital lobes and above the temporal lobe. They contain the somatosensory cortex and are involved in spatial perception and both memory for and planning of motor sequences.

Parkinsonism Usually, PARKINSON'S DISEASE. However, on occasion the term is used to refer generally to cases in which patients display some or all of the symptoms that characterize the classic disorder independent of the presence of the actual disease. Often written as *parkinsonism*.

Parkinsonism, drug-induced 1 A syndrome with many of the classic symptoms of PARKINSON'S DISEASE produced as side effects of long-term use of ANTIPSYCHOTIC DRUGS. It is treatable with antiparkinsonian agents. Also called *pseudoparkinsonism*. 2 Any of several disorders with Parkinson's-like symptoms caused by drugs or environmental factors. Implicated here are the street drug MPTP and chemicals such as manganese and carbon monoxide.

Parkinson-plus syndromes A group of neurological syndromes that have Parkinsonian features but are distinct from Parkinson's disease, including PROGRESSIVE SUPRANUCLEAR PALSY, CORTICO-BASAL GANGLIONIC DEGENERATION, and MULTI-SYSTEM ATROPHIES. All of these have generally poorer prognosis than Parkinsonism and do not respond to dopamine-replacement therapy. Also called *multi-system degenerative diseases*.

Parkinson's disease (PD) A neurological disorder named after James Parkinson, the English physician who first described it. The primary symptoms are a rapid, coarse tremor, a mask-like facial expression, loss of sensorimotor coordination, loss of the ability to initiate action and a general tendency toward exhaustion. There are also subtle cognitive deficits involving a general slowing of learning and memory and some loss in executive cognitive functioning that may be difficult to identify in individual cases. Speech difficulties are often observed, including dysarthria, imprecise articulation and an oddly accelerated speech rate in which words tend to run together. The disease is caused by dopamine deficiency in the basal ganglia. A substantial proportion of patients (perhaps a third) develop a pro-nounced depression. Also called *parkinsonism* (or PARKINSONISM – see for nuances), and, in older texts, *paralysis agitans* or sometimes simply *palsy*.

parophresia PAROSMIA.

parorexia Craving for strange, unusual foods. The term is applied only to truly pathological cases. See PICA.

parosmia Generally, any disorder in the sense of smell. Also called *parophresia*.

parotid glands The large salivary glands in the cheeks just below and in front of the external ears. It was the parotid glands of a dog which, under the orchestration of Ivan P. Pavlov, produced some of psychology's most important early data.

parous Pertaining to females who have borne at least one viable offspring.

paroxetine A SELECTIVE SEROTONIN REUPTAKE INHIBITOR that functions as an ANTIDEPRESSANT and a treatment for ANXIETY DISORDERS. Trade names: Paxil, Seroxat.

paroxysm 1 Specifically, a spasmodic fit or convulsion. 2 More generally, any sudden increase in the severity of a disease or of an emotional disorder. 3 Figuratively, any sudden rage or anger.

parse Generally, to analyse a complex stimulus into its constituent parts. In linguistics it refers to the process of breaking a sentence down into its grammatical parts (subject, verb, object), in vision to decomposing a visual scene into its elemental features.

parsimony, principle of A general *heuristic* which states that if two scientific propositions or two theories are equally tenable the simpler one is to be preferred. The principle is eminently reasonable, applying it is another matter. In practice it turns out that two equally tenable propositions or theories are about as rare as hens' teeth. Moreover, how tenable a theory is is typically judged by its effectiveness in accounting for known phenomena and not by any additional insights it may yield: the more complex of the competing theories may indeed turn out to have greater predictive validity. In psychology and other social sciences, the issue is further confounded because, unlike in some branches of the physical sciences and in pure mathematics (where the principle has its strongest role to play), determining the complexity of theoretical propositions is often impossible. Finally, there is the ever-present problem that this rational principle must be applied by the human scientist, a creature not known for its rationality. Nevertheless, the principle has merit and keeps reappearing in various guises; see LLOYD MORGAN'S CANON and OCCAM'S RAZOR.

part correlation SEMIPARTIAL *CORRELATION.

parthenogenesis From the Greek, meaning *virgin origin*, the production of a viable offspring from a female egg without male fertilization.

partial 1 adj. Pertaining to that which is less than the whole of some object, system or organization. **2** n. A PARTIAL TONE.

partial aim In psychoanalytic theory, any means of deriving sexual gratification prior to the development of the genital stage.

partial correlation CORRELATION, PARTIAL.

partial hospitalization A treatment programme for patients who only require hospital care part of the time, usually overnight or at weekends.

partial instinct In classical psychoanalytic theory, instincts are assumed to develop from the specific manifestations of a number of component instincts. These more molecular elements are the *partial* (or *component* or, simply, *part*) instincts. For example, the sex instinct is assumed to derive from the partial libidinal contributions of the oral, anal and genital.

partialism A PARAPHILIA marked by an individual's sexual interest being exclusively focused on a single part of the body.

partialization O. Rank's term for the process now referred to as DIFFERENTIATION (5).

partial out PARTIAL *CORRELATION.

partial regression (equation) REGRESSION, EQUATION; REGRESSION, MULTIPLE.

partial reinforcement A somewhat ambiguous synonym of INTERMITTENT *REINFORCEMENT. See SCHEDULES OF *REINFORCEMENT.

partial-reinforcement effect Behaviour maintained with partial or intermittent reinforcement has greater resistance to extinction than behaviour maintained with continuous reinforcement. Despite the preference for the term *intermittent reinforcement* over *partial reinforcement*, the latter is used in this case.

partial relations Relations between variables discovered by dividing a sample into subsets (or parts).

partial-report method An experimental procedure in which the subject is required to report only part of a stimulus display rather than the whole display.

partial tone Any of the separate tones produced by a vibrating body. The lowest and loudest is the *fundamental tone*, the rest form the *harmonic* or *overtone series*. Also called, simply, *partial*.

participant The American Psychological Association has recommended that this term be used to refer to an individual who participates in an experiment. Previously term of choice was SUBJECT (1), but many felt this demeaned those who volunteered their services in the name of science. Alas, all manner of difficulty has been created by this policy. Psychologists who run animals object to calling the focus of their researches participants since they do not participate in anything like the manner assumed by the APA. Volunteers whose behaviour is observed surreptitiously are surely not participants in the normal sense of the word and, as many have argued vociferously, there is not really anything wrong with the time-honoured sobriquet. In any event, many of the issues that have driven the APA to make its recommendation have already been acknowledged in the field. See the discussion under SUBJECT for more details.

participant observer In a study of a group, community or society, an observer who is simultaneously a full participant in the group. Often this role is taken by a psychologist, anthropologist or sociologist in order to examine group processes *in situ*.

participation 1 The taking of an active, sharing part in a game, a group, an experiment, etc. **2** By extension, the dynamic characteristic of a complex activity that results from the participation (in sense 1) of a number of interacting components. This sense is often expressed in Piaget's writings, particularly as it pertains to a young child's manner of thinking about external and internal realities.

participative management In industrial/organizational psychology, a form of management of an organization in which the employees are involved in managerial decision-making on issues that directly concern them.

particular complex In psychoanalysis, any individual or idiosyncratic complex as contrasted with those complexes assumed to be universal. See NUCLEAR COMPLEX, UNIVERSAL COMPLEX.

particularism An approach to social theory in which standards of conduct are developed with a recognition of the role of individual circumstances and possible mitigating contexts. Compare with UNIVERSALISM.

partile Any of the set of points that divide an ordered distribution of scores into a series of equal-sized divisions. The most common are *percentiles* or *centiles*, although logically any subdivision is possible, e.g. *quartiles, quintiles, deciles*. Note that sometimes these terms are used to designate the points themselves, as above, and sometimes to designate divisions between any two points. See the discussion under CENTILE for clarification of this often confusing usage.

part instinct PARTIAL INSTINCT.

partition measure Any measure or statistic that partitions off one part of a distribution of scores from another part or other parts. The most commonly used are PARTILES.

part-learning method WHOLE-LEARNING METHOD.

part object OBJECT, PART.

parturition The act of giving birth.

paruresis Inability to urinate in the presence of others. Generally regarded as a SOCIAL *ANXIETY DISORDER, it is found in men and women and known by a host of names including *pee shyness, bashful bladder* and *shy bladder (syndrome)*.

parvocellular system A neural pathway in the visual system that is composed of small, slowly conducting cells. It is responsible for the perception of colour, fine detail and high contrast. The system, which is found only in primates, is named after the evolutionarily newer parvo cells, which make up the parvocellular layers of the lateral geniculate nucleus. Also called the *P-system*. Compare with MAGNOCELLULAR SYSTEM and KONIOCELLULAR SYSTEM.

Pascal distribution DISTRIBUTION, PASCAL.

passing-stranger (effect) The often observed phenomenon of a person divulging the most private information about him- or herself to a perfect stranger – information that even the person's spouse or therapist may not be privy to. Sometimes it is called the *stranger-on-a-train effect*, because trains are a likely place for such encounters. The explanation seems simple enough: the stranger will probably never be seen again and so the cathartic release of unburdening oneself can take place without fear that the information will ever be used against one.

passive 1 Not active, at rest. **2** Characterizing a particular attitude or stance whereby one permits outside influences to control a situation. **3** Characterizing a submissive posture whereby one allows oneself to be controlled by outside influences or persons, particularly in matters sexual. See ACTIVE AND PASSIVE for Freud's use of the term and its opposite.

passive-aggressive Descriptive of patterns of behaviour in which aggressiveness is displayed but in a passive rather than in an active manner. It is commonly seen in persons in a relatively low power position in which overt aggressiveness would surely lead to reprisals.

passive-aggressive personality disorder A PERSONALITY DISORDER marked by a pattern of passive resistance to requests for appropriate social and/or occupational performance. An individual with the condition typically procrastinates, becomes sulky and irritable when asked to do things he or she does not wish to do, works slowly on jobs (in a seemingly deliberate manner) and avoids obligations or responsibilities. Also called *negativistic personality disorder*.

passive analysis PASSIVE *THERAPY.

passive avoidance AVOIDANCE.

passive-dependent personality DEPEND-
ENT PERSONALITY DISORDER.

passive learning INCIDENTAL *LEARNING.

passive therapy THERAPY, PASSIVE.

passive vocabulary VOCABULARY, PASSIVE.

pastoral counselling Psychological counselling carried out by members of the clergy
who have been trained to work with members of their congregation who seek help
with emotional problems.

past-pointing 1 The inability to place
accurately one's finger on some specified
part of the body. It is a sign of various neurological disorders. 2 The tendency to point
past a specific spot following rapid rotation
of the whole body. Unlike 1, this is normal
and a sign that one's vestibular system is
functioning properly.

patella The kneecap.

patellar reflex KNEE-JERK REFLEX.

paternal behaviour Collectively, all those
behaviours relating to or associated with
being a father. The caveats concerning
usage outlined under MATERNAL BEHAVIOUR
apply here as well. See also PARENTAL BEHAV-
IOUR.

paternalism 1 Specifically, a leadership
pattern in which males in positions of
authority use their power to provide protection and control in return for loyalty and
obedience. 2 More loosely, any relationship
in which adults are treated like children and
denied the right to personal control.

path 1 Simply, a line connecting two
points. More specifically: 2 In neurophysiology, a route formed by neurons along which
nerve conduction takes place. 3 In simple
learning experiments, a route through a
maze. 4 In K. Lewin's field theory, a topological metaphor for a route over which a person moves psychologically. 5 In sociometry,
a component in a theoretical model which
displays the hypothesized causal relationships between variables. In all these uses,
the synonym *pathway* may be used, particularly in 2.

path analysis A type of multivariate analysis that enables a researcher to discern the

causal relations that exist between several
variables. The relations are represented by
graphs called *path diagrams* that show the
various paths that these causal influences
travel.

pathergasia A. Meyer's term for the syndrome in which a personality or behaviour
disorder is associated with an anatomical or
structural abnormality.

pathetic fallacy ANTHROPOMORPHISM.

pathetism A rare synonym of HYPNOTISM.

pathic Pertaining to disease, disease-like.

-pathic Suffix used to indicate: 1 The experience of being affected, or feeling that one has
been affected, in a particular way, e.g. *telepathic*. 2 A diseased condition, e.g. the *cardio-
pathic*. 3 A general disorder, e.g. *sociopathic*.
4 A form of therapy or treatment, e.g. *osteo-
pathic*.

path(o)- Word element borrowed from the
Greek *pathos* and carrying essentially the original meaning of *suffering, disease* or, more
generally, *feeling*.

pathobiography The use of largely historical data to perform a psychoanalytic, biographical analysis on a person.

pathogenesis As the roots of the word suggest, the origin and development of disease.

pathognomic 1 Generally, capable of
recognizing emotions and feelings. 2 More
specifically, capable of recognizing and diagnosing disease. 3 A synonym for PATHOGNO-
MONIC.

pathognomonic Relating to a symptom or
group of symptoms that are diagnostic
'trademarks' of a particular disease or disorder. Occasionally used as a synonym of
PATHOGNOMIC.

pathological gambling GAMBLING, PATHO-
LOGICAL.

pathological intoxication ALCOHOL INTOXI-
CATION, IDIOSYNCRATIC.

pathology 1 An abnormal condition or biological state in which proper functioning is
prevented. The specific medical usage connotes an *organic* dysfunction or disease, not
a *functional* one. However, in clinical psychology and psychiatry, the usage has been

extended so that disorders for which there are no known biological components are included, hence the term *psychopathology*. **2** A general label for the scientific study of such conditions. **3** A suffix used to specify a particular scientific or medical field, e.g. *neuropathology*. Note, however, that the simple term *pathologist* is still reserved for a medical specialist who deals with organic tissue abnormalities. Other specialists are always referred to by appending a qualifying prefix. adj. (for 1), *pathological*.

pathomimicry The feigning of a pathological state, mimicking the symptoms of a disease. The term is a general one and is used to refer to conscious, deliberate MALINGERING and MÜNCHAUSEN'S SYNDROME as well as more subtle, unconsciously motivated HYPOCHONDRIASIS. See also FACTITIOUS DISORDER.

pathway Synonym of PATH (esp. 2).

-pathy 1 Suffix denoting *disease, suffering* or *feeling*. **2** Combining form used to denote names of systems or methods of treatment, e.g. *osteopathy*.

patient In medicine: **1** n. One who is receiving treatment for a diagnosed illness or injury. **2** n. One who is receiving medical care. Meaning 2 is more general and covers persons with no demonstrable illness who are undergoing tests for possible disease. In psychology: **3** n. An individual in psychotherapy.
    Meanings 1 and 2 are straightforward, meaning 3 is not. Within psychology the use of the term to refer to a person in therapy derives from the influential MEDICAL MODEL of psychological and psychiatric disorders, which assumes that a MENTAL DISORDER is a MENTAL DISEASE analogous to an organic, somatic disease. While there are good reasons for regarding many mental and behavioural disorders as diseases and for viewing those suffering from them as patients in the medical sense (e.g. a seriously deteriorated schizophrenic who requires hospitalization and is receiving antipsychotic drugs under the care of a psychiatrist), it is far from clear that the term should be applied to an individual who consults a psychiatrist or a clinical psychologist for weekly sessions to work through feelings of insecurity (see CLIENT) or to persons who are undergoing psychoanalysis (see ANALYSAND).

patriarchy A social organization using the male or the father as the base. The organization may be local and small such as a family, or large and inclusive such as a society with a complex, male-dominated structure. See MATRIARCHY.

patrilineal descent The passing on of the family name or inheritance through the male line.

pattern 1 A model or sample. **2** A configuration or grouping of parts or elements with a coherent structure. References to 'patterned behaviour' or 'patterning' carry meaning 1, with the connotation that the behaviour is modelled after or copied from another. See MODEL, MODELLING and OBSERVATIONAL LEARNING. The connotation of meaning 2 is that the separate parts of an array, although distinguishable, form a coherent, integrated whole which is emphasized and which is the pattern. See here CONFIGURATION, GESTALT, PATTERN PERCEPTION and PATTERN RECOGNITION. Both meanings have verb forms, hence *to pattern* means either to copy or model, or to integrate or organize the elements of a stimulus array into a conceptual structure.

pattern analysis A statistical technique whereby one attempts to discover the set of test items that 'belong together' and thus enable the tester to make a more successful prediction of some criterion. Note that in a pattern analysis, unlike an analysis based on MULTIPLE CORRELATION, the implication is that the discovered pattern of scores is interactive and representative of an underlying ability.

pattern discrimination The process whereby a PATTERN (2) is detected in a complex stimulus array, e.g. discriminating a melody rather than just a sequence of notes. The term is used roughly interchangeably with PATTERN RECOGNITION on the grounds that discrimination entails recognition of a pattern and recognition of a pattern entails discrimination of that which is recognized as being distinct from other things. See also PATTERN PERCEPTION, which is used as a cover term here, thus obviating these lexical difficulties.

patterning 1 Behaving so as to copy or model a PATTERN (1); see here MODELLING (preferred). **2** The act of imposing a coherent structure or a PATTERN (2). **3** The acquisition of a response to a PATTERN (2) rather than to any of its subelements. **4** A programme of physical therapy used in treating children with brain damage.

pattern learning A term often used synonymously with RELATIONAL LEARNING. But see the discussions under PATTERN PERCEPTION and PATTERN RECOGNITION for further detail and special meanings.

pattern perception Loosely and generally (and, alas, tautologically), the perception of a PATTERN (2). Actually, most of what is really interesting about PERCEPTION involves the perception of patterns. In fact, it is trivially true that *all* perception involves patterning in that even in the case of the simplest possible visual stimulus display, a single point of white light, there is a pattern in that the perceiver distinguishes the spot from the background (see here FIGURE–GROUND). Thus, *pattern perception* has come to be used in the technical literature as an umbrella term and may refer to any or all of the issues involved in the *detection, discrimination* and *recognition* of patterns.

pattern recognition The separate words define the phrase rather nicely: pattern recognition is the act of recognizing that a particular array of stimulus elements or sequence of stimulus events is representative of a particular PATTERN (2). The simple definition of the term, however, covers some very tricky theoretical issues, which can be illuminated by posing a few simple questions: How does one recognize that a particular collection of facial movements is a smile and not a frown? That a particular configuration of wood, cloth and stuffing is a chair rather than a sofa? That a particular four-legged, hairy beast is a domestic dog and not a wolf? And so on. Such questions have proven rather resistant to simple answers; see here the entries on CATEGORY et seq. and CONCEPT et seq. to see how various terminologies have been introduced in an attempt to deal with them. Note also that many authors will use *pattern recognition* interchangeably with PATTERN DISCRIMINATION; see this term for discussion on why this synonymity is attractive. See also PATTERN PERCEPTION, which serves as an umbrella term.

pause 1 Generally, any short interruption in an ongoing process. More specifically: **2** In operant analyses of behaviour, a momentary cessation of operant responding. **3** In normal speech, a break in the speech stream. Here, FILLED, HESITATION and SILENT *PAUSES are distinguished. **4** In the study of eye movements, a FIXATION PAUSE.

pause, filled In speech, a pause in the ongoing flow of words which is filled with 'verbal gestures' such as 'ah', 'um' and 'well'. Since silence is often a cue for turn-taking during conversation, filled pauses act like 'floor-holders' and keep the speaker from being interrupted.

pause, hesitation A short hesitation in the flow of speech. Although some use this term synonymously with SILENT *PAUSE, it seems better to reserve it for those short spots of silence which serve linguistic function; e.g. appreciate how different the meaning is in the following sentence depending on whether the speaker puts a hesitation before or after the word *not*: 'He was not surprisingly killed by the blast.' Distinguish from JUNCTURE, which is phonemic.

pause, silent A pause in the flow of speech, a short period of silence. Most silent pauses (as well as most FILLED *PAUSES) have a 'computational' or 'lexical selection' function. That is, they are pauses during which the speaker plans the next phrase or sentence, or searches his or her memory for a particular word. Some use the term as a synonym of HESITATION *PAUSE, a practice not recommended (see that term for reasons). Also called *unfilled pause.*

Pavlovian Of or pertaining to the empirical and theoretical work of the great Russian physiologist Ivan Petrovich Pavlov (1849–1936). Although Pavlov's researches took him from the study of the heart through a series of investigations of the physiology of digestion (for which he was awarded the Nobel Prize in 1904) to an extensive programme of experimentation on conditioned responses, in psychology it is in this last area of research that he is best known and it is this work that is denoted by the adjectival form of his name. For details on specifics of the Pavlovian approach see CLASSICAL CONDITIONING, CONDITIONED RESPONSE, CONDITIONED STIMULUS, CONDITIONING and PAVLOVIANISM.

Pavlovian conditioning A term often used to mean CLASSICAL CONDITIONING.

Pavlovianism A variation on the physicalist IDENTITY THEORY associated closely with the work of I. P. Pavlov. The doctrine maintains that psychological states and processes are identical with physiological states and processes in the brain and, by extension, that investigation of the physiology and neurology of the brain (through, for example, the study of conditioning) is the only approach to psychological understanding likely to prove scientifically fruitful. It is this last proposition that kept Pavlov from ever referring to himself as a psychologist, preferring instead to regard his work as quintessentially physiological. See also PAVLOVIAN.

pavor (diurnus and *nocturnus*) SLEEP TERROR DISORDER.

Paxil Trade name for PAROXETINE.

pay-off The outcome of a trial expressed in terms of costs and/or benefits associated with taking a particular course of action.

pay-off matrix A matrix or table that gives the various PAY-OFFS associated with each of the possible outcomes in a signal-detection experiment, a game, a decision-making experiment, etc. See e.g. PRISONER'S *DILEMMA.

PCP PHENCYCLIDINE THIOPHENE.

PDP models PARALLEL DISTRIBUTED PROCESSING (PDP) MODELS.

peak-clipping The cutting-off (i.e. clipping) of the high-amplitude portions (or peaks) of a speech wave. Peak-clipping produces strange-sounding speech but surprisingly little reduction in its intelligibility, particularly when compared with *centre-clipping*, although, to be sure, size of clip is an important factor.

peak-end rule A cognitive heuristic whereby a past experience is evaluated based on how pleasant or unpleasant it felt at its peak and at its end, disregarding other information. The resultant bias in information processing is called the *peak-end effect*.

peak experience A term coined by Abraham Maslow to characterize a profound moment in a person's life, an instance when they feel in harmony with all things, clear, spontaneous, independent and alert and often with relatively little awareness of time and space. Maslow was interested in the occurrence of such moments of reverie, particularly their relationship to the attainment of SELF-ACTUALIZATION.

peak shift In conditioning, a shift in maximum responding away from the original conditioned stimulus (CS). For example, condition an organism with a 1,000 Hz tone as the CS followed by the non-reinforced presentation of tones below 1,000 Hz. The organism subsequently will show a 'shift' in 'peak' responding to tones higher than 1,000 Hz.

Pearson chi-square (χ^2) tests Any of several variations on the basic CHI-SQUARE statistic used mainly to test GOODNESS-OF-FIT.

Pearson product-moment correlation PRODUCT-MOMENT *CORRELATION.

Peckhamian mimicry MIMICRY.

pecking order The term derives from studies of chickens in which the order of dominance and its attendant privileges and priorities are expressible in terms of which chicken pecks which chicken. The phrase is used quite generally as a metaphor to characterize any graded ordering of privilege quite independently of fowl. Actually, since the phrase has become so common in everyday language, psychologists now prefer the phrase DOMINANCE HIERARCHY.

P-E-C scale MEASUREMENT OF *AUTHORITARIANISM.

ped- PAEDIA-, PAEDO-.

pedagogy Broadly, the science and art of teaching. The latter aspect, being the ascendant one, stamps the lie upon the former.

pederasty Specifically, anal intercourse with a young boy. Occasionally, although not correctly, it is used to mean any anal intercourse between two males. See SODOMY.

ped(i)- Combining form meaning *foot*.

pedia- PAEDIA-, PAEDO-.

pediatric psychology PAEDIATRIC PSYCHOLOGY.

pedication A catch-all term for a host of unusual sexual practices including pederasty, bestiality and sodomy.

pedigree 1 A schematic representation of the structure of a family showing marriages, offspring, etc.; in short, a richly detailed family tree. **2** In genetics research, a complex system of notation has been adopted so that specific aspects of gene-linked conditions are represented in a pedigree.

ped(o)- PAEDIA-, PAEDO-.

peduncle Any of several stalk-like bundles of nerve fibres in the brain.

peduncular hallocinosis A disorder caused by damage in the upper brainstem and marked by visual hallucinations and, on occasions, sleep disturbances and agitation. Interestingly, the patient is aware that the hallucinations are not real.

peeping Tom A term that has wended its way from the common tongue to the technical. Simply, a *voyeur*; see VOYEURISM.

peer From the Latin for *equal*, an individual who may be regarded as equal with another or others with respect to some function (e.g. skill, educational level) or some situation (e.g. socioeconomic status). The term PEER GROUP is preferred by many.

peer group Any group the several members of which have roughly equal status within the confines and functions of the group. Age is no issue, the term being used with regard to children as well as adults. Note, however, that legal issues may often intrude, as a peer group may also be defined as those of equal rank or of equal standing before the law. The latter meaning may or may not encompass the former – and vice versa.

peer rating A rating by one's PEERS in the sense of members of one's PEER GROUP. See also PEER REVIEW.

peer review Quite literally, a review by one's PEERS or by the members of one's PEER GROUP. Hence: **1** In social psychology, a process whereby one's behaviour is analysed and evaluated by other members of one's social group. **2** In the actual functioning of science, a set of procedures whereby one's colleagues in a scientific field evaluate one's contribution in that field. In this sense, peer review is used to determine the publishability of scientific papers, to evaluate research proposals, to assess grant applications, etc.

pee shyness PARURESIS.

pegboard test Any of several performance tests of manual dexterity in which pegs must be placed in holes as rapidly as possible.

peg-word system A mnemonic technique in which the memorizer uses the components of a previously learned system as 'pegs' upon which to 'hang' new material. Perhaps the most common is the 'one-bun, two-shoe, three-tree', etc. rhyme, which, once learned, can be used to memorize a long list of new words by associating the first word with a bun, the second with a shoe, and so forth.

pellet A small, round bit of laboratory chow of standardized size, weight and nutritional content used as a reinforcement in animal experiments.

penalty As a simple extension of its standard meaning, the term is used in some experimental work to refer to the outcome of a trial in which the subject makes an error. The term is used in this sense as roughly equivalent to PUNISHMENT, although that term has additional meaning.

penetrance In genetics, the frequency of expression of a particular trait in a population of organisms all of which possess the genetic configuration for that trait.

penile Pertaining to the penis. Compare with PHALLIC.

penis The male copulatory (and, in mammals, urinary) organ. Distinguish from PHALLUS.

penis captivus A set of circumstances in which the penis is held within the vagina and cannot be withdrawn. It exists as a momentary normal component in the copulatory behaviour of some species but it is clinically unknown in humans.

penis envy The hypothesized envy of the penis. The primary usage is with regard to women who, according to the classical Freudian view, are universally afflicted with a repressed wish to possess a penis. This position, stemming as it does from Freud's characterization of women as incomplete men, has been vigorously criticized and is rarely taken completely seriously any more. The secondary usage is with respect to young boys, who often display envy of the adult male.

pentatonic Of a musical scale based on five tones.

pentobarbital A short-to-immediate-acting BARBITURATE.

peotomy Surgical removal of the penis. Distinguish from CASTRATION.

pepsin An enzyme secreted by the stomach that breaks peptide bonds and thus initiates the process of breaking the proteins in food into their constituent amino acids.

peptic Pertaining to the stomach and to digestion.

peptide A chain of AMINO ACIDS held together by PEPTIDE BONDS. Molecules made up of several peptides are called *polypeptides*, and when the chains extend to over 50 amino acids they are called *proteins*. Many peptides produced in the body function as NEUROTRANSMITTERS, NEUROMODULATORS and HORMONES.

peptide bond A bond between the amino group of one amino acid and the carboxyl of another.

perceive Simply, to be aware of the source of that which impinges on the sensory receptors. Usage, however, is far from simple; see PERCEPTION for discussion.

perceived self SELF, PERCEIVED.

percentile Any of the 99 numbered points that divide an ordered set of scores into 100 parts, each of which contains a hundredth of the total. This straightforward meaning unfortunately often gets lost in confusion; see CENTILE and PARTILE for discussion.

percentile score A score given as a percentile and representing the percentage of scores in a sample that fall below it. That is, a score at the 50th percentile indicates that 50% of the scores fall below it. Note that the highest possible percentile score is 99; a score of 100 makes no sense since a score cannot be greater than itself.

percept That which is perceived. Note that a percept should not be confused with either a physical object (see DISTAL STIMULUS) or the energy that impinges on a receptor (see PROXIMAL STIMULUS). In the final analysis, a percept is phenomenological or experiential; it is the outcome of the process of PERCEPTION.

perception 1 Collectively, those processes that give coherence and unity to sensory input. This is the most general sense of the term and covers the entire sequence of events from the presentation of a physical stimulus to the phenomenological experiencing of it. Included here are physical, physiological, neurological, sensory, cognitive and affective components. Because this use of the term is so broad, it should be seen as encompassing many of the more specialized and restrictive senses that follow. **2** The awareness of an organic process. This meaning focuses on perception as a conscious event, as the actual experiencing of a chain of (organic) processes initiated by some external or internal stimulus. **3** A synthesis or fusion of the elements of sensation. This usage is found in the approach of STRUCTURALISM (1). **4** An intervening variable; a hypothetical internal event that results directly from stimulation of sensory receptors and is affected by drive level and habit. This meaning, of course, is that expressed within BEHAVIOURISM. **5** An awareness of the truth of something. This sense is largely nontechnical and connotes a kind of implicit, intuitive insight. **6** A label for the field of psychology that studies any or all of the processes entailed in the above meanings.

Not surprisingly, the full range of connotations of the term envelops nearly every aspect of psychology, and existing theories of perception are far-reaching indeed. In essence, the study of perception always begins with recognition of the fact that what is perceived is not uniquely determined by physical stimulation but, rather, is an organized complex dependent upon a host of other factors. While there is no doubt that the incoming stimulus is an essential feature of what is ultimately perceived, the old structuralist argument that perceptions are built up entirely out of sensations is accepted by virtually no one today. The following is a quick review of the factors that determine what is perceived; terms of importance are treated in more detail elsewhere in this volume.

(a) *Attention*. For an event to be perceived it must be focused upon or noticed. Moreover, attention itself is selective, so that attending to one stimulus tends to inhibit or suppress the processing of others. See here ATTENTION, COCKTAIL-PARTY PHENOMENON, INFORMATION PROCESSING.

(b) *Constancy*. The perceptual world tends to remain the same despite rather drastic alterations in sensory input. A book seen from an angle is still perceived as rectangular although the retinal image is distinctly trapezoidal. See here CONSTANCY, UNCONSCIOUS INFERENCE.

(c) *Motivation*. What is perceived is affected by one's motivational state; hungry people see food objects in ambiguous stimuli that sated people do not. See here NEW LOOK, PERCEPTUAL DEFENCE, PERCEPTUAL VIGILANCE.

(d) *Organization*. Perception is not a simple juxtaposition of sensory elements, it is fundamentally organized into coherent wholes. See GESTALT and related entries.

(e) *Set*. The cognitive and/or emotional stance that is taken toward a stimulus array strongly affects what is perceived. See here ATTITUDE, SET (2).

(f) *Learning*. There are two issues here. One concerns the question of how much of perception is innate and how much is acquired from experience; see HEREDITY–ENVIRONMENT CONTROVERSY, NATIVISM. The other concerns the question of how learning can function to modify perception; see PERCEPTUAL *LEARNING.

(g) *Distortion and hallucination*. Strong emotional feelings can distort perceptions rather dramatically, and hallucinations can be produced by a variety of causes including drugs, lack of sleep, sensory deprivation, emotional stress and psychosis. These 'misperceptions' are an intriguing problem because the essential perception seems to come from 'inside the head' rather than from the environment. See HALLUCINATION.

(h) *Illusion*. There are many circumstances in which what is perceived cannot be easily predicted from an analysis of the physical-stimulus array. See ILLUSION.

There are, of course, other elements involved in both the study of perception and the impact of perceptual research on other areas of psychology. Many of these are dealt with in the entries below; others are found under the relevant modifying term.

perception, binocular Normal perception with both eyes such that the two retinal images fuse into a single percept. See BINOCULAR and DEPTH PERCEPTION.

perception, span of APPREHENSION SPAN, SPAN OF *ATTENTION.

perception, subliminal A curious phrase since *subliminal* means below the threshold for perception. The term actually refers not to PERCEPTION in the usual sense of that term (meaning 1), but to the effect of a below-threshold stimulus upon an individual's behaviour. There has been considerable scientific debate over the reliability and/or validity of the effects of subliminal stimuli, and extensive discussion of the ethical issues raised by even the possibility that such effects might be real and thus be used by unscrupulous advertisers or politicians. There are reliable effects here (see PERCEPTUAL DEFENCE, PERCEPTUAL VIGILANCE, SUBCEPTION), but they are small and there is no evidence that they can be used to modify attitudes or emotions.

perceptive Only loosely related to the meaning of PERCEPTION, *perceptive* is most commonly used as descriptive of persons who are sensitive in picking up important cues in social situations.

perceptron A label used of any of several neural network models of perception based on principles of CONNECTIONISM (2).

perceptual Pertaining to PERCEPTION. Almost always used in combined form, as the following entries exemplify.

perceptual anchoring Characterizing any process where what is perceived is dependent not so much on the physical properties of the stimulus but on one's frame of reference.

perceptual cycle A term used by U. Neisser to characterize his argument that a critical aspect of perception consists of a set of cognitive anticipations about to-be-perceived information. The full perceptual cycle consists of three components: (a) a set of cognitive schemata which direct perceptual processes; (b) a set of perceptual-exploration responses which sample information; and (c) the actual stimuli of the physical environment. The information thus picked up modifies the existing cognitive schemata, which affect the exploration processes, and so on round the cycle. The term is Neisser's but the general notion of feedback and adjustment is common to many theories of perception.

perceptual defence Operationally, perceptual defence is said to occur whenever the recognition threshold for a stimulus is raised. Evidence for such an effect was put forward by workers in the so-called NEW LOOK approach, in which tachistoscopically presented words with unpleasant connotations and taboo words had higher thresholds than neutral words. This was hailed as a significant demonstration of the role of emotional and motivational factors in perception – not to mention as support for psychoanalytic theory, which places considerable stress on unconscious defences. Enthusiasm was tempered somewhat when it was recognized that these early experiments did not clearly distinguish between *unconscious* perceptual defence and *conscious* response inhibition; to wit, is it perceptual defence that prevents a subject from seeing a taboo word, or response inhibition that prevents the subject from reporting that that 'dirty word' was, in fact, *really* presented by the experimenter? Some more recent studies run with proper controls seem to suggest that perceptual defence (and its opposite, PERCEPTUAL VIGILANCE) may be real phenomena, although their effects are very small. Contrast with SUBCEPTION.

perceptual field 1 A very general term used to refer collectively to all of those aspects of the physical stimulus that an individual is conscious of. Because of the factors discussed under PERCEPTION, the elements of the perceptual field rarely, if ever, correspond with those in the environment in any simple one-to-one fashion. **2** RECEPTIVE FIELD.

perceptual fluency PROCESSING FLUENCY.

perceptual induction An occasional synonym of EMPATHY.

perceptual learning LEARNING, PERCEPTUAL.

perceptual organization ORGANIZATION, PRINCIPLE OF *ORGANIZATION.

perceptual schema SCHEMA (1).

perceptual sensitization A phenomenon said to occur when the recognition threshold for a stimulus is lowered, i.e. the subject is more sensitive than usual. See PERCEPTUAL VIGILANCE for nuances in usage.

perceptual set EINSTELLUNG, SET (2).

perceptual structure Loosely, the overall cognitive-perceptual organization of a complex stimulus. See here GESTALT and related entries.

perceptual transformation A general term for any modification in a percept produced by (a) additions to, deletions from or alterations in the physical stimulus, or (b) novel interpretations of the stimulus, changes in set or attitude, or sudden insights concerning the material.

perceptual vigilance A synonym of PERCEPTUAL SENSITIZATION, which, although clearly preferred on semantic grounds, is not as common in the literature. The word *vigilance* is a little tricky here because it carries the connotation that the subject is actively, even consciously, looking for a particular stimulus event, and most of the theories of the phenomenon (and its opposite, PERCEPTUAL DEFENCE) assume that unconscious processes are responsible. Nevertheless, *vigilance* is kind of catchy and continues to be the term of choice for most psychologists.

perch An antiquated term for a FIXATION PAUSE in reading.

percipient 1 Generally, one who perceives, a perceiver. **2** In parapsychology, one who supposedly receives a telepathic message.

perfect correlation CORRELATION, PERFECT.

perfect pitch ABSOLUTE PITCH.

perforant path A neural pathway connecting the ENTORHINAL CORTEX with the DENTATE GYRUS of the HIPPOCAMPAL FORMATION.

performance In its broadest sense performance can be equated with behaviour; hence any activity or set of responses that has some effect upon the environment. However, there are nuances of usage found in specific contexts. To wit: (a) Performance is sometimes equated with *achievement* in the sense that some measure of the adequacy of the behaviour is involved. The point here is that performance is often viewed as behaviour in some particular situation requiring particular responses, as in a test. Distinguish this usage from PERFORMANCE TEST, which is specifically a test in which the role of language is minimized, or a test which involves only motor coordination. (b) Performance is often used in a general way to include only that which is overt. In this sense, one finds distinctions between *performance* and COMPE-TENCE (3) or between *performance* and LEARN-ING. In these cases *performance* refers to the overt, observable behaviour while *competence* or *learning* refers to the covert, hypothesized states or processes inside the organism.

performance anxiety A general label for any unusually high level of stress or anxiety felt when required to perform some activity. The anxiety is assumed to emerge from fears of failure, public humiliation and/or the sense that one has not lived up to expectations, personal or public. The term is used in a host of contexts including fears associated with behaving in public (see SOCIAL *PHO-BIA), test taking (TEST ANXIETY) and sexual functions.

performance test Any test designed to rely on nonverbal PERFORMANCE. There is a variety of such tests using form boards, mazes, picture completions, puzzles, etc. The correlations between scores on these tests and on standard verbal tests designed to evaluate the same processes are moderately positive, although, given our cultural orientations, it is not surprising that verbal tests have the higher predictive validity.

performative A SPEECH ACT in which, by its very utterance, the speaker performs something. Examples: judge to prisoner, 'I sentence you to five years in prison'; delegate at a political convention, 'I nominate Joe Blow for president.' Verbs typically used performatively: *appoint, order, urge, promise, guarantee, state, request, thank,* etc. See also COMMISSIVE and DECLARATIVE, which are other speech acts that can have performative properties.

peri- Combining form meaning *around, about, outside* or *beyond.*

periaqueductal grey (PAG) An area in the midbrain surrounding the cerebral aqueduct. It contains opiate-sensitive cells that play an important role in inhibiting pain through descending axons that synapse onto neurons in the lower brainstem and spinal cord that mediate *analgesia*. It also plays a role in control over aggressive behaviour and the female sexual response.

perimacular vision VISION, PERIMACULAR.

perinatal During the period just preceding, during or just following childbirth.

period 1 The duration of a complete oscillation of a cyclic (periodic) event. **2** The days of the menstrual flow. **3** The menstrual discharge itself.

periodicity theory of hearing THEORIES OF *HEARING.

periodic reinforcement A descriptive label for any reinforcement presented according to a regular time schedule. See SCHEDULES OF *REINFORCEMENT.

period prevalence In epidemiology, the total number of cases of a disease that occur within a specified time period. Compare with POINT PREVALENCE.

peripheral A multipurpose adjective used in a variety of circumstances when one wishes to distinguish between things, events or processes that are external or on the outside (i.e. on the periphery) from those which are internal or central. Thus, it is used to pertain to: **1** The surface or outer part of an organ or body. **2** The sensory (afferent) and motor (efferent) neurons connecting the surface of the body with the central nervous system, i.e. the *peripheral nervous system.* **3** Those psychological processes assumed to be intimately connected with that which is muscular, glandular, visceral, skeletal or sensory; that is, processes not considered to be intrinsic to the higher brain centres. This use, as many have noted, is highly arbitrary. Theorists who argue for PERIPHERALISM include many processes here that others would classify as central; e.g. Watson even considered *thinking* a peripheral process. **4** That which is of marginal or doubtful relevance or importance.

peripheral dyslexia DYSLEXIA, PERIPHERAL.

peripheralism A theoretical perspective that focuses on peripheral processes as explanatory devices. The strongest proponent of this point of view was the originator of radical behaviourism, John B. Watson, who took the arguments about as far as they could go – to the point of characterizing thinking as merely subvocal laryngeal movements and all emotions as mechanical glandular responses. From this orientation, conscious experience was regarded as epiphenomenal and without a causal role in determining behaviour. The WATSONIAN position was a reaction to STRUCTURALISM (2) and PSYCHO-ANALYSIS. It has no serious adherents today.

peripheral nervous system NERVOUS SYS-TEM.

peripheral route to persuasion ELABOR-ATION LIKELIHOOD MODEL.

peripheral vision VISION, PERIPHERAL.

periphery of the retina The outermost area of the retina, that farthest from the fovea. It is not sharply defined, but generally regarded as the area where the cones are effectively absent. Peripheral vision is relatively poor, low in acuity and strictly achromatic.

perirhinal cortex PARAHIPPOCAMPAL CORTEX.

periventricular hypothalamus HYPOTHA-LAMUS.

Perky effect A confusion between imagery and perception. In the basic procedure, the subject is asked to image an object, say an apple, on an initially blank screen. A very dim picture of an apple is then projected on the screen and the subject is often incapable of detecting that the real picture of the apple is other than the imaged apple.

permanent memory LONG-TERM *MEMORY.

permeable Capable of being permeated. In physiological work, descriptive of a membrane through which certain substances are able to pass. Somewhat more metaphorically, characterizing any boundary that can be penetrated.

permissiveness An attitude or characteristic of persons such that they tend to be liberal, granting considerable behavioural freedom and latitude to others over whom they have authority. Contrast with AUTHORI-TARIANISM.

pernicious trend Pernicious means *ruinous, harmful*, even *fatal*. Hence, this term is used as descriptive of any serious, regressive trend away from normal development. It is also used by researchers to describe a pattern in their data that consistently supports someone else's theory.

persecutory anxiety PARANOID ANXIETY.

perseverance PERSISTENCE.

perseveration Several uses are found, all deriving from the notion of a tendency to persist, to endure, although, unlike the base term *persevere*, its connotations are negative. It will be found denoting a propensity to continue with a dysfunctional pattern of behaviour, a tendency to repeat a word or phrase to a pathological degree and to the tendency for a particular memory or idea to recur without any detectable stimulus for it. Compare with PERSISTENCE. adj., *Perseverate*.

perseveration deficit DEFICIT, PERSEVERA-TION.

perseveration set A SET (2) that one carries over from one situation to another. The usual connotation is that such a set reflects an inability to shift strategies appropriately.

perseverative error 1 Any error made repeatedly. 2 More rarely, a response that is an error because it is a response to the previous rather than the current stimulus.

perseverative functional autonomy Allport's term for an extreme form of FUNCTIONAL *AUTONOMY displayed as inappropriate repetitions and ritualized acts. Compare with PROPRIATE FUNCTIONAL AUTONOMY.

perseverative trace TRACE, PERSEVERATIVE.

persistence Similar in meaning to PERSE-VERATION in that it reflects a behavioural tendency to persevere or persist, but with two important differences. First, the negative connotations of *perseveration* are generally not present; *persistence* suggests an admirable striving against opposition. Second, *persistence* typically refers to behaviour, while *perseveration* is generally suggestive of a tendency. In this sense *persistence* is used to refer to processes which continue in time after the stimulus that initiated them is no longer present. syn., *perseverance*.

persistence of vision ICONIC (2).

persistent Müllerian duct syndrome A congenital condition in which there is an absence of ANTI-MÜLLERIAN HORMONE receptors. In a genetic male it produces a hermaphrodite with both male and female internal sex organs.

persistent vegetative state VEGETATIVE STATE.

person Psychology, in one guise or another, concerns itself with entities that behave, act, think and emote and do so within the context of some social and physical environment. When such an entity is a member of the species *Homo sapiens* the term *person* is appropriately used as label.

persona From the Latin, meaning *person*. In classical Roman theatre, a mask which an actor wore to express his role. By extension of this notion, Jung used the term in his early formulations to refer to the role a person takes on by virtue of the pressures of society; that is, the role that society expects a person to play in life, not necessarily the one played at a deep psychological level. The persona is public, the face presented to others. Compare with ANIMA (2).

personal 1 Relating to some thing, event or characteristic that has the quality of a person. **2** Relating to some thing, event or characteristic that is intrinsic to a particular person. Meaning 1 is general, the reference being personhood; meaning 2 is specific, the reference being a single individual.

personal construct The central concept in George Kelly's theory of personality. The term is a cover for all of the ways in which a person attempts to perceive, understand, predict and control the world. Each of an individual's personal constructs functions like a hypothesis, a possible way of constructing the physical and social environment. It may be altered if conflicting information is perceived, or become fixed and incorporated as basic aspects of one's personality. See REP TEST.

personal determinant DETERMINANT.

personal disjunction The disparity between what one would ideally like to get from a situation (or from life in general) and what one actually expects to get. Note that the discrepancy is not between desire and reality, it is between what is wanted and a judgement of how likely it is that that want will be fulfilled.

personal disposition G. W. Allport's term for PERSONALITY TRAIT.

personal document Any self-produced document that provides information about an individual, e.g. a diary, personal essay, autobiographical sketch, letter or recording. The personal aspect is what makes it of interest. Because its creation is intrinsically motivated, unlike the responses to a questionnaire or an interview, a personal document presumably provides insights into those aspects of social and personal life that the writer/recorder regards as most salient.

personal equation A term coined by the 19th-century astronomer F. W. Bessel to refer to a procedure for correcting for differences in reaction time between two observers of stellar transit. Bessel proposed the 'equation' as a mathematical method to correct for the individual differences of astronomers so as to prevent such factors from contaminating astronomical research. By extension, it became a phrase used to mean any adjustment for difference in simple reaction times between any two subjects.

personal fitness In evolutionary biology, an individual organism's reproductive success. Also called *Darwinian fitness* and, simply, FITNESS (2).

personal identity 1 The phenomenological sense that one has of one's own intrinsic self independent of all others and transcending the biological and psychological emendations and amputations produced by a world in flux. See here SELF. **2** The fact that each person is a separate individual. Meaning 1 is the existentially more interesting one: it reflects the essential quality of selfness and if lost the continued existence of 2 hardly seems to make any difference.

personalism 1 Generally, an approach to psychological science that maintains that the individual personality is the central construct against which all else must be considered. **2** More specifically, the general principle that a person perceives and interprets the actions of another partly by reference to the extent to which those actions are directed personally at him or her. Thus, one reads of the personalisms of another's behaviours, meaning the degree to which they are seen as directed at the perceiver. **3** A synonym of PERSONALISTIC PSYCHOLOGY.

personalistic psychology The orientation that argues that psychological principles only have meaning when they are mapped into or shown to be reflections of personal life and personal experience.

personality One of the classic 'chapter heading' words in psychology. That is, a term so resistant to definition and so broad in usage that no coherent simple statement about it can be made – hence the wise author uses it as the title of a chapter and then writes freely about it without incurring any of the definitional responsibilities that go with introducing it in the text. Rather than repeat here the folly of several score unwise authors (G. W. Allport, back in 1927, was able to cull nearly 50 different definitions from the literature, and heaven only knows how many one could find today), we shall not characterize the term definitionally but rather according to its role in personality theory. This approach seems best, since each author's meaning of the term tends to be coloured by his or her theoretical biases and by the empirical tools used to evaluate and test the theory. The easiest procedure is to present a few of the most influential general orientations and outline how each characterizes the term:

1. *Type theories*. The oldest of these is that of Hippocrates, who hypothesized four basic temperaments: choleric, sanguine, melancholic and phlegmatic. The assumption here, as in all subsequent type theories, was that each individual was a representation of a particular balance of these basic elements. The most complete typological theory was that of W. H. Sheldon, who elegantly (but unconvincingly) argued that body types were intimately related to personality development. See CONSTITUTIONAL THEORY for a discussion. Carl Jung's approach, although belonging properly with the psychoanalytic theories (see below), is sometimes pigeonholed as a type theory because of his emphasis upon classifying individuals according to types, e.g. *introvert* vs. *extravert*.

2. *Trait theories*. All theories of this kind operate from the assumption that one's personality is a compendium of *traits* or characteristic ways of behaving, thinking, feeling, reacting, etc. The early trait theories were actually little more than lists of adjectives,

and personality was defined by enumeration. Other approaches have used the techniques of factor analysis in an attempt to isolate underlying dimensions of personality. Currently, the most influential model is FIVE FACTOR THEORY based on a cluster of five underlying dimensions although some earlier theories, such as that of R. B. Cattell based on a set of SOURCE *TRAITS also have adherents.

Note that the *type* and *trait* approaches complement each other and, indeed, one could argue that they are two sides of the same coin. Type theories are primarily concerned with that which is common among individuals, while trait theories focus on that which differentiates them. However, they certainly entail very different connotations of the base term *personality*.

3. *Psychodynamic and psychoanalytic theories*. A multitude of approaches is clustered here, including, among others, the classic theories of Freud and Jung, the social psychological theories of Adler, Fromm, Sullivan and Horney, and the more recent, somewhat unorthodox approaches of Laing and Perls. The distinctions between them are legion but all contain an important common core idea: personality for all is characterized by the notion of *integration*. Strong emphasis is generally placed upon developmental factors, with the implicit assumption that the adult personality evolves gradually over time, depending on the manner in which the integration of factors develops. Moreover, motivational concepts are of considerable importance, so that no account of personality is considered to be theoretically useful without an evaluation of the underlying motivational syndromes. syn., CHARACTER (2).

4. *Behaviourism*. The focus here has been on the extension of learning theory to the study of personality. Although there are no influential, purely behaviouristic theories of personality, the orientation has stimulated other theorists to look closely at an integral problem: how much of the behavioural consistency that most people display is due to underlying personality *types* or *traits* or *dynamics*, and how much is due to consistencies in the environment and in the contingencies of reinforcement? Not surprisingly, the points of view below, all of which were influenced to some degree by behaviourism, look beyond the person for answers here and,

to some degree or another, actually question the usefulness of the term *personality*.

5. *Humanism*. This orientation emerged as a reaction to what was perceived as the dominance of psychoanalysis and behaviourism in psychology. Thinkers such as Maslow, Rogers, May and Frankl focused on PHENOMENOLOGY, in which subjective mental experiences are paramount, on HOLISM, which rejects the reductionism of behaviourism, and on the importance of the drive toward SELF-ACTUALIZATION (2). Humanism's main problems concern the difficulty of testing scientifically many of its theoretical notions. Nevertheless, it has remained an important approach to the study of personality and has given rise to the HUMAN POTENTIAL MOVEMENT.

6. *Social learning theories*. Much of the theorizing from this point of view derives from the problem of balancing the impact of the environment with that of naturally given properties. However, the notion of personality is treated as those aspects of behaviour that are acquired in a social context. The leading theorist here is Albert Bandura, whose position is based on the assumption that although learning is critical, factors other than simple stimulus–response associations and reinforcement contingencies are needed to explain the development of complex social behaviours (such as *roles*) that essentially make up one's personality. In particular, cognitive factors such as memory, retention processes and self-regulatory processes are important, and much research has focused on modelling and observational learning as mechanisms that can give a theoretically satisfying description of the regularities of behaviour in social contexts.

7. *Situationism*. This perspective, championed by Walter Mischel, is derivative of behaviourism and social learning theory. It argues that whatever consistency of behaviour is observable is largely determined by the characteristics of the *situation* rather than by any internal personality types or traits. Indeed, the very notion of a personality trait, from this point of view, is nothing more than a mental construction of an observer who is trying to make some sense of the behaviour of others and exists only in the mind of the beholder. The regularity of behaviour is attributed to similarities in the situations one tends to find oneself in rather than to internal regularities.

8. *Interactionism*. This position is a kind of eclectic position 1. It admits of certain truths in all of the above, more single-minded, theories and maintains that personality emerges from interactions between particular qualities and predispositions and the manner in which the environment influences the ways in which these qualities and behavioural tendencies are displayed. It is far from clear from this perspective that personality can be said to exist as a distinct 'thing'. Rather it becomes a kind of cover concept for the complex patterns of interaction.

It is interesting to note that the above theoretical approaches can be seen as representing two distinguishable generalizations concerning the very term *personality*. For 1–3 the word represents a legitimate theoretical construct, a hypothetical, internal 'entity' with a causal role in behaviour and, from a theoretical point of view, with genuine explanatory power. For 4–8 it is a secondary factor inferred on the basis of consistency of behaviour – while other operations and processes play the critical causal roles in dictating behaviour – and, hence, a notion that has relatively little explanatory power.

The foregoing does not, of course, exhaust the theoretical approaches that have had their turn in the scientific spotlight (see e.g. EXISTENTIALISM, FIELD THEORY), but it should suffice to give a feeling for the diversity of forms of meaning that the term *personality* can express. The term is also found in a wide variety of combined forms, the more common of which follow.

personality disintegration Since many personality theorists regard *integration* as one of the key aspects of a normal, well-adapted, functioning PERSONALITY, this term is used to designate the circumstances in which the various components (behavioural, emotional, motivational) lose their integrated, structured quality. However, since various theorists propose various ways of conceptualizing the components of personality, there are similarly various ways of conceptualizing just what personality disintegration is.

personality disorder This term has served for a considerable length of time as an umbrella term for any of a number of psychological disorders. The primary difficulty in determining just what belongs under the umbrella and just how it is being used derives from the fact that several 'official' definitions have been 'traded in' for newer models over the past several decades. To wit: **1** Originally, any mental disorder manifested by maladjustments in motivation and maladaptive patterns of relating to one's social environment. This sense was used so broadly that it encompassed minor neuroses as well as full-blown psychotic disturbances. It also had a tendency to be applied rather arbitrarily to styles of social interaction that were outside the observer's particular perspective concerning what was right and proper. Because of this looseness of usage, this meaning was abandoned – and it is surely of interest that the term itself survived this (and a further) adjustment in denotation rather than simply succumbing to such excess. **2** A class of behavioural disorders, *excluding* the neuroses and psychoses, manifested as pathological developments in one's overall personality and marked by relatively little anxiety or distress. Within this general use of the term three subclasses of disorders were identified: (a) The *general personality disorders*, including COMPULSIVE, CYCLOTHYMIC, PARANOID and SCHIZOID PERSONALITIES. (b) The *sociopathic disorders*, characterized by a general lack of appropriate affect, little or no guilt following transgressions and an inability to form lasting emotional bonds with others. Included here were ANTISOCIAL, DYSSOCIAL, PSYCHOPATHIC and SOCIOPATHIC PERSONALITIES. (c) The *sexual deviants*, whose primary mode of sexual gratification was generally regarded as socially undesirable. This sense of the term was the dominant one until the third edition of the US DIAGNOSTIC AND STATISTICAL MANUAL in 1980, which revised the use of the term considerably. Many of the subcategories of personality disorder given in the following are carryovers from those in 2; however, the label *personality* which was attached to each disorder has been altered so that *personality disorder* is now the preferred term, e.g. *schizoid personality* is now *schizoid personality disorder*. **3** A mental disorder the essential features of which are deeply ingrained, enduring, maladaptive patterns of relating to, thinking about and perceiving the environment that are so extreme they cause impairment in social and behavioural functioning. Recent classification systems break this group into three 'clusters' based on the manner in which the behavioural aspects of the disorder are manifested. Specifically, there is a *dramatic* cluster including BORDERLINE, ANTISOCIAL, NARCISSISTIC and HISTRIONIC PERSONALITY DISORDERS all of which are characterized by overt, dramatic displays and personal styles; an *anxious* cluster including DEPENDENT, AVOIDANT and OBSESSIVE-COMPULSIVE PERSONALITY DISORDERS where the emotions and behaviours are characterized by excessive anxiety, and the quaintly named *odd* cluster which includes PARANOID, SCHIZOID and SCHIZOTYPAL PERSONALITY DISORDERS each of which is marked by socially inappropriate behaviours. Note that several of these subtypes are used with more than one of the focal meanings. See each for additional details. Personality disorders are generally recognizable in childhood or adolescence and continue through most of adult life. Note, however, if diagnosed before age 18, the proper diagnostic category is DISORDER OF *CHILDHOOD.

personality dynamics A general term for the study of the complex, interactive, dynamic aspects of motivation, emotion and behaviour. See DYNAMIC.

personality integration Generally, the coordination, organization or unification of the disparate traits, behavioural dispositions, motives, emotions, etc. that make up one's personality. See also PERSONALITY DISINTEGRATION and the core term PERSONALITY.

personality inventory A personality-assessment device based on a large number of items to which the subject responds by indicating those that apply to or are descriptive of him- or herself. Three types of inventory are common: in one the subject responds to statements with 'yes', 'no' or 'questionable'; in another the subject chooses from pairs of statements the one that best applies in each case; and the third uses the LIKERT SCALE. See e.g. MINNESOTA MULTIPHASIC PERSONALITY INVENTORY.

personality organization PERSONALITY INTEGRATION.

personality problem A basically nontechnical term used as a catch-all label for any minor, persistent or recurring behavioural, motivational or emotional pattern that makes a person unhappy.

personality, segmentalized A term borrowed from sociology for one who has developed, as a response to societal pressures, a diverse and inconsistent set of social roles and ways of behaving. It is argued by some that complex urban societies are more likely to produce this type of personality than small, more coherent, rural societies. Distinguish from MULTIPLE PERSONALITY.

personality sphere R. B. Cattell's term for the entire range of measurable human personality. In his model it is comprised of a large set of SURFACE *TRAITS and a smaller group of SOURCE *TRAITS derived by factor analysis.

personality, split A strictly nontechnical term used in popular parlance more or less appropriately for MULTIPLE PERSONALITY (see DISSOCIATED IDENTITY DISORDER) and more or less inappropriately for SCHIZOPHRENIA.

personality syndrome The original meaning of *syndrome* carried with it the notion of a characteristic pattern of symptoms of a disease. This meaning has been extended to the notion of personality such that *syndrome* here refers to a set of maladaptive behavioural characteristics that have been shown to be common to many persons. When the unqualified term is used, the 'disease' aspect is largely dropped, on the grounds that the causal factors are largely social and cultural rather than biological. However, when physiological factors are clearly implicated, the term ORGANIC *PERSONALITY SYNDROME is used.

personality syndrome, organic Any marked alteration in personality where a specific biological factor has been identified. Typical symptoms include socially unacceptable action, extreme emotional lability, loss of impulse control and lack of recognition of the consequences of one's actions. FRONTO-TEMPORAL DEMENTIA and FRONTAL-LOBE SYNDROME are used nearly synonymously. Note also that this diagnostic category is no longer listed in the *DSM*. See discussion under ORGANIC (5).

personality test Very loosely, any device or instrument for assessing or evaluating personality. Typically, *direct tests* (e.g. the MINNE-SOTA MULTIPHASIC PERSONALITY INVENTORY) are distinguished from *indirect* or *projective tests* (e.g. the RORSCHACH test).

personality theory PERSONALITY.

personality trait Loosely a TRAIT of personality. That is: **1** Some hypothesized underlying disposition or characteristic of a person that, in principle, can be used as an explanation of the regularities and consistencies of his or her behaviour. See, here, the discussion under PERSONALITY (esp. 2). **2** A simple description of an individual's characteristic modes of behaving, perceiving, thinking, etc. Meaning 2 is used descriptively without explanatory intent; meaning 1 is grounded in a particular approach to personality theory.

personality type Generally, any label used for classifying an individual's personality. There are many different typologies, each with its own categorization system. All, however, are predicated on the assumption that coherent patterns of behaviour or consistent styles of action exist which are sufficiently well defined that individuals may be classified as falling into one or more types. See PERSONALITY (esp. 1).

personalized instruction A general term for any educational programme designed with sufficient flexibility to be adapted to individual students of differing capabilities.

personal space The area immediately surrounding an individual. It may be a large area or a small one depending on a host of momentary factors (whom you are with, your mood, the nature of the interaction, etc.) and more permanent factors (cultural traditions, physical size, etc.).

personal unconscious Jung's term for an individual person's unconscious as distinguished from the transpersonal, COLLECTIVE UNCONSCIOUS. Jung conceived of the personal unconscious as consisting of repressed, suppressed, forgotten or even ignored experiences and treated it very much like Freud's PRECONSCIOUS in that material from it could and often did enter consciousness.

person-centred therapy An occasional synonym of CLIENT-CENTRED THERAPY.

personification 1 Generally, the imputing of human or personal qualities to some abstraction. The abstraction may be a social group or a social structure, an image or representation of some real person, or even something which is not human. See ANTHROPOMORPHISM and ANIMISM. **2** More specifically, a type of defence mechanism in which the individual attributes qualities or the blame for things to others as a result of personal frustrations. See here PROJECTION, of which personification is generally regarded as a form.

personnel 1 n. Specifically, the employees in an organization. **2** n. More generally, the human aspect in business and industry. **3** adj. Pertaining to either 1 or 2.

personnel psychology A general label for that aspect of industrial/organizational psychology concerned with (a) the selecting, supervising and evaluating of PERSONNEL, and (b) a variety of job-related factors such as morale, personal satisfaction, management–worker relations and counselling.

personology 1 The label Henry Murray applied to his herculean efforts to develop a comprehensive theory of personality. His viewpoint was strongly organic and holistic. He insisted that no isolated piece of behaviour could ever be understood without taking into account the fully functioning person. **2** Loosely, the study of personality. The preferred usage is the first.

person perception A general label for an area in social psychology concerned with the issue of how we perceive other persons. Although the basic principles of perception certainly apply, there are a variety of additional variables and factors which make other persons rather special objects of perception. To appreciate the kinds of issues involved here see ATTRIBUTION THEORY, IMPRESSION FORMATION and PREJUDICE.

person positivity bias A tendency to view individual persons more positively than the group which they represent. The most dramatic case is that of politicians, who collectively are viewed rather poorly, yet tend to be liked individually by many people, particularly their own constituents.

perspective 1 A mental view, a cognitive orientation, a way of seeing a situation or a scene. **2** The arrangement of the parts of a whole scene as viewed from some concep-

tual, physical or temporal vantage point. The implication is that this vantage point provides the proper point of view, the perception being more veridical than from some other. **3** The arrangement of objects on a flat surface such that the viewer receives the impression of a three-dimensional scene.

perspective-taking 1 In the Piagetian approach, the capacity of a child to view the environment from the position other than the one he or she is in. In the classical experiment to study the effect, a puppet is placed in a room away from the child, who is asked what the puppet can see. **2** In social psychology, the capacity to appreciate the point of view of another person with whom one is interacting. In this sense, it is an essential feature of smooth social relationships.

persuasion A process of inducing a person to adopt a particular set of values, beliefs or attitudes. Studies of this process have been far-reaching and have implicated a number of factors both rational and nonrational. See e.g. COGNITIVE DISSONANCE, CREDIBILITY, PERSUASIVE COMMUNICATION and ELABORATION LIKELIHOOD MODEL.

persuasive communication Quite literally, a communication that persuades. Identifying the set of factors that make up such a message is an important goal in social psychology. Both external aspects (the message itself, the arguments presented, the credibility of the source, the medium used, etc.) and internal aspects (the receiver's beliefs, credulity, etc.) are involved.

persuasive therapy An approach to psychotherapy based on the use of direct suggestion, the giving of specific advice and direct counselling.

pervasive developmental disorder DEVELOPMENTAL DISORDER, PERVASIVE.

perversion As derived from the Latin *perversio*, (meaning facing the wrong way), a perversion is any turning away from the right course, any distortion from the proper path to the proper end. With this general connotation, the term can be and is used to refer to thought processes, emotions, judgements or actions which are, in some sense, warped or distorted. However, the overwhelmingly common reference is to behaviours that are sexual – so much so that many use the term as if its sole semantic domain were sexual. In an effort to disabuse readers of this unnecessary restriction, the sexual aspect is given under the separate entry SEXUAL *PERVERSION.

perversion, sexual Any form of sexual behaviour that is a distortion of the 'proper goal' of sex (see PERVERSION). Ascertaining precisely what constitutes the proper goal and hence what characterizes perverted sexual behaviour has proven something of a problem. If one takes the point of view that procreation is the only proper goal, then anything other than heterosexual intercourse under the biologically appropriate circumstances is a sexual perversion; if one assumes that sexual pleasure is a legitimate and proper goal then it becomes difficult to exclude anything. Many psychiatric nomenclatures, deriving as they do from the early decades of the 20th century, list *homosexuality, voyeurism, exhibitionism, fetishism, sadism, masochism, bestiality, pederasty* and *sodomy* as sexual perversions. More modern (enlightened?) nosologies restrict the domain of the term to those sexual acts that violate the personal rights and desires of others, and hence include *exhibitionism, rape* and *child molesting*; modes of sexual expression such as *sadism* or *sodomy* are only regarded as perversions when they are imposed on an unwilling partner or a juvenile. In some nomenclatures PARAPHILIA is used synonymously.

Peter principle The notion that a person gets promoted through the ranks of an organization until he or she reaches his or her level of incompetence; that is, the level at which he or she can almost, but not quite, do the job well.

petit mal MINOR *EPILEPSY.

petrification R. D. Laing's term for a defensive reaction, used by the insecure when under severe psychological threat. An individual depersonalizes ('turns to stone') either the outside other who is the source of the threat or himself or herself.

peyote **1** Specifically, the peyote cactus (*Lophophora williamsii*), from which the psychoactive drug MESCALINE is derived. **2** Loosely, mescaline itself.

PGO spikes Bursts of activity originating in the pons (P), moving to the geniculate nucleus (G) and the occipital cortex (O), characteristic of REM SLEEP. Also called *PGO waves*.

PGR Abbreviation for *psychogalvanic response*. See GALVANIC SKIN RESPONSE.

phacoscope An instrument for observing the changes in the images reflected from the lens of the eye (see PURKINJE–SANSON IMAGES) during accommodation. var., *phakoscope*.

Phaedra complex From the myth of Phaedra, wife of Theseus, the incestuous desire of a mother for her son.

-phagia, -phagy Combining form from the Greek, meaning *eating*.

phagocytosis Lit., cell-eating. Used of the complex process in which particular cells in the body engulf and digest neurons that have died and, by extension, similar absorption of noncellular material such as food particles and other foreign substances.

phakoscope PHACOSCOPE.

phallic Pertaining to: **1** PHALLUS. **2** PENIS. Meaning 1 is preferred, particularly when symbolic reference is made; PENILE is best used for meaning 2.

phallic character An adult who compulsively displays behaviours which, according to psychoanalytic theory, are referable to the phallic stage of development. The dominant trait here is regarding sexual behaviour as a display of power and potency. Contrast with GENITAL CHARACTER.

phallic love In boys, love of the penis; by extension, in girls, love of the clitoris.

phallic phase PHALLIC STAGE.

phallic primacy In psychoanalysis, the focusing of erotic interest upon the penis or the clitoris during the early GENITAL STAGE.

phallic stage (or **level** or **phase**) In psychoanalytic theory, the stage of psychosexual development marked by great interest in (Freud called it a preoccupation with) one's penis or, by extension, in girls, one's clitoris. Theoretically, it follows the ANAL STAGE and is succeeded by the Oedipal stage (see OEDIPUS COMPLEX).

phallic symbol Anything that can be interpreted from a psychoanalytic perspective as symbolically representing a phallus. Most writers limit this class of objects to things pointed or upright, but this often underestimates the ingenuity of the interpreter.

phallic woman In psychoanalytic theory, the notion of a female with phallic traits. Theoretically, this is how the pre-Oedipal child views its mother. The idea of a phallic woman is also commonly found in folklore and myth and, according to some interpretations, is manifested in the (unconscious) conception of women in masochistic, submissive men.

phallocentric A sobriquet for the classical theory of psychoanalysis. The term was first applied by Ernest Jones as a critical comment upon the theory for placing so much emphasis on the penis and phallic symbolism, in particular the tendency to view the psychological development of the female as a reaction to the discovery that she does not have a penis.

phallus While *penis* is used as an anatomical term, the connotations of *phallus* are primarily symbolic. The reference, then, is the image or representation of the penis as a symbol of power. Jung is generally credited with the comment that nicely sums up the distinction: 'The penis is only a phallic symbol.'

phantasy FANTASY.

phantom 1 Generally, an image or semblance of something perceived but not physically present in the stimulus environment. See e.g. PHANTOM LIMB. **2** In psychoanalysis, an unconscious representation of a person.

phantom colours Colours perceived with achromatic stimuli. See BENHAM'S TOP.

phantom limb A subjective experience of sensations arising from a limb that has been amputated. Although the amputation of the limb removes the peripheral extremity itself, it does not destroy the neural representation of the limb, particularly in the cortex. When neighbouring cells begin to invade the cortical regions which are no longer receiving afferent inputs, feelings and sensations (often painful) are experienced as though coming from the nonexistent limb.

pharmacodynamics The study of drugs and their manner of action, particularly on specific receptors and receptor sites in the brain.

pharmacodynamic tolerance TOLERANCE, PHARMACODYNAMIC.

pharmacogenetics The study of the patterns of interaction between drugs and the genetic factors that influence their manner of action. Special attention is paid to individual differences in response to dosage levels and the metabolic actions that underlie them.

pharmacologic antagonism DRUG *ANTAGONISM.

pharmacology The science of the study of drugs. For its relevance to psychology, see PSYCHOPHARMACOLOGY.

pharmacopeia 1 Specifically, an authoritative treatise on drugs, including their preparation, chemical make-up and properties, recommended dosages and manner of administration. **2** More loosely, a full compendium of available drugs.

pharmacotherapy See DRUG THERAPY.

pharyngo- The combining form for PHARYNX.

pharynx The part of the oral cavity, including the surrounding muscles and membranes, connecting the mouth and nose with the larynx and oesophagus.

phase 1 An aspect of appearance or state of some thing or event which recurs as the thing or event passes cyclically through various modes or conditions. The key word in this definition is *recur*. Thus one sees references to the phase of a sound wave, the phases of the moon, the manic phase of manic-depression, etc. **2** A temporary *stage* in a person's life in which characteristic behaviours are observed. Strictly speaking, this usage is not proper, because the notion of recurrence is missing – unless one assumes that the recurrence is not within a single person but across many (all?) persons. It is frequently used in this latter sense in developmental and/or psychoanalytic works (e.g. *phallic phase*), and is particularly common in nontechnical writings with regard to periods during which children exhibit behaviours that their parents hope will soon cease. If a particular combined term with the word *phase* is not listed below, look under STAGE, which is preferred when the notion of recurrence is absent.

phase difference A difference in the phase relations of any two sound waves. When the phase difference is zero and the peaks and troughs occur simultaneously, the waves are said to be *in phase*. If the peak of one occurs simultaneously with the trough of the other, the waves are said to be *in opposite phase*. Phase differences are measured in phase angles, with 180° representing opposite phase. Phase differences are perceived as beats, as slight increases and decreases in intensity, and can be used as cues for the localization of a sound source.

phase locking In neurophysiology, the tendency of a cell to fire in a manner coordinated with particular portions of a cyclically repetitive stimulus. Many auditory fibres display this property, which was, interestingly, predicted by the *volley theory* of hearing long before it had been empirically identified. See THEORIES OF *HEARING.

-phasia Suffix meaning *speech disorder*, used with the implication that the disorder is due to a cortical lesion. See e.g. APHASIA.

-phemia Combining form meaning *speech disorder*, used with the implication that the disorder is due to psychological, i.e. nonorganic, factors.

phenazocine A synthetic OPIATE.

phencyclidine thiophene A hallucinogen chemically known as phenylcyclohexylpiperidine hydrochloride (PCP), with effects that are dose-related and range from a mild euphoria at low doses, through tenseness, palpitations, disorientation and hypertension as dosage is increased, to convulsions and possible death at high doses. Recovery from an overdose is not infrequently followed by an acute delirium, which may last for several days. PCP is a frequently abused drug with the street name of *angel dust*.

phenobarbital One of the more frequently prescribed long-acting BARBITURATES.

phenocopy A phenotypic syndrome that, owing to environmental factors, mimics a genetic syndrome.

phenomenal field Rather inclusively, absolutely anything that is in the total momentary experience of a person, including the experience of the self. The emphasis is on *experience* independent of physical stimuli; thus, those things imaged, emoted and thought are part of the phenomenal field even if not present physically, while those things present physically but not noticed or attended to are not. Also called *phenomenological field*.

phenomenalism 1 The philosophical point of view that knowledge and understanding are limited to 'appearances', to the ways in which objects and events are perceived, and that true reality outside of that which is phenomenological is unknowable. 2 A synonym of PHENOMENOLOGY, which is a somewhat different philosophy from 1. 3 A Piagetian term used to refer to the sense that if any two events occur in temporal contiguity then one of them must have caused the other; see PHENOMENISTIC THOUGHT.

phenomenalistic introspection A form of INTROSPECTION that is a free-flowing report of experience given in everyday language. As used by those with a phenomenological approach, it differs quite dramatically from the structured, systematic introspections of the *structuralists* and the *act psychologists*.

phenomenal motion APPARENT *MOTION.

phenomenal pattern That which is experienced or perceived as opposed to the objective, physical stimulus. For example, in a case of AMBIGUOUS *FIGURES, the objective stimulus remains constant but the phenomenal pattern changes.

phenomenal regression This term refers to the fact that neither the principles of perspective and geometry nor the principles of object constancy accurately predict what is perceived. The perceived size of a distant (and necessarily familiar) object tends to be slightly larger than geometric, line-of-sight estimates predict and somewhat smaller than if it were regarded as an object of constant size. The *regression* in the term is because, with practice, the perceived size tends to shift toward the predictions of the geometric principles.

phenomenal self SELF, PHENOMENAL.

phenomenistic causality PHENOMENISTIC THOUGHT.

phenomenistic thought A term used by Piaget to characterize the reasoning of a young child whose cognitive structures are predominantly organized round the physical appearance of the things in its environment. Phenomenistic thought gives rise to *phenomenistic causality*, in which simple physical co-occurrence is endowed with causal status; e.g. a child might remark, 'Trains go fast 'cause they're big.'

phenomenocentrism The tendency to accept one's own personal, immediate experience as revealing the true aspects of mind. It is a fallacy akin to ETHNOCENTRISM (1) and ANTHROPOMORPHISM. The phenomeno-centric perspective suffers from the general failure to recognize that immediate personal experiences, no matter how poignant and convincing they may seem, are still the products of social presuppositions and personal histories and cannot be taken as valid indicators of general mental processes.

phenomenology In simplest terms, a philosophical doctrine that advocates that the scientific study of immediate experience be the basis of psychology. As developed by Edmund Husserl, the focus is on events, occurrences, happenings, etc. as one experiences them, with a minimum of regard for the external, physical reality and for the so-called scientific biases of the natural sciences. Note that there is no attempt here to deny the objective reality of events; rather, the basic issue for a phenomenological analysis is to avoid focusing upon physical events themselves and instead to deal with how they are perceived and experienced. Real meaning for a phenomenologist is to be derived by examining an individual's relationship with and reactions to real-world events. Compare with PHENOMENALISM (1).

phenomenon From the Greek, meaning *an appearance, that which appears*. Hence: **1** Any perceptible change, any occurrence that is open to observation. This meaning, which is very general, embodies two aspects each of which is represented in the following more restricted senses. **2** A physical occurrence, a fact, a proven event. Note also that the term is often used in this sense without consideration of the causes of the happen-

ing. **3** An internal experience of which one is aware, the data of personal experience. This meaning is reflected in the perspective of PHENOMENOLOGY. **4** In Kantian terms, appearance or knowledge of events or objects interpreted through categories; phenomena here serve as the basis for inferring reality.

phenothiazines A major group of ANTI-PSYCHOTIC DRUGS used in the alleviation of severe psychological disorders, notably schizophrenia. Chlorpromazine, thiorida-zine and fluphenazine are the most frequently prescribed. All drugs of this group have important effects on the autonomic nervous system, including epinephrine- and norepinephrine-blocking at sympathetic receptors and acetycholine-blocking at postganglionic parasympathetic receptors. They depress sensory input to the reticular formation and raise the general threshold for such stimuli in the brainstem. As a result, all have a sedative effect, although this differs from that of the *barbit-urates* in that there is little *ataxia* and the patient can be aroused easily. They also alleviate the nausea and vomiting caused by other drugs and/or conditions (not, however, motion sickness). Side effects include disruption of temperature-regulation processes in the hypothalamus, some disruption of the endocrine system and a variety of motor disorders, including tremors from muscle weakness (see EXTRAPYRAMIDAL SYN-DROME) and, with long-term administration, TARDIVE DYSKINESIA.

phenotype The actual, physical, observable; the manifested structure, function or behaviour of an organism. For more detail see GENOTYPE.

phenylketonuria (PKU) A genetic disorder of amino-acid metabolism in which the enzyme *phenylalanine hydroxylase*, necessary for the oxidizing of phenylalanine, is missing. In most industrialized societies babies are screened for the disorder a few days after birth, and if it is diagnosed, a diet low in phenylalanine is instituted and untoward effects are prevented. If it is left untreated, the resulting build-up of phenylpyruvic acid causes severe and permanent mental retardation (called *phenylpyruvic oligophre-nia*). Pregnant women who were diagnosed with the condition in childhood must make appropriate adjustments in their diet to prevent damage to the foetus.

phenylpyruvic oligophrenia PHENYLKETO-NURIA.

pheromone A chemical substance used as a means of communication among members of a species. Pheromones serve a variety of functions in different species, such as signalling sexual receptivity or alarm and marking territory. See e.g. LEE-BOOT EFFECT, BRUCE EFFECT. Their role in human behaviour is controversial although some feel that the MCCLINTOCK EFFECT suggests that they play some role.

phi (φ) coefficient An index of the relationship between any two sets of scores, provided both can be represented on ordered, binary dimensions, e.g. male–female; married–single. Also called the *fourfold-point correlation*.

-philia Combining form meaning *love of, friend of, affinity for*.

phil(o)- Combining form meaning *loving, friendly*.

philology Lit., the love of words. Generally used as the name of a branch of linguistics concerned with the study of the origins and evolution of the meanings of words. Occasionally, in some older writings, a synonym of *linguistics* itself.

philosophical psychotherapy An approach to therapy predicated on the assumption that one's beliefs, attitudes and general *Weltanschauung* (overall outlook on life) have a profound impact on one's behaviour, feelings and ways of dealing with reality. The basic goal is to alter the client's philosophical attitude or posture. Phenomenological approaches like Rogers's client-centred therapy and Frankl's logotherapy have philosophical-psychotherapy components but the prototype of the approach is *existential therapy*.

philosophy In that most hackneyed of phrases, the search for the truth. There are various ways to conduct this search that properly belong within the discipline and various domains of nature into which it has, over the millennia, led. The most convenient division is to break philosophy into two broad subdisciplines: EPISTEMOLOGY and METAPHYSICS. The former encompasses efforts

to understand the origins, nature and limits of thought and human knowledge, the latter embraces similar attempts to comprehend the ultimate reality of existence. Other prominent branches are *aesthetics, ethics* and *logic*.

philosophy of mind MIND, PHILOSOPHY OF.

phi motion PHI PHENOMENON.

Phineas Gage GAGE, PHINEAS.

phi phenomenon 1 Specifically, a form of APPARENT *MOTION produced when two stationary lights are flashed successively. If the interval between the two is optimal (in the neighbourhood of 150 msec), then one perceives movement of the light from the first location to the second. **2** More generally, Max Wertheimer used the phrase to refer to the 'pure' irreducible experiencing of motion independent of other factors such as colour, brightness, size and spatial location. The phi phenomenon in the first sense was considered by Wertheimer to be a good example of the second sense and hence is sometimes called the *pure phi phenomenon*. While the term is primarily used for visual displays, there is an auditory analogue where a sound can be made to seem to move across space with appropriate timing of two separate sounds.

-phob- Combining form meaning *fear, dread* or *aversion*. The form *-phobe* is used to characterize a person displaying a fear, *-phobia* is used to refer to an actual condition, and *-phobic* serves an adjectival function.

phobia From the Greek for *fear* or *dread*. In keeping with this etymology, specific phobias are properly given Greek root qualifiers, e.g. *pyrophobia* = fear of fire, *nyctophobia* = fear of the night, etc. In standard psychiatric work, a reaction must be shown to display several factors before it can be properly classified as a phobia. Specifically, the fear must be persistent and intense, there must be a compelling need to flee or avoid the phobic object or situation, and the fear must be irrational and not based on sound judgement. Both the technical and the common terms for specific phobias can be found in Appendix A.

phobia, simple Any persistent fear of a specific stimulus object or situation. Specifically excluded from this category are SOCIAL·PHOBIA and a fear of having a PANIC ATTACK (see also PANIC DISORDER). The most common simple phobias involve animals, blood, closed spaces and heights; see Appendix A for a full list. Note that in the latest edition of the DSM, five distinct types of simple phobia are identified, an *animal type* (insects, mice), a *natural environment type* (heights, lightning), a *blood-injection-injury type* (any invasive medical procedure), a *situational type* (elevators, flying, enclosed spaces) and an *other type* (other objects or situations). Frankly, it is not clear to us what is gained by this excessively precise cluster of designations, but there they are. Also called *specific phobia*.

phobia, social An ANXIETY DISORDER marked by a persistent fear of particular social situations in which the individual is subjected to possible scrutiny by others and fears that he or she will act in some way that will humiliate or embarrass. The actual fear itself may be quite circumscribed, such as being unable to speak in public, choking on food while eating in the presence of others, having one's hand tremble when attempting to write in front of others, etc. Social phobias often coexist with PANIC DISORDER and any of various SIMPLE·PHOBIAS. Also called SOCIAL·ANXIETY DISORDER; see that entry for nuances on usage.

phobic anxiety The fear experienced by one with a phobia when presented with the phobic object or circumstances.

phobic character A psychoanalytic term for an individual who tends to deal with difficult or anxiety-provoking situations by adopting the simple expedient of avoiding them, usually by restricting his or her activities in life and seeking a protective environment.

phobic disorder Earlier nomenclatures used this term as a synonym of PHOBIA. It is rarely found in contemporary writing.

phobic neurosis A NEUROSIS manifested as a PHOBIA. The term is not used in contemporary nosologies.

phobic object An object or stimulus that elicits PHOBIC ANXIETY. Also called *phobic stimulus*.

phocomelia A birth defect characterized by incomplete development of the limbs.

phon A measure of the subjective loudness of a tone. The phon scale is based on comparisons with a 1,000 Hz standard.

phonation Generally, the production of speech sounds; more specifically, the production of speech sounds by the vibration of the vocal cords.

phone Any discrete speech sound the characteristics of which can be specified independently of its role in any specific language. Compare with PHONEME, which is language-specific. Phonetic elements are traditionally denoted by placement within square brackets, [ ]. See also INTERNATIONAL PHONETIC ALPHABET.

phoneme The minimal unit of speech in a given language that 'makes a difference' to the fluent speaker of that language. It is not really a discrete speech sound, but rather a *class* of sounds, and is represented in speech through one of its *allophones*. To use every linguist's favourite example, in English the classes of sounds denoted as /r/ and /l/ are two distinct phonemes while in Korean they are treated as allophonic variations of a single phoneme. Phonemic notation is traditionally given, as in the above example, between slashes, / /. There is a temptation to regard the letters used in alphabetic writing as representing phonemes. This should be resisted, for it completely misrepresents the role of the phoneme in language. Ultimately, phonemes are cognitive/perceptual abstractions and as such are independent of writing systems. To appreciate this point see ORTHOGRAPHY and related entries. Compare with PHONE.

phonemic Pertaining to: **1** PHONEME. **2** PHONEMICS.

phonemic restoration effect The phenomenon of a dramatically altered acoustic element in speech being extremely difficult to detect; e.g. replacing a /t/ with a click still sounds like proper speech. The listener fills in or restores the missing or distorted components through the use of other cues in the speech. The effect is not found in isolated speech sounds.

phonemics The study of the speech sounds

of a specific language. That is, the examination is focused on the *phonemic* patterns of a language, not the *phonetic*. For example, the English words *pan*, *span* and *nap* contain three different 'p' sounds, but a phonemic analysis treats them all similarly because they are allophonic variations of a single PHONEME, /p/. Compare with PHONETICS, which takes the differences between the three into consideration in its analysis.

phonetic Pertaining to: **1** PHONE. **2** PHONETICS.

phonetic alphabet INTERNATIONAL PHONETIC ALPHABET.

phonetic boundary The point at which a minor change in an acoustic property will result in perception of one PHONEME rather than another. See CATEGORICAL PERCEPTION.

phonetic method Any method of speech training that focuses on the relationship between movements of the articulators (tongue, lips, etc.) and speech sounds. Distinguish from PHONICS METHOD.

phonetics The study of speech sounds, including classification, transmission, production and perception of phonetic elements. Generally considered to consist of two subdisciplines: *articulatory phonetics*, which analyses the methods of production of speech sounds; and *acoustic phonetics*, which analyses their physical properties. The former is grounded in biology, the latter in physics. Compare with PHONEMICS, noting particularly that *phonetics* is language-free and *phonemics* language-dependent.

-phonia Combining form used to denote a vocal disorder.

phonic Of sounds, specifically speech sounds.

phonic(s) method A method of reading instruction in which the focus is on the relationship between letters and letter groups and the sounds of the language they represent. Compare with WHOLE-WORD METHOD. Distinguish from PHONETIC METHOD.

phonism A form of SYNAESTHESIA in which sounds are experienced when stimuli from other, nonauditory modalities are presented.

phon(o)- Combining form meaning *sound*, *voice* or *vocal*.

phonography Any writing system based on the sounds of the spoken language. See e.g. ALPHABET, SYLLABARY.

phonological alexia ALEXIA, PHONOLOGICAL.

phonological disorder In the latest edition of the DSM, the approved term for DEVELOPMENTAL *ARTICULATION DISORDER.

phonological dysgraphia DYSGRAPHIA, PHONOLOGICAL.

phonological dyslexia DYSLEXIA, PHONOLOGICAL.

phonological loop A form of WORKING *MEMORY in which auditory information is held in memory and rehearsed. In Baddeley and Hitch's model, it is composed of a phonological store that holds auditory information and an articulatory process so that it can be rehearsed. Linguistic inputs that arrive visually are assumed to be recoded and processed here; visual input is handled by the VISUO-SPATIAL SKETCHPAD. Also called *phonetic loop* and *articulatory loop*.

phonology A term used loosely to cover the study of the sound patterns of a language. It is not a particularly useful term since it fails to distinguish between the separate study of PHONEMICS and PHONETICS.

phonopathy A general term for any vocal disorder.

phonoscope Any device that converts sound energy into a visible form. See SPECTROGRAPH for the most commonly used variety.

phon scale PHON.

phoria Generally, the orientation of the two eyeballs while focusing on an object. Specifically, any abnormality in which there is a lack of coordination between the two eyes.

phorometry Measurement of the balance of the muscles that turn the eyeballs.

phosphenes Luminous images produced by mechanical stimulation of the eye or the visual cortex. They can easily be produced by gently pressing on the side of the eye with the lid closed or by a blow on the head. They also occur normally, but less dramatically, during *accommodation* and *convergence*.

phosphodiesterase CAFFEINE.

phot A unit of illuminance. Specifically,

that falling on a surface 1 cm from a point source of light of 1 candle.

photerythrous Descriptive of persons who have a heightened sensitivity to long-wavelength light.

photic Pertaining to light.

photic driving The use of a stroboscopic (i.e. rapidly flashing) light to accentuate or 'drive' brainwave patterns, particularly alpha waves.

photism 1 The hallucination of a bright light. 2 The experience of colours when stimuli from other, nonvisual modalities are presented; a form of SYNAESTHESIA.

phot(o)- Combining form meaning: 1 *Relating to light*. 2 *Of photography*.

photochromatic interval The range of luminous stimulus intensities sufficient to stimulate the *rods*, and thus produce a sensation of light, but not the *cones*, so that no hue is perceived.

photogenic epilepsy EPILEPSY, PHOTOGENIC.

photographic memory A nontechnical term for a perfect memory. As used in the common language it has no reference, for, as a look at MEMORY et seq. will show, such a perfectly recording memory is not to be found in creatures of organic origin. The closest thing to it is the phenomenon of EIDETIC IMAGERY.

photokinesis In lower organisms, a movement or general activity in response to light.

photoma A hallucinated flash of light.

photometer PHOTOMETRY.

photometric brightness LUMINANCE.

photometric measurement PHOTOMETRY.

photometry A general term covering the devices for, the procedures of and the theory of the measurement of the visual effectiveness of light. The essential problem in photometry is that the eye is not uniformly sensitive to all wavelengths; as a result all modern *photometers* have a set of built-in standards that are based on an internationally agreed-upon characterization of the normal human visual system.

photon An obsolete term for what is now called a TROLAND. The usage of *photon* in physics forced this change in terminology.

photophobia An abnormal sensitivity to light. Note, it is not a fear of light, as the root *phobia* seems to imply. Photophobia occurs in albinos, who lack pigmentation, and in a variety of other conditions.

photopic vision Normal daylight vision; vision under sufficiently high illumination conditions that the cones of the retina are functioning. Photopic vision has the following general properties: (a) hues are perceived; (b) the visual threshold is, relative to *scotopic vision*, high; (c) the *luminosity curve* shows maximum sensitivity to a wavelength of approximately 555 nm, with a rapidly decreasing sensitivity to longer and shorter wavelengths; and (d) because the fovea is entirely made up of cones, visual acuity is high. Compare with SCOTOPIC VISION.

photopigment Any of several light-sensitive chemicals found in the receptor cells (rods and cones) of the retina. Photopigments absorb light and undergo chemical changes that represent the first stage in the transduction of light energy to visual experience. See RHODOPSIN, the photopigment of the rods.

photoreceptor Any of the receptor cells of the retina that are stimulated by light energy and give rise to the experience of vision. See RODS and CONES for details.

phototaxis An orienting response with regard to light. *Positive* phototaxis is movement toward the source, *negative* away from it. The term is properly reserved for such movements in animals; *phototropism* is used for plants. *Heliotaxis* and *heliotropism* are occasionally found as synonyms. See TAXIS.

phototherapy The use of light in therapy. The most common use is in the treatment of SEASONAL AFFECTIVE DISORDER.

phototropism PHOTOTAXIS.

phrase 1 In linguistics, a group of words and morphemes arranged according to grammatical rules and functioning as a unit within a sentence. 2 In speech, a group of words and sounds spoken with an intonation contour that reflects the underlying meaningful structure of the unit. Note that a phrase in sense 2 is not necessarily a phrase in sense 1.

phrase-marker TREE (2).

phrase-structure grammar GRAMMAR, PHRASE-STRUCTURE.

-phrasia Combining form used to denote speech disorders.

-phren-, -phrenia, phreno- Combining forms meaning generally *mind, mental, mentality*.

phrenasthenia Lit., mental weakness.

phrenology Originally conceptualized by the anatomist Franz Joseph Gall as the science that studied the relationship between mental faculties or functions and specific brain areas. The practice of phrenology was based upon three assumptions: (a) that there was a clear relationship between specific brain areas and particular mental functions; (b) that the more developed a function was, the larger the relevant area of the brain was; and (c) that the shape of the skull conformed to the shape of the brain. On the basis of these, Gall developed the practice of 'reading' mental capacity, emotions and even personality from the bumps on the head. The first two assumptions were not terribly far off the mark (SEE LOCALIZATION OF FUNCTION, MODULARITY) although Gall's characterizations were far too extreme. The final one is just flat out wrong. There is no scientific basis for phrenology and current practitioners are frauds.

phylaxis 1 Specifically, the body's active defence against infection. **2** More generally, protection, defence.

phyl(o)- Combining form meaning *race* or *tribe* based upon kinship; by extension, any biologically defined group.

phylogenesis PHYLOGENY.

phylogenetic PHYLOGENY, GENETICS.

phylogenetic memory A memory or idea that is presumed universal in all individuals, reflecting an early phyletic stage. Phrased this way it is a rather empty concept; if one recasts the idea into the framework of *species-specific* behavioural tendencies, it is not quite so bizarre.

phylogenetic principle RECAPITULATION THEORY.

phylogeny (or **phylogenesis**) The origin and, by extension, the evolution, or evolutionary history, of a species or other form of animal or plant. Contrast with ONTOGENY, the origin and development of an individual organism.

phylum A primary division in the classification of animals and plants.

physiatrist A physician who specializes in the treatment and rehabilitation of someone who has suffered a physical disability. Physiatrists are often involved in pain management and the treatment of suffering from chronic pain. The associated field is called *physical medicine and rehabilitation* or simply *physiatry*.

physical 1 Pertaining to properties of matter, energy, etc.; in short, to the physical sciences. **2** By extension, pertaining to material elements of nature other than those peculiar to living matter, i.e. external to an organism, e.g. a *physical stimulus*. **3** Pertaining to the body, to *physique*; *somatic*. **4** By extension, vigorous, active. The mutually contradictory nature of 1 and 2 versus 3 and 4 actually causes less trouble than one might suppose; context typically determines the sense intended. ants., *biological* (1 and 2), *mental* (3 and 4).

physical dependence PHYSIOLOGICAL *DEPENDENCE.

physicalism The philosophical point of view that all scientific propositions can be expressed in the terminology of the physical sciences. The variety most influential in psychology is IDENTITY THEORY. See OPERATIONALISM and POSITIVISM, with which it is closely aligned.

physical stimulus A stimulus specified in terms of its properties of energy and energy changes. See the discussion under STIMULUS for details.

physio- Combining form from the Greek, meaning *pertaining to nature*. Given the breadth with which the term NATURE is used, this suffix can be taken to relate to that which is biological or to that which is material. In psychology, the reference is virtually always the former, so much so that *physio* is lab jargon for *physiological psychology*.

physiodynamic therapy A cover term for a

number of psychotherapeutic procedures, that directly target physiological processes including ELECTROCONVULSIVE THERAPY, INSULIN-SHOCK THERAPY, NARCOTHERAPY and PSYCHOSURGERY.

physiogenetic Characterizing that which originates in the body or in a part thereof.

physiognomic 1 Pertaining to PHYSIOGNOMY. **2** Characterizing an empathic reaction in which emotional qualities are interjected into perceptual/cognitive judgements; e.g. when someone says a brand-new car looks 'alert'.

physiognomic perception The perception of emotions and feelings. Gestalt psychologists maintained that it was as primary an aspect of perceptual experience as 'ordinary' qualities. For example, in music a melody is not heard as a sequence of notes but as an organized whole with emotive content.

physiognomy 1 The physical appearance of the face. **2** Specifically, the use of the face and facial expressions to judge mental abilities, character, emotional attitudes, etc. Meaning 1 represents a simple exercise in description; meaning 2 is sheer quackery – see e.g. LOMBROSIAN THEORY.

physiological age AGE, PHYSIOLOGICAL.

physiological antagonism DRUG *ANTAGONISM.

physiological dependence DEPENDENCE, PHYSIOLOGICAL.

physiological limit The theoretical asymptote or upper limit of performance as presumably dictated by biological factors.

physiological motive A generic term for any motive based on body needs or tissue needs, e.g. food, water, avoidance of noxious stimulation, etc. See here DRIVE and PRIMARY *DRIVE.

physiological nystagmus NYSTAGMUS, PHYSIOLOGICAL.

physiological psychology 1 A branch of psychology that is oriented toward description and explanation of psychological phenomena based on physiological and neurological processes. It shares much of its subject-matter and many of its techniques with biology and physiology and typically reflects either a *correlational* orientation, in which the search is for the physiological correlates of behaviour, or a *reductionistic* orientation, in which the final explanation for action and thought is sought in physiological principles. A number of synonyms and near synonyms are used for this field, including *biological psychology, biopsychology, psychobiology* and *psychophysiology.* **2** Wilhelm Wundt's term for what we would now refer to as 'experimental' or 'scientific' psychology. Wundt used the term to emphasize that his approach was, unlike philosophy, going to take a focused, scientific approach to the study of mind and mental life.

physiological zero The temperature which stimulates neither a response to warm nor a response to cold. All other things being equal, this point of thermal indifference corresponds to the temperature of the skin, or roughly 32°C (90°F). The zero point is not a true point but a small range of temperatures within which no thermal sensation is reported. Note also that the level of adaptation of the skin and the area of the body where stimulation occurs also affects the measured zero point.

physiology Broadly, the discipline within biology that studies the functions of cells, tissues and organs of living organisms.

physique The structure and anatomical organization of the body – usually, but not exclusively, the human body.

physostigmine An acetylcholine *agonist* that functions by inactivating *acetylcholinesterase.*

PI PROACTIVE *INTERFERENCE.

Piagetian Of the theories and perspectives of Jean Piaget (1896–1980) and his colleagues, who established the so-called *Genevan school* of developmental psychology. Piaget's work focused on the attempt to understand the development of cognitive functioning in children and is typically expressed in terms of his *stage theory*, in which a child is seen as passing through a series of cognitive periods, each displaying its characteristic modes of thought. See here CONCRETE OPERATIONS, FORMAL OPERATIONS, PREOPERATORY THOUGHT, SENSORIMOTOR INTELLIGENCE.

Piaget's original training was in zoology, and his interest in children derived from his concerns with epistemology – the origins, nature and limits of knowledge. His approach is often called GENETIC EPISTEMOLOGY, for it reflects his deep conviction that the development of intelligence can be seen as naturalistic and biological, the result of a dynamic interaction between a child and its environment. The Piagetian orientation, however, is not nativistic in the usual sense of NATIVISM; he did not conceptualize a child as emerging pre-equipped with *innate ideas*. Rather, he maintained, phylogenetic evolutionary pressures result in a neonate with very general regulatory mechanisms and modes of processing environmental inputs. It is the interplay of these (see e.g. ACCOMMODATION (3), ASSIMILATION (4), EQUILIBRATION (2)) that yields the modes of thought representative of the several stages.

pia mater Latin for *tender mother*. The term for the innermost of the three meninges covering the brain and spinal cord. The membrane is thin and highly vascular and closely envelops the underlying tissue.

piano theory of hearing THEORIES OF *HEARING.

piblokto A CULTURE-SPECIFIC SYNDROME found among Inuit. The primary symptom is an acute attack of screaming and crying and running uncontrollably through the snow. var., *pibloktoq*.

pica From the name of a genus of birds which includes the voracious magpie, a persistent eating of nonnutritive substances, e.g. chalk, clay, bits of trash, etc. It often accompanies mental retardation and in such cases is classified as a FEEDING DISORDER OF INFANCY OR EARLY CHILDHOOD. Also called *allotriophagy*. See also EATING DISORDERS.

Pick disease A dementia characterized by gradual changes in personality, stereotyped and inappropriate social behaviour, emotional instability and a progressive, unrelenting decline in cognitive function. First identified and determined to be a FRONTOTEMPORAL DEMENTIA by Arnold Pick in 1892. Also known as *Pick's disease*.

pico- Combining form meaning *a trillionth*.

pictogram A picture or symbol used to represent an object or a concept.

pictophilia A PARAPHILIA characterized by the deriving of erotic stimulation from viewing sexually oriented pictures or films to the extent that such viewing is necessary to maintain sexual arousal and to achieve orgasm. The term is reserved for those whose sexual behaviours are dependent on such pictures and is not used to refer to the normal arousal experienced by most people when viewing erotic material.

picture-arrangement test A test consisting of a series of cartoon-like pictures presented in a haphazard order. The subject's task is to arrange them as quickly as possible so that a coherent story is represented. Such tests are a common feature of intelligence tests.

picture-completion test A test in which incomplete pictures are presented to the subject (e.g. a picture of a person with a foot missing, a cow with only one horn), who must identify the omitted details.

picture-interpretation test A generic term for any test or part thereof in which the subject is given a picture and asked to interpret it.

pidgin A verbal communication system that develops when two different language communities make occasional contact with each other. A pidgin emerges when the contact is not general enough to motivate the learning of each other's language and a blend is devised. Note that pidgins are not usually classified as natural languages (see LANGUAGE) until or unless they become creolized (see CREOLE).

piecemeal activity, law of Thorndike's term for the generalization that a part of a learning situation may become prepotent and evoke responding even though other aspects of the situation are altered or removed.

pie chart A way of presenting proportional data in the form of a circle (the *pie*) with each category represented by a *slice*, the size of which reflects what proportion it is of the whole.

Pierre Robin syndrome A congenital syndrome marked by a small receding chin and a cleft palate. In cases with brain damage there may be mental retardation, although intelligence is usually normal. Poor respiration and feeding problems are common, and children with the disorder may fail to thrive.

pigment 1 Generally, any substance, usually in the form of nonsoluble particles, that differentially absorbs light of particular wavelengths and thereby gives colour or hue to a surface. That is, a red pigment is perceived as red because it contains particles that absorb more light of medium and short wavelength than light of long wavelength, which it reflects back to the viewer. **2** In physiology, any such substance in tissues that gives them colour.

pigment layer The first layer of the retina containing the pigmented cells.

pill-rolling Obsessive behaviour such that the person affected continuously rolls little balls (i.e. pills) of fabric or paper around.

pilo- Combining form meaning *hair*.

piloerection Of hair, standing on end.

pilomotor response Pimpling of the skin with accompanying piloerection; commonly known as *goose flesh* or *goose bumps*.

pilot study Common synonym of EXPLORATORY STUDY.

Piltz's reflex ATTENTION REFLEX.

pimozide An ANTIPSYCHOTIC DRUG used in the treatment of TOURETTE'S SYNDROME.

pineal body (or **gland**) A tiny structure located sufficiently close to the geographical centre of the brain for Galen to have believed that it regulated the very flow of thoughts and for Descartes to have hypothesized that it functioned as the locus of interaction between the body and the rational soul. Its actual functions are not completely known but are currently believed to be somewhat less cosmic. It does play an important role in the hormonal changes that occur during adolescence. During childhood it secretes a hormone, MELATONIN, that inhibits sexual maturation. When secretion diminishes during adolescence sexual development begins.

There is also evidence that the gland plays a role in sleep regulation in humans, and in various other species it has been implicated in exerting control over the full diurnal cycle. In some species, such as lizards, it contains light-sensitive neurons. Also called the *epiphysis cerebri*.

pink noise NOISE, PINK.

pinna The fleshy outer part of the external ear. It serves some sound-gathering functions.

pipeline techniques Any of several techniques used in social cognition to examine individuals' attitudes, beliefs and implicitly held knowledge by using an indirect 'pipeline'. The first of these to be developed was the *bogus-pipeline* in which devices like GSRs or ECGs are attached and subjects are warned not to be deceptive in their answers to upcoming questions because the devices will allow the experimenter to know if they are lying. In the *bona-fide pipeline technique* (also called the *evaluative semantic priming method*), attitudes toward an object or concept are assessed by presenting the target followed by an exemplar of a highly negative or positive category. For example, a subject is presented with the target 'computer' followed by 'sewer'. If the target has positive associations for the subject, the RT to 'sewer' will tend to be slower than if the associations are negative. The underlying principle is that concordant stimuli are responded to more rapidly because the affective mental component has already been primed (see PRIMING, esp. 3). All pipeline procedures use these 'round about' methods to assess attitudes; they are particularly useful when the topic is one that is culturally sensitive or one that the participants are likely to be less than open about. See also IMPLICIT ASSOCIATION TEST.

Piper's law A generalization which states that for moderate-sized, uniform areas of the retina outside of the fovea, the absolute threshold is inversely proportional to the square root of the area stimulated. Compare with RICCO'S LAW.

PI, release from A technique for measuring the build-up of PROACTIVE *INTERFERENCE (PI) in a learning task. It consists of giving the subject successive tasks with similar materials (which builds up PI) and then abruptly switching the type of materials. The performance with the new material relative to the performance with the old material gives a measure of the amount of PI 'released'.

pitch **1** The dimension of psychological experience that corresponds (roughly and complexly) with the frequency of an auditory stimulus. The typical range of the normal (and young) human ear is from approximately 20 to 20,000 Hz, with low-frequency tones sounding low in pitch and high-frequency tones sounding high. **2** In linguistics, a SUPRASEGMENTAL phonetic element which marks the fundamental frequency of a component of speech. The role of pitch is most easily appreciated by comparing the uttering of a simple sentence like 'That's a book' first with a flat pitch contour, which yields a simple declarative, and second with a rising pitch at the end, which produces a question.

Pitres' law (or **rule**) The generalization that a multilingual stroke victim with APHASIA will recover each language in the order of most frequent use prior to the injury.

pituitary gland The 'master gland' of the endocrine system, so called because of its role in regulating actions of the other endocrine glands. It is attached to the base of the brain by the infundibular stalk and divided into two lobes. The anterior lobe (*adenohypophysis*), which is connected to the *hypothalamus* via the hypothalamic-hypophyseal portal system, produces: *somatotrophic hormone* (STH), which regulates growth; *adrenocorticotrophic hormone* (ACTH), which controls the activity of the adrenal cortex; *thyrotrophic hormone* (TTH), which regulates activity of the thyroid gland; the *gonadotrophic hormones*, including, among others, *follicle-stimulating hormone* (FSH), which stimulates development of ovarian follicles in females and spermatogenesis in males; *luteinizing hormone* (LH) or *interstitial cell-stimulating hormone* (ICSH), which, in conjunction with FSH, stimulates secretion of oestrogens, ovulation and the development of the corpus luteum; and *lactogenic hormone*, which controls milk production in a mature mammary gland. The posterior lobe (*neurohypophysis*) secretes the *antidiuretic hormone*, which controls water metabolism, *vasopressin*, which induces contraction of the smooth muscles of blood vessels, and *oxytocin*, which strengthens uterine contractions and the milk-ejecting functions of the mammary glands. Also known as the HYPOPHYSIS.

pivot class (words) PIVOT GRAMMAR.

pivot grammar A grammar proposed as a description of the early two-word stage of language development. It is based on the division of a child's vocabulary into two classes of words: *pivot* (P) and *open* (O). The former includes a small number of high-frequency words that function by attaching other words to them to form utterances; all the other words are members of the latter. Utterances are hypothesized to be of three types: P + O (e.g. 'allgone milk'), O + P (e.g. 'Daddy there') and O + O (e.g. 'Daddy read'). Pivot grammars were vigorously criticized on many grounds, primarily for being overly simplistic, and are rarely taken seriously any more as valid generalizations of early child language.

PK Abbreviation for PSYCHOKINESIS (1).

PKMζ Abbreviation for *protein kinase M zeta*, an enzyme that appears to play a significant role in maintaining the persistence of long-term memories (see LONG-TERM POTENTIATION). Recent research shows that PKMζ inhibitors, when introduced into specific brain structures known to be important in LONG-TERM •MEMORY, disrupt the persistence of memories previously consolidated into stable long-term form.

PKU PHENYLKETONURIA.

placebo A preparation with no medicinal value and no pharmacological effects. In studies on the effects of a drug or other substance, a placebo control condition is invariably used (see DOUBLE-BLIND) to separate the true pharmacological effects from the psychological effects of subjects (or the experimenter) believing that a real drug is being administered.

placebo, active A PLACEBO that mimics the side effects of the drug under investigation but lacks its specific, assumed therapeutic effects. Employed in cases in which the side effects of the experimental drug could be used as clues by the subjects to enable them to identify whether they are in the experimental or the control group. Compare with DUMMY (2).

placebo effect Any observed effect on

behaviour that is 'caused' by a PLACEBO. Although the term was first introduced in the context of pharmacological research, it has been widely used and may be found in situations having nothing to do with the study of drugs. For more on the central issues here see DOUBLE-BLIND and EXPERIMENTER BIAS.

place cells Neurons in the hippocampus that respond to the specific location that an organism is in or moving toward.

place-learning LEARNING, PLACE.

placement Generally, the process of determining the appropriate position for a person. The term is used in educational settings, where it refers to placing a student in an appropriate class for instruction; in foster care, where it is used in reference to the settlement of a child with foster parents; and in industrial and organizational settings, where it refers to finding the optimum position for a worker.

placenta In mammals, an organ consisting of embryonic and maternal tissue to which the foetus is attached via the umbilical cord. The placenta is the 'life-support system' for the foetus: oxygen, food substances and antibodies enter through it, and metabolic waste products leave through it. In general, there is no admixture of maternal and foetal blood. The placenta also serves as an endocrine organ producing various hormones so that the uterus remains properly adapted during pregnancy.

place theory of hearing THEORIES OF *HEARING.

plain-folks technique A form of propaganda in which, in order to gain the support of others, a person attempts to persuade them that they are not of high station or great power but, rather, 'just plain folk' and 'one of us'.

plan 1 An outline or design for an experiment usually including a description of the nature and number of subjects to be used, the experimental and control groups that will be run, the procedures to be implemented and the data analyses to be carried out. **2** An articulated, verbalized statement about how some action or procedure is to be carried out. **3** A covert, mental, hierarchical operation that is assumed to exist 'inside the head' of an organism and to guide its behaviour. Note that when the organism is either nonhuman or nonverbal, the plan is not necessarily considered to operate in the same way as is assumed in sense 2. However, when the subject is verbal, there is a tendency to take meanings 2 and 3 as equivalent, with the assumption that 2 is merely the conscious expression of 3. To put it mildly, this equivalence is debatable.

plane A two-dimensional surface representing a slice, real or imaginary, through a body or organ. Planes are used as 'points' of reference for indicating various anatomical aspects of the organ or body under discussion. A plane is the result of a SECTION (2); see that entry for details of various kinds.

planned behaviour, theory of THEORY OF *REASONED ACTION.

planned comparison A PRIORI (OR PLANNED) TESTS.

planned parenthood The voluntary regulation of the size of a family by planning the spacing and number of children. The term is inclusive of any number of procedures that operate to prevent unplanned births. Also called *voluntary parenthood*.

planned tests A PRIORI (OR PLANNED) TESTS.

planning fallacy FALLACY, PLANNING.

planning, social A general term applied to any large-scale, organized effort to deal with current and projected problems of a society and to proposed solutions and goals.

planning, urban Social planning for an urban area.

planophrasia Erratic flight of ideas.

plantar reflex Toe flexion in response to a stroking of the sole of the foot.

plantigrade Characterizing a mode of walking in which the whole sole is placed on the ground. It occurs in infants around 6–10 months of age.

planum temporale A part of WERNICKE'S AREA. Abnormalities here have been implicated in developmental DYSLEXIA.

plaques Patches of abnormal tissue. There are various kinds of plaques including the fatty deposits that cause ATHEROSCLEROSIS, those that produce DEMYLINATION in multiple sclerosis and the AMYLOID PLAQUES found in Alzheimer's disease and Down syndrome.

plasticity Flexibility, modifiability, malleability, adaptability, teachability, etc. The term is used widely. For example: (a) in neurophysiology, the ability of brain tissue to subsume functions normally carried out by other tissue (see EQUIPOTENTIALITY (3)); (b) in education, a creative, flexible cognitive style; (c) in social psychology, nonrigid adherence to roles; (d) in the study of imagery, the ability to shift and modify images.

plastic tonus CATATONIC WAXY FLEXIBILITY.

plateau 1 A period of time during the learning of a response when no improvement is detected. **2** A period of time during an operant-conditioning experiment when no responses are made. In both cases the term derives from the fact that a plot of the data reveals a flat portion in the curve – the plateau.

Plateau's spiral A spiral that, when rotated, produces an illusion of expansion or contraction. When stopped an afterimage occurs where the spiral appears to move in the opposite direction and the expansion or contraction reverses.

Platonic Relating or pertaining to the philosophical doctrines of Plato (*c.* 427–347 BCE). Most typically this adjectival form is used in combination with other terms, as in the following entries. var., *platonic*.

Platonic idea Plato argued for a strong form of DUALISM in which mind and body were made up of different stuff and obeyed different laws. The mental was, for him, the supreme, and the general form – the idea – represented the true basis for reality. Platonic ideas were to be achieved through a kind of dialectic induction, making the apprehension of the idea a truly rationalist endeavour.

Platonic ideal The nonphysical manifestation of a thing apprehendable only through rational thought. See also PLATONIC IDEA.

Platonic love Friendship, affection, comradeship, love (the intensity of the emotion being a matter of debate) without sexual feelings. For Plato, this kind of attachment transcended the physical and reached the

contemplation of the spiritual ideal. The modern usage of the term, however, has debased it somewhat and it tends to be used to refer simply to a nonerotic heterosexual relationship.

platonize To make a thing PLATONIC. Specifically: **1** To render a relationship nonerotic. **2** To idealize. **3** To think rationally about a thing without carrying out any action. **4** In psychoanalysis, to use the defence mechanism of *platonization*. This mechanism is assumed to function in one of two ways: either through the process in 1, and here platonization is treated as very similar to SUBLIMATION; or through the processes in 2 and 3, where the mechanism is essentially identical with OMNIPOTENCE OF THOUGHT.

platoon-volley theory of hearing Another name for the *volley theory*; see THEORIES OF *HEARING.

platy- Combining form meaning *broad, flat.*

platycephalic Lit., flat-headed.

platykurtosis KURTOSIS.

play An *abridged* dictionary we consulted gave 55 distinguishable meanings for this term. At the core of all is the notion that somehow play involves diversion or recreation, an activity not necessarily to be taken seriously. For psychologists, the study of play is almost entirely within the realm of childhood (although, see ANIMAL *PLAY), and while diversion and recreation seem to be strong elements, it would be a mistake to conclude that such things are not taken seriously by the participants. Although many kinds of play have been studied and authors frequently create specialized terms for them, Piaget's three classes serve well as a general framework within which to view the current research: (a) games of mastery (building, copying, designing); (b) games with rules (marbles, war games, hide-and-seek, etc.); and (c) games of make-believe and fantasy. See following entries for other special forms.

play, animal Loosely, any activity of animals that seems to be PLAY, that is, behaviour that doesn't appear to have any specific adaptive value. The current view, however, is that the behaviours are adaptive and have a preparatory role; through them young animals learn many of the aggressive, protective, social and sexual behavioural skills needed later in life. See PRACTICE THEORY OF PLAY.

play, associative Play, typically seen in preschool children, where each child plays relatively independently although they may share toys and talk with each other. Compare with COOPERATIVE *PLAY and PARALLEL *PLAY.

play, cooperative Play, in which the individuals (usually children are the topic) interact with each other and share activities. Compare with ASSOCIATIVE *PLAY, PARALLEL *PLAY.

play, organized Play that is planned in advance and carried out under rules agreed upon by the participants.

play, parallel Play that is not coordinated with the activities of playmates. It is often observed in early childhood, when, according to Piaget, it results from a failure of a young child to accommodate playmates, a failure to decentre. Note, however, that although this side-by-side play is uncoordinated, presence of the other increases interest and activity. Compare with ASSOCIATIVE *PLAY, COOPERATIVE *PLAY. See here SOCIAL *FACILITATION. This quality is carried through to adulthood in games like golf.

play therapy The use of play situations in a therapeutic setting. There are a variety of sophisticated procedures involved in such therapy but they can all be grouped into two main classes: (a) diagnosis, in which a child's behaviour in a play situation reveals patterns that are indicative of his or her particular emotional and social-interactive difficulties; and (b) treatment, in which the play environment provides a forum within which pent-up emotions and feelings can be expressed freely. The first use is, in many respects, a real-life *projective* test, while the second is derived from the theoretical concept of *catharsis*.

pleasant 1 Characterizing an emotional experience which has positive, agreeable qualities. See PLEASURE. **2** Characterizing any environmental situation or stimulus conditions to which an organism will learn to make responses to bring them about and not learn to make responses that result in their termination. This, of course, is the behaviourist's usage. See also UNPLEASANT.

pleasure An emotional experience that many regard as fundamentally undefinable. Some treat it as though it were a pole on a continuum, its opposite number being either UNPLEASURE or PAIN. Those with a behaviourist bent eschew the subjectivity entailed by this device and typically regard pleasure as an internal state manifested by an organism's engaging in certain behaviours and avoiding other behaviours. Neither of these approaches is very satisfying: the use of a pleasure–unpleasure or a pleasure–pain continuum leaves more problems than it solves, as a look under PAIN will clearly show; and the behaviourist characterization somehow seems to miss the internal affective state that most people associate with the term. What is interesting about these lexicographic conundrums is that pleasure, by virtue of its undefinability, may simply be a fundamental emotional experience characterizable as a desire to have the stimulation that produced it repeated. If this is still unsatisfying, see the extended discussion under REINFORCEMENT, a term used rather differently but one which entails the same kind of definitional lexicographic problems.

pleasure centres A term coined by James Olds for areas in the brain which when stimulated with mild electric current produce what seems to be pleasure. Olds's work was with lower organisms and, in a flagrant display of anthropomorphism, he took the fact that his animals made large numbers of responses in order to receive the stimulation as evidence of the experience of pleasure. The specific areas implicated lie along a predominantly dopaminergic pathway from the brainstem through the lateral hypothalamus and other parts of the limbic system to the frontal lobes. See PLEASURE.

pleasure–pain principle One often sees this psychoanalytic term in its shortened form, *pleasure principle*. The reference here is to a hypothetical early and primitive id function that seeks to satisfy any need either by direct means or through hallucination and fantasy – with the implication that at this point in an infant's development there is a failure to differentiate the fantasy from the reality. However, this focus upon the 'pleasure' aspect is slightly misleading since, as the classical theory of psychoanalysis developed, the operations involved here were viewed not simply as strivings for pleasure but as coordinated strivings for gratification *and* withdrawals from or avoidances of the unbalanced tension and excessive affect of pain and/or unpleasure.

According to the standard Freudian model, the primitive, pleasure-seeking, pain-avoiding operations gradually become modified by the REALITY PRINCIPLE as ego functions are developed and the child comes to replace the fantasized wish-fulfilment with more appropriate and reality-oriented adaptive behaviour. Note also that the *pain* of the principle is different in meaning from the *pain* of the PAIN PRINCIPLE, which hypothesizes a striving *for* pain, not an avoidance of it. Note that the term *pleasure–unpleasure principle* is also used. See PAIN for reasons why *pain* and *unpleasure* are often interchanged within psychoanalysis.

pleasure principle PLEASURE–PAIN PRINCIPLE.

pleasure–unpleasure principle PLEASURE–PAIN PRINCIPLE.

-plectic -PLEGIA.

-plegia A suffix from the Greek, meaning *stroke*. It is used to connote paralysis or loss of function due to a stroke or other neural damage; for example, *hemiplegia* is a paralysis on one side of the body, *diplegia* involves both sides, *paraplegia* is a paralysis of both lower limbs, *monoplegia* of only one limb or a single muscle group, *facialplegia* involves the facial muscles. adj., *-plectic*.

pleio-, pleo-, plio- Combining forms meaning *more*.

pleiotropic Of a gene that influences more than one phenotypic trait. The majority of genes appear to function in such a manner. n., *pleiotropy, pleiotropism*.

plethysmograph A device for measuring volume, usually that of blood supply, in a part of the body.

plexus Any network of nerves or of blood or lymphatic vessels.

plosive A speech sound that is produced by a momentary stoppage of the flow of air followed by a sudden release of the articulators and a rush of air. Plosives may be *voiced* (e.g. *d, b, g*) or *voiceless* (e.g. *t, p, k*).

plot 1 vb. To present data in graphic form.

2 n. The result of such an operation. There is a tendency to reserve the term for scatter diagrams, although most use it for any form of graphic display.

pluralism 1 A philosophical point of view that ultimate reality consists of more than one form of basic substance or principle. Strictly speaking, DUALISM is a pluralism, although the terms are usually kept distinct; VITALISM, when appended to a dualistic approach, is another example. **2** The tendency to search for multiple causes. This sense is very general and characterizes any number of theoretical approaches that assume that psychological phenomena result from a multiplicity of causal factors. **3** The tendency for social groups to break up into smaller units. This usage is strictly descriptive. **4** A social-philosophical perspective that maintains that the diverse cultural characteristics of minority groups are important aspects of a whole society and that they should be encouraged by the more powerful majority. This usage is clearly prescriptive. The term *cultural pluralism* is often used to help distinguish this meaning from others.

pluralistic ignorance A term introduced by Floyd Allport to characterize the feeling that one's beliefs or attitudes are not shared by others when they actually are – but the others aren't talking. Allport suggested that sudden observed changes in societal mores may come about when all the silent ones begin to express their previously covert beliefs.

plurel A term used primarily in sociology and social psychology to refer to a category or class containing any number of persons greater than one.

plus-sum game ZERO-SUM *GAME.

PMAs PRIMARY MENTAL ABILITIES.

PMS PREMENSTRUAL SYNDROME.

pneumat(o)- Combining form meaning *pertaining to air* or *respiration*.

pneum(o)- Combining form meaning *lung*.

pneumogastric nerve Obsolete term for VAGUS NERVE.

pneumograph An instrument for recording breathing.

Poetzl effect The later appearance in dreams and waking imagery of parts of tachistoscopically presented pictures which were not reported as being perceived when actually presented. var., *Pötzl effect.*

Poggendorff illusion An illusion of discontinuity. The line in the drawing is straight.

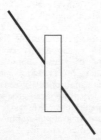

point-biserial correlation CORRELATION, POINT-BISERIAL.

point-for-point correspondence ISO-MORPHISM.

point-light display A visual display in which a scene is in total darkness except for small (point) lights. The technique is commonly used in studies of motion perception, specifically biological motion. Initially, lights were attached to the joints of a filmed actor to determine the minimal information needed by perceivers to identify the actions performed. Current research uses computer displays to explore these and other facets of motion perception.

point of regard REGARD.

point of subjective equality (pse) The point along a stimulus continuum at which two stimuli are perceived as indistinguishable from each other. Actually, the *point* here is a statistically derived one and represents one of the following: (a) the value of the comparison stimulus that is most frequently judged as indistinguishable from the standard; (b) the point at which either of two stimulus values is equally likely to be judged as being greater or lesser than the other; or (c) the value halfway between the upper and lower thresholds of the stimulus continuum.

point prevalence In epidemiology, the number of cases of a disease at a specific point in time. Compare with PERIOD PREVALENCE.

point scale In psychological testing, a scale that compares a person's performance to peers, rather than to a developmental or educational standard. The term is sometimes restricted to ability tests that have multiple subtests or scales.

point source A source of light sufficiently small in area for it to be regarded for photometric purposes (see PHOTOMETRY) as a single point.

point-to-point correspondence ISO-MORPHISM.

Poisson distribution DISTRIBUTION, POISSON.

polar continuum Any continuum the poles of which are opposites. Various hypothesized psychological continua are represented as reflecting this characteristic of polarity. Some are straightforward, such as psychophysical dimensions like light–heavy, loud–soft; others are less obvious, such as many of the personality traits like introversion–extraversion, dominance–submissiveness. See also POLARITY (1).

polarity 1 Generally, the property of having two poles or opposites. Magnets have polarity, as do various continua or series; see POLAR CONTINUUM. **2** In neurology, the property of a neuron such that ions of opposite charges are separated by the semi-permeable membrane of the cell. See ACTION POTENTIAL, DEPOLARIZATION. **3** The expression of opposite extremes of emotions, behaviours or traits, e.g. the polarized love–hate relationship many children have with their parents. **4** In a group setting, the focusing of attention on a single individual. See also BIPOLAR et seq.

polarization 1 The treatment of light such that all vibrations are confined to a single plane. **2** Concentration of electrical potential at one pole. **3** The equilibrium of electrically charged ions on either side of a cell membrane; see DEPOLARIZATION. **4** The adjustment of behaviours and opinions so that they are oriented or conform to one end of a POLAR CONTINUUM. **5** The state of a group in which its activities are focused on a central figure.

polar opposites Any two aspects of things

(such as behaviours, objects, events or feelings) that represent the extreme poles on a continuum. For example, The pair *hot–cold* would be considered polar opposites but the pair *warm–cool* would not.

poll The original meaning is *crown of the head*, and contemporary uses in the social sciences still reflect this sense in that a poll is a head count of opinions or attitudes. Note that modern polling no longer literally counts all the heads, rather it uses sophisticated sampling techniques to provide estimates of populations of individuals from relatively small samples of persons. See SAMPLING et seq.

Pollyanna mechanism A defence mechanism whereby one believes that all is well despite all evidence that it is not. The name comes from a character in an Eleanor Porter novel who was hopelessly and blindly optimistic.

poly- Combining form from the Greek, meaning *many*. Generally used in combination with words of Greek origin; words of Latin origin properly use MULTI-.

polyandry A mating (or, in humans, a marriage) system in which a single female may mate with (or marry) two or more males. Rare in humans, it tends to occur in species (such as seahorses) the males of which make the highest PARENTAL INVESTMENT. Compare with POLYGYNY.

polyandry, fraternal A form of polyandry in which a woman's several husbands must all be brothers.

polychromatic Having many colours.

polydactyl Possessing more than the usual complement of fingers.

polydipsia A general term for excessive drinking.

polydipsia, psychogenic A relatively rare psychological disorder characterized by the drinking of extreme amounts of water. It can, on occasions, prove fatal since sodium levels in the blood can be so severely reduced that coma and convulsions ensue.

polydipsia, schedule-induced Excessive drinking in experimental animals that emerges when small amounts of food are provided on an intermittent schedule.

polydrug dependence POLYSUBSTANCE DEPENDENCE.

polygamy A mating (or, in humans, a marriage) system involving the pairing of more than two individuals. For specialized forms, see POLYANDRY and POLYGYNY.

polygamy, serial A marriage system in which a person may have more than one legal spouse but only seriatim; that is, only one at a time. This most common of marriage systems is often called *serial monogamy*, although this term is not preferred in the technical literature because the prefix *mono-* clearly denotes *one*.

polygenic Characterized by many genes. The term is used most often to refer to traits or structures that are determined by many genes.

polyglot One who speaks many languages. Contrast with POLYLOGIA.

polygraph Lit., multiple graph. Hence, any apparatus that reports or graphs data from more than one system at a time. The most common is the multi-channel recorder that simultaneously collects data (typically presented on moving graph paper) on a variety of events such as breathing, heart rate, perspiration and galvanic skin response. Although used in a wide variety of laboratory situations, the polygraph has been so identified in the public eye with the LIE DETECTOR that *polygraph test* is often used synonymously with *lie-detector test*. This equivalence is unfortunate and surely misleading.

polygynandry A mating system in which each male may mate with two or more females and each female with two or more males. It is seen in species that live in troops, such as chimpanzees. The term *promiscuity* used to be applied to this situation, which, while accurate, had a bit of an edge on it. *Polygynandry* is clearly the euphemism of choice.

polygyny A mating (or, in humans, a marriage) system in which a single male may mate with (or marry) two or more females. It tends to occur in species (including many mammals) the females of which make the highest PARENTAL INVESTMENT. Compare with POLYANDRY.

polygyny, sororal A form of polygyny in

which a man's several wives must all be sisters.

polylogia Continuous, incoherent speech.

polymorphism 1 In biology, the presence of several types of physical characteristics or behavioural tendencies within a given species. **2** In genetics, the existence of two or more variants of a gene.

polymorphous Appearing in many forms or varieties.

polymorphous perverse A term often used in classical psychoanalysis to characterize the sexual nature of a young child, who is viewed as deriving sexual pleasure in a variety of erotic forms – oral, anal, etc. – which would be regarded (at least they were in Freud's time) as SEXUAL *PERVERSIONS in an adult.

polyneuritic psychosis An occasional synonym of KORSAKOFF'S SYNDROME.

polyonomy In linguistics, a situation in which a language has a large number of specific terms for the various aspects of a thing. For example, the Inuit languages have separate words for fresh snow, hard-packed snow, walk-on-able snow, light windblown snow, etc., all of which require extensive use of adjectives in English. The existence of polyonomy in a particular perceptual or conceptual area reflects a particular cultural/linguistic view of the world and helps to perpetuate it within the culture. Polyonomy has also been a focus of various theories concerning the interrelationship between language, perception and thought; see here WHORFIAN HYPOTHESIS. Contrast with POLYSEMY.

polyopia Lit., more than one image. The term is reserved for conditions in which, because of irregularities in the refraction of light by the lens of the eye and/or the cornea, more than one image is formed on the retina. Contrast with DIPLOPIA. var., *polyopsia*.

polypeptide PEPTIDE.

polyphagia Excessive eating; see e.g. BULIMIA.

polyphasic sleep A pattern of sleep consisting of several short sleep episodes throughout the day. Common in infants, it typically is replaced by the more usual pattern by school age.

polyphony 1 In linguistics, descriptive of single graphemes that are used to represent many different sounds, e.g. the English letter *s* as in *sin, sure, treasure* and *lose*. **2** In music, descriptive of having two or more melodies simultaneously.

polyphrasia A synonym for LOGORRHOEA.

polysemy Lit., many meanings. Used generally of single words with many distinguishable meanings, e.g. *rose* as a flower, the past tense of *rise*, a colour, etc. Note that in comparative linguistics, it is also used to refer to two or more words in different languages which have the same root.

polysubstance dependence A SUBSTANCE-RELATED DISORDER characterized by the use of three or more drugs, no one of which predominates. The term is not used when nicotine or caffeine are among the drugs. Also called *polydrug dependence*.

polysynaptic reflex arc Any reflex arc in which the basic neural pathway has two or more synapses. The simplest consists of an *afferent* neuron, an *association neuron* and an *efferent* neuron. Also called *multisynaptic reflex arc*.

ponderal Latin for 'of weight'.

ponderal index A measure of weight relative to height. Based on the cube of body length, it is used with infants to yield an index of relative chubbiness in studies of physical maturation. Differentiate from the BODY MASS INDEX (BMI) which uses the square of body height.

pons 1 Generally, tissue that connects two or more parts. **2** Specifically, a rounded prominence on the ventral side of the brain-stem connected with the cerebellum and linking the MEDULLA OBLONTAGA and the CEREBELLUM with various other brain structures through a host of ascending, descending and transverse fibres. It has roles in maintaining equilibrium and coordinating voluntary movements. Several of the cranial nerves have their origins at its borders. adj., *pontine*. Also known as *pons varolii*.

pons varolii See PONS (2).

pontine See PONS.

pontine-geniculo-occipital spikes See PGO SPIKES.

pontine nucleus Any of several nuclei in the PONS (2). They send information about intended movements to the lateral regions of the cerebellum.

pontocerebellar-angle syndrome A syndrome produced by a tumour that exerts pressure on the auditory-vestibular (VIIIth cranial) nerve. Because the nerve carries fibres that serve both audition and balance, the syndrome displays both movement disorders (ataxia with staggering gait, vertigo, hemiplegia) and hearing disturbances (tinnitus, progressive hearing loss). Occasionally the facial (VIIth cranial) nerve is involved as well, producing a facial anaesthesia and loss of the corneal reflex.

Ponzo illusion As depicted; also known, not surprisingly, as the *railway illusion*. Both horizontal bars are the same length.

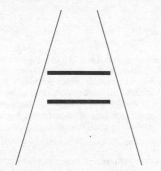

pooh-pooh theory THEORIES OF *LANGUAGE ORIGINS.

pooled variance A single measure of VARIANCE produced by pooling several independent measures.

pooling A term used in various contexts to express the notion of combining things, usually data. Thus: **1** Combining scores from several variables to produce a single measure; e.g. overall academic achievement as measured by pooling scores from all types of tests, grades on exams, papers, etc. **2** Combining data from more than one group of subjects; e.g. all 3rd- and 4th-grade children grouped together and compared with 5th and 6th graders as a separately pooled group. In both types of pooling, *weighting* procedures are usually required to prevent distortions.

pop out An experience that occurs when one particular part of a stimulus display is so distinctive that it automatically jumps out at the perceiver. On a page full of simple dashes, like –, a plus sign, +, will pop out. The effect occurs regardless of how many distractors are in the display.

population 1 All of the organisms of a specific kind (usually, but not necessarily, people) within a defined geographic area at a particular point in time. **2** In statistics, the total number of cases about which a specific statement can be made. Note that in this sense of the term, the population may be: (a) finite, existing and knowable (e.g. all the students enrolled in a particular school); (b) finite, existing but effectively unknowable (e.g. the population of the UK on the day of publication of this volume); or (c) infinite (e.g. all possible coin flips). Distinguish from SAMPLE, which is an observed or selected subset of a population. See also SAMPLING POPULATION.

population stereotype Loosely, any perceptual, cognitive or behaviour pattern that is common among a particular population of individuals. The population can be a group defined by almost anything, gender, ethnicity, religion, geography, etc. Some examples: in North America people typically open the right door of a double doorway; in Great Britain, they usually take the left; in North America and Europe people overwhelming select '3' or '7' if asked to pick a number from 0 to 9; in China they favour even numbers except for 4 which is avoided.

poriomania An extended period of confusion with subsequent amnesia resembling a FUGUE STATE.

pornography Lit., from the original Greek, *writing about prostitutes*. Contemporary usage has expanded the domain of the term considerably and it is typically defined today as any form of written or pictorial representation that either is obscene or has as its sole function the sexual arousal of the beholder. There are serious problems with both criteria. Equating pornography with that which is obscene merely shifts the definitional burden; see OBSCENITY for a discussion of semantic problems. Characterizing it by reference to that which is sexually arousing makes the definition dependent upon the sexual preferences of the beholder. There seems to be no simple solution here and the actual connotations of the term are invariably coloured by the writer's subjective point of view.

Porter's law FERRY–PORTER LAW.

position The core meaning here is *place* or *location*, and all specialized usages of the term reflect this. Specific meanings are: **1** In perception, a location of an object with reference to the point of view of an observer. **2** In sociology and social psychology, a place in a social class or a system of social relationships. Note that this meaning is similar to STATUS in that a social *position* entails social *roles*. **3** In ethology, a point in a DOMINANCE HIERARCHY. **4** In Lewin's field theory, a region in a LIFE SPACE where an event, fact, thing, etc. takes place. **5** In general, a point of view or attitude that one assumes.

position factor Generally, any effect of temporal or physical location of a stimulus on a response. See e.g. POSITION PREFERENCE.

position habit A learned POSITION PREFERENCE.

position preference Any preference, learned or otherwise, that an organism has for one temporal or spatial location over others. For example, a tendency to select the stimulus on the right over the one on the left in a two-choice discrimination experiment; or a tendency to select the first of the alternatives in a multiple-choice exam or questionnaire. Generally, such position factors need to be carefully controlled for by randomizing the positions of stimuli on test items.

positive Although the term enjoys wide currency and multiple meanings in everyday language, within psychology its use is almost always reserved to refer to the upbeat, sanguine, hopeful, encouraging aspects of events, situations, syndromes and outcomes. It is also found in an array of phrases where the author wishes to denote these 'positive' elements of whatever is being referenced. In the following entries we've given those whose meanings may not be obvious; for the others we leave it up to the reader. See NEGATIVE for a lexicographically similar state of affairs.

positive acceleration ACCELERATION.

positive adaptation ADAPTATION (1) when there is a gradual increase in sensitivity.

positive affect Loosely, a good feeling after achieving a goal or completing an action. The term tends to be used in technical writing when reporting that an individual 'felt good' just seems too pedestrian.

positive afterimage AFTERIMAGE, POSITIVE.

positive attitude change ATTITUDE CHANGE, NEGATIVE AND POSITIVE.

positive correlation CORRELATION, POSITIVE.

positive eugenics See EUGENICS.

positive feedback Descriptive of any FEEDBACK loop which accelerates or increases a process.

positive predictive value The proportion of people identified by a test who are 'true cases'. If a test identifies 86 people as *depressed,* and 70 of these really are depressed, then the positive predictive value of this test is $70/86 = 0.81$.

positive psychology An approach to clinical, social and personality issues that emphasizes mental health and well-being rather than pathology. In this approach, mental health is measured by happiness, optimism and such features rather than by the absence of mental illness.

positive punishment PUNISHMENT, POSITIVE.

positive recency In experiments on guessing and predicting, the tendency to identify the event that has occurred most recently. Contrast with NEGATIVE RECENCY.

positive regard Simply, a positive and supportive attitude toward another. Within Carl Rogers's theory of personality, being raised with *unconditional* positive regard from parents and significant others – being surrounded by supportive, loving and respectful caretakers regardless of shortcomings – made a rich, self-actualized life likely. On the other hand, *conditional* positive regard, whereby a child's actions only meet with support when they fit a particular set of standards, is argued to produce less well-adjusted adults with a higher likelihood of various psychological problems.

positive reinforcement REINFORCEMENT, POSITIVE.

positive schizophrenia SCHIZOPHRENIA, POSITIVE.

positive symptoms Symptoms of psychoses marked by the presence of bizarre behaviours and thoughts such as hallucinations and delusions. Compare with NEGATIVE SYMPTOMS.

positive transfer TRANSFER, POSITIVE.

positive transference TRANSFERENCE.

positivism A philosophical point of view generally cited as having been formulated by Auguste Comte, although he was clearly influenced by Francis Bacon and by the British Empiricists. The 'positive' is that which is given, that which is accepted as it is found. Comte argued against the attempts of metaphysicists and theologians to enquire after first causes and/or ultimate ends. He maintained it was not possible to go beyond the objective world given to observation. Hence, for the positivists, all knowledge is contained within the boundaries of science, and only those questions answerable from the application of the scientific method can be approached. The general perspective has emerged in a number of versions, including OPERATIONALISM. In psychology, the positivist approach is most closely associated with BEHAVIOURISM, with its focus on objective observation as the basis for the formulation of laws. Positivism is sublimely hard-headed and often praised for its common-sense approach. It is also, interestingly, occasionally defended on pragmatic grounds even by those who are unconvinced that all questions of knowledge can ultimately be reduced to scientific terms uncontaminated by metaphysics, mentalism and/or theology. It is also vigorously critiqued, even by dedicated contemporary scientists, on the grounds that it places too many sharp limitations on what can legitimately be included in a scientific programme.

positivism, logical A variant of POSITIVISM that had at its core the argument that any nontautological proposition that could not, in principle, be verified by empirical, observational means was utterly devoid of meaning. The focus was to relegate all nonempirical aspects of philosophy and science, such as metaphysics, theology, aesthetics and ethics, to the status of expressions of emotion and belief. The doctrine was ultimately hoist by its own petard for, among other difficulties, it was simply not clear that its own central principle of verifiability could be verified in the dictated manner.

positivity effect The tendency for older adults to have a better memory for positive events than for negative effects. In contrast, young adults tend to attend to and remember negative events better than positive events.

positron emission tomography (PET) A procedure that provides an analysis of the amount of metabolic activity taking place in various parts of the brain. To undergo a PET-scan the patient is injected with a radioactive glucose-like substance that is absorbed into the cells, particularly those that are metabolically active. The patient's brain is scanned in a manner similar to a CAT-scan. A beam of X-rays is passed through the head and the activities of the radioactive molecules are detected by a computer, which compiles a picture of the brain revealing the differential metabolic activity of various structures. See COMPUTERIZED AXIAL TOMOGRAPHY and MAGNETIC RESONANCE IMAGING.

possessive instinct The drive for power and control over others, which is considered by some psychoanalysts to be an instinct. The sucking and swallowing behaviour of the infant is assumed to be an early manifestation of it.

possessiveness Strictly speaking, this term can be used for any tendency to attempt to gain and hold ownership over things. The psychologically interesting aspect, however, arises when these things are people. In fact, some authors use the term so that its sole connotative domain is the tendency to maintain power and control over others, to treat them as though they were one's possessions. It is most commonly observed in parents' attitudes toward their children and husbands and wives toward each other.

post- A combining form meaning *after, later, behind.* There is little agreement on the spelling of compound terms with this prefix. Sometimes a hyphen is inserted, sometimes not. We have not discovered any systematic regularity, as per the following entries.

postcentral gyrus The GYRUS or ridge just posterior to the CENTRAL FISSURE containing the primary somatosensory cortex.

postchiasmatic visual defect Any visual defect produced by neural damage to the visual pathways after the OPTIC CHIASM.

postcognition The presumed capacity to know events that occurred in the past without using normal sensory systems. See PARA-PSYCHOLOGY for reasons why few take this seriously.

postconcussion disorder (or **syndrome**) A neurological disorder resulting from the widespread head trauma that accompanies concussion. It is usually caused by multiple concussions without sufficient time for recovery from earlier trauma. Symptoms include chronic depression, fatigue, difficulties with impulse-control, memory problems, diminished ability to concentrate and, in severe cases, early onset dementia. It is seen in women subjected to multiple batterings and is all too common in athletes who play high-contact sports.

postconventional level of moral development MORAL DEVELOPMENT.

post-encephalic amnesia AMNESIA, POST-ENCEPHALIC.

posterior In time, *following*; in space, *behind*. Contrast with ANTERIOR. In human anatomical terminology, *posterior* is frequently found as a synonym of *dorsal*, *anterior* as a synonym of *ventral*. Many brain structures have distinct posterior (and anterior) regions. Rather than list them all here, see the base term for information about location and function.

posterior commissure A band of myelinated fibres that connects the oculomotor structures of the midbrain of the two hemispheres.

posterior root SPINAL ROOT.

postformal thought A cover term for the varieties of cognitive function that characterize mature, adult thought. It is assumed to develop after Piaget's stage of FORMAL OPERATIONS and be critical for dealing with a world cluttered with ambiguities and contradictions, non-logical structures and organizations that malfunction. It allows adults to synthesize these often mutually contradictory messages into coherent wholes and integrate them with fleeting and fluctuating emotions of self and others.

postganglionic neurons Efferent neurons of the autonomic nervous system that synapse directly onto their target organs.

post-hallucinogen perception disorder An ORGANIC MENTAL DISORDER characterized by FLASHBACKS in which one re-experiences the perceptual disruptions of a hallucinogen following cessation of the drug. The term is only used when the symptoms cause psychological distress.

post hoc Latin for *after this*. The term is generally used to refer to hypotheses or explanations developed on the basis of contiguity or correlation. Such hypotheses are not necessarily valid, because they assume causality without proper verification. Note that the phrase is actually a shortened form of *Post hoc, ergo propter hoc* or, literally, *After this, therefore because of it*. A *post hoc* fallacy is the unwarranted presumption of causality of *x* on *y* simply because one has observed that *x* preceded *y*.

post hoc fallacy See POST HOC.

post hoc tests (or **comparisons**) Any of several statistical procedures for determining which specific comparisons in a multifactor experiment are significant. These comparisons are run after (*post*) a general procedure such as an analysis of variance or a regression analysis has shown overall significance. Two of the more frequently used *post hoc* tests are the TUKEY HONESTLY SIGNIFICANT DIFFERENCE TEST and the SCHEFFÉ TEST; others are the DUNCAN MULTIPLE-RANGE TEST and the NEWMAN–KEULS TEST. Also known as *incidental tests*. See also A POSTERIORI TESTS.

posthypnotic amnesia Generally, the inability to recall some event that occurred while one was hypnotized. It is a form of posthypnotic suggestion in which the subject is specifically told that he or she will, upon waking, not be able to remember a particular fact or event.

posthypnotic suggestion A general term for any suggestion given to a hypnotized subject that he or she will behave in a particular way after being woken. See HYPNOSIS.

postictal Following an ICTAL experience such as a stroke or an epileptic seizure. Postictal syndromes can be varied and unpredictable and may include fears and anxieties, memory dysfunctions, inappropriate aggression and dissociative disorders.

postnatal After birth; compare with PRENATAL.

postpartum Latin for *after childbirth*.

postpartum blues A minor episode of sadness and moodiness following childbirth. It is surprisingly common with some studies suggesting that up to 75% of mothers and more than a few fathers experience some form. Occasionally called, even in scientific work, *baby blues*. Distinguish from POSTPARTUM DEPRESSION.

postpartum depression Loosely, any acute depression occurring within four weeks following childbirth. If psychotic symptoms are present, such as delusions, hallucinations, marked illogical thought or loosening of associations, the term *postpartum psychosis* may be used. Note, the four-week criterion is not universally adhered to and a variety of time periods may be cited as diagnostically relevant. Although generally thought of as a disorder of the mother, fathers have also been known to display a version. Distinguish from POSTPARTUM BLUES.

postpsychotic depression of schizophrenia POSTSCHIZOPHRENIC DEPRESSION.

postremity (principle) The principle that the most probable response an organism will make in a particular situation is the last one it made in that situation. The principle played an important role in E. R. Guthrie's early CONTIGUITY THEORY of learning.

postrotational nystagmus NYSTAGMUS, ROTATIONAL.

postschizophrenic depression A major depressive episode that occasionally occurs during the residual phase of SCHIZOPHRENIA or SCHIZOPHRENIFORM DISORDER. Also known as *postpsychotic depression of schizophrenia*.

postsynaptic Of a cell that is on the receiving side of a synapse, the cell upon which the terminal buttons synapse.

postsynaptic potential (PSP) Generally, any change in the membrane potential of a postsynaptic neuron. PSPs are produced by transmitter substances released by the presynaptic terminal buttons. The *excitatory postsynaptic potentials* (EPSPs) are *de*polarizations, which lower the threshold of the neuron and increase its likelihood of firing; the *inhibitory postsynaptic potentials* (IPSPs) are *hyper*polarizations, which have the opposite effect.

post-test A general term for any test given at the end of an experiment, a training programme, a course of instruction or the like. By comparing the score on the post-test with that on the PRETEST (2), one gets a measure of the effectiveness of the procedure. Also called *end test*.

post-traumatic amnesia AMNESIA, POST-TRAUMATIC.

post-traumatic stress disorder (PTSD) An ANXIETY DISORDER that emerges following a psychologically distressing, traumatic event such as a natural disaster, a bad accident, war or rape. The syndrome includes re-experiencing the trauma in dreams, recurrent thoughts and images, a kind of psychological numbness with an accompanying lessening of feeling of involvement with the world around one, hypervigilance, and an exaggerated startle response. In psychiatric diagnosis, the term is not applied until the symptoms have continued for at least a month; prior to that the condition is called an *acute stress disorder*.

postulate An ASSUMPTION that is accepted as true for the purpose of further reasoning. Postulates are similar to AXIOMS in so far as neither is directly susceptible to proof or disproof, but, unlike axioms, postulates are not universally self-evident. Their apparent truth is limited to the confines of a particular theory. Postulates also differ from THEOREMS in that they are not logical deductions, and from HYPOTHESES in that they are not open to direct empirical evaluation.

postulational method A synonym of HYPOTHETICO-DEDUCTIVE METHOD.

postural Pertaining to posture. Used specifically with regard to the position of the body and, more metaphorically, mental attitudes or beliefs.

postural reflexes Collectively, the variety

of reflex-like responses responsible for maintenance of body posture.

postural set A body position preparatory to a particular response.

postural tremors Fine, rapid tremors, most commonly of the fingers and hands and occasionally of the head, mouth or tongue, that occur when the affected body part is held in a fixed posture, e.g. hands outstretched, mouth held open. A side effect of LITHIUM, they are regarded as a MEDICATION-INDUCED MOVEMENT DISORDER.

posture 1 The overall position of the body. **2** A mental attitude or belief.

pot Slang for *marijuana*. See CANNABIS (SATIVA) for details.

potency 1 Most generally, power. Some authors use the term to refer to actual manifested power although, properly, the central connotation is that of *latent* power. See POTENTIAL, which shares the same etymology. **2** Effectiveness, particularly that of a drug. **3** Sexual capability, specifically the relative ability of the male to 'perform' sexually. Potency in this sense is independent of fertility: a sterile man may have great sexual potency. See IMPOTENCE for more on usage. **4** One of the three hypothesized universal dimensions of *semantic space* in Osgood's theory of word meaning. See SEMANTIC DIFFERENTIAL.

potential 1 adj. Characterized by POTENCY. **2** adj. Relating to the condition of POTENTIALITY. Note, however, that *potential* is often used as a shortened form of *potentiality*, i.e. as a noun denoting this condition rather than an adjective relating to it. **3** n. In electricity, voltage or electrical pressure. With respect to the electrical changes associated with neural impulses, see ACTION POTENTIAL and EVOKED POTENTIAL.

potentiality A set of circumstances that suggests a latent ability; characteristics that are used to infer that some property or talent not currently manifested will develop or be learned (e.g. the faint hope that many parents cling to when they look at their children). See also POTENTIAL (2).

potentiation 1 The action by which stimulation increases the likelihood or magnitude of response to subsequent stimulation of the

same kind. For example, a pain-inducing stimulus will often increase the pain response to a later stimulus. **2** A type of DRUG INTERACTION where a second drug increases particular effects of another drug taken previously.

poverty A relatively low standard of living in terms of goods and materials. *Relative* here is characterized in terms of the general standard of living in a particular society, its distribution of wealth, a person's status within the society and his or her personal expectations. The term is also used more metaphorically to characterize a relative lack of mental functioning, e.g. a poverty of ideas.

poverty of the stimulus A phrase used for the theoretical argument that the stimulus environment within which an organism is raised is not sufficiently rich and/or well organized to allow easy learning of the structural features of that environment. The term is generally applied in a *domain-specific* manner. So, for example, Chomsky has argued that the speech heard by infants is IMPOVERISHED (2) in just this fashion. It's worth noting that many disagree with this position.

power The basic meanings are rather concrete: **1** In mathematics, either the product of a number multiplied by itself, or the exponent indicating the number of times the self-multiplication operation is to be carried out. **2** In optics, the magnification of a lens. **3** In physics, a measure of the rate of doing work. **4** Muscular strength. **5** SOCIAL *POWER. **6** STATISTICAL *POWER OF A TEST.

power analysis A statistical analysis that enables a researcher to estimate how many subjects will be needed in a planned experiment. It is based on an assumption about how large an EFFECT SIZE is expected and what particular statistical tests are to be used. When the assumed effect size is large and the tests are powerful (see here STATISTICAL *POWER OF A TEST) few subjects are needed. When a small effect size is anticipated and/or tests with little power are to be used, larger sample sizes are required.

power assertion A form of discipline whereby parents control the behaviour of their children by using or threatening to use punishments and rewards.

power-coercive strategy A label used for

any of a variety of strategies based on the use of political, economic or social power to bring about social change. Usually, only techniques utilizing some degree of coercive pressure are included here, e.g. strikes, boycotts, sit-ins. Compare with NORMATIVE-RE-EDUCATIVE STRATEGY.

power elite C. Wright Mills's term for the 'intricate set of overlapping cliques' within the government, the military and the business world the members of which make the basic decisions about national events.

power field(s) In Lewin's field theory, those regions in the life space over which the individual has control. They may be objects, events or other persons.

power figure An individual as an identifiable representative of authority and power. The authority and power may be real or imagined: the primary role of the power figure is that of being someone with whom one can identify.

power function 1 In statistics, an index of the power of a statistical test to reject, at a specified risk level, a false null hypothesis; see STATISTICAL *POWER OF A TEST. **2** In psychophysics, an equation that expresses a particular theoretical relationship between the magnitude of a physical stimulus and the intensity of the sensory experience it evokes. See POWER LAW.

power law A generalization, due primarily to the work of S. S. Stevens, that states that the psychophysical relationship between a physical stimulus, S, and the psychological experience of that stimulus, ψ, is given by the equation, $\psi = kS^n$, where n is the exponent or the power to which S must be raised that is characteristic of that particular continuum, and k is a constant. Compare with LOG LAW. See also METHODS OF *SCALING, PSYCHOPHYSICS and SCALES.

power law (of performance) A generalization about learning that states that the speed of performance of a sensorimotor task increases as the power of the number of times the task is carried out. In layperson's terms, practice makes perfect (or at least makes you faster!).

powerlessness A psychological state in which one feels deprived of power, control

or influence over events. The state may relate to feelings vis-à-vis social and political events or to feelings with respect to one's own personal psychological needs.

power of a test, statistical A measure of the probability that any given statistical test will detect a significant relationship when one actually exists in the data. Or, in the more usual phrasing, the probability that the test will correctly reject, at a given level of risk, the NULL *HYPOTHESIS of no relationship when, in fact, that hypothesis is false. The power of any statistical test increases as the sample size increases. See also STATISTICAL SIGNIFICANCE.

power, social Social psychologists and sociologists typically view power as the degree of control that a person or a group has over other persons or groups. Power is thus viewed in terms of relationships; maximum power is the ability to exert total control over others while remaining simultaneously immune from attempts by the powerless to do likewise. Such power may be manifested in any of a number of ways. Formal AUTHORITY carries with it formal, legal power, but surreptitious manipulations can often render it impotent. Physical force and coercion are obvious vehicles for exerting control but subtle and more genteel persuasions based upon deceit and deception are probably more common. Moreover, it must be recognized that an important aspect of social power is the degree to which one can compel another to act against his or her will. Thus, one means of wresting power from another is simply to withdraw one's emotional investment. This particular device is commonly observed in marital relationships and in the functioning of small social groups.

The more behaviouristically inclined have a rather simple and not inelegant way of expressing the components of social power: they view power as the degree to which one may dispense rewards and punishments to others while remaining unaffected by such attempts at dispensation by those others. Bertrand Russell remarked that the social sciences ought to follow through on their oft-stated desire to emulate the natural sciences and, as physics has done, make power the fundamental concept. Since there are few areas of psychology with more obvious relevance to the real world there are many who believe he was right.

power spectrum In acoustics, a graph of the mean square amplitude of a sound wave.

power test Any test that measures ability by determining the degree of difficulty of material that can be mastered with no time pressures on the subject. Compare with SPEED TEST.

practical intelligence See INTELLIGENCE, PRACTICAL and TRIARCHIC THEORY OF INTELLIGENCE.

practice An abridged dictionary we checked provided 21 separate definitions for this term and, without much stretching, one could find almost all of them represented in the psychological literature. However, the following four account for most of the term's use in psychology: **1** The repetition of an act or a series of acts. **2** The repetition of an act or a series of acts for the purpose of improving functioning. Meanings 1 and 2 are kept separate because of theoretical debates over the relationships between LEARNING and PERFORMANCE and the impact of repetitions of behaviours upon either or both. **3** Any habitually performed, ritualized behaviour. **4** Any behaviour that is customary or traditional, particularly within a particular culture. var., *practise*.

practice, distributed In the study of learning, circumstances in which practice trials are separated by rest periods or by periods of other activity. Compare with MASSED *PRACTICE, in which there are no such pauses. Also called *spaced practice*.

practice effect Basically, the effect of practice. The term is used to refer to a factor that needs to be carefully controlled in experimental work to take into account effects of experience that are not relevant to the situation under study. For example, re-using the same IQ test with a person may invalidate it as a device for measuring his or her intelligence because of the practice effect produced by taking the test the first time.

practice, massed In the study of learning, an arrangement in which subjects complete many trials with very short or no intertrial intervals. Learning under such conditions is generally slower than that with DISTRIBUTED *PRACTICE.

practice material Material given to a subject to familiarize him or her with the general experimental procedure prior to collecting the real data.

practice period 1 A period during which a subject works with PRACTICE MATERIAL. **2** A period during an experiment or test in which the subject is permitted to practice.

practice theory of play The generalization that play, particularly that observed in animals, is adaptive, in that it provides the opportunity to practice behaviours that will be of value as the organism matures. This hypothesis has also been applied to children's play but found to account for little of the observed data. See PLAY.

practice trials See PRACTICE PERIOD.

Prader-Willi syndrome A congenital syndrome typically, but not always, marked by mental retardation ranging from mild to severe. Physical characteristics include short stature, generalized obesity, underdeveloped genitalia and, occasionally, abnormal metabolism. Bizarre eating patterns are common. Also known as *hypotonia-obesity syndrome*.

prae- Variation of PRE-.

Praegnanz Variation of PRÄGNANZ.

pragmatic Concerned with the outcome rather than with the process; preferring that which is practical to that which is theoretical; favouring the concrete over the abstract.

pragmatics 1 As originally developed, the study of the relationship between signs (words, expressions, etc.) and their uses. **2** More recently, owing largely to the work of Austin and Searle in the 1950s and 1960s, a rather general endeavour encompassing philosophical, linguistic, sociological and psychological aspects of the use and effects of verbal signs and forms. Pragmatics differs from most other areas of linguistic endeavour in its emphasis on the function of various language forms rather than on the forms alone. Pragmatics is often equated with SPEECH ACT theory, although it should be noted that the latter is more properly only one theory of pragmatics.

pragmatism A philosophical doctrine in

which values, meanings and truths of propositions are taken as equivalent to the practical, empirical consequences derivable from them. Several of psychology's foremost early theorists were exponents of pragmatism, including John Dewey and William James.

Prägnanz A Gestalt principle of organization that holds that perceived or experienced forms tend toward a more coherent structure, i.e. they become better defined, more symmetrical, more stable, simpler and more meaningful. The term itself derives from the German word for *pregnant*, and this is, indeed, the core of the connotation. It is occasionally referred to as the *law of pregnance* or the *law of precision*.

prandial Relating to a meal, e.g. prandial drinking is drinking associated with eating.

-praxia A word element meaning *doing* or *practice*.

pre- A combining form meaning *before, in front of*. var., *prae-*.

preadolescence By convention, the 2 years before puberty.

preattentive processing Unconscious processing of information that takes place prior to awareness of what has been heard or seen.

precategorical acoustic store (PAS) An unnecessarily long synonym for ECHOIC *MEMORY. It tends to be used by theorists who emphasize that the material in the PAS has not been processed or categorized.

precausal thinking Piaget's term for a developmentally early form of thinking where natural events (rain, thunder) are viewed in terms of intentions and wills and interpreted anthropomorphically rather than physically.

precedence effect A phenomenon of perception. The first of two or more stimuli to be noticed attracts one's attention such that the other(s) is (are) not perceived as accurately. See also LAW OF *PRIOR ENTRY for a similar phenomenon.

precentral gyrus In the frontal lobes, the GYRUS or ridge just in front of the CENTRAL FISSURE containing the neural tissue that controls the skeletal muscles. Also known as the *primary motor cortex*.

precentre To provide a fixation point in the visual field prior to presentation of a stimulus. By having the subject focus on this point, the area of the retina upon which the stimulus will fall is controlled.

precipitating cause The factor or occurrence that is the immediate cause of some event. Like PREDISPOSING CAUSE it tends to be used of diseases, syndromes and clinical disorders.

precision, law of PRÄGNANZ.

precision of process (h) In statistics, the reciprocal of the variance; i.e. $h = 1/\sigma^2$. Just as σ^2 reflects the uncertainty associated with observations drawn from a population, h reflects certainty.

precocial Pertaining to species whose young are relatively independent at birth; specifically those capable of locomotion and, in many cases, feeding themselves. Compare with ALTRICIAL.

precocity Generally, premature, rapid development. Although the term is most often used with respect to the particularly early appearance of some intellectual or artistic ability, it can be applied to any early-maturing function. var., *precociousness*. adj., *precocious*.

precoding Determining the coding system to be used prior to the collection of data.

precognition The hypothesized paranormal ability to have knowledge of future events. The term is not used for well-reasoned inferences and predictions made on the basis of current knowledge. See PARAPSYCHOLOGY.

precommissural fornix FIMBRIA.

preconcept Piaget's term for the primitive concepts used by a preoperatory-stage child. Such concepts tend to be concrete and action-oriented; see TRANSDUCTIVE REASONING.

preconscious A psychoanalytic term for knowledge, emotions, images, etc. which are not in consciousness at any moment but are easily accessible. Sometimes called the *descriptive unconscious* or the *foreconscious*; distinguish from UNCONSCIOUS and compare with SUBCONSCIOUS.

preconventional level of moral development MORAL DEVELOPMENT.

precuneus An area of cortex in the medial surface of the parietal lobe, just in front of the CUNEATE NUCLEUS. It seems to be involved in a variety of cognitive functions, intriguingly those that are linked with consciousness. In particular, it is active when one is thinking about oneself.

precursor Generally, any thing that precedes another thing, with the implication that the first-occurring plays an essential role in the determination of the nature of the subsequent. The term is used most often with regard to various biochemical substances that play a role in the synthesis of other substances, e.g. *L-dopa* is a precursor of *dopamine*. Occasionally, a preliminary training programme and/or learning experience may be called a precursor of the acquisition of other, more complex, skills.

precursor load strategy A psychopharmacological treatment method for various psychiatric disorders in which the patient is given doses of the precursor for a needed substance. The strategy is used in cases in which the required substance does not cross the blood–brain barrier but the precursor does, e.g. the oral administration of L-dopa for Parkinson's disease.

predation A cover term for all those behaviours associated with an animal's hunting, attacking and seizing other organisms for food. *Predator* is used for the animal that carries out these behaviours, *prey* for the victim. adj., *predatory*.

predatory aggression AGGRESSION, PREDATORY.

predatory attack The kind of physical attack typically seen when an individual of a predatory species attacks one of its normal prey. The pattern of behaviour has been artificially elicited in experiments with cats by stimulation of the brain; under such conditions it is called, descriptively, a *quiet biting attack*.

predelay reinforcement (procedure) A variation on the DELAYED REACTION (PROCEDURE) in which the subject is reinforced in a particular place and then prevented from returning for various lengths of time before being permitted to attempt to go to the proper location.

predestination PREDETERMINISM.

predeterminism A philosophical point of view that maintains the full script for the universe has already been written and that all that happens is merely the acting out of the grand design; i.e. all that transpires is predestined. A curious thing about this doctrine, which its adherents never quite seem to understand, is that it makes absolutely no difference whether it is true or false. Distinguish from DETERMINISM.

predicate (or predicative) thinking Reasoning whereby two objects are assumed to be similar or even identical because they share the same predicate; that is, they possess the same attribute with respect to a subject. Many psychoanalysts argue that the *id* 'thinks' predicatively, and Piagetians consider predicate thinking a central aspect of preoperatory thought in the young child. Note, however, that the primitiveness implied by these usages is not the whole issue: predicate thought is also an element in cognitively sophisticated symbolism and symbolic thought, in which generalizations concerning concepts are made on the basis of shared features.

predication In logic (originally) and linguistics (more recently), a formal linking of a subject and a predicate. In simple terms, making a statement or proposition which attributes characteristics to a subject; e.g. 'Richard is a dirty rat' predicates of a person, Richard, a particular characteristic, dirty-rat-ness. Predication always involves the notion of linking or asserting.

prediction Simply, a statement about what will be observed before it actually occurs. In all scientific endeavours, prediction is a sophisticated operation involving detailed knowledge of the phenomena under consideration, including relevant facts and basic principles. Accurate prediction is usually regarded as the most stringent test of a scientific theory. In psychology, essentially all predictions are couched in forms probabilistic – although it should be recognized that this may be considered true in all sciences, the difference being that the probabilities are closer to 1.0 in some than in others.

prediction, clinical A term usually used in opposition to *statistical* or *empirical prediction*. The issue involves the question of whether predictions about an individual's behaviour are more accurately made on the basis of an essentially subjective understanding that results from close individualistic scrutiny (i.e. *clinical*) or from statistical judgements made by evaluating the person with respect to objective scales and population norms (i.e. *statistical* or *empirical*). Note that both procedures may use 'hard' and 'soft' data: the critical distinction is in how these data are combined, either subjectively and intuitively or objectively and mechanically.

prediction, differential Basically, any *either/or* prediction.

prediction, empirical CLINICAL *PREDICTION.

prediction, statistical CLINICAL *PREDICTION.

predictive efficiency A measure of the success of a test, a rule, a principle, a theory, etc. in making accurate predictions. Usually, in cases of relatively simple and well-defined situations, such as predicting who will succeed in an academic setting, the measure is given as a proportion of correct to total predictions.

predictive index INDEX OF *FORECASTING EFFICIENCY.

predictive validity VALIDITY, PREDICTIVE.

predictor Loosely, any variable that can be used to make predictions about an individual's future performance, health, mental state, etc.

predictor variable VARIABLE, PREDICTOR.

predisposing cause Any factor which, although not *the* PRECIPITATING CAUSE of an event, plays an important role in the manifestation of that event. The term is most frequently found with regard to diseases, hereditary syndromes and clinical disorders.

predisposition 1 Specifically, any genetic factor or set of factors that increases the likelihood of its possessor displaying a particular trait or characteristic. 2 More generally, a DISPOSITION.

preemie A PREMATURE INFANT.

preference Basically, a liking for one thing more than for another. In practice, many psychologists prefer to operationalize the term and it is often used with reference to a turning toward, or the actual selection of, one alternative over another; that is, *choice* is taken as the indicator of preference.

preference test 1 Generally, any experimental situation in which the subject must select the preferred of two or more alternatives. 2 Specifically, any of several tests of personal preference, e.g. the KUDER PREFERENCE RECORD.

preferential looking method An experimental design used primarily with infants and animals based on how long the subject looks at one display versus another. The utility of the procedure depends on an organism's preference for some feature of the display. Depending on the experimental design, the subjects will look longer at a display that is novel, at one that is more intrinsically interesting or one that violates an implicit or explicit expectation. Also called *visual preference method*.

preformationism In its earliest form, the doctrine that all traits and structures were present in the germ plasma. The usual assumption here was that a HOMUNCULUS (1), a miniature form of the organism, was present at the time of conception. The more modern variation holds that the characteristics and traits of an individual are present at conception in the form of a genetic code and that development is an unfolding of these 'preformed' patterns. Compare with EPIGENESIS. Also called *preformism*.

prefrontal Pertaining to the anterior part of the frontal lobes of the brain.

prefrontal cortex The region of cortex in the very front of the brain, rostral to the association areas of MOTOR CORTEX. Standard neuroarchitecture divides it into two parts, DORSOLATERAL PREFRONTAL CORTEX and ORBITO-FRONTAL CORTEX. Prefrontal cortex is involved in planning, control and execution of action. It plays important roles in evaluating the basic emotional inputs from other regions and in carrying out EXECUTIVE FUNCTIONS.

prefrontal lobotomy LOBOTOMY, PREFRONTAL.

preganglionic neurons Efferent neurons

of the autonomic nervous system that synapse on POSTGANGLIONIC NEURONS.

pregenital stage (or **level** or **phase**) In psychoanalytic theory, a stage of psychosexual development preceding the genital stage. An infant during this period is presumed to derive libidinal satisfaction from the oral and anal zones. Thus, the term is used so that it encompasses both the oral and anal stages.

pregnance, law of PRÄGNANZ.

pregnant 1 Pertaining to the state of pregnancy. **2** Pertaining to a figure or a Gestalt having the characteristic of PRÄGNANZ.

prehensile Capable of grasping.

prehension 1 The physical act of grasping. **2** Occasionally, the mental act of understanding. The connotation in both cases is that of a rather primitive kind of act.

prejudice 1 A prejudgement, an attitude formed on the basis of insufficient information, a preconception. In this literal sense, a prejudice can be either negative or positive in evaluative terms; it can be about any particular thing, event, person, idea, etc.; and it can even be an aspect of coherent scientific work, for a hypothesis formulated on little evidence can legitimately be called a prejudice. **2** A negative attitude toward a particular group of persons based on negative traits assumed to be uniformly displayed by all members of that group. **3** A failure to react toward a person as an individual with individual qualities and a tendency instead to treat him or her as possessing the presumed stereotypes of his or her socially or racially defined group. Meanings 2 and 3 are connotatively very different from meaning 1; they are also the more commonly intended ones.

Prejudice (2 and 3) is often popularly thought of as being characteristic of the members of the majority group in a society with respect to that society's minority groups. In fact, it tends to be an endemic attitude in many (all?) areas of social life. It should be differentiated from the notion of a *preconception* (see 1, above) largely because of the connotative element, the evaluative aspect. Contrast also with DISCRIMINATION, which tends to be reserved for behaviours while *prejudice* is more clearly reserved for attitudes – which may or may not have behavioural accompaniments.

preliterate Used synonymously with NON-LITERATE; distinguish from ILLITERATE.

prelogical thinking Any mode of thought that does not follow the principles of logic. The prefix *pre-* implies that logical thought is somehow within the range of an individual's cognitive potential but simply hasn't made its appearance yet. Hence, it is typically used of young children.

Premack principle The generalization put forward by David Premack that if any two behaviours differ in the probability of their occurrence at any particular moment, the opportunity to engage in the more probable will serve to reinforce the less probable. The principle presents REINFORCEMENT as relative, not absolute. For example, food will reinforce running for a hungry rat but running may be made to reinforce eating if the rat is fully satiated but has been physically confined for a time and deprived of the opportunity for exercise.

premature ejaculation Ejaculation during sexual intercourse which occurs too soon to satisfy the coital partner. Note that this functional definition has absolutely nothing to do with real time.

premature infant A viable foetus born prematurely. *Premature* in this context has been defined in a variety of ways over the years. Originally, the number of days since conception was used, with 250 days set as criterial for prematurity. Difficulties in obtaining accurate and objective data on conception led to a shift to birth weight as the critical factor, with the generally accepted criterion being 2.5 kg (approximately 5.5 lb). When date of conception can be reasonably well identified, the concept of *weight appropriateness* relative to gestational age is used, so that terms such as *small for date, preterm* or, in extreme cases, *very low birth weight* (usually restricted to infants below 1,000 g) are applied.

premenstrual dysphoric disorder A MOOD DISORDER in women that begins during the last week of the luteal phase (see MENSTRUAL CYCLE) and remits during the first few days of the onset of the menses. It is marked by emotional lability, periods of anxiety and/or depression and feelings of helplessness. The term is only used when the symptoms are so severe that they interfere with work, social activities or relationships. Distinguish from PREMENSTRUAL SYNDROME, where the mood swings are less dramatic and do not interfere with normal functioning. Also called *late luteal phase dysphoric disorder.*

premenstrual syndrome (PMS) Minor mood lability in women associated with the late luteal period. The irritability and mood swings typically disappear within a few days of the onset of menses. Distinguish from PREMENSTRUAL DYSPHORIC DISORDER.

premise In any argument, one of the propositions upon which another proposition (the conclusion) is based. See SYLLOGISM.

premonitory dream PROPHETIC DREAM.

premorbid Prior to the onset of a disorder. The term *premorbid functioning*, for example, is used to refer to the physical or psychological level of function before the disruptive effects of a condition or disorder; *premorbid estimation* refers to any of several procedures used to determine such functioning.

premorbid personality A loose term for an individual whose characteristic modes of behaviour and thought are taken as signs of a predisposition to a psychosis, notably schizophrenia.

premotor cortex MOTOR AREA.

prenatal Prior to birth.

prenatal influences Very generally, anything that has an effect upon the developing foetus. The term is used neutrally and should be distinguished from the doctrine of the INFLUENCE OF *MATERNAL IMPRESSION.

prenubile Pertaining to the period from birth to the onset of puberty.

pre-Oedipal stage (or **level** or **phase**) In psychoanalytic theory, the stage(s) of psychosexual development prior to the *Oedipal stage* (see OEDIPUS COMPLEX). During this period a child is conceptualized as rather single-mindedly devoted to the mother.

preoperational thought PREOPERATORY THOUGHT.

preoperatory stage (or **level** or **period**) In Piagetian theory, the stage of cognitive development following the SENSORIMOTOR STAGE. It is first detectable with the establishment of OBJECT PERMANENCE and ends with the emergence of CONCRETE OPERATIONS. During this stage, a child is characterized largely by dependence upon perceptual features of the world and thinking is intuitive in nature rather than logical, although the capability for some early forms of symbolic representational thought is present. Also called the *preoperational stage.*

preoperatory thought A term used by Piaget to refer to the kinds of cognitive capabilities manifested by a child during the PREOPERATORY STAGE.

preoptic area An area of the brain lying just rostral to the HYPOTHALAMUS and comprised of several distinct subareas. The *ventrolateral preoptic area* plays a role in sleep. Stimulation of the region suppresses alertness and promotes drowsiness; lesions cause insomnia. The *medial preoptic area* is the forebrain region most critical for male sexual behaviour. It contains the *sexually dimorphic nucleus* that plays a role in sexual behaviour of both sexes although it is far larger in males.

preorgasmic FRIGIDITY (3), ORGASM DISORDERS.

preparadigmatic Thomas Kuhn's term for the state of a science before a generally accepted PARADIGM (2) has become established. It has often been claimed that psychology is in just such a state compared with, say, physics. This seems a tad wrong-headed if only because psychology, by virtue of the wide range of its subject-matter and goals, is unlikely to ever have anything resembling a Kuhnian paradigm.

preparation **1** Most generally, the act of preparing, of getting ready to perform some behaviour. **2** The thing so prepared. **3** In problem-solving, the preliminary stage, during which the solver attempts to gather the relevant information needed for attempted solutions. **4** In physiological psychology, an organism prepared for examination or experimentation.

preparation, acute A PREPARATION (4) studied for a short period of time, specifically while the temporary (i.e. acute) effects of some drug or surgical procedure are being manifested by the experimental subject.

preparation, chronic A PREPARATION (4)

studied over an extended period of time. A common example in physiological work is the permanent implantation of an electrode in an animal's brain.

preparatory interval In experiments, particularly those in which *reaction time* is the major dependent variable, a short period of time between a 'ready' signal and the presentation of the stimulus for responding.

preparatory response A behaviourist term used by some learning theorists to refer to all the responses in a sequence of behaviours (except the very last response) leading an organism to a single reinforcement. Since, strictly speaking, only the very last of a chain of responses gets reinforced, the previous responses in the sequence are dubbed *preparatory*.

preparatory set SET, PREPARATORY.

preparedness A feature of particular organisms, such that they are biologically prepared to learn some associations more readily than others; a close synonym of BELONGINGNESS (1).

preperception 1 PREATTENTIVE PROCESSING. 2 A vague perceptual experience without any clear sense of the identity of a presented stimulus. It is often the first experience one has when confronted with an AMBIGUOUS *FIGURE.

pre-post Characterizing a common research design where each participant is tested or evaluated prior ('pre-') to carrying out a specific manipulation and then tested afterward ('post') to evaluate its effects. The term has become so common that it is not unusual to see it without the hyphen, *prepost*.

prepotent reflex (or **response**) Any reflex or response that takes precedence over any other potential reflex or response that an organism might make.

prepotent stimulus Any stimulus that takes precedence over all the others in the environment at a given point in time; the stimulus with the greatest attention-getting capacity.

preprogramming Technical jargon for the extent to which the behaviour of a species or individual organism is genetically programmed. Typically used with respect to the degree to which the neural patterns of

the brain are assumed to have been genetically 'prewired' for particular behaviours. See here HEREDITY–ENVIRONMENT CONTROVERSY.

prepsychotic Loosely, pertaining to behaviours or emotional or cognitive states that a clinician considers to be indicative of an incipient psychosis.

prepuberal stage A synonym of PREADOLESCENCE. Also spelled *prepubertal*.

prepulse inhibition The diminishing or inhibiting of a reflex by presenting a weak stimulus prior to the strong stimulus that would normally evoke the response.

presby- A combining form meaning *old, aged*.

presbyacusis Loss of sensitivity to sound stimuli with increasing age. The term is used specifically to refer to the common partial or complete deafness in the aged, although essentially everyone past childhood is somewhat presbyacutic, especially with regard to high-pitched stimuli (above roughly 15,000 Hz).

presbyopia A visual defect produced by a hardening of the lens. The rigidity of the lens, which is common in old age, causes a loss of accommodation such that the ability to focus on close objects is lost. Bifocals correct for the condition.

preschool 1 The period of life prior to reaching school age. 2 Any kindergarten and/or nursery school.

presenile dementia DEMENTIA, PRESENILE.

presenile onset PRESENILE *DEMENTIA, SENILE.

presenium The period of life before the age of 65.

presentation 1 Generally, any manner in which material is put before a person for learning or understanding. 2 In experimental work, the act of placing a stimulus before a subject. 3 The stimulus itself. 4 In psychoanalysis, the manner in which an instinctual drive is expressed. 5 In ethology, the sequence of behaviours engaged in by a female animal indicative of receptivity to coitus. 6 In social interactions, the manner in which a person expresses him- or herself; see e.g. PRESENTATIONAL RITUALS.

presentational rituals E. Goffman's term

for the many things we do to promote social interactions in a polite manner. He cites four classes of rituals: salutations, invitations, compliments and minor services. Presentation rituals and AVOIDANCE RITUALS together make up what he calls *deference behaviour*.

presenting symptom 1 A symptom that causes a person to seek medical or psychological therapy. **2** The symptom that a patient 'presents' as the initial one during the first intake work-up by a physician or a therapist. 1 and 2 may not be the same symptom.

presolution variability A term for the general observation that prior to the discovery of a solution to a complex problem there is typically considerable variability in behaviour as many different strategies are employed in an attempt to find the correct route to take.

press In Henry Murray's theory of personality, those aspects of the environment that are effective determinants of behaviour. Press are (note that Murray used the term in the plural) external and represent features of objects that have straightforward implications for the individual in his or her efforts to fulfil needs which are conceptualized as internal. In actual behaviour, a *press-need pattern* emerges which collectively represents the various actions taken to satisfy the needs produced by press. For example, the press of poverty may produce a need for financial security and the person may, according to circumstances, cheat, work hard, train for a lucrative profession, etc.

press-need pattern PRESS.

pressure The basic dictionary definition – exertion of force against something – is generally adequate in psychology. There are also a few specific uses, as follows: **1** The sensation experienced when physical force is applied to an area of the body; see PRESSURE SENSATION. **2** The emotional experience of feeling compelled to respond to someone's wishes or to external forces. **3** The use of coercion to persuade another to act in a particular manner. See also SOCIAL PRESSURE.

pressured speech Extremely rapid, frenzied speech. Seen in cases of mania.

pressure gradient The gradient of deflection of the skin away from the point where

the pressure is applied. This gradient is the critical stimulus for PRESSURE SENSATION, as can be shown by placing one's finger in a jar of mercury. Although there is considerable physical pressure everywhere, the only sense of pressure is where there is a gradient, at the surface.

pressure sensation The perceptual experience when sufficient tissue distortion to establish a detectable PRESSURE GRADIENT takes place. The phrase *tissue distortion* is used here to emphasize that, although in the normal course of affairs pressure is typically experienced when a stimulus deforms the skin inward, outward deflections are similarly perceived as pressure, as are tensions in muscles, joints, tendons and internal organs. Although there are many unresolved issues, there is evidence to implicate the *Pacinian corpuscles*, the *Meissner corpuscles* and the *free nerve endings* as pressure receptors.

pressure-sensitive spot Any small spot on the skin with lower threshold for the sensation of pressure than the surrounding area.

prestige Loosely, an attribute of being held in high regard by one's associates. Prestigious persons are generally influential in a group or society, although, since prestige may be limited to a specific area or field of endeavour, their influence may be tempered by limited credibility.

prestige suggestion The process of persuading others by associating prestigious persons with the point of view one is attempting to put forward. See PERSUASION and related entries.

prestriate cortex Visual association cortex that surrounds the primary visual cortex (see STRIATE CORTEX). It receives fibres from both the primary visual cortex and the superior colliculi (see COLLICULUS). Also called circumstriate cortex and EXTRASTRIATE CORTEX.

presupposition 1 Generally, a supposition made in advance, an assumption, a postulate. **2** In studies of language, an assumption that a speaker makes about the listener's knowledge in order that an utterance will make sense. For example, in uttering a simple sentence like 'Pat is sick too', the speaker presupposes that he and the listener share knowledge of a person named Pat and another unnamed person of their acquaintance whom they both know is sick.

presynaptic Of a neuron that synapses on another; the cell on the other side of the synapse from the POSTSYNAPTIC neuron.

pretest 1 A practice test, a number of trials or a period of time during which the subject in an experiment is familiarized with the materials to be used. **2** A preliminary test or series of trials given prior to the actual experimental manipulations. Scores on the pretest form a baseline against which to measure the effects of the manipulations. **3** A final run with a questionnaire or survey prior to full-scale implementation; a kind of last-minute shakedown to detect any existing problems in design, wording of questions, etc.

prevalence The frequency of occurrence of an event or condition in a specified population at a particular point in time. See INCIDENCE to appreciate a distinction based on timing. Both terms are often used so that the 'event' or 'condition' is a disease or a disorder.

preverbal A general term used to refer to the time prior to the acquisition of language.

prewiring PREPROGRAMMING.

priapism A chronically erect penis. The term is properly used of an abnormal and painful condition in which a persistent erection occurs without sexual arousal. It should not be used as a synonym of SATYRIASIS.

pricking pain PAIN, PRICKING.

pride The state of satisfaction with oneself for efforts made and gains accomplished.

pride, neurotic K. Horney's term for the neurotic condition in which a person's sense of self-worth far exceeds what the data actually warrant.

primacy Generally, the property of being first in any respect. In psychoanalytic writings, the meaning is often not a simple temporal or logical one but may connote *prepotence*. That is, a tendency which has *primacy* is one which is strong and can withstand regressive tendencies or other infantile id pressures. adj., *primary*.

primacy effect 1 In cognitive psychology, the common finding that in a free recall situation, the materials that are presented first in a series are better recalled than those that are presented in the middle. See also RECENCY EFFECT and SERIAL-POSITION EFFECT. Also called the *law of primacy* or the *principle of primacy*. **2** In social psychology, the finding that information about an individual presented early on has a greater impact on impression formation than information presented later.

primacy, law or principle of PRIMACY EFFECT.

prima facie Latin for *at first appearance, at first view*. In scientific work, the term refers to the circumstances in which a fact or an observation is put forward which is suggestive of a particular interpretation but requires further analysis or research before conclusions can be legitimately drawn. In *forensic* matters, it refers to evidence deemed indicative of an event having occurred and which, unless rebutted, is probably legally acceptable. Note that we find scientists here somewhat more conservative in their stance than lawyers and judges.

primal First in a temporal sequence, first in time. Often used as equivalent to *primitive* or *primordial*, particularly in psychoanalytic works.

primal anxiety In psychoanalytic theory, the anxiety experienced immediately after birth when the infant is expelled from the protective womb and thrust into the frenetic stimulation of the outside world. Otto Rank expanded on this notion with his concept of a BIRTH TRAUMA (1). See PRIMARY ANXIETY and SIGNAL ANXIETY.

primal fantasy In psychoanalysis, a fantasy used by children to make sense of sexual matters about which they have no direct knowledge, e.g. CLOACA THEORY.

primal father PRIMAL HORDE.

primal horde Freud's term for the primordial community hypothesized originally by Darwin in which social structure was organized around a dominant male (the *primal father*), a number of females whom he reserved for himself and the subordinate males whom he kept in subjugation. It should be appreciated that Freud's notions were based upon psychoanalytic theory, not archaeological or anthropological data, and that Darwin's original hypothesis was based upon the observation of nonhuman primates.

primal repression REPRESSION (1).

primal scene A recollected or confabulated scene from childhood of some early sexual experience, most commonly of one's parents copulating.

primal sketch In vision, an abstract representation that contains information about the contours and major shading of an object or scene. It is assumed in some theories to be the first step toward object and scene recognition. The primal sketch forms the foundation for computation of a more detailed perceptual sketch that includes some depth information. Some digital photography software allows one to transform a digital photograph into a primal sketch, thus mimicking the perceptual process.

primal trauma A term used very generally in psychoanalytic approaches to refer to some painful childhood experience. The experience of birth, an especially severe punishment, the death of a parent, witnessing parental coitus, the knowledge that your parents do not love you, etc. have been so labelled by various theorists.

primary First, in the broadest possible sense. The basic idea is that one thing is primary with respect to other things if all the things can be ordered in some logical, coherent fashion, e.g. according to time, spatial location, order of development, order of magnitude or relative importance. Note that distinctions between this term and its various partial synonyms are occasionally made. To wit: *prime* = first in importance, *primal* = first in a temporal sequence, *primitive* = first in a series of things of increasing complexity, *primordial* = first in an evolutionary or geological time sequence. Compare with SECONDARY. n., *primacy*.

primary abilities PRIMARY MENTAL ABILITIES.

primary amentia A mental deficiency assumed to be due to genetic factors.

primary anxiety In psychoanalysis, the emotional experience that accompanies the dissolution of the ego. In Freud's later theorizing about anxiety, he regarded this form as the basic, fundamental (i.e. primary) anxiety

and distinguished it from SIGNAL ANXIETY, which was conceptualized as having a protective, altering function. Distinguish from PRIMAL ANXIETY.

primary auditory cortex Areas in the temporal lobe, specifically the upper regions of the lateral fissure that separates the temporal from the parietal lobe, where auditory stimuli are represented cortically.

primary circular reaction CIRCULAR REACTION.

primary colour COLOURS, PRIMARY.

primary degenerative dementia DEMENTIA, PRIMARY DEGENERATIVE.

primary drive DRIVE, PRIMARY.

primary emotions EMOTIONS, PRIMARY.

primary factor FACTOR, PRIMARY.

primary gain 1 In psychoanalytic theory, the basic relief from anxiety that results from the initial development of a neurosis. **2** More generally, an initial gain achieved through the development of any disorder. Also called *paranosic gain*. Compare with SECONDARY GAIN and ADVANTAGE BY ILLNESS.

primary group GROUP, PRIMARY.

primary hue UNIQUE *HUES.

primary identification In psychoanalytic theory: **1** The total devotional identification an infant feels with its mother before an awareness of the existence of others develops. **2** More generally, identification with the same-sexed parent.

primary insomnia INSOMNIA, PRIMARY.

primary integration Freud's term for the initial recognition by a child that it is an integrated whole, separate and distinct from the rest of the environment. Piaget used the term SUBJECT–OBJECT DIFFERENTIATION in a similar manner.

primary memory MEMORY, PRIMARY.

primary mental abilities The basic, fundamental mental abilities that have been hypothesized as being the components of intelligence. The term derives from, and tends to be associated closely with, the factor-analytic studies of L. L. Thurstone, which yielded seven such abilities (verbal, word fluency, numerical, space, memory, perceptual and reasoning). abbrev., *PMAs*.

primary motivation Motivation that derives from basic, biological needs and which is assumed to be common to all members of a particular species. See the discussion under MOTIVATION.

primary motor cortex The region of the cortex located on the PRECENTRAL GYRUS. The cortical cells here are the final point for the activation of muscular contractions that control motor functions throughout the body. See MOTOR AREA and HOMUNCULUS (2) for more detail.

primary narcissism NARCISSISM, PRIMARY.

primary need NEED, PRIMARY.

primary object In psychoanalytic theory, the initial or first OBJECT (4) to which an infant relates, usually the mother or the breast.

primary process In psychoanalytic theory, mental functioning operative in the *id*. Primary processes are conceptualized as unconscious, irrational, ignorant of time and space and governed by the pleasure–pain principle. Compare with SECONDARY PROCESS.

primary progressive aphasia APHASIA, PRIMARY PROGRESSIVE.

primary quality PRIMARY AND SECONDARY *QUALITY.

primary reinforcement PRIMARY *REINFORCER.

primary repression REPRESSION (1).

primary sensory cortex A general term for those areas of the cerebral cortex that contain the primary inputs from one of the sensory systems. Typically modifiers are used to reflect the sensory modality under consideration, e.g. primary visual cortex, primary auditory cortex.

primary sex characteristics SEX CHARACTERISTICS, PRIMARY.

primary somatosensory cortex A region of cortex on the POSTCENTRAL GYRUS lying along the anterior PARIETAL LOBE just behind the central sulcus. Cortical cells here are the first stage of processing of tactile information. Input is received from the VENTRO-

POSTERIOR NUCLEUS of the thalamus and projections go to various locations throughout the parietal lobes. See HOMUNCULUS (2) for more detail.

primary tastes See TASTE (2).

primary visual cortex The region of the occipital lobes where the primary visual inputs from the *lateral geniculate nucleus* of the thalamus are represented. It is located on either side of the *calcarine fissure*. Also known as *striate cortex*, it is surrounded by *extrastriate cortex*, where further analysis of basic information is carried out. Primary visual cortex is also referred to as V1. See that term for additional information and for links between V1 and the other visual areas of the brain.

primary zone In psychoanalysis, the zone that provides maximum libidinal satisfaction at each particular stage of psychosexual development.

primate Any member of the Primates, an order of mammals. There are three suborders: Lemuroidea, Tarsioidea and Anthropoidea; the last counts our own species among its members.

prime 1 adj. Primary, in the sense of first in importance or quality. **2** n. A mark (') used to designate a variant of a symbol. **3** n. The fundamental tone, the first partial. **4** n. A prime number. **5** Any event that functions so that the phenomenon of PRIMING occurs. **6** vb. To make ready, to prepare.

priming 1 Generally, the process of presenting an event or episode (the PRIME (5)) that prepares a system for functioning. **2** In animal learning, the presentation of a specific experience that makes an animal more sensitive and/or responsive to a wider range of stimuli. **3** In cognitive psychology, the triggering of specific memories by a specific cue; e.g. *river* will prime one meaning of *bank* while *money* will prime another. Interestingly, this priming can take place outside of consciousness: one can fail to recall or even recognize words previously presented yet respond with them when 'primed' by something, such as the first three letters. See IMPLICIT *MEMORY.

priming, negative The reverse of regular PRIMING (3). Here, one typically finds slower and less accurate responding to an aspect of the stimulus display that the subject was previously told to ignore.

primipara A female who has borne offspring but once.

primitive 1 Loosely, undeveloped. **2** Characterizing or referencing the (theoretical) earliest stages of the development of man. **3** Pertaining to a NONLITERATE people or culture. The first two usages are fairly unambiguous (see PRIMARY); the third is not and fortunately is gradually dropping out of use. The issue here is that there is no reason to suppose, nor is there any evidence to support the view, that people who are primitive in sense 3 are primitive in senses 1 or 2.

primitivization A loose synonym of REGRESSION (1).

primordial PRIMARY.

primordial image UNCONSCIOUS IDEATION.

principal First, leading, of greatest importance. Distinguish from PRINCIPLE.

principal-component analysis A technique in factor analysis whereby a major axis representing a factor is first determined and a second axis that accounts for as much of the remaining variance as possible is located at right angles to it.

principle 1 n. A general, basic maxim; a fundamental truth. **2** n. A generally accepted rule of procedure, particularly scientific procedure. Some fine distinctions are drawn between *principles, canons, rules* and *laws,* the most common being that *law* should be reserved for cases in which uniformity and validity are beyond doubt, while the other terms serve for more problematical cases. In actual usage, the connotations of these terms overlap so much that distinctions often become academic. However, see SCIENTIFIC *LAW.* **3** The active ingredient of a substance. Distinguish from PRINCIPAL.

principle of continuity CONTINUITY, PRINCIPLE OF.

principle of proximity 1 LAW OF *PROXIMITY. **2** MINIMUM-DISTANCE PRINCIPLE.

principles and parameters A class of linguistic models developed in the spirit of GENERATIVE *GRAMMAR and based on the notion that all languages possess fundamental *principles* (e.g. sentences must contain a subject, even it is only implied) and a set of *parameters* that dictate the particular syntactic rules for any given language. The model, due largely to the work of Noam Chomsky and his collaborators, is argued to capture the underlying features of UNIVERSAL *GRAMMAR.

prion diseases Any of several devastating neurological disorders (e.g. CREUTZFELDT–JAKOB DISEASE) caused by self-replicating proteins known as *prions.*

prior entry, law of A generalization, first formulated by E. B. Titchener, that of two simultaneously presented stimuli the one upon which one's attention is focused will be perceived as having occurred first. See PRECEDENCE EFFECT for a similar phenomenon.

prism In optics, a wedge-shaped lens that bends and disperses light in accordance with its wavelength. Note that although the term is specifically optical, any wedge-shaped object may, on occasion, be called a prism; see e.g. HENNING'S PRISM.

prism diopter In optics, the unit of measurement of the strength of a prism given as 100 times the tangent of the angle through which the light is bent.

prisoner's dilemma DILEMMA, PRISONER'S.

prison psychosis GANSER SYNDROME.

private 1 adj. Generally, of an individual, with respect to a person, not shared, personal. **2** adj. Belonging to a single individual, e.g. private property. **3** Internal, subjective.

private acceptance The covert accepting of the opinions or beliefs of others, conforming to the attitudes of others. The term is used so that there is no entailment of behaviour; i.e. one who privately accepts the beliefs of others is not necessarily expected to act upon them. CONVERSION (1) is used synonymously. See CONFORMITY for more on this point. Compare with COMPLIANCE.

private opinion OPINION, PRIVATE.

private speech Synonym of EGOCENTRIC SPEECH.

privation A lack of satisfaction or the means to achieve satisfaction of one's needs. Compare with DEPRIVATION, which is the loss or removal of such means.

-privic A suffix used to denote *privation* or *deficit*; e.g. *glucoprivic* is a state characterized by a deficit of glucose.

privilege Any advantage accruing to some members of a group or society and not to others. In the context of social psychology, the term is restricted to advantages guaranteed by virtue of social status. In psychiatry and clinical psychology, it denotes the legal rights of patients to the confidentiality of what is divulged during therapy; see PRIVILEGED COMMUNICATION.

privileged access A phrase used to characterize the fact that one's own internal, phenomenal experiences are directly available to but one person, oneself.

privileged communication Generally any document, statement or other form of communication that is not open for public inspection. Within the confines of psychotherapeutic proceedings, material that emerges in the course of treatment is generally regarded as such – although the laws pertaining to what can and cannot be divulged in court differ from locale to locale.

pro- Combining form meaning: **1** *In front of, before*. **2** *On account of*. **3** *In favour of*.

proactive Generally, descriptive of any event, stimulus or process that has an effect upon events, stimuli or processes that occur subsequently. See e.g. PROACTIVE *INTERFERENCE. Compare with RETROACTIVE.

proactive inhibition PROACTIVE *INTERFERENCE.

proactive interference INTERFERENCE, PROACTIVE.

probabilism The philosophical perspective that maintains that events may be empirically and rationally predicted but only with some probability, $p < 1.0$. Actually, there are two varieties of this position. One argues that the probabilistic aspect is a result of the complexity of the phenomena under examination and of our current level of ignorance, which force us to be content with probabilistic estimates. The other maintains that the underlying reality is probabilistic in nature. See DETERMINISM for other issues and terms.

probabilistic functionalism A theory of perception and, by extension, a general theory of behaviour, due primarily to Egon Brunswik. The theory stresses that perception is a process of discovering which aspects of the stimulus provide the most useful or functional cues, i.e. those that produce the greatest probability of successfully reacting to the environment. See also ECOLOGICAL VALIDITY.

probability 1 In the simplest, nontechnical sense, the likelihood of an event. Specification of the number that corresponds, more formally, with that likelihood is determined by the ratio of the number of ways that that event can occur to the total number of possible events under consideration. Thus, the probability of any event *A* is a statement of the expectation of the proportional frequency of *A*s observed in the long run. **2** Somewhat more loosely, the state of being probable, of being likely to occur. **3** Shorthand for PROBABILITY THEORY.

probability, conditional The likelihood of an event, *A*, that is dependent upon the occurrence of some other event, *B*, denoted as $p(A|B)$.

probability curve Very generally, any graph of the probabilities of particular outcomes.

probability distribution DISTRIBUTION, PROBABILITY.

probability function Simply, a formal expression that gives the pairing of each event in a particular situation and the probability of its occurrence.

probability, joint The probability of a joint event, i.e. the likelihood that two (or more) events will occur simultaneously.

probability learning LEARNING, PROBABILITY.

probability mass function A graph (or its functional rule) of a discrete random variable with the values it may assume on the x-axis and the probability units on the y-axis.

probability matching In a PROBABILITY *LEARNING experiment, the correspondence between the probabilities, as predicted by the subject, of several events occurring and their actual occurrence. Compare with MAXIMIZING and OVERSHOOTING; see also MATCHING

LAW, a somewhat more ambitious-sounding term used in roughly the same fashion.

probability of response The frequency of occurrence of a particular response (or, more precisely, of the various instances of a *class* of responses) relative to the theoretical maximum frequency of occurrence of that (class of) response(s) under specified conditions. Strictly speaking, the term should be restricted to circumstances in which one knows the number of possible responses, in which the likelihood of each has been empirically determined and in which a mathematically meaningful probability may be calculated, e.g. in a two-alternative, forced-choice recognition experiment. One should, properly, resist the temptation to embellish one's research with bogus quantification by using the term otherwise. Workers in operant conditioning are often guilty of misuse of the term when they refer to the 'probability of a bar press' when what they really mean is the frequency of bar presses relative to some base rate: frequency alone does not a probability make.

probability ratio The ratio of the number of occurrences of an event of a specific class to the total number of occurrences of events in a specified set.

probability sampling SAMPLING, PROBABILITY.

probability space For any given, finite set of events, the specification of the probability of occurrence of each.

probability, subjective A belief about the likelihood of occurrence of some event or about its relative frequency of occurrence. Such beliefs are often not consciously held and people may have considerable difficulty in expressing specific values that reflect them. Nevertheless, people's behaviour often reflects strongly held subjective-probability estimates. See e.g. PROBABILITY *LEARNING.

probability theory The discipline within mathematics that deals with probability. The mathematical foundation of probability theory forms the basis for all the statistical techniques of psychology. Probability theory had its origins in gambling, in which, on the basis of a relatively small number of trials (roulette-wheel spins, dice throws, poker hands),

decisions need to be made about the likelihood of particular events occurring in the long run, given the basic assumption of the uniformity of nature and the mutual cancellation of complementary errors. The logic of modern statistical theory is entirely consonant with this notion: given a relatively small number of observations in an experimental setting, one needs to make decisions about the likelihood of such observations in the long run.

probable error ERROR, PROBABLE.

proband The individual who first comes to the attention of investigators and, because of his or her mental or physical disorder, prompts a detailed study of the genetic-transmission pattern within the family to determine if there is a pattern of disorders that might be genotypic in nature. Also called the *propositus* or the *index case*.

probe 1 vb. To penetrate with intent to explore. **2** n. An instrument or a stimulus used in such a manner. For example, in the so-called *probe technique* for the study of memory, a subject is given a list of stimulus items to memorize followed by a final stimulus, the probe; that is, a list like 7, 1, 6, 9, 5, 4, 8, 3, 5 might be followed by the stimulus 9, and the subject asked to recall the number that immediately preceded or followed 9 in the list.

problem Basically, a situation in which some of the attendant components are known and additional components must be ascertained or determined. Problems are of interest to psychologists when the unknown characteristics which can lead to solution are neither obvious nor easily ascertained. See PROBLEM-SOLVING.

problem behaviour Loosely, behaviour which may lead to psychological problems. Generally included are behaviours that are incomprehensible to others, and those that are antisocial, destructive, disruptive or broadly maladaptive. Distinguish from BEHAVIOUR PROBLEM.

problem box PUZZLE BOX.

problem check-list A self-report personality inventory which contains a list of typical problem situations (e.g. those having to do with money, sex, interpersonal relationships, achievement in school or at work). The subject checks off those that are germane.

problem child Loosely, a child whose behaviour is such that his or her parents, teachers, friends, etc. cannot deal effectively with him or her. Although this definition seems to put the burden on these other persons and not on the child, it really is the only accurate characterization of the situation.

problem finding Basically, discovering that there is a problem. Perhaps not surprisingly, the ability to find a problem is a skill that contributes significantly to acts of creativity and scientific discovery. It has been argued that this skill may be more important than PROBLEM-SOLVING (1), just as asking the right question can be the key to scientific or creative breakthroughs.

problem isomorphs Any group of problems that, despite superficial differences, can be solved using a similar set of operations. For example, the group of puzzles based on the principle that some operation that 'undoes' an earlier move must be used in order to make progress (see TOWER OF HANOI and the HOBBITS AND ORCS, both of which are in this group).

problem-solving 1 The processes involved in the solution of a problem. **2** The area of cognitive psychology that is concerned with these processes. For some examples of classic problems see ANAGRAMS, PUZZLE BOX and WATER-JAR PROBLEM. For some classic issues which emerge in the study of problem-solving, see FUNCTIONAL FIXEDNESS, INSIGHT and TRIAL-AND-ERROR *LEARNING.

problem space The conceptual space that represents all possible paths to solving some problem.

procedural knowledge KNOWLEDGE, PROCEDURAL.

procedural learning LEARNING, PROCEDURAL.

procedural memory MEMORY, PROCEDURAL.

procedural rationality RATIONALITY, PROCEDURAL.

procedural validity VALIDITY, PROCEDURAL.

procedure Generally, any technique for controlling the relevant factors for the purpose of examining some phenomenon. The term is used in a similar fashion to METHOD but with the connotation that a procedure is a concrete manipulation of specific conditions whereas a method generally suggests a broader orientation. For example, the phrase *experimental procedure* refers to the specific techniques used in a specific experiment, while *experimental method* refers to a general class of techniques used in doing experimental work.

proceeding H. Murray's term for any complex unit of psychologically significant behaviour involving interactions between persons and objects.

proceptivity Characterizing overt and active female behaviours that function to arouse a male's sexual interests. Distinguish from RECEPTIVITY (2) where the female role is passive.

process A term with a rather rich variety of meanings in psychology. Note, however, that in spite of the seeming diversity of usage, all derive from the Latin *processus*, meaning *a going forward*, and the underlying connotation is always that of a series of steps or a progression toward some aim or some goal. Hence: **1** Very generally, any change or modification in a thing in which directionality or focus can be discerned. The usual sense here is that the form or structure of an organism or object is relatively static or stable and that any systematic modification in it over time represents some underlying, meaningful process that leads to a different form or structure. *Process* here is regarded as *active, structure* as *passive*. This general meaning is applicable in almost any domain of the social sciences and, as many have argued, psychology is basically a study of processes. **2** The manner in which some change is brought about. The usual reference here is to some set of operations that produces a particular result, e.g. the *learning process*, the *extinction process*, the *therapeutic process*. **3** In cognitive psychology, any operation that is a component of the organizing, coding and interpreting of information. The so-called *cognitive processes* include memory, thinking, interpreting, problem-solving, creativity and the like. See here INFORMATION PROCESSING and related terms. Meanings 1–3 can all be conveyed by the verb *to process*, meaning to engage in or carry out any of the operations described. **4** In physiology, the underlying (causal?) operations of behaviour. The implication here is the indisputable fact that some physiological or biological *process* underlies all observed behaviour. **5** In anatomy, any slender extension or projection from an organ or cell; axons and dendrites are processes, for example. **6** In Titchener's structuralism, a conscious content without reference to its meaning, value or context.

process dissociation procedure A method used in the study of IMPLICIT *MEMORY developed by Jacoby. In the canonical experiment, participants first learn a list of words. Later they are asked to complete a series of stem completions (e.g. fill in the blank with the first word that comes to mind: MOT——) but never to use a word from the list. The standard finding is that subjects cannot help using words from the list even though they cannot consciously recall having seen them. The method, in principle, shows the dissociation between implicit and explicit memories.

processing error Any error introduced during the processing (i.e. analysing, organizing, reporting, etc.) of the data from an experiment.

processing fluency FLUENCY.

processing, parallel Information processing in which more than one sequence of processing operations is carried out simultaneously (i.e. in parallel). The processing may involve extremely low-level, non-symbolic components such as those used in the PARALLEL DISTRIBUTED PROCESSING MODELS and NETWORK MODELS (2), or it may be based on higher-level elements such as those used in retrieval of information about words, in which meaning, spelling, pronunciation and role in syntax are all accessed at virtually the same time. Compare with SEQUENTIAL *PROCESSING.

processing, sequential Information processing in which complex stimulus inputs are processed by the manipulation of pieces of information in series (i.e. sequentially). Most consciously controlled information processing is sequential in nature. As a simple demonstration, try attending to two conversations at the same time: the only way you will manage will be by shifting your atten-

tion rapidly back and forth so that the multiple processing is not really carried out at the same time but rather in a sequence of shifts of attention. Also called *serial processing*. Compare with PARALLEL *PROCESSING.

process observer In the study of groups, an individual who oversees, monitors and comments on the functioning of the group. The observer may be a member of the group or an outsider brought in for this express purpose.

process research Loosely, research into processing. However, the term is used almost exclusively to refer to psychotherapeutic processes and studies the factors, procedures, mechanisms and techniques used in therapy to ascertain their effectiveness.

process schizophrenia SCHIZOPHRENIA, PROCESS.

process study See PROCESS RESEARCH.

prochlorperazine A mild PHENOTHIAZINE introduced as an ANTIPSYCHOTIC DRUG but now used primarily for treatment of nausea.

procyclidine An ANTICHOLINERGIC DRUG used in the treatment of PARKINSON'S DISEASE.

prodigy From the Latin *prodigium*, meaning a *prophetic sign*. As such, its original meaning was as a reference to something extraordinary, something so unusual that it seemed to be an omen of things to come. Contemporary usage has narrowed the reference to a person with some extraordinary talent or power, specifically when this emerges at an early age. It's worth pointing out that children so labelled do not always (or even often) become extraordinary or especially gifted adults. What marks the child prodigy are rapid and efficient learning abilities which, while important, are not sufficient for innovation, artistic development, scientific discovery or other hallmarks of creative adults.

prodromal Pertaining to the earliest stages of an illness, the period between the occurrence of the very first symptom and the full manifestation of the disorder. n., *prodrome* = a premonitory symptom.

prodrop language A language which allows the pronoun form of a sentence's subject to be dropped, at least in written language. Italian, Spanish, Japanese and Welsh are all prodrop languages; English is not.

production In psycholinguistics, actual verbal output. A child's language-production capabilities are often compared with its *comprehension* of language, with the suggestion that the latter typically precedes the former.

production method A general label for any of several kinds of experimental procedure in which the subject is required to produce a response relative to a particular stimulus. The most common use is in psychophysical scaling, when the subject adjusts a stimulus to correspond to some value, e.g. adjusts a light so it is half as bright as a standard light. See METHODS OF *SCALING.

production systems A class of theoretical models of cognitive functioning based on the assumption that much of human thought is captured by a set of general 'if–then' rules. The classic model has a component that specifies the 'if–then' (or 'production') rules for a given setting, a working memory that holds relevant information about the situation and a control system that takes the information from working memory and 'recycles' it back to the production component. Production systems have been effective in modelling human activity in several problem-solving situations and can learn to play games like noughts and crosses (0s and Xs).

productiveness 1 PRODUCTIVITY, in the sense of the industrial psychologist. **2** A characteristic of behaviour that serves to increase the development and well-being of an individual and the groups of which he or she is a part. This latter meaning is quite general and encompasses creativity and originality as well as simple output.

productive vocabulary ACTIVE *VOCABULARY.

productivity 1 In industrial psychology, a measure of the effective output of some system. The system here may be an individual worker, a unit in a business or factory, an entire organization, etc. **2** In academia the term carries the additional connotation of originality or creativity. **3** The property of all natural languages that an unlimited number of distinct sentences can be generated by novel combinations of words.

product-moment correlation CORRELATION, PRODUCT-MOMENT.

profession Any occupation that requires a high degree of skill and extensive specialized training for the purpose of performing a specialized societal role. Professions tend to have their own codes of ethics and conduct within their practice and, owing to the high degree of specialization and the monopoly of knowledge and skills, they tend to be highly resistant to control or 'interference' in their affairs by outside groups.

professional manager In industrial and organizational psychology, one who is specifically trained for a managerial position, as distinguished from an owner–manager.

profile 1 A drawn or sketched outline of a thing. **2** A graphic display of a set of scores, usually in the form of a *histogram* or *bar graph*. **3** A PROFILE ANALYSIS.

profile analysis 1 A general presentation of an individual's personality traits and characteristics as displayed relative to a set of norms for the population as a whole. The analysis may take the form of a literal PROFILE (2), in which the data are presented in graphic form (educational profiles of students often use this method), or it may be a more general metaphoric profile in the sense of a general overview of the individual's characteristics or traits presented in summary form. **2** Any statistical analysis of the scores of one or more samples on multiple measures with the goal of determining whether scores vary across measures or whether the pattern of scores differs across groups.

profile-matching system A system of selecting personnel in which the profiles of each job candidate, including all of the variables deemed important for the position, are compared with the profiles of successful workers and personnel decisions are made on the basis of the closeness of the match.

profound mental retardation MENTAL RETARDATION, PROFOUND.

progeria (adultorum) WERNER'S DISEASE.

progesterone A hormone produced by the corpus luteum following ovulation and, during pregnancy, by the placenta. See also MENSTRUAL CYCLE.

progestin 1 A synthetic hormone with progesterone-like effects. **2** In older writings, PROGESTERONE.

prognathy An anatomical arrangement in which the jaw projects out in front of the cranium. Compare with ORTHOGNATHY.

prognosis 1 Specifically, the predicted (in the sense of the best-educated guess) eventual outcome of a disease or other disorder. **2** More generally, a prediction of the course and outcome of any process, be it educational, industrial, methodological, programmatic, etc. Tests designed to collect data for such projections are called *prognostic tests.*

prognostic test See PROGNOSIS.

program PROGRAMME.

programme 1 An extended plan of research. The term is used in this sense for the research of anything from a single individual to a whole institution and even to the abstract notion of the research activity of an entire field or discipline. **2** In genetics, the set of instructions coded in the DNA molecules. **3** A set of instructions to a computer for the purpose of having it perform specified operations. var., *program.*

programme assessment The application of social science research tools to assessing the extent to which a social, educational or behavioural programme is fulfilling its original aims and, by extension, whether it should be ended or continued, cut back or expanded, modified or maintained. The term is used in similar ways to OUTCOMES ASSESSMENT.

programmed instruction (or **learning**) A generic term covering the use of any machine or other device as a technological aid to learning. See PROGRAMMED TEXT and COMPUTER-ASSISTED INSTRUCTION.

programmed text Any text that presents the material to be learned in a series of small, graded steps.

programming In computer terminology, the operation of preparing the set of instructions for a computer to carry out a specific function or solve some problem.

progression 1 In mathematics, a series in which each item is related to the preceding by some specifiable constant relation. For example, 1, 4, 7, 10, 13…is an *arithmetic* progression derived by adding a constant; 1, 2, 4, 8, 16, 32…is a *geometric* progression derived

by multiplying by a constant. **2** Any advance or movement forwards. Used here to refer to simple locomotion (walking, running) as well as to more abstract forms, such as the *progression of knowledge* or *ideas.*

progressive 1 adj. Moving forwards, advancing. **2** adj. Pertaining to progress. **3** In medicine, characterizing the progression of a disease or disorder. Note that 1 and 2 both carry generally sanguine connotations while 3 carries a distinctly negative sense.

progressive education A general orientation toward educational theory and practice that derives primarily from the theories of John Dewey. The core of Dewey's thinking in philosophy, psychology and education stressed flexibility, function, holism and pragmatism, and, not surprisingly, the educational programme he espoused revolved round these principles. Most progressive education programmes (e.g. A. S. Neill's Summerhill) focus on the individual student and his or her intrinsic interests and needs, skills and desires. They reflect a generally experimental attitude, a corresponding vigorous denial of the values of dogmatism and a pragmatic ethic in which education is tied to functioning in the real world.

Progressive Matrices Test Any of several PERFORMANCE TESTS in which one is asked to complete a pattern by selecting the missing element from a set of alternatives. There are three different forms, each designed for use with a different population. The *Coloured Progressive Matrices* is for young children and individuals with special educational needs, the *Standard* form is for most others and the *Advanced* form is designed for above-average adolescents and adults. They are all called 'progressive' because each set of items becomes progressively more difficult. Also called *Raven's Progressive Matrices Tests* for their initial developer.

progressive-relaxation therapy RELAXATION THERAPY.

progressive supranuclear palsy A degenerative neural disease with Parkinsonian features (see PARKINSON-PLUS SYNDROMES), dementia and loss of volitional eye movements. Affected cortical pathways include the periaqueductal grey, the superior colliculus and various subthalamic nuclei, among others. Prognosis is poor, death usually occurring within 7 years of initial diagnosis.

progressive teleological-regression hypothesis A theory of schizophrenia that maintains that the disorder results from a process of active concretization, i.e. a purposeful returning to lower levels of psychodynamic and behavioural adaptation, which, while it may prove momentarily effective in reducing anxiety, tends ultimately toward repetitive behaviours and results in a failure to maintain integration. The term is Silvano Arieti's and was chosen because the disorder itself is viewed as *progressive*, the direction is *regressive* and the regression itself appears to function as though it had a purpose, i.e. it is *teleological*.

projection Standard dictionary definitions here all carry the basic idea of a jutting out or protruding; technical uses also reflect this notion but with the understanding that, in many uses, the projecting may be abstract and/or symbolic. To wit: **1** In classical psychoanalysis, the process by which one ascribes one's own traits, emotions, dispositions, etc. to another. Typically used here with the implication that there is an accompanying denial that one has these feelings or tendencies, that the projection functions as a defence mechanism to protect oneself from anxiety and that some underlying conflict has been repressed. **2** In other psychodynamic theories, the process of ascribing unwittingly one's beliefs, values or other subjective processes to others. This usage, which is typical of the Kleinian approach, has a different connotation. Here, the process is viewed as a normal aspect of psychological development and not necessarily reflective of neurotic tendencies. **3** The perceiving of events and environmental stimuli (particularly ambiguous ones) in terms of one's own expectations, needs, desires, etc. This meaning is completely neutral with regard to the issue of the pathological aspect of projection. Rather, it is accepted as axiomatic of the operation of the process itself and, hence, forms the theoretical basis for the use of PROJECTIVE TECHNIQUES. **4** The attribution of one's own faults and shortcomings to another. This sense of the term is the one generally assumed in everyday speech and is not technically correct, because of the limitation to faults and shortcomings, which is but one component of the technical meanings. In anatomy and physiology: **5** Any anatomical or neurological protuberance. **6** The efferent connection between the neurons in one specific cortical region and those in another. **7** The spreading out of the sensory fibres through the cerebral cortex after emerging from the spinal cord. The spatially separate areas in the cortex where the neural representations are mapped are called *projection areas*. **8** In factor analysis: the mapping or plotting of the factor loadings onto some surface, usually a sphere. **9** In perception and related areas of study, there are several distinct uses. See OPTICAL *PROJECTION, RETINAL *PROJECTION and VISUAL *PROJECTION.

projection areas PROJECTION (6, 7).

projection, optical **1** A point-by-point PROJECTION (9) of the information in a distal display onto the retina. **2** The functions of slide projectors.

projection, retinal A point-by-point PROJECTION (9) of visual information encoded in the retina to V1, the primary visual cortex. See RETINOTOPIC REPRESENTATION for additional detail.

projection, visual A term with a host of ambiguous and occasionally conflicting uses. It can be found used as a synonym of both OPTICAL *PROJECTION and RETINAL *PROJECTION.

projective device PROJECTIVE TECHNIQUE.

projective identification Similar to PROJECTION (1–3), but with a twist: the individual does not fully disavow what is projected. Instead, the person remains aware of his or her own feelings or impulses, but misattributes them and regards them as being justifiable reactions to the behaviour of the other persons involved.

projective play A general label for any of several projective techniques utilizing a play situation with children. With all such techniques, the assumption is that a child's repressed feelings, conflicts, attitudes, etc. will emerge in an unstructured situation. The most commonly used techniques revolve round dolls, houses and interpersonal interactions. See also PLAY THERAPY.

projective technique A cover term for any test, device or set of procedures designed to provide information about or insight into an individual's personality by allowing him or her the opportunity to respond in an unrestricted manner to unstructured or ambiguous objects or situations. As the name suggests, all of these procedures are based upon the general sense of PROJECTION, as captured by meanings 1, 2 and/or 3. Very roughly, one can identify four types of techniques here: (a) Those based on the assumption that there are deeply repressed, unconscious factors underlying personality which can be revealed through projection onto highly ambiguous stimuli. The prototype here, of course, is the RORSCHACH TEST. (b) Those based on the assumption that underlying patterns of needs are revealed by interpretations of stories or pictures. Murray's THEMATIC APPERCEPTION TEST (TAT) is the best known of these. Note that, as Murray characterized the TAT, it was not designed to probe the deep unconscious like the Rorschach but rather to provide a forum in which the needs, desires, beliefs and attitudes that are part of an individual's psychosocial make-up can be revealed. These need patterns may even be consciously known by the person, but without the ambiguity of the projective device they may never be articulated. (c) Those procedures based on the assumption that some ego defence, either momentary or firmly established, is blocking awareness and a projective procedure is needed to circumvent it. Projective-play techniques, picture-completion tests and the like are examples. (d) Those procedures used with children (or individuals with compromised cognitive or language functions) on the assumption that their poorly developed linguistic abilities prevent them from being able to verbalize conflicts or emotional disturbances. In this category are play techniques, puppet enactments and the like.

Note that there is vigorous debate over the use of projective techniques in all their forms. The points of contention range from the scientific issues of whether they have the reliability and validity required of psychological assessment devices, to the pragmatic issue of whether they are worth the time and expense when other, more objective, procedures exist, and the political/ethical question of whether they violate basic civil liberties and the right to privacy. (The last issue, of course, is only germane if the first two are

decided in the affirmative.) Also called *projective device*.

projective test A label for any of a variety of devices used in personality assessment and clinical psychology whereby an individual is presented with a standardized, unstructured set of stimuli and requested to respond to them in as unrestricted a manner as possible. Note, some authors use the term only to refer to a PROJECTIVE TECHNIQUE that has been standardized (e.g. the Rorschach *test*. the Thematic Apperception *Test*); others have abandoned it entirely on the grounds that the devices are not really tests since they do not provide *scores* and there is doubt about what they *measure*, and instead use the generic terms *projective technique* and *projective device*.

prolactin A hormone secreted by the anterior pituitary gland responsible for the onset and maintenance of lactation in mammals after the birth of young. Also called *lactogenic* or *luteotropic hormone*.

proliferation The root meaning is biological and relates to growth by cell division. However, its connotations have been extended to cover any rapid growth, e.g. of people, ideas, theories and, obviously, technical terms.

prolonged withdrawal syndrome WITHDRAWAL SYNDROME, PROLONGED.

promiscuous 1 Characterized by a rather jumbled, haphazard heterogeneity. **2** Lacking discrimination or selectivity, casual. From these original meanings we have ended up with the now dominant: **3** Unselective and haphazard sexuality.

promise A SPEECH ACT in which the speaker is understood to commit him- or herself to something. Promises are COMMISSIVES and are generally more cognitively complex and learned later by children than some other speech acts, such as DIRECTIVES.

prompt A hint, suggestion or act of help; the act of presenting such. Often used in experiments on memory, particularly as a measure of the degree of learning of verbal materials. For example, the fewer the prompts necessary during recall the better the learning of the material can be assumed to have been.

prompting method ANTICIPATION METHOD (2).

pronation 1 Lying face downward. **2** Turning one's arm so that the palm faces down. Opposite of SUPINATION.

pronomenalization A linguistic procedure whereby condensation of a message is achieved by substituting a simple expression (like a pronoun) for a more complex and longer one (like a full noun phrase).

pronoun A nominal form that can take the place of a noun. Once their reference is clear (see PRONOMENALIZATION), pronouns share the same privileges of occurrence in linguistic messages as nouns. How the young child learns this is a much-researched problem.

proof 1 Within a formal system, a proof of a conclusion, *C*, is a sequence of well-formed propositions, *P*, such that each follows from the initial set of axioms and preceding *P*s according to proper rules of inference and culminates in *P* = *C*. **2** Somewhat more loosely, any conclusionary proposition derived validly from true premises. **3** Even more loosely, any demonstration that provides logical or evidential support for a belief.

Properly, proof needs to be treated in several distinct fashions. Specifically, meanings 1 and 2 need to be distinguished from 3. Within axiomatic systems, proof amounts to a formal demonstration that a proposition follows inferentially and deductively. That is, one can, in Euclidean geometry, *prove* propositions concerning points, lines and spaces; within a system like general relativity theory, one can *prove* propositions concerning the bending of light in the neighborhood of large masses; and, within connectionist theory, one can *prove* that a system will establish particular representations given appropriate stimulus inputs. But *proof* here is no more than a statement that, *within the system*, the syntax of the sentence that forms the conclusion is proper and follows from premises. That is, it is proof in senses 1 and 2.

Sense 3 has different and problematical connotations; it extends the domain of the term into the realm of data and theory. It invites one to take, for example, Euclid's geometry as *proven* if it describes the three-dimensional world of our senses, relativity theory as *proven* if light bends while passing a star, or connectionism as *proven* if people form the same kinds of representations as the model. That is, all appear as evidential support for a belief about nature. Clearly, this kind of proof is a rather different kind of thing from that in senses 1 and 2 – so much so that in the technical literature meaning 3 is typically not found. Proof is properly dealt with here from the point of view of the failure of attempts at disproof; see here FALSIFICATIONISM.

proof-reader's illusion There is some confusion here because the term is used in two slightly different ways, neither of which is really representative of an illusion: **1** The failure to notice that written material does not make sense because one is doing low-level proof-reading, i.e. looking for typographical errors, misspellings, etc. **2** The failure to notice a low-level error in written material because one is concentrating on higher-level processing, i.e. comprehension, understanding, etc. The latter is the more common meaning.

propaedeutic Pertaining to or having the characteristic of being preliminary.

propaedeutic task 1 Specifically, a task or teaching aid used in the instruction of the retarded or the handicapped. Such tasks involve instruction in things that are preliminary to and necessary for future instruction. **2** More generally, any task that is designed to impart preliminary knowledge, e.g. memorizing the alphabet in order to read English.

propaganda Most broadly, a generic term covering any attempt to manipulate opinion. In practice, social psychologists find it useful to impose some conditions on the use of the term. Specifically, a message is regarded as propaganda only if it (a) represents a conscious, systematic and organized effort, (b) conceals the true nature of the debate by presenting only one side of the issues, and (c) is characterized by an attempt to disguise the fact that it is, indeed, propaganda. vb., *propagandize*.

propagation 1 Generally, reproduction. **2** The transmission of a neural impulse down the axon of a neuron. See ACTION POTENTIAL. **3** The dissemination or spreading of information, particularly through a group or society. Distinguish this last sense from PROPAGANDA.

propanediols A group of ANTIANXIETY drugs that depress the central nervous system and produce muscle relaxation (e.g. MEPROBA-MATE). They have been largely replaced by the BENZODIAZEPINES, which are less toxic and have fewer side effects.

propensity Any strong, persistent tendency for action. It is used broadly, and terms like DRIVE and DISPOSITION (2, 3) are rough synonyms. Note that some use the term with the clear implication that a propensity is innate; others are neutral on this issue.

prophetic dream Any dream that seems to contain elements about future events. Among all the frivolous claims made in PARA-PSYCHOLOGY, this is the most common. Also called *premonitory dream*.

prophylactic **1** n. Any measure or device that produces PROPHYLAXIS. **2** adj. Characterizing such a device or measure.

prophylaxis Generally, the use of any preventive measure. Specifically, the use of measures designed to prevent disease.

propinquity Latin for 'nearness' and used in both the geographic and social senses. People who are highly likely to meet and interact are said to be of high propinquity and, not surprisingly, it is a strong factor in the formation of interpersonal attraction. See also MERE EXPOSURE.

proportion **1** A ratio of magnitudes, either of one part to another or of a single part to the whole. Note that in the latter case the proportion can be expressed as a percentage. **2** In aesthetics, a pleasant balance between the parts of something.

proposition **1** Generally and inclusively, whatever can be stated, asserted, contended, supposed, presupposed, derived, negated or implied. That is, whatever can be expressed in the standard form of an indicative sentence. Various types of proposition are distinguished: **2** A *formal* proposition is a statement that relates objects, events and properties (or their symbolic representations) to each other in well-defined ways. Such propositions are ultimately neither true nor false: their truth value consists in their conforming to the principles of logic. The formal proposition 'Apples are red' is deductively true or false depending upon preceding propositions regarding apples, colour, perceptual principles, etc. **3** An *empirical* proposition is a statement of a similar kind but the elements consist of observable objects, events or operations (or their symbolic representations) and it can be tested empirically for its truth. The empirical proposition 'Apples are red' is demonstrably true or false based upon observations of apples and determination of their colour. **4** A *linguistic* proposition is a formal statement that represents a component of the underlying meaning of a sentence. Here, the sentence 'Apples are red' would be represented as (apple, all, red). The notion of truth here is irrelevant; the concern is with whether or not the proposition provides an accurate characterization of the underlying meaning of the sentence being analysed.

propositional attitudes Those particular stances that people take toward propositions, e.g. they may *believe* that a proposition is true, *wish* that it be true, *doubt* that it is true.

propositional content In linguistics, the full set of PROPOSITIONS (4) expressed by a sentence, paragraph or extended discourse.

propositus PROBAND.

propranolol A BETA BLOCKER that, in low doses, has found use in treating social phobias owing to its ability to diminish peripheral symptoms such as hand tremors and a quaking voice.

propriate functional autonomy Gordon Allport's term for a level of FUNCTIONAL *AUTONOMY which included personal interests, values, lifestyle, etc. Such behaviours are assumed to be learned and largely internally motivated. Compare with PERSEVERATIVE FUNCTIONAL AUTONOMY.

propriate strivings PROPRIUM.

proprio- Combining form meaning *one's own*.

proprioception The sense of the location, position, orientation and movement of one's body and parts thereof. One of the INTEROCEP-TORS, the system is based on one group of proprioceptors in the muscles, tendons and joints of the body (see KINAESTHESIS) and another group in the VESTIBULAR APPARATUS of the inner ear (see EQUILIBRIUM (2)).

proprioceptor Any of the sensory receptors that mediate PROPRIOCEPTION.

proprium A term coined by Gordon Allport to cover the full range of acquired functions that comprise the various elements of selfhood. Seven aspects of the proprium were hypothesized, from the sense of bodily self that appears in childhood to the sense of self as a reasoning, cognitive person capable of handling distant goals that emerges during adolescence. Other components dealt with self-image, self-identity, self-esteem, characteristic patterns of thought, cognitive style, etc. The term itself was chosen in an attempt to clarify some of the issues which had become muddled through the repeated reusing of terms like *self* and *ego*. See SELF (esp. 1, 2 and 5) to appreciate what these conceptual problems are.

prosaccade SACCADE.

prosencephalon The embryonic FOREBRAIN.

proso- Combining form meaning *forward*, *anterior*.

prosocial A general descriptive label for those social behaviours that are cooperative in nature. Usually included are friendship, empathy, altruism, helping behaviour, etc. ants., ANTISOCIAL, ASOCIAL.

prosocial aggression AGGRESSION, PROSOCIAL.

prosodic features Features of language such as stress, pitch, pitch changes, intonation, juncture and pausing. Prosodic features are generally treated as distinct from the SUPRASEGMENTALS in that they are not typically phonemic; that is, they serve to mark function or intention rather than to distinguish meaning. Specific examples of prosodic features are rising intonation contour, which generally cues a question; strong sharp stress, which can convey anger or an order; high pitch, which may signal insecurity or anxiety, etc. Note that some of these prosodic features may also be regarded as phonemic in some situations. See, for example, CONTENT.

prosody 1 All those aspects of language related to the use of PROSODIC FEATURES. **2** All those aspects of language related to the use of the prosodic features and the SUPRASEGMENTALS. Meaning 1 is preferred.

prosopagnosia A neurological disorder characterized by an inability to recognize faces (*prosopon* means 'face'). In serious cases it may include a failure to recognize one's own face. In most cases, discrimination of gender, race, age and emotional expression is preserved and, interestingly, IMPLICIT *MEMORY and IMPLICIT *LEARNING involving faces are normal. The disorder is associated with lesions in the inferior temporal lobe, usually bilateral, although cases in which the damage is restricted to the right hemisphere exist. Distinguish from FACE BLINDNESS, which has similar features.

prospective memory MEMORY, PROSPECTIVE.

prospective sampling SAMPLING, PROSPECTIVE.

prospect theory An influential theory of decision-making developed by Daniel Kahneman and Amos Tversky based on a complex set of relationships between risk and uncertainty, loss and gain and the psychological perspective that people have with regard to particular outcomes. The theory is grounded on the principle of RISK AVERSION and assumes that people are more motivated to avoid losses than to seek equivalent gains. The position has had a significant impact on psychology, economics and related disciplines and forced a rethinking of classic theory based on RATIONAL-ECONOMIC MAN.

prostaglandin A hormone first discovered in the prostate (hence the name). It sensitizes free nerve endings to histamine, thereby playing a role in pain perception. Aspirin's analgesic effects come from its ability to interfere with the production of prostaglandin.

prosthesis Any artificial device used in addition to or in place of a dysfunctional or missing body part.

protanomaly A visual condition in which there is a minor diminution in sensitivity to long-wavelength light. See also PROTANOPIA.

protanopia A form of DICHROMACY characterized by a lowered sensitivity to long-wavelength light. The Greek prefix *proto-*, meaning *first*, is applied to this condition because this form of colour-deficient vision is assumed to be due to a deficiency in the red-light-absorbing pigment in the retina, and red is considered to be the first primary colour. Compare with DEUTERANOPIA.

protected relationships Those professional relationships that enjoy certain legal protections concerning the confidentiality of records, statements or other information. Physician–patient, psychotherapist–client, lawyer–defendant are all relationships considered protected in this manner.

protective reflex Any reflex that evolved as a protective mechanism, e.g. limb withdrawal to heat, eye blink to a puff of air.

protein Any long-chain polymer of AMINO ACIDS. Proteins are integral components of the protoplasm of every cell, provide the amino acids that an organism cannot produce by itself and are an essential part of nutrition. The term 'complete protein' is used for those that contain all the essential amino acids needed for growth, maintenance and repair of bodily tissue.

protein kinase M zeta PKMζ.

protensity An archaic term used by Titchener to refer to the direct experience of the duration of sensation.

prothetic The basic meaning of the word connotes the addition of a thing without a change in the qualitative aspects of that to which it is added. It is used to characterize stimulus dimensions that do not change qualitatively with changes in physical intensity. For example, *weight* is prothetic because systematic increases in mass produce systematic increases in perceived heaviness; likewise for the loudness of sounds, brightness of lights, etc. Compare with METATHETIC continua, such as the wavelength of light or the concentration of some odours. By and large, prothetic continua produce *power functions* when scaled, metathetic continua do not.

proto- A common prefix from the Greek, meaning *first, original, primary, primitive*.

protocol 1 The original record of an experiment or other investigation made during or immediately after the event. **2** A set of procedures for carrying out formal arrangements, treaties or agreements. **3** A plan for a research study.

protoconcept A primitive CONCEPT (2),

such as displayed by infants and nonhuman animals.

protopathic 1 Generally, primitive and undifferentiating. Used most commonly with respect to cutaneous sensitivity. **2** See discussion under EPICRITIC (2).

proto-tool use TOOL USE.

prototype 1 The original, primitive type or form of a thing. **2** The most typical of a class or category of things. Note that a prototype, in this sense, is regarded as an abstraction based on shared features or functions of the members of a class or category. It is not treated as necessarily represented by any one instance. For example, a robin is regarded by most people as a more typical bird than, say, a chicken or a penguin; in fact many regard a robin as more bird-like than any other bird. This, however, does not mean that the robin is the prototype of the category *bird*; only that it is closer to the abstract, prototypical bird. This notion of a prototype plays an important role in many theories of memory and thinking; see e.g. CATEGORY, CONCEPT, NATURAL *CATEGORY.

Proustian memory MEMORY, PROUSTIAN.

pro-verb In linguistics, a verbal form which, once the reference is clear, can be used in place of a full verb phrase; e.g. *do so*.

proxemics The study of space and its use in different social and cultural situations. Major areas of interest include CROWDING, TERRITORIALITY and PERSONAL SPACE.

proximal From the Latin, meaning *near to, close*. Hence: **1** In anatomy, referring to points near the centre of the body, the centre of an organ or the point of attachment of an organ or other structure. **2** Touching or contiguous. Compare with DISTAL.

proximal response Any direct internal response, e.g. one that is muscular or glandular.

proximal stimulus The physical energy that actually impinges upon a receptor. The dog that just walked into the room is the DISTAL STIMULUS, the pattern of light reflected off the dog that stimulates your retina is the proximal stimulus.

proximate explanation In evolutionary biology an explanation of a species' behaviour in terms of the mechanisms and immediate circumstances that bring on that behaviour; e.g. explaining the mating behaviour of a male elephant seal by focusing on shifts in temperature that stimulate increased production of testosterone which in turn stimulates particular brain centres, etc. The focus is on environmental stimuli and physiological mechanisms. Compare with ULTIMATE EXPLANATION.

proximity, law of GESTALT LAWS OF ORGANIZATION.

proximodistad (or **proximodistal**) **development** CEPHALOCAUDAD DEVELOPMENT.

proxy variable VARIABLE, PROXY.

Prozac FLUOXETINE.

PRP PSYCHOLOGICAL *REFRACTORY PERIOD.

pruning The process by which the numbers of neurons and neural connections in the brain are reduced. The term is reserved for normal processes such as the *neural* pruning that occurs during development and the *synaptic* pruning that occurs as performance becomes efficient.

pseudaesthesia Generally, any sensory illusion. The term is usually used of illusions of location of stimulation, e.g. PHANTOM LIMB var., *pseudesthesia*.

pseud(o)- A prefix denoting *false, fake, counterfeit*. The connotation is that the 'pseudo' event or object is a copy of the real one.

pseudoangina A functional chest pain that resembles a heart attack.

pseudochromaesthesia An unnecessarily long synonym for CHROMAESTHESIA var., *pseudochromesthesia*.

pseudoconditioning An increase in the frequency of occurrence of a response to a stimulus which has not been systematically paired with an unconditioned stimulus. Pseudoconditioning can be observed most clearly just after a series of true conditioning trials have been run, when the subject will produce the 'conditioned' response to some neutral stimulus. It is presumably due to *sensitization* of the subject.

pseudocyesis False pregnancy. This can be a most compelling functional syndrome that

may include abdominal swelling and cessation of the menses.

pseudodementia A temporary drop in performance of intellectual functioning brought about by emotional conditions. It is observed in cases of depression and is usually temporary.

pseudohermaphroditism A congenital abnormality where the genitalia of one sex are present but with ambiguous morphology. In the most common cases the external genitals are present but compromised. Females may be masculinized with a large clitoris or labia that resemble a scrotum; males feminized with a small penis and a lack of testes. Occasionally cases occur with normal appearing external genitalia but internal structures of the other sex.

pseudoinsomnia Not a true INSOMNIA, but a condition in which an individual wakes up several times or dreams that he or she is lying in bed awake. Despite actually having a normal number of hours of sleep, the person wakes up thinking he or she has spent a sleepless night.

pseudoisochromatic charts A general term for any of several coloured plates designed to test colour vision. See e.g. ISHIHARI COLOUR PLATES.

pseudolalia Nonsensical babbling.

pseudomemory Lit., any false memory; see PARAMNESIA.

pseudomnesia A term occasionally used for a PSEUDOMEMORY that is severe or pathological.

pseudoneurological Characterizing symptoms of a neurological disorder with no known underlying pathology. Seen often in SOMATIZATION DISORDER.

pseudoneurotic schizophrenia SCHIZOTYPAL PERSONALITY DISORDER.

pseudoparkinsonism DRUG-INDUCED *PARKINSONISM.

pseudophone A device which transposes the spatial location of sounds so that those that would normally enter the right ear enter the left ear and vice versa. It was developed to study the process of sound localization.

pseudopsychology Lit., fake or false psychology. The term has two common uses: **1** As a label for those unscientific endeavours that are clearly fraudulent and the practitioners of which are obvious quacks, e.g. graphology, palmistry, phrenology. **2** As a characterization of the endeavours of one's scientific foes who insist on adhering to theoretical points of view that one knows are clearly unscientific. Everything from psychoanalysis to behaviourism to parapsychology has been called a pseudopsychology at one time or another. See PSEUDOSCIENCE.

pseudopsychopathic schizophrenia SCHIZOPHRENIA, PSEUDOPSYCHOPATHIC.

pseudopsychopathy ACQUIRED SOCIOPATHY.

pseudopsychosis FACTITIOUS DISORDER WITH PSYCHOLOGICAL SYMPTOMS.

pseudorandom numbers See RANDOM NUMBER GENERATOR.

pseudoretardation A syndrome often seen in intrinsically normal but culturally or socially deprived children who, because of a lack of stimulation, socialization or parenting, or through some emotional disturbance, show up initially as retarded on standard intelligence tests.

pseudoscience Generally, the improper use of the scientific method, a fake or false science. Most pseudoscience has the superficial trappings of real science but is contaminated by such factors as poor control over experimental conditions, improper analysis of data, illogical deductive reasoning and, occasionally, outright fraud.

pseudoscope An optical device that transposes the images to the two eyes such that light that would otherwise fall on the right retina falls on the left and vice versa. Depth relations are reversed in scenes viewed through one. Distinguish from REVERSING LENSES.

pseudosenility A reversible decline in cognitive functioning in the elderly that frequently accompanies stressful situations such as falls, surgery, malnutrition, depression or metabolic disorders.

psi (ψ) A Greek letter. When the letter itself is used it serves as an abbreviation for *psychology*; when spelled out in English it refers to the parapsychologist's *psi processes*.

psilocybin A hallucinogen extracted from a Mexican mushroom. It has actions similar to those of LSD and shows CROSS *TOLERANCE with that drug.

psi-missing In parapsychology, a situation in which a paranormal 'process' seems to be working in a negative 'fashion; e.g. rather than being able to predict the turn of a card with greater-than-chance probability, the subject makes many more errors than predicting with chance probability would produce. See PARAPSYCHOLOGY for a discussion of the general issue of such presumed phenomena.

psi process A general term of any individual paranormal ability, e.g. telepathy. See PARAPSYCHOLOGY for a discussion. Also called, simply, *psi*.

PSP POSTSYNAPTIC POTENTIAL.

psychalgia A cover term for disorders the dominant symptoms of which are pains of a mental origin, most commonly headaches or backaches, not due to any other psychiatric disorder and with no detectable organic dysfunctions.

psychasthenia Pierre Janet's term for a disorder characterized by anxiety, obsessions and fixed ideas.

psyche 1 The oldest and most general use of this term is by the early Greeks, who envisaged the psyche as the soul or the very essence of life. **2** More conventionally, the connotation is limited to *mind*. Although both of these meanings reflect a kind of DUALISM, 2 is considerably less problematical and is favoured over 1. It also carries the sense of the original meaning of *psychology*. **3** The SELF. adjs., PSYCHIC (1 or 3), *psychical*.

psychedelic An invented term constructed by combining the Greek words *psyche*, meaning *mind*, and *delos*, meaning *manifest* or *visible*; hence, *mind-manifesting*. It is used to distinguish the group of hallucinogenic drugs the dominant effects of which are specific and reliable changes in mood, perception and judgement from others that have hallucinogenic side effects independent of their primary use. Thus, *psychedelic* is used of drugs that are self-administered for the primary purpose of producing these experiences, e.g. *LSD, mescaline, psilocybin, marijuana.*

psychiatric classification/diagnosis See DIAGNOSTIC AND STATISTICAL MANUAL.

psychiatric social work A specialization within social work in which the social worker is trained for collaborative work with psychiatrists and clinical psychologists, or trained to do some of the same therapeutic work as these professionals.

psychiatrist A person trained in medicine who specializes in the prevention, diagnosis and treatment of mental and emotional disorders. The actual practices of the psychiatrist and the clinical psychologist overlap considerably, the primary difference being that the psychiatrist, by virtue of his or her medical licence, is legally authorized to prescribe drugs while the clinical psychologist typically is not. See PSYCHIATRY.

psychiatry A specialization within medicine encompassing prevention, diagnosis, treatment and research of mental and emotional disorders. Psychiatry, although parallel in many respects to CLINICAL PSYCHOLOGY, is historically and presently a branch of medicine, and psychiatrists hold an MD degree whereas a clinical psychologist holds a PhD or other professional degree. The historical issue here is more important than many realize, for psychiatry has traditionally taken the point of view that emotional and behavioural disorders are medical problems and that a person with a serious behavioural or emotional disability is mentally ill; see MEDICAL MODEL and MENTAL ILLNESS for more on terminology. As such, the psychiatrist is trained specifically in abnormalities and their prevention and cure, and little training is received in theories of normal behaviour, experimental design, collection and analysis of data, etc.

psychic 1 adj. Generally and loosely, pertaining to mind and that which is mental, and/or to person and the dimensions of personality – in short, a synonym of *psychological.* 2 More narrowly, pertaining to various aspects of PARAPSYCHOLOGY, usually mediumship and spiritualism. In this sense the noun form refers to one who claims to have supernatural powers. 3 Pertaining to psychogenic or functional disorders.

Although this meaning is fairly well rooted in usage (e.g. *psychic blindness*), it is, given meanings 1 and 2, misleading to many, and PSYCHOGENIC is generally preferred. var., *psychical* (particularly for 2).

psychical PSYCHIC (esp. 2).

psychic(al) research Research in PARAPSYCHOLOGY.

psychic anaphylaxis PSYCHOLOGICAL *ANAPHYLAXIS.

psychic ataxia MENTAL *ATAXIA.

psychic blindness 1 FUNCTIONAL *BLINDNESS. 2 AGNOSIA.

psychic determinism A form of DETERMINISM reflecting the point of view that all psychological processes are causally determined by antecedent factors. The term is used primarily by psychoanalytical theorists with respect to unconscious motives and causes.

psychic energy 1 In classical psychoanalysis, the assumed dynamic force underlying all psychological functioning. 2 In PARAPSYCHOLOGY, a mysterious form of energy that is assumed to pervade all living matter and be responsible for many purported paranormal phenomena.

psychic healing FAITH HEALING.

psychic impotence 1 IMPOTENCE which is psychogenic. 2 A temporary inability to carry out normal psychological processes.

psychic isolation ISOLATION (4).

psychic numbing A diminished responsiveness to the outside world, a numbing of one's emotions. Often seen in cases of POST-TRAUMATIC STRESS DISORDER.

psychic reflex PSYCHIC SECRETION.

psychic secretion I. P. Pavlov's original term for those first few drops of saliva elicited by a once-neutral stimulus. More generally, any conditioned salivary response. The more general term *psychic reflex* is also used here.

psychic trauma A general term used for any painful psychological experience. Typically used with the implication that the impact of the experience is long-lasting and that it interferes with normal functioning.

psychic vaginismus VAGINISMUS.

psychism PARAPSYCHOLOGY.

psycho Nontechnical slang for an individual suffering from a psychosis.

psycho- Combining form meaning pertaining to *mind*, *psyche* or *psychology*.

psychoacoustics A discipline within psychology concerned with sound, its perception and the physiological foundations of hearing. A hybrid field with contributions from physics, biology and applied areas in audiology and the speech sciences, it is now a fundamental part of many other areas, including the study of language, speech and music.

psychoactive Loosely, characterizing any compound that has an effect on mood, awareness, emotional tone or other psychological state. While not connotatively restricted, the term tends to be used for biological and biochemical substances (SEE PSYCHOACTIVE SUBSTANCE). See also PSYCHOTROPIC, a close synonym.

psychoactive substance (or **drug**) Generic terms for any substance or drug that affects consciousness, mood and awareness. At one time or another all of the antipsychotics, antidepressants, antianxiety drugs, stimulants, sedatives, psychedelics and hallucinogens have been so classified. Actually, this kind of categorizing doesn't help very much because essentially any drug could be placed in this group; aspirin, when it relieves a headache, can change one's consciousness and awareness. Nevertheless, the term has achieved a certain currency, although its application is properly restricted to substances that produce a marked psychological effect.

psychoactive substance abuse SUBSTANCE ABUSE.

psychoactive substance dependence SUBSTANCE DEPENDENCE.

psychoactive substance-induced organic mental disorders SUBSTANCE-INDUCED DISORDERS.

psychoactive substance use disorders A category of disorders marked by various cognitive and behavioural changes associated with the regular use of psychoactive substances that affect the nervous system. See SUBSTANCE-RELATED DISORDERS, the preferred term.

psychoanalysis **1** A theory of human behaviour. **2** A doctrine associated with this theory. **3** A set of techniques for exploring the underlying motivations of human behaviour. **4** A method of treatment of various mental disorders. Meaning 1 is typically used of the comprehensive theory due to Sigmund Freud (see FREUDIAN), although it may refer to any of a variety of related dynamic theories that are derivative of Freud's work even when quite distinct from the orthodoxy of classical Freudianism, e.g. Adler's individual psychology, Jung's analytical psychology. Note, some prefer the term *neopsychoanalysis* for these to prevent muddying the definitional waters. Meaning 2 refers to a cultural and social movement that has had an impact upon a variety of endeavours anthropological, political, aesthetic, literary and philosophical. It is a very loose doctrine that may or may not reflect Freudian purity; its application is detectable largely by the extensive use of interpretation, hypothesizing of unconscious motives and a search for deep causes. Meaning 3 covers the basic methods Freud developed over a period of several decades and which have been elaborated and extended by many others. The core components here are *free association, rich interpretation* and *transference*. In a nutshell, the subject free-associates while the analyst interprets the associations produced, the obstacles that bar others and the subject's feelings toward the analyst. Meaning 4 refers to an extension of the techniques covered by 3 in a systematic fashion to treat the psychoneuroses.

psychoanalyst **1** One who practises PSYCHOANALYSIS (4). Here application of the term is reserved for persons who have had psychoanalytic training at a recognized institute. They may have had any of a number of different forms of training prior to the psychoanalytical, e.g. an MD degree with a psychiatric residency, a doctorate or other advanced degree in psychology, or even a master's degree in social work or counselling. The term *lay analyst* is often used for practitioners who have not taken a medical degree. **2** One who is given to interpretations of events in accordance with psychoanalytic theory. This usage reflects those who use PSY-CHOANALYSIS in senses 2 and 3 of that term.

psychoasthenia Mental deficiency, mental retardation.

psychoasthenics The study of mental retardation.

psychobabble Thankfully, not a technical term, but one used all too often (and all too appropriately) to characterize extended displays of psychological nonsense dressed up with arcane psychological terminology to make the message sound profound. Perhaps not surprisingly, a new term NEUROBABBLE is appearing with increasing frequency.

psychobiography A biographical work that focuses on psychological factors, puts forward psychological profiles of the subject and interprets events in the person's life from a psychological perspective. The term is neutral as to the theoretical framework from which the biographer works. See PATHOBIO-GRAPHY and PSYCHOHISTORY.

psychobiology 1 Originally, a school of thought in psychiatry based on the theoretical orientation of Adolf Meyer, which stressed the mechanisms of integration of the biological, the psychological and the social experiences. **2** Contemporarily, a general term for the study of psychological process from a biological point of view. syn., *biopsychology* (for 2).

psychoceramics As conceptualized by the once and future Professor Josiah Carberry of Brown University, a highly specialized subdiscipline dealing with the crackpot in all his manifestations. The much-travelled Professor Carberry is said, like Freud, to have developed his theories largely from intensive self-examination.

psychodiagnosis Specifically, procedures for diagnosing psychological abnormalities, mental disturbances, etc. Somewhat more generally, the term is used of any psychological or personality assessment procedure. See DIAGNOSIS for more details on usage.

psychodrama A psychotherapeutic technique developed by J. L. Moreno in which the client acts out certain roles or incidents in the presence of a therapist and, often, other persons who are part of a therapy group. The procedures are based on the assumption that the role-playing allows the client to express troublesome emotions and face deep conflicts in the relatively protected environment of the therapeutic stage. Common variations are *group psychodrama*, in which all the actors are in the therapy group, and *family groups*, in which difficult domestic scenes are enacted.

psychodynamic 1 A label used freely for (a) all those psychological systems and theories that emphasize processes of change and development, and/or (b) those systems and theories that make motivation and drive central concepts. In short, psychological theories that deal with that which is DYNAMIC are all so labelled. **2** Occasionally, a synonym of *psychoanalytic*.

psychoendocrinology The study of the interactive role of the endocrine glands with various neurological processes, and their combined effects on thought, emotion and behaviour.

psychogalvanic response (PGR) GALVANIC SKIN RESPONSE.

psychogalvanometer A device for measuring the GALVANIC SKIN RESPONSE.

psychogenesis 1 The origin and, by extension, development of the psyche. In this sense the term is applied very generally to essentially any aspect of psychological functioning. **2** The origin and development of a specific psychological event within a particular organism. adj., *psychogenetic, psychogenic* (for 2).

psychogenetics 1 The study of the genetic basis of psychological processes; see BEHAVIOURAL GENETICS. **2** In some older texts, the study of PSYCHOGENESIS (1).

psychogenic 1 Psychological in origin. Used here primarily as a qualifier for disorders that are assumed to be functional in origin, i.e. those in which there is no known organic dysfunction. **2** Occasionally, pertaining to PSYCHOGENESIS (properly, only 2).

psychogenic amnesia DISSOCIATIVE *AMNESIA.

psychogenic disorder Any disorder for which there are no apparent organic bases; see FUNCTIONAL DISORDER.

psychogenic fugue FUGUE.

psychogenic pain disorder PAIN DISORDER.

psychogram **1** Generally, a profile of an individual on a variety of standard tests. See PROFILE ANALYSIS. **2** Specifically, H. Murray's term for a representation of an individual's pattern of needs and *press*.

psychohistory A general term for any literary work that attempts to understand historical events by providing a detailed psychological analysis of the characters involved. Compare with PATHOBIOGRAPHY and PSYCHOBIOGRAPHY.

psychoimmunology PSYCHONEUROIMMU-NOLOGY.

psychokinesis **1** The hypothesized parapsychological phenomenon of an individual supposedly influencing a physical event without direct intervention. Commonly abbreviated as *PK*. Also called *parakinesis* and *telekinesis*. **2** Occasionally, in psychiatric writings, manic behaviour.

psycholagny Sexual excitement brought about by the use of one's imagination, usually by forming mental images.

psycholepsy A sudden loss of mental alertness, a feeling of hopelessness, helplessness, depression.

psycholinguistics A field that was created and named during an interdisciplinary conference held in the USA in 1953. Despite protestations from one of the prominent participants, Roger Brown, that the name sounded more like a description of a deranged polyglot than a scientific field, it has become an important part of psychology. Most broadly, the focus is upon the study of any and all behaviours that are linguistic. Subfields include the acquisition of language, bilingualism, pragmatics, speech-act theory, studies of grammar, the psychology of reading and the relationship between language and thought. Because of the ubiquity of verbal behaviour in humans, many psycholinguistic issues emerge in other areas as well, including cognitive psychology, memory, information processing, speech and hearing sciences, sociolinguistics, neuropsychology and clinical psychology. Note, some use the term as though it pertains only to the approach to the psychology of language championed by Noam Chomsky

that focuses on syntax and makes assumptions about innate structures (see LAD). This denotative limitation is unfortunate. Compare with VERBAL LEARNING.

psycholinguistics, developmental A division of PSYCHOLINGUISTICS that focuses on the study of the acquisition of natural language by the child.

psychological **1** Pertaining to psychology in any and/or all of its manifestations. **2** Characterizing an event, process, phenomenon or theory so as to emphasize its role in psychology as opposed to any other connotations which it may have, e.g. psychological test, psychological warfare. **3** Pertaining to that which is mental in origin; see PSYCHO-GENIC (1). A very large number of compound terms exist that use 'psychological' as a modifier or a prefix. For those not found below, look under the nominal listing (e.g. *psychological distance* is under *distance, psychological*).

psychological environment Loosely, all aspects of the environment that are psychologically relevant to an individual at any point in time. Exactly what constitutes this environment, however, is viewed very differently by different writers. *Caveat lector.*

psychological factors affecting physical condition A cover term for those mental factors that play a significant role in PSYCHO-SOMATIC DISORDERS.

psychological moment MOMENT (1).

psychological present SPECIOUS PRESENT.

psychological space LIFE SPACE.

psychological test A cover term for all tests of a psychological nature. See TEST and related entries for discussion and definitions of various kinds of test.

psychological type TYPE (esp. 3).

psychological warfare Originally, the use of psychological manipulations in the waging of wars. Most attempts are essentially morale-boosters for one's allies and -depressors for the enemy. More recently, use of the term has been extended beyond the military domain and is found in the context of similar morale-manipulating techniques used in marriages, business, sports, etc.

psychologism A point of view that psychological phenomena are the critical ones for ascertaining truth. Those who defend this position argue that logic appears 'logical' because it reflects how human cognitive systems operate, that a word's meaning is given by the mental idea(s) that correspond with it or that truth of an empirical proposition is to be determined by its correspondence to a mental proposition. Some of these proposals are found in PHENOMENOLOGY and EXISTENTIAL-ISM but virtually no one currently supports the original position. Indeed, the term is used mainly derisively.

psychologist Determining to just whom this term applies is no simple matter. The difficulties stem from the fact that some who claim it do so because they *practise* psychology, others because they *apply* it, others because they *teach* it and still others because they *research* it. When a formal definition is provided, it is usually done so to satisfy some particular practical and/or legal issue. For example, many governmental bodies that regulate licensing of psychologists require that an applicant have completed an advanced degree (a master's minimally, often a doctorate) at a recognized institution, undertaken one or more years of a supervised internship or practicum and passed a written examination. Criteria of this kind are most often applied when a psychologist is defined as one who is recognized or qualified to undertake any of a number of professional duties, e.g. a clinical psychologist, consulting psychologist, forensic psychologist or school psychologist. However, when assessing whether one who teaches and/or does research in psychology 'deserves' this four-syllable mantle, things become less clear. For example, the standard characterization of a psychologist that is usually offered is that he or she is one who (a) holds at least a master's degree or preferably a doctorate and (b) studies psychological processes. The degree requirement presents problems. What degree counts? Whatever are we to call Erik Erikson, the great analyst and humanitarian who never received a university degree, or Herbert Simon, Nobel laureate in economics who was one of the leading theorists in the field of cognitive psychology, or Jean Piaget, who remade developmental psychology despite being trained in biology, or William

James, perhaps the greatest of them all, whose first course in psychology was the one he taught?

The other requirement, that a psychologist study psychological processes, is equally futile, for each new development in psychology implicates processes once thought to lie in other domains. This volume contains hundreds if not thousands of terms derived from sociology, anthropology, biology, physiology, medicine, philosophy, computer sciences, linguistics, mathematics, chemistry and physics; the scientists who studied these processes often did not presume to be studying psychology but they were. What shall we call them?

The bottom lexicographical line here is that the designation is 'awarded' by two different kinds of collective agencies. One is a legally constituted body: it determines who shall be called a psychologist according to governmentally regulated standards which have been designed to protect the public, to ensure that the 'psychologist' who offers his or her services does, in fact, possess the training and skills that one can legitimately expect him or her to have. The other is a loosely federated community of scholars and operates much less formally. It functions according to implicit criteria concerning an individual's accomplishments. Here, one who has taught, written, lectured and/or researched about those phenomena that fall within the confines of psychology will end up not only being called a psychologist but, in the long run, defining what it is those who are called psychologists (according to the former set of criteria) actually do. He or she may, and usually will, have a doctorate degree, and this will probably be in psychology, but these are not defining features of the label. Many who claim the label through the latter criterion would not qualify for it via the former. For more on these definitional issues, see PSYCHOTHERAPIST and, of course, PSYCHOLOGY; for distinctions concerning those persons with medical training, see PSYCHIATRIST and PSYCHIATRY.

psychologist's fallacy The tendency to project one's point of view or one's interpretation onto another – when committed by a psychologist; for example, a clinical psychologist who makes a fallacious inference about a client in therapy, or an introspectionist who reads unwarranted interpretations into an observer's reports.

psychology Psychology simply cannot be defined; indeed, it cannot even be easily characterized. Even if one were to frame a definition or characterization today, tomorrow would render the effort inadequate. Psychology is what scientists and philosophers of various persuasions have created to try to fulfil the need to understand the minds and behaviours of various organisms, from the most primitive to the most complex. Hence, it is not really a thing at all: it is about a thing, or about many things. It has few boundaries, and aside from the canons of science and the ethical standards of a free society it should not have any imposed upon it either by its practitioners or by its critics. It is an attempt to understand what has so far pretty much escaped understanding, and any effort to circumscribe it or box it in is to imply that something is known about the edges of our knowledge, and that must be wrong.

As a distinct discipline psychology finds its roots a mere century and a half or so back in the faculties of medicine and philosophy. From medicine it took the orientation that explication of that which is done, thought and felt must ultimately be couched in biology and physiology; from philosophy it took a class of deep problems concerning mind, will and knowledge. Since then, it has been variously defined as 'the science of mind', 'the science of mental life', 'the science of behaviour', etc. All such definitions, of course, reflect the prejudices of the definer more than the actual nature of the field. In the course of writing this volume, a rather strange metaphor has emerged that somehow seems to capture the essential quality of our discipline. It is like an amoeba, relatively unstructured but very much identifiable as a distinct entity with a peculiar mode of action by means of which it sends out a projection of itself toward some new technique, some novel problem area, some theoretical model, or even some other distinct field of science, incorporating it and slowly pulling itself clumsily into another shape. Not very flattering perhaps, but accurate. For more on the lexicographical problems here see PSYCHOLOGIST.

psycholytic Lit., mind-loosening. Used

occasionally of the hallucinogenic or psychedelic drugs.

psycholytic therapy A radical form of psychotherapy which is based, in part, on the administration of psychedelic drugs. There has been a good deal of controversy over its therapeutic value compared with more traditional approaches, and it is rarely used today.

psychometric Lit., pertaining to the measurement of that which is psychological. Hence: **1** Pertaining to mental testing in any of its facets, including assessment of personality, evaluation of intelligence and determining of aptitudes. **2** Pertaining to PSYCHOPHYSICS. **3** Pertaining to issues of the application of principles of mathematics and statistics to the data of psychology.

psychometric function Generally, a mathematical expression relating the values of a physical variable to the psychological experiencing of each value. See e.g. POWER LAW.

psychometrician Broadly, a specialist in the study of that which is PSYCHOMETRIC. Usually, however, the reference is to an individual who is an EXPERT (1), a specialist in the theory and/or practice of administering, scoring and interpreting the results of mental tests. The term is also used according to the other two senses of PSYCHOMETRIC, but somewhat less frequently.

psychometrics Collectively, the branches of psychology concerned with measurement. See PSYCHOMETRIC for details.

psychometrizing A paranormal process in which information about a person or event is supposedly obtained by touching or holding an object belonging to or related to the person or the event. See PARAPSYCHOLOGY.

psychometry **1.** The field that embodies PSYCHOMETRIC (generally 1) research. **2** PSYCHOMETRIZING. The use of the same label for two fields, one reasonable and the other not, is unfortunate.

psychomimetic Generally, of that which mimics or resembles a natural psychological process. See PSYCHOTOMIMETIC for a more specific reference.

psychomotor Loosely, pertaining to mental events which have motor effect or vice versa. See SENSORIMOTOR.

psychomotor agitation Excessive motor activity that is marked by nonproductivity and repetitiveness and associated with feelings of inner tension. Typical behaviours are an inability to remain seated, constant pacing, hand-wringing, tugging at and fussing over one's clothes, and rapid, complaining speech.

psychomotor epilepsy EPILEPSY, PSYCHOMOTOR.

psychomotor retardation A general slowing down of motor action, movements and speech. Seen as a common symptom of various disorders, notably depression.

psychoneural parallelism PARALLELISM, PSYCHONEURAL.

psychoneuroendocrinology An interdisciplinary approach that explores the links and interactions between the nervous system, the endocrine system and psychological functions.

psychoneuroimmunology An interdisciplinary science that studies the interrelationships of the psychological, behavioural, neuroendocrinal processes and immunology. Also called *psychoimmunology*.

psychoneurosis 1 A term used more or less interchangeably with NEUROSIS. It is preferred by many writers because etymologically it emphasizes the functional, nonorganic aspects. The original, but now largely obsolete, meaning of *neurosis* made reference to disorders of the nervous system and its actions, and the prefix *psycho-* was first appended to distinguish clearly between the *neurotic* and *neural*. **2** A diagnostic category comprising a group of disorders characterized by anxiety, including *conversion reaction*, the *phobias* and *obsessive-compulsive reaction*. Note, however, that this category is gradually being dropped from the diagnostic classification system of mental disorders – at least in the USA, where the DIAGNOSTIC AND STATISTICAL MANUAL no longer lists it. See NEUROSIS for more on contemporary terminology here.

psychoneurotic inventory NEUROTIC INVENTORY.

psychonomic 1 Relating to or concerned with that which is lawful in psychology. A psychonomic enterprise is one which searches for general principles and underlying lawful relationships. Although there are variations in use, the term generally characterizes an approach to psychology patterned after the natural sciences. **2** (obs.). Pertaining to environmental effects on psychological development.

psychooncology The study of how having cancer affects a person's psychology.

psychopath A term with two uses, both of which are falling out of favour. **1** A general label for a person with any severe mental disorder. This usage is now absent from technical writings but still occurs in popular literature. **2** An individual diagnosed as having a PSYCHOPATHIC PERSONALITY. Note, however, that that term has been largely superseded, first by SOCIOPATHIC PERSONALITY DISORDER and more recently by ANTISOCIAL PERSONALITY DISORDER.

psychopathic PSYCHOPATHY.

psychopathic personality An older term for one diagnosed with an ANTISOCIAL PERSONALITY DISORDER. The term is rarely used these days in the technical literature but is still found in the popular press.

psychopathology 1 The scientific study of mental disorders. Strictly speaking, the term refers to a scientific domain that includes the research work of, among others, psychologists, psychiatrists, neurologists, endocrinologists and pharmacologists, and is distinguished from the actual *practice* of clinical psychologists and psychiatrists in the treatment of those with mental disorders. adj., *psychopathological*. Distinguish from *psychopathic* (see PSYCHOPATH). **2** Loosely, any pattern of behaviour or thought viewed as dysfunctional.

psychopathy 1 Any abnormal mental condition of which the aetiology is unknown and a diagnosis has not been (or cannot be) made. In this sense, the term is an open admission of ignorance. Alternatively: **2** A forensic psychiatric term for the condition described under ANTISOCIAL PERSONALITY DISORDER. It is rarely used today.

psychopharmacology The study of drugs,

specifically with a focus on their psychological effects. It is a hybrid field deriving its foundations from biology, physiology, biochemistry, medicine and psychology.

psychophysical 1 Pertaining to PSYCHOPHYSICS. **2** Pertaining to the oft-hypothesized division between that which is mental and that which is physical. See e.g. DUALISM, PSYCHOPHYSICAL *PARALLELISM.

psychophysical function Generally, any mathematical function relating sensory experience with physical stimuli. The POWER LAW is a good example.

psychophysical law In his enthusiasm over his early discovery Fechner used this term for what is now called FECHNER'S LAW.

psychophysical measurement Generally, the process of determining some scale of measurement that relates the values of a physical variable with the psychological experiences associated with those values. See MEASUREMENT OF *THRESHOLD, METHODS OF *SCALING, SCALE OF MEASUREMENT and related entries for details.

psychophysical methods Broadly, any and/or all of those methods developed in the study of *psychophysics*. See MEASUREMENT OF *THRESHOLD, METHODS OF *SCALING and SCALES OF MEASUREMENT for details.

psychophysical parallelism PARALLELISM, PSYCHOPHYSICAL.

psychophysical scale PSYCHOLOGICAL *SCALE.

psychophysics An area of psychology concerned primarily with the quantitative relationships between physical stimuli and the psychological experience of them. The study of psychophysics began formally with the work of Gustav T. Fechner in the 1860s, although, in Fechner's mind, it was the larger science of determining the formal relationship between mind (psyche) and body (physics). As it developed, two broad classes of problems emerged: the determination of THRESHOLDS (1, 2) and the establishment of PSYCHOPHYSICAL *SCALES. See these and related entries for details on method and theory.

psychophysiological Pertaining generally to the relationship between physiological processes and psychological experience.

psychophysiologic disorder PSYCHOSOMATIC DISORDER.

psychophysiology PHYSIOLOGICAL PSYCHOLOGY.

psychoprophylactic method LAMAZE METHOD.

psychose passionnelle The relatively rare delusion that another person, usually one of high social status or a celebrity, is deeply in love with one. Also called *pure erotomania* and *de Clérambault's syndrome*.

psychosexual 1 Broadly, relating to all aspects of sexuality, the mental as well as the physical and physiological. **2** Relating to the mental components of sexuality, particularly in the context of their being considered more important than the somatic components. **3** Within psychoanalytic theory, pertaining to the notion that psychological processes originate in that which is sexual. For example, *development* in classical Freudian theory often means PSYCHOSEXUAL DEVELOPMENT, a term which incorporates all three meanings.

psychosexual development Within the classical psychoanalytic model, a series of stages of development characterized by the interaction between biological drives and the environment. According to the standard model, balanced, reality-oriented development takes place when there is a proper resolution of this interaction; unbalanced development with attendant conflicts and fixations results in psychological disturbances which may lie latent or be manifested as personality or behavioural disorders. The stages assumed by the theory are the ORAL, ANAL, PHALLIC, LATENCY and GENITAL; see each for details.

psychosexual disorder SEXUAL AND GENDER DISORDERS.

psychosexual dysfunction SEXUAL DYSFUNCTIONS.

psychosis 1 Originally, but now rarely, the total mental condition of a person at a specific moment. **2** A PSYCHOTIC DISORDER. pl., *psychoses*.

psychosis with cerebral arteriosclerosis MULTI-INFARCT *DEMENTIA.

psychosocial Generally, a grab-bag term

used freely to cover any situation in which both psychological and social factors are assumed to play a role.

psychosocial deprivation During childhood, the condition of getting less than appropriate psychological and social interaction, contact, experience, etc. The term is generally used to characterize an aberrant home environment in which there is inadequate parenting. The condition is suspected of being one of the primary causes of mild mental retardation, since in many cases enriching the environment causes tested IQ to rise sharply to normal levels.

psychosocial development A term that may be used loosely and literally to refer to an individual's psychological/social development but is more commonly associated with Erik Erikson's characterization of personality growth and development, which stresses the interaction between the person and the physical and social environments. See STAGES OF MAN for more details on the hypothesized process.

psychosomatic Generally, pertaining to that which is presumed to have both *psychic* (mental) and *somatic* (bodily) components. The usual implication here is that these two aspects interact, each having impact upon the other. See PSYCHOSOMATIC DISORDER and PSYCHOSOMATIC MEDICINE.

psychosomatic disorder A general label used for any disorder with *somatic* (bodily) manifestations that are assumed to have at least a partial cognitive and emotional aetiology, i.e. that are to some degree *psychological*. Several approaches can be taken to these disorders: the one chosen dictates the connotations of the term. From one widely held perspective, three subcategories of disorders can be distinguished: (a) those related to an individual's overall personality (e.g. highly anxious people show a relatively high incidence of respiratory disorders); (b) those intimately connected to a person's lifestyle (e.g. people in high-pressure, stressful occupations show a relatively high rate of hypertension and gastric dysfunctions); and (c) those manifested primarily by heightened reaction to substances and conditions (e.g. allergies, which, while stimulated by foreign substances, are differentially experienced depending on psychological factors).

However, there is another general point of view that is predicated on the assumption that the manifestation of *all* somatic disorders is psychological to some degree. This orientation suggests a rather different nosology. Here, the disorders are named and classified according to the organ system involved, e.g. gastrointestinal, respiratory, cutaneous. See also SOMATOFORM DISORDER.

psychosomatic medicine The branch of medicine concerned with the relationship between psychological states (conceptualized broadly) and somatic disturbances. While much of the focus is on PSYCHOSOMATIC DISORDERS, the basic operating hypothesis is that there are subtle but critical interactions between somatic and organic dysfunctions and psychological/emotional factors in *all* cases. Distinguish from SOMATOPSYCHOLOGY. See also SOMATOFORM DISORDER.

psychosurgery A general label for any surgical procedure performed on brain tissue for the purpose of alleviating psychological disorders. Procedures range from major surgical interventions (SEE PREFRONTAL *LOBOTOMY) to minor techniques that are carried out under local anaesthetic (see TRANSORBITAL *LOBOTOMY). Other techniques involve severing pathways that mediate limbic-system activity (see AMYGDALOTOMY) and the dramatic procedure of severing the fibres of the *corpus callosum* (see SPLIT-BRAIN TECHNIQUE). Increasingly common are highly localized, minute lesions made possible by developments in imaging and novel microsurgical techniques. However, in all cases psychosurgery remains, and most certainly should remain, controversial and used only when all other treatments have failed.

psychotechnician One trained specifically and only to administer certain kinds of psychological and educational tests.

psychotechnology A sometime synonym of *applied psychology*. Used rather loosely, its meaning depends upon the theoretical orientation of the author.

psychotherapeutic 1 Pertaining to PSYCHOTHERAPY. **2** Pertaining to that which has curative value in psychological disorders. These two meanings are not necessarily equivalent.

psychotherapist Generally, one who practises psychotherapy. Note, in fact, that in some locales the term has taken on a legal definition and may be formally distinguished from PSYCHOLOGIST. That is, some governmental bodies and professional licensing boards recognize a person with some special training as qualified to function as a licensed psychotherapist (e.g. one trained in social work or school or counselling psychology), while reserving the title *psychologist* for those with doctoral degrees and recognized internships.

psychotherapy In the most inclusive sense, the use of absolutely any technique or procedure that has palliative or curative effects upon any mental, emotional or behavioural disorder. In this general sense the term is neutral with regard to the theory that may underlie it, the actual procedures and techniques entailed and the form and duration of the treatment. There may, however, be legal and professional issues involved in the actual practice of what is called psychotherapy, and in the technical literature the term is properly used only when the treatment is carried out by someone with recognized training and using accepted techniques. For more on this issue see PSYCHIATRIST, PSYCHOANALYST, PSYCHOLOGIST and PSYCHOTHERAPIST. The term is often shortened to *therapy*, particularly when modifiers are appended to identify the form of therapy or the theoretical orientation of the therapist. Specific forms are listed in this volume by modifier.

psychotic 1 adj. Pertaining to a PSYCHOTIC DISORDER. Often used in combined form to mark a specific disorder when the symptoms are characteristic of or strongly resemble a psychosis, e.g. PSYCHOTIC *DEPRESSION. **2** n. One who has been diagnosed as having a psychotic disorder.

psychotic depression DEPRESSION, PSYCHOTIC.

psychotic disorders A general cover term for a number of severe mental disorders of organic or emotional origin. In contemporary psychiatric nosology, the defining feature of these disorders is gross impairment in REALITY-TESTING (2). That is, a patient makes incorrect inferences concerning external reality, makes improper evaluations of the accuracy of his or her thoughts and perceptions and continues to make these errors in the face of contrary evidence. Classic

symptoms include delusions, hallucinations, severe regressive behaviours, dramatically inappropriate mood and markedly incoherent speech. The standard clinical literature lists as psychoses: BIPOLAR DISORDER, BRIEF REACTIVE PSYCHOSIS, the SCHIZOPHRENIAS, various ORGANIC MENTAL DISORDERS and some of the MOOD DISORDERS.

psychotic episode BRIEF REACTIVE PSYCHOSIS.

psychotic surrender A term used occasionally to characterize a reaction in individuals who are seen as reaching a point at which they will 'throw in the towel', giving up on their battle to face reality and surrendering to a psychotic withdrawal.

psychotogenic Generally, characterizing events, circumstances or substances that produce psychotic states.

psychotomimetic Lit., mimicking a psychosis. First used of those psychotropic drugs with actions that were assumed to mimic psychotic disorders, specifically hallucinogens like LSD. This assumption has been found wanting and the term is now used loosely to characterize drugs that produce a state similar to or symptomatic of a psychotic disorder.

psychotropic Lit., mind-altering or mood-altering. Most often used to characterize drugs that affect psychological functioning, such as those used in drug therapy, like the antianxiety, antidepressant and antipsychotic drugs, as well as hallucinogens, such as LSD, mescaline, etc. Like its near synonym, *psychoactive*, the term tends to be used loosely.

P technique R CORRELATION.

ptosis Dropping, drooping. Used of organs or parts, e.g. the drooping of an eyelid as a result of paralysis.

PTSD POST-TRAUMATIC STRESS DISORDER.

puberal Pertaining to PUBERTY. var., *pubertal*.

pubertas praecox PRECOCIOUS *PUBERTY.

puberty The period of life during which the sex organs become reproductively functional. Onset in the female is fairly clearly marked by the menarche; in the male it is less obvious, but the growth and pigmentation of underarm hair is often taken as criterial. The end of puberty is difficult to specify and many authors simply select an arbitrary cut-off point based on age (e.g. 14 in the female and 15 in the male are often used), although it should be recognized that there is considerable variation in age of onset and rate of development, so such an approach is of questionable value.

puberty, precocious Lit., early puberty. The term is reserved for the abnormal condition in which, owing to pituitary malfunction, the normal maturational sequence is speeded up and the onset of puberty, including the maturation of the sex organs and the emergence of the secondary sex characteristics, occurs at an abnormally early age. Also called *pubertas praecox*.

puberty rites Generally, any cultural ritual concerning the passage into adult status. Note that although the term is most often used in anthropological discourses on tribal lore and tradition in preliterate societies, many modern social, ethnic and religious groups have similar practices. Compare with PUBIC RITES.

puberum dysphonia DYSPHONIA, PUBERUM.

pubes 1 n. sing. The hair or the entire hairy region of the lower abdomen and genital area. **2** n. pl. The pubic bones that form part of the pelvis.

pubescence The process of first reaching puberty.

pubescent Of one in the early period of puberty.

pubic Pertaining to the external genitals and the immediate genital area; pertaining to the pubes.

pubic rites Any ritual or ceremony involving the genitals. They may or may not be associated with PUBERTY RITES; e.g. circumcision is usually performed soon after birth.

public 1 adj. Open, unrestricted, available. **2** adj. Pertaining to the people or, by extension, the government of the people. **3** n. A large aggregate of persons. Note that this last use is generally broken down so that it may refer to: (a) the full complement of persons in a state or country, which is the meaning usually conveyed by the simple use of the definite article as in *the public*; or (b) a number of

persons who share a common set of interests, which is the meaning usually conveyed by the use of delimiting adjectives as in e.g. the *golfing public* or the *buying public*. Note that this particular use of the term is similar to that of *group* but without the connotation of *organization*. See GROUP for discussion.

publication bias FILE DRAWER PROBLEM.

public opinion OPINION, PUBLIC.

public self SOCIAL *SELF.

public-speaking anxiety ANXIETY, PUBLIC-SPEAKING.

pudenda The external genitals. sing., *pudendum*.

puerile Childlike. Usually used as descriptive of the behaviour of an adult that is inappropriately childish.

puerperal Pertaining to childbirth or to the weeks immediately following. Often used in phrases that relate to disorders accompanying childbirth, e.g. *postpartum depression* is also called *puerperal depression*.

puerperium The period following childbirth, often specified as 42 days.

Pulfrich phenomenon (or **effect**) An illusion of depth produced when viewing a pendulum swinging in one plane when one eye is covered with a dimming filter. Because the brain treats the mismatched inputs as binocular disparity, the natural interpretation is that the pendulum is swinging in three dimensions.

pulmonary Pertaining to the lungs.

pulse 1 Generally, any regular rhythmic throbbing. **2** Specifically, the beating produced by the rise and fall of pressure in the arteries resulting from heart-muscle action.

pulvinar An area of the thalamus that projects fibres to the visual association areas in the parietal and temporal lobes.

punch drunk DEMENTIA PUGILISTICA.

punctate Marked with or by points. A punctate stimulus is one applied to a point on the skin.

punctuated equilibrium A model of evolution which argues that new species evolve in rather rapid (geologically speaking) fashion rather than in the gradual manner depicted by the standard Darwinian model. The term connotes that evolution can be seen as periods of relative stability occasionally punctuated by the saltatory emergence of new species. Compare with DARWINISM.

punisher Any event that operates opposite in sign to a REINFORCER. That is, a *positive punisher* reduces the probability of responses that produced it and a *negative punisher* reduces the probability of responses that terminated it. See also NEGATIVE *REINFORCER, POSITIVE *RE-INFORCER.

punishment **1** The administration of some aversive stimulus contingent upon a particular behaviour. **2** The aversive stimulus itself. Behind these formal definitions of the term lie a variety of issues, and the exact connotations of the term depend on the manner of its use. To wit: (a) the aversive stimulus itself may be short, simple and well defined, as in most laboratory studies in which electric shock is used, but it may also be an extended, complex event, as when society incarcerates a legal offender; (b) the punishing event may be the presentation of some aversive stimulus (an electric shock, a spanking) or it may consist of the withdrawal of some desired or pleasant thing (a treat, a parent's love; (see NEGATIVE *PUNISHMENT, POSITIVE *PUNISHMENT)); (c) the punishment may be either for the performance of some response (a rat pressing the wrong bar, a felony) or for the nonperformance of a response (failure to press the bar, not studying for an exam). Moreover, some authors use the term so that the threat of punishment is considered to be a punishment. This extension is defended by the argument that the anxiety associated with the possibility of the infliction of the aversive stimulus is, in itself, punishing. Compare with and distinguish from NEGATIVE *REINFORCEMENT.

punishment by reciprocity Punishment that takes account of the nature and severity of the transgression and is logically related to it; punishment that 'fits the crime' and makes clear to the transgressor the implications of the offence. Older children tend to favour this over EXPIATORY *PUNISHMENT.

punishment, costly Punishment that carries negative consequences for the individual administering it.

punishment, expiatory Punishment that is painful in proportion to the seriousness of the transgression and not necessarily dependent on the nature of the offence committed. Younger children tend to favour this over PUNISHMENT BY RECIPROCITY.

punishment, negative Punishment where a positive or desirable stimulus is removed contingent upon some action. Compare with POSITIVE *PUNISHMENT.

punishment, positive Punishment where an aversive stimulus is presented contingent upon some action. Compare with NEGATIVE *PUNISHMENT.

punitive Pertaining to punishment, especially with the connotation of the use or threat of punishment to control the behaviour of others. Compare with IMPUNITIVE, INTROPUNITIVE and EXTRAPUNITIVE.

pupil **1** The adjustable opening in the iris of the eye through which light passes. **2** Any child in the elementary grades. **3** Any student being tutored.

pupillary reflex A change in the size of the pupil of the eye. Contraction of the iris muscle causes constriction of the pupil, relaxation produces a dilated pupil. The reflex is produced by a variety of stimuli, including changes in light level, changes in point of focus, and emotional aspects of the visual stimulus – although in the case of the last of these, changes in pupil size are probably conditioned responses and not true reflexes. Also called *iris reflex* and *iritic reflex*.

pure **1** Unadulterated, free from extraneous factors, homogeneous; e.g. a *pure tone* consists of only a single frequency, a *pure hue* of only one wavelength. **2** Uncontaminated, morally sound, virtuous. **3** Not applied. Here the term is used for research aimed at the accumulation of knowledge, understanding and explanation independently of possible applications. This is not to suggest that applications may not be made, only that such potential is not a motivation in the actual research itself. The term is widely used as a modifier. Specialized phrases can be found under the alphabet listing of the key term.

pure erotomania PSYCHOSE PASSIONNELLE.

pure research RESEARCH, PURE AND APPLIED.

pure word deafness AUDITORY *APHASIA.

Purkinje (Purkyně) afterimage The second POSITIVE *AFTERIMAGE, which occurs following a bright stimulus; it is in the hue complementary to the original.

Purkinje (Purkyně) cells Large neurons in the cerebellum. They are the major efferent projections from the cortex of the cerebellum to its deep nuclei. The cells have extensive dendritic processes that project to the molecular layer of the cortex.

Purkinje (Purkyně) effect (or **phenomenon** or **shift**) When the illumination of a multihue display is reduced, those hues toward the long-wavelength end of the spectrum (reds, oranges) lose their perceived brightness more rapidly than those toward the short-wavelength end (greens, blues). This shift is due to the fact that the rods, which have greater overall sensitivity than the cones, are also maximally sensitive to short wavelengths.

Purkinje (Purkyně) figures (or **network**) The perception of the network of interwoven blood vessels of the retina. Under the proper conditions (e.g. low room illumination, with a small, relatively bright light held just under the eye, staring at a blank wall) it can be seen.

Purkinje (Purkyně)–Sanson images Three distinct images of an object that a person is viewing that can be observed by looking at that person's eye under the proper conditions. One is from the surface of the cornea, one from the front of the lens and the third from the back of the lens.

purple A hue (or, better, a series of related hues) that results from mixtures of blue and red light. The purples are often referred to as *extraspectral* because there are no single wavelengths in the visible spectrum that produce them; hence they are defined by specifying the wavelength of their complements, e.g. the greens and yellow-greens in the neighbourhood of 550 nm.

purpose 1 The internally represented mental goal or aim which is set by an individual and which guides and directs his or her behaviour. **2** A hypothetical determiner of behaviour inferred from an organism's behaviour that reveals directedness, persistence and focused orientation toward some goal. Meaning 2 was introduced by E. C. Tolman to permit behaviourists to theorize about purpose in sense 1 without having to admit to it. See PURPOSIVE PSYCHOLOGY.

purposive psychology An orientation of psychological science that stresses the role of purpose in the determination of behaviour. The term was introduced by the neobehaviourist Edward Chace Tolman to characterize his theoretical position that behaviour could not be properly understood from the pure behaviourist perspective, which stressed only the mechanical chaining of reflexive, physiological processes. Note, however, that several other theoretical positions, while not necessarily labelled as *purposive*, make similar assumptions about behaviour, e.g. the hormic psychology of McDougall and virtually all of the depth or analytic approaches.

pursuitmeter Any device for measuring a subject's ability to follow (i.e. pursue) an erratically moving target. The most commonly used are the *pursuit rotor*, for a target that follows a rough and erratically varying circular path, and the *pursuit pendulum*, for a target that traces a varying pendular path.

pursuit movement Eye movement made while tracking a moving object. The eye moves relatively smoothly and in a manner such that the image remains on the fovea. Compare with SACCADIC MOVEMENT.

pursuit, ocular PURSUIT MOVEMENT.

pursuit pendulum PURSUITMETER.

pursuit reaction Generally, any set of movements that serves to keep an organism oriented with respect to a moving stimulus.

pursuit rotor PURSUITMETER.

push-down stack 1 In computer terminology, a temporally ordered list. This list is in the form of a limited-capacity storage system in which each new incoming stimulus occupies the topmost position in the stack, 'pushing down' the previously stored stimuli. When the capacity of the stack is reached, each new stimulus 'pushes out' the oldest of the stored ones. **2** In cognitive psychology, a metaphor for the mode of operation of human SHORT-TERM *MEMORY, which displays many of these properties.

putamen One of the large subcortical nuclei that comprise the BASAL GANGLIA.

puzzle box Generally, any experimental apparatus consisting of a locked box and an unlocking device which must be manipulated in the proper manner by the subject either (a) to obtain a reward locked in the box, or (b) to get out of the box in which it is locked. The unlocking device may be either a simple lever, bar or string or a complex mechanism, depending upon the cognitive sophistication of the subject in the experiment. See e.g. THORNDIKE PUZZLE BOX.

Pygmalion effect 1 Named after the play by G. B. Shaw, the oft-observed effect in which people come to behave in ways that correspond to others' expectations of them. See SELF-FULFILLING PROPHECY. **2** From the name of a king in a Greek myth (from which Shaw also borrowed the name), a pathological condition in which one falls in love with one's own creation. syn., *pygmalionism* (for 2).

pyknic Referring to a compact, thick body type. See CONSTITUTIONAL THEORY for more detail. var., *pyknik*.

pyramidal cells Multipolar cells with triangular-shaped bodies and extensive dendritic processes found in the cerebral cortex and the hippocampus.

pyramidal (motor) system PYRAMIDAL TRACT.

pyramidal tract A neural system consisting of a long monosynaptic pathway that rises in the primary motor cortex, the premotor area, the somatosensory area and areas of both the frontal and parietal lobes and runs to the motor neurons of the cranial-nerve nuclei and ventral horn of the spinal cord. Most of the fibres in the system decussate at the medulla, the others further down the pathway. It contains axons of the lateral and ventral *corticospinal tracts* (see CORTICOSPINAL PATHWAY). Also called *pyramidal motor system*.

pyramids Compact elevated bundles of nerve fibres in the medulla.

pyromania An IMPULSE-CONTROL DISORDER characterized by a recurrent failure to resist impulses to set fires and a deep fascination with watching them burn. A defining feature of the disorder is that the fire-setting is undertaken without obvious motivations such as monetary gain, revenge or political ideology.

pyrosis Heartburn.

Q

Q Abbreviation for: **1** QUARTILE DEVIATION. **2** When subscripted, a QUARTILE: Q_1, Q_2, Q_3 designate the first, second and third quartiles. **3** *Question*, as in *Q* and *A* (*answer*). **4** *Questionnaire*, used generally.

q The proportion of events in a population failing to exhibit a particular characteristic and thereby distinguishable from a mutually exclusive proportion of events, *p*, such that $p + q = 1$.

Q data Any data obtained from a questionnaire.

Q method A general term for the use of questionnaires in research.

Q sort A technique used in personality assessment based upon a series of statements and trait names which the subject sorts into categories such as 'most characteristic of me' to 'least characteristic of me'.

Q technique R CORRELATION.

Q test COCHRAN Q TEST.

quadranopia A POSTCHIASMATIC VISUAL DEFECT marked by blindness in one quadrant of the visual field.

quadrant **1** One of the four cells in a 2×2 table. **2** One of the four equal-sized areas of a plane created by subdividing it with intersecting perpendicular lines.

quadrigemina CORPORA QUADRIGEMINA.

quadriplegia Paralysis of all four limbs.

quale The singular of QUALIA.

qualia n., pl. The qualitative, subjective experience of something, e.g. the smell of fresh-ground coffee, the taste of vinegar, the pain of a headache. Qualia are presumed to constitute the irreducible, phenomenal character of experience; they are what something is *like*. As the argument goes, you may be an expert on colour vision, but if you are colour-blind you have no idea about what makes red *red*. Qualia were the focus of the introspectionism of early STRUCTURALISM (1) and are currently the topic of considerable debate in the philosophy of mind. Within REDUCTIONISM, qualia are thought of as natural consequences of neurological action; within DUALISM, the very phenomenological nature of these experiences is argued to render an explanation of them outside the tentacles of the physical or neurological sciences. sing., *quale*.

quality **1** Originally, in early forms of structuralism, a basic attribute of a sensation, an aspect of a thing that enabled it to be distinguished from other things. Qualities were expressed by names and labels, adjectives and modifiers, e.g. *pink*, $F^\#$, *hard*, etc. The point of this usage was to divorce the concept of quality from that of QUANTITY, the latter to be reserved for reference to differences in amount, degree or intensity of sensations and the former for differences in kinds of sensation. The distinction is not as easy to make as once thought. The term was used similarly to *quale*; see QUALIA. **2** A more-or-less quantitative assessment of the value or worth of a thing. Note, this meaning differs sharply from 1, having a distinctly quantitative connotation.

quality, primary and secondary A distinction first drawn by Democritus and revived several times by the likes of Galileo, Descartes, Newton and, most significantly, Locke, to the effect that the qualities that things possess may be separated into the primary and the secondary. The former encompasses those qualities that objects actually have (solidity, extension, shape, motion, number), while the latter covers those qualities that are only reactions to these (sounds, colours, tastes, etc.). The distinction is surely inviting and historically clearly robust, but it has turned out to be epistemologically problematic and is rarely made any more.

quanta Plural of QUANTUM.

quantal Pertaining to that which: **1** Changes in small discrete steps. **2** Occurs in small elemental units.

quantal hypothesis The hypothesis that continuous increments in a physical variable produce discrete (quantal) increases in sensation. The hypothesis has been extended to the neurological level, where it is called, not unexpectedly, the *neural quantal hypothesis*.

quantity An aspect or property of a thing that renders it countable or measurable in numerical terms. See and contrast with QUALITY (1).

quantum **1** In physics, the elemental unit of radiant energy. **2** More generally, any discrete amount of anything. pl., *quanta*.

quartile **1** One of the three points that divide an ordered distribution into four parts each containing one quarter of the scores. **2** One of the four parts of the distribution so divided. See the discussion under PARTILE and CENTILE for problems of usage encountered because of the inconsistency of meanings here.

quartile deviation One half of the difference between the third and first QUARTILES (1). Occasionally used as a 'quick and dirty' estimate of the variability of a distribution, particularly when the median is used as the measure of central tendency. Also known as the *semi-interquartile range*, it is, in a normal distribution, equal to the *probable error*.

quasi- A combining form used freely as an affix, an adjective or an adverb. The usual connotation is that the thing so qualified is but a resemblance of or only superficially similar to some other thing.

quasi-experimental research An umbrella term for any research carried out without full control over the independent variables. Much naturalistic social psychological research comes within this category,

such as analysis of people's reactions to natural disasters when the subjects are those who just happen to fall victim and are not selected by any controlled sampling procedure.

quasi group A sociological term often used to refer to an aggregate of persons with the, as yet unrealized, potential for forming into a true GROUP.

quasi need A term occasionally used for any nonbiological need.

quazepam A moderately potent BENZODIAZEPINE used mainly as a HYPNOTIC. It has rapid uptake accompanied by slow elimination leading to accumulation in the body and next-day sedation.

Queen's English KING'S ENGLISH.

queer Originally an epithet for *homosexual* (usually male), the term was co-opted by gay and lesbian activists who, by embracing it, turned it into an accepted and now widely used term. It is found in both lay and scientific writings and there are academic programmes in 'queer studies' and professional 'queer rights' activists.

questionary A rarely used synonym of QUESTIONNAIRE.

questionnaire Broadly, any set of questions dealing with any topic or group of related topics designed to be answered by a respondent.

Quételet index The original name of the BODY-MASS INDEX.

quetiapine An ATYPICAL ANTIDEPRESSANT DRUG used primarily in schizophrenia. In addition to blocking dopamine receptors, it blocks serotonin uptake. Common side effects are sedation and weight gain.

quick and dirty Laboratory slang for any simple technique for making a rough estimate. For example, 'eye-balling' a regression line, using the quartile deviation as a measure of variability, etc. Such procedures are called *quick* because they are, and *dirty* because they typically have a high error rate.

quickening The first foetal movements *in utero*. Typically felt between the 18th and 20th weeks of pregnancy, although earlier movements are not uncommon.

quiet biting attack PREDATORY ATTACK.

quintile 1 One of the four points that divide an ordered distribution into five parts each containing one-fifth of the scores. **2** One of the five parts of the distribution so divided.

quota control A way of establishing control over the sample of subjects selected for an investigation by using QUOTA *SAMPLING. See that entry for details.

quota sampling SAMPLING, QUOTA.

quotidian Daily, occurring daily.

quotidian variability Day-to-day variability.

quotient The result of the operation of dividing one number by another. Quotients are commonly used to express data in psychology, e.g. IQ = INTELLIGENCE QUOTIENT. When used in this way, their mathematical status as such is often misunderstood.

R

R A (sometimes confusingly) polyfunctional abbreviation. To wit: **1** *Response*, as in the common shorthand *S–R* for *stimulus–response*. **2** *Stimulus*, from the German word *Reiz*. The confusion once produced by these two conflicting uses is less these days as the latter use is now rare. **3** MULTIPLE *CORRELATION coefficient. **4** A general *reasoning* factor hypothesized by some to be a primary mental ability.

R$_c$ An infrequent abbreviation for *conditioned response*; *CR* is more common.

R$_G$ In Hull's theory, any goal-attaining response, e.g. eating, drinking.

R$_{1, 2, 3,...n}$ MULTIPLE *CORRELATION coefficient.

R$_P$ The probability of a response. This abbreviation is used little, *p* being the more common notation for probability, with the response under consideration usually being clear from context.

R$_u$ An infrequent abbreviation for *unconditioned response*; *UR* and *UCR* are encountered more often.

r **1** The PRODUCT-MOMENT *CORRELATION coefficient: see also R$_{xy}$. **2** In Hull's theory, the efferent reaction leading to an overt response. Also called a PURE-STIMULUS *ACT.

r$_{bis}$ The BISERIAL *CORRELATION coefficient.

r$_G$ In Hull's theory, a FRACTIONAL ANTEDATING GOAL RESPONSE.

r$_{12.34}$ PARTIAL *CORRELATION coefficient. It denotes the correlation between the variables to the left of the point (here, 1 and 2) after the influences of those to the right (here, 3 and 4) have been removed.

r$_2$ The square of the value of a PRODUCT-MOMENT *CORRELATION coefficient. It provides an estimate of the proportion of the variance in the data that can be attributed to the relationship. Occasionally written *r-squared*.

r$_t$ The TETRACHORIC *CORRELATION coefficient. Also denoted as r_{tet}.

r$_{tet}$ R$_T$.

r$_{xy}$ The PRODUCT-MOMENT *CORRELATION with the variables (*x* and *y*) that enter into its computation denoted.

race A term born in anthropological innocence and meant simply to designate the major subdivisions of *Homo sapiens*. A race was defined as any relatively large division of persons that could be distinguished from others on the basis of inherited physical characteristics such as skin pigmentation, blood groups, hair texture and the like. In actual practice, it is nearly impossible to classify or distinguish individual persons by such physical characteristics, for no specific set of them truly constitutes criterial features. If the concept has any residual meaning in this respect, it is only when the relative frequency of occurrence of physical traits in a population is assessed. For example, there are many 'blacks' with lighter skins than many 'whites', so skin colour cannot serve as a definitive criterion for any arbitrarily selected individual. However, among the population of persons who identify themselves as 'black' there will be a higher relative frequency of dark-skinned individuals than among the population of those who identify themselves as 'white'. Since the key criterion here is *identify themselves as*, it is clear that the working definition of race is one that is dependent upon a social–cultural–political identification and not one that can be unambiguously determined by genetic classification. See also RACE DIFFERENCES.

race differences Those characteristics that are supposedly distinctive of the members of one race and serve to distinguish them from those of other races. When large populations of persons are under consideration, a variety of physical traits can be identified and, with the proper caveats (see RACE), the use of the term in this domain is not disputed. The difficulties with it emerge when nonobvious characteristics such as intelligence and aptitudes for particular professions are examined with respect to possible differential distributions in different races. These difficulties come in two forms. First is the problem of the determination of the existence of racial differences on such psychological dimensions. Here the research is badly muddled because of the difficulties of measurement associated with factors like INTELLIGENCE (see which for discussion). Second is the problem of assignment of cause for any differences that may eventually emerge. Strictly speaking, the use of the term *race differences* does not necessarily entail the presumption of genetic differences since sociocultural differences associated with racial identification in a society may yield differences that emerge on standard tests. However, as the term *race* itself carries unambiguous genetic connotations, many authors use *race differences* with this implication as well.

It is an unhappy commentary that this phrase rates such an extensive entry in a contemporary lexicon of psychology. The focus on the assessment of differences to the neglect of that which is universal distorts issues of paramount social, political and individual importance.

race prejudice Any PREJUDICE based on race. See RACISM (esp. 2).

racialism RACISM.

racial memory MEMORY, RACIAL.

racial unconscious COLLECTIVE UNCONSCIOUS.

racism 1 A PREJUDICE based on race and characterized by attitudes and beliefs about the inferior nature of persons of other races. This sense is close in many ways to ETHNOCENTRISM (1). **2** A social/political doctrine that argues for differential social, economic, educational and legal treatment of persons based on their race. Sense 1 does not entail adherence to the doctrine of 2 nor to its programme of discriminatory practices; 2, however, assumes the attitudes of racial superiority of 1. See the discussions of RACE and RACE DIFFERENCES for more on the connotations of usage. var., *racialism*.

racism, aversive A form of racism in which little or no conscious prejudice is expressed verbally but behavioural evidence belies a discriminatory attitude. It is observed in individuals who express respect of persons of diverse backgrounds, yet favour their own when making decisions about friendship, entertainment or employment, or make unthinking remarks that are hurtful to a person of another race or ethnicity. Probably the dominant form of racism in contemporary society, it is generally unconscious and unrecognized by the persons exhibiting it. var., *aversive racialism*.

radial-arm maze A maze consisting of a central hub out from which a number of arms (usually six or seven) radiate.

radial glia GLIA.

radiance RADIANT ENERGY as measured by the rate of emission and the area of the source.

radiant energy Electromagnetic energy usually conceptualized as propagated in wave form. Although the full spectrum of radiant energy runs from the very long wavelengths (e.g. radio waves with peak-to-peak wavelengths of up to 3×10^{15} nm) to the very short wavelengths (e.g. cosmic rays, 3×10^{-9} nm), the area of roughly 400–750 nm is visible and generally called *light*.

radiation 1 Generally, the spread of energy from some source through space or matter. **2** Specifically, neural radiation, usually expressed as the spread of neural excitation. **3** The radiation of pain from a source. **4** RADIANT ENERGY.

radical The core meaning here is *pertaining to a root*. Thus: **1** In mathematics, a sign ($\sqrt{}$) signifying the operation of factoring the quantity under it into its roots. **2** In social/political terms, descriptive of any point of view or proposal that argues for basic, fundamental change. **3** A person who advocates such change. See RADICALISM.

radicalism 1 Generally, any sociopolitical point of view that advocates extreme, rapid and fundamental change. Radicalism is, strictly speaking, a nonconformist point of view with dramatic societal change as its aim and, thus, is not necessarily associated with either the left or the right poles of the political spectrum. However: **2** An extreme ideological perspective of the left.

rage A term usually taken to refer to the extreme end of the domain of emotionality denoted by ANGER, i.e. anger that has got out of control. It is usually identified by the same patterns of visceral and muscular responses as less extreme anger, but the pattern is more extreme and more intense, and an attack response is considered more likely.

railway illusion PONZO ILLUSION.

ramping A progressive moderate increase in some process, function or act. It is commonly used to refer to the slow progressive movements moderated by the basal ganglia (called *ramp movements*). Occasionally, it will be used to characterize gradual increases in neural activity (contrast here with BISTABILITY) and to progressive increases in a skill.

ramus 1 Any branch of a nerve or vein. **2** Any of the several branches of each of the spinal nerves.

random Most dictionaries attempt to define this term by listing synonyms or near-synonyms. The typical list includes words or phrases like *haphazard, by chance, occurring without voluntary control, aimless, purposeless*, etc. While it is true that *random* is used in ways that correspond to these (e.g. one frequently sees references to *random activity, random thinking*, etc.), such clustering of synonyms tends to miss the essential point. Randomness is a mathematical or statistical concept, and the term means simply that there is *no detectable systematicity* in the sequence of events observed. Strictly speaking, *random* refers not to a thing but to the *lack* of a thing, the lack of pattern or structure or regularity. For more discussion, see another often misunderstood term, CHANCE.

random activity The usual reference of this term is behaviour that is aimless or purposeless. Note, however, that it is not used to imply that the activity so labelled is intrinsically without aim, nor that it is acausal; rather it is used to label behaviour in which

the observer cannot discern any clear aim, purpose or eliciting stimulus. See RANDOM.

random dot stereogram JULESZ'S STEREOGRAM.

random effects model RANDOM *FACTOR.

random error CHANCE *ERROR.

random factor FACTOR, RANDOM.

random group RANDOM *SAMPLE.

randomization test One of the more powerful nonparametric statistical tests. It is based on the determination of the exact probabilities of an observed set of differences in scores between two matched samples and the assessment of just how likely such a difference would be under the null hypothesis of no difference in the underlying distributions.

randomize 1 To select or choose objects, events, experimental subjects, etc. in such a way that there are no detectible biases or systematic patterns. That is, to make one's selections so that each event has an equal and independent chance of being sampled. **2** To arrange a sequence or collection of events in such a way that there is no detectable pattern or systematicity. See RANDOM, RANDOM *SAMPLE.

randomized block design BLOCK DESIGN, RANDOMIZED.

random mating MATING, RANDOM.

random movement RANDOM ACTIVITY.

random noise WHITE *NOISE; see also NOISE (1).

random number The concept of a single random number makes no sense except in terms of the manner in which it was selected or chosen, i.e. a number that has been selected at random from a RANDOM NUMBER TABLE or a RANDOM NUMBER GENERATOR.

random number generator (RNG) Any device that functions to produce sequences of RANDOM NUMBERS. Some are based on physical effects such as those of subatomic particles that reflect processes of quantum mechanics. Most, however, are computer programs that generate 'pseudorandom' numbers that follow algorithms for producing sequences that, while not truly random, lack easily detectable patterns or structures.

random number table A large collection of digits tabulated in such a way that there is no statistically detectable pattern or systematicity in the table. In all practical cases, when a table consists of but several thousand digits, true randomness is only approximated. Such tables are common in text books; however, in research a RANDOM NUMBER GENERATOR is typically used.

random observation Any observation or series of observations made without any systematic pattern and without preconception about what is to be observed. Random observation is an important control procedure, particularly in naturalistic studies when periodic observations may produce biased data.

random ratio (**RR**) See SCHEDULES OF *REINFORCEMENT.

random sample SAMPLE, RANDOM.

random variable Any variable, the values of which are determined randomly. *Random* here refers to the manner in which the values are chosen, not to the variable itself. For more detail, see RANDOM.

random variation Those differences in the values of a variable that are due to chance. Also called *random error*.

range The standard dictionary meaning is basic to all uses in psychology: the extent to which, or the limits between which, variation can occur. Thus: **1** The interval or 'distance' between the highest and lowest scores in a distribution. **2** In statistics, a crude measure of the variability or dispersion of a set of scores. It is obtained by subtracting the lowest score from the highest. **3** In sociology and ethology, the physical area over which a particular group lives or a particular species is found. Compare with HABITAT. **4** In psychophysics, the domain or interval over which a particular sensory system functions, e.g. the *audibility range*.

range, audibility AUDIBILITY RANGE.

range, discriminating The range of scores on a test that have reliable predictive values. For example, the scores above roughly the 90th percentile on the Graduate Record Examination lie outside of this range since

there are no reliable predictive differences found between those students who score within this interval.

rank 1 n. In statistics, the position in an ordered series of scores. The rank of a score on some measure tells only where that score is relative to all others (i.e. 1st, 2nd, 3rd, ... n^{th}); it reveals nothing about the distance between the scores. Scores that are ranked form an ORDINAL *SCALE and, hence, only nonparametric statistics may be used in analysing them. **2** vb. To order or arrange scores, events, individuals, etc. in a graded (i.e. ranked) order.

rank-difference correlation CORRELATION, RANK-ORDER.

ranked distribution DISTRIBUTION, RANKED.

rank order Any ordering of scores according to RANK.

rank-order correlation CORRELATION, RANK-ORDER.

rank transformation A transformation of scores in a distribution where the actual values are replaced with ranks, usually for the purpose of carrying out nonparametric statistical tests.

Ranschburg effect Under tachistoscopic viewing conditions more individual stimuli can be recognized if all are different than if some are identical.

Ranvier, nodes of Small gaps in the myelin sheath of nerve fibres.

raphe 1 In anatomy generally, a crease or seam marking the joining of two halves. **2** Specifically, a complex of nuclei in the core of the brainstem. See RAPHE NUCLEI. var., *rhaphe*.

raphe nuclei A group of nuclei located in the midline of the RETICULAR FORMATION of the medulla, pons and midbrain. The vast majority of the brain's serotonergic neurons (see SEROTONIN) are found here and project widely to such areas as the thalamus, basal ganglia, hippocampus and neocortex. Some of these projections synapse on other neurons (see M SYSTEM), others release their serotonin diffusely (see D SYSTEM).

rapid-cycling bipolar disorder BIPOLAR DISORDER, RAPID-CYCLING.

rapid eye movements (REM) The rapid, jerky eye movements characteristic of one particular stage of sleep. For details, see REM SLEEP, SLEEP and related terms.

rapid serial (or **sequential**) **visual presentation (RSVP)** A procedure used in the study of perception whereby a series of visual stimuli are presented rapidly one after the other.

rapport 1 Generally, a comfortable, relaxed, unconstrained, mutually accepting interaction between persons, especially when the persons are a tester and a subject in psychological testing, a client and a therapist in therapy, or the like. **2** In *hypnosis*, the affective contract between hypnotist and subject so that the latter will 'accept' the suggestions of the former. **3** In *parapsychology*, the presumed relationship between a medium and his or her spiritual contact.

RAS (or **ras**) RETICULAR ACTIVATING SYSTEM.

rate 1 n. A ratio expressed as the number of occurrences or observations of some event within a specific period of time divided by either (a) the total number of possible occurrences of that event, or (b) a standardized number of units. For example, *annual birth rate* can be given as the number of births per year relative to either (a) the total number of women of child-bearing age, or (b) a standardized number of such women, e.g. 100, 1,000, 1,000,000. **2** n. The number of occurrences of some event within a specified time period; e.g. the *response rate* is a common dependent variable in operant-conditioning experiments and is usually given as the raw number of responses per minute or some other time unit. **3** n. Shorthand for RATE OF CHANGE. **4** vb. To assign a number or score reflecting ordinal position or RANK on some variable. **5** vb. To assign a RATING.

ratee A person being rated.

rate law In neurophysiology, the generalization that the strength of a stimulus is represented by the rate at which the axon of a neuron fires. See also ALL-OR-NONE LAW (1).

rate of change An expression that reflects the RATE (1 or 2) at which change is observed to occur. It is expressed as a ratio of the amount of change observed in a given time period to the value prior to the change.

rater One who carries out a RATING.

rater reliability INTERRATER *RELIABILITY.

rate score In timed tests, a score based on the number of problems or tasks completed per unit time.

rating 1 An estimate or evaluation of an object, event or person (including oneself, the so-called *self-rating*). Ratings are used commonly in social and personality research to measure qualities and characteristics that are subjective and for which no objective measurement techniques exist. See RATING SCALE et seq. **2** An occasional synonym of RANK (1). This semantic equivalence derives from the fact that rating procedures often utilize ORDINAL *SCALES which are based on ranks.

rating, behaviour The use of rating techniques in a fairly restricted manner such that only overt, objectively observable behaviours enter into the assessment. The term is used to refer to either an assessing of the degree to which specific behaviours are observed to occur or a simple recording of the presence or absence of particular behaviours.

rating scale Generally, any device used to assist a rater in making ratings. Social scientists have developed a rather impressive array of such devices: the more commonly used are listed below.

rating scale, bipolar Any rating scale of which the dimensions along which the ratings are made are specified by two opposing poles, with the scale itself laid out between these. A typical scale of this kind consists of a list of dimensions such as 'good–bad', 'pleasant–unpleasant', 'cooperative–uncooperative'; the respondent marks the point between, or at one of, the two poles which is appropriate for what or whomever is being rated.

rating scale, check-list A rating scale based upon a list of traits or characteristics in which the rater checks those that apply to the person being rated. Such scales are often used in self-reporting procedures.

rating scale, graphic Any rating scale that utilizes a graphic or pictorial format. The most commonly used is for an attitude statement, which is presented with a line marked from positive at one end, through neutral in the middle, to negative at the other end. The rater marks a spot on the line at the point that represents his or her attitude with respect to the statement.

rating scale, itemized A rating scale based on a series of ordered categories (e.g. most negative to most positive, most desirable to least desirable, most characteristic to least characteristic). The rater selects the one category that is most applicable to the item or person under consideration.

ratio A quotient, a relationship between any two magnitudes expressed as the product of division.

ratio estimation METHODS OF *SCALING.

rational 1 Relating to or suggestive of the use of reason, the process of reasoning or the property of being reasonable. **2** Pertaining to that which is correct or, at least, justifiable by reason, e.g. a rational decision. **3** Descriptive of an organism capable of high mental functioning; our own species is often called (seriously as well as in jest) the *rational animal*. **4** Connoting sanity or lucidity. **5** Primarily cognitive in nature as opposed to emotional.

rational authority AUTHORITY, RATIONAL.

rationale The reason or the grounds offered for an opinion, attitude, decision, etc. The usual implication is that a rationale is reasonable (see RATIONAL) and that it is consciously reached and expressible.

rational-economic man A general model of behaviour predicated on the assumption that the basic, fundamental principle underlying human nature is the rational (*sic!*) striving for self-interest, particularly economic and material gain. The term and the theory it denotes suffer from a variety of problems. Its core assumption is flawed in that people typically do not act rationally in their decision-making (see PROSPECT THEORY) and its entailments are suspect in that the world view it promotes can undermine SUSTAINABILITY, because each individual or organization that follows it attempts to maximize private, immediate gains.

rational emotive (behaviour) therapy A form of psychotherapy developed by Albert Ellis which focuses on the rational, problem-solving aspects of emotional and beha-

vioural disorders. Ellis's approach was highly directive (see DIRECTIVE THERAPY), consisting in large measure of telling the client what he or she must do in order to be happy and then 'encouraging' him or her, often through confrontation and encounter, to act and think accordingly. Although related in some ways to the behaviour therapies, the rational emotive approach is distinguishable from them in being strongly cognitive and emotive. In recent years Ellis took to calling the approach rational emotive *behaviour* therapy to emphasize the fact that while it has an emotive, cognitive base, the primary goal is to change behaviours.

rational equation EQUATION, RATIONAL.

rationalism Any of several philosophical perspectives all of which share the assumption that truth is to be ascertained through the use of reason, of rational thought. Older forms of rationalism (e.g. Platonic, medieval theological) maintained that *only* through reason could ultimate truth be discovered. More modern perspectives (e.g. Chomskyan linguistics) are not quite so totally antiempirical; rational deductions are generally treated as susceptible to empirical demonstration and test.

rationality A state characterized by reasonableness, a willingness to accept that which is well reasoned.

rationality, bounded 1 A particular characteristic of human decision-making under conditions of extreme complexity. **2** A theory of cognitive processes as they are displayed under such conditions. In either usage, the reference is to the notion that in the face of complexity one cannot behave in a totally rational manner, simply because one's information-processing capacities are too limited to encompass all the knowledge required for such ideal decision-making. The theory of bounded rationality describes individuals as decision-makers who circumscribe the situation by limiting (or bounding) the amount of information to be dealt with – often in creative and imaginative ways – and then behaving in a rational fashion with this limited knowledge base. The theory is most closely associated with the work of the American economist-philosopher-psychologist Herbert Simon, who was awarded the Nobel Prize in Economics for it.

rationality, procedural   RATIONALITY in decision-making based on the use of logical reasoning. Procedural rationality is process focused and is often contrasted with *substantive rationality* where the focus is on the nature of the final decision itself. Interestingly, procedurally rational processes can lead to nonrational outcomes if the ˙ ...al premises are flawed, and substantively rational decisions can be rational even if reached illogically.

rationality, substantive   See PROCEDURAL *RATIONALTIY.

rationalization 1 In general terms, the process through which things that are confusing and obscure and irrational (or, better perhaps, *non*rational) are made clear, concise and rational. **2** In psychoanalytic theory the term carries the general sense of 1 but with the additional connotation that the process serves as a DEFENCE MECHANISM to conceal the true motivations for one's actions, thoughts or feelings. **3** The outcome of the rationalization process in either of the above senses.

rational-legal authority   LEGAL *AUTHORITY.

rational problem-solving   The reaching of a solution to a problem through the use of logical, systematic reasoning. Because the emphasis is on the process, not the outcome, identical solutions arrived at using other means (e.g. insight) are not counted.

rational psychology   A cover term for any approach to psychology in which the overall theoretical structure for interpretation and understanding of psychological phenomena is grounded in a theological and/or philosophical framework. Note that the term really has a rather narrow reference in that defence of the position derives from the philosophical foundations of RATIONALISM. Rational psychology is, thus, usually contrasted sharply with empirical or scientific approaches to psychology.

rational types   In Jung's classification of personality types, individuals whose dominant mode of functioning is based on feeling and thinking. These types are contrasted with the so-called *irrational types*, who tend to utilize sensing and intuiting. Note that by *irrational*, Jung really meant *nonrational*. See also FUNCTION TYPES.

rational uniformity   Social uniformity based on the (rational?) assumption that it is usually easier and ultimately to one's advantage to conform to social norms. The term is used to characterize behaviour based not on one's true personal desires or values but on the belief that one can profit by going along with others.

ratio production   METHODS OF *SCALING.

ratio reinforcement   REINFORCEMENT, RATIO.

ratio scale   SCALE, RATIO.

rat man   In the psychoanalytic literature, the sobriquet for the man described by Freud in his classic analysis of an obsessive neurotic.

rauwolfia alkaloids   A group of drugs derived from an Indian climbing shrub that includes RESERPINE (see for more detail).

Raven's Progressive Matrices   PROGRESSIVE MATRICES TEST.

raw data   Data which have not been coded, transformed or analysed. See RAW *SCORE.

Rayleigh equation   A quantitative relationship between the proportions of red and green needed to match a given yellow. Typically, the subject is given a spectral green and a spectral red and required to mix them until they match the hue of a spectral yellow target. The resulting equation is a sensitive test for ANOMALOUS *TRICHROMACY.

reactance, psychological   An unpleasant drive state brought about by a threat to one's perceived freedom.

reactance theory   A point of view which maintains that, under the appropriate circumstances, people will react against attempts to restrict or control their choices and decisions. The theory makes two important predictions: (a) because the attractiveness or desirability of an object or activity is assumed to be related to the opportunity to choose it or engage in it, the more an individual perceives that others are attempting to limit his or her opportunities the more attractive the object or activity becomes; and (b) when an individual perceives that strong pressure is being exerted to force a particular decision or attitude, he or she will tend to become contrary and resist the pressure by selecting an opposing perspective. See also REACTIVE (3).

reaction 1 Basically, a 're-action', response, act, movement, etc. that an organism makes when stimulated. **2** By extension, a group or social response against social change. The connotation here is that this kind of reaction is politically or culturally conservative in the extreme, or *reactionary*. **3** In psychiatry, a cluster of behaviours or a syndrome characteristic of a particular disorder. Often the longer phrase *reaction pattern* is used; see also REACTION FORMATION.

reaction, false 1 Any response to an inappropriate stimulus. **2** A FALSE ALARM.

reaction formation The process through which unacceptable feelings or impulses are controlled by establishing behaviour patterns directly opposed to them. According to classical psychoanalytical theory, reaction formation operates by repressing the original impulse, which is assumed to continue to exist unconsciously in its original form and is, thus, likely to emerge under some circumstances. The concept has played an important role in theoretical analyses of various clinical cases, e.g. those in which a pattern of antisocial behaviour has precipitously emerged in a person with a past history of kindliness and solicitude.

reaction potential In Hull's learning theory, the likelihood of occurrence of a particular response.

reaction range In behavioural genetics, the limits on the expression of a *phenotype* that are imposed by the *genotype*. Compare with NORM OF REACTION.

reaction-specific energy ACTION-SPECIFIC ENERGY.

reaction time (RT) Generally, the time between the presentation of a stimulus and the subject's response to it. The RT is one of experimental psychology's oldest dependent variables and several specialized types have been studied; these are described in the following entries. Note that the term refers to the actual time that it takes a subject to respond as well as the experimental procedure that uses RTs as the basic data. When unqualified, the term refers to SIMPLE *REACTION TIME.

reaction time, associative In word association experiments, the time between the presentation of a stimulus word and the subject's verbal response.

reaction time, choice An extension of SIMPLE *REACTION TIME. In this case the subject is confronted with two (or more) stimuli and two (or more) corresponding responses.

reaction time, complex (or **compound**) Any reaction time when two (or more) stimuli and/or two (or more) responses are employed, i.e. all possible variations other than SIMPLE *REACTION TIME.

reaction time, discrimination A variation of CHOICE *REACTION TIME in which there are two distinctive stimuli and the subject is instructed to respond to just one of them and refrain from making a response to the other.

reaction time, disjunctive An umbrella term covering CHOICE, COMPLEX and DISCRIMINATION *REACTION TIME procedures.

reaction time, simple The minimum lag between a single simple stimulus (e.g. a light or tone) and the subject's making of a single simple response (e.g. pressing a button or releasing a switch).

reactivation of memory A term often used with respect to memories which have been triggered by some external cue or event. See e.g. PRIMING.

reactive 1 Very generally, a synonym of RESPONSIVE. However, there are two additional meanings of the term that are occasionally intended: **2** Pertaining to or characterizing an action that is a reaction. That is, of an action that is not internally motivated but rather occurs as a response to a particular stimulus or to particular actions of another. This is the sense intended in most of the compound terms containing this word given in the following entries. **3** Contrary. This usage amplifies the preceding by appending the notion that the reaction is an attempt to rescue one's personal freedom from attempts by others to restrict choice or direct behaviour. See REACTANCE THEORY.

reactive attachment disorder A disorder of childhood or infancy characterized by failure to develop normal social relatedness prior to the age of five. The disturbance is marked either by persistent failure to initiate or respond appropriately to social interactions or (in older children) by indiscriminate sociability particularly with strangers and other socially inappropriate individuals. The disorder is presumed due to grossly pathological early care marked by a lack of normal physical and social stimulation, since it has been observed even when there is good nutrition and sanitation. Note, the term is not used if there is evidence of mental retardation or any other pervasive developmental disorder. Also called *hospitalism*; see also ANACLITIC DEPRESSION and FAILURE-TO-THRIVE.

reactive depression DEPRESSION, REACTIVE.

reactive inhibition INHIBITION, REACTIVE.

reactive psychosis A psychosis that stems from strong environmental pressures and stresses. Also called *situational psychosis*. See BRIEF REACTIVE PSYCHOSIS.

reactive reinforcement In psychoanalysis, a hypothesized process whereby conscious attempts at emotion and affect bolster (i.e. reinforce) the opposite emotion at an unconscious level. Conscious aggression theoretically stimulates unconscious nonaggression and vice versa.

reactive schizophrenia SCHIZOPHRENIA, REACTIVE.

reactive type A general term applied to individuals whose primary mode of behaving is reacting to others.

readability 1 Loosely, a measure of the understandability of written text as given by an analysis of a variety of factors, including syntactic complexity, vocabulary, thematic expression and continuity of themes. **2** A measure of how readable a text is based on the average grade level of readers who can read and understand it.

These two usages are insidiously contradictory and lead to anomalous constructions like 'One would be advised to lower the readability of the school's text books.' What such a statement means in sense 2 is that the texts used for, say, 5th-graders, are written at too high a level for the average 5th-grade student. However, in sense 1 it connotes that the understandability of the text should be lowered, i.e. that it should be made harder to read. Since both meanings are used widely, caution is advised.

readiness 1 A position of preparedness in which an organism is set to act or to respond. **2** A state of a person such that they are in a position to profit from some experience. Depending on the type of experience, this state may be conceptualized as relatively simple and biologically determined (e.g. sexual readiness) or developmentally and cognitively complex (e.g. reading readiness).

readiness, law of In Thorndike's early theory of learning, the hypothesized principle that satisfaction was derived from the functioning of behavioural 'conduction units' (a notion that was never clearly specified) which were ready to function. This 'law' and its corresponding *law of unreadiness* (functioning is unpleasant if the unit is not ready) are now only of historical importance.

readiness potential An evoked potential that occurs roughly 300 msec before an individual claims to have 'just decided' to make a particular response. On the face of it, this potential is fascinating since it suggests that the brain has already 'decided' that the response is going to be made before the individual 'wills' it to be made. However, on closer inspection it is not quite so mysterious. If one factors in the time it takes for the brain to carry out the neural processes linked with knowing *when* the decision to respond was made, the anticipatory element becomes less clear. In fact, trying to analyse cortical functions in a linear fashion is almost certainly unwise. The neural processes are best viewed as complexly interwoven with each other rather than as beads on a string.

readiness test A general label for any test that assesses READINESS (2). Such tests are a common feature of educational programmes.

reading 1 In simplest terms, the process by which information is extracted from written or printed text. This process, in fact, is extremely complex and only partly understood, although two critical aspects of it deserve mention here. First, the process of reading is dependent on the written format, the ORTHOGRAPHY. To read an alphabetic system of writing like English requires that one decode the phonetic relationships that exist between the marks on the page (letters) and the sounds of the spoken language, whereas to read a logographic system like Chinese requires one to match the marks on the page (the ideograms) with the word or concept in the language that each represents. Thus, alphabetic systems carry an intervening stage of decoding of the phonetic component, a stage not involved in the use of logographic systems. The term *reading*, therefore, entails different cognitive and perceptual processes depending on orthographic form. Second, reading consists of both a phonetic/acoustic process and a semantic/syntactic process. Consider the hypothetical example of an illiterate Greek farmer and his English professor friend whose schooling has taught him how to pronounce all the Greek letters and letter combinations although he cannot speak a word of modern Greek. The professor pronounces what for him are the nonsense sounds from a Greek newspaper for his illiterate friend, who comprehends their meaning perfectly. Neither of the two can be said to be *reading*, yet between them they represent the skills that a reader must have. The purpose of raising these points here is to clarify for the reader the fact that many simplistic definitions of reading which characterize the process in terms of pronouncing words are misleading and blur the deeper, more important aspects of the process. It is likely that many of the problems involved in the teaching of reading derive from our failure as yet to understand fully these various processes.

2 By extension of the word *text* in the simple definition given above, the term is also applied to the extraction of information from Braille symbols, musical notation, patterns of lip movements, gestures, etc. **3** In parapsychology, the interpretations of a fortune-teller, phrenologist, palmist, etc.

reading age 1 The typical age at which a normal child is generally expected to begin to learn to read. This meaning is outmoded and simplistic; see the discussion under READING READINESS. **2** A score on a standardized reading test given in terms of *age equivalent* scores.

reading disability (or disorder) DEVELOPMENTAL *READING DISORDER.

reading-disabled child DEVELOPMENTAL *READING DISORDER.

reading disorder, developmental An ACADEMIC SKILLS DISORDER characterized by a marked failure in learning to read. The term is usually (but not always) reserved for a child who falls significantly (i.e. two or more grades) below the norms for his or her age and educational level (provided that he or she does not show any significant mental retardation and no obvious neurological pathology). See also DYSLEXIA.

reading readiness A term used to characterize the degree to which a child is prepared to profit from instruction in reading. Exactly what competences and skills define this preparedness are far from clear, but a variety of factors – perceptual, cognitive, emotional and motivational – have been implicated. The notion that chronological age is, in any sense, the indicator is misleading.

reading span Roughly, the amount of written text that can be perceived within a single FIXATION PAUSE. Although various values such as seven to ten letter-spaces are often cited as typical, several facts about the span must be noted: (a) the size of the span corresponds to foveal vision and the number of letter-spaces within this region depends on the size of the type used in the printing of the material and the distance at which the text is held from the eyes; (b) some information outside the foveal area can be used by a fluent reader during the course of normal reading, e.g. spaces between words, capital letters, etc.; (c) the fovea is circular and most measurements of reading span are made only linearly using a single line of text at a time. In normal reading, information from adjacent lines is also often picked up and used. Occasionally called *eye span* or *visual span*.

reafference A cover term for those sensory events that are produced by voluntary movements of a sense organ, e.g. those resulting from the movement of an image across the retina that accompany voluntary movements of the eye. They are contrasted with *exafference*, or those sensory events produced by changes in the stimulus itself, e.g. those resulting from movement of an image across the retina that accompany real displacements of the physical object.

real **1** Existing, actual, nonimaginary. **2** Empirical, as opposed to theoretical. **3** Physical, as opposed to mental; objective, as opposed to subjective.

real anxiety See OBJECTIVE ANXIETY.

real definition DEFINITIONS (esp. (c)).

realism **1** A philosophical point of view which argues that abstract concepts have a coherent real existence and are thus subject to empirical study. Contrast with NOMINALISM (1). **2** A philosophical point of view which maintains that the physical world has a reality separate from perception and mind. Contrast with IDEALISM (1). **3** An attitude generally characterized as the recognition that there are limits to the impact that one can have upon the world. Distinguish from CONSERVATISM, which resists change, and from IDEALISM (2), which ignores issues of pragmatics. **4** A term used by Piaget in some of his earlier writings to characterize a young child's belief that its perceptual perspective is shared by others; e.g. if a child can see a photograph held up by an adult, the child assumes that the adult can also see it. See here EGOCENTRISM, which is used more or less equivalently.

realistic anxiety ANXIETY, REALISTIC.

reality **1** Most restrictively, those aspects of the physical universe that are directly or indirectly measurable. In this sense, reality is objective and limited to what can be publicly and reliably measured. **2** By extension, the term may be used to refer to constructs that are inferable or interpretable from logical induction or theoretical analysis, but not measurable in the above sense; e.g. gravity, natural selection and personality would all be regarded as parts of reality according to 2, although they may be problematical for 1. **3** By yet another extension, the term is used by many to refer to all that which forms an integral part of what an individual believes to be REAL (1). Thus, free will, ghosts, God, etc. form a compelling part of reality for some but not for all. For an extension of this last meaning, see SOCIAL *REALITY.

reality adaptation In psychoanalytic theory, the process through which an infant gradually brings its perceptions, desires, needs, etc. into line with the external reality. It is often characterized as a trading-in of the pleasure–pain principle for the reality principle.

reality, contact with Perceiving and assessing the environment in ways coordinate with one's social and cultural schemes and values. Note that in this phrase the word *reality* is used in the sense of SOCIAL *REALITY and not necessarily in any of the other senses that it has; see REALITY.

reality, flight from Generally, the use of fantasy and imaginary satisfactions to avoid dealing with a harsh reality. It may be manifested in any number of ways, including excessive day-dreaming, inappropriate rationalization, resorting to drugs or alcohol and, in extreme cases, FUGUE. Also called *retreat from reality*.

reality monitoring A term coined by M. K. Johnson for the cognitive functions involved in paying attention to, coding and processing the events in one's life.

reality principle **1** In psychoanalytic theory, the recognition of the real environment by a child, the growing awareness of its demands and the need to accommodate to them. Normal development is seen here as the acquisition and strengthening of this reality principle to function as a brake on or modifier of the more primitive, unreal, pleasure principle. **2** In speech-act theory, the assumption that the speaker is talking about real things and events.

reality, social REALITY (3) that is dependent upon or, indeed, defined by the consensus of a group. The term is applicable to anything from a very small group to a whole society. Thus, the social reality shared by a small band of fanatics who are awaiting the end of the world on a mountain-top is as REAL (1) as the nearly universal belief in the value of education.

reality-testing **1** Very generally, any process by which an organism systematically assesses the limits on its behaviour imposed by the external environment. This meaning is inclusive of the following, more specialized uses of the term. **2** A set of perceptual, cognitive and sensorimotor acts that enables one to determine one's relationship with the external physical and social environments. This meaning is typically expressed with the connotation that one is determining just how far one can go in having an impact on the environment, in attempting to modify or alter events and processes. In childhood, this is viewed as an intimate aspect of cognitive growth and socialization. A breakdown of reality-testing in this sense in adulthood is taken as symptomatic of a PSYCHOTIC DISORDER. **3** In psychoanalytic theory, a set of ego functions that enable a child to distinguish between subjective impression and external reality and to adjust the primitive subjective components to the constraints of the objective environment. DELUSIONS and HALLUCINATIONS are viewed here as failures of reality-testing.

reality therapy THERAPY, REALITY.

real motion MOTION, REAL.

real self SELF, REAL.

reason **1** n. A rough synonym of *logical thought*. Originally, reason was viewed as an integral mental *faculty* which functioned in a purely *rational* manner. This meaning is rarely intended in contemporary writings. **2** n. A justification offered as an explanation (or apology) for one's actions, usually expressed in terms of one's motivations. **3** n. An objective cause for some event. **4** n. A logical, sound mind. **5** vb. To think rationally and logically.

reasoned action, theory of In social psychology, a theory that attempts to explain the link between attitudes that people have and the actual behaviours they display. It assumes that behaviour is ultimately the result of *behavioural intentions* and that these intentions are themselves the end product of an integration of: (a) attitudes toward specific behaviours, (b) the subjective perception of norms regarding specific behaviours, and (c) the perceived amount of control an individual feels he or she has over specific behaviours. Also called the *theory of planned behaviour*.

reasoning **1** In general, thinking, with the implication that the process is logical and coherent. **2** More specifically, problem-solving, whereby well-formed hypotheses are tested systematically and solutions are logically deduced. Note that the term is used with the sense that it is the cognitive processes that are of concern, not whether the correct outcome is achieved. Perfectly logical reasoning can easily lead to the wrong solution if one's initial assumptions are at fault.

reassurance A label for the myriad devices that psychotherapists use to instil confidence in their clients that the therapy really is worth all the trouble and that a favourable outcome is in the offing.

reattachment DETACHED AFFECT.

rebelliousness, neurotic One of Karen Horney's forms of what she called NEUROTIC *RESIGNATION. It is characterized by a continuous, active reaction on the part of the person displaying it. Horney hypothesized it as being directed either against outside persons and societal influences or toward one's own internalized regulations.

Reber's law This law, never before publicly articulated, was the outcome of work on this dictionary. It states, quite simply, that the closer anything is examined, the more complex it is seen to be.

rebirth fantasy In psychoanalysis, a fantasy of being born. Often expressed in symbolic form, e.g. a dream of emerging from water.

rebirthing Any of several techniques built around the dubious assumption that reliving one's birth, either by so-called hypnotic regression or focused reflection can be used therapeutically. See INNOVATIVE THERAPIES for reasons for maintaining a sceptical stance.

rebound (effect) **1** Generally, any phenomenon characterized by a distinct increase in some behaviour following a period during which it was depressed or inhibited, e.g. a physical rebound following an illness. **2** In the phrase *rebound effect*, however, the meaning is usually restricted to an increase in some physiological function following a period of inhibition or deprivation, e.g. an increase in *REM sleep* following one or more nights of REM deprivation.

rebound insomnia INSOMNIA, REBOUND.

rebus A writing format based on the notion that two words that are homophones (i.e. that sound alike) can be expressed using the same sign. Thus, we can cryptically render Shakespeare into a rebus orthography:

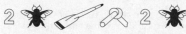

The rebus principle has been used as a teaching device in some reading curricula because it is a fairly painless way to introduce a child to the notion that, in alphabets and syllabaries, the marks on the page represent sounds and not meanings.

recall **1** The process of retrieving information from memory. Lest this definition appear disarmingly simple, the complexities lurking behind it can be appreciated by referring to MEMORY et seq. **2** An experimental procedure for investigating memorial processes whereby the subject must reproduce material previously learned. Compare with RECOGNITION.

recall, cued RECALL (1) that is triggered by a CUE (2). An experimental example would be reminding the subject in a list-learning study that names of animals were included in the list. A natural example is seeing your diary and remembering that you have to make a dental appointment.

recapitulation theory As embodied in the rather catchy phrase 'Ontogeny recapitulates phylogeny', the doctrine that the development of an individual organism is a microcosmic replaying of the evolution of its species. The theory has had two, not unrelated, manifestations: one which focused on biological and physiological factors (particularly the embryological), and one that focused on the development of cognitive and perceptual skills. Taken literally, the generalization does not have much value. For an anthropological variation on this theme, see CULTURE-EPOCH THEORY.

Received Pronunciation (RP) The phonetician's technical term for the idealized standard pronunciation pattern of British English. The term derives from the sense of *received* as 'accepted at court'. Hence, the phrase KING'S ENGLISH is also used of this speech pattern. See also STANDARD ENGLISH.

receiver In information theory, that which picks up a physical signal and converts it into a usable form. The term is used broadly and may refer to an electronic device, an organism's sensory-receptor system with its accompanying neural circuitry, or the organism itself, depending on context.

receiver-operating characteristic (ROC) curve A way of representing the data from a signal-detection experiment. The ROC curve plots the number of *hits* (trials in which the subject responds 'yes' and there is a signal) and *false alarms* (subject responds 'yes' but there is no signal) depending on the number of *catch trials* (trials in which there is, in fact, no signal). The result is a sensitive measure of the subject's true sensory sensitivity. See SIGNAL-DETECTION THEORY for more detail.

receiving hospital A hospital to which patients come for diagnosis, evaluation and preliminary treatment. Those deemed to require long-term care or hospitalization are referred elsewhere.

recency effect The common finding that in a free-recall experiment the items that are presented toward the end of a list (i.e. most recently) are more likely to be recalled than those in the middle. See also PRIMACY EFFECT and SERIAL-POSITION EFFECT. Also known as the *law* (or *principle*) *of recency*.

recent memory MEMORY, RECENT and REMOTE.

receptive aphasia WERNICKE'S *APHASIA.

receptive character Fromm's term for an individual who is excessively passive and requires a great deal of support and guidance from those about them. Also called *oral passive*.

receptive dysphasia DEVELOPMENTAL *LANGUAGE DISORDER.

receptive-expressive aphasia GLOBAL *APHASIA.

receptive field **1** With respect to any single cell in any part of the visual system, that area in the retina which, upon presentation of a visual stimulus, produces a reliable change (either excitatory or inhibitory) in that cell's pattern of firing. **2** By extension, an analogous region on the body surface.

receptive language disorder DEVELOPMENTAL *LANGUAGE DISORDER.

receptive vocabulary PASSIVE *VOCABULARY.

receptivity **1** Openness, acceptance, passivity. Note that, depending on the context, the term may have positive connotations, in that one who displays receptivity may be seen as nondogmatic, flexible and reasonable, or it may have negative connotations, in that the characterization is of one who is weak, passive and dependent (see RECEPTIVE CHARACTER). **2** The state in a female animal of willingness to copulate. Distinguish from PROCEPTIVITY.

receptor In most general terms, a specialized neural cell or part thereof that transduces physical stimuli into receptor potentials. That is, a cell that is responsive to a particular form of stimulation and which reliably undergoes a particular pattern of change. Such a definition is wide enough for all of the following to be properly regarded as receptors: (a) peripheral cells in the various sensory systems that respond to specific forms of physical energy, e.g. rods and cones in the retina, hair cells in the organ of Corti of the inner ear, pressure-sensitive cells in the skin, taste buds in the tongue; (b) proprioreceptors that respond to internal stimulation, e.g. the hair cells in the semicircular canals of the inner ear, the stretch receptors in the viscera, the kinaesthetic receptors in the joints and tendons; and (c) the postsynaptic neurons that respond to the release of neurotransmitter substances within the nervous system; see here RECEPTOR SITE.

Several systems for classifying receptors have been used over the years. Some are keyed to location of the receptors in the body, e.g. exteroceptors, interoceptors and proprioceptors; some are based on the specific modality served, e.g. visual receptors, auditory receptors; some are dependent on identification of the form of the physical stimuli to which the receptors are sensitive, e.g. chemical receptors, such as those serving taste and smell, mechanical receptors for pressure and audition, photic receptors in vision, temperature receptors for warm and cold; and others are keyed to the neurotransmitter substances that mediate the neural pathway that serves a particular receptor system, e.g. cholinergic receptors, dopaminergic receptors. Note that this last classification system is predicated on central-nervous-system considerations rather than on the specific sensory systems that initiate neural changes. Generally, the context within which particular receptors are discussed makes clear the classification system in use.

receptor potential A graded potential change in receptor cells that lack axons and, hence, do not produce action potentials. Receptor potentials are transmitted (chemically or electrically) to neurons with axons. They function by raising or lowering the likelihood of these axonal neurons firing. See also ACTION POTENTIAL and GENERATOR POTENTIAL.

receptor site A specific area of the membrane of a cell that is sensitive to a particular neurotransmitter or hormone. The presence of that substance will initiate a characteristic sequence of changes in the cell.

recess 1 A period of rest between periods of work or activity. **2** In anatomy, a small depression or cavity in an organ or structure.

recessive 1 Generally, not dominant, holding back, receding, not expressed. **2** In genetics, of one allele of a gene pair which is suppressed by the other and therefore is not expressed in the phenotype. **3** In genetics, characterizing a trait that only emerges in the phenotype when both parents contribute the recessive gene, a trait that remains latent if suppressed by the dominant gene. See here DOMINANCE (esp. 2); ant., *dominant*, but see that entry for specifics on usage.

recessive allele RECESSIVE (2).

recessive trait RECESSIVE (3).

recidivism From the Latin for *relapse*, a return to delinquency or crime. Most restrict the term to forensic matters: a recidivist is typically defined as one who has had a second (or further) conviction or incarceration. Some, however, extend the meaning to cover the recurrence of a mental disorder, although this is not generally recommended.

recidivism rate The proportion of persons in a sample who are incarcerated or institutionalized again within some specified period of time after discharge. It is often used as a measure of the effectiveness of treatment programmes.

reciprocal 1 n. In mathematics, a number the product of which when multiplied by another number is unity; the reciprocal of any number n is $1/n$. **2** adj. Descriptive of any relationship in which the elements operate in coordinated opposition to each other; see e.g. RECIPROCAL INHIBITION.

reciprocal altruism ALTRUISM.

reciprocal assimilation ASSIMILATION, RECIPROCAL.

reciprocal inhibition 1 The inhibition of the action of one neural pathway by the activity of another; see e.g. RECIPROCAL *INNERVATION. **2** The inability to recall a word, name or image owing to the activation of another word, name or image. This meaning is dropping out of use; see the discussion under INTERFERENCE (4, 5) for reasons. **3** The inhibition of one response by the occurrence of another mutually incompatible response. This meaning is the one expressed in RECIPROCAL INHIBITION THERAPY.

reciprocal inhibition therapy A form of behaviour therapy based on the notion of RECIPROCAL INHIBITION (3). Developed by Joseph Wolpe, it uses the technique of conditioning a new response that is incompatible with the response that is to be eliminated. For example, anxiety and relaxation are incompatible responses and a phobic disorder can be removed by conditioning a relaxation response to the stimulus that previously evoked an anxiety response. See DESENSITIZATION PROCEDURE for more detail.

reciprocal innervation INNERVATION, RECIPROCAL.

reciprocal roles ROLES, RECIPROCAL.

reciprocal translocation CHROMOSOMAL ALTERATIONS.

reciprocity There are several specialized uses of this term, all of which carry the underlying meaning of mutual exchange, the notion of equal give and take. To wit: **1** In sensory psychology, the generalization that the duration and intensity of a stimulus interact to produce sensation, the so-called BUNSEN–ROSCOE LAW. **2** In Piaget's theory of *cognitive* development, the cognitive process of recognizing that one can neutralize or control a factor for the purpose of studying a second factor and then later reintroduce the first. Such thinking does not emerge until the FORMAL OPERATORY STAGE. **3** In Piaget's theory of *moral* development, the attitude that one should return a favour in kind ('You scratch my back, I'll scratch yours'). See also PUNISHMENT BY RECIPROCITY. **4** In Heider's BALANCE THEORY, the principle that social

attraction is mutual: if I know you like me, it increases the likelihood that I will like you.

recoding Generally, any cognitive operation that systematically shifts the form of a memory; e.g. '106614921776' can be viewed as a random number sequence or 'recoded' as a series of historically important dates.

recognition 1 The awareness that an object or event is one that has been previously seen, experienced or learned. **2** An experimental procedure for the study of memory; see RECOGNITION PROCEDURE. **3** Acknowledgement, taken generally, e.g. of achievement, of the validity of a statement, of a kindness.

recognition memory MEMORY assessed by use of the RECOGNITION PROCEDURE.

recognition procedure (or **method**) An experimental procedure used in the study of memory in which the subject is required to respond to a series of test stimuli by stating whether or not they were among the stimuli presented in a learning session held earlier. Actually, there are many variations on this basic theme. The subject may be required to respond 'yes' or 'no' to each individual stimulus, to select previously seen stimuli from a large array, to sort new and old items, etc. Compare with RECALL.

recognition span An occasional, but slightly misleading, synonym of READING SPAN.

recognition test Any test which relies on differentiating old, previously seen material from new material. Most multiple-choice exams are of this type.

recognition vocabulary PASSIVE *VOCABULARY.

recognitory assimilation ASSIMILATION, RECOGNITORY.

recollection A general term for remembrance of things past.

reconditioning Conditioning again. Thus we get two confusing usages: **1** To renovate or improve a weakened response by reintroducing the unconditioned stimulus. **2** To condition a new response to an old stimulus and thereby *de*condition the old response. Most authors intend the former, reserving COUNTERCONDITIONING for the latter.

reconstruction 1 Generally, the act of restoring the original order or structure of a thing. 2 In psychoanalysis, a procedure whereby extensive biographical and autobiographical data on an individual are interpreted (i.e. reconstructed) to provide understanding of contemporary behaviour. 3 In the study of memory, a procedure whereby the subject is required to restore a disrupted stimulus sequence to its original form or order. See RECONSTRUCTIVE *MEMORY for further discussion.

reconstruction method RECONSTRUCTION (3).

reconstructive memory MEMORY, RECONSTRUCTIVE.

recovered memory MEMORY, RECOVERED.

recovery 1 Generally, the return to or re-establishment of the normal, original state of a person, an organ, a response, a neuron, etc. 2 The act of retrieving information from memory.

recovery time Generally, the time required for a system to recover its normal state after performing some function. The term is applied to neurons (see REFRACTORY PERIOD) and other physiological functions (see REFRACTORY PHASE).

recreational drugs Quite literally, drugs used for recreational purposes. However, the manner in which the term is used often carries the connotation that these are 'drugs of abuse'. While it is true that many psychoactive drugs that are used for recreation are abused, this semantic entailment appears to be more of a value judgement than a defining feature. See DRUG ABUSE for more on usage.

recruitment The neural process by which successive or prolonged stimulation increases the number of nerve cells excited. Also called *recruiting response*.

rectilinear Forming, characteristic of or characterized by a straight line. Used synonymously with LINEAR.

rectilinear distribution UNIFORM *DISTRIBUTION.

rectilinear regression LINEAR *REGRESSION.

recurrent brief depressive disorder BRIEF DEPRESSIVE DISORDER, RECURRENT.

recurrent (collateral) inhibition A neurological phenomenon in which a cell, upon firing, produces a self-inhibiting action. Some motor neurons, for example, have a *recurrent collateral* process which, via an inhibiting neuron (a *Renshaw cell*), synapses back on itself and produces an inhibitory postsynaptic potential that prevents the motor neuron from firing for a time.

recursion A process whereby a rule or operator is applied once and then reapplied to the result, which is then subjected to the rule, etc. Recursive operations are important in LOGIC, GENERATIVE GRAMMARS and models based on CONNECTIONISM (2).

red The PRIMARY *COLOUR experienced when the normal eye is exposed to wavelengths in the range 650–730 nm. Actually, the reds in this range are perceived as having a slight tinge of yellow or blue in them and to produce a 'pure' red a small quantity of short-wavelength light must be added.

red–green (colour) blindness The most frequently occurring form of partial colour blindness, in which reds and greens are not differentiated. See DICHROMACY.

redintegration 1 Generally, the re-establishing of a whole by the bringing together of its several parts, a reintegration. This meaning is common in clinical and health psychology where the reference is to re-establishing mental or physical well-being after a period of disordered functioning. 2 More specifically, the capability of one aspect of a complex stimulus to evoke a response originally associated with the whole stimulus. 3 The recalling of many (or all) of the details of a complex memory upon presentation of one detail; see REDINTEGRATIVE *MEMORY. Also called *reintegration*.

redintegrative memory MEMORY, REDINTEGRATIVE.

red nucleus A group of nerve cells in the tegmentum that forms part of the extrapyramidal motor system. It is an important link in the transmission of information along the corticorubrospinal system, which runs from the cortex through the red nucleus to the spinal cord.

red-sighted 1 Heightened sensitivity to

long-wavelength light, to the reds. **2** A tendency to see objects tinged with red.

reduced cue Any diminished or partial CUE. Generally, after extensive learning or conditioning, a reduced cue can evoke the response originally associated with the full cue.

reduced score Any score or datum from which a constant has been subtracted.

reductio ad absurdum The reducing of a proposition to an absurdity. Generally used of arguments which disprove a proposition by showing that it leads to an absurd conclusion. Note that in logic the phrase also refers to an indirect method of proving a proposition by showing that the denial of that proposition leads to a demonstrably false conclusion.

reduction division The type of cell division that occurs in MEIOSIS.

reductionism Stated broadly, a philosophical point of view which maintains that complex phenomena are best understood by a componential analysis that breaks down the phenomena into their fundamental, elementary aspects. The core of the reductionist's position is that greater *insight* into nature is derived by recasting the analyses carried out at one level into a deeper, more basic level. As such, the issue of reductionism in science is really an issue of degree, of pragmatic considerations and of that mysterious quality, elegance. The degree of reductionistic endeavour espoused by a theorist typically has little to do with the stated, 'pure' arguments of reductionism, such as final demonstrations of adequacy or underlying causal explanations of reality; rather it turns on pragmatic issues, and the debates that ensue are invariably over questions of the richness and depth of understanding provided by ceasing the effort at one point or another. This latter point is a subtle one and some examples may help.

No one doubts for a moment that neurological and biochemical factors ultimately underlie all behaviour, but many question whether significant insights into psychological phenomena could ever emerge by characterizing them in such terms. The history of psychology abounds with such debates. The early structuralists attempted to reduce perception to elementary sensations; the Gestalt theorists countered by arguing that to do so *lost* explanatory power, for the perceived whole was not equivalent to the sum of its parts. Behaviourists sought to reduce all complex acts to stimulus–response terms; cognitive theorists countered that images, thoughts, plans, ideas, etc. existed as entities with causal roles to play in behaviour the reality of which was distorted by a recasting into an S–R format. Personality theorists argue that personality is composed of distinguishable traits, or that types of individuals can be identified; proponents of organismic and humanistic approaches insist that such an analysis does violence to the integrity of the whole person. In each of these cases, the debate is typically not over whether the more molecular components *exist*: it is over whether or not greater insight into the underlying nature of the phenomena under consideration can be achieved by reaching down to them. To borrow an analogy, we know that all of mathematics can be ultimately reduced down to the notions of set and set-inclusion, but this fact is of no pragmatic value to one who is attempting to establish an algorithm to solve a set of simultaneous equations.

reduction screen In its simplest form, a large piece of cardboard that blocks the visual field except for that which can be seen through one (or two) tiny, clean-edged pin holes punched in it. The device is used in experiments in which contextual cues provided by the background need to be excluded from the visual field.

reduction sentence DEFINITIONS (esp. (f)).

reductive interpretation Jung's term for an analytic interpretation in which a particular piece of behaviour is evaluated as an indicator of the existence of some unconscious process.

redundancy In information theory, the degree to which a message is constrained. One usually speaks of the amount of redundancy in terms of the predictability of the letters or words based upon what has gone before. For example, in the message 'Today is Anne's birthday, she is ten years—', the last word is essentially perfectly predictable and hence is utterly redundant. However, if the message is 'My phone number is 386 847–', there is no way to come up with the last digit other than guessing, hence there is zero redundancy in the message. See also ENTROPY, INFORMATION THEORY and related entries.

reduplicative paramnesia PARAMNESIA, REDUPLICATIVE.

re-education 1 A true 're-'education, in the sense that a lost skill or capability is reacquired or relearned. **2** A learning of a new set of adaptive habits to replace maladaptive ones. Sense 1 is generally found in discussions about persons recovering from disabling injuries or mental disorders, sense 2 in discussions about criminals, delinquents and, under some governmental systems, wrong-thinkers.

re-enactment Loosely, any re-experiencing of the feelings, actions, images or thoughts of an early event in one's life. The usual connotation is that the important feature of a re-enactment is the emotional, that the process has value in the alleviation of anxiety. See ABREACTION.

reference axes In factor analysis, the axes of two orthogonal (independent) factors which are used as the frame of reference for the location of other factors.

reference group Any group with which a person feels some identification or emotional affiliation and which he or she uses to guide and define his or her beliefs, values and goals. The term is used even though the individual may not belong, nor even wish to belong, to the group; indeed, his or her perceptions of the group's values may be wildly distorted. Also called *positive reference group* to distinguish it from NEGATIVE *REFERENCE GROUP.

reference group, aspirational Any reference group of which an individual aspires to membership. The implication is that such a group has a more compelling impact on a person's beliefs and values than a simple REFERENCE GROUP in that the aspirational component demands a greater conformity to the ideals of the group.

reference group, negative A reference group which an individual uses as a countervalent balance point in guiding and defining his or her values. The group's values serve as a

motivator for oppositional opinions and beliefs.

reference memory SEMANTIC *MEMORY.

reference vector In factor analysis, the set of axes that define the basic coordinate space into which the various relations between factors given in the correlation matrix can be placed. In normal Euclidean space the CARTESIAN COORDINATES represent the reference vector.

referent The entity in the real world that is indicated or picked out by word, phrase or expression. Strictly speaking only concrete objects or events can be considered as referents, although some authors stretch the term to cover abstractions which can be operationalized.

referential signals In animal communication, signals that have specific referents. A cry indicating pain wouldn't qualify. Several species use distinct signals for the presence of a predator on the ground, a predator in the air, food, water and the like. It is tempting to treat these as the beginnings of symbolic representational capacity, which, of course, they may be.

referral 1 The act of sending a patient or client to another physician, therapist or clinic for treatment. **2** The person so sent.

referred pain PAIN, REFERRED.

referred sensation Generally, any sensory experience that is subjectively localized at a point other than the one actually stimulated; see e.g. REFERRED *PAIN.

reflected colour The colour reflected off an object, its SURFACE *COLOUR.

reflection 1 The core meaning is that of a rebounding, a casting back or returning of a thing, and the term is used freely in the technical literature with this general meaning. There are also three more specialized uses: **2** A synonym for INTROSPECTION. **3** Thinking about a thing, particularly with the notion of meditation upon a previous experience or event and its significance. **4** In factor analysis, changing of the signs of one (or more) columns or rows in a correlation matrix.

reflection of feeling A technique used in nondirective therapy in which the therapist rephrases what the client has said with an emphasis on the emotional aspects.

reflection spectrum SPECTRUM, REFLECTION.

reflectivity–impulsivity A hypothesized dimension of COGNITIVE STYLE based on the observation that in the solving of problems some people tend to be rather impulsive and react quickly on the basis of the first thing that comes to mind, while others are more reflective, more systematic, and tend to think a problem through before acting.

reflex **1** Generally, any relatively simple mechanical response. Reflexes are usually regarded as species-specific, innate behaviours which are largely outside of volition and choice and show little variability from instance to instance. This is the preferred meaning in the technical literature. **2** An unlearned stimulus–response relationship. This sense merely extends 1 by including within the definition the stimulus conditions for evoking the reflex. **3** More metaphorically, any unthinking, impulsive act. This sense extends 1 and 2 considerably and, although common, is not recommended.

Many authors interchange *reflex* and *response* despite the fact that the term *response* carries none of the species-specific, innate connotations of *reflex* (at least in its preferred meaning). Hence, many compound terms have ended up in the literature under either or both general headings, e.g. the so-called *startle response* is often called the *startle reflex*. For terms not found below, see RESPONSE (R) or the modifying term.

reflex arc The hypothesized neural unit representing the functioning of a reflex. This abstract arc is schematically represented by a sensory (afferent) neuron stimulated by physical energy and a motor (efferent) neuron to which the impulse is transmitted via an intermediary neuron. Also called *reflex circuit*.

reflex association V. M. Bekhterev's term for CONDITIONED RESPONSE; see REFLEXOLOGY.

reflex circuit REFLEX ARC.

reflex facilitation An increase in the magnitude of a reflex as a result of the presentation of another stimulus that would not, by itself, produce the reflex. The classic example

is an increase in the knee-jerk reflex stimulated by grasping and squeezing an object.

reflex inhibition The inhibition of one reflex by a mutually incompatible one. See RECIPROCAL INHIBITION.

reflex latency The time between the presentation of an eliciting stimulus and the appearance of a reflex.

reflexology A mechanistic, behaviouristic point of view that argues that all psychological processes may be represented as reflexes and combinations of reflexes. The label is generally associated with the Russian physiological approach, beginning with I. M. Sechenov and developed further by I. P. Pavlov and V. M. Bekhterev, the last being credited with coining the term.

reflex reserve A term originally used by B. F. Skinner to refer to the hypothetical reservoir of responsiveness remaining after reinforcement had terminated; operationally it was given as the number of responses made by an organism during experimental extinction. Although occasionally used as a synonym of OPERANT RESERVE, it should really be restricted to cases of classical conditioning.

reflex sensitization An approximate synonym of PSEUDOCONDITIONING.

reflex time REFLEX LATENCY.

refraction **1** Generally, the bending or changing of direction of a wave of light, sound or heat as it changes speed when passing obliquely from one medium into another. **2** In vision, the ability of the eye to focus light to form an image on the retina. The ability in 2 is, of course, dependent on the principle of 1, in the context of which the cornea and lens are the refractive media.

refraction, error of An umbrella term covering a variety of conditions in which the refractive characteristics of the eye are such that the image that falls on the retina is out of focus.

refraction, index of A measure of refraction, a value that expresses the degree to which a ray of light is bent when passing from one medium to another.

refractoriness **1** An occasional synonym of

SATIATION (2). **2** The state of a neuron during the various *refractory periods*.

refractory Stubborn, unmanageable, unresponsive. Clearly, a term with these meanings is going to have considerable currency in a field like psychology. It is used of people (especially children) who are unmanageable, of abnormal conditions that resist attempts at therapy, of diseases that are difficult or impossible to cure, of neurons that do not respond to stimulation, etc.

refractory period, absolute A very brief period of time during which neural tissue is totally unresponsive. It corresponds to the period of actual passage of the neural impulse along the axon, and, depending on the properties of the cell, ranges from 0.5 to 2 msec.

refractory period, psychological (PRP) A short period of time during the processing of and responding to one stimulus when the processing of and responding to a second stimulus is slowed.

refractory period, relative A brief period of time following the ABSOLUTE *REFRACTORY PERIOD during which the excitation threshold of neural tissue is raised and a stronger-than-normal stimulus is required to initiate an action potential. This period lasts for a few milliseconds before the threshold returns to normal.

refractory phase The period immediately following orgasm during which sexual arousal and orgasm are not possible. It is species-specific and shows considerable gender variation within species. In humans it occurs only in males and shows dramatic age effects becoming longer with increasing age. Failure to distinguish this term from REFRACTORY PERIOD can lead to amusing (or embarrassing) confusions.

regard That which can be seen or that which is being looked at; e.g. the *point of regard* is the fixation point, the *field of regard* is the visual field with the head held stationary.

regeneration From the Latin, meaning *a making over, producing anew*. Thus: **1** Generally, an emotional or intellectual renewal. **2** In biology and physiology, the restoration of a neuron, organ or other bodily part.

region **1** An area, a physical space. **2** In K. Lewin's topological *field theory*, a psychological area in one's life space defined by present and contemplated acts, facts, feelings and thoughts and enclosed by boundaries. Lewin hypothesized a host of such regions with a variety of functions. They are primarily of historic interest today.

regional cerebral blood flow Literally, blood flow in the brain. See BOLD for how it is used as a brain imaging technique.

region of rejection In statistics, an interval of values sufficiently extreme for any result falling within it to be so unlikely under the assumptions of the null hypothesis that one can feel secure in rejecting the null hypothesis in favour of the alternative hypothesis. A result within this preset region (or region*s* if a TWO-TAILED TEST is being used) is considered to have STATISTICAL SIGNIFICANCE. Also called the *critical region*.

Registrar General's scale/categories HOLLINGSHEAD SCALES.

regnancy H. A. Murray's term for the 'totality of brain processes occurring during a single moment'.

regression A richly polysemous term in psychology. The core meaning which underlies its various specialized uses is that of reverting, a going-backward, a retreating; the opposite of *progression*. Thus: **1** A reverting to an earlier, more primitive or more child-like pattern of behaviour. When the term is used in this sense, the individual so characterized may or may not have ever actually engaged in the exhibited primitive behaviour; e.g. a 12-year-old child may show regression by thumb-sucking even though he or she never sucked their thumb as an infant. Contrast here with RETROGRESSION (2). Moreover, the connotation of *relapse* is always present; *regression* is not used of primitive behaviours that have never been lost. Contrast here with FIXATION. It should be appreciated that this meaning of the term has different evaluative connotations in different areas of usage: (a) in psychoanalytic theories, it has a negative implication, i.e. the notion that stress or anxiety is causing the individual to flee from reality into a more infantile state, but (b) in cognitive/developmental theories, it refers to a temporary falling-back upon an earlier form of thinking in order to begin to learn how to deal with new complexity, and regression is viewed as a way station in an ultimately progressive development of cognitive processing. **2** In statistics, a relationship between the selected values on one variable (x) and the observed values on a second variable (y). When the REGRESSION EQUATION for a set of data is worked out, the most probable value of y can be predicted for any value of x. The term in this sense is actually a shortened form of REGRESSION TOWARD THE MEAN. **3** In genetics, the LAW OF *FILIAL REGRESSION. **4** In reading, any eye movement back over material already read. The frequency of such regressions is related to the difficulty of the material and the reading skills of the individual. **5** In conditioning studies, the reappearance of a previously acquired response. Such regression to a response lower on the HABIT HIERARCHY is most frequently observed during punishment of the dominant response. Many behaviourists take the effect here as a laboratory analogue of regression in sense 1. adjs., *regressive, regressed*; vb., *regress*.

regression analysis 1 Generally, any statistical use of REGRESSION (2) to analyse data. **2** Somewhat more restrictively, the use of qualitative ratings on one variable to make quantitative predictions on another variable.

regression coefficient In a linear REGRESSION EQUATION, the constant that represents the rate of change of one variable (y) as a function of variations in the other variable (x). When the *regression line* is plotted graphically, the coefficient represents the slope of the line and is thus a measure of its steepness.

regression curve The smooth curve fitted to a set of paired entry data from a correlation table. If the regression is linear, the curve is a straight line; if it is quadratic, there is a single inflection point; etc.

regression, curvilinear Any nonlinear regression wherein the regression equation for changes in one variable (y) as a function of changes in another (x) is a quadratic, cubic or higher-order equation. It should be appreciated that although it is always possible mathematically to have a regression equation that fits every wiggle in the curve, most of these perturbations are due to sampling or measurement error and nothing is

gained by such a perfect fit. Whether a curvilinear regression is appropriate for a set of data is not always easy to determine, although there exist statistical tests for determining whether each higher order of equation increases significantly the goodness of fit for a given set of data.

regression equation The equation representing the relationship between the values of one variable (x) and the observed values of another (y). The equation is, thus, a formula which permits the prediction of the most probable values of y for any known value of x. Linear regression equations are of the form $y = ax + b$, quadratic of the form, $y = ax^2 + bx + c$, etc.

regression, hierarchical multiple A form of MULTIPLE *REGRESSION in which individual predictor variables or sets of variables are entered in an order determined by the person performing the analysis, hopefully based on careful consideration of some underlying theoretical model.

regression, hypnotic Regression produced by the use of hypnosis. The phenomenon has been vigorously debated, some arguing that a true REGRESSION (1) actually takes place, others that the hypnotized subject merely acts out (i.e. mimics) the immature state suggested.

regression line The line (or curve) that best fits a set of data points. It will be the graphic form of the REGRESSION EQUATION for those data.

regression, linear Any regression that is represented by a linear REGRESSION EQUATION. Linear regressions are always represented by straight lines; compare with CURVILINEAR *REGRESSION.

regression, logistic A variety of DISCRIMINANT ANALYSIS that uses variables that are discrete, dichotomous or continuous to predict a singular outcome. It is useful in cases such as determining whether or not an individual has a disorder or falls into one of two dichotomous categories.

regression, multiple A statistical technique that is an extension of simple REGRESSION and allows one to make predictions about performance on one variable or measure (called the CRITERION *VARIABLE) based on performance on two or more other variables (called the PREDICTOR *VARIABLES). If the regression equation is in standard score form, then the relative weights or contributions of each of the predictor variables may be assessed. The basic term *multiple regression* is often used with the understanding that the regressions are linear. See also MULTIPLE *CORRELATION.

regression of y on x A phrase used to characterize the typical REGRESSION EQUATION whereby values of *x* are used as the basis for making predictions about the most likely values of *y*.

regression, stepwise Any of several MULTIPLE *REGRESSION techniques in which the independent variables are deleted or entered into the REGRESSION EQUATION one at a time. Some techniques allow for the entry or removal of more than one of the variables, but in all cases some criterion must be defined in advance of applying the technique.

regression time The amount of time spent in making regressive eye movements during reading. See REGRESSION (4).

regression toward the mean A generalization, stated simply, that given any standard score on one variable, *x*, the optimal linear prediction of the standard score on another variable, *y*, will be closer to the mean of all the *y*-scores than *x* was to the mean of all the *x*-scores. The phenomenon is a result of the statistical assumptions built into the use of REGRESSION (2) as a means of making predictions and should not necessarily be viewed as a feature of nature.

regression weight A synonym of REGRESSION COEFFICIENT.

regret Generally, the feeling that, in retrospect, one might have behaved differently in the past or that things might have turned out better had events gone differently. See also ANTICIPATORY *REGRET.

regret, anticipatory A feeling that often accompanies decision-making when various alternatives are considered. It is essentially a vague sense of worry about the negative elements that might result if a given choice is actually made, a kind of 'I will regret this action tomorrow' feeling.

regulatory behaviour 1 In biology, any behaviour that serves to maintain balance or equilibrium. The term is used here in the sense of the maintenance of HOMEOSTASIS. 2 By extension to psychological systems, daily rituals and habits that help maintain emotional stability.

regulatory drive DRIVE, REGULATORY.

rehabilitate 1 To restore to good form or proper functioning condition. 2 To restore to a previous condition or status. Note that meaning 1 is not necessarily equivalent to meaning 2, In psychological writings the usual connotation is that of 1.

rehabilitation Loosely, restoring or renewing. The term is used widely, usually with a modifier to specify the type of rehabilitation, e.g. *cognitive* rehabilitation for those with brain injuries, *physical* rehabilitation for stroke victims with motoric difficulties. Often used in the abbreviated form, *rehab*.

rehearsal 1 Practice of an act in anticipation of a time when its performance will be required. 2 Repetitive review of material previously learned with an eye toward a later need to recall it. In some contexts the process is viewed as a rather shallow cognitive process dealing primarily with the surface, physical form of the material and not necessarily with its underlying meaning. In this sense, it is hypothesized by some as the procedure for keeping information in SHORT-TERM *MEMORY.

Reid Technique A set of interviewing and interrogation guidelines that is frequently used by law enforcement agencies. In the initial structured interviewing step, questions are asked to elicit signs of truth-telling vs. falsehood. If this step reveals suggestions of deception, then a structured series of interrogation tactics is utilized to elicit a confession. Because of the highly adversarial nature of the technique and its high false confession rate, use of the technique with minors is prohibited in Great Britain.

reification Literally, according to its Latin roots, '*thing-a-fying*', i.e. the making real and concrete of that which is abstract and/or hypothetical; or, better, the acting as if one believed that the abstract or hypothetical were real. From a purely rationalistic perspective reification is a cognitive/emotional act of children and other unsophisticated folk; in reality, it is one of the more seductive ways in which social scientists distort and misrepresent the status of many of their hypothetical entities and constructs. In the latter case it is called the *reification fallacy*.

reification fallacy REIFICATION.

reinforce 1 To shore up, to strengthen, to solidify a thing. **2** To present a REINFORCEMENT or (more properly) a REINFORCER. See both of these terms for details.

reinforcement There is considerable diversity in the usage of this term. Most of the definitional variations, however, stem from theoretical issues in learning theory about what reinforcement is and how it functions. At the core of them all is a relatively simple meaning: **1** The operation of strengthening, supporting or solidifying something, or the event that so strengthens or supports it. Since the term is most commonly found in the literature on conditioning and learning, the something strengthened is generally considered to be a learned conditioned response or the bond between that response and a stimulus. **2** In classical conditioning, the unconditioned stimulus (US) when it is presented either simultaneously, overlapping with or shortly following the conditioned stimulus (CS). The US in these circumstances clearly functions as a reinforcer of the CS–US 'bond' in sense 1, since if it is omitted extinction of the CR occurs.

These first two meanings are relatively uncontroversial: 1 is a harmless tautology ('reinforcement reinforces') and 2 is a description of an empirically demonstrable state of affairs. The difficulties with the term emerge when definitions are offered which contain theoretical assumptions about the mechanisms involved, particularly when operant or instrumental behaviours are under consideration. To wit: **3** Any set of circumstances that an organism finds pleasurable or satisfying. While it is probably true that pleasurable or satisfying events 'reinforce' behaviour, this definitional effort only serves to pass along the problem. Since *pleasure* and *satisfaction* are no more definitionally tractable terms than *reinforcement*, nothing is gained here. Compare this usage, however, with that of REWARD, which some authors treat as a synonym of *reinforcement* in this sense. **4** Any event or act which serves to reduce a drive. This is, of course, not a definition so much as a theoretical statement about the mechanism of reinforcement; see here DRIVE-REDUCTION HYPOTHESIS. As such, it has been largely abandoned because of a failure to find evidence for the operation of drive reduction in all those cases in which reinforcement effects (in sense 1) are observed. **5** A termination or modification of a particular stimulating condition. This definition derives from CONTIGUITY THEORY, which maintains that the last act performed in a situation is the one learned. Actually, as the defenders of this point of view were quick to note, it is no definition at all but rather an attempt to do away with the term *reinforcement* altogether. **6** Any behaviour with higher momentary probability of occurrence than some other behaviour. This meaning is expressed by the so-called PREMACK PRINCIPLE (see for details), which emphasizes the relativity of reinforcement. **7** Knowledge of results, feedback about the correctness or appropriateness of one's behaviour. This sense is the one intended in essentially all areas of psychology in which human beings are the primary experimental subjects.

This array of partially overlapping and, on occasion, contradictory definitions pleases no one, least of all psychologists, who find themselves often trapped lexicographically into the use of the term. In a very real sense, part of the difficulty results from attempts to treat the concept as if it represented a single fundamental principle that operated in all circumstances. Somehow, this seems rather wrong-headed: it appears unlikely that the same principles pertain when a hungry rat is fed after a bar press as when a Nobel prize is awarded for a brilliant scientific discovery – yet both reinforce behaviour, in that the rat returns to press the bar and the scientist to the laboratory to work on other problems. Moreover, physical pain functions as reinforcement for the masochist, punishment may reinforce confession in one who experiences a deep sense of guilt, altruism is reinforcing for the noble, and abdication of responsibility will serve for the authoritarian personality. The range and diversity of things which can function as reinforcement (in sense 1) is essentially without bound and the failure to discern any unitary underlying mechanisms has led to: **8** Any event, stimulus, act, response or information which, when made contingent upon the response that preceded it, serves to increase the relative frequency or likelihood of occurrence of that response. This is the so-called neutral definition, because it begs no theory and makes no presumptions about the underlying action or role of reinforcement. It is also inherently circular: the existence of reinforcement is predicated upon the observation of increased responding, and increased responding is, perforce, evidence of the existence of there having been some reinforcement. Many have railed against this definition and with good reason. This kind of semantic bootstrapping is a feeble definitional basis for such an important one of psychology's most used constructs. Nevertheless, it is the dominant meaning, it reflects fairly accurately the way in which the term is most often used and thus, for now, it will have to suffice.

Note, in all of the senses outlined the term itself may be found referring to (a) the procedure of presenting or removing the reinforcing event, (b) the theoretical process that is presumed to be involved in its action, or (c) the actual event or act itself. It is recommended that *reinforcement* only be used for the first two and *reinforcer* serve for the last.

Finally, there are uses of the term that do not touch upon the various disputes of meanings 1 to 8: **9** In studies of reflexes, the operation whereby one reflex strengthens or increases the operation of another reflex; e.g. the magnitude of an eye-blink response is reinforced by heightened muscle tone. **10** In dream analysis, the process whereby the theme of a dream is amplified and supported by a secondary dream within the primary one.

reinforcement-affect theory A model of social attraction that maintains that attraction (or lack of it) between two individuals can be produced directly and simply by association. Whenever positive events occur during an interaction they increase mutual attraction, while negative events diminish it.

reinforcement, contingent Quite literally, reinforcement that is contingent upon some response. In the vast majority of uses of the unqualified term REINFORCEMENT, this is the intended meaning. Compare with NONCONTINGENT *REINFORCEMENT.

reinforcement, continuous A SCHEDULE OF *REINFORCEMENT in which every response is reinforced. abbrev., *crf* or *CRF*.

reinforcement, differential **1** The reinforcement of only one response to a particular stimulus. All other responses made to that stimulus either are not reinforced or are punished. **2** The reinforcement of a response to only one of several stimuli. Responses made in the presence of the other stimuli either are not reinforced or are punished. **3** A label for a class of SCHEDULES OF *REINFORCEMENT all of which are dependent upon responses being emitted at specified rates, e.g. *differential reinforcement of low rate*.

reinforcement gradient (effect) A generalization that the closer a given previously unreinforced response is to a reinforced response, the more it is strengthened. Note that 'closeness' here may depend on spatial, temporal and/or structural conditions.

reinforcement, intermittent An umbrella term for all those SCHEDULES OF *REINFORCEMENT in which some of the responses made go unreinforced. That is, all those schedules of reinforcement other than CONTINUOUS *REINFORCEMENT and EXTINCTION. Also called *partial reinforcement*.

reinforcement, interval Any SCHEDULE OF *REINFORCEMENT based on time intervals.

reinforcement, negative 1 Any procedure or method of training that uses a negative reinforcer. **2** Any event, stimulus or behaviour which, when its removal is made contingent upon a response, increases the frequency or likelihood of that response. See here NEGATIVE *REINFORCER, which is the preferred term for this meaning. Contrast with PUNISHMENT, which is the presentation of an aversive stimulus, and with POSITIVE *EXTINCTION, where reinforcement (of any kind) is no longer presented.

reinforcement, noncontingent Reinforcement which occurs independently of any behaviour. For a sense of the role that such reinforcement can play in the development and maintenance of behaviour, see SUPERSTITIOUS BEHAVIOUR.

reinforcement, periodic Any SCHEDULE OF *REINFORCEMENT based on varying time intervals.

reinforcement, positive 1 A procedure or method of training which uses positive reinforcers. **2** Any event, stimulus or behaviour which, when made contingent upon a response, serves to increase the frequency or likelihood of occurrence of that response. See POSITIVE *REINFORCER, which is the preferred term for this meaning.

reinforcement, ratio Any SCHEDULE OF *REINFORCEMENT in which reinforcements are delivered on the basis of some number of responses.

reinforcement, schedules of Quite literally, any of the schedules under which reinforcements are presented to a subject dependent upon some spatial, temporal or sequential aspect of the response. In what follows, it is assumed that *operant* behaviour is under consideration: although some of the schedules have been used in classical conditioning (e.g. *continuous reinforcement*), the use of the term *schedule of reinforcement* is rare in those contexts.

The fascination that many psychologists, particularly *Skinnerian* behaviourists, have with schedules of reinforcement derives from the simple fact that the reinforcement of behaviour in day-to-day living is typically irregular and nonuniform. Gamblers do not collect after every bet, not every seed planted grows and many a political speech ends without persuasion of a voter. Yet gamblers continue to lay wagers, farmers to plant crops and politicians (alas) to give speeches. Hence, there has been considerable effort invested in the examination of the effect that the schedule with which reinforcements appear has upon the development and maintenance of behaviour. The following list includes the most thoroughly studied schedules of reinforcement. The classification system used here is more or less standard, although others may be found in the technical literature: first the 'simple' schedules, in which there is a single type of contingency between responding and reinforcement, are presented; next the 'compound' schedules, in which two or more simple schedules are in force, are described; finally the 'special' schedules, which do not fit neatly into either of the preceding classes, are outlined.

It will be clear, in practice, to anyone who plods through the following outline that the range of possibility is nearly without bound. The reader may also get the feeling that much of the research is little more than an exercise in esoterica. Even Skinnerians are occasionally beset with such intimations. Recovery from such self-doubt usually takes the form of listing the various applications in educational, industrial, organizational and therapeutic settings that have been made (which, admittedly, are many).

I. *Simple schedules.* All of the following are schedules in which there is but one, constant, contingency between the response and the occurrence of the reinforcer. **1** *Continuous reinforcement* (*crf* or *CRF*). Quite simply, every response is reinforced. **2** *Extinction* (*ext* or *EXT*). No responses are reinforced. **3** *Fixed ratio* (*FR*). A class of schedules in which the ratio between responses and reinforcements is fixed, i.e. reinforcement is contingent on a fixed number of responses being made since the preceding reinforcement. Thus, *FR 10* means that every 10th response is reinforced. Note, according to this usage, CRF is actually a fixed ratio schedule, specifically *FR 1.* **4** *Variable ratio* (*VR*). A class of schedules in which the ratio between responses and reinforcements varies in some random or semi-random fashion but with a specific mean value. Thus, *VR 10* means that on average every 10th response is reinforced. **5** *Random ratio* (*RR*). A variation on the VR schedule in which a ratio specifies the probability that any given response will be reinforced. In an *RR 10*, for example, there is a 0.10 probability that any given response will be reinforced, independent of the number of responses made since the previous reinforcement. **6** *Fixed interval* (*FI*). Time-contingent schedules in which the last response made after a given interval of time since the preceding reinforcement is reinforced. Usually the notation is given in minutes: *FI 3* means *fixed interval 3 minutes*. **7** *Variable interval* (*VI*). Time-contingent schedules in which reinforcements are 'set up' on a random or semi-random sequence of intervals with a specific mean value. Thus, *VI 3* means that on the average the interval between potential reinforcements is 3 minutes. Note that VI schedules tend to produce very regular response rates while FI schedules tend to produce bursts of responses followed by periods of few or no responses. **8** *Fixed time* (*FT*). A class of schedules in which, like FI schedules, reinforcements are delivered at fixed time intervals but, unlike FI schedules, independently of any responses made or not made by the subject. **9** *Variable time (VT)*. Like FT schedules but here the time between reinforcements varies. **10** *Differential reinforcement of low rate (drl or DRL)*. A class of schedules based on a specified rate of response which must not be exceeded for reinforcement to occur. Thus, in *DRL 10* (seconds), 10 seconds must pass between responses or no reinforcement is delivered; a response made too soon 'resets' the clock and another 10 seconds without a response must pass. **11** *Differential reinforcement of high rate (drh or DRH)*. In contrast to DRL, here the rate must exceed some set value for reinforcement to occur. *DRH 1* (second) means that the interresponse time must be less than 1 second. **12** *Differential reinforcement of paced responses (drp or DRP)*. A class of schedules that combines aspects of both DRL and DRH in that the rate of responding must fall within certain limits in order for reinforcement to occur. **13** *Differential reinforcement of other behaviour (dro or DRO)*. A schedule which reinforces the failure of a specific response to occur. Thus, *DRO 30* (seconds) means that reinforcement will occur after 30 seconds provided that the response under consideration has not occurred during that interval; in effect, all other behaviours emitted during the interval are being reinforced.

II. *Compound schedules*. The following are schedules in which two or more simple schedules are combined into compound form. They may be either 'sequential', in which case one component of the schedule must be satisfied before the other(s) is in effect, or they may be 'simultaneous', in which case two or more schedules are in effect concurrently. **1** *Tandem (tand)*. A sequential schedule in which reinforcement depends upon the successive completion of two or more simple schedules. Thus, in *tand FI 2 FR 5*, the FI 2 component must be satisfied before responses count toward the FR 5. The full sequence is carried out without discriminative cues to the subject about which component is in effect at any point in time. **2** *Chained (chain)*. A sequential schedule similar to *tand* except that a discriminative stimulus is associated with each component. **3** *Mixed (mix)*. A sequential schedule in

which two or more simple schedules are presented either alternating or at random. As with *tandem* schedules, no discriminative cues are used. **4** *Multiple (mult)*. The same as a *mixed schedule* with the addition of discriminative stimuli to mark off each of the components. **5** *Alternative (alt)*. A simultaneous schedule in which satisfying any one of the components produces reinforcement. After reinforcement, the schedule 'resets'. Thus, in *alt FI 5 FR 50* reinforcement occurs either after the 50th response if it is made in under 5 minutes, or after the 1st response at the end of the 5-minute period following the last reinforcement. **6** *Conjunctive (conj)*. Similar to *alternative* except that here all components must be satisfied before reinforcement is delivered. **7** *Concurrent (conc)*. A general label used to cover all situations in which two or more schedules that are set up independently of each other operate simultaneously.

III. *Special schedules*. These schedules have time or rate components that do not easily fit into the above categories. **1** *Interlocking (interlock)*. A class of schedules in which reinforcement is delivered upon completion of a given number of responses but this number is changed as a function of the time since the last reinforcement. For example, a linear reduction in number of responses might be programmed so that the longer the subject waits the fewer the number of responses required for reinforcement. **2** *Adjusting (adj)*. A class of schedules in which the requirements for reinforcement are adjusted systematically as a function of the subject's performance. For example, an FR may be increased or decreased depending upon whether the latency of the first response after a reinforcement is greater or less than some predetermined value. **3** *Conjugate (conjug)*. A schedule in which the intensity level of some reinforcing stimulus increases or decreases with the rate of responding, e.g. the brightness of a TV screen changes systematically with response rate. **4** *Interpolated (inter)*. A schedule in which a small block of reinforcements on one schedule is introduced, without discriminative stimuli, into a different ongoing schedule.

There are others but enough is enough. See CLOCK, COUNTER, CUMULATIVE RECORDER, OPERANT CONDITIONING, REINFORCEMENT, SHAPING, SKINNERIAN, TIME OUT and related terms.

reinforcement, social Broadly, any social event which serves to increase the likelihood or frequency of some behaviour which preceded its presentation.

reinforcement theory Loosely, any theory that attempts to explain the process of REINFORCEMENT. See SKINNERIAN and HULLIAN for classic examples of the genre.

reinforcer Any event or behaviour which functions as a REINFORCEMENT, which has reinforcing properties. Note that although *reinforcement* and *reinforcer* are often used interchangeably (including in this volume), the former is best reserved for the operation or the process, the latter for the event or stimulus.

reinforcer, conditioned A reinforcer with properties not intrinsic to it but due to association with another reinforcer; a learned (i.e. conditioned) reinforcer. Money is, of course, the classic example. See HIGHER-ORDER CONDITIONING, and compare with PRIMARY *REINFORCER. Also called *secondary reinforcer*.

reinforcer, negative A REINFORCER that functions by its *removal*. Note that events that are negative reinforcers, if *presented* contingent upon a behaviour, function as POSITIVE *PUNISHMENT.

reinforcer, positive A REINFORCER that functions by its *presentation*. Positive reinforcers, if *removed* contingent upon a behaviour, function as NEGATIVE *PUNISHMENT. If discontinued they result in EXTINCTION.

reinforcer, primary Basically, any event or behaviour the reinforcing properties of which are a naturally occurring result of the intrinsic characteristics of the species under consideration. In classical conditioning, the unconditioned stimulus (US) is such a natural event, as its presence under the proper conditions (see CLASSICAL CONDITIONING for these) reinforces the conditioned response (CR). In operant conditioning, the situation is somewhat more complex. While it seems clear that some events are manifestly primary reinforcers by virtue of the physiology of a species (e.g. food, water, moderate temperatures, sex), in many cases no simple way of making the determination exists. Compare with CONDITIONED *REINFORCER.

reinforcing stimulus A term used more-or-less synonymously with REINFORCEMENT (8) and REINFORCER.

reintegration REDINTEGRATION.

Reissner's membrane The delicate membrane in the cochlea that separates the cochlear canal from the scala vestibuli.

Reiz German for *stimulus*. In some older works where the term was borrowed straight from the German it was abbreviated *R*, which caused no end of confusion since English-speaking psychologists were using this abbreviation for *response*.

rejection The core meaning is a failure or refusal to assimilate or to accept. Thus, a body can reject an organ transplant or a food substance, a parent can reject a child, an adult a lover, a committee an idea, a society a cultural value, etc. In all cases there is an implied system or structure that refuses or fails to incorporate a thing.

rejection, parental A parent's rejection of a child. There is no simple term for the reverse.

reject-then-retreat technique A two-stage process for obtaining compliance in which an initial, inflated, request is made. When the request is denied (as expected), the individual 'retreats' to a smaller request, closer to what was originally desired. Compare with the THAT'S-NOT-ALL TECHNIQUE.

relapse Generally, a falling-back into a previous state or into an earlier behaviour pattern. The term is used rather freely in moral, mental, physical and medical cases.

relation 1 Generally, a relationship between two or more events, objects or persons. The precise nature of the connection may vary considerably. Usually one of the following is intended: 2 A connection between two variables such that variation in one is accompanied by variation in the other; see CORRELATION. 3 A connection between propositions such that the truth or falseness of one implicates the truth or falseness of (an)other(s). 4 A connection between events such that one serves as an antecedent condition for (an)other(s). Note that one can, in a sense, order these last three meanings along a dimension that reflects the strength of relation, with 4 suggesting a strong, causal connection that is only hinted at in 3 and logically absent from 2. **5** A RELATIVE (4).

relational aggression AGGRESSION, RELATIONAL.

relational learning LEARNING, RELATIONAL.

relational problems A loose term for difficulties in a relationship that are sufficiently serious to become the focus of clinical attention.

relationship 1 = RELATION. **2** = KINSHIP.

relationship, primary In interpersonal relations, a basic, long-lasting relationship founded upon strong emotional ties and a reciprocal sense of commitment. Unlike SECONDARY *RELATIONSHIPS, primary relationships tend to be rather diffuse, covering a variety of roles, behaviours and situations; they are generally not bounded by strict rules of interaction and the persons involved generally know each other extremely well. A primary relationship is such that one member cannot simply replace the other with a new person.

relationship, secondary In interpersonal relations, a relatively short-lived relationship between persons characterized by limited interaction, rather clear rules for relating and fairly well-defined social roles. Unlike a PRIMARY *RELATIONSHIP, secondary relationships rarely have much in the way of emotional involvement and one member can rather easily replace the other.

relative 1 adj. Loosely, characterizing a condition in which an event or datum is regarded as having a RELATION to another event or datum. **2** adj. Not ABSOLUTE (1); dependent upon other data, events or considerations for meaning. The value, effectiveness or even the very nature of a relative event or datum is derived by taking into consideration its relationship with other events or data. **3** adj. Partial, incomplete. For example, a response may be referred to as relative when it is but a part of the full response that might potentially be made. **4** n. A person with a particular KINSHIP relation to another person.

relative deprivation/gratification The generalization that the rewards one receives are not valued absolutely but as relative to one's expectations. Being promoted to the post of general manager in a company may be viewed as relatively gratifying to a person whose expectation was an assistant manager's post but as relatively depriving for one who anticipated a vice-presidency. Note that a social/cultural element is generally implied in the use of the term in that one's expectations are often established relative to what other persons, particularly one's peers, value and achieve.

relative infertility INFERTILITY (2).

relative refractory period REFRACTORY PERIOD, RELATIVE.

relative risk The ratio of the INCIDENCE of a particular disorder or condition to the number of individuals exposed to the predisposing conditions. Relative risk is an important factor in recommending particular treatments that have known side effects or carrying out studies that have some potentially harmful consequences; it allows one to estimate whether the gains are worth the risk.

relativism RELATIVITY.

relativity (or **relativism**) A general principle that maintains that all experimental and physical events have meaning only with respect to their relationships to other events. From a relativistic perspective, events have no intrinsic meaning independent of other events or of a general framework within which they may be viewed. The principle, in some form or another, is found in nearly every branch of science.

relaxation 1 Most generally, the state of low tension in which emotional level is diminished, especially the level of emotions such as anxiety, fear and anger. **2** The process used to bring about this state; see RELAXATION THERAPY. **3** More specifically, the return of a contracted muscle to its normal resting state.

relaxation therapy Generally, any psychotherapy that emphasizes techniques for teaching the client how to relax, to control tensions. The procedure used is based upon E. Jacobson's *progressive relaxation techniques*, in which the client learns how to relax muscle groups one at a time, the assumption being that muscular relaxation is effective in bringing about emotional relaxation. Jacobson's techniques are often used in various forms of behaviour therapy; see DESENSITIZATION PROCEDURE.

relearning 1 Simply, learning again material that has been forgotten or responses that have undergone extinction. **2** A procedure for studying memory or retention in which the effort required to learn material a second time is compared with the effort needed in the initial learning experience.

release from proactive interference (PI) See PI, RELEASE FROM.

releaser In ethology, any SIGN STIMULUS that serves a communicative function and initiates social behaviours. In older texts, this notion is captured by the term *object of instinct*.

release therapy Generally, any therapeutic procedure based on the assumption that there is therapeutic value in the releasing of deep, pent-up emotional conflicts. The client is invited, indeed encouraged, to express openly and actively anger, hostility, aggression, etc. Such techniques are often used in *play therapy*, *psychodrama*, *Gestalt therapy* and others. See also CATHARSIS.

reliability 1 Very generally, dependability. **2** In personality assessment, a characteristic trustworthiness; a reliable person is a responsible person, one who can be counted upon. **3** In psychological testing (and in measurement generally), a generic term for all aspects of the dependability of a measurement device or test. The essential notion here is *consistency*, the extent to which the measurement device or test yields the same approximate results when utilized repeatedly under similar conditions. Compare here with VALIDITY. The degree to which a procedure is reliable can be assessed in a number of ways: the more commonly used are listed below.

reliability, alternate forms A method of determining the reliability of a test by developing two (or more) parallel sets of items of similar types and difficulty and correlating the scores obtained from one form with those from the other(s). Also called *equivalent* or *parallel forms reliability*.

reliability, coefficient of A correlation coefficient expressing the degree of relationship between two sets of scores in which these sets of scores are the results from two

testing sessions with the same instrument. The coefficient is then used as a quantitative expression of the RELIABILITY (3) of the testing instrument or measurement procedure. There are several different coefficients of reliability depending on the particular scores that are being compared. For example, a *coefficient of stability* is obtained in the *test–retest* method (see TEST–RETEST *RELIABILITY), a *coefficient of equivalence* provides an estimate of reliability when *alternate* or *parallel* forms of a test are used (see ALTERNATE FORMS *RELIABILITY), a *coefficient of internal consistency* is obtained from intratest manipulations such as the *split-half* procedure (see SPLIT-HALF *RELIABILITY).

reliability, index of A statistic that provides an estimate of the correlation between the actual scores obtained from a test and the theoretical true scores. The index is given as the value of $\sqrt{r}$, where r is the calculated COEFFICIENT OF *RELIABILITY.

reliability, interrater The degree to which two or more independent observers agree in their assessment of behaviour. Whenever one is dealing with data that are dependent on highly subjective interpretations of situations, for example where shifts in facial expression of people in a conversation are being studied, high interrater reliability must be shown before the data can be accepted as valid. Also called *rater reliability*.

reliability, item The reliability of a test determined by the degree to which the items in the test measure the same construct. Also called *scale reliability*.

reliability, sampling Any evaluation of the degree of consistency of two samples of scores taken from the same population. See SAMPLING and related entries.

reliability, scale ITEM *RELIABILITY.

reliability, split-half A general label for several methods of determining the reliability of a test by evaluating the test's overall internal consistency. The methods are logically similar to the equivalent forms procedure (see ALTERNATE FORMS *RELIABILITY): the single test is split into two forms and a COEFFICIENT OF *RELIABILITY between the two is obtained. The two halves of the test may be produced in any way provided the result is two comparable forms. Some common procedures are to put the odd-numbered items on one form and the even on the other, to alternate blocks of items from form to form or to assign items to forms on a random basis.

reliability, test–retest A method for determining the reliability of a test by administering it two (or more) times to the same persons and obtaining a COEFFICIENT OF *RELIABILITY between the scores, on each testing. Usually a reasonably long period of time is allowed between the test and the retest, for obvious reasons.

religion Basically, a system of beliefs with either an institutionalized or a traditionally defined pattern of ceremony. Religion is regarded by many as a cultural universal which emerges invariably as an outcome of the need to understand the human condition. Most, although not all, religions share certain characteristics, notably the concept of a (or several) supreme being(s), the promise of a pathway to an ideal existence and an afterlife.

religion, comparative An interdisciplinary field that encompasses the work of sociologists, anthropologists, philosophers, social psychologists and theologians. The primary foci are: (a) those universal needs of human existence which (presumably) stimulate the development of religions; and (b) comparisons between the various theological and cultural factors which have given rise to the diversity of forms in which contemporary and past religions appear.

religion, psychology of A subdiscipline within psychology concerned with the origins of religions, their role in human existence, the nature of religious attitudes and experiences, etc.

religiosity Involvement, interest or participation in religion. Although the term is used by some authors to denote a high degree of religious involvement, it properly refers to a continuum of degree of participation in religious ritual and practice, and one may also correctly characterize a person as displaying low or moderate religiosity.

religious instinct An assumed INSTINCT (see that term for a discussion of the caveats involved in its use in a context like this) in *Homo sapiens* for religious beliefs.

Most authorities do not assume a single 'instinct' here but identify a number of perceptual and cognitive tendencies that predispose humans to think and believe in ways that give rise to religious convictions.

religious trance TRANCE, RELIGIOUS.

REM RAPID EYE MOVEMENTS.

REM behaviour disorder A PARASOMNIA characterized by a loss in the muscle paralysis that marks normal REM SLEEP. Patients display often wild, erratic and occasionally violent behaviours as they apparently 'act out' their dreams. Occurring primarily in males over the age of 50, it is usually treated with sedatives, commonly the antianxiety drug *clonazepam*.

remedial Of a training or educational programme designed to correct deficiencies and to elevate the student or trainee to an acceptable (i.e. median) level. n., *remediation*.

remember To recall, recollect, retrieve, reinstate or reproduce an earlier experience, event, stimulus, etc. See MEMORY and related entries.

remember–know distinction Quite literally, the distinction between remembering something where one is recalling an actual episode and knowing something independent of any particular experience, e.g. I *remember* having cake for dessert last night. I *know* the Eiffel Tower is in Paris.

remembrance The act or product of remembering; see REMINISCENCE for more detail.

reminiscence 1 The general meaning is similar to that of REMEMBRANCE except that reminiscence is often regarded as the unconscious recall of information while a remembrance is considered to be the result of a conscious effort to retrieve information. 2 A rambling, sequential recalling of information about some earlier experience. In this sense, the connotation is that the process is a rather leisurely and enjoyable one. 3 Simply, a synonym of RECALL (1). The unconscious aspect is absent from 2 and 3. See OBLIVISCENCE, the loss of information from memory.

remission A cessation of the symptoms of a disorder or disease. The connotation of CURE is entirely absent from this term; the disorder or disease is still assumed to be present even though there are no apparent symptoms. The term is often used with the (guarded) connotation that the symptoms are not expected to reappear; distinguish, on these grounds, from INTERMISSION.

REM latency The period of time between the onset of sleep and the first period of *REM sleep*. There are suggestions that unusually short REM latency is a symptom of depression.

remote Distant, removed, far away. The term is used in a variety of contexts, as given in the following entries.

remote association ASSOCIATION, REMOTE.

remote conditioning A relatively rare synonym of TRACE CONDITIONING.

remote dependency Any statistical relationship between nonadjacent events. For example, in a pattern-learning experiment the stimulus that appears on trial n may be made to depend upon the stimulus that appeared on some remote, earlier trial $n - y$, where $y > 1$.

remote masking MASKING, REMOTE.

remote memory MEMORY, RECENT and REMOTE.

remote perception Perception of a stimulus object through some intermediary device not normally used for the gathering of such stimulus information, e.g. the perception of the shape of an object by probing with a stick or cane while blindfolded.

remote viewing CLAIRVOYANCE.

REM sleep A stage of sleep named for the rapid eye movements which are among its most salient characteristics. For more detail, see SLEEP.

REM storm Extremely vigorous episodes of rapid eye movements (REM) during sleep. During such bursts the eye movements have very large amplitude and are often accompanied by facial movements, brow-raising and eye-opening. They are relatively common in neonates up to about 5 weeks of age and less frequent thereafter.

renal Pertaining to the kidney.

renifleur A *paraphilia* in which erotic stimu-

lation is derived from odours, specifically from the smell of the urine of others.

renin A hormone of the kidney. Release of renin is produced by sympathetic stimulation or by a reduction in blood flow in the kidneys. When released, renin causes angiotensinogen in the blood to convert to angiotensin, which, in turn, produces thirst as well as stimulating the adrenal cortex, resulting ultimately in sodium retention.

Renshaw cell A small neuron with a short axon that functions as an inhibitor of motor neurons. See RECURRENT INHIBITION.

renunciation A tricky term with three related but different usages: **1** In common parlance, a surrendering of self, will, title, inheritance, etc. **2** In the psychology of religion, the surrendering of one's personal will or desires to what one perceives to be the will of one's god. **3** In psychoanalysis, the *refusal* of the ego to surrender to either the primitive demands of the id or the unrealistic restrictions of the superego.

reorganization theory The theory that the primary process involved in learning is the altering or modifying of existing mental structures. This generalization appears most frequently in research in cognitive and perceptual processes and, as with the base word, ORGANIZATION, the term's meaning derives from the assumptions of GESTALT THEORY. Reorganization theory stands in strong opposition to associationistic theory, which assumes that learning is essentially the appending of new responses without structural reorganization; see ASSOCIATIONISM. The term is used in a variety of contexts and it is not infrequently found in studies of personality and social psychology, where the link with Gestalt theory is not always apparent.

repair mechanism In interpersonal communication, any statement or utterance designed to correct (i.e. repair) a misunderstanding. Repair mechanisms are of particular interest during early language development, when a parent must frequently correct a child's miscommunications caused by using linguistic forms beyond its competence or by a lack of attention.

reparation In psychoanalysis, the reduction of guilt by the doing of good works. In

Melanie Klein's approach, reparation was considered a nonneurotic defence mechanism used to resolve ambivalent feelings toward objects and persons.

repeated measures 1 An experimental design in which subjects are measured using the same test or instrument two or more times. This sense of the term is generally used only for designs where a measure is applied at least three times. 2 Any statistical procedure for analysing differences in scores across repeated tests that have the same theoretical properties, generally with the aim of identifying changes attributable to such factors as the passage of time, growth, development or an experimental intervention. Although a variety of procedures exist, the term is typically used when there are three or more measurement points and the implication is that an ANALYSIS OF VARIANCE is used to assess the effects.

repertoire The full compendium of behaviours of an organism or a species. Some authors restrict the term to those behaviours which a given organism can currently perform, others use it more generally to include potential behaviours that a member of a particular species may perform. The latter meaning is more often the intended one.

repetition 1 The practising or repeating of some act. When this operation functions merely to *hold* information in memory, the term is essentially synonymous with REHEARSAL: when it functions to *improve* performance, the meaning is synonymous with PRACTICE. 2 Any replica or reproduction. 3 A single trial in an experiment. The repetitive aspect is missing in this meaning.

repetition blindness REPETITION EFFECTS.

repetition compulsion 1 Generally, a common form of compulsion in which there is an irrational and rather irresistible desire to repeat some behaviour. 2 In psychoanalytic theory, the impulse to re-enact emotional experiences from early life independent of any advantage that may be derived from so doing.

repetition effects Quite simply, the effects on perception and memory of repeating a stimulus. Depending on conditions of presentation and testing, one may observe *repetition priming* (see PRIMING), in which re-presentation of a stimulus increases the likelihood of its being perceived or recalled in a subsequent test, or *repetition blindness*, in which, perhaps surprisingly, the second of two rapid presentations of a visual stimulus is often not noticed.

repetition, law of LAW OF *FREQUENCY.

repetitive transcranial magnetic stimulation TRANSCRANIAL MAGNETIC STIMULATION.

replacement sampling SAMPLING WITH REPLACEMENT.

replicate To reproduce, to duplicate. Specifically, to duplicate an experiment as precisely as possible to see if the same results are obtained as on the first occasion; to run a REPLICATION (1).

replication A term commonly used in discussions of experimental methodology but with two different (although semantically related) meanings: 1 An experiment that reproduces or replicates an earlier experiment. 2 Each of the subdivisions of an experiment which contains all of the basic parametric variations of interest. Note that some use the term in sense 2 to refer to the operation of subdividing an experiment; in this case, the term *replica* is used to denote each part.

replication therapy A technique used in some behavioural-therapy approaches whereby an attempt is made to reproduce real-life situations or to encourage reactions in the client which are similar to those made in real-life situations.

represent 1 To stand for, in the sense of a symbol or substitute. See here REPRESENTATION, REPRESENTATIVE. 2 To present again; often spelled *re-present* to distinguish from 1.

representation A thing that stands for, takes the place of, symbolizes, or represents another thing. In studies of perception and cognition one often sees reference to the *mental representation* of a stimulus event, which, depending upon theoretical orientation, may be characterized as a direct mapping of the stimulus (see DIRECT REALISM), an elaboration of the stimulus (see CONSTRUCTIVISM), a mental code of it (see IDEA, IMAGE) or an abstract characterization of it (see PROPOSITION). In psychoanalytic theory, dreams, memories, fantasies and the like are also called representations of unconscious factors and repressed impulses.

representative Having the characteristic of being able to take the place of a thing or to be substituted for it without disrupting the overall structure or introducing systematic bias. See e.g. REPRESENTATIVE *SAMPLING, REPRE-SENTATIVE SCORE.

representative measure REPRESENTATIVE SCORE.

representativeness A COGNITIVE *HEURISTIC in which decisions are made based on how representative a given individual case appears to be independent of other information about its actual likelihood. For example, when people read about a man who is conservative, enjoys mathematical games, tends to wear white, short-sleeve shirts and has little interest in politics, they are more likely to believe he is an engineer than a lawyer – and will continue to believe this even if told that he was selected randomly from a group composed of 70 lawyers but only 30 engineers. Representativeness is one of the reasons why people commit the BASE-RATE FALLACY.

representative sample SAMPLE, REPRESENTA-TIVE.

representative score A single score or number which, within recognized limits of confidence, can be taken as representative of a large number of scores. The term is most frequently used of the *mean* as a measure of central tendency that best characterizes (i.e. represents) all the scores from which it is calculated. Also called *representative measure* and *representative value*.

representative value REPRESENTATIVE SCORE.

repress 1 Outside of psychoanalytic theories the term is used in ways similar to the common sense, i.e. to hold or put down, to suppress, to keep from occurring. **2** Within psychoanalysis, to engage the operations of the defence mechanism of REPRESSION; see meaning 1 of that term for details.

repressed Loosely, characterizing any mental element that has been relegated to or maintained in the unconscious. Thus we have repressed wishes, repressed complexes, repressed desires, etc.; see REPRESSION (esp. 1) for a discussion of usage.

repression The basic meaning derives from the root verb, *to repress*, which in various contexts means to put down, suppress, control, censor, exclude, etc. Hence: **1** In all depth psychologies from the classical Freudian model onward, a hypothesized mental process or operation that functions to protect the individual from ideas, impulses and memories which would produce anxiety, apprehension or guilt were they to become conscious. Repression is considered to be operative at an unconscious level; that is, not only does the mechanism keep certain mental contents from reaching awareness, but its very operations lie outside of conscious awareness. In classical psychoanalytic theory, it is regarded as an ego function and several processes are included under it: (a) *primal repression*, in which primitive, forbidden id impulses are blocked and prevented from ever reaching consciousness; (b) *primary repression*, in which anxiety-producing mental content is forcefully removed from consciousness and prevented from re-emerging; and (c) *secondary repression*, in which elements that might serve to remind the person of that which has been previously repressed are themselves repressed. An important corollary of this analysis is that that which is repressed is not deactivated but continues to have a lively existence at the unconscious level, making itself felt through projections in disguised symbolic form in dreams, parapraxes and psychoneuroses. Within these analytic psychologies, the term has a fairly clear referential domain and should be contrasted with other seemingly synonymous terms such as SUPPRESSION and INHIBITION. **2** In sociology and social psychology, the limitations of a group's or an individual's freedom of expression and action by a dominant group or individual.

repression, organic A vaguely misleading term for the inability to recall past events owing to organic dysfunction, brain damage, etc. The word *repression* is misused here since the term is properly restricted to those conditions with an organic basis, whereas REPRESSION is used very differently. See AMNESIA, which is preferred, especially ANTEROGRADE *AMNESIA.

repression–sensitization scale A personality-assessment scale designed to evaluate an individual's defensive reactions against threatening stimuli. *Repressors*, as compared with *sensitizers*, have difficulty with threatening stimuli, often tending not to notice them. They also show poorer memory for threatening materials they have learned, and have lower overall awareness of anxiety and a more positive self-image.

reproduction 1 Generally, the process of re-producing a thing, or the product of such a process. **2** The process that produces a new organism from one (asexual reproduction) or two (sexual reproduction) parents.

reproduction method (or **procedure**) **1** In the study of memory, any procedure in which a subject is required to reproduce as completely and accurately as possible all of the stimulus materials originally learned. **2** In psychophysics, a synonym of the *method of adjustment*; see here METHOD OF *SCALING and MEASUREMENT OF *THRESHOLD for details.

reproduction theory A theory of mental imagery or ideation that maintains that an image is a copy or point-by-point reproduction of the original stimulus. The last word on this discredited theory was provided by William James in 1890, who dubbed such a faithful mental image or ideal 'as mythological an entity as the Jack of Spades'.

reproductive assimilation ASSIMILATION, REPRODUCTIVE.

reproductive facilitation An increase in the ability to reproduce previously learned material caused by the interpolation of some other unrelated activity or material between the learning and the time of recall. This facilitation effect seems to result from a release of proactive interference; see RELEASE FROM *PI.

reproductive function A biological term for those activities of organisms that result in new organisms. Note that both sexual and asexual reproduction are included.

reproductive images ANTICIPATORY IMAGES.

reproductive interference A decrease in the ability to reproduce previously learned material resulting from the interpolation of some other activity or material between the learning and the time of recall. The effect seems to result from RETROACTIVE *INTERFERENCE.

reproductive isolation ISOLATION (2).

reproductive memory MEMORY, REPRODUCTIVE.

reproductive ritual Any cultural ritual that centres on sex, sexuality, sex roles or other factors relevant to reproduction. Generally included are puberty rites, male or female initiation rites, elaborate taboos (as, for example, those surrounding menstruation), birth practices such as couvade, and the like.

Rep Test A personality-assessment test designed by George Kelly to facilitate the process of coming to know how an individual views his or her world. The full name of the instrument is *Role Construct Repertory Test*, and it is used for diagnosing or assessing *personal-role constructs*, which, in Kelly's theory, are essential components of personality. See PERSONAL CONSTRUCT for more detail.

Rescorla–Wagner theory A generalization about conditioning due to R. Rescorla and A. Wagner that is founded on the premise that organisms do not merely respond to the *co-occurrence* of the conditioned stimulus (CS) and the unconditioned stimulus (US) but rather are sensitive to the actual *covariations* that exist between them. The point is that conditioning only occurs when a particular CS is a good predictor of the US. The theory provides an answer to the question 'Why didn't Pavlov's dogs salivate to Pavlov since he was the one who administered the food?' The reason is because Pavlov was also there when the food was *not* delivered. Thus, unlike the bell, he was not a reliable predictor of the arrival of food: he merely co-occurred with it.

research Theodorson and Theodorson, in their *Modern Dictionary of Sociology* (New York, 1969), provide one of the best comments on this term we've seen: 'Any honest attempt to study a problem systematically or to add to [our] knowledge of a problem may be regarded as research.' No more really needs to be said: if more is wanted see SCIENTIFIC *METHOD for how most research is carried out in psychology as well as the other sciences.

research, pure and applied Research that focuses on issues that emerged from considerations that were primarily scientific in nature will often be termed *pure*. Research where the considerations derived from issues of the utilization of knowledge will frequently be termed *applied*. The distinction is in the initial aim of the scientist and not the ultimate end to which the findings are put. Applied researchers often solve pure scientific problems and those who do pure research frequently find that there are applications for their discoveries.

reserpine An alkaloid of the Indian shrub *Rauwolfia serpentina*, this was the first ANTIPSYCHOTIC drug to be used widely. In low doses it has a marked calming and sedative effect, in large doses it may cause seizures and, on occasion, severe depression. These side effects make it no longer a legitimate choice as an antipsychotic, the PHENOTHIAZINES being favoured. It is, however, still used in small doses for hypertension because of its marked effects in reducing blood pressure and heart rate.

reserve **1** A reluctance to participate in social interactions. **2** That which is kept back, that which remains; see COGNITIVE RESERVE, OPERANT RESERVE and REFLEX RESERVE.

residual **1** Generally, characterizing that which is left over or remains behind after some operation or event has occurred. **2** Pertaining to the perceptual function remaining following an accident, injury or operation, e.g. *residual vision*. **3** In factor analysis, characterizing that portion of the variance that remains after that accounted for by all of the factors has been extracted. n., *residual*. **4** In statistical regression, the difference between the data points and the regression line.

residual marker MARKER, RESIDUAL.

residual phase That phase of an illness or disorder that occurs after appearance of the initial symptoms that mark the full disorder.

residual schizophrenia SCHIZOPHRENIA, RESIDUAL.

residue pitch VIRTUAL PITCH.

resignation Generally, an attitude of acquiescence, a giving up of the 'good fight' and accepting, with vague negative feelings, one's fate. However, note that Karen Horney differentiated between DYNAMIC *RESIGNATION and NEUROTIC *RESIGNATION.

resignation, dynamic Horney's term for a conscious, planned resignation in a situation in which a person feels that it is momentarily unfavourable to make further efforts on his or her part. It characterizes a situation in which the individual does not admit defeat and is alert for changes in the situation that may turn things in his or her favour. Compare with NEUROTIC *RESIGNATION.

resignation, neurotic Horney's term for a psychoneurotic withdrawal from a conflict. Horney hypothesized three different forms which the condition could take: PERSISTENT *RESIGNATION, SHALLOW LIVING and NEUROTIC *REBELLIOUSNESS. See each of these for details and distinguish this class of reactions from DYNAMIC *RESIGNATION.

resignation, persistent A form of NEUROTIC *RESIGNATION manifested by inertia, ennui, passivity and a generalized lack of initiative in dealing with the ordinary conflicts and decisions of daily living.

resilience The capacity to maintain effective psychological and behavioural adjustment in the face of factors that normally put individuals at risk for poor adjustment. The term is used without implications about the source. An individual can show high resilience because of a basic TEMPERAMENT or HARDINESS, by having learned specific ways of dealing with stress, or by living in a social environment that provides sources of support. In the study of personality development, the terms *ego-resilience* and *resiliency* will be used to extend the reference to the person's ability to shift behaviours and search for viable and healthy responses to both traumatic and daily events. This usage implies the operation of EXECUTIVE FUNCTIONS in a way that the general meaning does not. ant., *vulnerability*.

resistance **1** Generally, any action of a body that opposes, withstands or strives against (i.e. resists) a force. **2** In electronics, the opposition of any circuit or body to the passage of an electric current. **3** In biology, the ability of a body to resist infection or stress. **4** A personality trait typified by a reluctance to follow orders, respond to group pressures, etc. **5** In psychoanalysis, opposition to making what is unconscious conscious. Note that some psychoanalysts also use the term somewhat more pragmatically to refer to the opposition to accepting the interpretations made by the analyst. In either case the resistance is generally regarded as caused by unconscious factors. It is also regarded as universal in psychoanalysis.

resistance, conscious Deliberate (i.e. conscious) refusal to divulge information by a client in a therapeutic situation. Distinguish from RESISTANCE (5), but appreciate that some theorists argue that unconscious resistance is the motivator of this conscious form.

resistance stage The second stage in the GENERAL ADAPTATION SYNDROME.

resistance to extinction The extent to which a learned response continues to be made after experimental extinction procedures have begun. It is used as a measure of the strength of conditioning, particularly in comparing the effectiveness of various SCHEDULES OF *REINFORCEMENT in maintaining operant behaviour.

resistance to temptation Quite literally, the ability to resist temptation, specifically the temptation to engage in forbidden or taboo behaviours. Within psychoanalysis it is commonly interpreted as a measure of superego functioning.

resolution Generally, the solution of a problem by the coordination of all relevant elements and/or the taking of a novel but workable perspective. This meaning is applied broadly in the study of problem-solving, in decision-making and in psychotherapy, where 'resolution of a conflict' is often taken as the key to establishment of normal, nonneurotic functioning. vb., resolve.

resolving power 1 Generally, in optics the ability of a lens to produce separate images of distinct but spatially proximate objects. 2 Specifically, a similar ability of the eye. 3 Metaphorically, the cognitive capability to make subtle discriminations between situations.

resonance 1 Sympathetic vibration in a body produced in response to an external vibration. 2 Metaphorically, a property of a situation in which two or more people are in agreement about the emotional aspects of a situation. This latter meaning, although basically nontechnical, has worked its way into the literature, particularly in the writings of humanistic psychologists.

resonance theory (of hearing) THEORIES OF *HEARING.

resonance-volley theory (of hearing) THEORIES OF *HEARING.

resonator Any device that uses the principle of RESONANCE (1) to amplify a tone.

respiration rate Breathing rate. Commonly used as a measure of emotionality and arousal by comparing relative amounts of time spent on inspiration and expiration; see I/E RATIO.

respondent 1 n. Any behaviour that is elicited from an organism by a specific stimulus; a classically conditioned response. 2 adj. Characterizing such a behaviour. See, and compare these two meanings with, OPERANT. 3 n. Loosely, any organism that responds to a stimulus – although this meaning is virtually always restricted to a person responding to items on a questionnaire.

respondent conditioning Skinner's term for CLASSICAL CONDITIONING.

response (R) There are real problems with defining this term. The difficulties are caused by its ubiquity and by the fact that in most contexts it is used with qualifiers. Considering it as a 'pure' term, one can identify several denotative domains, as follows: 1 Any reaction of an organism to, or in the presence of, a stimulus. This usage is utterly general and utterly inclusive. 2 Any muscular or glandular reaction or process made to, or in the presence of, a stimulus. This meaning was favoured by early behaviourists. 3 Any answer to any question. This sense is mostly found in research work using questionnaires and survey techniques. 4 A unitary process that serves as a theoretical category representing all behaviours that share sufficient similarity to be regarded as functionally equivalent for the topic or issue under consideration. This meaning, although rarely specified, underlies all of the above. It is a necessary aspect of any definition of the term, since individual responses differ from instance to instance: no two bar-presses are identical, all gaits are different, repeated utterances of even simple sentences may vary in their own ways as much as interpretations of a Beethoven sonata, and so on. This issue is made explicit in the Skinnerian definition of the term: **5** A class of behaviours all of which have the same effect. Note, however, that in this context one further distinguishes operant responses (*operants*) and reflexive responses (*respondents*).

Note, finally, that there are a large number of partial synonyms, e.g. *reaction, behaviour, act, movement, process*. Just how synonymous each is depends on the context and the biases of the writer. Generally, one can get away with almost any interchanging of these terms.

response amplitude In studies of conditioning, the magnitude of a response measured along some set dimension. See RESPONSE MAGNITUDE.

response attitude RESPONSE *SET.

response bias Generally, any preference for making one particular response over any of the other alternatives available when that preference is exhibited independent of the relevant stimulus conditions. Response biases often pose difficult problems in research. For example, in experiments on absolute THRESHOLD (1), subjects who are rather liberal with their 'Yes, I detected it' responses produce substantially different data from those with a more conservative bias, even though presumably their sensitivity to the stimuli is about the same. See CATCH TRIAL and SIGNAL-DETECTION THEORY. Difficulties stemming from response biases also emerge in social and personality inventories and questionnaires; see FORCED-CHOICE TECHNIQUE. They can also pop up in the most innocent way in research, such as subjects showing a bias for the item on the left, the stimulus at the top of the monitor, the first (or last) item presented in a list, etc. Great care needs to be taken to ensure that such biases do not contaminate one's data.

response class A term occasionally used to clarify the meaning of RESPONSE when the author is using that term in sense 4 or 5.

response competition Literally, the set of circumstances where more than one response is elicited by a stimulus. For a classic case, see STROOP TASK.

response differentiation DIFFERENTIATION (esp. 4 and 5).

response generalization GENERALIZATION, RESPONSE.

response hierarchy Essentially a synonym of HABIT HIERARCHY, although *response hierarchy* probably has greater currency since *habit hierarchy* is tinged with specific connotations from its use in Hullian theory.

response latency LATENCY, RESPONSE.

response learning LEARNING, RESPONSE.

response magnitude In studies of conditioning, any characteristic of a response that reflects its underlying response strength. Various measures have been proposed such as response latency, intensity and the like. None work terribly well and the best measure is probably the response's RESISTANCE TO EXTINCTION.

response-operating   characteristic RECEIVER-OPERATING CHARACTERISTIC CURVE.

response probability PROBABILITY OF RESPONSE.

response rate 1 The number of responses per unit of time. It is a commonly used measure of learning in operant-conditioning experiments. **2** In survey research, the ratio of completed surveys returned to surveys distributed. It is used as a rough measure of the representativeness of the sample and, during pilot testing, as a possible indicator of problems with the instrument that make it unlikely to be completed and returned.

response set SET, RESPONSE.

response-shock interval TEMPORAL AVOIDANCE CONDITIONING.

response strength 1 Quite literally, the strength of a response as reflected by its magnitude; see RESPONSE MAGNITUDE. **2** More abstractly (but more correctly), the degree to which a response continues to be made after extinction procedures have been instituted; see RESISTANCE TO EXTINCTION.

response time The time required for a response to be made. See also REACTION TIME, RESPONSE *LATENCY.

response topography A full characterization of the pertinent components of a behavioural response. For example, an operant response of a rat in a Skinner box might be called a 'bar press'. But its topography could differ depending on whether it is a forceful press or a gentle one, made slowly or quickly, with the left paw or the right, etc. With selective reinforcement the topography of the response can be modified.

response variable Basically, the DEPENDENT *VARIABLE in an experiment.

responsibility, diffusion of Quite literally, the diffusion of one's sense of responsibility to act in a particular situation owing to the presence of many other persons all of whom may be viewed as potentially responsible for acting. See also BYSTANDER INTERVENTION EFFECT.

responsive Characterizing: **1** Any organism or part thereof that makes a response to a particular stimulus. **2** Any organism that gives evidence of being prepared to respond or capable of responding. **3** A person who provides pertinent and appropriate responses to questions or requests.

rest **1** A state of not responding (relatively speaking). **2** A state of relaxation; the term is typically used in this sense with the connotation of a recuperative or rehabilitative function.

rest-activity cycle BASIC REST-ACTIVITY CYCLE.

resting potential The electrical potential of a neuron at rest. See and compare with ACTION POTENTIAL.

restless leg syndrome An ORGANIC *SLEEP DISORDER characterized by rhythmic limb movements during sleep, typically the legs. Often accompanied by daytime feelings of limb twitchiness or discomfort and a compulsion to change limb positions repetitively while resting, particularly in the evening. A majority of sufferers also experience NOCTURNAL MYOCLONUS. Also called *Ekbom's syndrome* or, more colloquially, *Jimmy legs*.

restoration effects Any of several perceptual phenomena where an incomplete or disrupted stimulus is 'restored'. The effects are due to TOP-DOWN PROCESSING where the missing information is restored based on prior knowledge (e.g. PHONEMIC RESTORATION EFFECT) or basic perceptual principles (e.g. CLOSURE).

Restorff effect VON RESTORFF EFFECT.

restricted code B. Bernstein's term for the speech mode adopted when one is speaking with peers with whom one shares close identification, similar views and common backgrounds and knowledge. Under such conditions, especially when the topic under discussion is in the 'here and now', the discourse is rapid, relatively simply planned and relatively predictable and often contains in-jokes and shorthand expressions. Compare with ELABORATED CODE.

restricted learning LEARNING, RESTRICTED.

restructure **1** Quite literally, to modify or adjust an existing structure. Generally used here with respect to the internal (mental) structure of an image, a memory, a situation, etc. **2** In FIELD THEORY, to alter in fundamental ways the relationships between the various aspects of a field.

retardation **1** Generally, a slowing of any process. **2** More specifically, a slowing of mental, intellectual or scholastic progress. See MENTAL RETARDATION for details on usage.

retarded depression DEPRESSION, RETARDED.

retention **1** Generally, the process of holding onto or retaining a thing. Most commonly used with respect to issues surrounding the retention of information, where the basic presumption is that some 'mental content' persists from the time of initial exposure to the material or initial learning of a response until some later request for recall or reperformance. See MEMORY et seq. and FORGETTING for more details. **2** In physiology, the retaining either voluntarily or involuntarily of faeces or urine.

retention curve A label applied to any of a number of possible graphic representations that present the course of retention of material over time.

retest reliability TEST–RETEST *RELIABILITY.

reticular From the Latin, meaning *net, network*.

reticular activating system (RAS) That component of the RETICULAR FORMATION that was once assumed to function as an activating centre and that when stimulated aroused the rest of the brain. Although the LOCUS COERULEUS in the reticular formation does play a role in some aspects of sleep (particularly REM sleep), there is no compelling reason to think of it or any other structure in the brainstem as functioning as the brain's activating system.

reticular formation A complex system of over 90 nuclei and a diffuse network of neurons with complex and extensive axonal and dendritic processes. It occupies the central core of the brainstem from the medulla to the upper part of the midbrain, receiving input from various ascending pathways and projecting fibres to the spinal cord, the thalamus and ultimately the cerebral cortex. It plays a role in attention, movement, sleep, arousal and various reflexes.

reticular membrane A membrane formed by the plates at the termini of supporting cells in the organ of Corti in the cochlea of the inner ear.

reticular nucleus A thalamic nucleus that relays information from the cortex to the reticular formation.

reticulospinal tract One of the VENTROME-DIAL PATHWAYS. It runs from the RETICULAR FOR-MATION to the grey matter of the spinal cord and controls the muscles responsible for postural movement.

reticulothalamic tract (or **system**) An offshoot of the SPINOTHALAMIC TRACT that carries afferent information about temperature and pain.

retifism See FOOT FETISH.

retina The innermost of the membranes of the inner surface of the posterior portion of the eye. Although extremely complex neuronally, with up to ten layers or zones identifiable, it is divided according to the usual description into three major layers, from front to back: the *ganglion-cell layer*, the *bipolar-cell layer* and the *photoreceptor layer*. The last of these contains the approximately 115 million RODS and 6 million CONES which serve as the primary visual receptors. The cones, which are responsible for colour vision and perception of fine details, are packed into the rod-free FOVEA and thin out toward the periphery of the retina (see here PHOTOPIC VISION). The rods, which handle low-illumination vision, begin just outside the fovea and increase in relative proportion toward the periphery (see SCOTOPIC VISION). pl., *retinas* or *retinae*.

retinal 1 n. A small molecule derived from vitamin A which, along with *opsin*, makes up the basic chemical constituents of photopigments. See RHODOPSIN for more detail. Also called *retinene*; distinguish from RETINOL. **2** adj. Pertaining to the retina.

retinal bipolar cells Straightforwardly, BIPOLAR CELLS in the retina. They receive inputs from the rods and cones and transmit signals to the amacrine and ganglion cells. Those that serve the rod system are distinct from those that serve the cones and are often denoted as the *rod* bipolars and the *cone* bipolars respectively.

retinal densitometry A technique for measuring the amount of light absorbed by the rods of the retina. The basic principle involves the reflecting of light off the dark choroid sheath behind the retina. The light passes through the retina twice and whatever is absorbed by the retinal pigments is absent in the final measurement.

retinal disparity DISPARITY, RETINAL.

retinal field The pattern or array of retinal receptors stimulated by a stimulus field. Distinguish from RECEPTIVE FIELD (1).

retinal fusion BINOCULAR RIVALRY.

retinal image IMAGE (2).

retinal light IDIORETINAL LIGHT.

retinal projection PROJECTION, RETINAL.

retinal projection area V1.

retinal receptive field RECEPTIVE FIELD (1).

retinal rivalry BINOCULAR RIVALRY.

retinal zones COLOUR ZONES.

retinene RETINAL (1).

retinex (**theory**) Edwin Land's theoretical model of colour vision. He hypothesized three separate visual systems (retinexes): one responsive primarily to long-wavelength light, one to moderate-wavelength light and the third to short-wavelength light. Each is represented as an analogue of a black-and-white picture taken through a particular filter, producing maximum activity in response to red, green and blue light for the long-, moderate-, and short-wavelength retinexes respectively.

retinitis pigmentosa A progressive disease

of the retina marked by atrophy of the photo-receptors. Because the rods are affected more than the cones, the primary symptoms are NYCTALOPIA and TUNNEL VISION.

retinol Vitamin A; it is an essential precursor for the synthesis of RETINAL (1).

retinotectal projection area VI.

retinotopic representation The topological representation of the retina on the visual cortex. It is not a linear representation, since the fovea, which is physically a small spot on the retina, provides roughly 25% of the cortical representation, but it does maintain the spatial code, that is, stimulating two neighbouring regions on the retina produces excitation of two adjacent areas on the cortex. Also called *retinotopic map, retinotopy, visuotopic representation* or *visuotopy.*

retinotopy RETINOTOPIC REPRESENTATION.

retreat from reality FLIGHT FROM *REALITY.

retrieval This term, absent from older lexicons of psychology, has become one of the more common – even voguish – words for the process of recalling information from memory. See RECALL and MEMORY et seq. for discussion.

retro- Combining form meaning *behind* or *backward in time* or *in space.*

retroactive Generally descriptive of any event, stimulus or process that has an effect on the effects of previously occurring events, stimuli or processes. Compare with PRO-ACTIVE.

retroactive association In serial-learning experiments, an association between an item on a list and any preceding item.

retroactive facilitation FACILITATION, RETRO-ACTIVE.

retroactive inhibition RETROACTIVE *INTER-FERENCE.

retrograde 1 Generally, moving backwards, retreating, retiring. 2 With respect to the orderings of events, reversed or inverted. 3 In biology, showing degeneration or deterioration.

retrograde amnesia AMNESIA, RETROGRADE.

retrograde degeneration DEGENERATION (1).

retrogression 1 A synonym of REGRESSION (1). Used in this sense by some authors who wish to avoid the psychoanalytic connotations that often accompany *regression.* 2 A reverting to an earlier form of behaviour that was actually engaged in by the individual. Lewin stressed this meaning, and many others use it as well; it should, unlike meaning 1, be contrasted with REGRESSION.

retrospection Lit., inspecting and reporting on that which has passed. There was an interesting debate among the early structuralists, some of whom argued that *retrospection* needed to be contrasted with *introspection* (observing and reporting on present experience), while others maintained that the processes were equivalent. Auguste Comte put forward this latter position succinctly: 'In order to observe (introspect) your intellect must pause from activity and yet it is this activity you want to observe. If you cannot effect the pause you cannot observe, if you do effect it, there is nothing (present) to observe.'

retrospective falsification Unconscious modification and distortion of previous experiences so as to make them conform with present needs. See also CONFABULATION, which may or may not have the connotation of *unconscious.*

retrospective sampling SAMPLING, RETRO-SPECTIVE.

Rett's syndrome (or disorder) A developmental disorder characterized by normal development for the first six months followed by a gradual loss of purposive hand movements with accompanying stereotypic hand-washing movements, a failure of normal head and trunk growth, ataxia, and marked delay and impairment of language development. Some classify it as a PERVASIVE *DEVELOPMENTAL DISORDER, others consider it to be an AUTISTIC SPECTRUM DISORDER although it's worth noting that, unlike other forms of ASD, it is diagnosed more often in girls than boys. Also called *Rett syndrome.*

reuptake The reabsorption of a substance. A term used commonly of transmitter substances that are taken up again by the terminal buttons from which they were liberated.

reuptake inhibitor Any substance that

inhibits or otherwise reduces the ability of a presynaptic neuron to reabsorb a neurotransmitter it has released. See SELECTIVE SEROTONIN REUPTAKE INHIBITORS for an example of an important group of such compounds.

revelation effect A type of false memory in which certain types of cognitive activity lead to an illusion of familiarity for items or events which were not actually experienced before. For example, after solving a number of anagrams, a new word might be falsely 'recognized' as having been previously encountered.

reverberating circuit In Donald O. Hebb's theory, a CELL ASSEMBLY that, functioning as a whole unit, continues to respond after the original stimulus that initiated its response has been terminated. Also called *reverberatory circuit*.

reverie A rather unstructured, relatively purposeless mental state characterized by aimless mental meanderings and fantasies. As the term is typically used, the connotation is that the state is a distinctly pleasant experience.

reversal In psychoanalysis, the turning-about of an instinct, e.g. sadism changes to masochism. Anna Freud argued that REACTION FORMATION as a defence mechanism occurred because of the capacity for reversal. Also called *reversal of affect* and occasionally used as a synonym of INVERSION OF AFFECT, particularly when no psychoanalytical connotation is intended.

reversal error REVERSALS.

reversal formation An occasional synonym of REACTION FORMATION.

reversal learning LEARNING, REVERSAL.

reversals (or **reversal errors**) Errors made in reading and writing characterized by the reversal of symbols. Such errors are most often single-letter reversals (e.g. *b* and *d*) or reversals of letter order (e.g. *was* for *saw*), although occasionally word-order errors are also called reversals. Note that the technical term *strephosymbolia*, which literally means the *twisting of symbols*, is dropping out of usage here and, for once in science, an easily understood term is replacing an awkward one.

reversal shift REVERSAL *LEARNING.

reverse anorexia A BODY DISMORPHIC DISORDER marked by a desire to increase body size, particularly muscle mass accompanied by excessive intake of calories, constant muscle-building exercise and unhappiness with body image. The term is relatively new and unfortunate for it misuses ANOREXIA. Hopefully a more lexicographically appropriate synonym will emerge.

reverse scoring In testing, the 'reversing' of the score on an item. For example, an instrument that assesses *attachment style* using a binomial response scale, would normally have each item endorsed by a respondent receive a score of '1' and each not endorsed a score of '0'. However, an item such as 'I feel uncomfortable in close relationships' would have to be 'reverse scored' so that the answer would be consistent with higher levels of a secure attachment style.

reverse tolerance TOLERANCE, REVERSE.

reversibility The property of a series of operations such that reversing their order restores the original state. In Piaget's theory, apprehension of this principle is an element in the establishment of *conservation*.

reversible figure FIGURE, REVERSIBLE.

reversible perspective ALTERNATING PERSPECTIVE.

reversing lenses (or **prisms**) Lenses which, when worn, reverse the visual field. They have been used in research on perceptual learning and relearning. See DISPLACED VISION for more detail.

reversion 1 Generally, the act of reversing. 2 In genetics, the reappearance of a recessive genetic trait which has not been present in the phenotype for one or more generations. 3 Loosely, REGRESSION (1).

revival 1 Generally, bringing back to life. 2 In the study of memory, the process of recall in the sense that a dormant memory has been triggered or resuscitated (i.e. revived).

reward Loosely, any pleasurable or satisfying event or thing that is obtained when some requisite task has been carried out. The similarity between this notion and that of REINFORCEMENT (esp. 3) has led some authors to treat the two terms as synonyms. For the meaning of compound terms using *reward* in this fashion, see the equivalent term following *reinforcement*: e.g. for *primary reward* see PRIMARY *REINFORCER. However, most prefer to distinguish the terms in a manner best expressed by the following example. 'For the children in the study, a reward of 1 penny served as the reinforcement for each correct response.' It is possible to split many a hair over the subtle semantic overlaps between *reward* and *reinforcement*; see the extended discussion under REINFORCEMENT for a few of them.

reward expectancy In Tolman's learning theory, the internal process that occurs when an organism recognizes that it is in a circumstance that has been previously associated with a reward.

rewrite rule In linguistics, a rule that specifies how one linguistic form is to be altered to produce a grammatical phrase or sentence; e.g. NP → Art + N is a rewrite rule that specifies that a noun phrase (NP) can be rewritten as → an article (Art) plus a noun (N).

Rey–Osterrieth figure COMPLEX FIGURE TEST.

RGB system A system for specifying colours; see COLOUR EQUATION for details.

Rh Abbreviation for *rhesus*, a species of monkey. See RH BLOOD GROUP.

-rhage Combining form meaning *discharge, bleeding*.

rhaphe RAPHE.

Rh blood group A blood group found in roughly 80% of all humans, the name of which is derived from the rhesus monkey, in which it was first discovered. The presence of the rhesus factor is noted as Rh+ (or Rh positive), its absence as Rh– (or Rh negative). If the factor is introduced into someone who is Rh– it causes the production of antibodies (anti-Rh agglutinin), and subsequent transfusions of Rh+ blood cause serious reactions. During pregnancy an Rh– woman may become sensitized if the foetus is Rh+, making subsequent pregnancies with Rh+ foetuses potentially dangerous because Rh antibodies in the maternal blood may cross the placenta and destroy foetal blood cells. Evidence suggests that offspring from such pregnancies are at higher risk of schizophrenia. Also called RhD group.

-rhea Suffix meaning *flow*.

rheo- Combining form denoting *flowing, fluidity* or *current*.

rheobase In neurophysiology, the threshold of excitability of neural tissue. It is given as the minimum direct current which, if applied indefinitely, is sufficient to produce excitation. See also CHRONAXIE.

rheotropism An orienting response to the flow of water.

Rh factor RH BLOOD GROUP.

rhinal fissure A small fissure that marks the boundary between the HIPPOCAMPAL FORMATION and the neocortex.

Rhine deck ZENER CARDS.

rhinencephalon Lit., the smell (or olfactory) brain. It includes the olfactory bulb, olfactory tract, pyriform area, parts of the pyriform cortex and parts of the amygdaloid complex.

rhino- Combining form meaning *nose, nasal*.

rhizotomy A neurosurgical procedure where a nerve root in the spinal cord is severed. Because the procedure is irreversible it is only used in the most extreme circumstances such as cases of unrelievable spastic cerebral palsy or intractable pain.

rho (ρ) The symbol for a correlation coefficient resulting from an analysis of rank-order data on two variables.

rhodopsin The photopigment of the rods. It consists of rod OPSIN and RETINAL, and its breakdown in the presence of light is the first part of the long chain of events in the transduction of light energy to visual experience. Retinal has two forms: a bent form (called *11-cis retinal*) and a straight form (*all-trans retinal*). Only the 11-cis form can attach to rod opsin. The 11-cis form is, moreover, very unstable and exists only in the dark. Hence, when rhodopsin is exposed to light, the 11-cis form straightens out to become the all-trans form and rhodopsin breaks down into its constituents, which causes the photoreceptor to hyperpolarize.

rhombencephalon The HINDBRAIN.

rhythm 1 Any regular pattern of events or fluctuations as, for example, those found in BIORHYTHMS. **2** Regular recurrence of a pattern of events, particularly with a uniform system of beats, accents or grouped sequences. Rhythm and rhythmic structures are important as mnemonic aids; e.g. a 7-digit telephone number like 2794762 is often encoded rhythmically as '279 (long pause), 47 (short pause), 62 (drop in emphasis)'.

RI Abbreviation for RETROACTIVE *INTERFERENCE (or retroactive inhibition).

ribonucleic acid (RNA) A large, complex molecule made up of a sequence of four nucleotide bases (*adenine, guanine, cytosine* and *uracil*) attached to a sugar-phosphate 'backbone' (specifically, *ribose*, hence the name) *Messenger RNA (mRNA)* is copied from one strand of DEOXYRIBONUCLEIC ACID (DNA) and delivers genetic information from part of a chromosome to a ribosome, where *transfer RNA (tRNA)* coordinates the assembling of the proper amino acids into enzymes for cell specialization.

ribosome A small structure found in all cells that functions as a site for protein synthesis.

Ribot's law The generalization that the progressive memory loss seen in various forms of neurological disease follows evolutionary lines such that those processes dependent on phylogenetically older structures are spared impairment. See JACKSON'S PRINCIPLE, which is more general.

Ricco's law A generalization that states that for very small areas of the retina (i.e. less than 10 minutes of arc) the absolute threshold is inversely proportional to the area stimulated. Compare with PIPER'S LAW. Ricco's law also holds reasonably well for thermal thresholds on the skin.

rich interpretation Extended and expanded interpretation of a text, a discourse, a dream, etc. that brings to bear all that is known about the culture, the persons involved and existing theoretical models about the processes under examination. The term is found in psycholinguistic studies of a person's understanding of textual material, in discourse analysis involving interpretations that go beyond the information literally contained in the material, in dream analysis when the latent content of a dream is deeply interpreted, and the like. Also called *deep interpretation*. Compare with DECONTEXTUALIZATION.

rickets A bone-development disease in children caused by insufficient vitamin D.

right and wrong cases, method of MEASUREMENT OF *THRESHOLD.

right-associates learning An obsolete term for PAIRED-ASSOCIATES *LEARNING.

righting reflex Quite as it says, a reflexive reaction of an organism to being tipped off balance or turned over by which the organism attempts to regain normal posture.

rigid Inflexible, unyielding, nonpliant, etc. The term is used in a wide variety of contexts, e.g. to characterize thinking that is invariant, muscles that are tense, attitudes that are inflexible and unmodifiable. The usual connotation is distinctly negative.

rigidity 1 In physiology, a state of strong muscular contraction. **2** In personality theory, a trait characterized by cognitive, perceptual and/or social inflexibility. Distinguish from PERSEVERATION.

Ringelmann effect The generalization that each new member added to a group contributes proportionally less to achieving the group's goals than previously added members. The reasons are found in phenomena such as SOCIAL LOAFING.

risk 1 Any action that places something of value in jeopardy. Here the focus is on the action and one speaks of taking a risk or engaging in risky behaviour. **2** The probability of loss of something of value as a consequence of some action or event. Here the emphasis is on the likelihood of loss. For more on usage see AT RISK, CHOICE SHIFT, GAME et seq., UTILITY and VALUE (1, 3).

risk aversion The general tendency to be afraid of taking risks even when they also carry substantial potential gain. To take a classic case: when offered a choice between (a) a sure gain of $3,000 and (b) an 80% chance of a gain of $4,000 and a 20% chance of gaining nothing, almost everyone chooses (a). However, if asked to choose between (a) a sure loss of $3,000 and (b) an 80% chance of losing $4,000 and a 20% chance of losing nothing, most people choose (b). That is, most people are risk aversive and choose so as to avoid taking risks when looking for some gain: they submit to risky propositions only when attempting to avoid a sure loss.

risk factor Any characteristic that increases the likelihood that an individual will develop a disorder or disease. The term is used freely for genetic, behavioural or environmental factors.

risk-taking A hypothesized personality dimension reflecting the degree to which an individual willingly undertakes actions that involve a significant degree of risk.

risky-shift CHOICE SHIFT.

risperidone An ATYPICAL *ANTIPSYCHOTIC DRUG used to treat a variety of psychoses, including schizophrenia and bipolar disorder in children, and to augment the action of SELECTIVE SEROTONIN UPTAKE INHIBITORS. Trade name Risperdal.

Ritalin METHYLPHENIDATE.

rite 1 A culturally directed format for a ceremony. **2** Occasionally, a RITUAL (2), but see that term and CEREMONY for distinctions in usage.

ritual 1 Generally, any sequence of actions or behaviours that is highly stylized, relatively rigid and stereotyped. **2** A culturally or socially standardized set of actions dictated by tradition (usually religious, magical or nationalistic), rather precisely defined and revealing little or no variation from occurrence to occurrence. Occasionally the term is treated in this sense as a partial synonym of RITE or CEREMONY, although *ceremony* is often taken as a more general term, several rituals comprising a ceremony. **3** An oft-repeated pattern of behaviour which tends to occur at appropriate times, e.g. the morning ritual of washing, grooming and dressing. **4** A fairly elaborate, stereotyped set of behaviours that perhaps had functional origins which are no longer apparent. The term *routine* is also used in senses 3 and 4. **5** Irrational, repetitive behaviours often observed in the OBSESSIVE-COMPULSIVE DISORDER.

It should be appreciated that some authors use the term with the connotation that all rituals, no matter how mundane their mani-festation, have some symbolic role to play either in a culture or in the psychological make-up of an individual.

rivalry A state of interaction between two or more entities (which may be persons, groups, institutions, biological structures, etc.) such that they are in a competitive pursuit of the same goals or things. The term is used generally, and the participants in the interaction may either be in direct contact with each other or pursue the goals separately. *Competition* is a common synonym in cases of direct contact but is generally not used when contact is indirect.

rivalry, sibling A popular term for the often aggressive, contentious interactions between siblings. The term has little technical value since it is used so inclusively that almost any competitive interaction is so labelled, no matter what the initiating cause or underlying dynamics may be.

RL An old abbreviation for *absolute* THRESHOLD (1); it comes from the German *Reizlimen*, meaning stimulus threshold.

RMS ROOT-MEAN SQUARE.

RNA RIBONUCLEIC ACID.

RNG RANDOM NUMBER GENERATOR.

Robbers' Cave study A classic experiment carried out by M. Sherif and colleagues in which two groups of 11-year-old boys attending a summer camp were allowed to form distinct group identities and manners of dress. After discovering the existence of each other, they were invited to engage in a variety of competitive activities including various games and athletic events. The competition between them quickly escalated into a mini-war, with all of the prejudices and distrust seen in larger societies. It took all the researchers' skill to overcome the mutual animosity and restore peace. Interestingly, the technique that worked best was to establish superordinate goals that required that both groups work together.

robust 1 Generally, strong, sturdy, resistant. **2** In statistics, characterizing a statistical test that remains useful even when some of its basic assumptions are violated.

ROC curve RECEIVER-OPERATING CHARACTERISTIC CURVE.

rod and frame test A test used primarily in measuring FIELD DEPENDENCE. The subject is presented with a rectangular frame and a rod within the frame. The orientation of the frame is changed from trial to trial and the subject attempts to set the position of the rod to the true vertical. The amount of error and its relationship to the orientation of the frame yield a measure of the subject's field dependence.

rod-cone break See DARK ADAPTATION.

rods The achromatic photoreceptors in the retina. Rods have lower thresholds than CONES and function under conditions of low illumination; see SCOTOPIC VISION. There are no rods in the fovea, where maximum acuity is found. Scotopic vision is both colour-blind and lacking in fine detail. Rods contain a single photopigment, RHODOPSIN (see which for more detail).

rod vision SCOTOPIC VISION; vision under low-illumination conditions, specifically below the threshold for CONES.

Rogerian Of or pertaining to the theories and clinical practices of Carl Rogers. For details, see CLIENT-CENTRED THERAPY and HUMANISTIC PSYCHOLOGY.

Rolandic fissure CENTRAL FISSURE.

role A word derived from the early French theatre, where a *rôle* was the roll of paper upon which an actor's part was written. In social psychology, it refers generally to any pattern of behaviour involving certain rights, obligations and duties which an individual is expected, trained and, indeed, encouraged to perform in a given social situation. In fact, one may go so far as to say that a person's role is precisely what is expected of him or her by others and ultimately, after it has been thoroughly learned and internalized, by the person him- or herself. Roles may assume rather wide manifestations: they may be momentary, e.g. the winner of a game; they may be indefinable in time, e.g. child, parent, spouse; or they may be essentially permanent, e.g. male, female, black. The term is also used in a variety of specialized ways, as the following entries show. See also STATUS and STEREOTYPE, which are used in ways that may overlap subtly.

role, achieved Quite literally, any role that

has been achieved or earned, e.g. corporation president. Contrast with ASCRIBED *ROLE.

role, ascribed A role ascribed to one, a role handed to one at birth (e.g. male, upper-class) or at some point later in life (e.g. adult).

role, assumed Loosely, any ROLE taken on in an effort to fill a position in a social group that the individual feels the group expects them to assume.

role conflict A situation in which a person is expected to perform in two or more roles that conflict in fundamental ways with each other. The classic example here is the situation confronted by a military chaplain. The term may refer to either the circumstances or the emotional state produced by the circumstances.

Role Construct Repertory Test REP TEST.

role, counterfeit Any role assumed falsely, usually to protect oneself from the social stigma of the truth, e.g. the divorced person who plays the role of widow or widower.

role diffusion Erik Erikson's term for a developmental stage, characteristic of childhood and early adolescence in which there is neither commitment to particular values and roles nor active exploration of alternative values and roles.

role discontinuity A situation where a sudden and often dramatic shift in one's primary role is necessitated. The recent retiree is a good example.

role distancing The process of playing out a role without really meaning it, without actually accepting the role but rather doing it with some other motive in mind. *Distancing* conveys the sense that the internalization process, normally regarded as central to the adoption of a ROLE, is missing.

role-enactment theory A theory of hypnosis which argues that the hypnotized person is basically acting out a role. The point of interest here is that the subject is not assumed to be in an altered state but merely so deeply involved in the enactment of the suggested role that his or her actions take place without conscious intent.

role model MODEL (2).

role-playing 1 The acting out or performing of a particular role. As a procedure, it has rather wide currency in psychotherapy, in education and even in industrial settings. **2** The acting out in an appropriate fashion of the role one perceives as properly characteristic of oneself. Note that 1 and 2 conflict in meaning. Those who use the term in sense 2 generally use the phrase *playing at a role* in sense 1.

role rehearsal The preliminary playing-out of an adult role by a child. The phenomenon is extremely common and is generally taken as an important component of socialization whereby a child identifies with an adult and mimics the adult's role behaviour. It is also seen in various infrahuman species, particularly primates.

role reversal A reversing of the social roles of two persons involved in a RECIPROCAL *ROLES relationship; e.g. the teacher becomes the pupil and vice versa, the dominant member of a pair becomes the submissive and the submissive the dominant.

role set Within the study of organizational behaviour, a term preferred by many over the more general term GROUP. The point here is that *role set* emphasizes the notion that a functioning group of individuals within an organization is defined primarily by the *role* relationships that exist between a *set* of individuals. The term was first used by the sociologist R. K. Merton in his analysis of social status and social structure.

roles, reciprocal Roles that are defined by the relationship between persons, particularly those in which the relationship produces an inseparable intertwining of the roles. Husband–wife, teacher–pupil, mother–daughter, etc. are examples.

rolfing Named after originator I. P. Rolf, a system of soft tissue manipulation presumed to enhance vitality. While there is evidence for its efficacy as a physical therapy, there is no evidence of its psychological effectiveness beyond that explained by a placebo effect.

romantic love LOVE, ROMANTIC.

Romberg's sign The inability to maintain body balance when standing with eyes shut and feet close together. It is a sign of neurological damage.

Romeo and Juliet effect The increase in the attractiveness between two people resulting from an attempt on the part of their parents or others to keep them apart.

root **1** n. In mathematics, any number which when multiplied by itself a given number of times yields a given quantity; e.g. 2 is the second (or square) root of 4, the third (or cube) root of 8, the fourth root of 16, etc. **2** n. In linguistics, a morpheme that serves as the basis of an inflectional paradigm; e.g. *talk* is the root of *talks*, *talked*, *talking*, *talker*, etc. **3** n. The embedded base of a growth such as a hair, nail or tooth. **4** n. A collection of nerve fibres entering or leaving the central nervous system. **5** adj. Primary or basic; e.g. the root cause, the root idea.

root conflict (or **problem**) In the depth psychologies, the underlying conflict that is assumed to be primarily responsible for an observed psychological disorder. Compare with NUCLEAR COMPLEX (or CONFLICT), a term which tends to be used in broader fashion.

rooting reflex A sequence of head-turning and mouthing movements elicited in an infant by a gentle stroking of the cheek.

root-mean square (**RMS**) $\sqrt{(\Sigma X^2/N)}$, where X represents each of the scores in the calculation and N is the number of scores. In the special case in which X = deviation of a score from the mean of the distribution, RMS = STANDARD *DEVIATION.

Rorschach ranking test A simplified variation on the RORSCHACH TEST in which the subject is given each of the ten inkblots along with a list of nine possible responses and asked to rank the responses as to their values as adequate descriptions of each inkblot.

Rorschach test The grandfather of all PROJECTIVE TESTS, designed and developed by the Swiss psychiatrist Hermann Rorschach. The administration of the test consists of a structured interview using a series of ten standardized, bilaterally symmetrical inkblots. Five of the blots are achromatic, two have some colour and the other three are in various colours. Each blot is presented to the subject, who is requested to state freely what he or she sees either in the blot as a whole or in any part of it. Extremely complex scoring and interpretation systems have been developed and lengthy training is required to become proficient in the test's use. According to the classical interpretation, responses to colour are supposedly reflective of emotional responsiveness to the environment; form and location responses are taken as indices of overall orientation to life; movement responses are assumed to reflect tendencies toward introversion; originality theoretically reflects intelligence but bizarre originality is seen as indicative of neurotic tendencies; etc.

There is a certain fascination with this test that affects all, professional and layperson alike. In some ways, particularly among lay people, it is seen as a symbol of psychology itself and keeps finding itself on the covers of textbooks. It reflects that strange belief which many have that psychologists and psychiatrists can somehow tell you something about yourself that you would never be able to ascertain on your own, as if they possessed some mysterious ability to read through the veils of defences and posturings which are opaque to all but these shamans and their testing procedures. Among the professionals its magnetic qualities are equally strong. The literature on the Rorschach is simply enormous and literally dozens of other PROJECTIVE TECHNIQUES have been developed based on similar theoretical principles. Yet, in the midst of all of this activity, devotion and fascination, there is little evidence that the test's numerous indexes exhibit strong or practically useful levels of validity. Nevertheless its supporters display an almost religious fervour in its defence and their claims often read like theological discourses rather than scientific analyses. Its attackers, on the other hand, are merciless and maintain that it is totally worthless and may even be harmful because it can lead the clinician astray.

When debates of this intensity and polarity occur between honourable people there are likely to be elements of truth on both sides. The following is a personal view. It seems not unreasonable to assume that the test can be of value in a clinical setting, but perhaps not necessarily because of any intrinsic property of the Rorschach itself nor of the manner of its administration. Rather, it is probably the case that the test provides an opportunity for an extended, unbounded interaction between client and therapist with the inkblots acting as the vehicle for the interaction. Given such an intensive, open setting, particularly when the client believes the test has a valid psychological role to play in the ongoing dialogue, the perceptive clinician can gain insight into the personality characteristics of the client. Thus, the usefulness of the Rorschach depends upon the sensitivity, empathy and insightfulness of the tester totally independently of the test itself. An intense dialogue about the wallpaper or the carpet would do as well provided both parties believed.

Rosanoff list (or **test**) KENT–ROSANOFF LIST.

Rosenthal effect A term derived from the extensive research of Robert Rosenthal on the manner in which one's beliefs, biases and expectations can have an impact on the phenomena under investigation. For special instances of the effect see DEMAND CHARACTERISTICS, EXPERIMENTER EXPECTANCY EFFECT, SELF-FULFILLING PROPHECY.

rostral Lit., toward or pertaining to the beak. Hence, toward the head or the front end of a body.

rotary-pursuit procedure PURSUITMETER.

rotation 1 Generally, any movement about some central point. **2** In FACTOR ANALYSIS, the operation of moving the axes so as to find the orientation that maximizes the loading. Such rotations may be *oblique*, when the angles between the FACTOR AXES are acute, indicating that they are correlated with each other and that a *second-order factor* exists, or they may be *orthogonal*, when the axes meet at right angles, indicating that the factors do not correlate with each other.

rote learning LEARNING, ROTE.

rote memory ROTE *LEARNING.

round window A small, round, membrane-covered opening in the COCHLEA of the inner ear which vibrates back and forth, functioning to alleviate the pressures set up by the vibrations of the OVAL WINDOW.

routine The kinds of RITUALS discussed under meanings 3 and 4 of that term are often referred to as *routines*, on the grounds that whatever symbolic elements the behaviours once had have been lost. The connotation is that somehow a routine is a more mundane, stereotyped behaviour pattern than a ritual. See also CEREMONY.

RP RECEIVED PRONUNCIATION.

RR Abbreviation for *random ratio*. See SCHEDULES OF *REINFORCEMENT.

R–R conditioning Conditioning of a series of responses in which each response is the precondition for the next response.

-rrhagia, -rrhea Combining forms used to denote *discharge, eruption, bursting forth*, with the connotation that it is an abnormal or unusual condition.

R–R laws Conditioning principles based on underlying response relationships. Although not all authors are consistent in their notation, many reserve the upper-case for overt responses and use *r–r* for discussions of covert or mental responses. Compare with STIMULUS–RESPONSE THEORY.

R–S interval TEMPORAL AVOIDANCE CONDITIONING.

r strategy In evolutionary biology, a type of reproductive breeding utilized by many species in which many offspring are born at a time. The r strategy involves the expenditure of little or no energy or effort in the rearing of the offspring and is usually accompanied by relatively short periods between one birthing and the next. Most insects utilize this strategy, as do other species such as sea turtles and many fish. Also called *r selection* or *r selection strategy*. Compare with K STRATEGY.

RSVP RAPID SERIAL VISUAL PRESENTATION.

RT 1 REACTION TIME. **2** RESPONSE TIME. Usually 1 is intended.

rubber hand illusion An illusion produced by having an individual sit with one hand unseen in their lap while looking at a rubber hand on a table in front of them. If the real hand and the rubber hand are stroked simultaneously the person will have a compelling sense that the rubber hand is theirs. The illusion is so compelling that hitting the rubber hand with a hammer will often produce a cry of pain.

rubella A relatively mild disease with one serious complication. During the first two or three months of pregnancy, it can produce a number of foetal anomalies including mental retardation, cataracts, heart disease and deafness. The dangers are greatest during the first month and lessen thereafter. Also commonly called *German measles*.

Rubin's figure The common ambiguous figure which is seen as either a vase or as two faces in profile. It is named after E. Rubin, who studied such reversible figures extensively.

rubrospinal tract The efferent nerve tract running from the red nucleus to the spinal cord.

rudiment 1 A basic element, a first principle. **2** A beginning, a first emerging appearance of a thing. **3** In biology, an organ or part of an organ that is incompletely developed or arrested in development, or that no longer serves any identifiable function; a vestige.

Ruffini corpuscle An encapsulated, branching nerve ending in subcutaneous tissue, suspected of mediating the sense of warmth. Also called *Ruffini cylinder*.

Ruffini end organ A branching nerve ending in subcutaneous tissue, suspected of functioning as a mediator of the response to constant skin indentation and thus playing a role in the sense of pressure. Also called *Ruffini papillary ending, Ruffini plume* or *Ruffini ending*.

rule A formal expression that codifies and specifies a particular set of relations. In this sense, the term is used in ways surprisingly close to CONCEPT. Indeed, many *concept learning* experiments are also referred to as *rule learning* experiments. The point of commonality here is the notion that as a concept is defined by some rule, to learn the concept is to display knowledge, albeit implicit, of the rule. See CONCEPT et seq.

rule learning LEARNING, RULE.

rule of inference TRANSFORMATION (3).

rule of thumb HEURISTIC.

rumination disorder of infancy A serious eating disorder characterized by repeated regurgitation of food. In the typical syndrome, partially digested food is regurgitated by an infant and either ejected or chewed and reswallowed. There is no nausea, retching or obvious gastrointestinal malfunction. Also called *merycism*.

rumour An unverified and typically inaccurate report, story or characterization which travels through a community usually by word of mouth. Rumours tend to arise during periods of societal stress and are usually concerned with persons or events in whom or which there is considerable interest but about whom or which there is little concrete, verifiable information. With propagation, rumours tend to undergo both *levelling* (becoming shorter and simpler) and *sharpening* (emphasizing particular details and neglecting others).

rumour-intensity formula A formula proposed by G. Allport and L. Postman that captures the generalization that the intensity of rumours tends to be a function of the importance of the subject and its ambiguity, i.e. $R = ia$, where R is the intensity of the rumour, $i =$ importance and $a =$ ambiguity. Note that a multiplicative relationship is assumed: if either i or a is zero, there is no rumour.

run 1 vb. To carry out an experiment or a single trial in an experiment. **2** n. The experiment or trial itself. **3** n. A sequence of identical symbols, e.g. AAAA is a run of As of length four.

runs test A nonparametric statistical test that determines whether a single data sample is significantly different from random by analysing the pattern of RUNS (3) that is observed. See also WALD–WOLFOWITZ RUNS TEST, which is used to evaluate differences between two samples.

runway Any straight alley maze or a longish straight in a maze.

rupture Any failure or breakdown of communication or interaction between client and therapist that occurs during a psychotherapy session. Such ruptures are of interest primarily for the way in which they are handled or repaired.

Rush chair A wooden chair into which a psychiatric patient would be quite thoroughly strapped with leather belts around arms, legs, chest and head held in a wooden block. It was invented by Benjamin Rush in the late 1700s. Rush, who is regarded by many as the founder of psychiatry as a medical speciality, promoted the chair on the grounds that it kept violent patients subdued and made bloodletting, which he was a devotee of, easier. Also called, oxymoronically, *tranquillizer chair*.

rut 1 In lower animals, a seasonal period of sexual excitement. See OESTRUS, HEAT (2). **2** In animals, copulation.

S

S Abbreviation for: **1** *Stimulus*; see s^D, s^Δ, s^+, s^-, s-r. **2** *Subject*. **3** In some older writings, *sensation*. This last use is generally restricted to instances in which *R* is used for stimulus; see REIZ. **4** In psychophysics, STANDARD (2).

'S' The pseudonym (his real name was Solomon Shereshevskii) of a *mnemonist* studied extensively by Alexander Luria. A man of average intelligence, S's seemingly inexhaustible memory capacity was aided by his use of a variety of mnemonic devices and coding schemes, a remarkable ability to form associations between things and a most unusual and bizarrely developed *synaesthesia*.

S^c, S_c CONDITIONED STIMULUS; *CS* is preferred.

S^D DRIVE STIMULUS.

S^D Abbreviation for DISCRIMINATIVE *STIMULUS. In operant-conditioning studies, S^D denotes the stimulus in the presence of which responses are reinforced and S^Δ the stimulus in the presence of which responses go unreinforced. Compare with s^+, s^-.

S^Δ See discussion under s^D.

S^+, S^- In discrimination-learning experiments, the positive stimulus (responses to which are reinforced) is generally denoted as S^+ and the negative stimulus (responses to which go unreinforced) by S^-. In this sense, $S^+ = s^D$ and $S^- = s^\Delta$. Note, however, that in some circumstances S^- is used to denote a stimulus in the presence of which responses are punished. In these cases, S^- has a distinct negative component that S^Δ does not.

S^u, S_u UNCONDITIONED STIMULUS; *US* and *UCS* are more common.

s 1 Sensation. **2** The standard deviation in a data sample. **3** Any variable stimulus. This use is generally restricted to the area of psychophysics.

s^g A FRACTIONAL GOAL STIMULUS.

s^2 VARIANCE.

$s_{\bar{x}}$ STANDARD ERROR OF THE MEAN.

SAC STIMULUS AS CODED.

saccade A quick eye movement, a jump of the eyes from one fixation point to another. Saccadic movements are seen most clearly during reading and the scanning of visual displays. The eye was once thought to be functionally blind during a saccade: it is now known that some vision does occur although fine details are not picked up. Saccades toward an object are sometimes termed *prosaccades*, those away, *antisaccades*. They may be either voluntary or automatic. vb., *saccade*.

saccadic dysmetria OCULAR DYSMETRIA.

saccule The smaller of the two vestibular sacs in the inner ear. Like the UTRICLE, it is approximately round in shape and has a layer of receptors on its 'floor' that respond to changes in orientation of the head.

sacral Pertaining to the area around and including the SACRUM.

sacral division A division of the AUTONOMIC NERVOUS SYSTEM.

sacred Characterizing aspects of a society that are treated with great respect. They may be physical objects (e.g. a cross, an ark), or they may be spiritual, supernatural or even emergent ideas derived from the shared values of a society (e.g. patriotism). In the social sciences the term encompasses more than the religious or the divine; in fact, it can be taken to refer to anything which is not to be taken frivolously.

sacrifice To terminate the life of an experimental animal for the purpose of carrying out a post-mortem examination.

sacrum The triangular bone at the lower end of the spine that connects with the hip-bones to form the dorsal part of the pelvis. adj., *sacral*.

SAD SEASONAL AFFECTIVE DISORDER.

sadism 1 The association of sexual pleasure with the inflicting of pain upon another. Note that *pain* here may take many forms other than the purely physical. As the term is used, causing psychic pain, humiliation, debasement, exploitation, etc. may all be regarded as sadistic acts. The term covers the actual derivation of sexual satisfaction as well as cases in which the sadistic behaviour serves as an arousal function as a prelude to further sexual action. When sadism is necessary for sexual gratification, it is classified as a PARAPHILIA. The term derives from the rather singular sexual orientation of the notorious essayist, novelist and revolutionary Donatien Alphonse François, the Marquis de Sade. **2** Somewhat more generally, the derivation of pleasure from the inflicting of pain and suffering on others. As with 1, *pain* may take forms other than the purely physical. In this usage, the sexual connotation may or may not be present. adj., *sadistic*; n., *sadist*. See also MASOCHISM.

sado-masochistic 1 A hybrid term reflecting the oft-noted tendency for sadistic and masochistic manifestations to occur together in the same person. **2** Characterizing a relationship between persons in which one enacts the role of sadist and the other the role of masochist. See SADISM and MASOCHISM.

safety device Horney's term for any of the techniques one uses for defending and protecting oneself from the difficulties of life. The usual usage is with respect to neurosis and the devices used by neurotics.

safety motive 1 Generally, any desire for or tendency to strive for safety and security. **2** A tendency to avoid failure or the threat of failure by withdrawing from a situation or by lowering one's level of aspiration or one's goals. Note that the first usage is a simple

description of a state of affairs; the second is a hypothesized explanatory mechanism.

sagittal 1 From the Latin for *arrow*, pertaining to the arrow-shaped suture joining the two parietal bones of the skull. **2** Pertaining to the plane passing through the long axis of the head which schematically divides the body into symmetrical right and left halves, or to any other plane parallel to this one.

sagittal axis The line of reference from the centre of the retina through the centres of the lens and pupil to the visual field.

sagittal fissure The fissure that separates the two cerebral hemispheres. Also called the *longitudinal fissure*.

sagittal section SECTION (2).

salience Distinctiveness, prominence, obviousness. The term is widely used in the study of perception and cognition to refer to any aspect of a stimulus that, for any of many reasons, stands out from the rest. Salience may result from simple physical characteristics of a display such as size or intensity but it may also be caused by emotional, motivational or cognitive factors. adj., *salient*.

salience map An abstract neurosensory representation of a perceptual space that captures the relative SALIENCE of the several elements in a display. For example, if the display contains four red objects and one blue, the map will reflect the conspicuousness of the latter, distinctly coloured object. A salience map would not represent colour, only that one object is distinct.

Salpêtrière school The psychiatric institute at the Salpêtrière Hospital in Paris was long a significant institution. Its fame began with the administration of the facilities by Philippe Pinel in 1793 and continued through the guidance of Jean Martin Charcot and Pierre Janet. The specific school of thought noted by the term, however, is that associated with the point of view of Charcot, who developed the so-called clinico-anatomical approach to mental disorders, whereby neurological diseases were associated with and classified according to the anatomic and pathological conditions, outlined a general theory of psychopathology based on neurological principles and proposed a theory of hypnosis based on the assumption that it was a pathological state rooted in a neurological disorder and associated with hysteria. This last theoretical position was vigorously criticized by the NANCY SCHOOL.

salpingectomy The surgical procedure of cutting, tying off or removing the Fallopian tubes. It is the simplest of the various surgical contraceptive procedures in women. See also VASECTOMY, the analogous procedure in men.

saltatory Characterized by leaps, discontinuous, quantal. n., *saltation*.

saltatory conduction The conduction of action potentials in myelinated neurons when the potential jumps from one NODE OF *RANVIER to the next.

salty One of the five primary qualities of TASTE (2). Sodium chloride is the best stimulus although other substances that ionize such as lithium, potassium and arginine, an amino acid, have similar tastes. The receptor appears to be a simple channel on a TASTE CELL that depolarizes when sodium enters. Salt is essential for life but, since it is not produced by the body, a specific system for detecting it is not unexpected.

sample 1 n. A part of a POPULATION selected (usually according to some procedure and with some purpose in mind) as representative of the population as a whole. **2** vb. To take such a selected part of the population. The term is frequently qualified to specify the kind of sample or the sampling procedure under discussion; the more frequently used of these are given below. When unqualified, a RANDOM *SAMPLE is generally meant. Note that *sample* and *sampling* are often interchangeably, especially in compound forms. If a term is not found immediately below, see those following SAMPLING.

sample, adequate A sample of sufficient size that the intended level of accuracy can be achieved. Note that the term pertains only to size and has no connotations concerning representativeness.

sample bias Any factor that decreases the likelihood of a REPRESENTATIVE *SAMPLE being drawn.

sample distribution The distribution of scores on some variable that is found in a

particular SAMPLE. Distinguish from SAMPLING *DISTRIBUTION.

sample, matched Any sample selected so that it reflects the same characteristics as another sample. See e.g. MATCHED-GROUPS PROCEDURE.

sample, nonrepresentative Any sample the characteristics of which do not reflect those of the population from which it has been drawn.

sample, random A sample which has been drawn such that each member or object in the population has an equal (and independent) probability of being selected. See RANDOM *SAMPLING.

sample, representative Any sample which is an accurate reflection of the population from which it has been drawn; an *unbiased sample*. All systematic sampling procedures are designed to yield representative samples.

sample space The totality of events which are potential candidates for any sample; in other words, the *population*.

sample, time Any sample based on the taking of observations at specified times or during specific time periods. Ideally the times are selected in an unbiased fashion and the sample data are the behaviours exhibited during them. See BEHAVIOUR *SAMPLING.

sampling The operation of drawing a sample from a population. If the term is unqualified, it is safe to assume that RANDOM *SAMPLING procedures are being used. Note, in many cases, particularly in the many compound terms, *sample* and *sampling* are used interchangeably: for terms not found below see those following SAMPLE.

sampling, accidental Sampling events or elements of which are drawn essentially by accident and without regard for representativeness. Such samples are almost always *biased*. The typical person-on-the-street polls that radio and television stations are so fond of taking are of this kind.

sampling, area Generally, any sampling method based on selection of subjects from geographical regions.

sampling, behaviour A recording of the behaviour exhibited by a subject during specific time periods. These periods are chosen so that the behaviour observed during them (the sample) can be taken as representative of the overall patterns of behaviour the subject displays.

sampling, biased Any sampling procedure in which some events or elements have a greater or lesser chance of being selected than they should given their frequency in the population. Biased samples are nonrepresentative and hence inferences from them will contain systematic errors.

sampling, block A sampling procedure in which the elements to be sampled are broken into groups (or blocks) and separate samples are taken from each. See e.g. AREA *SAMPLING, STRATIFIED *SAMPLING.

sampling, controlled A generic term covering any sampling procedure whereby some measure of control is exerted over the manner in which the sample is selected. See e.g. MATCHED *SAMPLE, STRATIFIED *SAMPLING.

sampling, convenience Sampling based not on representativeness but on convenience. Despite statements to the effect that the subjects in such and such a study were selected 'at random', most experimental psychology with human subjects is based on samples drawn not from the population at large but from a convenient subset of it – usually students taking Introductory Psychology. Also called *opportunistic sampling*.

sampling distribution DISTRIBUTION, SAMPLING.

sampling, domal A form of AREA *SAMPLING where restrictions are placed on who is sampled. For example, only every fifth house (*domal* = domestic, or household) may be chosen and only the head of the household is used in each sample.

sampling error ERROR, SAMPLING.

sampling fraction The percentage of the full population that is in a given sample.

sampling, horizontal Sampling of subjects from within a single social or socioeconomic class. Contrast with VERTICAL *SAMPLING.

sampling, nonprobability Sampling in which the probability of each event or element being drawn is not known; see e.g. ACCI-DENTAL *SAMPLING, QUOTA *SAMPLING. Compare with PROBABILITY *SAMPLING.

sampling, opportunistic CONVENIENCE *SAMPLING.

sampling population Strictly speaking, the population from which a sample is drawn. However, this may not, in actual practice, correspond with the real, theoretical population. For a simple, omnipresent exemplary case, consider that almost all psychological experiments that investigate the cognitive processes of normal human beings are performed on samples of college undergraduates. The theoretical inferences made are based on the presumption that this sampling population is representative of the true population or *universe* (i.e. all cognitively normal human beings). There are, obviously, many reasons for questioning this extension. Hence, although many authors use *population* and *sampling population* as synonyms, there are subtle but potentially important reasons for keeping their denotative domains separate. See POPULATION (esp. 2) for more details on usage.

sampling, probability Sampling in which the events or elements are drawn according to some known probability structure. Note that RANDOM *SAMPLING is a special case of probability sampling in which the probability structure is one which specifies that all elements are equally likely to be chosen. Compare with NONPROBABILITY *SAMPLING.

sampling, prospective Sampling where the cases are selected based on suspected risk factors or other variables that, compared with a control group, are expected to show particular features or syndromes. Compare with RETROSPECTIVE *SAMPLING.

sampling, quota A variety of STRATIFIED *SAMPLING in which a specific number of cases (the quota) are selected from each stratum.

sampling, random The classic procedure for drawing a sample in which each event or element in the population is independent of every other and each is equally likely to be included in the sample.

sampling reliability RELIABILITY, SAMPLING.

sampling, representative Sampling which yields a truly REPRESENTATIVE *SAMPLE.

sampling, retrospective Sampling where individuals are selected because they have been exposed to some risk factor or other circumstance. They are then followed over time and compared with a control group. Compare with PROSPECTIVE *SAMPLING.

sampling, snowball Sampling in which each person in the sample is asked to provide the names of several other persons, who are then added to the sample and asked to provide names, and so on.

sampling, stratified Sampling in which the population as a whole is separated into distinct parts (or strata) which are drawn from separately. Contemporary political polling uses this type of sampling, as it helps to ensure that the full population is properly represented.

sampling, systematic Sampling based on a systematic rule such as 'every 10th case' or 'every other element'. Many experiments which report random sampling actually use this procedure, particularly studies in which the first subject who shows up goes into one group, the second into the second group, the third into the first group, etc.

sampling theory A branch of mathematical statistics concerned with the principles and applied techniques for drawing representative and adequate samples from populations such that valid inferences can be made. See also PROBABILITY THEORY, which lies at the core of sampling theory and, indeed, all statistical procedures.

sampling unit Loosely, any element that forms the basis for selecting a sample. The 'units' could be people, groups, political parties, countries, age brackets, etc.

sampling validity VALIDITY, SAMPLING.

sampling variability The variability of successive samples drawn from a population evaluated relative to what a truly random sample would reflect.

sampling, vertical Sampling of subjects from two or more social or socioeconomic classes. Compare with HORIZONTAL *SAMPLING.

sampling without replacement Sampling in which the selected elements are not replaced in the sample set and are thus not available for future sampling. Compare with SAMPLING WITH REPLACEMENT.

sampling with replacement Sampling in which the selected elements are placed back in the sample set so that they are available for future sampling. Compare with SAMPLING WITHOUT REPLACEMENT.

samsara From the Sanskrit for *transmigration*, the doctrine of the continuous cycle of death and rebirth. See also METEMPSYCHOSIS.

sane (and **sanity**) Terms which, despite their high frequency of usage in both the technical and popular literatures, really have no clear, agreed-upon definitions outside of the legal domain. Presumably, a sane person is one who is NORMAL (see which for a discussion of usage) and capable of adequate, adaptive functioning on a day-to-day basis. For the legal issues involved here, see INSANITY.

sanguine Lit., bloody. Used typically to label a person of rather optimistic temperament with an air of hopefulness and warmth. The origins of the term go back to the ancient classification of personality types based upon the presumed bodily humours.

Sanson images PURKINJE (PURKYNĚ)–SANSON IMAGES.

Sapir–Whorf hypothesis See WHORFIAN HYPOTHESIS. Edward Sapir, as Whorf's teacher and collaborator, often has his name attached to this theory.

Sapphism From the Greek lyric poet Sappho, of the island of Lesbos, female HOMOSEXUALITY.

saralasin SUBFORNICAL ORGAN.

SAT SCHOLASTIC ASSESSMENT TEST.

satellite cell A cell that functions to support neurons in the peripheral nervous system; see e.g. SCHWANN CELL.

satiation 1 SATIETY. **2** A state of dramatically reduced sensitivity to new stimulation resulting from fatigue from immediately preceding multiple stimulations. syn., *refractoriness*.

satiety A state of an organism in which desire or motivation for a thing no longer exists because the need has been satisfied.

satiety centre A term used occasionally for the ventromedial area of the HYPOTHALAMUS.

satiety mechanism Any mechanism that operates to alert the body that some need has been satisfied. The interesting feature of such mechanisms is that they operate in anticipation of the tissue needs being fulfilled. For example, your thirst is quenched after drinking a glass or two of water even though the water has not yet had a chance to replace that which is missing from your cells.

satisfaction An emotional state produced by achieving some goal. Interestingly, early behaviourists (e.g. Thorndike) used this term freely, despite its inescapable mentalistic qualities. See SATISFIER for Thorndike's attempts to circumvent this difficulty.

satisfice To accept a choice or judgement as one that is good enough, one that satisfies. According to Herb Simon, who coined the term, the tendency *to satisfice* shows up in many cognitive tasks, such as playing games, solving problems and making financial decisions, when people typically do not or cannot search for the optimal solutions. ant. MAXIMIZE.

satisfier As originally used by the early behaviourist Edward Lee Thorndike, any stimulus possessing pleasant or desirable properties. Defined operationally, a satisfier is a stimulus which an organism will approach or learn some behaviour to obtain. See REINFORCER and REINFORCEMENT.

saturation 1 In the study of colour, the dimension that reflects purity or richness. A highly saturated colour is vivid and rich, a poorly saturated one is faded or washed out. **2** In factor analysis, the extent to which any particular factor is correlated with a test.

satyriasis An exaggerated sexual desire in males. The term derives from the satyrs, Greek deities who displayed a fondness for erotic revelry. Compare with NYMPHOMANIA and EROTOMANIA. Also called *Don Juanism*.

savant From the French, meaning *knowledgeable*. The term is used of persons who display special, indeed occasionally extraordinary, mental capabilities, such as individuals who have had no formal musical training but are able to play on the piano any piece heard but once, or those who display a computer-like capacity to perform arithmetic calculations or are able to calculate the day of the week on which any given date in the future will fall. Such persons were once called *idiot savants* because they often have rather limited overall social and/or mental capabilities; fortunately, this term is falling out of use.

savings, method of A procedure for studying memory developed by Ebbinghaus in the 1880s. The subject is required to relearn old material, and a comparison is made between the number of trials (or the time) needed for the relearning and the number of trials (or the time) required for the original learning. Comparison between the two yields a *savings score*.

savoury See UMAMI.

S–B STANFORD–BINET SCALE.

Sc CONDITIONED STIMULUS; *CS* is preferred.

scaffolding An interactive behavioural process whereby structure is provided by one person in the form of behaviours that another person can respond to. As the second person becomes more and more adept at making appropriate contributions, the first individual loosens or modifies the structure, thereby increasing the demands on the second until both have learned the full system. Often seen in developmental settings, particularly when a parent is teaching a child a new game. Also called *formatting*.

scalability To make a long story short, the property of being representable in an ordered series of some kind. To make this short story long, see SCALE OF MEASUREMENT and METHODS OF *SCALING.

scala media COCHLEA.

scalar analysis An analysis that yields information about where on a known scale a particular item or variable falls.

scala tympani COCHLEA.

scala vestibuli COCHLEA.

scale 1 Generally and inclusively, any procedure or device that is used for the purpose of arranging objects or events in some progressive series. This meaning, which is the dominant one, entails the notion that in each and every case there exists some rule for assigning numbers or values to the objects or events to be scaled. The rule(s) applicable in individual cases are what reflect the meaning that the scale values have. **2** Any progressive numerical arrangement that can be used to assign magnitudes to events or objects. The primary difference between 1 and 2 here is between the abstract and the concrete. For example, a thermometer is a scale in sense 2 but it reflects the temperature scale in sense 1. **3** A testing instrument which has items or tasks arranged along some dimension. The dimension may be any of several, such as *difficulty*, as is typical in *intelligence scales*, or *preferences*, as in *attitude scales*. Note that these concrete scaling devices may yield various kinds of measurement scales. vb., *to scale*, meaning to assign numbers to events according to some rule.

scale, absolute A RATIO *SCALE. The term *absolute* is occasionally used here because the establishment of the true zero point permits the conversion of an interval scale into a ratio scale, and *true zero* is also called *absolute zero*.

scale, additive An INTERVAL *SCALE. The term is derived from the fact that the most powerful arithmetic operation one can carry out with such scales is addition.

scale, difficulty A general term for any scale or test with the items marked in order of difficulty.

scale, interval A scale that reflects precise statements about the differences between observed magnitudes, i.e. the *interval* of measurement is specified. The classic examples here are the everyday temperature-measurement scales (in Fahrenheit or Celsius), on which the interval between, e.g. 40° and 30° is the same as that between 20° and 10°. However, while the intervals are specified, the numbers used in measurement are arbitrary, i.e. the zero point on such a scale is not a true zero.

The statistical operations of addition and subtraction can be carried out with interval scales, and means and standard deviations can be calculated. The major limitation is that proportions cannot be specified, e.g. 80° is most assuredly not twice as warm as 40°. See and compare with NOMINAL *SCALE,

ORDINAL *SCALE and RATIO *SCALE. Also called *additive scale*.

scale, nominal The most primitive of the possible scales of measurement, this is essentially a system of notation for identifying, classifying and naming observations. In fact, some authorities maintain that the term *scale* is misapplied here since quantification and magnitude are not relevant. The numbers on athletes' uniforms, the taxonomy of biologists and psychiatric nosologies, are examples. The only statistic permissible is the mode. Also called *categorical scale*. See and compare with INTERVAL *SCALE, ORDINAL *SCALE and RATIO *SCALE.

scale of measurement A cover term for any of the SCALES (1) that can be used for measuring some quantity. It is worth noting that a number of mathematical assumptions are always made, either implicitly or explicitly, when actually measuring something along some scale – and not all things are or can be measured in the same manner. For details of the various scales of measurement that are in common use in psychology, see the four most important – NOMINAL *SCALE, ORDINAL *SCALE, INTERVAL *SCALE and RATIO *SCALE – as well as the less-used ORDERED METRIC *SCALE.

scale, ordered metric A scale of measurement that lies in power and degree of generality between an ORDINAL *SCALE and an INTERVAL *SCALE. The basic assumption is that an ordered metric scale results when measurement techniques permit the ordering of the magnitudes of intervals between measured objects.

scale, ordinal A scale with order properties in the specific sense that it is a ranking of observations along some dimension. The assignment of a larger number to one ordinally scaled observation than to another means that there is more of the thing being measured in the first case than in the second. Examples are the hardness scale for minerals, the order of finish in a race and the pleasantness rankings of odours or tastes. Such scales are limited in that true magnitude cannot be expressed, only relative magnitude. This formally limits the kinds of statistical operations that can be performed. However, because so many important psychological factors are actually measured on ordinal scales (e.g., intelligence, personality dimensions, attitudes), a certain statistical legerdemain is needed so that means and standard deviations can be calculated. The standard trick is to assume that the underlying theoretical dimension is normally distributed. Compare with INTERVAL *SCALE, NOMINAL *SCALE and RATIO *SCALE.

scale, psychological Essentially any scale that specifies some kind of system or device for measuring a psychological variable. Note that some authors differentiate between *psychophysical scales*, on which there is a known physical variable to which the psychological one is related (e.g. frequency of a tone or pitch), and *psychological scales*, which have no counterpart in the physical domain (e.g. intelligence).

scale, ratio A scale of measurement on which ratios of magnitude of those observations being scaled can be expressed. Most of the measurement scales in the physical sciences have this property, e.g. the scale of weight, according to which an object weighing 10 g is twice as heavy as one weighing 5 g. The fundamental property of a ratio scale is the existence of a true zero point, the one property that INTERVAL *SCALES lack. They are the most powerful of scales, and all mathematical and statistical operations are permissible on observations measured on ratio scales. They are actually relatively rare in psychological measurement, although psychophysical methods exist for establishing ratio scales for some basic sensory systems (e.g. the *sone* scale for loudness – see METHODS OF *SCALING). It is worth noting that the measurement of observations has often moved upwards from scale to scale as new techniques and theories have been developed. For example, temperature measurement was on an *ordinal scale* when only subjective sensations of 'warmer' or 'cooler' were available; it moved onto an *interval scale* with the invention of the thermometer, and onto a *ratio scale* with the extrapolation of the absolute zero point based on the thermodynamics of ratios of gases. Also called *absolute scale*. See and compare with NOMINAL *SCALE, ORDINAL *SCALE and INTERVAL *SCALE.

scale reliability ITEM *RELIABILITY.

scaling Scale construction and utilization, most commonly the former. Typically in the social sciences, the construction of a scale consists of the evaluation of subjective psychological experience and the development of a numerical system for its measurement. To take as examples some seemingly trivial but actually rather fundamental and important questions answerable by principles of scaling: Does a 10 kg weight *feel* twice as heavy as a 5 kg weight? Does doubling the power output of a radio make it *sound* twice as loud? Does 10 minutes *seem* twice as long as 5 minutes? In each case the answer can only be obtained by constructing a scale along a psychological dimension (heaviness, loudness, time) which is mathematically related to some known physical dimension. For further discussion of related terminology, see METHODS OF *SCALING, MULTIDIMENSIONAL SCALING, SCALE and SCALE OF MEASUREMENT.

scaling, indirect A cover term for those methods of scaling based on indirect evaluations of experience, such as *bisection* or the *method of adjustment*. They are to be contrasted with the more direct scaling methods, such as *magnitude estimation*. See the discussion under METHODS OF *SCALING for descriptions of these and other procedures.

scaling, methods of Simply, procedures for SCALING. Although a century and a half of research on the construction of psychological scales has produced dozens of variations, the most common procedures can be summarized under three general classes: **1** *Interval scaling*. Here subjects are requested to judge stimuli on the basis of intervals or differences. In *bisection*, the subject must adjust a stimulus so that it lies halfway between two other stimuli; in *categorical estimation*, different stimuli are grouped into a small number of categories; in the *method of equal-appearing intervals*, stimuli are sorted into groups so that the intervals between them are subjectively equal. **2** *Ratio scaling*. Here the subject estimates the subjective experience by assigning numbers either directly or indirectly to stimuli so that they reflect his or her judged experiential magnitude. In *magnitude estimation*, each stimulus is assigned a number that reflects its proportionate intensity relative to some standard; e.g. if the standard is called 10, a stimulus subjectively twice as great is assigned 20, one half as great is assigned 5, etc. In the *method of production*, the subject is asked to produce a stimulus that corresponds to some proportional value of a standard, e.g. twice as bright, one-third as loud; this procedure is also called the *method of adjustment*. In *cross modality matching*, the magnitudes are arrived at indirectly, e.g. the loudness of a tone is adjusted so that it sounds as loud as a given weight feels heavy. **3** *Nonmetric scaling*. These are procedures for dealing with psychological variables that are *nonmetric*, i.e. those that cannot be simply dealt with in interval-scale form, such as scaling of preferences, tastes and value judgements. Participants are given pairs of stimuli and asked to judge them in terms of desirability or preference, e.g. 'Would you rather have a cheese sandwich or a ham sandwich?' Several mathematically sophisticated procedures exist whereby these ordered judgements can be made to yield true interval scales. See also MULTIDIMENSIONAL SCALING.

scallop A term used in operant-conditioning studies as reflective of the shape of the graph of cumulative responses typically produced by an organism run for some time on a fixed-interval schedule of reinforcement. The scallop pattern is produced by the fact that relatively few responses occur immediately after a reinforcement, with the number increasing dramatically toward the end of the interval.

scalogram analysis GUTTMAN SCALING.

scan 1 vb. To produce a picture of a slice through the soft tissue of a body, most commonly the brain. **2** n. The picture itself. **3** n. The procedure that produces the picture. The four most frequently used scanning or IMAGING procedures are COMPUTERIZED AXIAL TOMOGRAPHY (CAT-scan), MAGNETIC RESONANCE IMAGING (MRI-scan), FUNCTIONAL MAGNETIC RESONANCE IMAGING (fMRI-scan) and POSITRON EMISSION TOMOGRAPHY (PET-scan). **4** In perception, sweeping a receptor across a stimulus space or display. The most common use of the term is when the eyes pass back and forth across a visual scene.

Scanlon Plan A group incentive plan used in many industries and other organizations. It is based on notions of learning theory and the social needs of workers. In it workers are encouraged to offer suggestions for improving working conditions and procedures and if these are successfully implemented the savings are returned to the workers as percentage increases in pay.

scanning speech ATAXIC SPEECH.

scanning techniques IMAGING (TECHNIQUES).

scapegoat *Scape* is an archaic form of *escape*, the goat is the animal upon which, in ancient Hebraic practice, the accumulated sins of the people were placed on Atonement Day. The goat thus symbolically burdened was then driven into the wild. Hence, scapegoating is the act of blaming a convenient (but innocent, as was the goat) person or group for one's own frustrations, grievances, guilts, etc. This phenomenon is found as a defence mechanism in individuals as well as a deliberate form of propaganda in governments.

scatological 1 As derived from the Greek word for *dung*, referring to excrement or to an abiding interest in excrement. **2** More loosely, characteristic of obscene language independent of faecal references.

scatter 1 n. The degree to which a set of scores (or the data points representing them – see SCATTER DIAGRAM) is clustered about some central score, typically the *mean*. In this sense the term is a synonym of VARIABILITY or DISPERSION. **2** n. The degree to which there is high variability in scoring, particularly intrasubject variability on a particular test. Persons who obtain high scores on some parts of a test but low on others, or students who achieve high grades in some subjects but low in others, are said to show high scatter. vb., *scatter*, used in either sense.

scatter diagram (or **plot**) A diagram, plot or table of two-valued data points such that all the *x*-scores are plotted with their respective *y*-scores. When presented in graphic fashion and fitted with a regression line, it provides a pictorial sense of the amount of SCATTER (1) in the data.

scedasticity From the word meaning 'tendency to scatter', the relative variability displayed in rows and columns of a scatter diagram. *Homoscedasticity* is the condition in which the measures of variability (usually the *standard deviation* or *variance*) lie within the range expected of chance variability; *heteroscedasticity* is the condition in which they are greater than would be expected by chance.

scepticism Generally, any philosophical position that argues that nothing can be known with complete certainty and that all knowledge is ultimately subjective and private. Varieties of scepticism have been proposed from the early Greek scholar Pyrrho of Elis through various medieval thinkers with the fullest and most reasonable expression of the position usually credited to David Hume. A modern approach that captures some of the principles is DECONSTRUCTIONISM although it would be a stretch to call contemporary deconstructionists 'Humeans'. var., *skepticism*.

schedule 1 A plan or organization used particularly with respect to a series of operations that are repeated. **2** An outline or a form, especially one set up for a questionnaire or for conducting an interview.

schedule-induced polydipsia POLYDIPSIA, SCHEDULE-INDUCED.

schedule of reinforcement REINFORCEMENT, SCHEDULES OF.

scheduling theory A general theory concerned with the mathematically complex problems of scheduling a large number of individual operations or processes that must be carried out to perform some complex task. Originally developed by computer operations theorists, it has been applied by industrial and organizational psychologists in handling problems in industry and by cognitive scientists as a basic model of how the brain allocates priorities and schedules various cognitive processes in the performance of complex tasks.

Scheffé test A common POST HOC TEST used to test specific comparisons after an analysis of variance or other statistical test has shown overall significance. It is a conservative test that tends to err on the side of underestimating the significance of differences between means, and it deals well with the problem of unequal numbers of cases in particular cells.

schema 1 A plan, an outline, a structure, a framework, a programme, etc. In all or any of these meanings the assumption is that the schemata (or schemas) are cognitive, mental

plans that are abstract and that they serve as guides for action, as structures for interpreting information, as organized frameworks for solving problems, etc. Thus, we find references to a linguistic schema for comprehending a sentence, a cultural schema for interpreting a myth, a prehensile schema for a child learning how to grasp an object, a means–end schema for solving logical problems, etc. A schema is more than a SET (2) because it is more elaborate and less restricted to a particular situation; it is more ideational or implicit than a STRATEGY (1) and conceptually richer than a HYPOTHESIS (2). **2** A general framework or structure within which data or events can be recorded, particularly one that emphasizes the overall relationships between major effects and downplays fine details. **3** By extension, a model or organized outline touching on the main or primary elements of a system. Compare with SCHEME.

schema, anticipatory Ulric Neisser's term for the SCHEMA (1) invoked when preparing to enter a particular situation. For example, knowing that one is going to the doctor brings up a schema with elements like a waiting room with chairs and magazines, a nurse, a doctor, particular smells and emotional reactions. One does not typically image chain saws or giraffes.

schematic 1 Usually, diagrammatic; presented in skeletal form. **2** Less often, pertaining to a SCHEMA or a SCHEME.

schematize To present in schematic form.

scheme An organized plan. Some use this term interchangeably with SCHEMA; others reserve *scheme* for the more concrete kinds of cognitive structures that are formed consciously. This distinction is particularly true of Piaget's use of the terms.

schizo- A combining form meaning *splitting, separating, cleavage*.

schizoaffective disorder A psychosis marked by either a major depressive episode or a manic episode concurrent with classic symptoms of SCHIZOPHRENIA, such as delusions, hallucinations, lack of volition and disturbed speech patterns.

schizoid A term with a tortured pattern of usage. **1** Pertaining to or descriptive of

SCHIZOPHRENIA or of an individual diagnosed as schizophrenic. Here the reference is clearly to a PSYCHOSIS. **2** Resembling some of the behavioural and cognitive characteristics of schizophrenia but displayed in a manner that is merely eccentric and not the least psychotic. See SCHIZOTHYMIA. **3** Shorthand form of SCHIZOID DISORDER OF CHILDHOOD OR ADOLESCENCE. **4** Shorthand form of SCHIZOID PERSONALITY DISORDER. Meanings 3 and 4 are, in contemporary writings, the ones usually intended. Meanings 1 and 2 have been dropped by most authorities because of the confusions involved in using the same term for a psychotic disorder and a simple pattern of eccentric but normal behaviour.

schizoid disorder of childhood or adolescence A childhood disorder marked by a lack of ability to form friendships with peers, a lack of interest in doing so and a decided lack of pleasure derived from such inter-actions when encouraged or arranged by others. Such children are withdrawn, aloof and seclusive and typically react negatively to demands from others for social inter-action. They display, however, none of the signs of a psychosis such as loss of reality-testing. If the disorder continues into adulthood it is termed SCHIZOID PERSONALITY DISORDER.

schizoid personality disorder A person-ality disorder characterized by an emotional coldness, secretiveness, solitude, withdrawal and a general inability to form intimate attachments to others. It is not regarded as a form of schizophrenia and is diagnostically differentiated from a SCHIZOTYPAL PERSONALITY DISORDER (see which for details).

schizophrasia A term occasionally used to refer to disconnected speech such as that observed in some forms of schizophrenia.

schizophrenia A general label for a number of psychotic disorders with various cogni-tive, emotional and behavioural manifest-ations. The term originated with Eugen Bleuler, who offered it in 1911 as a replace-ment for DEMENTIA PRAECOX. It literally means *splitting in the mind* and was chosen by Bleuler because the disorder seemed to reflect a cleavage or dissociation between the func-tions of feeling or emotion on one hand and those of thinking or cognition on the other. That is, the split is horizontal, not ver-

tical: a vertical dissociation yields MULTIPLE PERSONALITY, a decidedly different psychiatric syndrome.

Although there are various distinguishable schizophrenias which display differing aetiologies and have distinguishable progno-ses, certain features are taken as hallmarks of all: (a) deterioration from previous levels of social, cognitive and vocational functioning; (b) onset before midlife (roughly 45–50 years of age); (c) a duration of at least six months; and most tellingly, (d) a pattern of psychotic features including thought disturbances, bizarre delusions, hallucinations (usually auditory), disturbed sense of self and a loss of reality-testing.

The borderline that distinguishes schizo-phrenia from other disorders is fuzzy, and differential diagnosis is problematical. For details see BORDERLINE *SCHIZOPHRENIA, SCHI-ZOAFFECTIVE DISORDER, SCHIZOID PERSONALITY DISORDER, SCHIZOPHRENIFORM DISORDER, SCHIZO-TYPAL PERSONALITY DISORDER. Note also that, although many authorities are convinced that a relatively straightforward (although still largely unknown) neurochemical cause exists for the disorder, it is not given as a diagnostic label when there is evidence of an ORGANIC MENTAL DISORDER. Schizophrenia shows familial patterns of incidence, and there is strong evidence that there is a genetic predisposition for individuals to display the disorder.

A number of terms have been and are used as equivalent to *schizophrenia*; they include *schizophrenic disorder, schizophrenic reaction* and *schizophrenic psychosis.* The various forms of schizophrenia that have been labelled at one time or another are given in the following entries. Those that are part of the contemporary psychiatric nosology (that is, that are recognized by either the DIAGNOS-TIC AND STATISTICAL MANUAL or the INTERNATIONAL CLASSIFICATION OF DISEASES are marked with an *.

schizophrenia, borderline A vague classi-fication used of persons who display some of the features of schizophrenia but do not fit the full profile of the psychosis. The preferred diagnostic label for such cases is SCHIZOTYPAL PERSONALITY DISORDER.

schizophrenia, catatonic (type)* A type of schizophrenia characterized by a tendency to remain in a stupor-like state during which the patient may hold a particular posture, sitting or lying in the same position for extended periods of time, sometimes for weeks or even months. Mutism, waxy flexibility and mindless stereotypy are also common. Frequently the catatonic state gives way to short periods of frenetic activity during which the patient is capable of considerable damage to others as well as to him- or herself. Note that there is a school of thought that views this syndrome not as a schizophrenia but as an AFFECTIVE DISORDER. Also called *schizophrenic disorder, catatonic type.*

schizophrenia, childhood Simply, schizophrenia occurring in childhood. Many experts question whether this is in fact a category of disorder separate from any of several others that occur during childhood. See e.g. INFANTILE *AUTISM.

schizophrenia, chronic A diagnostic label for any schizophrenia the symptoms of which have continued for an extended time and proven relatively refractory to therapeutic intervention.

schizophrenia, deficit (type)* A diagnostic label recently suggested for a subtype of schizophrenia in which the clinical picture is dominated by enduring, disabling NEGATIVE SYMPTOMS in the absence of disorganized behaviour, speech, or affect.

schizophrenia, disorganized (type)* A type of schizophrenia which is, in a sense, the prototype of the disorder. The primary symptoms are the erratic speech, strange, often childish mannerisms and general bizarreness of behaviour that are regarded as hallmarks of the psychotic. A variety of other symptoms are often, although not always, noted, including hearing voices, elaborate fantasies (including the belief that one is someone else), withdrawal from day-to-day realities, delusions of grandeur and/or persecution, and strange bodily feelings (including the delusion that vital organs are missing). This is the single most common diagnostic category in Western mental institutions. Also called *hebephrenia, hebephrenic schizophrenia* and *schizophrenic disorder, disorganized type.*

schizophrenia, hebephrenic DISORGANIZED (TYPE) *SCHIZOPHRENIA.

schizophrenia, iatrogenic A mental disorder with a diverse set of symptoms including those also seen in other forms of schizophrenia. As the name suggests, it results from medical practices or procedures, in particular the long-term use of antipsychotic drugs. See TARDIVE DYSMENTIA.

schizophrenia in remission A diagnostic label for cases in which the patient has had a history of schizophrenia but currently is symptom-free. The term is used whether or not the patient is taking medication for the disorder. Just how long a person should remain free of symptoms before the diagnostic label is dropped is a matter of dispute among authorities.

schizophrenia, negative Loosely, any form of SCHIZOPHRENIA marked by NEGATIVE SYMPTOMS such as withdrawal and diminished affect. These types are, perhaps surprisingly, more difficult to treat than the POSITIVE *SCHIZOPHRENIA forms.

schizophrenia, paranoid (type)* A type of schizophrenia characterized primarily by delusions of persecution or grandiosity or hallucinations with persecutory or grandiose content. Delusional jealousy is often part of the disorder and any of a number of associated symptoms may be found, including unfocused anxiety, anger, argumentativeness, doubts about gender identity, a stilted, formal quality and aloofness. Unlike many other forms of schizophrenia, the patient is usually of relatively normal appearance and clean in habits, and if the delusions are not acted on impairment in functioning may be minimal. Also called *paraphrenic schizophrenia* and *paraphrenia*. Distinguish from PARANOIA, PARANOID PERSONALITY DISORDER and DELUSIONAL (PARANOID) DISORDER.

schizophrenia, positive Loosely, any form of SCHIZOPHRENIA marked by POSITIVE SYMPTOMS such as bizarre behaviour, thoughts and hallucinations. Compare with NEGATIVE *SCHIZOPHRENIA.

schizophrenia, positive paranoid (type) A relatively new label suggested for the subtype of schizophrenia known as *paranoid (type) schizophrenia*. The term emphasizes the positive aspects of the disorder; see PARANOID (TYPE) *SCHIZOPHRENIA to appreciate this point.

schizophrenia, process A term used

loosely to refer to chronic schizophrenias attributed more to organic causes than to environmental. These are marked by gradual onset and generally poor prognosis and distinguished from the so-called REACTIVE *SCHIZOPHRENIA. Also called *nuclear schizophrenia*.

schizophrenia, pseudopsychopathic A disorder once thought of as a form of SCHIZOPHRENIA but where the psychotic behaviours and cognitions are masked by behaviours with psychopathic features including inappropriate aggression, sexual deviations and pathological lying. Individuals displaying this cluster of symptoms are now classified as SCHIZOTYPAL PERSONALITY DISORDER or BORDERLINE PERSONALITY DISORDER.

schizophrenia, reactive A term used loosely to refer to schizophrenia marked by abrupt onset and relatively short duration. As the word *reactive* suggests, the disorder is generally attributed to predisposing factors and/or precipitating environmental events. The prognosis is regarded as favourable. Contrast with PROCESS *SCHIZOPHRENIA.

schizophrenia, residual (type)* A psychiatric category for cases in which the patient has a history of at least one episode of schizophrenia, currently displays no prominent psychotic symptoms, but still manifests evidence of maladaptive behaviour, such as unusually low or inappropriate affect, erratic or illogical thinking, strange associations and social withdrawal.

schizophrenia, simple A form of schizophrenia characterized by an extreme lack of what are considered normal emotional reactions to the real world. Emotions such as joy, sadness, anger and resentment are missing, ambition and initiative likewise; apathy, indifference and resignation dominate. With social and economic impoverishment, vagrancy often results. This diagnostic label goes back to the mid-19th century. The latest edition of the *DSM* recommends SIMPLE DETERIORATIVE DISORDER as a replacement.

schizophrenia, undifferentiated (type)* A diagnostic category for clinical cases considered to be schizophrenic because they display some of the classic symptoms of the disorder, such as delusions, hallucinations, incoherence and disorganized behaviours,

but fail to display any one cluster of these symptoms clearly enough to meet the criteria for any of the other types.

schizophrenic episode, acute A relatively brief episode (lasting a few weeks or months) of schizophrenic symptoms: typically, clouding of consciousness, emotional turmoil and disorganized thought. Also called REACTIVE *SCHIZOPHRENIA, but see that term for further discussion of usage.

schizophrenic thought disorder SCHIZOPHRENIA.

schizophreniform disorder An acute psychotic disorder with symptoms similar to that of schizophrenia except that social and occupational functioning is usually not seriously impaired. Compare with BRIEF PSYCHOTIC DISORDER, where the symptoms last less than a month. If the condition continues past six months or so, the diagnosis is shifted to SCHIZOPHRENIA. Note, this condition has caused all manner of terminological confusion. The French call it *bouffée délirante*, in the *ICD* it is listed as *acute polymorphic psychotic disorder* and both *acute delusional psychosis* and *acute hallucinatory psychosis* are also found.

schizophrenogenic Generally, pertaining to any factor hypothesized to be causally related to the development of schizophrenia. Two broad classes of factors have been identified, *genetic* and *environmental*, leading to three broad theoretical models of the aetiology of the disorder: (a) the *specific gene theory*, which assumes that the disorder is caused by one or more faulty genes that produce metabolic disturbances; (b) the *environment theory*, which views schizophrenia as a reaction to a stressful environment rife with anxiety-producing conditions (see SCHIZOPHRENOGENIC PARENT); and (c) the *constitutional-predisposition theory*, which combines these two, arguing that a variety of disparate dispositions are inherited but that the emergence of a diagnosable schizophrenic disorder is dependent upon the degree of these dispositions and the extent to which they are encouraged by particular kinds of environmental conditions. This last point of view has the largest number of adherents among specialists: few today put much stock in the purely environmental model.

schizophrenogenic parent A term for a parent who is cold, rejecting, distant and aloof but dominating. Theoretically, such a parent puts a child in a hopeless double-bind by simultaneously fostering and rejecting dependency. Whether such a parenting style can actually cause a child who is not genetically predisposed to become schizophrenic is a highly debatable question.

schizotaxia A hypothesized neurological integration deficit that some argue marks a biological predisposition for schizophrenia.

schizothymia The tendency to display erratic patterns of thought and behaviour. A schizothymic is regarded as a quite normal individual, merely eccentric. See also SCHIZOID (2).

schizotypal personality disorder A personality disorder characterized by markedly eccentric and erratic thought, speech and behaviour and a tendency to withdraw from other people. The disorder is characterized as similar to but less severe than SCHIZOPHRENIA, although it is occasionally called *borderline schizophrenia*. This diagnostic category is used in the *DSM* as roughly equivalent to the *ICD*'s SIMPLE *SCHIZOPHRENIA. Distinguish from SCHIZOID PERSONALITY DISORDER, in which the eccentricities of thought, speech and behaviour are not present.

Schmerz PAIN (3).

Scholastic Assessment Test (SAT) In the US, the most widely used of the college admissions tests. It consists of one reasoning test (with separate reading, writing and mathematics sections) and a series of subject achievement tests. Formerly called the *Scholastic Aptitude Test*.

school Outside of the obvious, a loosely organized group of scholars or researchers whose approach to a field of study is rather doctrinaire and structured around a particular theoretical point of view. Frequently the school is tied in with the theory of one person, e.g. the Freudian school; often, however, the orientation prevails without eponym, e.g. the Gestalt school.

school phobia 1 Irrational fear of school or the school situation. **2** Another term for SCHOOL REFUSAL. This usage is not recommended, as is explained under that entry.

school psychology A subdiscipline of educational psychology. School psychologists are concerned with counselling and advising primary and secondary schoolchildren, assisting in curriculum development and testing for and assessing potential emotional and/or learning disabilities.

school refusal Refusal on the part of a child to attend school or, by extension, go away to camp, stay at a friend's house, etc. It is generally taken as one of the hallmark features of SEPARATION-ANXIETY DISORDER. Note that some authors use the term as a synonym of SCHOOL PHOBIA. This equivalence is not recommended: strictly speaking, a refusal to go to school may be caused by a school phobia but most school refusals are due to separation anxiety. In a true school phobia a child will show the phobic reaction even if his or her parents are present.

Schröder staircase STAIRCASE ILLUSION.

schwa (Ə) In phonetics, a common mid-central neutral vowel. It plays an important role in the sound patterns of English, appearing as a reduced, unstressed vowel between syllables that are stressed or accented; e.g. in most English dialects, the phrase '*a* moment *ago*' is pronounced so that the italicized a, e and a are all schwas.

Schwann cells The cells that make up the NEURILEMMA, the membrane that covers the myelin sheath of axons in the peripheral nervous system. They are a form of oligodendroglia (see GLIA) and aid in regeneration of damaged axons by guiding the route of regrowth.

Schwann sheath NEURILEMMA.

SCID STRUCTURED CLINICAL INTERVIEW FOR THE *DSM*.

science 1 A body of knowledge, particularly that which has resulted from the systematic application of the SCIENTIFIC *METHOD. **2** A branch of study or a discipline focused on the derivation of basic principles and general laws. **3** A system of methods and procedures for the investigation of natural phenomena based upon scientific principles.

scientific attitude (or **approach**) Simply, that orientation toward the study of phenomena that presumes that basic understanding is best achieved through the systematic application of the SCIENTIFIC *METHOD.

scientific law LAW, SCIENTIFIC.

scientific method METHOD, SCIENTIFIC.

scientific psychology Basically, the pursuit of psychological knowledge using the SCIENTIFIC *METHOD. Given the breadth of procedures and interpretative laterality involved here, the term covers essentially all of psychology.

scientism A term typically used in a critical vein of those who, in the eyes of the critic, place too much emphasis on science to provide solutions to problems and understanding of phenomena.

scientist-practitioner model An approach to the training of clinical and other applied psychologists that focuses on both the scientific foundations of the field and the applied skills of the practitioner. It is also called the *Boulder model* from a 1959 conference held in that Colorado city when these principles were developed. Both terms are used primarily in North America, and the approach to training is more common there than elsewhere.

sciosophy Any body of beliefs about the natural or supernatural systematized by tradition or imagination independently of scientific thinking or scientific methods.

sclera The thick, fibrous, white, opaque outer covering of the eyeball. Also called the *sclerotic coat* or *layer*.

sclerosis Generally, a pathological hardening of tissue.

sclerotic coat (or **layer**) SCLERA.

scoliosis An abnormal lateral curvature of the spine, usually consisting of two curves in opposite directions.

scope The domain within which some action takes place.

-scope Combining form meaning *device* or *instrument for viewing*.

-scopia, -scopy Combining forms meaning *examination, viewing, scrutiny*.

scopic Measured or evaluated by direct (visual) observation as opposed to by the use of instruments.

scopolamine (hydrobromide) An alkaloid obtained from plants of the nightshade family. Once used as a sedative and, in combination with either phenobarbital or morphine, to produce 'twilight' sleep. Despite the fantasies of spy novelists, it is not a truth serum.

scopophilia The deriving of sexual pleasure from visual sources, e.g. watching others make love, nudity, pornographic pictures or films. Most people are scopophilic: only if an individual requires such activity for sexual arousal is the condition classified as a PARAPHILIA; see VOYEURISM. vars., *scotophilia*, *scoptophilia* (neither is recommended).

-scopy -SCOPIA.

score A number or other quantitative value used to represent: **1** An individual *response*, i.e. any measurable act of a subject. **2** A summed or totalled value based on a number of individual scores (in sense 1). This meaning is usually found in testing, a final score frequently being composed of several subtest scores. The term is typically used in combined form with qualifiers which specify the kind of score under consideration: the more common are given below.

score, cutoff A score above which one action is taken, and below which another is taken. Often used in *diagnostic tests*, such that an obtained score above the cutoff will result in a diagnosis and in education where cutoffs mark grade boundaries. Sometimes the reference will be to scores 'above' and other times as 'at or above' the cutoff. Take care: the two meanings can make a difference in classification.

score, difference Generally, any score that results from calculating a difference between two measures taken at different times or under different conditions.

score, gross Any score presented in the original units of measurement.

score, raw The originally observed and recorded value; a score that has not been subjected to any transformation or statistical analysis. Compare with DERIVED SCORE. Also called *obtained score, observed score, crude score*.

score, standard 1 Generally, any derived score that is based on the STANDARD *DEVIATION.

2 More specifically, and more commonly, a Z-SCORE.

score, transformed Any score that is derived from a transformation in which the original score is mapped onto and expressed in a different scale.

score, true The value of a population statistic. All observed scores from samples are assumed to be made up of a true score plus or minus some ERROR. In theory, since sampling errors are assumed to be random they cancel each other out, and with increasingly large databases the observed values approach the true values. In actual practice, the mean of the observed scores, within its standard error, is taken as an unbiased estimate of the true score. Also called *true value.*

scoring Generally, procedures for assigning values, for making measurements. Usually one distinguishes between *objective scoring* and *subjective scoring*: the former is used for situations in which some unambiguous rule or code essentially guarantees that any competent observer will arrive at the same conclusion concerning the scores, the latter for situations in which complex and sophisticated evaluations are made based on often nonspecifiable and subjective procedures. Multiple-choice examinations are scored by the former, essay examinations by the latter.

scoterythrous A loss of colour sensitivity to the long-wavelength lights; see PROTANOPIA.

scoto- Combining form meaning *dark, darkness.*

scotoma 1 A totally or partially blind area of the retina in the visual field. It may be caused by damage to cells in the retina or to lesions anywhere along the visual pathways. The term is generally reserved for pathologies, although some authors refer to the normal *blind spot* as *physiological scotoma.* Often qualifiers will be appended to specify location, form or cause of the scotoma. pl., *scotomata*; adj., *scotomatous.* **2** More metaphorically, a gap or blind spot in an individual's psychological awareness.

scotomization A defence mechanism whereby a person develops blind spots (metaphorically speaking) to certain kinds of emotional or anxiety-producing situations or conflicts.

scotophilia 1 SCOPOPHILIA. **2** Preference for darkness or night-time; also called *nyctophilia.*

scotopic adaptation DARK ADAPTATION.

scotopic vision Twilight vision, vision under conditions of low illumination such that visual experience is that provided by the rods of the retina. Scotopic vision has the following general properties: (a) hues are not seen, vision is in terms of black and white; (b) the brightness threshold, compared with that of PHOTOPIC VISION, is low; (c) the luminosity curve shows maximum sensitivity to a wavelength of approximately 510 nm with rapidly decreasing sensitivity to longer and shorter wavelengths; (d) because the rods exist only outside of the fovea, visual acuity is poor.

scratch reflex A reflexive scratching response elicited from an animal by a sharp stimulus such as a pinch on the back or the flank.

screen 1 n. Any device for blanking out part of the visual field. **2** n. A device upon which a stimulus is displayed. **3** n. In psychoanalytic theory, any event or object that serves a defensive function and prevents a person from realizing the underlying meaning of an event, a symbol, a dream, etc. **4** vb. To select a small subset of events or things from a larger population. These events or things may be stimuli, in which case an observer is said to *screen* (or to *filter*) *out* some while attending to the others, or they may be persons applying for a position, in which case certain candidates are said to be *screened out* of the selection process. Note that, in these usages, while the rejected items or persons are referred to as having been *screened out*, the others are said to have *passed the screening* or to have *passed through the screen.*

screen memory A psychoanalytic term for the memory of events dating from early childhood, fleeting, elusive memories that have managed to filter through the ego's defensive efforts at repression. The usual interpretation is that such memories function as 'covers' for other emotionally dangerous information which, in fact, they help to repress. Hence, a common synonym is *cover memory.*

script 1 In sociology and social psychology, a scenario, a characterization of the events that occur in a particular social setting. **2** In the cognitive sciences, an individual's knowledge of such events in terms of appropriate behaviour to be carried out, knowledge of who does what, when, to whom and why. Usually scripts are qualified to specify the setting or circumstances, e.g. a restaurant script, a night at the theatre script. **3** Cursive handwriting.

S-curve S-SHAPED CURVE.

SD STANDARD *DEVIATION.

SDT SIGNAL-DETECTION THEORY.

SE STANDARD ERROR.

seance 1 A sitting, as a session of a learned group or a class for the purpose of discussion or deliberation. **2** A sitting for the purpose of communicating with spirits. The second meaning has, unfortunately, become the dominant one.

search In cognitive psychology: **1** vb. To scan through one's memory for some specific fact or other piece of information. **2** n. The process of making such a scan. The following entries give the various kinds of memory searches that have been hypothesized; note that most of them derive their names from work in INFORMATION PROCESSING and ARTIFICIAL INTELLIGENCE and hence have a kind of computer-like character to them.

search, exhaustive A memory search in which all possible alternatives are considered. Compare with SELF-TERMINATING *SEARCH.

search, parallel Any memory-search process in which more than one type of scanning goes on simultaneously. See also PARALLEL *PROCESSING.

search, self-terminating A memory-search process in which one considers alternatives until the searched-for target has been found. Compare with EXHAUSTIVE *SEARCH. Note that most theories of memory that hypothesize a self-terminating search routine assume that it has a time component; i.e. if the target is not found within some period of time, the search terminates and the individual is said to have forgotten the material. See FORGETTING for more on usage here.

search, serial A memory search in which pieces of information are examined one at a time in a series. See also SEQUENTIAL *PROCESSING.

Seashore tests A series of tests of auditory and musical ability developed by Carl E. Seashore.

seasickness MOTION SICKNESS.

seasonal affective disorder (SAD) The most common form of SEASONAL MOOD DISORDER. Characterized by depression, lethargy and sleep disturbances, it typically occurs during the winter months and can often be treated by regular exposure to bright full-spectrum lights. Also called *mood disorder with seasonal pattern*.

seasonal mood disorder An umbrella term for any MOOD DISORDER that shows a regular temporal pattern, such as recurring every summer or every winter. See also SEASONAL AFFECTIVE DISORDER.

secondary 1 Second, particularly in importance, rank or significance. The fundamental idea is that a thing is considered secondary with respect to other things when the things can be ordered in some way – in time, in space, in magnitude, etc. **2** Dependent on something else; based on or derived from a primary thing. The term enjoys wide currency in combined phrases; see the following. Contrast with PRIMARY.

secondary advantage SECONDARY GAIN.

secondary circular reaction CIRCULAR REACTION.

secondary (or second-order) conditioning HIGHER-ORDER CONDITIONING.

secondary drive A learned or ACQUIRED *DRIVE.

secondary elaboration A psychoanalytic term for the tendency to fill gaps, make inferences and reorganize one's memory of dreams upon awakening.

secondary emotions EMOTIONS, SECONDARY.

secondary extinction EXTINCTION, SECONDARY.

secondary gain 1 Generally, any continuing gain derived from being ill. **2** More specifically, the advantages derived from a neurosis, e.g. avoidance of conflict and lessening of anxiety. Compare with PRIMARY GAIN. See also ADVANTAGE BY ILLNESS. Also called *epinosic gain*.

secondary group GROUP, SECONDARY.

secondary identification Identification with someone other than the usual parental figure.

secondary integration Freud's term for the integration of the psychic elements of the pregenital stage into a coherent psychosexual identity.

secondary memory See PRIMARY *MEMORY.

secondary motivation Motivation that derives from learned incentives, ones with cognitive or social features that have no underlying biological components, e.g. NEED FOR ACHIEVEMENT.

secondary motor cortex See MOTOR AREA.

secondary narcissism NARCISSISM, SECONDARY.

secondary personality In cases of multiple personality, the aspect that separates off from the main personality.

secondary process In psychoanalytic theory, mental functioning which is conscious, rational and logical. Secondary processes are conceptualized as intimately linked with the ego and the reality principle. Compare with PRIMARY PROCESS.

secondary quality PRIMARY AND SECONDARY *QUALITY.

secondary reinforcer CONDITIONED *REINFORCER.

secondary relationship RELATIONSHIP, SECONDARY.

secondary repression REPRESSION (1).

secondary reward See CONDITIONED *REINFORCER.

secondary sex characteristics SEX CHARACTERISTICS, SECONDARY.

secondary somatosensory cortex An area of cortex in the PARIETAL LOBE just above the LATERAL FISSURE. It receives inputs from the PRIMARY SOMATOSENSORY CORTEX and regions in

the anterior parietal lobe. Efferent pathways project to the posterior parietal lobe and to several regions that serve motor functions.

secondary symptoms 1 Symptoms of a disorder that are frequently observed but are not distinctive features of that disorder. Bleuler used this term in this manner to designate symptoms found in schizophrenia that were also observed in other disorders. **2** Symptoms that are incidental to a disorder, e.g. social withdrawal resulting from stuttering.

secondary visual system Collectively, those parts of the visual system that lie outside of PRIMARY VISUAL CORTEX. The neural substrates are evolutionarily old and the vision modulated has poor acuity but is sensitive to motion and localization, particularly in the periphery.

second-generation Characterizing treatments, drugs or other procedures that were developed later and, presumably, improved on the effectiveness of the ones that came before.

second messenger Generally, any chemical within a cell that initiates a series of steps involved in synaptic transmission. Such chemicals are called *second messengers* with the understanding that the NEUROTRANSMITTERS are the *first*.

second moment The VARIANCE of a distribution. See also MOMENT (2).

second-order conditioning HIGHER-ORDER CONDITIONING.

second-order factor FIRST-ORDER *FACTOR.

second-signal system In the PAVLOVIAN approach, stimuli or signals are separated into two domains: those that are due to direct physical events (the *first-signal system*) and those that are generated internally, inside the organism (the *second-signal system*). Pavlov viewed speech and language as the primary vehicles for the functioning of the second-signal system, but other Russian theorists have extended the domain to include all forms of ideational, mental, imaginal and mediational activity.

secrete 1 v. To discharge a substance. Usually the reference is to such secretion from cells and glands into other parts of the body (a synaptic gap, blood). **2** n. The substance itself, although the preferred term is *secretion*.

sect A group that espouses a particular set of religious beliefs and practices. A sect is generally viewed as a separate, exclusive entity, with abstract ideals, existing within another, larger religious organization. Compare with CULT.

section 1 Generally, a subdivision or the act of creating a subdivision. **2** More specifically, a slice of tissue or the cutting or slicing of tissue. Various types of section are commonly made in physiological work: (a) *Transverse sections* are cut straight across the longitudinal axis at right angles to it. Note that other terms are used to specify particular kinds of transverse section: *cross-section* is used generally, *frontal section* when the cut is made toward the front of the organ and *coronal section* when it is made toward the rear. (b) *Horizontal sections* are cut parallel to the ground. (c) *Sagittal sections* are cut perpendicular to the ground.

sectioned A patient is described as sectioned when it has been determined that he or she is certifiable as suffering from a severe mental disorder and may be committed to a mental institution. The term is common in Great Britain, where it derives from the holding of the individual under the appropriate *section* of the Mental Health Act. See also CERTIFIABLE and COMMITMENT.

secular 1 Originally, observed but once in a century or an age. Generally descriptive of processes that evolve slowly, e.g. cultural change. **2** More commonly, worldly, temporal, as opposed to religious or spiritual.

secure attachment ATTACHMENT STYLES.

security A sense of confidence, safety, freedom from fear or anxiety, particularly with respect to fulfilling one's present (and future) needs.

security operations 1 H. S. Sullivan's cover term for all those efforts engaged in by individuals to maintain or increase security and avoid anxiety. **2** In Fromm–Reichmann's approach, *security operations* is essentially synonymous with *defence mechanisms*.

sedative, hypnotic or **anxiolytic amnestic disorder** An AMNESTIC DISORDER brought about by prolonged, excessive use of any sedative, hypnotic or anxiolytic drug.

sedative, hypnotic or **anxiolytic withdrawal** An organic mental disorder resulting from the cessation of prolonged, moderate or heavy use of a sedative, hypnotic or anxiolytic drug. The symptoms of nausea, weakness, anxiety, irritability and the like are similar to those of ALCOHOL WITHDRAWAL. This disorder is often called *uncomplicated* to distinguish it from cases in which *delirium* is one of the symptoms.

sedative, hypnotic or **anxiolytic withdrawal delirium** Similar to SEDATIVE, HYPNOTIC OR ANXIOLYTIC WITHDRAWAL, but with delirium, vivid hallucinations and marked autonomic hyperactivity, including tachycardia and sweating. The disorder is typically not seen unless the drug has been used heavily for five or more years prior to withdrawal.

sedatives A class of drugs all of which produce drowsiness and are prescribed most frequently in cases of insomnia. Sedatives are usually classified into the BARBITURATES (of which there are several – see that entry for details) and the *nonbarbiturates*; the latter group includes CHLORAL HYDRATE, ETHINAMATE, METHAQUALONE and PARALDEHYDE. All of these drugs function similarly to depress, nonselectively, central-nervous-system functioning. Depending on the size of the dose, they produce mild sedation, 'hypnotic' sleep (see HYPNOTICS), anaesthesia, coma or death from respiratory failure. All are subject to build-up of tolerance, so that increasing doses are needed to maintain the same effect, and all produce drug dependence. They also diminish sensorimotor skills and interact strongly with many other drugs, significantly alcohol. Other drugs are occasionally included in the category of sedatives, in particular ANTIHISTAMINES, which have drowsiness as a side effect, several ANTICHOLINERGIC DRUGS (e.g. *scopolamine*) and some ANTIANXIETY DRUGS.

segmentation 1 Generally, the process of dividing up a whole into its component parts or segments. **2** In linguistics, the dividing of the surface structure of a sentence into its constituents and phonetic elements.

segregation 1 In Gestalt theory, the perceptual process whereby the coherent, organized figure is seen as phenomenologically distinct from the rest of the field (the ground); see FIGURE–GROUND. **2** By extension from perception to cognition, the compartmentalization of thought processes. **3** An ecological process whereby particular demographic units – usually cities – become subdivided into distinct, functional/cultural districts, e.g. industrial, residential, upper-income, slum, high-rise, ethnic. **4** A subdividing of the residential areas of a city and their accompanying services – schools, shopping facilities, transportation, churches, theatres, etc. – such that their availability to persons is controlled and determined by racial, ethnic or religious characteristics. In this context see RACISM and PREJUDICE and compare with DISCRIMINATION. Note that meaning 4 is, in a sense, included in the more general and neutral meaning 3, although 4 has become the dominant sociopolitical meaning. **5** In genetics, the process of reduction division (see MEIOSIS) in sexual reproduction such that only a single gene from each gene pair is in a gamete.

seizure 1 Generally, any sudden attack of a disorder or malady. **2** More specifically, a convulsion.

seizure disorder A term often used synonymously with EPILEPSY.

selected group GROUP, SELECTED.

selection 1 Broadly, choice. The term is used freely with respect to any operation whereby some individual, group, subject, item, etc. is chosen to be included in a sample, an experiment, a group, etc. **2** In evolutionary biology, the process whereby individual organisms, possessing particular genetic characteristics which make survival and reproductive success in their environmental niches more likely, cause a progressive sequence of changes in the genes of their species. Strictly speaking, it is the *genes* themselves that are selected for by this process, although it is the success of their associated phenotypes that is the causal process. Note that this definition focuses on selection pressures on single organisms and is known generally as *individual selection*. Other evolutionary mechanisms function in ways that impact on larger groups. See here, GROUP •SELECTION. See also NATURAL SELECTION. **3** In operant-behaviour analysis, the process

whereby particular behaviours become part of an organism's repertoire of responses by virtue of the particular consequences of those behaviours. Meanings 2 and 3 are analogous except in the context of 2 features of species are selected for while in the context of 3 behaviours of individual organisms are. See also SHAPING.

selection, group In evolutionary biology, those mechanisms that operate to select forms and functions that impact on the survival and reproductive success of groups of individuals. Such processes operate in most species but are most compellingly seen in those that form groups (humans, chimpanzees) or developed social, colonial lives (bees, termites). Behaviours that favour ALTRUISM and COOPERATION are examples.

selection index A formula for assessing the power of a particular test or an item in a test in discriminating individuals from each other.

selection, individual See SELECTION (2).

selection, kin In evolutionary biology, a type of GROUP •SELECTION for traits that function to increase likelihood of survival and reproductive success of an individual organism's close relatives. See also PERSONAL FITNESS and INCLUSIVE FITNESS.

selection, social An obsolete term used originally as a sociological analogue of *natural selection*. Social selection was the basic principle hypothesized to operate in SOCIAL DARWINISM.

selective adaptation ADAPTATION, SELECTIVE.

selective attention ATTENTION that results from controlled decisions to focus on a particular aspect of a display. While a variety of factors can attract one's attention without any conscious intention (movement, especially in the periphery is an excellent stimulus), when the modifier *selective* is used it marks situations where internal decisions determine where one's attentional resources will be utilized.

selective breeding Controlled mating for the purpose of producing offspring with particular characteristics.

selective inattention 1 A lack of conscious

attending to some aspect of a stimulus. **2** A synonym of PERCEPTUAL DEFENCE.

selective learning LEARNING, SELECTIVE.

selective mutism Quite literally, selecting not to speak. Classified as a childhood disorder, it is characterized by a failure to speak in specific social situations in which speech is expected, such as school. Also called *elective mutism*.

selective serotonin reuptake enhancers (SSREs) A novel group of antidepressants that, unlike the commonly prescribed SELECTIVE SEROTONIN REUPTAKE INHIBITORS, operate by enhancing the reuptake of serotonin thereby making less of it available to function as a neurotransmitter. They are still regarded as experimental drugs and are not available in all countries.

selective serotonin reuptake inhibitors (SSRIs) An important group of ANTIDEPRESSANT DRUGS all of which function by reducing the reuptake of the neurotransmitter SEROTONIN thereby increasing its availability to function as a neurotransmitter. Currently they are the drugs of choice for depressive disorders because they appear to be more effective and have fewer side effects than either the TRICYCLIC COMPOUNDS or the MONOAMINE OXIDASE INHIBITORS. Note that, despite the name, many of the drugs included in this category also block the reuptake of the monoamine NOREPINEPHRINE.

self One of the more dominant aspects of human experience is the compelling sense of one's unique existence, what philosophers have traditionally called the issue of personal identity or of the *self*. Accordingly, this term finds itself rather well represented in psychological theory, particularly in the areas of social and developmental psychology, the study of personality and the field of psychopathology. The diversity of uses, not surprisingly, is extremely broad and rather unsystematic, and the meaning intended is often confounded by the fact that the term may be used in ways which interact subtly with grammatical forms. To appreciate this problem, see the separate entry for the combining form SELF-.

The following are what appear to be the six primary intentions of the users of the term *self*: **1** Self as inner agent or force with controlling and directing functions over motives, fears, needs, etc. Here the self is a hypothetical entity, an assumed aspect of the psyche with a particular role to play. This meaning is found in Adler's notion of the CREATIVE *SELF, in Sullivan's SELF-SYSTEM and in Jung's early writings. **2** Self as inner witness to events. Here, self is viewed as a component of the psyche which serves an introspective function. This self presumably can scan and introspect upon the self expressed in meaning 1. William James pointed out in 1890 that these two meanings might best be spoken of as the *me* and the *I*, the *me* being the self known, the self as object as in 1, and the *I* being the knowing self, the self as subject as in 2. **3** Self as the totality of personal experience and expression, self as living being. Here the term is used inclusively and relatively neutrally, and other terms like *ego*, *person*, *individual* and *organism* are acceptable synonyms. **4** Self as synthesis, self as an organized, personalized whole. This meaning is similar to 3 but with the additional connotation that one is concentrating upon the integrated aspect. Those who refer to self in this fashion often present it as a logical construct which is inferred indirectly by an individual's experience of personal continuity despite changes over time. Thus, generally, the term PERSONALITY is an acceptable synonym in this sense (but consult that entry for a discussion of the difficulties in usage). **5** Self as consciousness, awareness, personal conception; self as identity. Gordon Allport's term PROPRIUM is an appropriate synonym here. **6** Self as abstract goal or end point on some personalistic dimension. This meaning is embodied specifically in the later writings of Jung, in which self became conceptualized as the ultimate archetype lying between consciousness and the unconscious, the achievement of self thus being the final human expression of spiritualistic development. Maslow also expressed this meaning but only tangentially in the combined term SELF-ACTUALIZATION. Note that self, in senses 1–5, is regarded, in one form or another, as an existing aspect of one's personhood: in sense 6 is not – it is, rather, a potential of one's personhood.

self- A reflexive prefix used in a rather impressive array of psychological terms, as the following entries show. There are several grammatical forms of it which are not always immediately apparent, and the manner of use of each carries subtle connotations concerning the presumed meaning of the root word SELF. For example, in phrases like *self-control*, the subject is treated as essentially identical with the object – the self controls the self; in phrases like *self-actualization*, the subject has an indirect-object-type relation – the self becomes actualized; in phrases like self-consistency, there is an adverbial relation with the subject – the self acts consistently; in phrases like *self-evident*, the whole combined form is treated as an adjective modifying some other proposition. The number of combined terms with this prefix is almost without bound. In the following entries we tried to limit coverage to those in fairly common use and whose meanings are not obvious.

self, abandoned A term used by William James to refer to an attempted identity, a model characterization of oneself that one has given up. Often used in the plural under the assumption that most people have several of these littering their lives.

self-abasement 1 An act of self-deprecation; the term is used here with the connotation that the critical self-evaluation is inappropriately excessive. 2 Submission of will or of independent action to another.

self-abuse A perfectly ludicrous term for *masturbation* which has its origins in puritanical attitudes toward sex and sexuality. As several critics have pointed out, it is a uniformly inappropriate term misrepresenting both of the base words, *self* and *abuse*.

self-acceptance Quite literally, an acceptance of oneself. The term is used with the specific connotation that this acceptance is based on a relatively objective appraisal of one's unique talents, capabilities and general worth, a realistic recognition of their limits and a rich feeling of satisfaction with both these talents and their boundaries.

self, actual Horney's term for the momentary psychic totality. The term is really a shorthand expression for referring to everything psychological about a person at a moment in time, including unconscious elements. See also IDEALIZED *SELF (2) and REAL *SELF.

self-actualization 1 A term originally introduced by the organismic theorist Kurt Goldstein for the motive to realize all of one's potentialities. In Goldstein's view self-actualization was the master motive – indeed, the only real motive a person has, all others being merely manifestations of it. 2 In Abraham Maslow's theory of personality, the final level of psychological development that can be achieved when all basic and meta needs are fulfilled and the actualization of the full personal potential takes place. Meanings 1 and 2 are similar. For Goldstein self-actualization was a motive and for Maslow it was a level of development; for both, however, roughly the same kinds of qualities were expressed: independence, autonomy, a tendency to form few but deep friendships, a philosophical sense of humour, a tendency to resist outside pressures and a general transcendence of the environment rather than a simple coping with it.

self-affirmation theory A theory of how dissonance is handled. It maintains that circumstances that arouse dissonance are also seen as threats to one's self-concept. Consequently, they can be (and in real life often are) ameliorated by engaging in self-affirming actions.

self-alienation ALIENATION.

self-appraisal Quite literally, the process of providing an appraisal of oneself. The term is used in a somewhat more neutral fashion than SELF-ESTEEM, which has an evaluative connotation.

self-awareness Generally, the condition of being aware of or conscious of oneself – in the sense of having a relatively objective but open and accepting appraisal of one's true personal nature. Compare with SELF-CONSCIOUSNESS (1).

self-concept One's concept of oneself in as complete and thorough a description as is possible for one to give. Contrast with SELF-ESTEEM and its emphasis on evaluative judgements.

self-consciousness 1 Generally, SELF-AWARENESS, but with a twist – the additional realization that it is possible that others are similarly aware of oneself. 2 Specifically, a sense of embarrassment or unease that derives from the sense expressed in 1 when the individual suspects that the awareness of others contains critical evaluative aspects that are incompatible with one's own personal self-assessment or reveal one to be inadequate.

self-consistency 1 Generally, the characteristic of any system when its several parts all display or reflect a pattern of broad-based compatibility between all of its elements. When the system under consideration is a questionnaire or a test, the term INTERNAL CONSISTENCY is used. **2** By extension, a pattern of behaviour of a person that reflects this characteristic. The term tends to be used here with the additional assumption that the displayed consistency is determined by internal factors of a psychological nature rather than by external, environmental factors.

self-construal Generally, the way in which the self is experienced, the manner in which one 'construes' oneself. The term is often found in cross-cultural psychology where the self is depicted as having two components, one based on INTERDEPENDENCE and one on INDEPENDENCE (esp. 4), with the manner in which one leans toward one or the other as the key factor.

self-control Quite literally, control of self. The term is generally reserved for the ability to control impulsiveness by inhibiting immediate short-range desires; its dominant connotation is that of repressing or inhibiting.

self-correlation In testing, the correlation between the scores from two administrations of a test (see TEST–RETEST *RELIABILITY) or between two forms of a test (see ALTERNATIVE FORMS *RELIABILITY).

self, creative In Adler's personality theory, the prime mover of behaviour, the inner striving for superiority which acts to give meaning to life.

self-criticism Basically, criticism of oneself by oneself with the connotation that such a critical evaluation is an objective and realistic appraisal of one's strengths and weaknesses, talents and shortcomings, etc. Such an analysis of self is part of a healthy self-acceptance. Note that some authors distinguish between *externally* imposed self-criticism, which focuses on failure to live up to societal standards, and *internally* imposed self-criticism, which focuses upon personal standards.

self-deception The deceiving of oneself in the sense of the inability to have accurate insights into one's limitations; a self-deceiver cannot display SELF-ACCEPTANCE.

self-defeating personality disorder A PERSONALITY DISORDER characterized by a pervasive pattern of self-defeating behaviour, including avoiding or undermining pleasurable experiences, being drawn into situations with a high likelihood of failure, seeking out relationships that are likely to be unrewarding, and preventing others from providing help. Also called *masochistic personality disorder*. This disorder was hotly debated in psychiatric circles over a period of several years because of possible gender bias and is no longer included in the *DSM*.

self-demand (schedule of) feeding Feeding upon request. The term is used in animal experimentation synonymously with AD LIB (feeding) and in child-rearing studies to refer to a flexible feeding arrangement whereby an infant is fed whenever it shows signs of hunger. Also called *demand feeding*.

self-denial The practice of deliberately forgoing pleasures and satisfactions. Typically adopted by those who value asceticism, who argue that they forsake superficial and trivial pleasures for greater psychological or spiritual gain.

self-desensitization In behaviour therapy, the use of the DESENSITIZATION TECHNIQUE by an individual in everyday situations as a way of dealing with anxiety.

self-determination Roughly, internally controlling one's behaviour, acting on the basis of personal beliefs and values rather than on the basis of social norms or group pressures. Some theorists, particularly those with an existentialist orientation, maintain that self-determination is an integral component of the optimal functioning of a person, while others, notably Skinnerian behaviourists, regard it as an illusion. See also SELF-DIRECTION.

self-development 1 Generally, growth of self, movement toward emotional and cognitive maturity. **2** In Maslow's model, progress toward SELF-ACTUALIZATION (2).

self-direction A rough synonym of SELF-DETERMINATION but used more neutrally; that is, *self-direction* does not invite the theoretical disputes that underlie the connotations of its approximate synonym.

self-discipline 1 Usually, control over one's behaviour, particularly over immediate impulsiveness. Essentially a synonym of SELF-CONTROL. **2** Occasionally, self-punishment.

self-dynamisms In H. S. Sullivan's theory of personality, an umbrella term for all of the basic motivational aspects of the self, i.e. the biological as well as the social and the learned as well as the unlearned. See SELF-SYSTEM.

self-effacement 1 Generally, modesty or humility. **2** Specifically, in Karen Horney's theory, a neurotic pattern in which one comes to idealize and identify with the originally least admirable characteristics of one's personality.

self-efficacy Bandura's term for an individual's sense of their abilities, of their capacity to deal with the particular sets of conditions that life puts before them.

self-embedded sentence Any sentence with a relative clause between the subject and the verb of the main clause, e.g. 'The man who wore the purple snow boots has already left.' Single embedded sentences such as this one are relatively easy to comprehend: double, triple and more highly embedded ones seriously strain one's interpretative and memorial capabilities.

self, empirical One of William James's alternative terms for the ME; see SELF (1, 2).

self-enhancement Any cognitive or behavioural process that serves to increase the SELF-ESTEEM of oneself and/or the groups with which one identifies. Self-enhancement functions by: (a) emphasizing the positive features of oneself and one's groups; and/or (b) by reinterpreting the less-than positive aspects so as to put them in a better light. There are cultural differences in the extent to which the emphasis is upon the individual or the group. Societies that favour individualism lean toward the former; those that are more collectivist focus on the latter. The term refers to the *processes* used to increase esteem, not the results.

self-esteem The degree to which one values oneself. Note that although the word *esteem* carries the connotation of high worth or value, the combined form, *self-esteem*, refers to the full dimension and the degree of self-esteem (high or low) is usually specified. Contrast with SELF-APPRAISAL, from which the evaluative component is absent. Note that the referential domain of the term is sometimes extended to include the esteem of a group with which one identifies or is a member of. See here, SELF-ENHANCEMENT.

self-evaluation SELF-RATING.

self-evident Characterizing any proposition, statement, principle, etc. the truth of which is evident on the face of it and requires no independent demonstration. It should be recognized that there is an oft-hidden connotation to the term that the evidentiary aspect is to be appreciated only by one who really understands the situation; therefore, vigorous debates over the self-evident status of particular propositions are more common than the definition would lead one to expect.

self-expression 1 The acting-out of one's inner feelings, beliefs, attitudes, etc. In many contemporary psychotherapeutic orientations, such a display is assumed to have therapeutic value. **2** Any behaviour carried out for the sheer pleasure and satisfaction that it provides for the individual. This meaning is what lies behind the presumption of the therapeutic value expressed in sense 1.

self-fulfilling prophecy A term used to refer to the fact that frequently things turn out just as one expected (or prophesied) that they would – not necessarily because of one's prescience but because one behaved in a manner that optimized these very outcomes. A teacher who predicts that a student will ultimately fail tends to treat that student in ways that increase the likelihood of failure, thus fulfilling the original prophecy. See also the related concepts DEMAND CHARACTERISTICS and EXPERIMENTER BIAS.

self-handicapping Engaging in behaviours that sabotage one's own ability to function in particular situations, thereby providing a convenient subsequent excuse for failure. Classic cases: a student neglects to set the alarm clock the night before an examination, an actor fails to rehearse a part before an audition, a lexicographer forgets to set the spell-checker.

self-help Essentially, helping oneself. The term is used mostly to refer to non-traditional approaches to psychotherapy that encourage personal growth and self-reliance, often in *self-help groups* that function mainly to provide mutual support, develop friendships and encourage change.

self, idealized 1 Generally, a perfected and lofty characterization of self in the sense of what one would like to become. When used this way, the term refers to a kind of personalistic goal of a well-adjusted individual. **2** In Karen Horney's theory, a neurotic self-image in the assumption of which one comes to believe that one has indeed achieved this glorified state.

self-identification The process whereby one develops affection and admiration for another person who possesses qualities and traits which resemble one's own. That is, one sees (i.e. identifies) oneself in the other; the term carries no connotation of confusion in personal identity, however.

self-image Generally, the image one has of oneself, the SELF (3, 4) one supposes oneself to be. Negative self-image is, not surprisingly, associated with a variety of dysfunctions and self-defeating behaviours; positive self-image is linked with psychologically salubrious outcomes. As Karen Horney noted, the important issue is not one's self-image per se but the inevitable disjunction between it and the real self.

self-inventory Any self-evaluation device (most commonly in the form of a questionnaire) with which the subject checks off those personality traits or characteristics which pertain to him- or herself. See also SELF-REPORT INVENTORY.

selfish gene The term refers metaphorically to a hypothesized characteristic of a species genotype. In simplest terms, the behaviour of any organism is hypothesized to maximize the survival of its genes, which are then passed on to future generations. Hence, the genes are 'selfish': they appear to function so that the organism of whose behaviour they are an important determiner will survive and breed and thereby ensure their survival.

The notion was introduced by Richard Dawkins and has had considerable impact on contemporary theorizing in SOCIOBIOLOGY and EVOLUTIONARY PSYCHOLOGY.

self-justification theory A theory that seeks to explain why many people are motivated to justify and maintain the status quo even, despite the paradox, when the current state is one of change or incipient change. The model posits a variety of cognitive and emotional antecedents (e.g. need for order) that contribute to such motivations and tries to explicate individual differences in self-justifying motivations and behaviours.

self-love A general term for any form of extreme love of oneself, e.g. NARCISSISM and EGOISM.

self-monitoring 1 Sensitivity to social cues and expectations combined with a willingness to adjust one's self-presentation in response. Usually spoken of as a *trait*, with all that entails. **2** A technique used in psychotherapy where the client is encouraged to keep a diary or an ongoing record of specific behaviours, emotional reactions to events and the like.

self-observation 1 Simply, observation of one's behaviour, observation of oneself. **2** More specifically, a synonym of INTROSPECTION.

self, perceived 1 The SELF of which one is aware. **2** The self as represented in SELF-PERCEPTION THEORY.

self-perception theory A theoretical point of view which argues that people's attitudes, beliefs and self-characterizations are, to a considerable degree, determined by observation of their own behaviours. The underlying principle is simple: just as we tend to judge the feelings of others by what we see them do, so we infer our own attitudes by self-observation. See also ATTRIBUTION THEORY, which is related.

self, phenomenal 1 The self as known through direct, unmediated experience. Generally the phenomenal self is presumed to derive from the environment (or, more precisely, from the interaction between the individual and the environment), and its ultimate expression is through one's direct, conscious, noninferential perception. See PHENOMENOLOGY. **2** The PERCEIVED *SELF (1).

self-presentation Quite literally, the process of presenting oneself in relationship to socially and culturally accepted modes of action and behaviour. The connotation is that the process is based on the use of specific strategies designed to shape what others will think of one.

self-preservation An umbrella term for any behaviours which function to increase the survival chances of an organism. It covers a wide range of processes, from the rather primitive aggressive behaviours and flight responses to sophisticated operations like the defence mechanisms for handling anxiety.

self psychology A generic label for any approach to psychology that makes the self the central concept against which all other events and processes are interpreted.

self-rating Any evaluation of oneself. The term is generally used with respect to personality-assessment devices in which the individual supplies information about him- or herself. Also called *self-evaluation*.

self, real In Karen Horney's system, a hypothesized font of psychic energy which can be utilized to orient a person toward a normal, nonneurotic life. Compare with ACTUAL *SELF and IDEALIZED *SELF.

self-realization More or less nontechnically, the fulfilment of one's potential. Generally used to refer to fulfilment in one domain, in contrast to SELF-ACTUALIZATION.

self-reference effect The phenomenon of having better memory for material that is relevant to oneself than for material that is not.

self-regard 1 Observing oneself. **2** High self-esteem. **3** Concern for one's personal interests.

self-report In personality and behavioural assessment, statements or answers to questions made by individuals about their beliefs, behaviours, opinions and feelings (e.g. SELF-REPORT INVENTORY). They are used primarily when the interest is on internal states and

perceptions not easily assessed by external observation. However, because such reports rely on self-awareness and personal honesty, there is only moderate agreement between them and the ratings of others, particularly in personality assessment. Contrast with COLLATERAL REPORT.

self-report inventory Any instrument that uses SELF-REPORT techniques to assess personality characteristics. Most use lists of traits or statements with which the individual indicates his or her level of agreement, or sets of imagined situations where the test-taker identifies those characteristic of oneself.

self-schema Quite literally, a SCHEMA (1) about oneself. It is typically composed of a set of coordinated personal beliefs about oneself that guide action and the processing of information relevant to oneself.

self-selected groups design A research method whereby subjects in effect select themselves by virtue of having particular characteristics or demographic properties.

self-sentiment See EGO COMPLEX.

self-serving bias Quite simply, any bias in interpreting events that operates so as to bolster its holder. Our (indeed most professors') favourite example: a student who did well on an exam feels that the test was a good measure of ability; one who failed insists that it was a poorly written exam or one that didn't accurately assess his or her knowledge.

self, social A general term used in several ways, all of which reflect some aspect of the 'interface' between society and self. **1** Those aspects of self that are largely determined by societal values and social influences. **2** The (usually delimited) aspects of one's self or personality which are readily perceived by other persons in social interactions. **3** Those components of personality that an individual regards as important in social interactions. **4** The general characterization of one's self that an individual perceives as being perceived by others. See also PERSON PERCEPTION, SELF-PERCEPTION THEORY.

self-stimulation Lit., stimulation of oneself. The term is used in various situations, e.g. of infants who, when left in relatively uniform environments, babble and wave their hands in an effort to provide their own varied stimulation, and of animals in studies of electrical brain-stimulation which can deliver stimulation to their own brains by making an operant response. Some researchers have argued that a class of behaviours common in *autism* (e.g. rocking, hand-waving) are forms of self-stimulation.

self-system Harry Stack Sullivan's term for the SELF-DYNAMISM that is composed of a set of tendencies that function to protect one from anxiety and to provide security so that one can behave effectively. As Sullivan viewed it, this self-system, like the defence mechanisms of the more orthodox psychoanalytic theorists, can have serious drawbacks: by protecting the individual from anxiety it may also prevent growth and productive change.

self-terminating search SEARCH, SELF-TERMINATING.

self-transcendence The condition where one transcends the self and becomes absorbed by one's work, by a desire to help others or a focus on social causes. In Frankl's humanistic vision, such a commitment to goals beyond the self was regarded as a high ideal.

self-verification The process whereby one attempts to verify one's SELF-CONCEPT. Typically this is achieved either by limiting one's activities to things that can be carried out in ways that validate the sense of self, or in efforts to persuade others that they should acknowledge and accept one's view of self.

semantic component 1 SEMANTIC FEATURE. 2 In some linguistic theories, that aspect of a grammar which contains the formal rules and procedures for representing meaning. Distinguish from SYNTACTIC COMPONENT.

semantic conditioning The conditioning of meaning. The term is used to refer to either (a) the simple association of a word with its referent, or (b) the more complex association of some other response to a particular meaning. When a child learns to associate a spoken word like *sheep* with a real sheep, (a) has presumably occurred; if a person shows a response originally associated with *sheep* to a semantically similar word such as *lamb*, (b) has occurred. Note that the occurrence of (b) is, in effect, a demonstration that the conditioning in (a) was really semantic.

semantic confusion Any confusion over which stimulus was presented, based upon semantic factors. Remembering *wolf* when the actual stimulus was *fox* is an example. Compare with ACOUSTIC CONFUSION.

semantic dementia DEMENTIA, SEMANTIC.

semantic differential A technique due to Charles Osgood and his co-workers for evaluating the connotative meanings of individual words. A subject rates the meaning of each of a series of words along a number of polar dimensions such as hot–cold, weak–strong, tense–relaxed and rough–smooth. Factor analyses of the data generally reveal three primary factors underlying connotative meaning: *activity*, *potency* and *evaluative*.

semantic feature Broadly, any defining characteristic of the meaning of a word which serves to distinguish it from the meaning of other words; e.g. *widow* is distinguished from *widower* by the semantic feature *female*. In discussions of child language, the term *semantic primitive* will often be found to refer to the basic or primitive features that children tend to learn first. That is, for a two-year old 'train' might have the features 'big, noisy, black' even though in adult language these would not be regarded as true semantic features of the word.

semantic generalization GENERALIZATION, SEMANTIC.

semantic memory MEMORY, SEMANTIC.

semantic network (model) A class of theoretical models of the structure of human LONG-TERM *MEMORY. Such models assume that information is stored in the form of words, concepts or propositions as independent units which are interconnected by links or relations. For example, the concept *cat* is assumed to be represented by links such as 'has fur', 'is domestic' and 'is a mammal'. The network formed by the central node and all of its associated links constitutes the memorial representation of the concept.

semantic primitive See SEMANTIC FEATURE.

semantics The study of meaning in any and all of its manifestations.

semantic satiation A curious phenomenon best explained by example: repeat any word (e.g. *giraffe*) over and over (10 or 15 times will do). The curious sense of loss of meaning of the word that you experience is called semantic satiation. Nobody has yet presented a compelling explanation of how or why it happens.

semantics, generative An approach to the study of language that focuses on the development of a grammar that generates underlying meanings of sentences and transforms the meanings into actual sentences.

semantic space A term used metaphorically to refer to the mental representation of word meaning in theories of SEMANTIC •MEMORY that hypothesize a kind of spatial model of the memorial form. See e.g. SEMANTIC NETWORK (MODEL).

semantic therapy A technique used in a number of therapies in which the focus is on getting the client to reinterpret distorted connotations of emotionally tinged words.

semasiography A primitive writing system based on the use of iconic symbols to represent meaning. See ORTHOGRAPHY.

semeiology 1 SEMIOTICS. **2** The study of the signs (i.e. symptoms) of disease.

semeiotics SEMIOTICS.

semen 1 The cloudy, viscous fluid in which the male sperm are suspended. **2** The sperm themselves. Typically the former is intended. adj., *seminal* (used much more generally, e.g. a seminal idea).

semicircular canals The three semicircular tubes that are part of the labyrinth of the inner ear. Each consists of a membranous canal filled with endolymph. They lie roughly at right angles to each other and approximate the three planes of the head. Movement of the head causes movement of the endolymph, which produces a shearing of the hair cells of the crista (the organ containing the receptors) in the ampulla (the enlargements at one end of each canal).

semi-interquartile range QUARTILE DEVIATION.

seminal vesicles The two sacs at the base of the bladder in males that store semen.

semiology SEMIOTICS.

semiotics Broadly, the study of patterned communication in all modalities. The focus is on SIGNS (4, 6) and the manner in which their combinatorial patterns of use convey meaning. The philosopher C. S. Peirce was the first to emphasize the notion that true meaning emerges from the patterns of relationships amongst signs, a notion embraced by proponents of STRUCTURALISM (3, 4). Thomas Sebeok extended the domain of the field by distinguishing between *anthroposemiotics*, the study of systems primarily linguistic in nature and specific to humans, and *zoosemiotics*, which includes examination of paralinguistic and nonverbal systems characteristic of communication in all species. var., *semeiotics*. Also called *semeiology* and *semiology* (the term Peirce used).

semipartial correlation CORRELATION, SEMIPARTIAL.

semi-structured interview Any interview that sets the topics to be covered, while affording the interviewer some latitude to adapt the interview to the interviewee in terms of wording and/or organization, particularly if further clarity or explication is warranted. Also called *patterned interview*.

semi-tone A half-tone; see TONE (2).

semi-vowel A speech sound with some basic vowel-like qualities on account of the air passage being relatively unobstructed but with more friction, e.g. /w/ in *wit*. Unlike vowels, semi-vowels cannot form syllables without support from other speech elements.

senescence 1 Old age. **2** The process of becoming old. **3** The years during which one becomes old. At one time the term was used as a rough synonym of *senility* but this meaning is no longer found; see SENILITY and SENILE.

senile 1 Aged; used particularly with respect to those patterns of thought and behaviour characteristic of old age. Note that, although this definition is basically evaluatively neutral, the term has taken on negative connotations, specifically: **2** Characteristic of those patterns of thought and behaviour that show the deterioration often, although not universally, observed in the aged. Many use the term with a strict criterion of age 65; thus *senile onset* is reserved for conditions that first appear after age 65 and *presenile onset* for conditions before age 65. Compare with the more neutral term SENESCENCE.

senile dementia DEMENTIA, SENILE.

senile dementia of the Alzheimer's type (SDAT) ALZHEIMER'S DISEASE.

senile onset SENILE.

senile plaques AMYLOID PLAQUES.

senile psychosis DEMENTIA, SENILE.

senility 1 SENESCENCE, in the neutral sense of that term. **2** The state of being, or the period of life when a person is, SENILE.

senium The period of life after the age of 65.

sensate focus 1 Generally, developing and maintaining the focusing of attention upon particular sensory inputs. **2** Specifically, such a focusing on sensual experiences. **3** By extension, a technique of sex therapy designed to overcome the fears and anxieties that accompany many forms of orgasmic dysfunction by gradually building up a recognition of, and ability to focus on, pleasurable sensual experience.

sensation 1 Any unelaborated, elementary experience of feeling or awareness of conditions within or outside the body produced by the stimulation of some receptor or receptor system; a *sense datum*. This definition has represented a kind of operating principle for a variety of theories of sensory experience and tends to be what is presented in most introductory textbooks, where *sensations* are usually distinguished from *perceptions*, the latter being characterized as resulting from interpretation and elaboration of sensations. It should, however, be appreciated that many psychologists dispute the very notion that one can have any experiential sense at all without elaborating, interpreting, labelling or recognizing what the experience is. **2** In Titchener's structuralism, one of the three basic elements of consciousness (along with *feelings* and *images*). **3** The process of sensing. **4** A label for the field of psychology that studies these basic processes of sensory experience. The focus is primarily on the examination of physiological and psychophysical principles.

sensation level The sensed or experienced level of intensity of a stimulus, e.g. how loud a particular sound is heard as, how bright a light is seen to be, etc. It is measured by using the individual's own absolute threshold as the reference level.

sensation-seeking A dimension along which individuals may be rated according to the degree to which they search out and enjoy partaking in activities with high levels of sensation.

sensation threshold THRESHOLD (1).

sensation type One of Jung's hypothesized personality types; see FUNCTION TYPES for details.

sense 1 n. A subjective category of sensory impressions grouped together on the basis of shared experiential features; a sense modality, e.g. the sense of hearing, of smell, of vision. **2** n. A similar classification but with the defining feature being a common receptor system rather than common experience. This usage often appears in qualified phrases like 'sense organ for hearing'. These two meanings are not as synonymous as they may initially appear. One may have a sense according to meaning 1 without a true receptor organ for it according to meaning 2, as with the phenomenon of the PHANTOM LIMB; one may have two or more senses according to meaning 1 with but one sense according to meaning 2, as with SYNESTHESIA; or one may have a single sense (meaning 1) with several anatomically different receptor organs for it (meaning 2), as is the case with pressure on the skin and muscles. **3** n. A classification of subjective experiences not clearly linked in a simple way with any particular sense (as in meanings 1 and 2) but coordinated in some complex fashion with a dimension of the physical world, e.g. a sense of time, a sense of space. **4** n. A form of awareness of some abstract quality or concept, e.g. a sense of humour, a sense of fair play, a sense of justice. **5** n. A summary of the general meaning of a thing, the gist of some event, episode, story, etc. **6** n. A well-considered or intelligent judgement, as in 'she showed good sense'.

In addition to these noun forms there are several verb forms: **7** To experience by virtue of a categorical judgement made with reference to a sensory modality. **8** To experience by virtue of the direct stimulation of a receptor system. Note that 7 is the verbal form of 1, and 8 of 2. **9** To have an emotional or cognitive experience that reflects one's judgement about an event or episode, e.g. 'I sense unhappiness behind his smile.'

There are also many combined phrases based on these meanings, and in many instances any of the following derived forms may be found. Although there is something less than universality in usage, generally speaking SENSORY is preferred when referring to those which are based on meanings 1, 2, 7 and 8, i.e. those dealing with sensation and the sensory processes; while SENSITIVE (1, 2) and SENSITIVITY are preferred when referring to those based on meanings 3, 4, 5, 6 and 9, i.e. those dealing with the emotional, judgemental and intellectual functions. SENSIBLE is, unfortunately, used rather haphazardly for both domains but is becoming increasingly rare in these contexts in the technical literature. For combined forms not found following one of these terms, see the others.

sense datum SENSATION (1).

sense illusion An obsolete term for a perceptual illusion.

sense impression Generally, any piece of sensory data. The term was a favourite among some early behaviourists, who wanted to theorize about perception and perceptual processes without admitting it.

sense limen THRESHOLD (esp. 1).

sense modality MODALITY.

sense organ Syn. of RECEPTOR.

sense perception A somewhat confusing term originally used to refer to the processes by which perceptual experiences are derived from sensory inputs. The inextricable relations now known to exist between sensation and perception have rendered the term relatively useless.

sense quality QUALITY (1).

sense, special A cover term used for those senses for which the receptors are in the head: usually vision, audition, smell and taste (although, of course, the VESTIBULAR APPARATUS should also be included).

sensibility The capacity for being SENSIBLE in any of the meanings of that term – although meanings 4 and 5 are usually the intended ones.

sensible An adjective which reflects the several meanings of SENSE: **1** Pertaining to that which is an effective stimulus for a sensory receptor, an above-threshold stimulus. **2** Pertaining to any stimulus object or event that is apprehended through the senses. **3** Pertaining to an individual who shows the capacity for responding to stimulation. **4** Having meaning. **5** Displaying good judgement. **6** SENSITIVE (1 or 2). Meanings 4 and 5 are the more common in contemporary writings.

sensing The process whereby one becomes cognizant of a stimulus which has impinged upon one's sensory organs. See SENSATION and PERCEPTION for discussions of the complexities involved in this process.

sensitive **1** adj. Generally, pertaining to sensitivity. **2** adj. Characteristic of one who is emotionally labile, easily moved by events. **3** n. One who presumably possesses certain paranormal abilities in communication and perception; see PARAPSYCHOLOGY.

sensitive period **1** CRITICAL PERIOD. **2** A loosely defined period of time during which an organism is sensitive to particular forms of stimulus inputs and physiologically and psychologically ready for the acquisition of a particular response or a particular type of knowledge. Unlike CRITICAL PERIOD, which, unhappily, some authors use synonymously, the connotation is that the time period is quite flexible. Sense 2 is much less sharply specified than 1; for example, one speaks of a sensitive period for acquiring language which can range from the age of a few months to puberty.

sensitive zone Any bodily area with a particularly high sensitivity to certain classes of stimulation, e.g. the erogenous zones.

sensitivity **1** Generally, susceptibility to stimulation. **2** More specifically, responsiveness to weak stimuli, having a low threshold. **3** Cognizance of the feelings of another, particularly an awareness based on relatively minor cues. **4** A personal vulnerability whereby one is easily hurt or offended. **5** In statistics, the ability of a test to detect an effect that is in fact present.

sensitivity training A generic term for a variety of quasi-therapeutic group procedures developed originally in the 1940s by

Kurt Lewin and Ronald Lippitt. They served as forums for the members of a group or organization to develop greater awareness of group dynamics and their own roles within the group. The techniques later merged with others from the *human potential movement*, losing much of their original scientific focus along the way. Also known as *T-group training.*

sensitization The process of becoming highly sensitive, usually with the implication that one is not uniformly sensitive to all stimuli but only to specific events or situations. See DESENSITIZATION for the opposite process.

sensor That which senses, hence: **1** An individual receptor, e.g. a free nerve ending, a retinal rod or cone. **2** A receptor organ, e.g. the eye, the ear. The former is the more common denotation; see RECEPTOR.

sensorimotor **1** Generally, pertaining to those processes which are theorized as being essentially made up of afferent (sensory) and efferent (motor) mechanisms. Although it is trivially true that virtually all behaviours, from the most primitive reflexive acts to the most complex cognitive processes, are in some sense sensorimotor, the term is typically reserved for those acts which are predominantly so; e.g. an infant reaching for a toy is so characterized, but the movement of a chess piece in a game is not. **2** More specifically, the neural circuit from a receptor to the central nervous system and back to a muscle. Often the variation *sensory-motor* is used synonymously, although its original meaning was restricted to **2**.

sensorimotor intelligence A general term used to refer to the types of cognitive capabilities exhibited by children during the SENSORIMOTOR STAGE. According to Piaget, such thinking is characterized by the differentiation and elaboration of the basic action schemas such as grasping, sucking and looking.

sensorimotor memory MEMORY, SENSORIMOTOR.

sensorimotor rhythm A moderately rapid (12–14 Hz) brainwave which can be recorded from the scalp over the sensorimotor areas of the cortex.

sensorimotor stage (or **level** or **period**) In Piagetian theory, the stage of cognitive functioning beginning at birth and continuing until the development or establishment of OBJECT PERMANENCE and the beginnings of symbolic thought.

sensorium Loosely, those areas of the brain that handle conscious registering and processing of incoming sensory information.

sensory Pertaining very generally to the senses, the sense organs, the sense receptors, the afferent neural pathways, sense data, sensation, etc. Contrast with MOTOR. See also SENSE (1, 2) and SENSATION (1).

sensory acuity ACUITY, SENSORY.

sensory adaptation ADAPTATION (1).

sensory aphasia WERNICKE'S *APHASIA.

sensory aprosodia APROSODIA.

sensory area(s) Most generally, those areas of the central nervous system that are the termini of ascending sensory neurons. Particular areas are typically specified by the name of the sensory modality they serve, e.g. the visual area, the somatosensory areas. Also called *sensory projection areas.*

sensory ataxia ATAXIA, SENSORY.

sensory automatism AUTOMATISM, SENSORY.

sensory conditioning SENSORY PRECONDITIONING.

sensory cortex SENSORY AREA(S).

sensory deprivation A term descriptive of a situation, either natural or experimentally arranged, in which there is a marked reduction in incoming sensory information. Relatively short periods of time in sensory deprivation are mildly pleasant and relaxing: long periods are extremely aversive and produce time-sense distortions, as well as bizarre thoughts, images and hallucinations.

sensory discrimination Essentially, a synonym for DISCRIMINATION (1 and/or 2).

sensory drive A drive for some specific sensation.

sensory field **1** = PERCEPTUAL FIELD. **2** = RECEPTIVE FIELD.

sensory gating GATING.

sensory homunculus HOMUNCULUS (2).

sensory information store (SIS) A memory system of extremely short duration. Immediately after the removal of a stimulus a sensory representation of the stimulus seems 'suspended' in the mind for a brief time – of the order of one or two seconds. The capacity of SIS is limited by the information that can be apprehended in one short exposure to a stimulus; the form of the memory is essentially a direct match of the stimulus.

Material is assumed to be lost from SIS either by DECAY (2) of the neural trace or by being disrupted by MASKING. Also called *sensory memory* and, occasionally, *sensory register*.

sensory memory See SENSORY INFORMATION STORE and MEMORY, SENSORY.

sensory modality MODALITY.

sensory-motor SENSORIMOTOR.

sensory nerve An afferent nerve, one that conveys sensory information to the central nervous system.

sensory neuron Any individual afferent neuron.

sensory organization Generally, the process of coordination and organization of the sensory input. See ORGANIZATION et seq. for more details.

sensory preconditioning An experimental procedure in which two neutral, non-generalizable stimuli are repeatedly presented together followed by the conditioning of one of them to a particular response. Sensory preconditioning is said to have occurred if the other, nonconditioned stimulus evokes the conditioned response on a test trial. Also called *sensory conditioning*, but *preconditioning* is more accurate.

sensory process Loosely and inclusively, any process conceptualized either physiologically or psychologically which relates to sensation, sense data, sensing, etc.

sensory projection areas SENSORY AREA(S).

sensory psychophysiology That aspect of the field of PHYSIOLOGICAL PSYCHOLOGY that is concerned with sensory systems and their manner of functioning.

sensory quality QUALITY (1).

sensory register SENSORY INFORMATION STORE.

sensory-seeking motives Generally, those motives to increase stimulation and heighten arousal and tension, e.g. the desire to engage in sporting events, parties, rides in amusement parks. See also SENSATION-SEEKING.

sensory stimulus A distinctly redundant term used by some authors to refer to stimuli that are above threshold; that is, stimuli that evoke a sensation.

sensory substitution The replacing of sensory input from one modality with input from another. For example, visual inputs can be replaced by tactile sensations by having a camera project its image onto a dense set of vibrating pins placed on a sensitive area, such as the tongue. The principle was applied by Paul Bach-y-Rita who developed several devices that allow blind individuals to 'see' and those with bilateral VESTIBULAR DYSFUNCTION to recover a sense of balance.

sensory transduction TRANSDUCTION (2).

sensual Generally, pertaining to gratification of the senses. In practice, usage is restricted to the carnal and erotic. syn., *sensuous*.

sentence A self-contained, grammatical, linguistic unit consisting of one or more words syntactically and semantically related to each other such that some assertion, question, command, etc. is expressed. In the written format, sentences are usually marked by appropriate punctuation: in the spoken format, they are rather less clearly marked, although there is generally a phonetically distinguishable pattern of stress, pitch and pausing. The sentence has become the primary unit of analysis of modern linguistics and, by extension, an important component in the study of psycholinguistics.

sentence-completion test (or **method**) **1** A procedure in which one is given partial sentences and required to complete them. Often used as a technique for assessing linguistic knowledge. **2** INCOMPLETE-SENTENCES TEST.

sentience 1 The state of being capable of sensing. **2** A fairly primitive, undifferentiated state of consciousness; 'pure' sensation without interpretation. Compare with SENTIENT.

sentient Following from the general meaning of SENTIENCE: **1** Capable of responding to stimuli. **2** Capable of a minimal consciousness of awareness of stimulation. But, by further extension: **3** Capable of awareness of or conscious recognition of the perception of detail; in short, intelligent. This last meaning, which goes much further than the other two, is now the dominant one.

sentiment Although etymologically this term is derived from SENSE, it tends to be used much more broadly. To wit: **1** A complex disposition based upon one's feelings toward a person, situation, idea, etc. A sentiment is more general and more complex than an *attitude* or a *judgement*, and behaviour is typically implied. That is, a given sentiment is more than just a complex affective state, it implies action; e.g. a person with a strong nationalistic sentiment is likely to defend his or her country vigorously. **2** R. B. Cattell's term for a learned, dynamic trait structure which focuses and mediates attention and reaction to classes of objects in characteristic ways.

sentimentality Emotionality which is shallow, maudlin, romantic and, in some respects, suspect in its veracity. Distinguish from SENTIMENT.

separation anxiety 1 In psychoanalysis, the hypothesized anxiety on the part of an infant or child concerning possible loss of the mother object. **2** By extension, anxiety over the possible loss of any other person or object upon whom one has become dependent. See SEPARATION-ANXIETY DISORDER.

separation-anxiety disorder An anxiety disorder of childhood in which the dominant feature is excessive and inappropriate anxiety on separation from the primary attachment figure(s) (usually one or both parents) or from the home environment. Common manifestations are unrealistic worries about harmful things happening to the attachment figure(s) while away, persistent fears of being lost, kidnapped or even killed if separated, social withdrawal and SCHOOL REFUSAL.

separation-individuation Margaret Mahler's term for a child's awareness of its discrete identity, its individuality, its separateness from the mother. In Mahler's theory, this awareness develops following the *symbiotic stage*, during which the mutually reinforcing relationship between mother and child is dominant.

septal area A region in the forebrain containing the septal nuclei (see nucleus accumbens for details) and the *septum pellucidum*, which separates the anterior horns of the lateral ventricles. It has several neural connections with the hypothalamus and hippocampus and is regarded as a component of the LIMBIC SYSTEM.

septum A dividing wall or membrane separating two cavities of an organ or other structure; e.g. the nasal septum separates the nostrils. pl., *septa*.

septum pellucidum SEPTAL AREA.

sequela Any residual condition that persists after a disease, illness or event. Examples include chronic weakness following a stroke, nightmares and depression following a traumatic event, and heightened anxiety after child abuse. pl., *sequelae*.

sequence 1 A consecutive ordering of events, numbers, etc. in some seriated fashion usually in time or space, or with respect to some dimension such as size or magnitude, etc. **2** In mathematics, a quantitative series in which each element is derived from the preceding by the application of a particular operation. adj., *sequential*.

sequential analysis Statistical analysis of data performed at a particular point in an extended study to determine whether enough data have been collected to evaluate properly the hypothesis under consideration, or whether to collect more. Such analyses are frequently used in large-scale *clinical trials*.

sequential marriage SERIAL *POLYGAMY.

sequential reaction time SRT TASK.

serendipity The finding of one thing while engaged in a search for something else. The term was first used with respect to scientific discovery by the physiologist Walter Cannon. It entered the language via Horace Walpole, who coined it in 1754, basing it on *The Three Princes of Serendip*, a tale by a 16th-century Venetian writer named Michele Tramezzino. The princes travelled the earth searching fruitlessly for certain things but always managing through careful observation and subtle logical reasoning to make other unanticipated but exciting discoveries. Serendipitous findings of import are, thus, not just a matter of random good fortune: it takes a shrewd and insightful person to understand the significance of some event 'stumbled across'. Probably every person who has ever owned a dog has seen it salivate in response to a nonfood stimulus such as a can opener, but it took the genius of Pavlov to recognize the magnitude of that *psychic secretion*, as he first called it when it happened to occur in his laboratory during the course of another experiment.

serial-anticipation method An experimental procedure in which each stimulus in a list is a cue for a response to follow. The subject's task is to make the proper response before being prompted with it.

serial association Generally, any association between one item on a list and the next. See SERIAL *LEARNING.

serial behaviour Generally, behaviour that consists of a series of responses or acts of which the order in which they are carried out is a critical feature. See CHAINING for behaviourist and cognitivist perspectives on such behaviour.

serial exploration, method of MEASUREMENT OF *THRESHOLD.

serial learning LEARNING, SERIAL.

serial monogamy SERIAL *POLYGAMY.

serial polygamy POLYGAMY, SERIAL.

serial-position curve A graphic display of the probability of a correct recall of an item plotted against the serial position of the item during presentation. The classic curve is bow-shaped with high probabilities for the first few and last few items. See SERIAL-POSITION EFFECT for more detail.

serial-position effect The generalization that in a free-recall experiment the likelihood of an individual item from a list being recalled is a function of the location of that item in the serial presentation of the list during learning. Items which are toward the beginning of the list (the *primary* items) and those toward the end (the most recent in

time at the point of recall) are more likely to be correctly recalled than those in the middle. The full serial-position effect is, thus, composed of two more local effects: the PRIMACY EFFECT and the RECENCY EFFECT; see each for details.

serial reaction time SRT TASK.

serial recall An experimental procedure used in memory research in which the stimulus materials are presented to the subject in a fixed order and must be recalled in that particular order. Compare with FREE RECALL.

serial search SEARCH, SERIAL.

seriation Arrangement in a series, in a consecutive order.

series An arrangement of items in succession such that by using some principle (temporal, spatial or logical) the items can be represented by number.

serotonergic Characterizing or pertaining to pathways, fibres or neurons in which SEROTONIN is the *neurotransmitter*.

serotonin A NEUROTRANSMITTER found in neural pathways of peripheral ganglia and in the central nervous system. Also known as *5-hydroxytryptamine* or *5-HT*, it is an inhibitory transmitter the actions of which have been implicated in various processes, including sleep, pain and the psychobiology of various affective disorders, specifically depression and bipolar disorder (see SELECTIVE SEROTONIN REUPTAKE INHIBITORS). At the time of writing, at least fifteen distinct types of SEROTONIN RECEPTORS have been identified. Interestingly, while serotonin is involved in mediating many important behaviours, only some 1–2% of the body's serotonin is found in the nervous system: most is in the mucous membranes of the gastrointestinal system and blood platelets.

serotonin and norepinepherine reuptake inhibitors (SNRIs) A class of antidepressant drugs (e.g. VENLAFAXINE) that were designed to inhibit the reuptake of both SEROTONIN and NOREPINEPHERINE.

serotonin-receptor agonists Compounds that increase the likelihood of SEROTONIN being available to its various receptors. Some, such as the SELECTIVE SEROTONIN REUPTAKE INHIBITORS, function indirectly by blocking reuptake thereby making more serotonin available; others (the TRIPTANS) operate directly by modifying features of the receptor sites.

serotonin receptors A class of receptors that bind or are sensitive to SEROTONIN. They are found in the brain, the peripheral nervous system, the gastrointestinal tract and smooth muscle. Currently some 15 types have been identified, each with different patterns of action with distinct forms of serotonin. The separate receptors are denoted as '5-HT' with an identifying subscript (e.g. 5-HT_{1A}, 5-HT_{2A}, 5-HT_{1B}).

serotonin reuptake inhibitors SELECTIVE SEROTONIN REUPTAKE INHIBITORS.

serotonin syndrome A relatively rare reaction to excess amounts of SEROTONIN. The syndrome is quite variable, but generally includes confusion, agitation, rigidity and flushing. Isolated symptoms of serotonin excess are not uncommon in individuals taking various antidepressant drugs, but the severe and potentially life-threatening combination of symptoms is infrequent.

sertraline A SELECTIVE SEROTONIN REUPTAKE INHIBITOR used for depression, particularly that accompanied by anxiety. Trade name Zoloft.

servomechanism Any device used to control a system which functions by sensing the difference between the actual state of the system and the desired state and acting so as to minimize this difference. The simplest example is a thermostat.

SES SOCIOECONOMIC STATUS.

set 1 n. A classification, aggregate or series of things sharing some defining property or properties such that they can be regarded collectively. This general meaning encompasses a variety of uses, from the purely mathematical characterization embodied in set theory to the more commonsense denotations, such as the *set* of respondents to a questionnaire, the *set* of stimulus items in an experiment, the country-club *set* in upper-class society, etc. Note that sets may be infinite in size (the set of integers), finite (the set of correct answers on a multiple-choice test), empty (the set of immortal persons) or poorly defined (the set of all young persons – see

here FUZZY SET). **2** n. Any condition, disposition or tendency on the part of an organism to respond in a particular manner. Note that the term *respond* here may encompass a number of acts. Thus, one may have an attentional or PERCEPTUAL SET for particular kinds of stimuli (see EINSTELLUNG), a task-oriented set for a problem (see AUFGABE), a functional set which directs the manner of use of objects (see FUNCTIONAL FIXEDNESS), a muscular set in which a particular motor act is optimized (PREPARATORY *SET), etc. To distinguish among these various uses, many authors use qualifiers, as in some of the following entries. It should also be recognized that the term is generally used with the connotation that the set under consideration is a temporary (although potentially recurring) one, and, that being so, its meaning is contrasted with that of terms like HABIT and TRAIT, which refer to enduring dispositions or conditions, and distinguished from that of SCHEMA (1), which is used to refer to more general orientations to situations. The longer term *determining set* is often used synonymously in the context of meaning 2, particularly of sets that exert some measure of control over how an organism is to respond. adj., *set*; vb., *set* (for 2).

set, hypnotic A term roughly equivalent in meaning to POSTHYPNOTIC SUGGESTION; see also HYPNOSIS.

set, motor 1 A preparatory readiness to perform a particular motor response. **2** The actual pattern of muscle tone accompanying such a state of readiness.

set, objective A readiness in which one is prepared to perceive a stimulus as a physical event in the external world, a set that is as free of interpretative, subjective bias as possible. See SET (2).

set point The desired value in a servomechanism: when departures from it are detected, compensatory activities ensue to reduce them. Various biological systems operate using a set point in roughly this fashion, e.g. THERMOREGULATION.

set point theory Loosely, any theory that assumes that a system functions as though there were an optimal SET POINT for it to be in and then makes adjustments to maintain this point. There is no single theory to which this term applies; versions of it are found in a variety of contexts including the study of body mass and maintenance of weight, drug tolerance and drug dependencies, and the maintenance of attachment between a growing child and his or her parents.

set, preparatory Any stance or posture which prepares an organism for a particular response. The term is usually used with respect to motor responses; see MOTOR *SET.

set, response A readiness to respond to a stimulus. For example, in a simple reaction-time experiment, the subject is in a set that calls for the making of a response as rapidly as possible as soon as the stimulus is sensed. Occasionally called *response attitude*. Contrast with STIMULUS *SET.

set, stimulus A readiness to sense a stimulus. Generally the term is used in situations in which there are two or more possible stimuli and the subject is set to react to them differentially. For example, in a choice reaction-time experiment, the subject is in a set in which one of two responses must be made depending upon which of two stimuli occurs. Occasionally called *stimulus attitude*. Contrast with RESPONSE *SET.

set-theoretical model Generally, any model which treats the units or entities under consideration as elements arranged in sets and formally represents the relations between the elements in terms of set theory. Such models have been applied to the study of semantic features, word meaning and human long-term memory.

SEU SUBJECTIVE EXPECTED UTILITY.

seven plus or minus two (7±2) George A. Miller's 'magical number'. The term denotes the approximate number of discrete pieces of information that can be held in short-term memory at one time. Note that this limit is based on the conceptualization of these pieces of information as 'chunks' or coded aggregates and not merely as a summing-up of the total amount of information in each. Note that Miller's early estimate appears to be a bit high. Recent research suggests that FOUR PLUS OR MINUS ONE may be more accurate.

severe mental retardation MENTAL RETARDATION, SEVERE.

sex 1 adj. Pertaining to those biological distinctions which differentiate female from male. This form of the term is used broadly and can encompass the functional, reproductive aspects as well as the specific organs, hormones and structures that anatomically differentiate female from male. When used in combined forms and phrases, however, the usual reference is to properties and characteristics that are functional and biological and not to those that involve either the amorous or the erotic – the form SEXUAL is properly reserved for these cases. For example, one has *sex hormones* but not *sexual hormones* and one engages in *sexual intercourse* but not in *sex intercourse*. In those instances where both forms are found, their meanings are (or should be) appropriately distinguished. Thus, *sex dominance* refers to a broad pattern of dominance of one sex over the other, while *sexual dominance* refers to the dominance of one individual over another during sexual activity. Similarly, *sex roles* refers to encompassing patterns of behaviour and affect of persons relating to their maleness or femaleness, one component of which is those persons' *sexual roles*. Note also that the term *gender* has become increasingly common as a synonym of *sex* in this adjectival sense. Although the original meaning of *gender* restricted its use to grammar, its connotative neutrality has made it the euphemism of choice for many contemporary writers, particularly when social or cultural issues are the focus. For combined terms not found below, see those following GENDER. **2** n. Either of the two forms biologically present in most (but not all) species, distinguished as male (the sperm-cell producer) and female (the egg-cell producer). **3** n. By extension of 2, the totality of characteristics that may be used as diagnostic features for identification of male or female. **4** n. The process, considered broadly, of reproduction. **5** n. Those organic and/or physiological pleasures and satisfactions associated with sexual activities.

sex- Combining form meaning: **1** *Sex*. **2** *Six*.

sex anomaly Any individual case in which the sex organs differ dramatically from the normal, e.g. a *hermaphrodite*. Also called *geni-*

tal anomaly. Distinguish from SEXUAL ANOMALY.

sex assignment The sex or gender assigned at birth. In cases of genital anomalies the assignment may be problematic.

sex change SEX REVERSAL.

sex characteristics Very generally, those characteristics or traits that are strongly associated with one sex relative to the other. The term is used uniformly of biological and behavioural features. Also called *sex characters*.

sex characteristics, primary Those genetically determined sex traits that are differentially associated more strongly with one sex than with the other and are intimately, biologically bound up with the functions of reproduction, e.g. the genitals, the organs of reproduction. Also called *primary sex characters*.

sex characteristics, secondary Those genetically determined sex traits that are differentially associated more strongly with one sex than with the other but are not functionally necessary for normal reproduction, e.g. body hair, fundamental pitch of the voice, patterns of musculature. Also called *secondary sex characters*.

sex chromosomes CHROMOSOMES.

sex differences Those differences that are statistically distributed in the population such that when large numbers of individuals are considered they can be used as distinguishing features between males and females. There are three potential referential domains here: (a) those differences expressed as PRIMARY *SEX CHARACTERISTICS; (b) those differences expressed as SECONDARY *SEX CHARACTERISTICS; and (c) those differences expressed as distinguishable mental, emotional and social-behaviour patterns. The divergences between the sexes diminish as one moves from (a) to (c). No one disputes the differences in primary sex characteristics, but the term is rarely, if ever, used in this sense. The differences observed in secondary sex characteristics are now known to be not quite so large nor so unequivocal as some had thought, but generally they are not disputed as existing and, like those in (a), are to a considerable extent genetically determined. The

difficulties with the term emerge only in the case of (c), and it is here that we find the domain of reference in virtually every case in which the term *sex difference* is used.

The problems that arise in applying the term to the factors included in (c) are due in large measure to the varying tendencies on the part of various authors to extrapolate from the known genetic determinants in domains (a) and (b) – this despite the fact that the term itself is neutral with respect to genetic factors and their entailment is a theoretical step, not a definitional one. The underlying causal factors for those sex differences that can be observed in category (c) have yet to be unequivocally determined. Many authors, in an effort to avoid the need to distinguish between the domains of (a) and (b) on one hand and (c) on the other, use the term *gender differences* for (c), thereby defusing, at least partially, the genetic-determination issue that is so problematical here.

sex distribution The distribution of males and females in a population. See SEX RATIO.

sex education 1 Broadly, education in all aspects of sex and sexuality including the physiological, reproductive, performative, emotional and interpersonal. **2** More narrowly, education in only the physiological and reproductive aspects of sex.

sex identity One's learned identity as it pertains to one's sex. See GENDER IDENTITY for more detail.

sex-influenced character (or **gene**) A genetic characteristic that is dominant in one sex and recessive in the other.

sexism A prejudice based on sex. As the term is used, its meaning goes beyond this simple definition in two ways. First, a prejudice is generally treated as an attitude or belief, while the term sexism (like the related term *racism*) generally connotes differential action and behaviour toward persons which discriminates between them on the basis of their sex. Second, the term is nearly always used with respect to discrimination against females, a unitary focus that derives from the objective data of society but which unfortunately limits the meaning of the term.

sex-limited character (or **gene**) A genetic

characteristic that is expressed in only one sex.

sex-linked character (or **gene**) A genetic characteristic that is controlled by genes located on the sex chromosomes.

sex object **1** A SEXUAL OBJECT toward which or upon whom sexual activities are focused. **2** Popularly, a person responded to in such a fashion that sex and sexuality are the primary aspects of the interaction – typically, a woman so treated by a man, although this limitation is social and not definitional. Note that being a sex object in sense 2 does not necessarily entail sense 1: you may treat someone as a sex object (2) without any of the specific sexual intentions connoted by meaning 1.

sex offender In legal parlance, one who has violated local statutes concerning sexual behaviour. Since laws differ from community to community and country to country, it is not possible to provide a precise definition of the term, although rapists and child molesters are almost universally so classified.

sexology The scientific study of sex and sexuality.

sex ratio The proportion of males or females in a population. Usually presented as the number of males (or females) per 100 persons.

sex reassignment A cover term for the legal, personal, behavioural and surgical actions involved in the reassignment of sex identity.

sex reversal A surgical procedure, with accompanying hormonal treatments, for changing a person's sex.

sex rivalry In classical psychoanalytic theory, the hypothesized competition between a child and the same-sexed parent for the affections and attentions of the other parent.

sex role The full complement of behaviours and attitudes of one's role in life as it is associated with one's sex. See GENDER ROLE and ROLE for further discussion.

sex-role inversion TRANSSEXUALISM.

sex-role stereotype The typical beliefs concerning the particular patterns of behav-

iour that are expected of persons according to their sex.

sex therapy A general term used to cover any therapeutic enterprise aimed at the relief of sexual dysfunctions or disturbances. Included are therapies aimed at altering a person's attitudes toward sex and sexual behaviour so as, for example, to relieve irrational fears or guilt feelings which inhibit performance and enjoyment; therapies specifically concerned with identifiable dysfunctions such as impotency, premature ejaculation or orgasmic dysfunctions; and 'family' therapies which focus on communication and interactive difficulties that a couple may be experiencing.

sexual **1** Characterizing reproduction by the union of two sex cells, one provided by a female and one by a male of the same species. Contrast with ASEXUAL (2). **2** Relating to, in a very general way, the behavioural and affective component of SEXUALITY. Compare with SEX (1).

sexual abuse Sexual mistreatment of another person. As the term is used it virtually always refers to the abuse of a child by an adult. See also SEXUAL HARASSMENT.

sexual aim The goal of the release of sexual tensions by orgasm. AIM is used here synonymously with GOAL rather than with OBJECT or TARGET: see these several terms for the distinctions implied. See also, and compare with, SEXUAL OBJECT.

sexual anaesthesia Loosely, the lack of erotic sensation during sexual activity.

sexual and gender disorder An umbrella classification for disorder of gender and of sexual behaviour and functions that have no identifiable organic cause. Included are the GENDER IDENTITY DISORDERS, PARAPHILIAS and SEXUAL DYSFUNCTIONS.

sexual anomaly Generally, any sexual practice that is 'anormal', i.e. outside the generally accepted practices of a society. Many authors use this term specifically to denote any of a variety of sexual behaviours that are statistically anomalous when they wish to be clear that no connotation of pathology or perversion is intended; e.g. they call homosexuality or fetishism sexual anomalies. For more on this point see SEXUAL *PERVER-

SION. The term should not be used as a synonym of SEX ANOMALY, which is reserved for the biological and anatomical.

sexual anorexia ANOREXIA, SEXUAL.

sexual apathy A general term for any unusually low interest in sex and sexuality. Also called *erotic apathy*.

sexual arousal disorders Those SEXUAL DYSFUNCTIONS characterized by a lack of the appropriate physiological responses that accompany sexual excitement, including FEMALE SEXUAL AROUSAL DISORDER and MALE ERECTILE DISORDER. Like SEXUAL DESIRE DISORDERS, the term is only used when the condition causes marked distress or interpersonal difficulties.

sexual aversion disorder A SEXUAL DESIRE DISORDER marked by persistent or recurrent aversion to and avoidance of genital sexual contact with a sexual partner. Note that some use the term more broadly to encompass any kind of sexual contact.

sexual desire disorders Those SEXUAL DYSFUNCTIONS marked by absent or diminished interest in sex and sexual activity, including HYPOACTIVE SEXUAL DISORDER and SEXUAL AVERSION DISORDER. Sexual desire is a personal thing and this label is used only when the condition causes marked distress or compromises interpersonal interactions. Many people have low libido and are quite content to be that way. Also called *inhibited sexual desire*.

sexual dimorphism Dimorphism means *two forms*, hence: relating to the circumstances in which a species has two distinct forms differentiated on the basis of sex characteristics.

sexual disorders See SEXUAL AND GENDER DISORDERS.

sexual drive LIBIDO.

sexual dysfunctions A subclass of SEXUAL DISORDERS marked by inhibition of arousal or of the psychophysiological aspects of the sexual response cycle. The term is only used when there is no evidence of an organic disorder that might cause the symptoms. Separate criteria are used for males and females. Included are the SEXUAL AROUSAL DISORDERS and the SEXUAL DESIRE DISORDERS. Occasionally called *psychosexual dysfunctions*.

sexual harassment *Harass* comes from Old French for *to set a dog on*, and generally means persistently to disturb, pester, plague or torment. The term applies to cases in which such badgering has a sexual component to it, particularly when there is a power imbalance between the parties. Overwhelmingly, such cases involve men harassing women. The term is not used for cases that involve children; see SEXUAL ABUSE.

sexual identity One's identity with respect to sexual orientation. The term is usually restricted to labelling oneself as hetero-, homo- or bisexual. Note that the term is used so that it does not necessarily encompass sexual behaviours; there are, for example, many persons who express a strong personal homosexual identity but who not infrequently engage in heterosexual activity and vice versa. See SEXUAL ORIENTATION.

sexual instinct 1 In psychoanalysis this expression originally stood as a cover term for the impetus assumed to underlie any pleasure-seeking. This remarkably inclusive meaning derived from Freud's early characterization of sexuality as the foundational motive for all pleasure. More recent usage puts boundaries on the term in that a hint of sexuality needs to be present for it to be applied. 2 In ethology, the underlying drive to engage in patterns of behaviour oriented around courtship and sexual union.

sexual intercourse 1 A synonym of COITUS. 2 By extension, other forms of genital interaction, although typically these are signalled by qualifiers, e.g. anal intercourse, homosexual intercourse.

sexual inversion INVERSION, SEXUAL.

sexual involution INVOLUTION.

sexuality 1 Generally, all those aspects of one's constitution and one's behaviour that are related to sex. Some authors use this meaning with a clear restriction to sex, others use it so that dispositions toward love and deep affection are included, even if not associated with the sex organs *per se*. Typically, the former is intended. 2 The state of having sex and sexual functions; the quality of being sexual. Note that this usage is occasionally amplified by the notion of excessiveness; that is, sexuality to some authors is not just the quality of being sexual but the quality of being too sexual. This evaluative component of the term is less common than it once was.

sexual latency LATENCY PERIOD.

sexually dimorphic nucleus A region in the *medial* PREOPTIC AREA that is considerably larger in males than females.

sexually transmitted disease (STD) Any disease that can be transmitted by sexual contact. To date, more than 20 such diseases have been identified; some are caused by bacteria and treated with antibiotics (e.g. gonorrhoea), others by viruses (e.g. herpes, HIV). Also called *venereal diseases*, although there is a tendency to restrict that term to gonorrhoea and syphilis.

sexual masochism Sexual behaviour that is linked intimately with suffering physical and psychological pain, humiliation and abuse. When used as a psychiatric label the term is restricted to circumstances where the masochism is an integral part of an individual's sexual activities, not merely their fantasies, and where the pain experienced is real and not simulated. See MASOCHISM.

sexual maturation Biological maturation of the organs of reproduction to a functional level. See MATURATION.

sexual object The individual or thing toward which sexual actions are directed. Distinguish from SEXUAL AIM and see also SEX OBJECT.

sexual orientation A term used to identify a person's sexual attraction toward persons of a particular gender. Those sexually attracted to the opposite sex are said to display a *heterosexual* orientation, those attracted to the same sex, a *homosexual* orientation and to both, *bisexual*. This term is the most encompassing of several near synonyms currently in use such as SEXUAL PREFERENCE and SEXUAL IDENTITY although, as noted under these terms, there are nuances of use and reference.

sexual pain disorders A class of SEXUAL DYSFUNCTIONS marked by physical pain during sexual intercourse, including DYSPAREUNIA and VAGINISMUS.

sexual perversion PERVERSION, SEXUAL.

sexual preference The preferred sex of one's sexual partner(s). The term was intro-

duced in response to the rapidly accumulating data that indicate that relatively few persons are purely heterosexual or homosexual, the more common pattern being to have had some experiences or feelings of both kinds but with a marked preference for one or the other. However, the term is falling out of favour because of its implication that sexuality is a choice. See SEXUAL IDENTITY and SEXUAL ORIENTATION.

sexual prejudice Literally, any display of prejudicial behaviours based on gender or sexual orientation. While this broad sense is etymologically correct, the term is virtually always used with regard to gay, lesbian and transgendered persons. The term does not carry connotations of fear as does HOMOPHOBIA and, since it tends to be displayed on an individual basis, it is not a true synonym of HETEROSEXISM which is reserved for societal or institutional level ideology and practices.

sexual reproduction The activities and processes of organisms which result in the production of new organisms through the union of sex cells. Compare with ASEXUAL (2) reproduction, in which new organisms are produced by grafts, spores or the fission of a single cell.

sexual sadism Sexual behaviour that is linked intimately with the inflicting of psychological or physical pain on another who may or may not be a willing partner. When used as a psychiatric label the term is restricted to circumstances where the actions are an integral part of an individual's sexual activities, not merely their fantasies, and where the pain inflicted is real and not simulated. See SADISM (1) and SADO-MASOCHISTIC.

sexual selection In evolutionary biology, the selection of particular traits or characteristics displayed by one sex by mates or potential mates of the other sex. The traits may have little to do with actual sexual behaviour or function but have come to signal fitness for that particular species. For example, female swordfish display a marked sexual selection for males with longer swords. Sexual selection is a powerful factor in evolution and can push the emergence of specific forms and functions in relatively short time periods. See also MATE SELECTION.

sexual trauma 1 Generally, any trauma of a

sexual nature. **2** More specifically, a disturbing or anxiety-producing childhood event related to sex that has a lasting effect on sexual adjustment.

s factor SPECIFIC *FACTOR.

shadow 1 n. In Jung's approach, one of the archetypes: a complex of undeveloped feelings, ideas, desires and the like – the 'animal' instincts passed along through evolution to *Homo sapiens* from lower, more primitive forms that represent the negative side of personality; the human species' 'alter ego'. **2** vb. To follow; see SHADOWING.

shadowing 1 Following a spoken message by repeating it as rapidly and accurately as possible what is said. It is used extensively as a control procedure in experiments on attention, since shadowing a message commandeers one's attentional focus so thoroughly that little or no attention can be directed toward any other stimulus that may be present. **2** A research procedure in which a relatively small number of participants are selected for in-depth study, which usually involves their being followed (i.e. shadowed) through their day. Most often, this form of data collection is used to supplement larger-scale (i.e. involving more participants) forms of collection, such as surveys.

shadow syndrome SUBSYNDROMAL.

shallow living One of Karen Horney's three forms of NEUROTIC *RESIGNATION, manifested by a hectic lifestyle in which the individual compulsively engages in so many activities that only the surfaces of things are dealt with and deep conflicts can be avoided.

shaman A practitioner of magic, particularly one who attempts to use magic, spiritualism and, almost invariably, psychoactive substances to heal. In popular jargon, a *medicine man* or *witch doctor*.

shame An emotional state produced by the awareness that one has acted dishonourably or ridiculously. The term is usually reserved for situations in which one's actions are publicly known or exposed to real or potential ridicule. Distinguish from GUILT.

sham feeding (procedure) A surgical procedure in which an oesophageal fistula (i.e. a tube) is implanted so that whatever is swallowed exits without reaching the stomach.

shamming Faking, feigning. Used as a protective device in some species; see e.g. DEATH FEIGNING.

sham rage A pattern of behaviour mimicking a rage reaction, produced by artificial means. Two procedures have been studied: in one the entire cortex of an experimental animal is removed; in the other, areas of the hypothalamus are stimulated in an intact animal.

sham surgery Surgery in which all procedures are carried out save the one under specific experimental study. It is used as a control procedure in animal experiments involving surgery to protect against the possibility that any effects observed could be caused by the trauma of the surgery.

shape The physical form of something. The shape of a stimulus is perceived and, hence, 'defined' by its contours or boundaries, the locus of points where there are sharp gradations in texture, shading, colour, brightness, etc.

shape constancy The tendency to perceive the shape of a rigid object as remaining fixed despite alterations in the viewing conditions. A swinging door looked at head-on is still perceived as rectangular despite the fact that as it is opened and closed its retinal projection changes from rectangular to trapezoidal.

shaping The gradual building-up of an operant behaviour by reinforcing successive approximations. Shaping functions by the selective use of reinforcement to convert existing simple behaviours into more complex patterns of responding. Also called *approximation conditioning* and *conditioning by successive approximations*.

shared paranoid disorder In older classifications this term was used for INDUCED PSYCHOTIC DISORDER. In the most recent edition of the DSM, both are subsumed under SHARED PSYCHOTIC DISORDER.

shared psychotic disorder In the most recent edition of the *DSM*, INDUCED PSYCHOTIC DISORDER is now known by this name. The diagnostic description is the same.

sharpening See LEVELLING.

sheep-goat effect In PARAPSYCHOLOGY, the

assumption that those who believe they have paranormal powers ('sheep') do better on tests of PSI than those who are sceptical ('goats'). The distinction was a kind of 'last gasp' effort of Gertrude Schmeidler to try to explain the fact that well-controlled studies with large samples revealed no evidence of psi.

shenkui A CULTURE-SPECIFIC SYNDROME reported in Chinese men. It is marked by anxiety and panic with accompanying somatic complaints, such as dizziness, backache, sexual dysfunctions and insomnia, that have no physical basis. Prevailing folk wisdom attributes it to excess loss of semen through frequent intercourse or masturbation.

shimmer The apparent dancing or jitter of a visual display that is the result of SACCADES. We are generally aware of this phenomenon only when trying to study extremely fine visual details or grids.

shock 1 A clinical syndrome that accompanies disruption of the oxygen supply to tissues, particularly brain tissues. Shock, to some extent, accompanies every injury although it is generally detectable only when there has been a major trauma, such as serious injury, surgery, an overdose of certain drugs or an extremely strong emotional experience. **2** The result of passing an electric current through the body. Severe shock in sense 2 can produce shock in sense 1. See also SHOCK THERAPY.

shock phase The first part of the *alarm reaction* stage in the GENERAL ADAPTATION SYNDROME.

shock–shock interval TEMPORAL AVOIDANCE CONDITIONING.

shock therapy A general term covering the use of shock-inducing procedures for the treatment of emotional disorders. The most commonly used of these procedures is ELECTROCONVULSIVE SHOCK; other procedures, which were once popular, such as *insulin shock*, are now little used. See ELECTROCONVULSIVE THERAPY for a discussion.

shoe anaesthesia GLOVE *ANAESTHESIA.

short-circuit appeal A propaganda technique designed to arouse by appealing to emotional rather than cognitive or rational considerations.

short-term memory (or store) MEMORY, SHORT-TERM.

shotgunning Lab slang for a broad-based hit-or-miss approach to a problem – rather like letting loose a shotgun blast in the hope that some pellets will be on target.

shoulds Karen Horney's term for the elaborate set of internalized demands upon one's behaviour. Although all persons are certainly replete with these internal pressures, Horney reserved the term for those excessive and irrational pressures and internal standards that contribute to neurotic obsessive and compulsive behaviours.

shrink Popular US slang for a psychiatrist or clinical psychologist.

shut-in personality A semi-technical term for an extremely withdrawn person.

shuttle box An experimental apparatus consisting of a box divided into two halves. Typically the subject must move from one side to the other to receive a reward, avoid an aversive stimulus, etc.

shwa SCHWA.

shy bladder (syndrome) PARURESIS.

shyness A general pattern of social reticence and inhibition assumed to be due to self-consciousness and anxiety. Signs are physiological arousal in social situations, worries about social evaluation, and social cautiousness. The term is used for children more often than adults. There has been a tendency to pathologize the term, a move that is not appropriate; shyness lies well within the range of normal behaviour. Compare with AVOIDANT DISORDER OF CHILDHOOD AND ADOLESCENCE and SOCIAL *PHOBIA. adj., *shy*.

sib 1 Short for SIBLING (1). **2** In anthropology, a kin group composed of all the lineal descendants of a single person. Usually a sib can be either matrilineal or patrilineal, although some authors use *clan* for matrilineal cases, *gens* for patrilineal and *sib* as a generic term.

sibilant In phonetics, any speech sound produced by the turbulent passing of air between two articulators, e.g. **s**ure, **ch**ur**ch**, **j**eer.

sibling 1 n. Generally, one of two or more offspring in a family, a brother, a sister. Some reserve the term for cases in which the parents of both siblings are the same, using *half-sibling* when there is only one common biological parent. **2** adj. In biogenetics, characterizing two species which are genetically very closely related. **3** n. In perception studies that use MORPHED STIMULI, the morphed by-products of the original stimulus.

sibling rivalry RIVALRY, SIBLING.

sibship All the brothers and sisters in a given family.

Sidman avoidance TEMPORAL AVOIDANCE CONDITIONING.

SIDS SUDDEN INFANT DEATH SYNDROME.

sight VISION.

sighting line VISUAL AXIS.

sight method WHOLE-WORD METHOD.

sight vocabulary VOCABULARY, SIGHT.

sigma:
Σ A symbol denoting *summation*, e.g. Σ*X* means 'Add up all the *X* values.' The symbol is read as 'sum of', not 'sigma', which is reserved for the lowercase form, σ.

σ A symbol denoting STANDARD *DEVIATION. In some older texts it may be seen as an abbreviation for *millisecond*.

σ$_m$ Denotes STANDARD ERROR OF THE MEAN.

σ$_{(m)}$ Denotes STANDARD ERROR OF MEASUREMENT.

sigma score Z-SCORE.

sign 1 n. Most generally and inclusively, an indicator, a hint, a clue. When a sign is a characteristic element of some thing or event, it is often referred to as a *natural sign* or a SIGNAL; e.g. fire is a natural sign that something is burning. When a sign has an arbitrary social or cultural component, it is generally referred to as a *conventional sign* or SYMBOL; e.g. fire, in some cultures, is a conventional sign of life. **2** n. By extension, an event or an action that serves as a signifier of something with meaning or manifestations beyond its own self. For example, to an archaeologist a pottery shard is a sign of human habitation, to a clinician tightly clenched fists are a sign of tension or anxiety in a client. This use, in discussion of pathologies, is similar, although not identical, to the use of SYMPTOM. Compare, for example, the meanings in 'A fever is a sign of infection' and 'A fever is a symptom of infection.' **3** n. An event which, by virtue of temporal and spatial contiguity with some other event, becomes capable of substituting for that event in eliciting a response. In Pavlov's original classic conditioning experiments, for example, the bell became a *sign* for salivation after being paired with food. Note that although the bell–food relationship here is arbitrary and learned, the term *symbol* is generally not used because the arbitrariness is not within the experimental subject's domain. **4** n. A physical gesture, especially a characteristic sequence or pattern of hand movements, used to stand for a word or a concept, as in SIGN LANGUAGE. **5** n. A mathematical expression which stands for a particular operation or set of operations, e.g. a + sign. Note, however, that *sign* and *symbol* are often interchanged here; a + sign is referred to as an example of a mathematical symbol, although the latter term is typically reserved for the generic. **6** n. In linguistics, a word considered as a *symbol* of a thing. Here, the sign is the concrete element that represents the abstract or symbolic. Used synonymously with SIGNIFIER (1). **7** n. One of 12 divisions of the zodiac. **8** vb. To indicate a thing or to communicate about a thing by use of signs (in any of the senses above). Compare here with the verb *to signify*, which means either (a) to show or indicate a thing using signs, or (b) to have meaning.

signal 1 n. Most generally, a SIGN (esp. 1) that serves to communicate something. **2** n. More specifically, an agreed-upon event or object that functions as an occasion for some action. **3** n. A stimulus, particularly as in SIGNAL-DETECTION THEORY. **4** n. In neurological work, any event that is transmitted along neural pathways. **5** n. Any transmitted event, e.g. a radio signal. See here INFORMATION THEORY. **6** vb. To indicate or denote a thing. adj., *signal*.

signal anxiety In his later writings about anxiety, Freud hypothesized a mechanism that served an alerting, protective role. This so-called *signal anxiety* was seen as a response to threats to the equilibrium of the ego and served as a warning device to prevent the devastating experience of PRIMARY ANXIETY, which accompanied ego dissolution.

signal-detection theory (SDT) A mathematical theory of the detection of physical signals. It is based on the assumption that sensitivity to a signal is not merely a result of its intensity but is also dependent upon the amount of noise present, the motivation of the subject and the criterion which the subject sets for responding. The essential nature of the theory is captured in the figure below. Another assumption is that the amount of neural stimulation is normally distributed and that the subject's decision to respond 'yes' (i.e. 'I detected a signal') is given by whether the *total* stimulation contributed either by noise alone or by noise plus signal exceeds the set-response criterion. The criterion is easily adjusted by changing the PAY-OFF MATRIX so that the costs and benefits associated with *hits* and *false alarms* are modified. The proportion of *hits* to *misses* in any given situation yields a measure of the subject's sensitivity (see D') independent of the criterion set or other possible bias. Also called, simply, *detection theory* because the principles apply to any situation, e.g. detecting a flaw in parts coming off a production line, detecting an abnormal feature in a patient's X-ray.

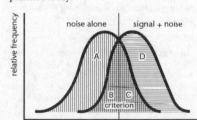

amount of neural stimulation

Key
A: Correct 'no' responses
B: Misses; incorrect 'no' responses
C: False alarms; incorrect 'no' responses
D: Hits; correct 'yes' responses

signalling system A term often applied to the communication systems of nonhuman species. It is preferred in these contexts to LANGUAGE. See also SEMIOTICS.

signal-to-noise ratio Quite literally, the ratio of the energy in the signal to which one is attending to the energy in the background noise. abbrev., *s/n*.

signature LOCAL SIGN.

sign Gestalt (expectation) E. C. Tolman's term for a cognitive process involving a stimulus environment, a particular response and the anticipation that that response in that situation will lead to the fulfilment of the organism's expectations. See also EXPECTANCY and MEANS–ENDS READINESS.

significance Importance, meaning, the quality of having importance or meaning. See e.g. STATISTICAL SIGNIFICANCE.

significance level An arbitrary value used as a criterion for determining whether a given data set departs sufficiently from what would be expected were only chance factors operating for the departure, or difference, to be classified as statistically significant. The usual level adopted in the social sciences is 5% or, as it is usually denoted, *p* <0.05, where *p* is the probability of observed results or more extreme results occurring by chance alone. Often called the *alpha level*. See also STATISTICAL SIGNIFICANCE.

significant difference STATISTICAL SIGNIFICANCE.

significant other 1 H. S. Sullivan's term for any person who is important in affecting an individual's development of social norms, values and personal self-image. **2** More generally, a spouse or person with whom one has an intimate relationship.

signifier 1 In linguistics, a SIGN (6). **2** In Lacan's psychoanalytic approach, a symbol that represents an element of an individual's unconscious.

signify SIGN.

sign language A language based on gestural communication. Typically the term refers to the rich, elaborate and fully grammatical manual system used by the deaf. Note that *finger spelling*, although it is an integral part of such communication since it is necessary for signing names, novel words and specialized terms which have no manual sign, is generally regarded as a separate component of communication by sign and not as part of the sign language itself.

sign learning E. C. Tolman's term for learning that consists primarily of acquiring an appreciation of the relations between signs, their references and the outcomes of behaviour emitted with respect to them.

sign stimulus In ethology, a species-specific stimulus that is effective in triggering a FIXED ACTION PATTERN. Occasionally called a RELEASER, although properly a releaser is but a particular kind of sign stimulus. See also INNATE RELEASING MECHANISM.

sign test A nonparametric statistical test useful for situations in which the data consist solely of whether the observed scores exceed (+) or fail to exceed (–) some theoretical values or some other scores. The test compares the observed proportions of plus and minus signs against what would be expected by chance.

sign tracking An occasional synonym of AUTOSHAPING.

silent pause PAUSE, SILENT.

silent speech SUBVOCALIZATION.

Simenon's syndrome An erotic delusion that one is loved by and has had a sexual liaison with a famous person. Similar to CLÉRAMBAULT'S SYNDROME but with an emphasis on the sexual component.

similarity A dimension of sameness, resemblance. Generally used with respect to the notion of shared features or shared principles: the more features or principles two things have in common the greater their similarity.

similarity, law of 1 The generalization that thoughts, images, words, etc. are more likely to elicit similar thoughts, images, words, etc. than dissimilar. **2** See GESTALT LAWS OF ORGANIZATION.

Simon effect Named after J. R. Simon, the phenomenon that one reacts faster when the locations of the response and the stimulus are congruent – even though location is irrelevant to the task. Subjects told to press the left button if they see a green light, no matter where it appears, show the fastest reaction times when the light is on the left side.

simple causation CAUSATION.

simple cell A cell in the STRIATE CORTEX that responds to a stimulus in the centre of its RECEPTIVE FIELD in a manner opposite to a stimulus in the surrounding area. Such cells respond maximally to stimuli such as edges or ends of bars. The visual cortex also contains *complex cells* that respond to particular relationships between elements of the visual input to the field, in particular differential contrast, orientation and direction and *hypercomplex cells* that respond to lines of particular lengths and corners that are part of moving displays. The discovery of these highly specialized cells by David Hubel and Torsten Wiesel was a major development in understanding the visual system.

simple correlation CORRELATION, SIMPLE.

simple deteriorative disorder In the latest edition of the *DSM* this term has been proposed to replace SIMPLE *SCHIZOPHRENIA on the grounds that it captures an essential feature of the disorder, its progressive deterioration of function.

simple phobia PHOBIA, SIMPLE.

simple reaction time REACTION TIME, SIMPLE.

simple schizophrenia SCHIZOPHRENIA, SIMPLE.

simple structure In factor analysis, the stage in which the factor rotation has yielded an arrangement in which the factors are located such that the sum of the number of factors required to describe each test is a minimum.

simple tone PURE *TONE.

simulate 1 Generally, to mimic, to assume the appearance of, to copy. **2** In psychiatry and clinical psychology, to malinger, to engage in a conscious attempt to pretend to be suffering from a mental disorder.

simulator Generally, an apparatus designed for training that mimics real-life situations. Airline pilots' training programmes, for example, make extensive use of simulators.

simultanagnosia An APPERCEPTIVE *AGNOSIA in which the patient can recognize individual elements of a complex picture one at a time but cannot appreciate the overall sense of the scene.

simultaneous conditioning An experimental conditioning procedure in which there is simultaneous presentation and termination of the conditioned and unconditioned stimuli. Compare with DELAY CONDITIONING and TRACE CONDITIONING.

simultaneous contrast CONTRAST.

sine wave A wave-form characterized by regular oscillations with a set period and amplitude such that the displacement amplitude at each point is proportional to the sine of the phase angle of the displacement. A pure tone is propagated as a sine wave.

single-blind An experimental technique in which the participants are ignorant of the experimental conditions but the researcher running the experiment knows them. The procedure helps to reduce expectation effects but does not control for possible experimenter-bias effects as well as the DOUBLE-BLIND.

single-cell recording SINGLE-UNIT RECORDING.

single-channel model The conceptualization that for the most part one can attend fully to only one sequentially structured stimulus input at a time.

single-loop learning LEARNING, SINGLE-LOOP.

single photon emission computer tomography (SPECT) A functional neuroimaging technique that, like a *PET-scan*, uses radioisotope tracers to monitor cortical activity.

singleton 1 An only child, one without siblings. **2** Any mammal born alone, with no litter mates.

single-unit recording In neurophysiology, a recording of the electrical activity of a single neuron taken using microelectrodes (with a tip diameter of less than 10 μ). Also called *single-cell recording*.

single-variable principle The empirical principle that when but one factor is permitted to vary while all others are held constant, any observed systematic effects must be due to the single variable being manipulated. See CONTROL.

sinister From the Latin, meaning *left* or *unfavourable*. The original use was with reference to omens that appeared on the left side, which were always thought to be portents of evil. The derived forms used in science today deal only with the notion of sideness, the evaluative meaning having been discarded. Thus, *sinistrad* is toward the left, *sinistral* refers to the left side of the body or to left-handedness, etc. Contrast with DEXTER, which

still retains the old meaning of favourable in both the technical and popular language, as well as the notion of right-sided.

sinistrality Any marked preference for the left side of the body. See SINISTER.

sinus From the Latin for *hollow* or *curve*, any cavity with a relatively narrow opening.

sinusoid(al) Pertaining to: **1** a sine wave; **2** a sinus.

SIS SENSORY INFORMATION STORE.

-sis A suffix from the Greek, meaning *state* or *condition*. Depending on the vowel that precedes it, it may take any of several forms: *-asis*, *-esis*, *-iasis* or *-osis*.

situation 1 Simply, a place, locale or position. This meaning, restricted largely to circumscribed physical domains, is actually rather uncommon in technical writing. **2** A complex whole representing the multiple stimulus patterns, events, objects, persons and affective tone existing at some point in time. In this sense the term is close in meaning to *state of affairs* or *set of circumstances*. In essentially all combined forms (see below) this is the meaning intended. adj., *situational*.

situational analysis The study or analysis of events and phenomena in natural surroundings as opposed to a laboratory setting. This term has been largely replaced by NATURALISTIC OBSERVATION, particularly when the subject of analysis is nonhuman.

situational approach An approach to group management and group leadership which stresses that there is no single personal profile or particular set of skills that makes for optimal leadership in all situations; rather, that different situations and circumstances require different skills and, therefore, that the types of people who are best qualified to take managerial and leadership roles vary.

situational attribution DISPOSITIONAL *ATTRIBUTION.

situational determinant DETERMINANT.

situational homosexuality HOMOSEXUALITY, SITUATIONAL.

situationalism A general perspective on behaviour that focuses on the role of the environment, the situation, the immediate and the enduring social circumstances of one's life rather than on 'internal' factors such as personality traits or characteristics. Originally championed by Kurt Lewin, its basic principle, in one form or another, is now acknowledged by virtually all. Also known as *situationism*.

situational psychosis REACTIVE PSYCHOSIS.

situational stress reaction A minor cognitive and personality disorientation in response to the stress of encountering difficult, new life experiences, such as a new job or moving to a new city or country. The duration of the disorder is typically brief as most people soon adjust to the novel circumstances.

situational test A contrived and necessarily disguised test in which the person being evaluated is put in a situation which simulates a particular slice of real life to determine whether he or she makes the appropriate response; for example, testing an applicant for a proof-reader's job by handing him or her a form with several typographical errors in it.

situation, defining the The process of examining, evaluating and assessing a particular situation prior to making decisions about how to behave in an appropriate fashion.

situation type phobia SIMPLE *PHOBIA.

situs inversus Reversal of the usual patterns of hemispheric dominance. In such cases the left hemisphere is dominant for spatial functions and the right for language.

16 PF SIXTEEN PERSONALITY FACTOR QUESTIONNAIRE.

Sixteen Personality Factor Questionnaire A personality assessment inventory developed by Raymond Cattell based on the 16 personality factors or SOURCE *TRAITS that emerged from his factor analyses of a wide range of SURFACE *TRAITS. The test itself consists of self-report statements concerning personality traits, e.g. 'sober vs. happy-go-lucky'. Also called the *16 PF*.

sixth sense Colloquially and erroneously, the paranormal sense. The problems with this term surround the question of its existence (see the discussion under PARAPSYCH-

OLOGY) and the number used, which implies that there are but five normal senses (hearing, vision, taste, smell and touch), thereby grossly misrepresenting the true situation, since kinaesthesis, equilibrium, the sensing of warmth (and coldness), at least two varieties of pain, etc. are omitted by this count.

size constancy The tendency to perceive the veridical size of familiar objects despite the fact that the size of the retinal image undergoes dramatic variation owing to changing conditions of viewing, most significantly the changing distance of the object from the perceiver.

size–weight illusion The tendency to estimate the weight of large objects as less than that of small ones of identical physical mass. Also called *Charpentier illusion*.

Skaggs–Robinson hypothesis The generalization that little or no similarity between stimuli causes both little or no interference and little or no facilitation in processing them.

skeletal From the Greek for *dried up*, pertaining to the skeleton, the body framework composed (in humans) of 206 separate bones.

skeletal age CARPAL *AGE.

skeletal muscle STRIATE *MUSCLE.

sketchpad VISUO-SPATIAL SKETCHPAD.

skepticism SCEPTICISM.

skew correlation CURVILINEAR *CORRELATION.

skewness The degree to which the curve of a frequency distribution departs from perfect symmetry. Skewness is described as *positive* (or *to the right*) or *negative* (or *to the left*) depending upon whether the tail of the distribution extends toward those values relative to the mode. Skewness is the third MOMENT (2) of a distribution.

skill The capacity for carrying out complex, well-organized patterns of behaviour smoothly and adaptively so as to achieve some end or goal. Although the term was originally used largely with respect to motor activity, it is now common to see references to verbal and social skills.

skin The external covering of the body. Consisting of epidermis, dermis and subcutaneous tissues, it is an extremely complex and vital organ involved in the mediation of the senses of temperature, pressure and pain and playing important roles in protection and temperature regulation.

skin conductance response (SCR) GALVANIC SKIN RESPONSE.

Skinner box An experimental apparatus named after its inventor, B. F. Skinner. Although there are an almost limitless number of variations, the basic design is simplicity itself: a small enclosed chamber with two essential components, a manipulandum (a button, bar, key, lever, etc.) which the experimental subject can operate, and a device which delivers reinforcements (a food hopper, water tube, etc.). Other common components are projectors and speakers for presenting visual and auditory stimuli, an electrifiable grid floor for studying aversive conditioning, additional manipulanda for investigations of choice behaviour, etc. The apparatus has become the prototypical device for the controlled laboratory study of OPERANT behaviour.

Skinnerian Pertaining to or characteristic of the general theoretical point of view of the great American advocate of BEHAVIOURISM Burrhus Frederic Skinner. The Skinnerian position embodies a strong POSITIVISM with its attendant OPERATIONALISM, a denial of the usefulness of hypothesizing unobservable mental acts, an eschewing of formal theory (although Skinner himself was seemingly irresistibly drawn to informal theorizing) and a denial of the explanatory value of concepts such as freedom, will and dignity. Like most comprehensive orientations, the Skinnerian has its own set of procedures (see OPERANT CONDITIONING, SCHEDULES OF *REINFORCEMENT, SKINNER BOX), its own technical journal (*Journal of the Experimental Analysis of Behavior*) and its own, often arcane, terminology (for some of the more unusual see AUTOCLITIC, MAND, PERCH, SCALLOP, TIME OUT).

Skinnerian conditioning OPERANT CONDITIONING is occasionally so referred to in honour of B. F. Skinner.

skin potential The electrical potential of the skin, which is measured as the GALVANIC SKIN RESPONSE.

skin potential response (SPR) GALVANIC SKIN RESPONSE.

skin resistance response (SRR) GALVANIC SKIN RESPONSE

skin senses Those senses for which the receptors are in the SKIN.

skin writing Tracing of a letter or number on the skin, usually the palm of the hand, and asking the individual to name it.

sleep Basically, a particular loss of consciousness characterized by a variety of behavioural and neurophysiological effects. In modern psychology sleep and the various stages of sleep are typically defined and characterized by particular physiological events, in particular brainwave patterns as recorded by an electroencephalograph, metabolic processes, muscle tone, heart and respiration rates and the important presence or absence of rapid eye movements (REMs). The typical division is into *REM sleep* and *NREM* (or *non-REM*) *sleep*. REM sleep is characterized by its primary defining feature, the rapid eye movements, and several less detectable but important factors, including a lack of delta waves (slow, large-amplitude brainwaves), flaccid musculature, fluctuating heart beat, erratic respiration, genital changes and, significantly, dreaming (in approximately 80–85% of cases studied, subjects awakened from a REM period report dreaming). NREM sleep is usually divided into four separate stages based on the proportion of delta waves observed: Stage 1 shows essentially 0% of the total brain activity as delta (but with no REM), Stage 2 has up to 20% delta, Stage 3 between 20 and 50% delta, Stage 4 over 50%. Not surprisingly, Stages 3 and 4 are often referred to collectively as *slow-wave sleep* (SWS). These stages also show a progressively deeper and deeper sleep and all are characterized by a lack of REM, a regular heart beat, rhythmic respiration, low levels of metabolic activity and moderate-to-high muscle tone. Although dreaming is strongly associated with REM sleep, there is roughly a 15% chance that dreams will be reported by persons woken from NREM sleep, although these dreams lack the clear imagery, emotional tone and structure of REM-sleep dreams. However, a variety of atypical sleep phenomena, such as SOMNAMBULISM and SLEEP TERROR DISORDER, tend to occur during Stage 4.

See also DREAM, DREAM ANALYSIS, HYPNAGOGIC IMAGERY. Note that many authors prefer the notations D *SLEEP and S *SLEEP for REM and NREM sleep respectively; see those entries for reasons.

sleep apnoea APNOEA.

sleep attack An overwhelming urge to sleep. Much more compelling than mere sleepiness, it occurs in SLEEP DISORDERS such as NARCOLEPSY.

sleep centre A term once applied to an area of the hypothalamus thought to control sleep. It is now known that there is no such identifiable neural centre: brainstem and forebrain structures have both been implicated in control over the complex sleep–waking cycle.

sleep, D A common synonym of *REM sleep*. The notation *D* is favoured by some because REM sleep shows a *d*esynchronized EEG pattern and because it is usually accompanied by *d*reaming. See SLEEP for more detail. Compare with S *SLEEP.

sleep disorder An umbrella term for any significant departure from the normal sleep–waking cycle. Contemporary terminology distinguishes between the ORGANIC *SLEEP DIS-ORDERS, which are caused by neurological or physiological factors, and the NONORGANIC *SLEEP DISORDERS, which are regarded as primarily psychogenic. The latter category is subdivided into the DYSSOMNIAS, which include disorders in the amount, quality or timing of sleep, and the PARASOMNIAS, which include disorders marked by abnormal events occurring during sleep. See each of these terms for more detail.

sleep disorder, nonorganic Any sleep disorder of which emotional factors are deemed to be the primary cause. See DYSSOMNIA and PARASOMNIA for details.

sleep disorder, organic Any sleep disorder of which organic, nonpsychogenic factors are deemed to be the primary cause, including NARCOLEPSY, APNOEA and NOCTURNAL MYO-CLONUS.

sleep, disorders of initiating and maintaining (DIMS) INSOMNIA.

sleep epilepsy NARCOLEPSY.

sleeper effect 1 Originally, Carl Hovland's term for the fact that attitude changes produced by a message often do not become evident until a period of time has passed. **2** More specifically, the phenomenon of a message from a low-credibility source that, to begin with, has no effect on people's attitudes, showing an effect after some time has passed. People remember the message but forget the source. See SOURCE *MEMORY. **3** In developmental psychology, an early event or circumstance that does not produce an effect until some time has passed.

sleep inertia A period of diminished functioning immediately after waking. Decision-making is impaired, reactions are slow and error rates high. It can last up to an hour but the impairments are worst in the first few minutes. The optimal remedy is a cup of coffee.

sleeping sickness The common name for the infectious disease *Encephalitis lethargica*, characterized by increasing drowsiness, lethargy and apathy.

sleep learning HYPNOPAEDIA.

sleep paralysis The temporary inability to move when the muscle flaccidity and accompanying paralysis typical of REM sleep intrude on an awake period. Such episodes usually occur immediately before or after sleep and can be mildly frightening.

sleep, pathological A general term for any abnormal pattern of sleep. See SLEEP DISORDER et seq.

sleep, S A common term for *NREM sleep*. The notation *S* is used to denote the fact that the EEG of a person in NREM sleep is characterized by *s*low waves, is *s*ynchronized and shows sleep *s*pindles. See SLEEP for more details. Compare with D *SLEEP.

sleep, slow-wave A term occasionally used for the sleep in Stages 3 and 4, in which a sleeper's EEG displays large-amplitude, slow, delta waves. See SLEEP for more detail. abbrev., *SWS*.

sleep spindles Short (about 1 sec.) bursts of rapid (12–14 Hz), low-voltage brainwave activity. They are observed in Stages 2, 3 and 4 of SLEEP (see which for details).

sleep terror disorder A sleep disorder marked by repeated episodes of waking in what appears to be a state of intense anxiety with dilated pupils, sweating, rapid breathing and a rapid pulse. After the agitation subsides, the sufferer usually reports a vague sense of terror with fragmentary dream-like images. Typically there is no memory of the event in the morning. The disorder generally begins in childhood and, unlike DREAM ANXIETY DISORDER, occurs during Stages 3 and 4 of sleep and not during REM sleep. Also called *pavor nocturnus* or, when occurring during daytime naps, *pavor diurnus*.

sleep, twilight The delirium-like state produced by an injection of scopolamine, morphine and phenobarbital.

sleep–wake schedule disorder A type of SLEEP DISORDER marked by a mismatch between a person's natural (*circadian rhythm*) sleep–wake cycle and that which is enforced by his or her environment (e.g. the demands of a job). The most common form is DELAYED SLEEP-ONSET INSOMNIA, in which the person tosses and turns, often for hours, before falling asleep. Also called *circadian rhythm sleep disorder*.

sleepwalking SOMNAMBULISM.

slip of the tongue PARAPRAXIS.

slippery slope A term used to characterize an argument in which, if a particular first step is taken, one can find oneself unhappily forced into accepting positions counter to one's initial stance. Slippery slopes appear most often in considerations of moral and ethical issues. For example, opponents of assisted suicide argue that it is the first step on a road that logically leads to legitimizing murder.

slope With respect to curves, the tangent of the angle made by a straight line drawn from a point on the curve by the *x*-axis. See also ACCELERATION.

slow Basically a nontechnical term used to characterize: **1** A child whose development is retarded relative to the norm. **2** Any person with below-normal intellectual functioning. See also terms beginning with BRADY-.

slow learner 1 A mildly retarded child. **2** A child with normal intellectual potential who, for any number of reasons, takes longer to learn material than is typical for his or her age. See MENTAL RETARDATION to appreciate the distinction between these two meanings.

slow-to-warm-up child See DIFFICULT CHILD.

slow (twitch) muscle MUSCLE TWITCH (1).

slow-wave sleep SLEEP, SLOW-WAVE.

small group By arbitrary convention, a group of individuals numbering approximately ten or fewer. Most small-group research involves the study of such small numbers of persons in face-to-face contact in either laboratory settings or natural environments.

small-sample theory The mathematical/statistical theory and accompanying techniques that permit the derivation of inferences from relatively small samples to larger populations.

smell 1 n. The sense modality of *olfaction*, that sense for which the stimuli are particular classes of chemicals in gaseous form. See OLFACTION, OLFACTORY and related entries. **2** n. A sensation produced by stimulation of the olfactory receptors and nerves. **3** vb. To process information in the olfactory modality, to perceive via the stimulation of the olfactory receptors and nerves. **4** vb. To emit an odour (despite the famous anecdote concerning Dr Johnson).

smoothed curve A curve in which erratic variations in slope have been evened out so that the general trend can be more easily seen. The fitting of a smooth line by a *least-squares* procedure is a commonly employed method.

smooth muscle MUSCLE, SMOOTH.

s/n SIGNAL-TO-NOISE RATIO.

Snellen chart A chart used as a rough test for measuring visual acuity. Letters are printed in various sizes on the chart, which is placed at a fixed distance from the viewer. The letters are based on a scale of 5 × 3 minutes of visual angle, with the size of the letters adjusted for the viewing distance.

snout reflex An abnormal reflexive pursing of the lips when the upper lip is tapped. It is suggestive of diffuse neurological damage, although it was once thought to be indicative of frontal lobe lesions.

snowball sampling SAMPLING, SNOWBALL.

snow blindness An impairment of vision, typically temporary, caused by exposure to extremely high-intensity light such as that reflected off a snow field under a bright sun. Complete blindness is rare: more commonly acuity is dramatically reduced and objects have a reddish tinge for a time.

SNRIs SEROTONIN AND NOREPINEPHERINE REUPTAKE INHIBITORS.

SOA STIMULUS ONSET ASYNCHRONY.

SOAR An acronym for *State Operator And Result*, a computer-implemented theory of human (and artificial) cognition developed by Allen Newell. SOAR's cognitive architecture is based on a PRODUCTION SYSTEM model and uses feedback loops to adjust and modify knowledge so that the system learns and can solve problems.

Sobel test A statistical test used to determine whether a variable functions as a MEDIATING *VARIABLE in a large sample. Also called *Sobel's z*.

sociability The tendency to have and make personal relationships; friendliness.

sociability index (or **rating**) A rating that expresses one's sociability. A SOCIOGRAM, for example, yields, among other measures, an assessment of the sociability of the various members of a group.

social A splendidly broad adjective which can safely be used for any situation involving two or more conspecifics (members of a species). Note that this is really the appropriate definition. Although the vast majority of uses of the term involve the species *Homo sapiens*, it is also used freely by comparative psychologists, ethologists and sociobiologists. As the many following entries suggest, it is rarely used as a free-standing term but generally qualified to narrow and specify its intended meaning. For combined terms and phrases not found here, see those in which CULTURAL or GROUP is the base term.

social accommodation ACCOMMODATION (4).

social action Any organized, concerted effort on the part of a group of persons to change or reform some (usually political or institutional) aspect of society.

social adaptation ADAPTATION (2).

social adjustment ADJUSTMENT (1).

social-adjustment theory A theoretical approach to the study of attitudes and attitude changes as social-adjustment operations. It draws upon basic principles of experimental psychology, especially psychophysics, to assess the processes involved in the establishment and modification of evaluative judgements. There are two general models: ASSIMILATION–CONTRAST THEORY and ADAPTATION LEVEL THEORY; see each for details.

social anchoring A form of ANCHORING in which personal decision-making and attitude formation are dependent primarily upon an external group's decisions or attitudes. A person is said to anchor decisions on those of some reference group. The effect is presumed by some theorists to be sufficiently strong to account for such social phenomena as dramatic shifts in the stock market and the bandwagon effect in politics, in which the candidate perceived to be ahead suddenly attracts the support of the undecided voters, who take their cue from the majority.

social anxiety Feelings of unease and discomfort in social settings typically accompanied by shyness and social awkwardness. If intense it can become a SOCIAL ANXIETY *DISORDER. Distinguish from SOCIAL *PHOBIA.

social anxiety disorder ANXIETY DISORDER, SOCIAL.

social atmosphere SOCIAL CLIMATE.

social attitude **1** The attitude which underlies a person's tendency to behave in a particular fashion toward other persons. **2** A particular pattern of beliefs common to a group of persons or a society. **3** Any personal belief which is acquired as a result of socialization processes.

social behaviour **1** Loosely, any behaviour of an individual which has social components. That is, behaviour that is influenced by the presence, attitudes or actions of others; behaviour that influences the presence, attitudes or actions of others; or behaviour learned primarily as a result of social factors. **2** More specifically, GROUP BEHAVIOUR or that behaviour which takes place in and is primarily determined by a group. The term is used without any species limitations.

social being A more or less nontechnical term for any organism or species the intrinsic nature and behaviours of which are dependent on the presence of and interactions with others.

social bond See BOND (3), BONDING.

social-breakdown syndrome Those symptoms of various mental disorders that are the result of conditions and facilities of treatment and not primary components of the psychiatric disorder itself. Generally included as contributing factors here are labelling (see LABELLING THEORY), learning the role of sick person (see ADVANTAGE BY ILLNESS), atrophy of social skills and identification with the sick.

social casework SOCIAL WORK.

social category A collection of persons who are classified together by virtue of societal criteria but do not form a group or an organization, e.g. adolescents, secondary-school teachers, unemployed persons. Compare with SOCIAL CLASS.

social change Generally, any alteration in the social organization or structure of a society. In practice, the term is typically reserved for major, significant changes in a society as a whole and is not applied to minor perturbations or to changes in subgroups within a society.

social class A social category in a stratified society which is usually defined by its members having roughly equivalent SOCIOECONOMIC STATUS. There is some debate as to the generality of this criterion of socioeconomic status. Some authorities stress that less obvious factors such as lifestyle, prestige, attitudes, identifications, etc. are better descriptive measures, and many use the notion of LIFE CHANCE(S) as the primary defining feature. Others, notably those with a Marxist orientation, stress that the means of production in a society dictate social class sufficiently strongly to outweigh other factors. Usage, thus, follows theory.

social climate A more or less nontechnical term for the general tenor or inclination of any society, or segment thereof, that has effects on the attitudes and actions of its individual members. Also called *group climate* or *social* (or *group*) *atmosphere*.

social climbing A nontechnical term for which we provide here a technical definition: behaving so as to attempt to move from *social class n* to social class *n + j*, where *n* and *j* are integers and the various social classes may be represented on at least an ORDINAL *SCALE.

social clock A temporal framework within a given culture that lays out the approximate times for various age-related events, e.g. when to start school, get married, have children, retire.

social code A general term for any set of rules, mores or regulations, formal or informal, which exerts control over the conduct of persons in a group or society.

social cognition A subfield that is essentially a blending of social and cognitive psychology and which focuses on how individuals perceive, recall, think about and interpret information about the actions of themselves and others.

social cohesion The tendency for any group or society to maintain itself, to hold together its several components. The degree of cohesion of a group is usually reflected by its resilience to disruption by outside forces.

social comparison The use of others as a basis for comparison in evaluating one's own judgements, abilities, attitudes, etc.

social comparison theory A model developed by Leon Festinger that maintains that when objective scales are missing (which is usually the case) people evaluate their abilities and attitudes by making comparisons with others. Implicit in the theory is that individuals tend to choose those with similar abilities and attitudes as the comparison group.

social consciousness **1** Generally, the awareness that one has of one's social nature and of one's role in a group or society. **2** Somewhat more specifically, the recognition that one's needs, feelings, attitudes and beliefs are not utterly unique but are shared by others, particularly those with similar social backgrounds. **3** A synonym of *group consciousness*, *collective consciousness* or GROUP MIND.

social constructionism The approach, akin to postmodernist thought, that all knowledge, including scientifically obtained knowledge, is a construct of culture, language and social roles and has no claim to final truth. Distinguish from *social constructivism* (see CONSTRUCTIVISM (2)) which represents a more moderate point of view, and compare with DECONSTRUCTIONISM.

social constructivism CONSTRUCTIVISM (2).

social contagion The rapid spread of attitudes, ideas or moods through a group or a society, as, for example, through *rumour*.

social control The control that a society exerts upon the individuals within it. The form that this control takes is embodied primarily in the socialization process and the resulting internalization of the norms and values of the society. The term is generally not used to refer to the use of personal or group power to effect exploitative or selfish control over others, although, to be sure, by the very nature of society such forms of social control do exist. Most social theorists find it useful to distinguish between *negative* social control, which functions through disapproval, ridicule, punishment, the threat of punishment, etc., and *positive* social control, which operates through rewards, approval, tangible benefits, etc.

social Darwinism The theory that social and cultural development could be explained by analogy with the Darwinian theory of biological evolution. The basic principle here, first articulated by the British philosopher Herbert Spencer, is that society functions primarily through competition and conflict, and that the fittest survive and prosper while the weak and poorly adapted are eliminated. The theory is indefensibly simplistic but has, unfortunately, been used by some as a defence of a rather ugly form of *laissez-faire* economics which ignores the importance of social class and related factors in affecting one's chances of success.

social desirability 1 Those characteristics generally approved of socially and which, if one possesses them, make one a socially attractive person. **2** A bias or set that inclines one to respond to self-evaluative questions in a socially approved manner so as to appear more socially desirable either to oneself or to others.

social determinism CULTURAL DETERMINISM.

social differentiation Collectively, the processes through which a society becomes divided into various statuses, classes, groups, strata, roles, etc.

social dilemma DILEMMA, SOCIAL.

social distance Generally, the degree of separation of groups or individuals in a society. Social distance is a complex concept and reflects patterns of personal and social interaction, the degree of intimacy and the mutual sympathy for values and ideals between persons in a society. It has been characterized in various ways, ranging from the extent to which a given stratum of a society is accessible to persons from another stratum, to the internal sense of disparateness an individual feels with respect to a particular segment of society, and the degree to which a person will willingly associate with another from a distinct social group. Note also that the terms *horizontal* and *vertical* are often used to characterize social distance between persons of the same and different socioeconomic classes respectively.

social distance scale Any sociometric instrument designed to measure SOCIAL DISTANCE. The most commonly used is the one developed by Emory Bogardus in which respondents are asked to indicate the degree to which they would willingly have interactions with individuals from other social, racial, ethnic or national groups. The scale is graded from 'exclude from my country' to 'admit to my family through marriage'.

social drive Loosely, any drive for social interaction, a drive with interpersonal aims rather than physical or material aims. Distinguish from SOCIALIZED DRIVE.

social dyad DIAD, SOCIAL.

social dynamics 1 Loosely, the processes that underlie social change. **2** Any approach to social psychology or sociology that is primarily concerned with the study of social change. Compare with GROUP DYNAMICS.

social ecology ECOLOGY, SOCIAL.

social equilibrium EQUILIBRIUM (3).

social-exchange theory A model of social structure based on the principle that most social behaviour is predicated on the individual's expectation that his or her actions with respect to others will result in some kind of commensurate return.

social facilitation A general phenomenon that demonstrates that activity is increased (i.e. facilitated) by the presence of CONSPECI- FICS. Examples abound. Fully satiated chick- ens will eat if placed among chickens who are eating hungrily, athletes perform better if an audience is watching, children play more enthusiastically if a playmate is near by, even if only engaged in parallel play, and even cockroaches will run a maze faster if watched by other roaches. Compare with SOCIAL INHIBITION and see SPECTATOR EFFECTS.

social factor Broadly, any variable that has an impact on behaviour in a social setting.

social fission The splitting apart of a group or other social unit. See FISSION.

social fixity/flexibility SOCIAL MOBILITY.

social heritage The compendium of folk- ways, mores, traditions, institutions, laws, customs, etc. passed on within a social sys- tem from generation to generation. Thus, the term captures the same essential mean- ing as the term CULTURE.

social history An overview of the primary social events in an individual's life, including such factors as marriage(s), divorce(s), job(s), education and drug or alcohol use patterns. Taking a social history is a routine part of many clinical interviews.

social identity One's IDENTITY (1) in the pub- lic, social domain. Not surprisingly, one's publicly construed self, group identities and overt social behaviours are not always in concert with one's private, personal iden- tity.

social identity theory The hypothesis that the social groups to which we belong can have significant impacts on our self-esteem. In general, identifying (or being identified) with groups that are held in high public esteem enhances one's self-esteem.

social immobility SOCIAL MOBILITY.

social impact theory A theory of the degree to which social influences are mani- fested. In general, the impact of social forces on an individual is given by how many other persons there are, how strong the impact of

each is, and how 'far away' (both physically and psychologically) they are. In mirror fash- ion an individual's impact on others is given by his or her personal influence over them, how many people he or she is influencing, and how 'close' he or she is to them.

social indicators Generally, those aspects of group or social behaviour that can be used as cues to general societal trends.

social influence A cover term for all those processes through which a person, group or class influences the opinions, attitudes, behaviours and values of other persons, groups or classes.

social inhibition A general effect where the presence of others interferes with or inhibits the carrying out of actions. Compare with SOCIAL FACILITATION and see SPECTATOR EFFECTS.

social insects Any of several species of insect with a mode of existence that is fun- damentally social, particularly those the hives or nests of which are hierarchically structured so that duties and behaviours are delegated to particular groups or classes.

social instinct Gregariousness, the ten- dency to seek out and form social contacts. Use of the term is ill-advised: the word INSTINCT is loaded with species-specific, gen- etic connotations that are far from giving the whole picture here. See SOCIAL DRIVE.

social institution INSTITUTION (1, 2).

social integration INTEGRATION, SOCIAL.

social interaction INTERACTION.

social interference SOCIAL FACILITATION.

social isolate A person who forms relatively few interpersonal ties. The causes may be either internal or external.

sociality SOCIABILITY.

socialization **1** Generally, the process whereby an individual acquires the know- ledge, values, facility with language, social skills and social sensitivity that enable him or her to become integrated into and behave adaptively within a society. Strictly speaking, this definition applies uniformly to persons of all ages, and, in a very real sense, socializa- tion is a lifelong experience. However, the dominant usage of the term is with respect to the processes by which a child becomes inculcated with society's values and with his or her own social roles. **2** The process of the taking-over by the state of the services, industry and other institutions of a society for the (ostensible) benefit of all members. **3** In industrial/organizational psychology, the process whereby a new recruit of an organization learns to adapt to that organization's norms and roles; in the layperson's terms, learning the ropes. **4** The respective outcomes of any of the above processes.

socialize 1 To bring about SOCIALIZATION (1, 2). **2** To interact freely with other persons. **3** To encourage such interactions in others.

socialized drive Any primary drive which has had its mode of manifestation shaped by social learning so that its satisfaction is achieved through socially accepted behaviours. Distinguish from SOCIAL DRIVE.

social lag CULTURE LAG.

social learning theory An approach to the study of social behaviour and personality due primarily to the work of Albert Bandura and Richard Walters. The theory is based upon the role of observation and the mimicking or imitating of behaviours observed in others, usually referred to as models. For more details on specifics of the theory see MODEL, MODELLING and OBSERVATIONAL *LEARNING.

social loafing The tendency for individuals to reduce the effort that they make toward some task when working with others. The effect has been found in a wide variety of circumstances: people put less effort into pushing a car or to solving cognitively complex problems when these tasks are carried out in a group.

social man A perspective on humankind that assumes that the basic principle underlying human nature is a complex set of social and interpersonal needs. The term is an unhappy one since it seems to exclude more than half of the individuals whose behaviour it seeks to explain.

social maturity Loosely, a measure of the degree to which an individual's social behaviours match the norms of age-matched peers. Some scales (e.g. VINELAND SOCIAL MATURITY SCALE) produce a *social quotient* which, analogous to an *intelligence quotient*, is a ratio of one's measured social age to one's chronological age.

social meaning The meaning of a situation, event or other social phenomenon as given by the shared understandings and interpretations of those present. Social meaning is derived from shared attitudes and beliefs of the persons in a group or a larger society.

social mind 1 GROUP MIND. **2** The dominant opinion within a group or society.

social mobility 1 A dimension that characterizes the degree to which individuals in a particular society can move along the social scale. Rigid, fixed social systems are characterized by social immobility such that a person's hereditary role largely determines his or her life chances: open, more democratic systems are typically characterized by somewhat greater social mobility. **2** The movement from class to class of individuals in a society. Although the term can, strictly speaking, cover both upward and downward movement, it is generally applied only to upward. Also referred to as *social fixity/flexibility*.

social mores MORES.

social motive Generally, any learned motive. Social motives are typically not essential for life, are learned through social interaction and are satisfied by social outcomes. Originally these 'secondary' motives were contrasted with the 'primary', physiologically based motives, but it is, in practice, often difficult to separate them; for example, sexual motivation is inextricably tied to both aspects.

social movement Loosely, any systematic, organized endeavour in which individuals work in a concerted manner toward some social goal. The term is used both for efforts designed to bring about social change as well as those directed toward resisting change and maintaining the status quo. It is applied to small local reformist efforts as well as to large, revolutionary movements.

social need Generally, any NEED with a social basis, e.g. NEED FOR AFFILIATION.

social network The structured set of social links an individual or group has with other persons or groups. See SOCIOGRAM for an approach to the study of such systems.

social neuroscience An approach to the study of social functions and processes that seeks to integrate behaviours and thoughts that have social elements with their underlying neurological foundations. Methods include the use of IMAGING TECHNIQUES and assessment of endocrine and immune system function and linking these measures with behaviour in socially relevant contexts.

social norm Any pattern of behaviour that occurs so often within a particular society that it comes to be accepted as reflective of that society and taken as sanctioned by the members of that society. Sometimes called *group norm*, although that term is probably best reserved for behaviour in smaller social units. See MORES.

social object An OBJECT that is a person or a group of persons.

social order 1 The totality of the institutions and structures that make up a society; usually preceded by the word *the*. **2** A relatively stable condition in a society in which things are harmonious and major conflicts are rare.

social organization ORGANIZATION, SOCIAL.

social pathology SOCIAL PROBLEM.

social perception Broadly, any aspect of PERCEPTION that has a social element. The term is generally used with respect to an individual's awareness of the behaviours of others which are revealing of their motives or attitudes. See here PERSON PERCEPTION; compare with SELF-PERCEPTION THEORY.

social phobia PHOBIA, SOCIAL.

social power POWER, SOCIAL.

social pressure The collective coercive influences of others, particularly when they are acting as a coordinated group. The term is usually used only when such patterns of pressure lie outside the formalized value systems of society. See PRESSURE (2, 3).

social problem An umbrella term for any situation which, from the point of view of a significant number of persons in a community, is deemed to constitute a problem of sufficient severity to require reform. Typic-

ally included here are drug abuse, juvenile delinquency, poverty, gangs, unemployment and the like.

social psychiatry Loosely, any approach to psychiatry or clinical psychology that focuses on social factors in the aetiology and treatment of mental disorders.

social psychology That branch of psychology that concentrates on any and all aspects of human behaviour that involve persons and their relationships with other persons, groups, social institutions and society as a whole. Gordon Allport captured this general sense in his now classic definition of social psychology as the discipline that 'attempts to understand and explain how the thought, feeling or behaviour of individuals are influenced by the actual, imagined or implied presence of others'. Social psychology exchanges freely ideas, models and methods with other social sciences, particularly SOCIOLOGY. In recent years the field has broadened its domain, incorporating methods and analytic strategies from other areas such as cognitive psychology SOCIAL COGNITION, the neurosciences (SOCIAL NEUROSCIENCE) and evolutionary biology (EVOLUTIONARY PSYCHOLOGY).

social pyramid A term for the vertical model of the social classes in a society which, if schematically represented with the size of each stratum reflecting the number of persons in it, has a pyramidal shape with the numerous lower classes at the base and the less numerous elite classes at the apex.

social quotient SOCIAL MATURITY.

social reality REALITY, SOCIAL.

social recognition A general term for a number of processes that relate to the ability of an individual to recognize particular social attributes and characteristics of other individuals or groups. Included here are such processes as recognition of species identity, group membership, sexual receptivity, social status, reproductive status and genetic relatedness. The term is used in reference to humans as well as other species.

social referencing Seeking out what others are feeling and how they are reacting to an unfamiliar event or object. The knowledge gained then shapes one's own emotional or behavioural reactions.

social reinforcement REINFORCEMENT, SOCIAL.

social role ROLE.

social sanction *Sanction* has several meanings, the ones carried by this term focus on the approval or disapproval of actions of individuals by the society within which they occur, with emphasis on *dis*approval.

social scale The various social classes ordered according to some set of criteria. Any number of social scales may be formed; the most common are those based on SOCIO-ECONOMIC STATUS or SOCIAL CLASS.

social selection 1 A term, first used by those espousing SOCIAL DARWINISM, for a hypothetical process by which certain individuals, groups or classes survived and prospered while others did not. The presumption was that social systems could be viewed as analogues of biological systems, with social selection operating as did NATURAL SELECTION. This meaning is obsolete. **2** More loosely, the role of social factors in determining the differential survival of individuals. From this point of view, SEXUAL SELECTION may be regarded as an example of social selection in many species in that interactions between individuals in attracting and maintaining a mate are important components in reproductive success.

social self SELF, SOCIAL.

social sensitivity SENSITIVITY (3). *Social* is often appended to distinguish this meaning of sensitivity from the others.

social space A region with both geographical and social boundaries which represents the social, interactive domain of an individual. One's social space may shift over time as new relationships are formed and old ones dissolve, as group membership changes and as one's social perceptions are modified. Compare with PERSONAL SPACE.

social status STATUS, SOCIAL.

social stratification The alignment of a society into social classes.

social structure The relatively stable, organized pattern of interrelated roles, statuses, norms and institutions characterizing a group or a society at a point in time.

social studies Generally, those aspects of a school curriculum which touch upon social issues, social problems, etc.

social support Generally and loosely, all those forms of support provided by other individuals and groups that help an individual cope with life.

social tension TENSION (4).

social therapy Loosely, any form of psychotherapy that utilizes social settings or social structure, e.g. MILIEU THERAPY.

social time TIME, SOCIAL.

social transmission CULTURAL TRANSMISSION.

social trap See SOCIAL *DILEMMA.

social value VALUE (2).

social welfare (programmes) Any of the programmes of formal agencies, private and public, which are designed to assist the disadvantaged in a society.

social work A professional field which bridges community psychology, clinical psychology and sociology. Social work is concerned broadly with the application of social-science principles to social problems. Although the field is difficult to circumscribe, particularly because new problems, theories and procedures tend to extend its domain, it is typically divided into three broad areas: (a) social casework, with a focus on individual and family therapy; (b) group work, with emphasis on work with gangs, youth, churches, etc.; and (c) community relations, with an orientation toward local organizations, neighbourhood groups, institutions, etc.

societal Pertaining to society or to that which is social in nature.

society 1 Inclusively, all of humankind taken as a whole. This meaning is rare these days. **2** A collection of persons with: (a) a recognized set of norms, values, roles and institutions which forms the basis of a common culture; (b) a relatively well-circumscribed geographical region which they populate; (c) a sense of unity; and (d) a feeling of belongingness or relatedness to the cultural norms and customs in (a). **3** Any organized, relatively long-lasting group of organisms of a species. This last definition, in a sense, encompasses 2, but it is deliberately vague so as to include species other than *Homo sapiens*. That is, one might wish to state that bees have a society in sense 3 but surely not in sense 2. **4** Any organized group of individuals bound together by common goals or sets of interests.

socio- A combining form meaning *social* or *societal*.

sociobiology A science that focuses on the study of the biological basis of social behaviour. The dominant paradigm in the field is the application of the principles and theoretical framework of evolutionary biology in an attempt to explain those structural and behavioural aspects of organisms as they pertain to social behaviour. Compare with EVOLUTIONARY PSYCHOLOGY.

sociocentre The person who lies at the centre of a SOCIOGRAM, the one to whom most of the arrows point.

sociocentrism 1 The perspective of a person that his or her social group represents the ideal standards of behaviour, opinions etc. against which the worth of other groups is judged. Like EGOCENTRISM and ETHNOCENTRISM, it implies a lack of sensitivity to the values and practices of others. **2** For some authors, a synonym of ETHNOCENTRISM, although the latter usually connotes a larger scope.

sociocultural mental retardation MENTAL RETARDATION, CULTURAL-FAMILIAL.

sociocultural perspective (or **theory**) Loosely, any model that emphasizes the role of social and cultural factors over the biological and genetic as causal factors in behaviour. Such approaches are found widely, particularly in approaches to mental health, psychopathology, education and, most significantly, developmental and social psychology. The most influential of these approaches is Lev Vygotsky's in which development is viewed as a process through which the child's own 'natural' cognitive abilities are shaped through interaction with the various personal and social elements in the environment.

sociocusis Hearing loss due to cultural factors such as street noise, aging and, increasingly in young adults, loud music.

sociodrama PSYCHODRAMA, but with an emphasis on role-taking in groups.

socioeconomic status (SES) Quite literally, a rating of the status of an individual's position in a stratified society based on a variety of social (e.g. family background, social class, education of parents, education of self, values, occupation) and/or economic (income of family, of self) indices. The HOLLINGSHEAD SCALES are an example. See also SOCIAL CLASS.

sociofugal Characterizing environments arranged to minimize intimacy among their users. Public places like waiting rooms in hospitals and train stations, where the furniture is set in rows, are good examples. Compare with SOCIOPETAL.

sociogenic 1 In sociology, pertaining to the origins of society. **2** More generally, characterizing the social origins of various behaviours, e.g juvenile delinquency is usually regarded as a sociogenic problem. var., *sociogenetic*.

sociogram In SOCIOMETRY a diagrammatic representation of the structure of interactions between the members of a group. The typical procedure is to represent the interactions by arrows connecting individuals, with each arrow marked for attraction or antagonism. Also called *Morenogram* to honour Jacob Moreno who developed the technique.

sociolect A DIALECT spoken by members of an identifiable social group.

sociolinguistics A field of study predicated on the principle that language normally functions in a social context and focused on the investigation of the broad range of interaction between language behaviour and social behaviour. Generally included are the study of linguistic variations, particularly those which are related to social class, ethnic groups and geographic regions, the interaction between linguistic variation and child-rearing patterns, the role of gesture and other paralinguistic devices in communication, the study of nonverbal communication, and the like. See PSYCHOLINGUISTICS and related entries.

sociology A discipline that focuses on the study of human behaviour from the perspective of the social dimension. Sociology concentrates relatively less upon the individual as a separate entity than does SOCIAL PSYCHOLOGY, tending to view behaviour as it occurs in social interactions, in groups, etc.

sociometric analysis (or test) A social rating analysis in which each member of a group is asked to select which other members of the group she or he likes or dislikes, would or would not be willing to work with, spend time with, etc. In the original format, the ratings were usually based on the liking and disliking dimension; however, many variations on the procedures are now used, often for rather specific purposes, such as the selection of committees, work groups, social organizations, etc., and so questions of liking are often deemed less important than other factors, such as work-oriented compatibility. The results of a sociometric analysis are typically displayed diagrammatically as a SOCIOGRAM.

sociometrics Loosely, any attempt to measure, quantify or formalize interpersonal relationships. The most developed is J. Moreno's SOCIOMETRY.

sociometry 1 Lit., the measuring of things social. **2** Specifically, the techniques and theory due largely to the work of Jacob L. Moreno that form the basis of the most oft-used procedures. Moreno's techniques consist primarily of laying out the network of interrelationships that exist between the various members of a group. The procedure for establishing a set of relationships is the SOCIOMETRIC ANALYSIS (OR TEST) and the resulting schematic diagram is called a SOCIOGRAM.

sociopath One with a SOCIOPATHIC PERSONALITY.

sociopathic personality A personality disorder characterized by disturbed, maladaptive social relationships, particularly those that reflect clear antisocial behaviours.

The term was introduced as a replacement for PSYCHOPATHIC PERSONALITY and, while the change was adopted by many, several near synonyms remained in wide use including, *psychopathy, psychopathic personality* and *sociopathy*. Hoping to clean up this lexicographic clutter, the latest edition of the DSM has recommended ANTISOCIAL PERSONALITY DISORDER as the 'official' diagnostic term. Caveat lector.

sociopathy The condition described under SOCIOPATHIC PERSONALITY.

sociopetal Characterizing environments arranged to increase intimacy among their users. In most homes, for example, the furniture is arranged so that people face each other. Compare with SOCIOFUGAL. var., *sociopedal*.

sociotechnical model An approach to the study of social systems that is predicated on the notion that all productive social organizations (or parts thereof) are dynamic products of their *technology* and their particular *social systems*. Technology is characterized broadly here and includes the physical layout, any apparatus or other technical devices that may be in use, the specific requirements of those persons involved in the organization, etc.; the social system is viewed as the dynamic interrelationships between those persons involved in the organization. The approach emerged from the work of the London-based Tavistock Institute in the 1950s and 1960s.

sociotherapy An umbrella term for any form of therapy in which the emphasis is on the socioenvironmental and interpersonal aspects rather than on the intrapsychic. Various forms of group therapy, psychodrama and the like are included.

sociotropic Socially oriented.

sodomy 1 Originally, as characterized in Genesis, anal intercourse. **2** More generally, bestiality or zooerasty. **3** In some legal instances, any 'unnatural' sex act; a PARAPHILIA. See SEXUAL *PERVERSION for a discussion of the problems involved in definitions such as this.

soft data Laboratory jargon for subjective data, e.g. impressions, ratings, clinical case studies, interviews, projective test analyses, etc. Compare with HARD DATA.

soft drug A nontechnical term for any drug that either has no clear PHYSIOLOGICAL *DEPENDENCE associated with it (e.g. marijuana) or is legal (e.g. caffeine, nicotine).

softening of the brain Obsolescent term

for the deterioration of brain tissue caused by advanced syphilis; see PARESIS (2).

softness A perceptual quality which is used to characterize a variety of perceptual experiences. In tactile perception, it is a characteristic of objects that yield readily to the touch; in vision, of objects the colours of which are low in saturation and brightness; in audition, of tones that are low in intensity and/or pitch.

soft palate PALATE.

soft psychology Laboratory jargon for those areas in psychology that focus on the social-science as opposed to the natural-science aspects; e.g. personality, abnormal psychology, developmental psychology, social psychology. See HARD PSYCHOLOGY for more discussion on terminology.

soft (neurological) sign Any of a number of minor abnormalities that either emerge in childhood or develop as a result of cortical injury. They are widely used as diagnostic indicators of minimal brain damage. Classic examples include *dysdiadochkinesis*, or difficulty in carrying out alternating movements (like tapping) with one's fingers or hands, and *synkinesis*, in which attempts to move one body part produce involuntarily movements elsewhere. Soft signs can be subtle and difficult to detect reliably; when they emerge in childhood, they tend to run their developmental course with no clear locus of origin and are not regarded as indicators of any specific neurological disease. The qualifier *soft* comes from the difficulties of interpretation and the uncertain association with structural brain damage.

soft spot FONTANEL.

software In computer terminology, the program. Contrast with HARDWARE.

soldier's disease (or **sickness**) A term coined to refer to addiction to opiates reportedly common among American Civil War veterans. Actually, there is little or no evidence to support the claim of widespread dependence on opiates among soldiers or veterans. Nevertheless, the term, which was introduced decades after the war, stuck and is still used, particularly by those who argue against the use of opiates for treating pain associated with trauma.

solidarity SOCIAL COHESION, but the term is used with the connotation of a collective, cooperative effort toward group goals.

solipsism The philosophical position that holds that the only thing of which one can be certain is one's own personal experience and, by extension, that one's experiences represent all of reality – the outside world existing only as an object of one's consciousness. An extreme variation of IDEALISM (2) rarely held these days.

solitary nucleus A cluster of cells in the solitary tract located in the medulla of the brainstem. It receives visceral and taste information from the VIIth, IXth and Xth CRANIAL NERVES. Neural projections go to the hypothalamus where they play a role in mediating acceptance and rejection of foods and the gag reflex and to the cingulate gyrus and other nuclei in the brainstem that are involved in the control of visceral motor and respiratory functions. Also called *nucleus of the solitary tract*.

solitary tract A pathway made up of myelinated neurons that runs through the SOLITARY NUCLEUS.

solution In order of specificity: **1** The value(s) that fit the conditions of an equation. **2** The answer to a question or problem. **3** The resolution of a set of difficulties or conflicts. Meaning 1 derives from logic and mathematics; 2 is the usual sense in the study of thinking, problem-solving, concept formation, etc.; 3 is the intended meaning in the study of personality, social psychology and clinical psychology and psychiatry.

solution learning A neobehaviourist term for TRIAL-AND-ERROR *LEARNING.

soma **1** The cell body of a neuron. **2** The body, taken as a whole and represented as distinct from the mind. **3** All of the cells in the body except the germ cells, *somatoplasm*. adj., *somatic*.

soma- Combining form meaning *body, bodily*. var., *some-*.

somaesthesia The sense associated with body contact; the skin senses, kinaesthesis and internal sensitivity taken collectively. vars., *somesthesia, somataesthesia, somatesthesia*.

somasthenia Chronic bodily weakness; syn., *somatasthenia.*

somataesthesia SOMAESTHESIA.

somatasthenia SOMASTHENIA.

somatesthesia SOMAESTHESIA.

somatic 1 Pertaining to the body. Hence, contrasted with either the *environment* or the *mind* (or with both, depending on the author's intentions). 2 Pertaining to all the cells except the germ cells. 3 Pertaining to all of the body except the nervous system. This meaning, confusing as it is given 1 and 2, is still found; see e.g. SOMATIC DISORDER (1). Note that in some combined forms the 'c' will be dropped (*somatization, somatisation*), in others 'o' will replace 'ic' (*somatoform*).

somatic delusion DELUSIONAL DISORDER, SOMATIC TYPE.

somatic disorder 1 Generally, any non-neurological disorder, i.e. a disorder of the body. 2 More specifically, an ORGANIC DISORDER. Generally, meaning 2 is intended.

somatic nervous system NERVOUS SYSTEM.

somatic obsession Quite literally, an obsession with some part of the body, characterized by constant checking that part of the body by touch or in mirrors and continual searching for reassurance from others. It is a key symptom of BODY DYSMORPHIC DISORDER and occasionally seen in cases of OBSESSIVE-COMPULSIVE DISORDER.

somatic therapy A cover term in psychiatry for those forms of therapy that are founded on the biological rather than the psychological, e.g. electroconvulsive therapy and the use of psychopharmacological agents.

somatization disorder A SOMATOFORM DISORDER characterized by a history of recurrent and multiple physical symptoms for which there are no apparent physical causes. The disorder virtually always begins in the teens or twenties and has a chronic but fluctuating course involving a wide variety of complaints concerning organic dysfunctions, including vague pains, allergies, gastrointestinal problems, psychosexual symptoms, palpitations and conversion symptoms.

somato- Combining form meaning SOMATIC.

somatoform disorders A class of mental disorders in which there are clear and present physical symptoms that are suggestive of a somatic disorder but no detectable organic damage or neurophysiological dysfunction that can explain them, leading to a strong presumption that they are linked to psychological factors. See AUTONOMIC AROUSAL DISORDER, BODY DYSMORPHIC DISORDER, CONVERSION DISORDER, HYPOCHONDRIASIS, NEURASTHENIA, SOMATIZATION DISORDER and PAIN DISORDERS. Cases with volitional symptoms (e.g. FACTITIOUS DISORDER) are specifically excluded.

somatoform disorder, undifferentiated Quite as it says, a SOMATOFORM DISORDER without a clearly differentiated set of symptoms. The term is used for cases involving physical complaints such as fatigue, loss of appetite, and intestinal and urinary complaints associated with psychological factors of stress and conflict.

somatogenic need Any biological or tissue need, a PRIMARY *NEED.

somatoparaphrenia A general term for a variety of neurological disorders all of which display a delusion about one side of the body. This can range from a disavowal of a specific body part, e.g. the patient refuses to accept that his right leg is, indeed, his, to more complex denials concerning an entire side of the body.

somatopsychic An occasional synonym of PSYCHOSOMATIC.

somatopsychology An approach that explores the psychological factors that accompany medical and physical disabilities. The term is little used these days, the field of study having been tucked under the larger umbrella of HEALTH PSYCHOLOGY.

somatopsychosis 1 Any psychosis the primary symptoms of which involve delusions about one's own body. 2 Any psychosis the mental disorder of which is a symptom of a bodily disease. Both uses are rather loose.

somatosenses Collectively, those sensory systems that mediate the various touch receptors, e.g. pressure, tickle, warm, cold, vibration, limb position, limb movement, pain. Generally classified into the *cutaneous*, the *kinaesthetic* and the *visceral* senses.

somatosensory Pertaining to the SOMATO-SENSES.

somatosensory areas Those cortical areas that respond to stimulation of the SOMATO-SENSES. The *primary* somatosensory areas are located along the POSTCENTRAL GYRUS where the body's sensory system can be mapped. This SOMATOTOPIC REPRESENTATION is contralateral and the distribution of cells devoted to each area of the body corresponds nicely with the overall sensitivity (see HOMUNCULUS (2) for more details.). A *secondary* area is located on the lateral surface of the parietal lobe.

somatosensory system Loosely, the entire system of receptors, afferent pathways, nuclei and cortical areas that are responsible for mediating the SOMATOSENSES. The system arises in the various peripheral receptors that respond to touch, pressure, temperature and positional change; the afferent pathways enter the spinal cord through the dorsal roots, ascend to the thalamus and are relayed to the SOMATOSENSORY AREAS.

somatostatin An inhibitory hormone. It is produced in the hypothalamus, where it inhibits the release of growth hormone, and the pancreas, where it inhibits the secretion of glucagon and insulin.

somatotonia One of the three classic components of temperament assumed by CONSTITUTIONAL THEORY. The somatotonic is characterized by highly developed physical abilities.

somatotopic representation The orderly mapping of the somatic sensory system onto the cerebral cortex. The body surface is represented in a point-by-point fashion along the SOMATOSENSORY AREAS on the postcentral gyrus.

somatotopy See SOMATOTOPIC REPRESENTATION.

somatotrophic hormone GROWTH HORMONE.

somatotype Lit., body type. The term is virtually always found in the context of CONSTITUTIONAL THEORY relating physique to temperament.

some- Var. of SOMA-.

somesthesia SOMAESTHESIA.

somnambulism Sleepwalking. Interestingly, sleepwalking tends to occur during the deepest stages of NREM sleep and not during REM sleep, when most dreaming occurs; see SLEEP for details. If recurrent and disruptive it is classified as a SLEEP DISORDER.

somniferous Sleep-inducing; SOPORIFIC.

sonant A voiced speech sound.

sone The basic unit of a ratio scale of loudness. It is defined as the experienced loudness of a 1,000 Hz tone at 40 db above absolute threshold.

sophistry The deliberate use of nonvalid argument with the intention of deceiving others. Most effective sophistry embeds the fallacy in convoluted syllogistic form, giving it the surface illusion of rigorousness and/or profundity.

soporific Sleep-inducing. Used with respect either to drugs, such as the barbiturates and narcotics, or to boring, dull experiences. syn., *somniferous*.

S–O–R A modification of the early classic S–R characterization of behaviour. Whereas S–R THEORY focused primarily on the stimulus (S) and the resultant (R), the modification explicitly put the organism (O) into the equation.

sororate The custom whereby an unmarried sister of a deceased woman marries the widower.

sorting test A general label for any test or task in which the subject is required to sort stimulus items according to some given principle.

Sotos syndrome A genetic disorder marked by rapid early growth leading to heavy features, a long, large head, a large, protruding jaw, wide-set eyes and large, broad hands. Mild to moderate degrees of mental retardation or other learning problems are typical. Also called *Sotos cerebral gigantism*.

soul Outside of the realm of theology: **1** An obsolete term for psyche or mind. See DUALISM. **2** Popularly, the affective, emotional domain of one's personality as opposed to the analytical, intellectual aspects.

soul-image Jung's term for the remote, unconscious domain of mind which he hypothesized to be composed of the ANIMA and ANIMUS.

sound 1 In physics, a pattern of energy represented as condensation and rarefaction of molecules in an elastic medium. **2** In psychology, that sensory experience resulting from the physical energy in 1 stimulating the auditory and neurological mechanisms of an organism – with the proviso that these mechanisms are sensitive to the frequency and intensity characteristics of the energy: a sound (sense 1) of 40,000 Hz will be a sound (sense 2) for a bat but not for a human. Note that appreciating the distinction here permits one to answer that hoary philosophical puzzle, 'If a tree falls in the forest and there is no one about to hear it, does it make a sound?' For related terms see the following entries, also ACOUSTIC, AUDITORY and combined terms with these as a base.

sound intensity 1 In physics, the power of a sound wave, typically expressed in dynes per square centimetre (dyn./cm^2). **2** In psychological terms, an occasional synonym of LOUDNESS.

sound-level meter A device for measuring the sound level at various frequencies. Such meters do not give 'raw' sound levels but contain weighting networks which adjust the power at each frequency in accordance with the known properties of the spectral sensitivity of the average human ear.

sound-pattern theory (of hearing) THEORIES OF *HEARING.

sound perimetry A procedure for determining the boundaries of the auditory space for an individual subject.

sound-pressure level (SPL) The physical intensity of a sound stimulus as specified against an objective standard. The standard typically used is 0.0002 dyn./cm^2, which corresponds approximately to the absolute threshold of the normal human ear for a 1,000 Hz tone.

sound, sensation level of The pressure level of a sound given in decibels above threshold.

sound shadow A region in a field in which sound is reduced owing to an object which blocks, obscures, absorbs or reflects the physical energy. The sound shadow produced by one's head serves as a cue in the location of sounds of relatively high frequencies.

sound spectrograph The full, proper name for what is more generally referred to as a SPECTROGRAPH.

sour One of the five primary qualities of TASTE (2). It is associated mainly with acids and appears to result from a binding of receptor cells in TASTE BUDS to hydrogen ions in acids.

source 1 Generally, the original location of some process or event. **2** In communication theory, the entity (typically an organism but occasionally a machine) that emits a signal. **3** In psychophysics, the device that puts out a stimulus. **4** In psychoanalysis, the underlying condition that initiates an instinct. **5** In social psychology, the locus of a socially important message, e.g. a rumour, a news story.

source amnesia AMNESIA, SOURCE.

source factors In PERSUASIVE COMMUNICATION, those factors that can be attributed to the source of a message such as the source's credibility, prestige and attractiveness.

source memory MEMORY, SOURCE.

source monitoring Cognitive tracking and storage (see SOURCE *MEMORY) of information about where and when particular events occurred or when and how particular information was acquired.

source, primary An original source of information. In the social sciences, any original document or firsthand report such as a diary, paper or tape recording that provides data for analysis.

source, secondary Any source of information based on a PRIMARY *SOURCE. Secondary sources include reviews, interpretations, revisions and summaries of primary sources.

source trait TRAIT, SOURCE.

sour-grapes mechanism From Aesop and his famous fox, a term used to characterize a defence mechanism whereby one devalues goals which one cannot obtain.

space 1 Fundamentally, space is an abstraction, a geometric characterization of a system of location of *m* objects in *n* dimensions. In the classic model of physical space, *m* is finite and *n* = 3. This so-called *Euclidean space* is such a compelling aspect of human experience that it has often been presented as a nativistically given form and *space* is often taken as denotatively equivalent to Euclidean space. However, such a limitation is inappropriate: any mathematical representation of *m* objects in *n* dimensions will satisfy the definition, and although it may not be as natural, one can conceptualize and formalize a two-dimensional plane space, a spherical space, a saddle-shaped space, etc. **2** In social psychology and environmental psychology, the experiential space in which one lives and functions. This sense of space is often contrasted with the raw physical space in the classical Euclidean sense; see e.g. PERSONAL SPACE. **3** In factor analysis, the conceptual space containing all the factors that emerge from the data analysis. This meaning is usually expressed by the phrase *factor space* to keep it distinct from other senses. See FACTOR ANALYSIS et seq. for details. **4** In multidimensional scaling, an abstract representation of an *n*-dimensional space that characterizes the hypothetical psychological character of the stimuli being scaled. For details, see MULTIDIMENSIONAL SCALING and METHODS OF *SCALING (3). Note that in senses 3 and 4 the number of dimensions may, and typically does, exceed three and the formal representation need not be, and typically is not, Euclidean. See, for a common example, SEMANTIC SPACE. **5** In K. Lewin's field theory, the representation of an individual in terms of a topologically complex LIFE SPACE (see which for details). **6** The area around something. **7** The distance between two things. adj., *spatial*.

spaced practice PRACTICE, DISTRIBUTED.

space error (or **bias**) Generally, any systematic bias in choice behaviour, discrimination learning, maze learning, etc. toward some spatial location or direction. Also called *location error* (or *bias*).

space factor A hypothesized underlying factor which presumably is what accounts for the several SPATIAL ABILITIES.

space perception Quite straightforwardly, the perception of SPACE (typically 1 and 2). The reference can be to either the physical

space surrounding an individual or the more subjective, experienced sense of space within which one behaves. The term is, thus, used rather freely to cover depth perception, spatial relations, real movement, apparent movement, personal space, etc.

space psychology The application of psychological principles and methods to the study of space-related issues. Much of the work involves extensions of the techniques of personnel selection and the study of human factors in the highly specialized circumstances surrounding space flight and living in outer space.

spandrel In evolutionary psychology and biology, a trait or function that derives its adaptive value from being linked with other traits or functions. That is, a trait that did not itself evolve because it had a specific adaptive role, but because it was a necessary consequence of other forms that did have adaptive functions. The term was introduced by S. J. Gould and R. Lewontin as a metaphor. They took the term from architecture, where spandrels are surfaces between arches that are there, not because they have any role to play, but because they are a necessary consequence of the physical form of arches. See EXAPTATION for more detail.

span of apprehension APPREHENSION, SPAN OF.

span of attention ATTENTION SPAN.

span of consciousness An obsolete term for the number of objects that can be apprehended simultaneously. For a more contemporary point of view on this topic, see SEVEN PLUS OR MINUS TWO, SHORT-TERM *MEMORY and SUBITIZING.

spasm Generally, any sudden, convulsive muscular movement. Spasms may be *clonic* (alternating contraction and relaxation) or *tonic* (continuous contraction); and they may involve skeletal (striated) muscle or visceral (smooth) muscle.

spasmophemia Any speech disorder caused by spasms. Occasionally used as a synonym of *stuttering*.

spastic 1 Pertaining to or resembling a spasm. **2** Characteristic of a disability caused by spasms. **3** A person suffering from any disorder with spasms as a primary symptom, e.g. cerebral palsy. This last meaning is not recommended as this sense of the term has taken on insulting connotations.

spasticity PARALYSIS.

spastic paralysis PARALYSIS.

spastic speech The erratic, jerky speech of persons with spastic conditions of the muscles involved in speech production.

spatial Pertaining to *space*. For combined terms not found below, see those following SPACE.

spatial abilities Those perceptual/cognitive abilities that enable one to deal effectively with spatial relations, visual-spatial tasks, orientation of objects in space, etc. Frequently *visual* and *nonvisual* spatial abilities are distinguished.

spatial cognition A loose term used to refer to the general ability to find one's way in a complex environment.

spatial discrimination 1 Loosely, the capacity to distinguish between the locations of objects in a spatial array. **2** In older texts, a somewhat confusing term for the ability to detect two disparate points of stimulation on the skin. See here TWO-POINT THRESHOLD.

spatial disorders A loose group of neurological disorders that impair an individual's capacity to deal with situations that call on spatial representation, judgement, orientation and memory, e.g. CONSTRUCTIONAL *APRAXIA.

spatial frequency See FREQUENCY (3).

spatial memory MEMORY, SPATIAL.

spatial neglect A form of NEGLECT where the disability is primarily in dealing with spatial information. In a typical case the patient may be unaware of an individual approaching from the left or be unable to image an object in the left visual field (neglect is virtually always a right hemisphere disorder).

spatial orientation 1 The ability to orient oneself in space relative to objects and events. See here FIELD DEPENDENCE. **2** Awareness of self-location.

spatial summation SUMMATION, SPATIAL.

spatial threshold TWO-POINT THRESHOLD.

spay To sterilize a female animal by ovariectomy.

speaking in tongues GLOSSOLALIA.

Spearman–Brown formula 1 A technique for predicting the reliability of a full test made up of two separate subtests when the reliability of each of the subtests is known. **2** A technique for estimating the gain in reliability of a measure with an increase in the number of observations. Occasionally called the *Spearman Brown prophecy formula* (for 1).

Spearman rank correlation CORRELATION, RANK-ORDER.

special-aptitude test APTITUDE TEST.

special case 1 Generally, any instance in a category that somehow stands out from the others. **2** Any exemplar of a category isolated for special treatment or analysis for some particular reason.

special child A child with emotional, social, physical or mental problems. The term has been adopted by many as the euphemism of choice for a handicapped, retarded or autistic child. Occasionally confusion is created, for some authors also use the term to refer to a child who is well above the average or shows special talents, while others use GIFTED CHILD for such cases. See also EXCEPTIONAL CHILD, the other common euphemism, which suffers from similar problems. Currently, the favoured term seems to be *child with special needs*.

special class (or **school**) SPECIAL EDUCATION.

special education 1 The area within the field of educational psychology that is concerned with the SPECIAL CHILD. Some aspects are highly theoretical and focus on issues of cognitive and perceptual competence: other components are more applied and focus on the problems of education. **2** Loosely, any educational programme, class or school for the education of special children.

special factor(s) GENERAL FACTOR.

special sense SENSE, SPECIAL.

speciation The process of the emergence of a new species.

species 1 In biology, a classification immediately below GENUS (1). It is the smallest category commonly used and is generally (and rather loosely) identified on the grounds of commonality or mutual resemblance of organisms. When possible, the criterion of the ability to mate among themselves and produce viable and fertile offspring is used. Thus, species is treated as a category of organisms that forms a reproductively isolated group the genes of which are freely admixed but not with those of other species. This criterion, however, cannot always be applied. It often fails with species of bacteria and various plants and when two species are genetically closely related. pl., *species*. **2** In Aristotelian logic, a category or class that differs from other categories within a larger class or GENUS (2) with regard to specified characteristics. When the terms *species* and *genus* are used in this fashion they carry no biological implications, although it is clear that the biological meaning derives from the Aristotelian.

species-specific adj. Of the behaviour of virtually all the members of a given species under roughly equivalent circumstances. The term is used to characterize those behaviours of a given species that are specific to that species, and approximates to the original usage of the more common term INSTINCT. However, see that term for nuances in usage and problems with connotations, and note that as is outlined there, many contemporary authorities prefer *species-specific* and its synonym *species-typical* and have dropped *instinct* from their technical lexicons. Although the term, like *instinct*, tends to carry the connotation of innateness, such an inference is not logically implied.

species-typical SPECIES-SPECIFIC.

specific 1 Pertaining to a SPECIES. **2** Distinctive, outstanding, highly detectable. **3** By extension, in factor analysis, uncorrelated with other things or factors. **4** Relating to a particular subject; peculiar.

specific ability In theory, any ability that is specific to a particular kind of task; in practice, any ability that is identified by factor-analytic techniques as one that shows little or no correlation with other abilities. Compare with GENERAL ABILITY.

specific developmental disorder DEVELOPMENTAL DISORDER, SPECIFIC but note that in

the most recent edition of the *DSM*, these disorders are classified as either COMMUNICATION DISORDERS or LEARNING DISORDERS.

specific developmental dyslexia DYSLEXIA.

specific energies doctrine SPECIFIC NERVE ENERGIES, DOCTRINE OF.

specific phobia SIMPLE *PHOBIA.

specific hunger HUNGER, SPECIFIC.

specificity 1 Preciseness, uniqueness. The term is used in this sense with the connotation that a thing characterized as possessing this quality is relevant to but a single phenomenon or event. For example, stimuli are said to display specificity when they are only associated with a single response, adaptive structures show specificity when their functions have not generalized beyond specific boundaries. **2** In sociology, a narrow pattern of expected behaviour in a particular situation; specificity is displayed when only a small aspect of one's full social role emerges in a given social context. **3** In factor analysis, the proportion of the variance not correlated with the main factors. **4** In epidemiology, the correct classification of cases that do not have a particular disease or condition, expressed as the probability that one will be identified as not having a condition when, in fact, one does not have that condition.

specific language disability LANGUAGE DISABILITY.

specific learning disability A synonym of LEARNING DISABILITY. The 'specific' was added because in many cases the problems only emerge in particular circumstances. For example, a child may experience difficulties in learning to read but have no problems with arithmetic.

specific nerve energies, doctrine of The generalization originally put forward by Johannes Müller that the various qualities of experience derive not from differences in the physical and environmental stimuli that impinge upon us but from the specific neural structures that each excites.

specious present The psychological sense of the present, of 'nowness'. This notion of a true *present* in the measurement of time has about the same status as the notion of a *point* on a line or in space does in geometry: it exists as a locus relative to other loci. It is the point that divides past from future, what has happened from what is still to happen. Yet, introspectively, this is not very satisfying, nor does it feel intuitively correct: this 'timeless moment', as it has been called, seems to have temporal duration – brief, perhaps, but most palpable.

SPECT SINGLE PHOTON EMISSION COMPUTER TOMOGRAPHY.

spectator effects Collectively, the various effects that spectators can produce on individual behaviour. Generally, when the actions to be carried out are well-learned and the individual is confident in his or her abilities, the presence of spectators is positive, producing SOCIAL FACILITATION; lack of skill or low confidence usually has the opposite effect, SOCIAL INHIBITION. Also called *audience effects*.

spectral Pertaining to or related to a SPECTRUM.

spectral-absorption curve A curve of the relative absorption of each wavelength of light for the particular substance under examination.

spectral colour The colour or (more accurately) the *hue* of any visual stimulus the dominant wavelength of which is within the visible spectrum.

spectral-emission curve In optics, a curve showing the relative number of quanta emitted by a light source as a function of wavelength.

spectral hue SPECTRAL COLOUR.

spectral-sensitivity curve A curve that displays the sensitivity of a receptor system across the full range of a particular spectrum. Such a curve for the human auditory system, for example, would show a peak sensitivity around 4,000 Hz, with diminishing sensitivity for higher- and lower-pitched tones. For the visual system there would be several distinct curves, corresponding to the ABSORPTION *SPECTRUM of each PHOTOPIGMENT.

spectro- Combining form meaning *appearance, image*.

spectrograph A device that provides a vis-

ual representation of sound. The resultant *spectrogram* is a display that presents all three acoustic dimensions of sound: *time* is represented on one axis of a two-dimensional display, *frequency* is given on the other, and the *intensity* of the sound at each frequency and point in time is represented by the darkness of the display (see FORMANT). Spectrographic analyses are primarily used in the study of speech production and perception. Their use in courts of law has created a lively controversy, with proponents arguing that *voiceprints* (as they are often called) can be used to identify individuals, and critics maintaining that the procedures lack reliability. So far the critics' case appears the stronger and few courts permit their use.

spectrophotometer In vision, a device for determining the ABSORPTION *SPECTRUM of a translucent substance.

spectrum Generally, a range of components of some energy source (e.g. a light wave, a sound wave) separated and arranged along some dimension (e.g. wavelength, frequency). Note that there is a strong tendency to use this term as though it pertained only to the physical dimension of radiant energy and the visual modality. This restriction is not accurate, although properly the term should be used with qualifiers to specify the particular spectrum under consideration, e.g. ABSORPTION *SPECTRUM, AUDITORY *SPECTRUM, VISUAL *SPECTRUM, pl., *spectra* (preferred) or *spectrums*.

spectrum, absorption In optics, the proportion of incident light absorbed by a body as a function of wavelength; see SPECTRAL-ABSORPTION CURVE.

spectrum, auditory The sound frequencies that are within the normal range of human hearing, i.e. those ranging from approximately 20 Hz to roughly 20,000 Hz.

spectrum, reflection In optics, the proportion of incident light reflected off of a body as a function of wavelength.

spectrum, visual (or **visible**) The wavelengths of light to which the normal human eye is sensitive, i.e. those ranging from approximately 380 nm to roughly 740 nm.

speculative psychology An approach to psychology that begins with empirical studies and known facts about behaviour and proceeds in an attempt to elaborate a speculative conceptualization of the nature of the human mind or the human condition. As an accepted discipline in psychology it has few self-proclaimed practitioners; as an unacknowledged practice it lurks, often unrecognized, behind nearly every theoretical advance in the field – despite the publicly articulated allegiances to pure formalisms, positivisms, hypothetico-deductivisms, logical behaviourisms and the like.

speech act An occurrence of an utterance in a language such that the person who utters it can be viewed as intending, with his or her words, to communicate something, to make something happen or to get someone to do something. Common speech acts are COMMISSIVES, DECLARATIVES, DIRECTIVES, EXPRESSIVES and REPRESENTATIVES; see each for details. The study of speech acts is usually regarded as part of the larger field of PRAGMATICS. syn., *illocutionary act.*

speech block A momentary inability to speak, a form of *stuttering.*

speech centre BROCA'S AREA.

speech disorder A cover term for a number of abnormalities in speaking. There is precious little agreement on exactly which language disabilities belong in this category and how they should be classified. Some authorities differentiate between *functional* or *psychogenic disorders* (e.g. many cases of STUTTERING) and those with an organic basis (e.g. the APHASIAS); some distinguish between those that affect linguistic functioning (e.g. DYSARTHRIA) and those that affect voice quality without disturbing communicative performance (e.g. the VOICE DISORDERS); and some keep the language-reception abnormalities (e.g. ALEXIA) in a separate diagnostic category whereas others include them, arguing that pure receptive disabilities showing no deficit in language production are rare.

speech disorder, acquired Any speech disorder that appears as a result of some event occurring after birth, e.g. an APHASIA.

speech disorder, congenital Any speech disorder due to an abnormal condition present at birth, e.g. as associated with cerebral palsy or a cleft palate.

speech impediment Loosely, anything that disrupts, inhibits or prevents normal fluent speech.

speech-retarded child A child who learns to speak at a later age than the norm. Note that the retardation is a literal slowing and the term *retarded* carries no connotations concerning eventual levels of performance: the typical child ultimately shows normal language ability but achieves it relatively late. The preferred terms are *speech-delayed child* and *child with language delays.*

speech synthesizer Any machine that can produce intelligible, speech-like sounds. The output of such a device is called *synthetic speech*, and recent advances in computer technology and acoustics have seen the development of sophisticated synthesizers with a quality of speech sufficiently 'human' for use in generating stimuli for many experiments on language and hearing as well (alas) as for wide application in business and industry.

speech therapy Loosely, any therapy aimed at correcting a speech disorder.

speed/accuracy trade-off The generalization that when speed is of the essence accuracy decreases and vice versa, hence there is a trade-off in functioning between them.

speed reading Since the average fluent reader reads somewhere between 100 and 140 words per minute (depending on the nature of the material), speed reading is defined simply as reading at rates significantly in excess of these norms. An issue of interest here (particularly in view of the popular and expensive programmes that claim to teach this skill) is whether such rapid rates can be achieved without sacrificing comprehension. The problem is a complex one but the evidence available indicates that they cannot.

speed test A general term for any test that measures ability by determining the number of problems that can be dealt with successfully within a fixed time period. Also called *speeded test*. Compare with POWER TEST.

spelling dyslexia DYSLEXIA, WORD-FORM.

sperm 1 Semen, the male ejaculant containing spermatozoa. **2** Spermatozoa, the mature male sex cells.

spermatozoa The plural of SPERMATOZOON.

spermatozoon A mature, male sex cell.

spheraesthesia Occasional synonym of GLOBUS HYSTERICUS. var., *spheresthesia*.

spherical aberration ABERRATION, SPHERICAL.

sphincter Any circular muscle which constricts during muscular contraction, thereby closing an orifice.

sphincter control Control over the sphincter muscles of the urinary and anal passages.

sphincter morality A psychoanalytic term for a pattern of attitudes and behaviour hypothesized to result from early, abrupt toilet training.

sphygmo- A combining form meaning *pulse*.

sphygmograph A device for measuring and recording the shape and force of the pulse.

sphygmomanometer A device for measuring arterial blood pressure.

sphygmometer SPHYGMOGRAPH.

spicy A class of olfactory qualities typified by spices. Early researchers (see HENNING'S PRISM) included it as a component of the gustatory sense; current physiological models of TASTE (2) do not, treating it simply as a mark of highly flavoured foods.

spike In the recording of the electrical activity of a neuron, the conspicuous tracing that is indicative of the rapid reversal of membrane potential of the ACTION POTENTIAL. Or, put more simply, the sharp peak in the record that indicates that the neuron has fired.

spina bifida See NEURAL-TUBE DEFECTS.

spinal Pertaining to or characteristic of the backbone (the spine) or the spinal cord.

spinal accessory nerve The XIth CRANIAL NERVE. A motor nerve to the trapezius and sternomastoid muscles of the neck and the pharynx. The accessory portion joins the vagus (Xth cranial) nerve supplying motor and cardioinhibitory fibres.

spinal animal An experimental preparation in which the neural pathways between the spinal cord and the brain have been severed. In such an animal, whatever control still exists over the muscles and sensory receptors of the periphery is that which is mediated by the spinal cord alone.

spinal canal The canal, containing cerebrospinal fluids, that runs through the vertebral column.

spinal column The vertebral column, more commonly referred to as the *backbone*. It encloses the spinal cord and consists of 33 vertebrae: 7 cervical, 12 thoracic, 5 lumbar, 5 sacral (fused to form a single bone) and 4 in the coccyx (also fused to form one bone).

spinal cord The long column of neural tissue running through the spinal canal from the 2nd lumbar vertebra up to the medulla.

spinal fluid CEREBROSPINAL FLUID.

spinal ganglia Enlargements on the dorsal root of each spinal nerve made up principally of the cell bodies of somatic and visceral afferent neurons.

spinal nerves Nerves arising from the spinal cord. In *Homo sapiens* there are 31 pairs: 8 cervical, 12 thoracic, 5 lumbar, 5 sacral and 1 coccygeal. Each is attached to the cord by two SPINAL ROOTS, one dorsal (or posterior) and one ventral (or anterior).

spinal reflex Any reflex mediated entirely at the spinal level. A spinal reflex can be elicited even in a SPINAL ANIMAL, in which the controlling influence of the brain has been removed.

spinal root Collections of neural fibres through which the SPINAL NERVES are attached to the spinal cord. Spinal roots occur in pairs: the *dorsal root* of each pair carries afferent fibres, the *ventral root* carries efferent fibres. Each pair fuses to form one of the spinal nerves.

spindle tendon GOLGI TENDON ORGAN.

spinocerebellum PALEOCEREBELLUM.

spinoreticulothalamic tract SPINOTHALA-MIC TRACT.

spinothalamic tract (or **system**) A complex ascending neural pathway that runs through the spinal cord to the thalamus.

Actually the term is slightly misleading, for in reality only a small proportion of the fibres ascend directly to the thalamus, most of them synapsing at lower levels in the brainstem, specifically in the reticular formation. See RETICULOTHALAMIC TRACT. The pathway is a major carrier of pain fibres from the periphery. Also called *spinoreticulothalamic tract*.

spiral aftereffect MOTION AFTEREFFECTS.

spiral ganglion A spiral-shaped collection of myelinated bipolar neurons located in the bony hub of the cochlea. The axonal processes of these cells run toward the organ of Corti and innervate the hair cells.

spiral test Generally, any psychometric instrument in which the several kinds of item (e.g. quantitative, verbal, general knowledge) are presented in a repeating series in which each new cycle 'spirals' upwards in difficulty.

spirometer A device for measuring breathing.

SPL SOUND-PRESSURE LEVEL.

splanchic Pertaining to the viscera.

split-brain technique The severing of the CORPUS CALLOSUM (and, on occasion, the OPTIC CHIASM), thus eliminating the exchange of information between the cerebral hemispheres. The procedure is used in humans only in cases of severe and intractable epilepsy. Those who have undergone the operation serve as natural laboratories for the study of LATERALITY.

split-half correlation CORRELATION, SPLIT-HALF.

split-half reliability RELIABILITY, SPLIT-HALF.

split-litter method A control procedure in which litter mates are divided into experimental and control groups. It serves as a partial control over genetic factors and has advantages over random assignment of either individual animals or whole litters to different groups.

split-off consciousness William James's term for those aspects of consciousness which are relatively well organized and structured but exist more or less independently of the rest of consciousness. The term is rarely used today.

split personality See DISSOCIATIVE IDENTITY DISORDER and MULTIPLE PERSONALITY.

splitting A defence mechanism whereby one deals with conflict and stress by compartmentalizing (i.e. splitting) the positive and negative aspects of oneself or others. Use of the mechanism is marked by a tendency to view oneself and others in alternating polar opposites, switching back and forth between highly positive and highly negative images.

spongioblast A cell that develops from the embryonic neural tube and is a forerunner of ependymal cells and astrocytes. See here GLIA.

spontaneity test Moreno's term for that aspect of a PSYCHODRAMA in which the individual is in a very life-like situation and must spontaneously act out feelings with respect to the others present.

spontaneity therapy A general label occasionally applied to J. L. Moreno's PSYCHODRAMA procedures, which emphasize roleplaying, emotional expression, empathy, etc.

spontaneous 1 Natural, unconstrained. 2 Not premeditated. 3 From within, endogenous, personal.

spontaneous discharge Generally, any neural impulse not directly initiated by a known external stimulus. Also called *spontaneous firing*.

spontaneous memory See INVOLUNTARY *MEMORY.

spontaneous recovery The reappearance of an extinguished conditioned response following a rest period.

spontaneous regression Sudden age regression in which the individual relives poignant memories of childhood.

spontaneous remission The lessening or abatement of the symptoms of a disease or disorder independent of any therapeutic intervention. See REMISSION.

spoonerism The exchanging of the initial phonetic elements of two (or more) words in a single phrase or sentence. The term honours the Rev. W. A. Spooner of Oxford, who had a rather extraordinary penchant for such confusions. Of the countless incidents attributed to the good reverend, our favourites are his attempted reference to Victoria Regina as 'our queer old dean', and his tongue-lashing of an inattentive student, 'You have tasted the whole worm.'

sport (and **exercise**) **psychology** A branch of psychology concerned (obviously) with sport and exercise. It is a diverse field with elements that incorporate the study of personality, social psychology, motor function, imagery, kinesiology, physiology and genetics and has applications in education, the study of childhood and clinical psychology.

SPR Abbreviation for *skin potential response*. See GALVANIC SKIN RESPONSE.

spreading activation 1 In cognitive psychology, the tendency for the activation of a memory to spread to conceptually associated memories, making them likely to be themselves activated. 2 In neurophysiology, a hypothesized set of neural processes that, in principle, underlies the kinds of effects given in 1.

spreading depression The phenomenon of a stimulus applied directly to the surface of the cortex producing a depression of electrical activity that spreads from the locus of stimulation and inhibits cortical responses to other stimuli.

spread of effect EFFECT, SPREAD OF.

spurious 1 Not genuine, not authentic. 2 Having superficial resemblance to something but with deeper, more important differences.

spurious correlation CORRELATION, SPURIOUS.

spurt Generally, any sudden increase in performance, growth, learning, etc.

SQ 3R method A reading/study method based on the presumption that information from a text can best be learned by *S*urveying the material first, *Q*uestioning the basic issues, *R*eading thoroughly, *R*eciting the basic points and then *R*eviewing the material once more.

SQUID SUPERCONDUCTING QUANTUM INTERFACE DEVICE.

squint STRABISMUS.

S–R STIMULUS–RESPONSE.

S–R learning LEARNING, S–R.

S–R psychology STIMULUS–RESPONSE PSYCHOLOGY.

SRR Abbreviation for *skin resistance response*. See GALVANIC SKIN RESPONSE.

S–R theory STIMULUS–RESPONSE THEORY.

SRT task An abbreviation for *sequential reaction time task*, in which participants are asked to respond as quickly as possible (usually by pressing a button on a panel) to each of a series of stimuli (typically a light flashing at one of several locations on a computer monitor). In the classic experiment, the sequence of lights follows a complex pattern. Learning is revealed by a systematic reduction in RTs to successive lights as subjects learn to anticipate the location of upcoming events. The procedure is commonly used in the study of IMPLICIT *LEARNING.

SS STANDARD *SCORE.

S-shaped curve OGIVE.

S–S interval TEMPORAL AVOIDANCE CONDITIONING.

S–S learning LEARNING, S–S.

S sleep SLEEP, S.

SSREs SELECTIVE SEROTONIN REUPTAKE ENHANCERS.

SSRI discontinuance (withdrawal, cessation) syndrome A syndrome that occurs within one week of discontinuance or reduction of SELECTIVE SEROTONIN REUPTAKE INHIBITORS. Symptoms range from the inconsequential (e.g. dry mouth) through the disconcerting (dizziness, rapid weight gain) to the alarming (suicidal thoughts). Individual expression is highly variable. Symptoms can be avoided by gradual tapering of medication. If experienced, symptoms generally ameliorate within a few weeks, although cases persisting for over a year are not unknown.

SSRIs SELECTIVE SEROTONIN REUPTAKE INHIBITORS.

SST STIMULUS-SAMPLING THEORY.

stabilimeter A device for measuring stability. It measures bodily sway while the subject, who is usually blindfolded, attempts to stand perfectly still.

stability 1 In physics, the relative lack of motion of a body compared with the motion of the surroundings. **2** In genetics, the relative invariances in genetically determined factors over generations. **3** In personality theory, a trait characterized by a lack of excessive emotional change. Here the qualifier *emotional* is often used. **4** In statistics, the reliability and consistency of a statistic. See STATISTICAL STABILITY. **5** In psychometrics, long-term TEST–RETEST *RELIABILITY where 'long-term' typically means test–retest gaps of months or even years.

stability, coefficient of COEFFICIENT OF *RELIABILITY, TEST–RETEST *RELIABILITY.

stabilized (retinal) image An image (or, more properly, a proximal stimulus) that has been stabilized or fixed so that it falls on the same spot on the retina regardless of the movements of the eye (see NYSTAGMUS and SACCADE for characterizations of these). There are several techniques for accomplishing this. One common one is to provide the subject with a contact lens with a small mirror attached; the stimulus is reflected off the mirror onto a screen via a series of other mirrors which control orientation. The resulting image is stabilized because no matter how the eye moves the image also moves and the area of the retina onto which the stimulus is projected is fixed. Under these conditions the perception fades rapidly, presumably from fatigue of the retinal receptors. Also called *stabilized retinal image, fixed image* and *stopped image.*

stable **1** Characterizing an individual whose behaviour is relatively reliable and consistent. ant., *unstable* (1, 2). **2** Characterizing a statistical result which is significant. See STATISTICAL STABILITY.

stage An identifiable period in an extended, ongoing process; specifically, one that appears to have its own internal coherence and so stands out from other, similarly identifiable periods. Compare with LEVEL, which is reserved for a particular point in the process or on a continuum, and with PHASE, which connotes cyclicity.

stages of man In Erik Erikson's characterization of personality, the life of man (generically speaking) is viewed as a sequence of eight periods during which an individual either resolves or fails to resolve a characteristic set of behavioural and emotional issues.

Each stage is conceptualized as an either/or configuration, reflecting Erikson's notion that at any point in one's life one may or may not be strong enough to accept the potential hazards of the current stage. The stages are: (1) trust vs. mistrust, (2) autonomy vs. shame and doubt, (3) initiative vs. guilt, (4) industry vs. inferiority, (5) identity vs. role diffusion, (6) intimacy vs. isolation, (7) generativity vs. stagnation, (8) ego integrity vs. despair. The first four correspond roughly to the Freudian stages up to adolescence, stage 5 encompasses late adolescence and early adulthood, stage 6 is the so-called 'prime of life' period, 7 corresponds to middle age and the last to old age.

stages of sleep SLEEP.

stage theory A label applicable to any theory of development that characterizes growth, be it physical, sensorimotor, cognitive, moral, etc., as a progression through a sequence of stages. Stage theories tend to be either *maturational* or *interactionist*, i.e. they view growth as basically biologically determined or as resulting from interactions between the biological and the experiential. Standard criteria of scientific adequacy dictate that a stage theory have at least four critical properties. First, it must predict qualitative differences in behaviour over time and with experience. Second, it must assume invariance of the sequence of stages – the rate of sequencing may be accelerated or retarded but the order must remain the same from individual to individual. Third, it must assume structural cohesiveness of a stage; that is, the behaviours within a stage must share a common conceptual base. Fourth, there must be hierarchical integration of structures from stage to stage so that a later stage incorporates and expands upon the structures from an earlier stage. Exemplary theories here are Gesell's for sensorimotor development, Piaget's for cognitive development, Kohlberg's for the development of morality and, somewhat more loosely, Freud's theory of psychosexual development and Erikson's stages of man.

stain To apply a pigment to tissue for histological examination.

staircase illusion As depicted on p. 768. Stare at the figure: the perspective will reverse so that the staircase will be seen from above or from below. Also called *Schröder's staircase*.

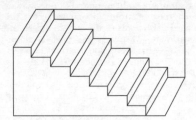

staircase method UP-AND-DOWN METHOD.

staircase phenomenon TREPPE.

stammering STUTTERING.

stance reflex A general term for the variety of postural adjustments, taken collectively, that an organism makes to maintain proper orientation and normal stance.

standard 1 Generally, a basis for comparison for making evaluative judgements or measurements. **2** In physics, a fixed unit for standardizing international scientific measurement, e.g. a standard metre, a standard candle. **3** In scaling, an arbitrary stimulus that serves as the basis for making estimates of psychological magnitudes; see METHODS OF *SCALING. **4** In the social sciences generally, any socially agreed-upon and expected behaviour within a society. Distinguish from NORM.

standard deviation DEVIATION, STANDARD.

standard difference The difference between two means divided by the standard error of that difference. Also called the *standard ratio*.

Standard English In the USA, the idealized form of spoken American English. References to Standard English are found primarily as a basis for comparison with other dialects, e.g. BLACK AMERICAN ENGLISH. Perhaps the only time, however, that one hears true Standard English spoken is by trained elocutionists and some radio and TV commentators. See also KING'S ENGLISH and RECEIVED PRONUNCIATION for similar terms used in Britain.

standard error The standard deviation of a theoretical sampling distribution. It provides an estimate of the variability which can be expected in the actual samples drawn from the underlying theoretical population and is, thus, a population PARAMETER. See also STANDARD ERROR OF THE MEAN. abbrev., *SE*.

standard error of estimate An estimate of the degree of error likely to occur when one uses a regression equation to predict (or estimate) the values of one variable from the values of another correlated variable. It is derived from a formula based on the standard deviation of the dependent (or predicted) variable, the correlation coefficient between the two variables and the size of the sample. The chances are about 0.67 that any actual value will lie within one standard error of its predicted value.

standard error of measurement An estimate of the degree to which a particular set of measurements obtained in a given situation (e.g. a test or one of several parallel forms of a test) might be expected to deviate from the true values. Denoted $\sigma_{(M)}$ or SE_M.

standard error of the mean The standard deviation of the theoretical sampling distribution of the mean. In practice it is used as an estimate of the degree to which the obtained mean of a sample may be expected to deviate from the true population mean. Denoted σ_M.

standardization The processes and procedures of finalizing a test and establishing a set of norms for a test.

standardization group A selected group of persons used to develop and/or STANDARDIZE (3) a test during the *try-out* phase of test development. Whether this group ends up as the *norm group* depends on the degree of change that needs to be made before the test is finalized.

standardize 1 Generally, to adjust something so that it is brought into some standard frame of reference; see e.g. STANDARD *SCORE. **2** To establish a set of norms or standards. **3** In testing, to establish the set of procedures for the administration of a particular test, the scoring techniques to be used and the methods of evaluation and interpretation of obtained scores.

standardized test TEST, STANDARDIZED.

standard measure STANDARD *SCORE.

standard observer In the study of sensory

statistical dependence

processes and perception, the hypothetical observer whose sensory receptor systems function ideally.

standard ratio STANDARD DIFFERENCE.

standard score SCORE, STANDARD.

standard stimulus STANDARD (3).

Stanford–Binet Scale (or **Test**) The first test of intelligence known by this name was the one prepared by L. M. Terman and his associates at Stanford University in 1916. It was designed to be a revision of the Binet–Simon Scale of 1911 (see BINET SCALE) for American culture and language, but it introduced so many changes that it was essentially a new test. Several revisions have appeared over the years which incorporate a large number of modifications, including extensive norms and the scales for measuring adult IQ.

stanine From *standard nine*, a statistical unit representing exactly one ninth of the full range of scores in a distribution.

stapedius muscle A muscle in the ear attached to the *stapes*. It contracts as a response to loud noises, pulling the stapes away from the oval window and thereby dampening the vibration passed on to the receptive cells in the inner ear. Spasms of this muscle can cause TINNITUS. Also called *stapedial muscle*.

stapes One of the AUDITORY *OSSICLES.

startle reflex STARTLE RESPONSE.

startle response (or **reaction**) A complex, involuntary reaction to a sudden, unanticipated stimulus. There is a flexion of most skeletal muscles and a variety of visceral and hormonal reactions. Occasionally it is called the *startle reflex*, although, except in newborns, the magnitude and patterned complexity of the reaction make this term somewhat inappropriate.

stasis A stable, unchanging state. adj., *static*.

state 1 A condition of a system in which the essential qualities are relatively stable. Note that it is the *qualities* of features that are unchanging; the features themselves may, in actuality, be dynamic. Thus, references to a *hyperactive state* or a *state of flux* are not uncommon. 2 A form of organized society with legitimate sovereignty over a geographical area, political authority and a central government.

state anxiety See TRAIT *ANXIETY.

state-dependent learning LEARNING, STATE-DEPENDENT.

state-dependent memory MEMORY, STATE-DEPENDENT.

static Stable, unchanging. Contrast with DYNAMIC.

static ataxia ATAXIA, STATIC.

static equilibrium A stable, unchanging condition.

static reflex (or **response**) Any posture-adjusting or orienting response. The *stance reflex* maintains proper posture under normal conditions, the *righting reflex* regains normal posture; both are examples of a static reflex.

static sense EQUILIBRIUM (2).

statistic 1 Generally, any value derived from mathematical or statistical manipulations. 2 More specifically, a value summarizing a characteristic of a sample and theoretically reflecting the population from which the sample was drawn; e.g. a sample mean, which is an estimate of the true population mean, is a statistic. The population mean is a PARAMETER (2). adj., *statistical*.

statistical artifact ARTIFACT, STATISTICAL.

statistical association Any statistical relationship between two or more variables such that change in one is accompanied by change(s) in the other(s). Such associations are captured by correlational analyses; see CORRELATION et seq.

statistical attenuation A term used to refer to the fact that all correlations based on sample data are theoretically reduced (i.e. attenuated) to some extent through errors of measurement. There are procedures for estimating the size of the attenuation and thus for estimating the maximum true correlations that theoretically could exist in the population under consideration.

statistical control CONTROL, STATISTICAL.

statistical dependence DEPENDENCE (1).

statistical error A general term for any inaccuracy in the sampling, recording or analysis of data. Large statistical errors can make it impossible to draw valid conclusions.

statistical inference The process of drawing generalizations about a population on the basis of sample data. See INFERENTIAL *STATISTICS.

statistical interaction INTERACTION.

statistical law LAW, STATISTICAL.

statistical learning LEARNING, STATISTICAL.

statistical-learning theory A term introduced in the early 1950s by W.K. Estes to cover a variety of attempts to formulate and quantify basic principles of learning theory. See e.g. STIMULUS-SAMPLING THEORY.

statistical power POWER OF A TEST, STATISTICAL.

statistical psychology An obsolescent term for the use of statistics and statistical principles to derive general laws and principles in psychology. Note, the term does not refer to the use of statistics to evaluate empirical data for the purpose of testing hypotheses. The broader term MATHEMATICAL PSYCHOLOGY now encompasses this field.

statistical significance The degree to which an obtained result is sufficiently unlikely to have occurred under the assumption that only chance factors were operating, and therefore the degree to which it may be attributed to systematic manipulations. The degree itself is typically specified and denoted as a probability; e.g. $p < 0.05$ means that the results obtained (or more extreme results) could only have occurred by chance in fewer than 5 cases in 100. The smaller the p value, the more significant the results; that is, the less likely that they occurred by chance. See SIGNIFICANCE LEVEL.

statistical stability An occasional synonym of STATISTICAL SIGNIFICANCE. The connotation of the term is that any statistically significant result is stable, in the sense that if the experiment were repeated one could confidently expect similar results.

statistical test Any procedure whereby sample data are evaluated statistically to determine an estimate of the probable truth of a hypothesis about a population.

statistics 1 Very generally, the branch of mathematics, pure and applied, which deals with collecting, classifying and analysing data. **2** Sets of procedures developed to describe and analyse particular types of data and enable a researcher to draw various kinds of conclusions on the basis of those data. This sense is the one commonly found with qualifiers that identify the specific class of statistics under consideration, e.g. *descriptive statistics*, *inferential statistics*. The most often used in psychology are given below. **3** Loosely, in popular usage, numbers used to represent facts or data.

statistics, correlational A general label for all those statistical procedures which are based on CORRELATIONS. Note that most consider these procedures to be part of DESCRIPTIVE *STATISTICS.

statistics, descriptive A general label for statistical procedures used to describe, organize and summarize samples of data. Basically, a descriptive statistic is a number that represents some aspect of a sample of data. The most common are measures of CENTRAL TENDENCY, measures of DISPERSION (or VARIABILITY) and measures of CORRELATION – although some authorities treat the last category separately.

statistics, inferential Statistical procedures used to make inferences. Basically, they utilize the mathematics of probability theory to infer or induce generalizations about populations from sample data. See STATISTICAL INFERENCE and PARAMETRIC STATISTICS and compare with DESCRIPTIVE *STATISTICS. Also known as *inference statistics* and *inductive statistics*.

statistic, sufficient A statistic that makes use of all of the available data in a sample in providing an estimate of a population parameter.

statoacoustic nerve Another name for the VIIIth CRANIAL NERVE; more commonly called the AUDITORY NERVE.

statokinetic response Any of the many postural responses or reflexes that maintain stable posture while the body is in motion.

stat rat (or subject) Short for *statistical rat*

(or *statistical subject*), a sort of laboratory slang for a theoretical experimental subject the hypothetical behaviour of which is generated by a computer or other device. In the most common situation, a computer is programmed to behave (metaphorically speaking) like a theoretical rat (or other subject).

statue of Condillac The subject of a thought experiment of the 18th-century philosopher Étienne Bonnot de Condillac. His fantasized statue was of marble and in human form. Condillac imagined it to be endowed, one by one, with the several normal human senses, first smell, then taste, followed by hearing, vision and finally touch. He argued that each of the components of human consciousness, thought, memory, feelings, etc. could thus be seen as fundamentally sensationalistic in nature.

status 1 Generally, a state of affairs, a condition. **2** A reasonably well-defined standing in the social order of a group or a society. Status, here, may be characterized in one of two ways: (a) in terms of rights, privileges, prestige, power, etc. relative to others in the social hierarchy; (b) in terms of roles, the patterns of socially accepted and expected behaviours. The former tends to emphasize position or location in a social structure and is often called *social status*, the latter tends to emphasize the obligatory behaviours of persons in particular positions. See ROLE, SOCIAL CLASS. **3** In medicine, a pathological or abnormal condition. Here the term comes straight from the Latin and is usually italicized.

status, achieved Any status that is acquired by effort, competition, knowledge, special skills, etc. Examples are the occupational statuses of physicians, professors, artists, etc. Compare with ASCRIBED *STATUS.

status, ascribed Any status based on inherited factors rather than individual ability, skills, etc. Compare with ACHIEVED *STATUS.

status epilepticus A rapid succession of convulsive epileptic seizures without the patient gaining consciousness in the intervals. *Status epilepticus* is a neurological emergency which, if left untreated, may be fatal.

status group 1 A group of persons classified together on the basis of social status, shared patterns of behaviour and privileges, and a sense of awareness of their group membership, e.g. a caste. **2** Any number of persons classified together because of a sharing of social status and lifestyle but not necessarily forming a group, e.g. factory workers.

status grouping A grouping of persons according to equivalent statuses.

status need A need to achieve a high social position.

status sequence A succession of statuses that occur in a set pattern. The classic example is the sequence medical student–intern–practising physician.

status, social STATUS (2).

status symbol More of a popular term than a technical one, used to refer to any visible mark, activity or affectation of behaviour that conveys one's membership in a particular status group or one's status aspirations. Application of the term is typically restricted to symbols of high-status groups and aspirations.

status validity CONCURRENT *VALIDITY.

STD SEXUALLY TRANSMITTED DISEASE.

steady state A general term for any unchanging condition. See HOMEOSTASIS.

stearic acid FATTY ACID.

stellate cell Generally, any cell with a star-like shape; specifically, such a cell in the cerebral cortex, particularly the fourth layer, and in the molecular layer of the cerebellum.

stem-completion task Any task in which the respondent is given a verbal or visual prompt and asked to complete the prompt. Most commonly, the participant is given a word stem (e.g. MOT...) and asked to complete it with the first word that comes to mind. Also called *word completion task* and *word stem-completion task*.

stenin A protein found coating the membrane of synaptic vesicles.

stenosis Any narrowing of a passage. The term is typically used with a modifier, e.g. *spinal stenosis* for a narrowing in the spine which restricts nerve function, *carotid stenosis* for a narrowing of the carotid artery which restricts blood supply to the brain.

step function Any function with discrete, quantal increments or decrements.

step interval An occasional synonym of CLASS INTERVAL.

stepwise phenomenon In Gestalt theory, the sense that a sequence of discrete steps along a continuum is an organized, smooth progression. For example, a sequence of lights of increasing brightness is seen as a stepwise progression. However, a sequence of lights of increasing wavelength is not so perceived; it is seen, rather, as a discontinuous progression moving through various hues. The stepwise phenomenon occurs with PROTHETIC continua but not with META-THETIC.

stepwise regression REGRESSION, STEPWISE.

stereo- A combinatory form from the Greek, meaning *solid*. By extension, it also means *heavy*, *deep* and *three-dimensional*.

stereochemical theory (of smell) A theory of olfaction that assumes that the physical forms, electrical charges and orientation of molecules of odorous substances give rise to particular olfactory experiences. The theory is a variety of the classic LOCK-AND-KEY MODEL which presumes that specific receptor sites are activated by substances with just the right physical properties. Seven primary odours are assumed (camphorous, musky, floral, minty, ethereal, pungent and putrid), all other odours being represented as combinations of these.

stereocilia In the inner ear, the shorter hairs projecting from the surface of the cells of the semicircular canals. See also KINO-CILIA.

stereognosis Perception – or, more literally, knowledge – of objects derived through touch.

stereogram A two-dimensional visual image that produces a compelling three-dimensional percept when viewed with slightly offsetting retinal images. The effect exploits the fact that RETINAL *DISPARITY is a reliable binocular cue to depth. Early stereograms were paired identical images that were slightly offset and, when viewed through a *stereoscope,* yielded compelling three-dimensionality. In the late 1800s, ANA-GLYPHS used colour filters to sort out the images that went to each eye. Both *single-* and *dual-image random-dot stereograms* (often called *Julesz* stereograms to honour Béla Julesz, who developed them) appeared in the 1960s using what appear to be random dots or blotches but yield three-dimensional figures when viewed using FREE FUSION. *Auto-stereograms,* which use the same principle, have become popular outside the laboratory because of the beautiful three-dimensional images that can emerge from fusing what appear to be abstract coloured designs. *Dynamic, random-dot stereograms* present random-dot stereograms sequentially at a fast pace and produce the perception that the three-dimensional object is moving. Also spelled *random dot,* without the hyphen.

stereopsis 1 Loosely, stereoscopic vision; vision through a stereoscope. **2** Specifically, the displacement of two objects in the third dimension; see RETINAL *DISPARITY for details. **3** The extent to which objects may be discriminated in three dimensions. See STEREO-SCOPIC *ACUITY.

stereoscope Any device for viewing two-dimensional pictures (stereograms) so that the perception of depth is produced. There are several such devices using different principles, but all function so that the perception of depth arises from having one eye view a scene from a slightly different perspective from the other eye. See RETINAL *DISPARITY.

stereoscopic acuity ACUITY, STEREOSCOPIC.

stereoscopic depth constancy A CON-STANCY in which the sense of depth of a scene remains the same despite a variety of changes in conditions of illumination.

stereoscopic vision VISION, STEREOSCOPIC.

stereotactic 1 Generally, characterizing or descriptive of circumstances that have a solid, three-dimensional component to them. **2** Specifically, referring to the three-dimensional features of an organ, most often the brain. var., *stereotaxic.* n., *stereo-taxis, stereotaxy.*

stereotactic atlas An atlas or map of an organ, usually the brain, presented in a coordinated three-dimensional format that depicts structures, nerve tracts and other key features.

stereotaxic STEREOTACTIC.

stereotaxis 1 STEREOTROPISM. **2** A method for precisely locating areas in the brain. It is used in both experimental research on lower organisms and in certain neurosurgical procedures on human patients. A stereotaxic instrument permits the positioning of another instrument (e.g. an electrode for recording electrical activity of neural tissue) guided by features of the skull and a detailed, three-dimensional atlas of the brain.

stereotropism Generally, any orienting response to a solid object.

stereotype This term derives from its use in printing, where it refers to a solid printing mould or plate which, once cast, is difficult to change. In keeping with this etymology, the term has typically been used in the social sciences to stand for: **1** n. A set of relatively fixed, simplistic overgeneralizations about a group or class of people. Here, negative, unfavourable characteristics are emphasized, although some authorities regard positive but biased and inaccurate beliefs as components of a stereotype. Given the ubiquity of this meaning it is of interest that empirical studies of people's attitudes toward social groups and classes other than their own have not supported the theory invited by this definition, particularly with regard to the notions of rigidity and inaccuracy. Hence: **2** n. Within a culture, a set of widely shared generalizations about the psychological characteristics of a group or class of people. This rather more neutral definition is preferred, as it (a) allows for stereotypes to change, as we know they do, (b) permits the inclusion of positive and accurate characteristics, and (c) emphasizes that stereotypes are widely shared – somehow, when a set of beliefs is held by only a few the term hardly seems justified. **3** vb. To form or utilize such sets of beliefs, to classify or categorize an individual on the basis of them. See also PREJUDICE.

stereotyped behaviour Rigid, inflexible behaviour that tends to be adhered to despite changes in the context and outcomes which would reasonably be expected to lead to modifications in behaviour. See also STEREO-TYPED MOVEMENT and STEREOTYPY.

stereotyped movement A persistent postural, gestural or verbal response that is with-out apparent meaning and tends to recur inappropriately.

stereotype threat Any threat that activates a stereotype about one's self-identified group (usually based on race, ethnicity or gender) and leads one to perform in a manner consistent with that stereotype. For example, being 'reminded' that women tend to do poorly in mathematics tends to disrupt women's performance on mathematics tests.

stereotypic movement disorder A MOVE-MENT DISORDER characterized by nonfunctional repetitive behaviours such as rocking back and forth, hitting, biting or scratching parts of one's body, repetitive vocalizations, etc. It is associated, especially in its more pronounced forms, with severe or profound mental retardation and often accompanies *autism*. Also called *stereotypy/habit disorder*.

stereotypy Generally, any condition characterized by a high degree of stereotyped behaviour and movement. Note, however, some authors restrict usage to psychopathological or neuropathological conditions; others apply it to the normal recurrent mannerisms of those who are free of disorder. The connotations of the term clearly depend on how it is used.

stereotypy/habit disorder STEREOTYPIC MOVEMENT DISORDER.

sterile 1 Not fertile, having the condition of STERILITY. **2** Free from microorganisms, free from contamination. **3** Impoverished or barren in thought and ideation; unimaginative, uncreative.

sterility A condition of being unable to serve as one of the partners in sexual reproduction; in the female the inability to become pregnant, in the male the inability to impregnate. Sterility can result from a truly remarkable variety of causes, physiological, anatomical and psychological. See and compare with INFERTILITY.

sterilization 1 The process of destroying the ability of an individual to reproduce, the act of rendering a person STERILE (1). It can be accomplished through the surgical removal of the testes or ovaries (see CASTRA-TION), by irradiation, which inactivates the germ-producing tissue, or by tying off or removing portions of the reproductive ducts (see VASECTOMY in the male, SALPINGECTOMY in the female). **2** The process of destroying all microorganisms on a substance or object; the act of rendering a thing STERILE (2).

Sternberg task A simple procedure developed by Saul Sternberg to study human memory. The subject is given a small set of items (four or five will do) to memorize. Then a single item is presented and the subject must say, as rapidly as possible, whether that item is a novel one or one from the original set.

steroids Hormones made up of small, fat-soluble molecules that are readily absorbed into cells, where they attach themselves to receptors in the nucleus. Steroids such as the sex hormones secreted by the testes and ovaries and those secreted by the adrenal cortex have *anabolic* properties and, consequently, are often abused by individuals seeking additional muscle mass. It should be noted that steroid abuse has a number of unhappy side effects, including sexual impotence.

Stevens' power law POWER LAW.

sthenia From the Greek, meaning *strength*. ant., ASTHENIA.

sthenometer Any device for measuring muscular strength.

stigma Greek for *mark* or *brand*. Hence: **1** Any mark or spot on the skin. Typically, this meaning is restricted to cases in which the blemish itself is benign but thought to be symptomatic of a degenerative condition. **2** In genetics, a criterial feature of a genetic disorder. **3** Figuratively, a mark or blemish on one's reputation. pl., *stigmata* or *stigmas*; vb., *stigmatize*.

Stiles–Crawford effect A term for either of two closely related effects. **1** Light that enters the eye through the centre of the pupil appears brighter than light that enters near the edge. This effect is related to the distribution of cones in the retina: clustered as they are near the centre in the fovea, they are less likely to be affected by light striking at an angle than by light arriving head on. The effect does not occur in the dark-adapted eye and hence is not due to rod action. **2** When monochromatic light enters the

eye, oblique rays entering off-centre result in the experiencing of hues slightly different from those produced by light entering through the centre. The effects holds even when the stimuli have been equated for brightness. With short and long wavelengths there is a slight positive shift (e.g. oblique long wavelengths look 'too red'), while in the middle-wavelength region there is a negative shift (e.g. an oblique 540 nm stimulus looks 'too yellow').

Stilling test A test for colour deficiencies consisting of numbers arranged in complex dot patterns on complexly arranged dot-pattern backgrounds. The saturation and brightness of the dots are carefully controlled, leaving only hue as a feature for detecting each number. The colour-weak eye will see only the random dots. The predecessor of the ISHIHARI COLOUR PLATES.

stimulant Any drug with arousing, altering, stimulating properties. Included in this large category are the powerful AMPHETAMINES, METHYLPHENIDATE, COCAINE and many common, less potent substances such as CAFFEINE and NICOTINE. All produce, in varying degrees, alertness, talkativeness, enhanced physical performance of gross sensorimotor acts, increased confidence and a diminution of appetite. To some extent all have an associated DRUG *DEPENDENCE. The primary medical uses are in the treatment of OBESITY, NARCOLEPSY and childhood HYPOKINESIS.

stimulation 1 Broadly, any event that arouses an organism, or the actual arousal itself. **2** More specifically, a particular event that, when applied to a sensory receptor or receptor cell, causes it to become active. Note that in 1 the term can be applied to either the event or the arousal; in 2 it only refers to the event, the term EXCITATION (1) serving to cover the resulting state of arousal. vb., *stimulate*.

stimulation-seeking Characterizing a personality disposition to seek out arousing situations and activities. Note that arousal here is in the eye of the beholder. Many people who would be classified as high in stimulation-seeking such as skydivers and rock climbers report their activities as joyful rather than arousing or dangerous.

stimulus (S) 1 Any thing (i.e. any event, any

occurrence, any change in a thing, any percept or concept, internal or external) that has some impact or effect on an organism such that its behaviour is modified in some detectable way. Although the following definitions all attempt to delimit the referential meaning of the term in some degree or fashion, in the final analysis this utterly inclusive definition represents the connotative meaning that the term almost invariably has. Note, however, that like RESPONSE it is often used with qualifiers in an attempt to specify the limits of applicability. **2** Any event or change in an event that alerts or arouses an organism. This meaning is preferred by some because it carries with it the original sense of the term STIMULATION (2). **3** Any change that is sufficient to excite a receptor or receptor system. This meaning is most commonly found in studies of sensory processes and occasionally in the study of perception. **4** A signal for action. Here the definitional focus is on the role of a stimulus as a sign or initiator of behaviour. **5** Some mental or internal event that provokes or prods an organism on, an *incentive*. This meaning is rare in technical writing but common in popular texts. **6** The environmental circumstances regularly present at the time of occurrence of a particular response. This definition is favoured by Skinnerian behaviourists because the focus is on the objective, physical environment; see DISCRIMINATIVE *STIMULUS, which reflects this meaning. Note that in all of these cases certain connotations hold. Specifically, (a) a stimulus must be characterized or in principle characterizable in physical terms – a ghost cannot be a stimulus, (b) it must fall within the range of receptivity of the relevant organism – a 40,000 Hz tone may be a stimulus for a bat but not for a human, (c) it must evoke some response from a receptor or some action from an organism and, (d) it must be external to an organism or to some internal but circumscribable part of the organism.

stimulus, adequate Any stimulus that produces a response in a receptor or receptor system. As the term is used, such a stimulus necessarily has two properties: (a) it is above the threshold for the sensory system under consideration; and (b) it is an appropriate energy form for the sense concerned. Compare with INADEQUATE *STIMULUS.

stimulus as coded (SAC) A stimulus characterized in terms of how it was processed or coded by the subject. While it is trivially true that all physical stimuli are of this kind, the term is reserved for circumstances where the difference between the objective and the encoded stimuli is dramatic, e.g. FUNCTIONAL *STIMULUS.

stimulus attitude STIMULUS *SET.

stimulus-bound 1 Generally, characteristic of situations in which what is perceived is determined virtually entirely by the physical properties of the stimulus. As pointed out in the discussion under PERCEPTION, this is usually not the case. **2** In personality research, characteristic of persons who tend to be rather rigid and inflexible and who tend to react on the basis of external stimuli rather than on reflection or interpretation of a situation.

stimulus continuum Generally, the underlying dimension that represents a continuous variable that any individual stimulus is a part of. For example, any given achromatic light represents a particular point along the black–white stimulus continuum.

stimulus control Loosely, the extent to which behaviour can be said to be under the control of environmental stimulus conditions. The term is applied to specific, overt behaviours as well as to differences in characteristics of behaviours. In studies of *operant conditioning*, learned behaviours will often be characterized as 'having been brought under stimulus control'.

stimulus differentiation DIFFERENTIATION (esp. 4 and 5).

stimulus, discriminative In operant-conditioning studies of discrimination learning, any stimulus in the presence of which responses are reinforced and in the absence of which they are not. abbrev., S^D.

stimulus element ELEMENT (3).

stimulus equivalence EQUIVALENCE.

stimulus error ERROR, STIMULUS.

stimulus field A very general term for the totality of stimuli impinging upon an organism at any point in time. Typically, it is reserved for reference to external stimuli: if mental or covert aspects are under consideration, the qualifier *internal* is usually appended.

stimulus, functional The stimulus, or the aspect of the stimulus, which is, in reality, functioning to exert some control over responses. For example, if several bright, coloured, moving objects are used as stimuli for a pigeon and a cat in a discrimination-learning experiment, the movements are likely to be the functional components of the stimulus for the cat while the hue and brightness will serve as the primary functional components for the pigeon. Similarly, an English-speaking subject given the non-sense syllable MIF in a memory experiment may code it as an acronym for 'my intimate friend', which then becomes the functional stimulus. See also STIMULUS AS CODED, which speaks to the same general issue. Also called, on occasion, *effective stimulus*.

stimulus generalization GENERALIZATION, STIMULUS.

stimulus, inadequate A confusing and, fortunately, obsolescent term for any stimulus the energy form of which is not normally effective for a particular sensory modality. For example, slight pressure on the side of the eyeball produces a visual sensation, and in some older texts is called an inadequate visual stimulus. A better term here is *anomalous stimulus*. See also ADEQUATE *STIMULUS. Compare with INEFFECTIVE *STIMULUS.

stimulus, ineffective Quite literally, a stimulus that is ineffective in producing a response or in exciting a receptor. The lack of functional effectiveness may stem from any of several conditions; e.g. the stimulus may be below threshold, it may be outside the range of receptivity of the organism's sensory system, or the organism's attentional focus could be directed elsewhere. Compare with INADEQUATE *STIMULUS.

stimulus, neutral 1 In operant conditioning, all environmental events that have no effect upon behaviour at a given point in time. **2** In classical conditioning, any stimulus that does not naturally elicit the conditioned response and, as a result, can serve as a conditioned stimulus.

stimulus object A loose term for any object that functions as a stimulus for some behaviour. *Object* may be taken here to stand for

things, persons or even abstractions, depending on the context.

stimulus onset asynchrony (SOA) The time between the onsets of two stimuli. The term is often used in studies of MASKING, in which the SOA is the time between the onset of the target and the onset of the masker. Compare with INTERSTIMULUS INTERVAL.

stimulus pattern Generally, any complex stimulus that functions as a whole in which the separate elements form a structured array. In a reductionistic sense, all but the most primitive unidimensional stimuli are stimulus patterns, but the term is typically applied only to situations in which it is the pattern itself which is the functional coded stimulus. The classic example is a melody. See FUNCTIONAL, *STIMULUS, PATTERN, STIMULUS AS CODED et seq.

stimulus population In STIMULUS-SAMPLING THEORY, the full complement of independent elements that make up the stimulus present on a given trial in an experiment.

stimulus pre-exposure effect LATENT *INHIBITION.

stimulus–response Of or representing the bond between a stimulus and its associated response. The term is used as a shorthand expression for a particular approach to psychology, specifically that predicated upon conditioning principles and affiliated with the general position of ASSOCIATIONISM, and it serves as an all-purpose adjective for phenomena, hypothetical mechanisms and general theories that are based on this bond. See e.g. STIMULUS–RESPONSE PSYCHOLOGY, STIMULUS–RESPONSE THEORY. Often referred to by the abbreviation, *S–R*.

stimulus-response compatibility Literally, the degree to which a given stimulus and response are compatible with each other, with 'compatibility' being broadly and functionally determined. See SIMON EFFECT for an example.

stimulus–response learning S–R *LEARNING.

stimulus–response psychology Loosely, that approach to psychology that views the STIMULUS–RESPONSE bond as the foundation of behaviour and conceptualizes the goal of a scientific psychology as the discovery of the functional relationships between stimuli and responses.

stimulus–response theory Loosely, any of the associationistic learning theories that have as their theoretical foundation the forming of a bond between a stimulus and a response. Often referred to by the shorthand *S–R theory*. See S–R *LEARNING.

stimulus-sampling theory A mathematically formal theory of learning due largely to the work of William K. Estes. Each stimulus is assumed to be made up of elements. On each trial of a learning experiment the subject samples some proportion of these elements and makes a response. When that response is reinforced, those elements become conditioned to it. Hence, the probability of that response on any given trial can be specified by the proportion of all stimulus elements conditioned to that response.

stimulus set SET, STIMULUS.

stimulus situation The full complement of environmental stimuli in the presence of which an organism behaves. The term connotes holistic and contextual effects as opposed to the atomistic, objective analysis preferred by the behaviourists.

stimulus–stimulus learning S–S *LEARNING.

stimulus trace Hull's term for the sensory aftereffects of a stimulus which are represented in the nervous system after the physical stimulus has been terminated. See ICONIC for a slightly different perspective on the same issue.

stimulus value A loose term for any quantitative aspect of a stimulus.

stimulus variable Any of the INDEPENDENT VARIABLES in an experiment that can be characterized as a change in a physical stimulus. For example, children of varying ages might be asked to read words of varying length. Both age and word length would be independent variables but only word length would be a stimulus variable.

stimulus word Loosely, any word used as a stimulus. Most often, a word presented to a subject in a word-association study or a reaction-time study or a word used as the stimulus in paired-associates learning.

stirrup STAPES, AUDITORY *OSSICLES.

stochastic From the Greek, meaning *skilful in guessing*, characteristic of any process or any sequence of events that can be described by using probability theory. Used roughly synonymously with *nondeterministic* and *probabilistic*.

stochastic resonance A perceptual phenomenon where adding NOISE to an input enhances detection and intelligibility of a SIGNAL (3, 5). For example, adding carefully designed noise to an already noisy aeroplane cabin can actually make speech easier to understand.

Stockholm syndrome An emotional bond between hostages and their captors which is frequently observed when hostages are held for long periods of time under emotionally straining circumstances. The name derives from the occasion on which it was first publicly noted, when a group of hostages was held by robbers in a Stockholm bank for five days.

stocking anaesthesia GLOVE *ANAESTHESIA.

stooge A person who poses as a subject in an experiment but who is actually a *confederate* of the experimenter.

stop consonant A speech sound produced by a momentary complete closure of the mouth, e.g. the /p/ in *pan*, /t/ in *tan*.

stopped image STABILIZED (RETINAL) IMAGE.

storage A synonym of *memory*. The term is very common in cognitive psychology. See MEMORY et seq. for details on contemporary terminology.

storage capacity As borrowed from computer sciences, the upper limit on the amount of information that can be stored in memory. Typically used with regard to limited-memory systems such as SHORT-TERM *MEMORY.

store 1 n. MEMORY. **2** vb. To commit to memory.

strabismus From the Greek, meaning *squint*, a lack of coordinated fixation between the two eyes due to muscular disorders. The condition may be *unilateral*, when the same eye always deviates, *alternating*, when either eye may deviate while the other fixates, *convergent*, when the deviant eye turns inward, *divergent*, when it turns outward, or *vertical*, when it turns downward.

straight-line processing Loosely, linear, sequential thinking.

straight-line sensory system A phrase used occasionally to refer to the primary afferent neural pathways from the peripheral sensory receptors to the brain.

strain 1 n. Generally, the state of a system when severe demands are placed upon it. This general meaning comes from the Old French for *bind* or *draw tight* and appears in a variety of contexts, typically with the connotation that the system is deformed in some way by the stress. Thus, references to muscular strain, the straining of a joint or tendon, psychological strain, eye strain, etc. are common. **2** n. The line of reproductively isolated members of a particular species. Common laboratory rats and wild rats represent two strains of a single species. This meaning derives from the Old English for *acquire*. **3** vb. To pass through a filter. **4** vb. To injure by the placing of excessive demands or severe stress. **5** vb. To engage in excessive efforts to accomplish something.

strange situation An experimental procedure developed by Ainsworth to study ATTACHMENT (2, 3) in which a young child is placed in a series of increasingly stressful situations and his or her emotional reactions are observed. The situations range from those involving minimal stress, e.g. the child plays with a parent, through those that are moderately stressful, e.g. a stranger enters the room in which the child is playing, to those involving considerable stress, e.g. the parent leaves the child alone in the room. The procedure is most commonly used with one- and two-year-olds.

strategy 1 As derived from the Greek for *generalship*, a plan of conduct or action, a consciously arrived-at set of operations for solving some problem or achieving some goal. **2** Occasionally, particularly in psychoanalytic writings, an unconscious programme of operation. References to the 'id's strategies for circumventing the ego' reflect this meaning. **3** In ethology and sociobiology, a species' collective pattern of adaptive behaviour, e.g. *survival strategy, reproductive strategy*. Note the rather different ways in which the question of consciousness is handled here. In meaning 1 the clear connotation is that a strategy is conscious, in 2 it is generally taken as an unconscious process, in 3 the question is irrelevant.

stratification In sociology and social psychology, the arrangement of the social classes in a society into a horizontal, layered arrangement such that the roles, statuses and life chances of those in each layer are relatively differentiated from those in other layers.

stratified sampling SAMPLING, STRATIFIED.

Stratton's experiment The term honours G. M. Stratton, who in 1896 published the original experiments with special prisms which invert the perceived visual field by rotating it through 180° of arc. See DISPLACED VISION for more detail.

streaming TRACKING (2).

stream of action The behaviouristic, functionalistic analogue of James's STREAM OF CONSCIOUSNESS.

stream of consciousness 1 As introduced by William James, a term used to emphasize the notion that consciousness is not a static thing made up of discrete elements, as conceptualized by the defenders of STRUCTURALISM (1), rather a confluent, continuous, multifarious succession of images, ideas, feelings, memories and thoughts. **2** A phrase used to characterize speech and/or writing which has an unedited quality, so that 'whatever worm makes it to the top, pops out'. It is not used of the speech or writing of those with diagnosed mental disorders, rather of the spoken or written output of those whose minds are 'normal' but whose verbal styles are eccentric.

strephosymbolia From the Greek, meaning *twisting of symbols*: **1** Left–right reversal of the location of symbols, e.g. reading *sag* as *gas*. **2** Left–right reversal of the orientation of symbols, e.g. reading *b* as *d*. The first meaning is the one usually intended. See also REVERSALS.

stress 1 Generally, any force that when applied to a system causes some significant modification of its form, usually with the connotation that the modification is a deformation or a distortion. The term is used with respect to physical, psychological and social forces and pressures. Note that stress in this sense is a *cause*; it is the antecedent of some effect. **2** A state of psychological tension produced by the kinds of forces or pressures alluded to in 1. Note that stress in this sense is an *effect*; it is the result of other pressures. When meaning 2 is intended, the term *stressor* is typically used to refer to the causal agent. **3** In linguistics, the emphasis placed on syllables and words. Here several levels of stress may be differentiated.

stress-induced analgesia ANALGESIA, STRESS-INDUCED.

stress interview Quite literally, an interview in which the person being interviewed is deliberately put under considerable emotional stress to evaluate their ability to handle such tension in real-life situations. It is one form of STRESS TEST.

stressor STRESS (2).

stress reaction, gross A general label for a situational reaction brought on by extreme stress, such as that of combat in war or of a major civilian disaster such as an earthquake, fire or accident. See also POST-TRAUMATIC STRESS DISORDER.

stress test Generally, any test that is carried out under real-life or simulated real-life conditions of considerable stress. The term is used of both the psychologically stressful, such as a STRESS INTERVIEW, and the physiologically stressful, such as a treadmill test for evaluating cardiovascular fitness.

stretch receptor A proprioceptor in muscle or tendons that is stimulated by pulling or stretching of tissue.

stretch reflex A reflexive muscle contraction in response to a pulling of the tendon of the responding muscle. Such reflexes are important in the maintenance of posture. Also called *myotactic reflex*.

stria atrophica The medical term for what are more commonly called *stretch marks*.

striate From the Latin for *striped*, marked by stripes or streaks. var., *striated*.

striate body CORPUS STRIATUM.

striate cortex The primary visual cortex, the region surrounding the CALCARINE FISSURE

and often referred to as Brodmann's area 17. The term *striate* is applied because this area contains a layer of cells that show up as dark stripes under histological examination.

striate muscle MUSCLE, STRIATE.

stria terminalis A fibre bundle that runs between the medial amygdala and various regions in the forebrain, including the *medial* PREOPTIC AREA.

striato-nigral degeneration A MULTI-SYSTEM ATROPHY whose symptoms closely mimic that of Parkinsonism (see PARKINSON-PLUS SYNDROME). Patients display muscle rigidity, a flat expressionless face, slowness of movement, poorly articulated speech and difficulty swallowing. Irritability and intense anxiety are common. It responds poorly to drug treatment.

striatum A part of the BASAL GANGLIA involved in movement and EXECUTIVE FUNCTIONS.

strident In phonetics, a DISTINCTIVE FEATURE (2) characterizing sounds produced with a distinct turbulence, e.g. /s/, /z/, /ch/.

string Generally, any concatenated series of stimuli. Thus, sentences are strings of words, written words are strings of letters, etc.

strip Goffman's term for any particular sequence of occurrences or actions in a larger FRAME (2) to which one wishes to draw attention.

striped muscle MUSCLE, STRIATE.

stroboscope Any device that presents a series of still pictures in rapid succession. When the time interval between the stills is appropriate, the viewer experiences motion. The standard motion-picture projector is, in effect, a stroboscope. See STROBOSCOPIC EFFECT.

stroboscopic effect 1 Generally, a type of APPARENT *MOTION perceived when two or more stationary stimuli are illuminated in rapid succession. The classic examples are motion pictures and advertising marquees. **2** More specifically, the variations in the perception of real motion produced by changing the rate at which a flashing light illuminates it. The classic example here is changing the perceived rotation of a spoked wheel from forwards to stationary to backwards by changing the rate of the intermittent light.

stroboscopic motion MOTION, STROBOSCOPIC.

stroke **1** Generally, any sudden severe attack. **2** More specifically, such an attack produced by a cerebrovascular accident, e.g. the rupture of a blood vessel in the brain.

Strong–Campbell Interest Inventory See STRONG INTEREST INVENTORY.

Strong Interest Inventory An instrument designed to assess and evaluate an individual's interests and make predictions about the likelihood of success in particular occupations. It is based on a series of several hundred items involving activities, occupations, descriptions of various kinds of individuals and self-descriptions which the test-taker marks according to how well they 'like' or 'dislike' each. The current version is a revision of the *Strong–Campbell Interest Inventory* which, itself, was an updating of the original *Strong Vocational Interest Blank* developed in 1927 by Edward K. Strong.

strong law of effect See LAW OF • EFFECT.

Strong Vocational Interest Blank See STRONG INTEREST INVENTORY.

Stroop effect See STROOP TASK.

Stroop task A procedure developed in 1935 by J. R. Stroop for studying verbal processes. The standard form of the test consists of a series of colour names (e.g. *blue, red, green*) printed in nonmatching colours; that is, the word *red* may be printed in blue ink. Most people find it extremely difficult to attend to the ink colour alone when asked to name the colour in which each word is printed, because of an automatic tendency to read the words, which produces interfering information. The general procedure has proven highly adaptive and a variety of different versions of 'the Stroop' (as it is commonly called) are used, for example asking an individual to count the words in a display of three words, each of which is spelled 'two' or requiring subjects to name pictures of animals when each is marked with a label giving the name of another animal. In the *Emotional Stroop Test*, the respondent must identify the colours of words which have either depressive or neutral content. The term *Stroop effect*

refers to the increase in reaction times and errors observed in any of these task variations.

Stroop test The term refers, not to a particular test, but to any of a variety of procedures based on the STROOP TASK. Because this task involves executive functions and is sensitive to interference effects, it has proven to be a sensitive device for evaluating disorders as diverse as ADHD, SCHIZOPHRENIA and, perhaps surprisingly, EATING DISORDERS. The anterior cingulate cortex in the frontal lobes has been implicated as playing an important role in the task.

structural Pertaining to STRUCTURE. Compare with FUNCTIONAL, DYNAMIC and BEHAVIOURAL.

structural equation modelling An advanced statistical technique most frequently used in circumstances where the effects of constructs that cannot (under existing conditions) be directly measured are evaluated by approximating their effects through other measures assumed to be functioning in a similar manner.

structuralism There are several theoretical and philosophical orientations that have been given, or have assumed, this label. All share a concern with the structure or organization of those phenomena under consideration. However, since the phenomena that are and have been the focus of investigation, as well as the presumed form of the underlying structure, differ sharply from orientation to orientation, the term is found denoting approaches that differ from each other, often dramatically. The following are those that have been most frequently designated as structuralist and which are of importance in the social sciences.

1 The system in experimental psychology closely associated with the writings and empirical findings of Edward B. Titchener. The approach was (the past tense is called for here since this particular approach effectively expired with Titchener) based on the presumption that all human mental experience, no matter how complex, could be viewed as blends or combinations of simple processes or elements. The experimental method used was INTROSPECTION, and the attempt was made to discover all of the basic elements of sensation and affection which went into making up mental life, and hence to reveal the underlying structure of mind. This approach was rather vigorously and effectively attacked by many: by behaviourists for its excessive mentalism, by Gestaltists for its unwarranted reductionism, by psychoanalysts for its insistence on studying only conscious awareness, by functionalists for its failure to appreciate the role and functions of mind, and by various others for excluding the study of animals, children, the mentally disturbed, social groups and any other subject that could not use introspection. **2** The theory of cognitive development of Jean Piaget. The focus here is very different from that of 1. The structure presumed is that of the mental representations which underlie intelligent, adaptive behaviours, and it is characterized as a sequence of quasi-logical and logical stages through which a child progresses to the end of a logically formal operatory level. See PIAGETIAN for more detail. **3** Any of several sociological/anthropological approaches, such as that of Claude Lévi-Strauss. Here the focus is on social organization and societal structures and the manner in which they are learned and reacted to by members of the society under examination. The emphasis is on the use of such organizational structures as the empirical basis for theoretical induction concerning personal and group conceptualizations of the structure of the world, from both the psychological and the physical standpoints. **4** The approach to the study of language developed by Swiss linguist Ferdinand de Saussure who argued that languages are closed systems in which meaning is derived, not through external referents, but from analysis of the structured patterns and relationships of signs and symbols. Saussure's key argument lay in his rejection of the standard notion that the meaning of a sign, a gesture or a word was derived from its links to specific external events and objects. Rather, he maintained, all meaning was dependent upon the manner in which signs, gestures and words are used in combination with other signs, gestures and words. The approaches outlined in meanings 2 and 3 had considerable impact on 20th-century philosophy, literary criticism, and the study of topics such as religion, mythology and art. Eventually they led to the postmodernist movement and the emergence of DECONSTRUCTIONISM.

structural mere exposure effect MERE EXPOSURE EFFECT.

structural psychology STRUCTURALISM (1).

structure 1 n. An organized, patterned, relatively stable configuration. The term is certainly one of the most freely used in all of psychology and is found with reference to the purely physical (stimulus structure), the biological (brain structure), the mental (the structure of memory), the social (group structure), the abstract (linguistic structure), etc. Generally, the term is used to convey the notion that the entity being characterized, taken as a whole, has intrinsic organization and that this organization is, in fact, one of its most salient aspects. Frequently, *structure* is used as though the author intends it to be an antonym of FUNCTION, PROCESS or even BEHAVIOUR. The difficulty here is that, more often than not, the functional, behavioural processes themselves have structure in that they too are organized, patterned and relatively stable. Approximate synonyms: include CONFIGURATION, GESTALT, ORGANIZATION and SYSTEM; see each for details. **2** n. Any complex system that is regarded from the perspective of the whole, e.g. the structure of science. This use reflects the notion that the *structure* exists only when the totality is under consideration. **3** vb. To organize or construct a relatively stable configuration from many elements.

Structured Clinical Interview for the DSM (SCID) A structured interview consisting of a set of questions that a clinician can use to reach a psychiatric diagnosis based on the classification system of the *DSM*. There are two distinct interviews, one focusing on Axis I and the other on Axis II (see AXIS I–V for more detail).

structured interview Any interview with a preset organization in which the topics and questions and their order of use are all determined in advance.

structured stimulus Generally, any stimulus with a salient, well-articulated and well-defined organization. The term appears most often in contrast with *unstructured stimuli*, which refers classically to the Rorschach ink blots. However, the distinction here is not simply a matter of pure structure versus the lack of it: it has more to do with the extent to which the perceiver contributes to the structure. In the case of a simple, well-organized stimulus like a triangle, the primary source of structure can be regarded as the physical stimulus itself and there is little interpersonal variation in what is perceived: in the case of a complex, ambiguously organized stimulus like an ink blot, the perceiver invests the display with a great deal of interpreted structure, and there are large individual differences in what is perceived. See also the discussion under AMBIGUITY.

structure from motion FORM FROM MOTION.

structure-of-intellect model J. P. Guilford's term for his three-dimensional model of intellectual functioning. It classifies intellectual traits along: (a) a set of *operations* – what a person *does*, including memory, cognition, divergent and convergent production, and evaluation; (b) a set of *contents* – the nature of the materials upon which operations are carried out, including those that are figural, semantic, symbolic and behavioural; and (c) a set of *products* – the forms in which information is processed, including units, classes, relations, systems, transformations and implications. The original model predicted a total of 120 factors underlying intelligence, a more recent version predicts 150. Neither version has received much empirical support.

STS Abbreviation for *short-term store*; see SHORT-TERM *MEMORY.

Student's distribution The T *DISTRIBUTION. See also STUDENT'S TEST.

Student's test The T TEST. The name Student is a pseudonym. It was adopted in 1908 by the test's developer, William S. Gosset, a chemist for the Guinness brewing company, which would not allow him to publish his findings under his real name.

study 1 n. Generally, a field of investigation or a branch of science, e.g. the study of psychology. **2** n. More specifically, an experiment or investigation. Occasionally the term is used here somewhat more loosely, in that the strict controls assumed to be present in those investigations called experiments are not always present in those called studies. **3** n. Popularly, any attempt to learn material. **4** vb. To engage in or carry out any of the above.

stump hallucination PHANTOM LIMB.

stupor 1 A general condition characterized by extreme unresponsiveness, lethargy and loss of orientation. **2** (obs.) Inability to speak, mutism.

stuttering A cover term for a number of SPEECH DISORDERS characterized by disruptions in the flow of speech. The most common of these disfluencies are blocking or stammering, repetition of particular sounds and prolongation of certain sounds, syllables or words. There is compelling evidence that it is a neurological condition and not the result of poor parenting, inappropriate language training, sexual anxieties or any of the other myriad causes that have been put forward over the years. Recent therapies using ATYPICAL ANTIPSYCHOTIC DRUGS such as OLANZAPINE are showing some success.

sub- Combining form meaning *under, beneath, inferior, in small quantity.*

subception The use of information extracted from a stimulus exposed too rapidly or too faintly to be consciously perceived and reported. The term is little used today. See SUBLIMINAL et seq. and THRESHOLD (esp. 1, 2) for details on current terminology.

subclinical 1 Referring to the period prior to the appearance of the symptoms of a disease or disorder. Contrast with SUBSYNDROMAL. **2** Referring to the existence of signs or symptoms of a disorder in the absence of full diagnostic criteria. For example, one might feel sad and anhedonic, yet not display sufficiently severe, persistent or numerous symptoms to warrant a diagnosis of MAJOR DEPRESSIVE EPISODE; hence, one would be cited as displaying *subclinical depression.*

subconscious 1 n. In psychoanalytic theory, a level of mind through which material passes on the way toward full consciousness. Note that, in fact, most purists eschew the term as overly popularized and imprecise, preferring PRECONSCIOUS. **2** n. More generally, an information store containing memories that are momentarily outside of awareness but which can easily be brought into consciousness. **3** adj. Characterizing information that is not part of one's momentary awareness but which can, given the proper circumstances, be made conscious. **4** adj. Descriptive of information or stimuli that are at the margins of attention, of events that one is only vaguely aware of. *Subconscious* should not, in any circumstance, be used as a synonym of UNCONSCIOUS.

subcortical Pertaining to the neural structures and associated functions of cerebral tissue lying below the cortex.

subculture The culture of a well-defined segment of a society. It is assumed to reflect the dominant cultural patterns of the society but to have, in addition, special, different values, norms and customs. The term tends to be used rather subjectively since it is virtually impossible to determine just how distinct these cultural patterns must be before the label is applicable. Some authors restrict its application to large, identifiable ethnic or religious groups, but others use it to refer to rather noncohesive segments of a society.

subcutaneous Lit., under the skin. Commonly used to refer to the receptors found in and below the skin or to preparations introduced just under the skin.

subdoxastic Descriptive of processes and states that are not explicit concepts and not integrated with consciously held concepts and beliefs. Used often in discourse on the philosophy of mind.

subfornical organ An area of the brain just below the fornix. Involved in the control of drinking, it appears to function as the site of action of *angiotensin* (RENIN) in that injections of this hormone stimulate drinking while injections of *saralasin* (which blocks angiotensin receptors) inhibit drinking.

subgoal An intermediary goal selected as an aim toward which one works when directed, ultimately, toward a final goal.

subiculum A part of the *hippocampal formation* the outputs of which project to the anterior thalamic nuclei and the mammillary bodies.

subitize To apprehend directly the number of dots or other small objects in an unstructured stimulus display without counting them. The limit on this process is about seven or eight.

subject 1 n. An organism (human or otherwise) which serves as a participant (willingly or otherwise) in an experiment. Several other terms are occasionally used interchangeably here, for which there are usually historical and/or traditional reasons. For example, *observer* was (and occasionally still is) used for the subject in an introspection experiment or a psychophysical investigation; *respondent* is often used in questionnaire or survey studies; *interviewee* in interviews; *testee* in tests; *patient* in medicine; *patient* and/or *client* in psychiatry and clinical psychology. By and large, one can use *subject* for the participant in any study; the other terms tend to be restricted to specific formats. For more on contemporary patterns of usage, see PARTICIPANT. **2** n. The topic of an investigation, the thing to which one refers or about which one speaks or writes. **3** adj. Liable to or having a propensity for a particular disease or disorder. **4** vb. To influence, dominate, control.

subjective 1 Loosely, characteristic of or dependent on an individual, a SUBJECT (1). Embedded in this core meaning of the term are three subthemes, each reflecting a different sense of the dependency: (a) *Private* – that which is subjective is internal, personal, not available for public scrutiny. This is found in meanings 2, 3 and 4 below. (b) *Mental* or *cognitive* – the subjective is experiential as opposed to physical or somatic. See here meanings 5, 6, 7 and 8. (c) *Individual* – the subjective is singular, only one person is involved. See meaning 9. The following, more specialized compound terms are commonly found in the social sciences and can be seen as reflecting one or more of these senses of the term. **2** Not directly public, not knowable to anyone else. The sense here is that the fundamental nature of an event can only be experienced internally, privately, and that the experience can never be publicly known but only inferred; e.g. weight is *objective*, heaviness is *subjective*; the acoustic wave form of a spoken sentence is *objective*, the meaning of the sentence is *subjective*. **3** Not directly verifiable by others, not determinable by the public in any straightforward manner. Here *subjective* is very close in meaning to *intuitive* or *implicit*; see the discussion under CLINICAL *PREDICTION for a classic example of the contrast between the *objective* and the *subjective* in this sense. **4** By extension of 2 and 3, unreliable, biased, contaminated by personal, emotional evaluations. This meaning is primarily found as an epithet used against one whose subjective assessments in sense 3 differ from one's own; there is no *logical* reason why the subjective ought to be less reliable or trustworthy than the objective. Consider the nature of aesthetic judgements to appreciate this point. **5** Of judgements made without the use of instruments or other devices. **6** Internal to the body or, more commonly, to the mind. Here *subjective* is nearly synonymous with *mental*. **7** By extension of 6, sensed or experienced as internally localized; e.g. experiences such as fatigue, in which there is no simple, determinable external stimulus, are regarded as subjective. **8** By still further extension, of experiences based on illusory or hallucinatory phenomena; imaginary. **9** Personal, pertaining to a single individual, to a specific person.

subjective attribute ATTRIBUTE (1).

subjective colours Colours (or more precisely, *hues*) experienced when the visual stimulus is in fact monochromatic. The phenomenon is well-studied (see BENHAM'S TOP, FECHNER'S COLOURS) but poorly understood.

subjective contour CONTOUR, SUBJECTIVE.

subjective doubles A DELUSIONAL MISIDENTIFICATION DISORDER characterized by the belief that a double of oneself is roaming about the world carrying out actions.

subjective error ERROR, SUBJECTIVE.

subjective expected utility (SEU) The personal value of an event or an outcome to an individual. The SEU of any choice between alternatives is given by the sum of the chooser's *subjective probability estimates* of each alternative times the *utility* of each. An assumption of many theories of choice behaviour and gambling is that people behave as if they maximized SEU.

subjective frequency SUBJECTIVE PROBABILITY.

subjective idealism IDEALISM (1).

subjective organization The grouping and classifying of words, pictures or events according to perceived similarities and interrelationships. For example, the set of animals *weasel, rabbit, lion, canary, cat* could be subjectively organized into any of several pairs of contrasting categories: predator vs. prey, pet vs. nonpet, etc. See also CLUSTERING.

subjective probability (or **frequency**) The intuitive sense of the probability or frequency of occurrence of some event or events. The term is used with respect to judgements made without recourse to counting or other mathematical calculation.

subjective psychology An occasional label for introspective or phenomenological approaches to psychology. Compare with OBJECTIVE PSYCHOLOGY.

subjective scoring Generally, any assessment of performance made by subjective means. The term is typically restricted in application to such scoring of tests as made by persons expert in the task. Projective tests like the Rorschach are scored subjectively, as are essay examinations in school.

subjective sensation Generally, any sensory experience that is produced internally and not as a direct result of physical energies impinging on one's receptors. The classic example is *tinnitus* (ringing in the ears).

subjective test Any test marked or scored using SUBJECTIVE SCORING, i.e. a test for which there are no standardized, objective assessment procedures.

subjective threshold THRESHOLD (2).

subjective vertigo VERTIGO.

subjectivism In ethics, the point of view that there are no absolutes in designation of right and wrong, that morality is derived from personal preferences and personal judgement. There are variations on this theme, from the naïve '*X* is right because I like to do it' through '*X* is right because most people like to do it' to the more sophisticated '*X* is right because it has properties *a*, *b*, *c*, all of which I have a preference for.' Contrast with OBJECTIVISM.

subjectivity 1 The quality of dealing with objects and events as phenomenological, subjective experiences. **2** An approach to phenomena characterized by internal interpretation. Contrast with OBJECTIVITY.

subject–object differentiation PRIMARY INTEGRATION.

sublimation 1 In classical psychoanalysis, the process whereby primitive, libidinous impulses are redirected and refined into new, learned, 'noninstinctive' behaviours.

Typically, the term is used with the understanding that the learned behaviours are socially acceptable whereas the deep, primitive impulses are not. Classical theory regards creative and artistic tendencies as manifestations of sublimation. **2** Generally, and more loosely, any redirection of energy from the socially unacceptable to the acceptable.

subliminal Lit., below the LIMEN, below the absolute THRESHOLD (1, 2). Note that the term, particularly in the phrase *subliminal perception*, is used in two distinct ways, often without distinguishing which meaning is intended. For example, some call a stimulus subliminal if it is so weak that it cannot be detected at all; others use the term to describe stimuli that can be detected but are too weak for the perceiver to be able to determine their identity. Needless to say these two meanings are very different and refer to very different stimulus intensities. See also SUBLIMINAL *PERCEPTION, SUBCEPTION and THRESHOLD (esp. 1 and 2) for further discussion of usage.

subliminal learning Learning of which one is not conscious. The term is often used with the connotation that the lack of consciousness is temporary and that when learning has proceeded sufficiently the individual will be become aware of it. This seems fundamentally wrong, since extensive learning often takes place totally removed from awareness, e.g. learning the rules that enable one to speak a language. A better term here is IMPLICIT *LEARNING.

subliminal perception PERCEPTION, SUBLIMINAL.

subliminal priming See PRIMING (3).

subliminal stimulus See SUBLIMINAL.

submission **1** Generally, yielding to others, to their demands, orders and needs; conformity. Compare with DOMINANCE (4) and ASCENDANCE. **2** In ethology, a pattern of behaviour exhibited by the loser of a conflict that displays to the victor a clear sign that the vanquished animal submits and will withdraw from the arena. The victor permits the loser to leave without further harm. The classic example is provided by wolves: the loser of a fight exposes its neck, its most vulnerable spot, and is allowed to with-

draw unmolested. Also called *appeasement behaviour*. Compare with DOMINANCE (3).

submissiveness A tendency to yield to others, to conform to their orders and their leadership. ant., *dominance* (4).

subnormal Less than NORMAL, below the average.

subordinate **1** n. An organism generally under the control of others. The term is used loosely and is found in research on the structural characteristics of human organizations and in ethological studies exploring the manner in which many animal species establish hierarchical social structures. **2** adj. Characterizing such an individual or animal. **3** adj. Characterizing a concept or category that is a member of a subclass of a larger concept or category; e.g. *rose* is a subordinate category of *flower*.

subordination **1** Accepting orders, allowing oneself to be dominated. **2** Classifying a thing into a lower subcategory or subclass.

substance **1** The heart of a matter, the central, most meaningful aspect of a situation or a communication. **2** In metaphysics, the essential nature of a thing or event. **3** A drug. This meaning often, although not necessarily, carries the connotation that the drug is psychoactive and one that is frequently abused. See following entries.

substance abuse A SUBSTANCE-RELATED DISORDER characterized by a maladaptive pattern of substance use such that the user experiences clinically significant cognitive and behavioural impairment or emotional distress that has an impact on work, school or the home. The term is only used in cases in which there is no evidence of SUBSTANCE DEPENDENCE. The drug or substance involved is typically specified, e.g. ALCOHOL ABUSE. See also DRUG ABUSE.

substance dependence A SUBSTANCE-RELATED DISORDER characterized by a maladaptive pattern of substance use such that the individual experiences clinically significant impairment or distress as manifested by the development of DRUG *TOLERANCE and WITHDRAWAL SYMPTOMS. The drug or substance involved is typically specified, e.g. alcohol dependence. See also DRUG *DEPENDENCE.

substance-induced amnesia AMNESIA, SUB-STANCE-INDUCED.

substance-induced disorders An umbrella term for any ORGANIC MENTAL DIS-ORDER that is intimately related to excessive and/or chronic consumption of a substance that has direct effects on the central nervous system. Most commonly these disorders are caused by psychoactive drugs taken nonmedically to alter mood or behaviour, e.g. alcohol, barbiturates, amphetamines, cannabis, opiates, cocaine. A host of specific substance-induced disorders can be found in the clinical literature, e.g. *substance-induced anxiety disorder, substance-induced psychotic disorder*, etc. For the meanings of each, look under the entry for the form of the disorder and treat it as though the condition were brought about by substance abuse. In cases where the condition lasts for a considerable length of time, the word 'persistent' is often inserted, e.g. *substance-induced persistent amnesia*.

substance P A NEUROPEPTIDE found in both central and peripheral nervous systems. It is found in the *dorsal-root ganglia* where it plays a role in the modulation of pain, in the *hypothalamus* where it has been implicated in sexual behaviour and in peripheral tissue where it functions as a vasodilator.

substance-related delirium DELIRIUM, SUB-STANCE RELATED.

substance-related delusion DELUSION, SUB-STANCE-RELATED.

substance-related disorders An umbrella term for those disorders associated with chronic and/or inappropriate use of or exposure to drugs or other substances, including SUBSTANCE ABUSE, SUBSTANCE DEPENDENCE and SUBSTANCE-INDUCED DISORDERS. It is preferred to *substance-use disorders* and *psychoactive substance abuse disorders* because these are terms for disorders that may, on occasion, be caused by agents that are not psychoactive and not abused (e.g. some environmental toxins).

substance-use disorders SUBSTANCE-RELATED DISORDERS.

substantia gelatinosa The portion of the tip of the dorsal horn of the spinal cord grey matter that functions to integrate afferent information.

substantia nigra A darkly pigmented layer of cells in the pons that is connected to the neostriatum by the nigrostriatal pathways. Dysfunctions in the dopamine projections from the substantia nigra are implicated in PARKINSON'S DISEASE.

substantive rationality See PROCEDURAL *RATIONALITY.

substantive universals LINGUISTIC *UNIVER-SALS.

substitute In older writings, a synonym of *conditioned*.

substitute valence VALENCE, SUBSTITUTE.

substitution 1 Generally, the replacing of one thing with another. Thus, more specifically: **2** Replacing one goal with another when the first has been blocked or removed. **3** In reading, writing or speaking, replacing a word, syllable, letter or phoneme with another. **4** In psychoanalysis, a defence mechanism whereby socially acceptable goals replace unacceptable ones.

substitution hypothesis 1 ALTERATION HYPOTHESIS. **2** SYMPTOM SUBSTITUTION (HYPOTH-ESIS).

substitution test Any test in which the subject must systematically replace each symbol in an array with another symbol, e.g. the CODE TEST.

subsyndromal Characteristic of a psychiatric condition in which only a few of the standard criteria for diagnosing the disorder (i.e. those listed in the DSM) are present. Such syndromes are also referred to as *subthreshold* or *shadow syndromes*, or *subclinical*.

subtest Any division or part of a larger test or test battery.

subthalamic nucleus A group of cells lying below the thalamus and linked anatomically and functionally to the BASAL GANGLIA. Also called *nucleus of Luys*.

subthreshold disorder SUBSYNDROMAL.

subtraction method Any of several methods for measuring the time it takes for particular psychological processes to occur. The best known is that developed by the

Dutch physiologist F. C. Donders, who studied three kinds of task: (a) SIMPLE *REACTION TIME; (b) DISCRIMINATION *REACTION TIME; and (c) CHOICE *REACTION TIME. By subtracting the time it took his subjects to carry out task (b) from the time it took to carry out (c) he obtained an estimate of how long it took to make a choice; by subtracting (a) from (b) he obtained an estimate of discrimination time.

subtractive mixing COLOUR MIXING.

subvocalization The 'speech' that sometimes goes on during reading. The term may be used to refer to: (a) a nearly audible whisper; (b) subtle movements of the lips, tongue and jaw; (c) minute patterns of muscular tension in the larynx detectable only with electromyographic recording devices; or (d) purely implicit, covert, mental processes unobservable by physical means. A variety of synonyms exist, e.g. *subvocal speech, implicit speech, silent speech, covert speech, silent articulation.*

subvocal speech SUBVOCALIZATION.

success, fear of A term coined by Matina Horner for a fear of accomplishing one's goals or of succeeding in society's eyes. She originally argued that women displayed this fear more than men, since striving for success places a woman in a conflict between a general need for achievement and social values that tell her that she should not achieve 'too much'. More recent research seems to indicate that men are just as likely to show this hypothesized fear. It should be pointed out, however, that it is far from clear how thoroughly one can divorce this fear from a *fear of failure,* particularly when each new success in life carries with it the potential for greater failure.

successful aging A relatively new term used to describe aging that is characterized by good physical and mental health, an optimistic outlook on life and a positive adaptation to increasing age. The term strikes us as a bit odd and we are confused about what its antonym could be.

successful intelligence INTELLIGENCE, SUCCESSFUL.

successive approximations, conditioning by SHAPING.

successive contrast CONTRAST.

successive reproductions, method of A procedure for investigating long-term memory of material which the subject is required to reproduce in several widely spaced reproduction trials.

succinylcholine A muscle relaxant used in ELECTROCONVULSIVE THERAPY to minimize complications.

succorance need H. Murray's term for the need to receive aid, assistance and guidance from others.

succubus An evil spirit which has sexual intercourse with its victim during sleep. The female form is *succuba.* See INCUBUS.

succus Any bodily fluid or secretion.

sucking **1** Generally, any oral suction. **2** More specifically, a reflex-like response observed in newborn and nursing mammals in which the nipple is grasped and milk drawn from it into the mouth.

sucking pad The fatty mass in the cheeks; it is particularly prominent in infants, where it aids in sucking.

suckling **1** The sequence of reflex-like behaviours in mammals including rooting, grasping the nipple, sucking on it and swallowing the milk **2** The act of presenting the breast and nipple to the nursing newborn. **3** Any newborn or young mammal still in the nursing period.

sudden infant death syndrome (SIDS) This term is used to cover any sudden and inexplicable death of an infant or a very young child. There are a number of hypotheses about the cause of such deaths, with sleep APNOEA being the most frequently cited, but, if this explanation is correct, what precipitates the drop in natural control over breathing is not completely understood. Particular classes of neonates are at risk, including premature and low-birthweight infants. Also called *crib death* or *cot death,* SIDS is one of the leading causes of death in the first few months of life.

sudoriferous Sweat-producing.

sufficient condition CONDITION.

sufficient statistic STATISTIC, SUFFICIENT.

suffix effect A phenomenon in the study of memory. An extraneous stimulus (called the suffix) presented just after the full list of to-be-recalled materials has the effect of depressing the recall of the materials, particularly those toward the end of the list.

suggestibility The condition of being readily responsive to suggestions from others.

suggestion **1** The process of inducing someone to behave in a particular way, accept a particular opinion or believe in something, through indirect methods. The term is only used when no force, argument, command or coercion is used to bring about the desired effect. **2** The actual verbal or pictorial communication used in this process.

suicidal ideation Recurrent thoughts about suicide. They may be simple and unelaborated or complex and involve detailed plans about how to take one's life. Such thoughts are common in cases of depression, post-traumatic stress disorder and bipolar disorder and, while they typically do not lead to actual suicide, they are signals that mental health workers cannot ignore.

suicide **1** A person who intentionally kills himself or herself. **2** The act of taking one's life. Émile Durkheim, the first to study suicide systematically, distinguished three different types, depending on what motivates the act of self-destruction: *altruistic, anomic* and *egoistic*; definitions of each are found below.

suicide, altruistic Durkheim's term for suicide based on sacrificing oneself for the good of others. The soldier who hurls himself upon a grenade to save others, and ritual suicide, such as hara-kiri, intended to save one's family from shame, are classic examples.

suicide, anomic Suicide that results, in Durkheim's analysis, from the sense that life no longer has meaning, from a sense of anomie, loneliness, isolation and loss of contact with the norms and values of society. Also called *normless suicide*.

suicide clusters CLUSTER SUICIDES.

suicide, egoistic In Durkheim's classification system, suicide resulting from a sense of deep personal failure, a feeling that one is personally responsible for not living up to societal and personal expectations.

sui generis Latin for *of its own particular kind*; a unique instance or example.

sulcus Generally, a shallow groove or furrow, especially on the surface of the brain. Sulci separate the elevated convolutions, the *gyri*. Occasionally used synonymously with FISSURE, but see that term for a distinction.

summated rating scale A general format in testing in which multiple items are presented and each is rated using a LIKERT SCALE format. The test-taker responds to each item on a scale representing the degree of endorsement and the responses are summed to yield a final score.

summation **1** In statistics, the act of cumulating or totalling a series of numbers. See Σ (under SIGMA). **2** Generally, cumulative action, a combination of effects. This sense is typically found in combined phrases in which the specific properties of the summation are noted, e.g. SPATIAL *SUMMATION, TEMPORAL *SUMMATION.

summation curve OGIVE.

summation, sensory Generally, an increase in experienced intensity or magnitude of sensory input as produced by either of two neurological processes: SPATIAL *SUMMATION or TEMPORAL *SUMMATION.

summation, spatial The funnelling of neurological impulses from two or more closely spaced loci of stimulation such that their net effect is greater than the effect of any of them taken separately.

summation, temporal The accumulating neurological effect of stimulation occurring over time. For example, a subthreshold stimulus such as a very dim light will, because of the action of temporal summation, become visible if it is flashed very rapidly or if it is left on continuously for a period of time.

summation tone COMBINATION TONE.

sundowning An increasing confusion seen around dusk in patients with dementias or acute confusional states.

sunk-cost fallacy The phenomenon in which people will persist longer in a disliked activity (e.g. sitting through a boring concert) for which they have paid than in one where they are participating cost-free. It is termed a 'fallacy' because if you really don't like the performance, you might as well leave early whether or not you paid for the tickets. Indulgence in this fallacy seems to reduce over the course of adolescence, but is still definitely present during adulthood.

super- Combining form meaning *beyond, above, superior.*

superconducting quantum interface device (SQUID) Currently, the most sensitive devices for measuring magnetic fields, they are used in MAGNETOENCEPHALOGRAPHY. See IMAGING (TECHNIQUES) for more detail.

superego In the Freudian tripartite model of the psyche, the hypothetical entity associated with ethical and moral conduct and conceptualized as responsible for self-imposed standards of behaviour. The superego is frequently characterized as an internalized code or, more popularly, as a kind of *conscience*, punishing transgressions with feelings of guilt. In the classical psychoanalytic literature, the superego is assumed to develop in response to the punishments and rewards of significant persons (usually one's parents), which results in a child becoming inculcated with the moral code of the community. Whereas the ID is conceptualized as concerned with the pleasurable and the EGO with the actual, the superego is viewed as being concerned with the ideal.

superego lacuna Lit., a gap in the superego, an area of conduct in which one's internalized moral code fails to function.

superficial 1 On or confined to the surface, particularly the surface of the body (the skin) or an organ, e.g. a superficial cut. **2** Shallow, cursory, not thorough, dealing only with the trivial. **3** Secondary or tangential. Here the reference is usually to personality characteristics that are regarded as rather unimportant in a person's overall make-up.

superficial reflex A reflexive muscular contraction in response to a light, gentle stimulus, such as stroking the skin with a feather or a piece of cotton.

superior 1 Above, higher, better. **2** In charge of or in command of. **3** In anatomical descriptions, particularly of brain structures, above (or dorsal) to an inferior (or ventral) structure.

superior colliculus COLLICULUS.

superior intelligence An arbitrary designation usually taken to apply to those who score in the top 15% on an intelligence test.

superiority complex The conviction that one is better than or superior to others. Although there are (indeed, must be) persons who are in fact superior in various ways and who recognize their talents, the term is typically not used for them. Rather, it is reserved for those who have an exaggerated and unrealistic sense of themselves, a condition generally interpreted as a defence against deeper feelings of inferiority. Also known as *superiority feelings*. See and compare with INFERIORITY FEELINGS and INFERIORITY COMPLEX and note that the problems of interpretation produced by the interchanging of the terms *feelings* and *complex* discussed there hold here as well.

superiority feelings SUPERIORITY COMPLEX.

superior olivary nucleus OLIVARY NUCLEUS, SUPERIOR.

superior temporal gyrus A *gyrus* on the upper part of the temporal lobe. The posterior portion is often called WERNICKE'S AREA, and lesions in the dominant hemisphere have been implicated in various forms of aphasia.

supernatural Beyond or outside the natural order. The term is typically used to refer to events or phenomena that are not explicable given the existing characterizations of nature. Occult phenomena and extrasensory perception are examples. See PARAPSYCHOLOGY for further discussion.

supernormal Above or exceeding the normal. Distinguish from SUPERNATURAL.

superordinate category CATEGORY, SUPER-ORDINATE.

superordinate goals Goals that can only be achieved by cooperation among many individuals. Peace is a good example.

superordination Classifying in a higher or superior rank or category. The connotation is that when a person is so categorized relative to others, the ranking carries with it the right to order or direct the actions of others of lower classifications. Compare with SUBOR-DINATION.

supersonic 1 ULTRASONIC. **2** Pertaining to speeds in excess of that of sound, i.e. about

1,192 k.p.h. (741 m.p.h.) at sea level with an air temperature of 0°C (32°F).

superstition Any notion or belief held in the absence of what one not holding that notion or belief would consider to be adequate evidence to substantiate or support it sufficiently to maintain it. Many superstitions have their roots in one or other theological system or religious tradition (indeed, some authors restrict application of the word to such cases), others exist uncritically as unexamined beliefs. Beliefs about the left side of the body (see SINISTER) are examples of the former, the common practice of carrying good luck charms is an example of the latter. Some authorities treat superstitions as descendants of primitive attempts to understand the inexplicable, to make sense out of a complex and confusing world; others, notably behaviourists, see them as natural consequences of a failure to recognize the existence (or lack of existence) of cause-and-effect relationships between one's own behaviour and subsequent occurrences in the world about us. For an illustration of this latter point of view, see SUPERSTITIOUS BEHAVIOUR.

superstitious behaviour Behaviour that results from and is maintained by adventitious reinforcements which are, in reality, not specifically coordinated with it. The easiest way to demonstrate such behaviour is to put an organism like a pigeon in a Skinner box and programme the feeding mechanism to deliver reinforcements on a variable schedule independently of the behaviour of the animal. When the first reinforcement occurs, the pigeon will be doing something, perhaps raising one of its wings. This wing-raising behaviour is thus reinforced and will increase in frequency of occurrence and hence be more likely to be occurring when the next reinforcement arrives, which, of course, will strengthen the response even further. Over time the pigeon will display a highly developed superstitious wing-raising response, a response that has, in reality, no direct relationship to reinforcement received. The point of the demonstration is to show that the notion of a contingency between response and reinforcement is in the mind of the beholder and that a true assessment of cause and effect is not necessary for highly developed behaviour. The argument is also made, not entirely convincingly, that such a demonstration reveals the ontogeny of sophisticated human superstitions.

supertaster Linda Bartoshuk's term for an individual who has particularly intense taste experiences. The exact mechanism responsible is unknown but it is assumed that it is related to biophysical properties, most likely a relatively large number of taste buds. The condition appears to have genetic roots with women being more likely to be supertasters than men and people of European descent to be less likely than those from other regions.

supervalent thought THOUGHT, SUPERVALENT.

supervenience In philosophy, a set of properties of one kind, A, is said to supervene on another kind, B, when those in A are in A precisely because they all share property B. The notion has interested psychologists who study mind and consciousness on the basis that mental acts and states can be seen as supervening on physical states. The argument is related to, but subtly different from, that of REDUCTIONISM.

supervisory attentional system A hypothesized network, presumably in the frontal lobes, that is responsible for control over nonroutine tasks that require attentional resources.

supination 1 Lying flat on one's back, supine. 2 Turning one's arm (or leg) so that the palm (or sole) is upward. Opposite of PRONATION.

supplementary motor area MOTOR AREAS.

support 1 n. Generally, the furnishing of that which is needed or lacking, providing for well-being or improvement. In this broad sense, theories receive support from corroborative evidence, political positions receive support from large numbers of adherents, etc. 2 n. More specifically, the furnishing of another person with comfort, recognition, approval, encouragement, etc. This is the meaning usually intended in the term SUPPORTIVE THERAPY. vb., *support*.

support group A therapeutic group that functions like a SELF-HELP group except that a supervisor or counsellor is present to provide support and guidance.

supportive therapy Very generally, any

form of therapy or any therapeutic procedure in which direct help is provided. Such support may be largely psychological in nature, taking the form of ego-bolstering, compliments, encouragement, positive evaluations and the like, or it may be more direct and objective, such as in helping to plan specific courses of action, giving unambiguous advice with problems, or working on behaviour-modification programmes. Supportive therapy avoids probing the individual client's deeper conflicts and works with the more cognitive and behavioural aspects.

supposition A rough synonym of POSTULATE.

suppression 1 In physiology, the complete cessation of some natural organic process; e.g. *amenorrhoea* is often called 'suppression of the menses' if a woman has had one or more normal periods. **2** Broadly, conscious, voluntary elimination of some behaviour. This sense can be found with respect to oneself (suppression of a bad habit) or to others (suppression of ideas, of a revolt, of a book). **3** In psychoanalysis, conscious exclusion of impulses, thoughts and desires that are felt to be unacceptable to the individual. The classic theory distinguishes suppression from REPRESSION in that the former is a conscious process and the latter unconscious. Despite some nagging similarities in connotation, *suppression* should also be distinguished from both EXTINCTION and INHIBITION.

suppression, monocular Suppression of the information from one eye even though, physiologically, the mechanism functions properly. The condition typically occurs when there is a failure of normal binocular fusion and only the input from one eye is used.

suppressor variable A variable (or, more accurately, a test) which functions to improve the overall predictive validity of a battery of tests by suppressing irrelevant variance in another test. For example, a test battery for selecting industrial mechanics may include three tests: (a) a general background factors evaluation; (b) a mechanical-insight test; and (c) an academic-type test of mechanical principles. Now, suppose that the criterion of job success correlates zero with (c) but very highly with (b). If (c) is treated as a suppressor variable and assigned 'negative' weight, the overall validity of the test battery

will be improved since those persons who might score highly on (b) purely through the application of academic principles, but lack the basic mechanical know-how, will be screened out.

supra- Combining form meaning *above, over, superior, in large quantities*.

suprachiasmatic nucleus A tightly packed nucleus of cells in the hypothalamus that appears to play a role in the monitoring of the light–dark cycle and is thought by many to be the primary biological clock – at least in the species that have been carefully studied, such as the rat.

supraliminal Above THRESHOLD.

supraordinate stimulus In operant conditioning, a stimulus that serves to indicate to an organism which aspects of a complex environment are the relevant ones for a particular task.

suprarenal ADRENAL.

suprasegmentals In linguistics, any of several phonemic elements which are conceptualized as superimposed on the consonant and vowel phonemes. Typically included are STRESS (3), JUNCTURE and PITCH (2). Note that these are usually treated as distinct from PROSODIC FEATURES, although some writers blur the distinction.

surdity Deafness.

surface alexia ALEXIA, SURFACE.

surface colour COLOUR, SURFACE.

surface dyslexia DYSLEXIA, SURFACE.

surface pain ACUTE *PAIN.

surface structure In linguistics, the sequence of elements (phonemes, syllables, words, phrases, sentences) that comprise an actual message as written or spoken. Compare with DEEP STRUCTURE.

surface trait TRAIT, SURFACE.

surgency A hypothesized personality trait characterized by ebullience, sociability, trustworthiness and the like.

surrogate 1 Generally, a person who takes on the role and function of another; e.g. a woman who carries to term the *in vitro* fertilized ovum of another woman is referred to as a *surrogate mother*. **2** More specifically, a person who takes on the parental role and functions for another person's child. The classic example here is the teacher who becomes a student's parent surrogate. As used here, the connotation is that the child is unaware of the relationship. **3** Loosely, any role substitute. Harry Harlow referred to the wire and/or cloth dolls he used in his studies of maternal attachment in monkeys as *surrogate mothers*.

surround 1 Broadly, the immediate environment within which one functions. It may include the internal and mental as well as the external and physical. **2** In perception, the stimulus that literally surrounds another stimulus; the latter is called the TARGET or *centre*.

survey 1 n. A general evaluation, an inspection. **2** n. An examination or inspection carried out with specific aims in mind, a search for particular kinds of information. This sense is carried in a number of specific kinds of research designs in which questionnaires, inventories or interviews may be employed to gather information about attitudes, opinions or preferences in a society or some segment of it.

survey, normative A survey designed to determine the norms of some variable or test or the performance levels of some behaviour in a large population. See NORMATIVE.

survey research Very broadly, the use of surveys typically carried out using questionnaires, polls or other sampling techniques to assess public opinion.

survey tests Tests constructed to yield general information about the distribution of levels of performance on some factor(s) in a group or population.

survival analysis An analysis of the history of specific cases or instances in terms of how long each persists in a particular state (i.e. how long they survive). Such analyses are common in medicine (how long illnesses last), in demography (life expectancies), in organizational psychology (the survival rate of small businesses), etc.

survival value The degree to which a particular biological structure or pattern of behaviour contributes to the likelihood of survival. The term is used with respect to the survival of an individual organism and to the survival of a whole species.

survivor guilt A deep sense of guilt often experienced by those who have survived some catastrophe which took the lives of many others. It was first noted and subsequently studied in those who survived the Holocaust in the Second World War and has subsequently been seen in other circumstances, including wars, famines, earthquakes, fires, etc. Part of the sense of guilt experienced by those who have survived derives from a feeling that they somehow did not do enough to save others who perished; another part of it comes from feelings of being unworthy relative to those who died.

survivor syndrome A term introduced by Lifton for a pattern of reactions frequently observed in those who have survived some terrible ordeal, such as an earthquake, a flood or a war. Symptoms are similar to those of POST-TRAUMATIC STRESS DISORDER and may include SURVIVOR GUILT.

susceptible Yielding easily to. Used in discussions of VULNERABILITY to suggest that an organism might be more reactive to environmental conditions in general, rather than simply reactive to adverse conditions.

suspicion 1 A general attitude of doubt, a sceptical orientation, particularly with respect to the sincerity of other persons. **2** SUSPICIOUSNESS.

suspicion probe A measure of what the participants in a study thought the study was about. It is common in experimental social psychology where deception is often an element and it becomes important to know if subjects were suspicious of or had figured out what the study's goals were.

suspiciousness A hypothesized personality trait characterized by a general tendency to be untrustful and doubting and to withhold emotional commitment out of a fear of being hurt.

sustainability The state and process of not consuming more resources than are needed to maintain the same or similar standard of living over future generations. Of concern in psychology because one of the keys to sustainability is the (admittedly) difficult task of persuading people to change their consumer behaviour.

sustentacular cell Generally, a supporting cell. There are several kinds of cell that serve this kind of function, such as those found in the acoustic macula, the organ of Corti and the testes.

susto A CULTURE-SPECIFIC SYNDROME found in Latino cultures. The term means *soul loss* and the disorder is assumed to result from the loss of the soul owing to a frightening experience. Symptoms include general malaise, sadness, disturbed sleep and feelings of low esteem. The condition resembles a MAJOR *DEPRESSIVE EPISODE.

Sutton's law A principle of diagnosis named after the notorious bank robber Willie Sutton who, when asked why he robbed banks, quipped, 'Because that's where the money is.' The principle, when applied to clinical diagnosis, states that one should look for a disorder where or in whom it is most likely to be found. It captures the generalization that all diseases and disorders have groups of predisposing factors.

sweet One of the five primary qualities of TASTE (2). It is elicited by sugars such as glucose or fructose. Of the various primary tastes, sweetness is the most pleasant which, from an evolutionary perspective, is not surprising since sugars are the immediate source of cellular energy.

Sydenham's chorea A childhood disease that usually appears between the ages of 5 and 15 and is typically associated with rheumatic fever. Symptoms include spastic involuntary movements of muscles of the limbs and trunk and occasional impairment of cognitive functions such as speech and memory. Recovery is usually complete in two or three months, but relapses may occur.

syl- SYN-.

syllabary A form of writing in which the basic signs in the system correspond to the primary syllables in the spoken language. Modern Japanese is written (partly) using a syllabary. See ORTHOGRAPHY for further discussion.

syllable A segment of speech consisting of a vowel or a continuant uttered alone or with one or more consonants and produced as part of a single pulse of air. Syllables are identified by a concentration of acoustic energy in the speech stream.

syllogism In logic, a valid deductive argument comprising three propositions, two serving as premises and the third as the conclusion. In the classic case, in which there are only three propositions, the syllogism is properly called a *categorical syllogism*; e.g. all dictionaries are boring, this book is a dictionary, therefore this book is boring. When at least one of the premises is a hypothetical proposition, one has a *hypothetical syllogism*; e.g. if poets ever lie to us we are in trouble, poets have been known to lie, therefore we are in trouble. When at least one proposition is a disjunction, one has a *disjunctive syllogism*; e.g. the mayor is either a crook or a fool, the mayor is honest, therefore the mayor is a fool. See also VALID.

Sylvian fissure LATERAL FISSURE.

sym- SYN-.

symbiosis 1 From the Greek, meaning *living together*, a relationship between members of two different species which live together in a mutually beneficial manner. In a true symbiotic relationship, neither of the two parties could survive without the other; e.g. in the symbiosis of the fig tree and the fig wasp, the wasp is dependent on the tree as a place to deposit eggs and the tree upon the wasp as its medium for fertilization. **2** Somewhat more loosely, any relationship between individuals in which interdependencies exist. Sadomasochistic relationships are sometimes described as symbiotic, as are extremely interdependent parent–child relationships. When the term is used in this manner the connotation is that the relationship is pathological; this connotation is entirely absent in sense 1. Note also that some authors use *symbiosis* to refer to relationships which have nonmutual benefits, in which one party profits at the expense of the other. This practice is not recommended: such patterns of interaction are best described as *parasitic*, not symbiotic.

symbiotic psychosis An obsolescent term now largely replaced by PERVASIVE *DEVELOPMENTAL DISORDER. The term was ill-advised on two counts: this category of childhood disorders bears little relationship to standard adult psychoses and the symbiotic relationship between parent and child hypothesized to play a causal role has not been shown to be the primary factor in its aetiology.

symbiotic stage SEPARATION-INDIVIDUATION.

symbol 1 Most generally, anything that represents, signifies or indicates something else. In the philosopher Charles Peirce's phrase, 'A symbol is a sign which is constituted a sign merely or mainly by the fact that it is used and understood as such.' In all of the following, more restrictive uses of the term this notion of symbol as arbitrary convention can be seen. **2** In linguistics, any language form (usually the *word* is the form under consideration) which can be used to represent a thing, event, person, etc. The word *apple* is a symbol for a real apple. **3** In mathematics and (symbolic) logic, a mark or a SIGN (esp. 5) which is used to represent an operation; e.g. Σ is the symbol for summation. Note the interesting relationship between meanings 2 and 3. Whereas both definitely reference things that are *symbolic*, 2 denotes the expression of things in words as symbols while 3 denotes the converting of words into symbols, particularly those of mathematics and logic. **4** An action, event, device or utterance (particularly a verbal slogan) that is intended to signify ideas or principles beyond that specific action, event, device or utterance. Compare with SIGN (1), which is used when the significance is limited to the thing itself. For example, fire as a *sign* of something burning as compared with fire as a *symbol* of life. **5** In Piaget's approach, an internal, private, endogenous representation. Here the term is clearly distinguished from SIGN (esp. 1 and 2) in that Piagetians regard *signs* as arbitrary, publicly shared representations and *symbols* as internally produced by the individual.

In psychoanalytic theory several variations on the term are found. All depend on the notion that the symbol is an unconscious representation which disguises or distorts the thing represented such that what is perceived consciously is a misrepresentation of the real meaning. In this fashion: **6** A conscious image or idea that represents some deeper, repressed desire or impulse. This meaning is the one generally intended in the literature on dream symbols. **7** An action or behaviour that is representative of some unconscious wish or impulse. The classic example here is the so-called Freudian slip (see PARAPRAXIS). **8** Any object which, because of some measure of perceived similarity with one's unconscious needs, represents those needs and is taken as a symbol of one's deep conflicts. For example, a tower is interpreted as a phallic symbol. **9** Any emotional symptom, such as nervousness or anxiety, which may be interpreted as representing a deeply repressed conflict.

symbol-digit test CODE TEST.

symbolic interactionism A theory, due primarily to G. H. Mead, that argues that the social domain, with its interplay of symbolic reactions and interpretations of language, action and behaviour of oneself and others, leads to the establishment of a basic self-concept and has an ongoing role in cognitive, emotional and interpersonal functioning. Mead's position is in sharp contrast with other approaches, especially the psychoanalytic, which posit that the inner psychological workings are primary and produce the patterns of social interaction.

symbolic mode See ENACTIVE REPRESENTATION.

symbolic play PLAY that transcends the concrete, so called because it presumes the use of mental SYMBOLS. It can be as simple as pushing a block along the floor while saying 'choo-choo' or as complex as a historical re-enactment. Developmental psychologists generally view the emergence of symbolic play as an indication that REPRESENTATIONAL THOUGHT is developing.

symbolic process Generally, any mental process based on the use of symbols, symbolization or symbolic representation. The term is found frequently in the writings of both cognitive psychologists and those with a psychoanalytic orientation. The former use it to refer to processes such as concept-formation, problem-solving, thinking, language and creativity; the latter typically use it to denote psychodynamic operations whereby repressed needs and conflicts are dealt with in disguised forms. See SYMBOL for more detail on usage.

symbolic representation 1 Loosely, any mental representation based on symbolic encoding. **2** A particular form of such representation in J. Bruner's theory of development. See ENACTIVE REPRESENTATION for details.

symbolic reward Any reward whose value is derived from the meaning it has for the one who receives it and not from any intrinsic value it may hold. Service awards from one's peers in the community, academic honours, honorary degrees and the like are examples.

symbol, individual In psychoanalytic theory, a symbol the repressed referent of which is specific to a particular individual and not presumed to represent any deep or universal symbolization. Compare with UNIVERSAL *SYMBOL.

symbolism 1 Generally, the act or the practice of using symbols. As in the case of the root term SYMBOL, the manner in which the term is used varies considerably, although this basic meaning is always present. **2** In essentially all forms of complex communication (e.g. language, art, music), the use of some arbitrary thing to represent or stand for some other thing. In the simplest case the word *chair*, be it spoken or written, is symbolic of some prototypical, abstract chair. In more complex circumstances, the symbolism may be less direct. Metaphor and simile in language are based on such symbolisms, e.g. 'He has a mind like a sieve.' In aesthetics, symbolism is the very heart of communication in that emotion or affect is symbolically conveyed in artistic forms such as painting, music and dance. **3** Within psychoanalytic theory, the unconscious process whereby repressed desires or wishes are transformed or disguised so as to be dealt with on a conscious level without psychic disturbance. Several theorists, notably Jung, have argued that this process forms the very foundations for all art, myth and religion. Note that meaning 3 denotes a *process* while 1 and 2 denote *practices*. Some of the confusion produced by these different usages can be avoided by using, as many do, the term *symbolization* for 3, thereby freeing *symbolism* for the others.

symbolization SYMBOLISM (3).

symbol-substitution test CODE TEST.

symbol, universal In psychoanalytic theory, a symbol that is assumed to represent the same referent universally. The argument is made that such symbols reflect basic, primordial components of the human psyche. See UNIVERSAL for a discussion of this issue from a general philosophical point of view. Compare with INDIVIDUAL *SYMBOL.

SYMLOG An acronym for *SY*stematic *M*ultiple *L*evel *O*bservation of *G*roups, it is as it says, an observational system for the study of groups. Designed by Robert Bales, it is based on measurements along three dimensions: (a) dominance–submissiveness; (b) friendly–unfriendly; and (c) accepting–opposing task orientation. It has enjoyed wide use in organizational settings to assess the values expressed by individuals as they function within groups and has been extended into clinical settings to examine therapy groups and family therapy.

symmetric (or **symmetrical**) Having the property of SYMMETRY.

symmetry 1 The property of correspondence of the size, form, shape and overall arrangement of parts on both sides of some dividing line or plane or point. **2** In mathematics, the property of a relation such that if it is valid for $x = y$ then it is also valid for $y = x$. **3** By extension of 2, any general correspondence between polar terms such that their relationship is reversible, e.g. good–bad, black–white. **4** Metaphorically, the property of being well proportioned, balanced. ants., *asymmetry*, SKEWNESS (used in statistics).

symmetry, bilateral Symmetry about a midline such that the left and right halves are mirror images of each other. The human body displays (roughly) such symmetry.

symmetry, radial Symmetry about a central point or axis such that all parts radiate from it equally. A wheel displays such symmetry.

sympathectomy A general term for any surgical excision of a portion of the sympathetic division of the autonomic nervous system.

sympathetic apraxia APRAXIA, SYMPATHETIC.

sympathetic chain The connected sequence of spinal sympathetic ganglia. See AUTONOMIC NERVOUS SYSTEM.

sympathetic ganglion Generally, any of

the ganglia of the sympathetic division of the AUTONOMIC NERVOUS SYSTEM.

sympathetic induction INDUCTION (2).

sympathetic nervous system AUTONOMIC NERVOUS SYSTEM.

sympathetic vibration RESONANCE.

sympathomimetic drug Any drug that imitates the effects of stimulation of the sympathetic nervous system.

sympathy 1 Lit., from the Greek roots SYN- and PATHO-, feeling with. Hence, the sharing in the feelings of another. Typically, owing to the original Greek usage, the term is only used of painful or unpleasant emotions. **2** A sense of compassion or understanding which allows one to interpret or justify the actions and/or feelings of another. In meaning 1 the clear connotation is that of a feeling *with* another, in 2 it is closer to a feeling *for*. The term is thus used in ways that can lead to real confusion. The difficulty derives from the tendency of English-speakers to use it in sense 1 and the French (where the word is a cognate) to use it in sense 2. In the technical psychological literature, 1 is usually what is intended; in popular writing or in literary criticism, 2 is more common. For further discussion on the general topic of shared affect, see EMPATHY.

symphorophilia A PARAPHILIA in which the individual derives sexual gratification by either (a) arranging a simulation of an elaborate disaster (*symphos* is Greek for disaster) or (b) manages to be at risk in such an orchestrated disaster. Typically the person masturbates as it occurs or afterward using imagery.

symptom 1 From the Greek for *occurrence*, any event or change in state in a system that tends to occur with another event or change of state and hence can be taken as an indicator or predictor of it. **2** In medicine and clinical psychology, any such occurrence which can be used as an indicator of the existence of or changes in a pathological condition.

symptomatic act In psychoanalysis, any ordinary act, such as PARAPRAXIS, that, under particular circumstances, can be interpreted as resulting from some unconscious process.

symptom bearer SYMPTOM WEARER.

symptom cluster SYNDROME (2).

symptom formation In psychoanalysis, one of the complex processes through which neurotic symptoms are assumed to develop. The classic analysis is as follows: when a substitute object is found for an unacceptable id impulse, occasionally the substitute itself also turns out to be unacceptable but, because it permits some psychic satisfaction, the behaviour associated with it persists and is manifested as a neurotic symptom.

symptom neurosis A loose term used descriptively of a neurosis that does not reflect any particular syndrome but in which clearly neurotic patterns of behaviour are present. The term *neurotic disorder* is used roughly equivalently, but see the extended discussion under NEUROSIS for explication of meaning and usage.

symptom substitution (hypothesis) The hypothesis that if only the superficial behavioural manifestations of a neurosis are treated in psychotherapy the unresolved underlying conflict will erupt elsewhere and new (and potentially more serious) symptoms will emerge. The hypothesis derives from the assumption that psychological disturbances are analogous to medical disturbances (see MEDICAL MODEL) and that they can only be treated by removal of the root cause of the disorder. The hypothesis is often invoked critically by classically trained psychotherapists as a warning against the dangers of a pure BEHAVIOUR THERAPY, which deals only with maladaptive behaviour and does not concern itself with underlying psychic conflicts.

symptom–symbol hypothesis The hypothesis that a particular symptom may be viewed as a symbol of a particular underlying psychological conflict. The hypothesis is common among the psychoanalytically oriented but is regarded as highly questionable by clinicians of other persuasions.

symptom wearer (or **bearer**) An individual in a complexly structured group (like a family) who manifests the symptoms of a mental disorder while the other group members do not. A careful analysis sometimes shows that there is a complex pattern of interactive behaviour in the group that is seriously maladaptive but that the psychic burden of this tends to fall mostly on one person. Also called IDENTIFIED PATIENT.

syn- From the Greek, a combining form meaning *with, along with, together with, joined together.* vars., *syl-, sym-, sys-*.

synaesthesia A condition in which a sensory experience normally associated with one modality occurs when another modality is stimulated. To a certain extent such cross-modality experiences are perfectly normal; e.g. low-pitched tones give a sensation of softness or fullness while high-pitched tones feel brittle and sharp, the colour blue feels cold while red feels warm. However, the term is usually restricted to the unusual cases in which regular and vivid cross-modality experiences occur, such as when particular sounds reliably produce particular colour sensations. See e.g. CHROMAESTHESIA. var., *synesthesia*.

synapse From the Greek for *juncture* or *point of contact*, the junction between the terminal button of the axon of one neuron and a part of the somatic or dendritic membrane of another neuron. The term itself was introduced at the turn of the last century by the great English physiologist Sir Charles Sherrington. A number of different types of synapse have been identified. They are usually denoted either by their anatomical characteristics (e.g. *axodendritic*) or by the neurotransmitter involved (e.g. *cholinergic*). They can be found in this volume under the relevant qualifying term. adj., *synaptic*.

synaptic button TERMINAL BUTTON.

synaptic cleft The small (roughly 20–30 nm across) space between the terminal button of the presynaptic neuron and the membrane of the postsynaptic neuron across which the neurotransmitters flow.

synaptic pruning PRUNING.

synaptic transmission A general term used for the process of transmission of information from one (presynaptic) neuron to another (postsynaptic) neuron. For more details see NEUROTRANSMITTER, POSTSYNAPTIC POTENTIAL and SYNAPSE.

synaptic vesicles Small capsule-like packages in the terminal buttons of presynaptic neurons that contain neurotransmitters.

synaptogenesis The growth of new synapses.

synchronicity The notion, championed by Carl Jung, that events that occur at the same time are, on occasion, causally joined in significant ways despite their lack of physical proximity. Jung, unfortunately, failed to appreciate the difference between *co-occurrence* and COVARIATION resulting in considerable confusion in various quarters. Not surprisingly, parapsychologists embraced the notion, delighted to be in such august company.

synchronized menstruation See MᶜCLINTOCK EFFECT.

syncope (*sin-co-pee*) A temporary loss of consciousness following a drop in blood flow to the brain, a fainting, a swoon.

syncretic thought SYNCRETISM (2).

syncretism 1 Generally, a bringing together of various disparate aspects in a more or less coordinated manner so as to produce a more unified single system. The connotation is that the resulting system may lack coherence and contain contradictions and/or inconsistencies. **2** In Piaget's developmental theory, a type of cognitive processing in which events are assimilated into global and largely unstructured schemas; that is, a rather nebulous classification system. Contrast this meaning with the Piagetian usage of JUXTAPOSITION (2). **3** In sociological analyses, the union of disparate elements from different social systems into a new structure. **4** In linguistics, the fusion of forms from different languages into a new form. **5** In religion, the reconciliation (or attempts thereat) of opposing principles or practices into a novel, coherent system.

syndrome 1 Generally, a number of characteristics, features, events or behaviours that seem to go with each other or are believed to be coordinated or interrelated in some way. **2** More specifically, in medicine and clinical psychology, a cluster of symptoms that occur together and can be taken as indicative of a particular disease or other abnormality. Individual syndromes are listed in this volume by qualifying term.

synecdoche A form of METONYMY where a

part is taken to represent a whole, e.g. *hand* stands for *worker*.

synesthesia SYNAESTHESIA.

synergic SYNERGISTIC.

synergistic 1 Generally, working together, cooperative. **2** In physiology, characteristic of organs, muscles or the various elements of a large, coordinated system which function together in combination toward some unified aim. Synergistic muscles function together to effect a particular movement, synergistic drugs combine effects cooperatively, and so forth. Contrast with ANTAGONISTIC. var., *synergic*.

synergistic drugs Any two drugs the conjoint effects of which are greater than the sum of the effects of the two taken separately.

synkinesis 1 Generally, an involuntary movement of one bodily part that occurs simultaneously with a voluntary movement of another part. **2** Specifically, an involuntary movement in healthy muscle that accompanies an attempt to move a paralysed muscle on the opposite side of the body.

synonym A word that has the same meaning as another word, or a very similar one. Two words are said to be synonymous if one may be replaced by the other in a sentence without modifying the meaning of the whole sentence. Although to some extent many such synonymous relationships exist between words, and in this volume many pairs of technical terms have been so labelled, it should be pointed out that there are many compelling arguments suggesting that no two words or phrases can ever be truly regarded as synonyms in the sense that no semantic violence whatsoever is done by replacing one with the other.

synopsia A type of SYNAESTHESIA where particular hues give rise to the experience of specific tones.

syntactic aphasia APHASIA, SYNTACTIC.

syntactic component In some contemporary linguistic theories, that aspect of a grammar that contains the formal rules and procedures for producing sequences of elements (usually morphemes or words). Contrast with SEMANTIC COMPONENT (2).

syntagmatic association PARADIGMATIC *ASSOCIATION.

syntax That aspect of grammar that deals with the rules for combining morphemes and words into sentences. adj., *syntactic*. See also GRAMMAR, SEMANTIC and related terms.

syntaxis 1 Use of complex syntax. **2** H. S. Sullivan's term for a mode of thinking and communicating in which the concepts used are objective and publicly observable. See PARATAXIS (2) and PARATAXIC DISTORTION.

synthesis 1 The process of combining elements such that the resulting fusion, integration or organization results in a unified whole. **2** The whole thus formed. Note that the connotation here is that the emergent whole has properties or qualities that are the result of the synthesis and not necessarily derivable from an analysis of the several elements. See CREATIVE SYNTHESIS. adj., *synthetic*, which can also carry the additional connotation of artificiality. Contrast with ANALYSIS.

synthetic language 1 In linguistics, any language that tends to express grammatical relationships by the use of inflections. In synthetic languages, unlike ANALYTIC LANGUAGES, word-order rules are relatively free. Also called *fusional language*. **2** Any artificial language constructed for empirical investigation. Compare with NATURAL *LANGUAGE.

synthetic speech Any speech produced by a mechanical device. Modern SPEECH SYNTHESIZERS produce remarkably human-sounding outputs.

synthetic trainer Any training device that simulates real-world conditions for the purpose of aiding the learning of a particular skill, a SIMULATOR.

synthetic validity VALIDITY, SYNTHETIC.

syntonia A general syndrome characterized by displays of a high degree of reactiveness to the surrounding environment. Some regard a syntonic as a well-adjusted person in harmony with the world, others hold onto the possibility that such reactiveness may be indicative of a proneness to bipolar disorder. With this kind of connotative conflict, this is a good term to avoid.

syphilis An infectious, chronic venereal disease caused by the spirochete *Treponema pallidum*, which enters the system through any break in the skin or a mucous membrane, most commonly during sexual intercourse. The disease has three stages. The primary stage is characterized by the tell-tale chancre that appears roughly two to four weeks after infection and some lymph-node enlargement. The secondary stage occurs about six weeks later and may be manifested in a number of symptoms, including a rash, skin lesions, headaches, fever and further lymph-node enlargement. Some, all or none of these may emerge in a given case. The tertiary stage occurs later, often years later, and is the dangerous one. The heart, blood vessels and entire central nervous system are frequently involved. The symptoms of syphilis in its latter stages are so varied that it has become known medically as 'the great imitator', since without the proper tests it can easily be mistaken for any of a number of other diseases. Neural damage may be severe enough for a variety of psychotic behaviours to occur; see PARESIS.

systaltic Alternately contracting and dilating; pulsating.

system 1 From the Greek, meaning *organized whole*. This sense is carried along in all of the many specialized contexts in which the term is found. Actually, because of the breadth and diversity of usage, the term is rarely found in isolation but is typically modified or qualified by other (one or more) terms or phrases, e.g. circulatory system, dynamic system, open system, nervous system. **2** A more or less well-structured set of ideas, assumptions, concepts and interpretative tendencies which serves to structure the data of an area of science, e.g. the Copernican system in astronomy or any of the several schools of psychology, such as behaviourism or structuralism. **3** Somewhat more restrictively, a particular arrangement of interconnected things (objects, machines, stimuli, etc.); a CONFIGURATION.

systematic 1 Characterized by reflecting the structure and organizational integrity of a SYSTEM (1). **2** Identified with a particular theoretical SYSTEM (2). **3** By extension, orderly, predictable, regular. Distinguish from SYSTEMIC.

systematic desensitization Joseph Wolpe's term for the form of behaviour therapy described under DESENSITIZATION PROCEDURE.

systematic distortion Any regular change in the manner in which memories of preceding events or stimuli are modified. The term is quite general and is used by Gestalt psychologists to refer to the filling-in of gaps in incomplete pictures when they are recalled some time after presentation, by psychodynamically oriented theorists to refer to the altering of memory of past events by defensive or repressive operations, and by cognitive theorists to refer to the constructive and interpretative processes that change the nature of material held in long-term memory.

systematic error CONSTANT *ERROR.

Systematic Multiple Level Observation of Groups SYMLOG.

systematic sampling SAMPLING, SYSTEMATIC.

systematized delusion DELUSION, SYSTEMATIZED.

systemic 1 Generally, pertaining to a SYSTEM (1). **2** More specifically, pertaining to the whole body rather than to any isolated part or organ. Distinguish from SYSTEMATIC.

systemic lupus erythematosus LUPUS.

systems analysis Generally and collectively, the processes and operations involved in the designing, implementing and coordinating of the various components of any complex system. More specifically, the use of systematic analytical procedures derived from industrial/organizational psychology, assisted by the techniques of computer science, to understand the workings of complex organizations, to identify problems and sources of error and to make recommendations for more efficient and effective structures.

systems perspective An approach to clinical research that views pathological behaviours as developing in dynamic social settings. Individuals are seen as developing patterns of behaviour as reactions to the complex interplay of interpersonal factors among members of their families, their friends, their colleagues and the society around them.

systole The contracting phase of the heart cycle.

T

T 1 Temperature. **2** Time.

ₛTᵣ In Hull's notational system, reaction time. Elsewhere *RT* is used.

t 1 A symbol used for denoting the ratio between a statistic and the measure of its standard error. See *t* TEST and *t* *DISTRIBUTION. **2** Abbreviation for *time*.

tabes 1 Generally, any progressive degeneration found in chronic disease. **2** More specifically, degeneration of the posterior columns of the spinal cord. syn., *tabes dorsallis* (for 2).

table A collection of scores or other data arranged in tabular form.

taboo 1 Any banned or prohibited act, object or behaviour. **2** The act of prohibition. The term comes from the Polynesian *tabu*, meaning *sacred, inviolable*, and was originally associated with objects set aside for religious practices and customs and forbidden for general use. Contemporary usage is much broader. adj., *taboo, tabooed*.

tabula rasa Latin meaning *blank tablet*. The term refers to the philosophical view that humans came into this world unencumbered (and unassisted) by particular innate ideas. Espoused strongly by the early British empiricists, this view formed the basis of the theory that learning and experience are the critical factors in the human condition: the environment writes its message upon the pristine mind.

tach Laboratory slang for TACHISTOSCOPE.

tachistoscope An instrument that presents visual materials under conditions of very brief exposures. A sophisticated variety may have up to three or four separate screens (the images from which may be superimposed upon each other in any combination), an extremely precise timing system that can present materials for extremely short durations (less than 1 msec.) and illumination controls to adjust the brightness of the display. Also called *T-scope, tach*.

tach(y)- Combining form meaning *rapid, fast, swift*.

tachycardia A general term for any abnormally rapid heart action.

tachylalia Unusually rapid speech.

tachyphasia Very rapid or highly voluble speaking.

tachyphrenia Rapid mental functioning.

tachyphylaxis Rapid, acute development of tolerance to a particular drug resulting from frequent, repeated administration. See DRUG *TOLERANCE. syn., *acute tolerance*.

tacit 1 Unspoken or silent. **2** Inferred or understood. **3** Unconscious. See also IMPLICIT.

tacit knowledge KNOWLEDGE, TACIT.

tact One of the categories of verbal behaviour proposed by Skinner in his analysis of language. Tacting is verbal behaviour that is under the control of its antecedents and makes contact with the external world. Naming is a classic tact. See AUTOCLITIC and MAND.

tact- Combining form meaning *touch*.

tactic TAXIS.

tactile Pertaining or relating to touch, tactual. Some use it as a synonym of HAPTIC, but see that term for a distinction.

tactile agnosia AGNOSIA, TACTILE.

tactile receptors MEISSNER'S CORPUSCLES, MERKEL'S DISCS.

tactile (sensory) aid Generally, any device that uses the sense of touch to compensate for other sensory disabilities. See SENSORY SUBSTITUTION for such a device that converts incoming stimuli into vibratory patterns.

tactoagnosia TACTILE *AGNOSIA.

tactual TACTILE.

Tadoma method A method for communicating used by the deaf and the deaf-blind by placing the fingers on the speaker's neck and cheeks and thumb on the mouth.

TAG An acronym for *talented and gifted*; TAG programmes are educational programmes designed specifically for the GIFTED CHILD.

tag question Any interrogative formed by appending a tag onto a declarative sentence. For example, in 'It's raining, isn't it?' the phrase 'isn't it?' is a tag. English has the interesting rule that the tag must be negative if the base sentence is affirmative and affirmative if the base is negative.

taijin kyofusho A CULTURE-SPECIFIC SYNDROME seen in Japan. It resembles a SOCIAL *PHOBIA marked by the distinctive sense that one's individual body or its parts or functions offend or displease others.

tail In statistics, the extended portion(s) of a distribution which, when presented graphically, appear(s) as the part(s) of the curve that tail off. Exactly where the tail(s) of a distribution begin(s) and the body of the distribution leaves off is only subjectively determinable. See TWO-TAILED TEST. .

tail flick Quite as it says, a flick of the tail. The latency of a tail flick in a laboratory animal after a painful stimulus has been applied is used as a measure of sensitivity to pain. The procedure is useful in testing analgesics.

Talbot-Plateau law The generalization that when a light flickers at a high enough rate to appear steady it has a perceived brightness that is the mean of the periodic impressions. For example, if the flickering is composed of equally long on and off periods the steady state has one-half the brightness of the on phase. This fused brightness is called *Talbot brightness*.

talent A high degree of ability for a particular skill. This term is particularly tricky in

that it is used by many authors to connote a genetic basis for skill. This genetic issue is theoretical and not lexical; properly the term is neutral with regard to issues of heredity vs. environment. See also ABILITY.

talion principle The principle of retribution, 'an eye for an eye and a tooth for a tooth'. In psychoanalysis, the primitive fear that injury, real or intended, will be repaid in kind.

talk Speech, speaking, uttering. *Talk* is also used as a technical term to refer to normal, everyday speech by writers who wish to be clear that they are making reference to such ordinary language as distinct from the often artificially constrained language and speech that is the focus of much of the laboratory-based research on language.

talking cure A half-joking term for psychoanalytic therapy making fun of the way a person seems to be cured of his or her neuroses simply by talking to an analyst. The usage has extended beyond pure psychoanalysis and is occasionally applied to other therapies based on having the client talk through problems. The term was not coined by an analyst but by a most famous patient, ANNA O.

talking out The full and spontaneous discussion of one's emotional and behavioural problems. Usually the term is restricted to the therapeutic setting but it is flexible enough to be applied in other situations, e.g. with a counsellor, a friend, a teacher.

talk turn TURN-TAKING.

tandem reinforcement SCHEDULES OF *REINFORCEMENT.

tangentiality A psychiatric term for a manner of speaking in which questions are answered in inappropriately oblique and irrelevant ways. Compare with CIRCUMSTANTIALITY.

tangential speech A style of speaking in which the speaker tends to drift off the topic.

tantrum A violent and uncontrolled display of anger.

tanyphonia A weak, thin, tinny-sounding voice.

tapetum A reflective layer of tissue behind

the retina in the vertebrate eye. By reflecting light back onto the retina it increases the ability to see at low-illumination levels. It is also responsible for the way in which eyes appear to shine when viewed at a certain angle, an especially striking effect in some species, such as cats.

tarantism The name for a disorder of the Middle Ages characterized by melancholy, stupor and, surprisingly, an uncontrollable desire to dance. The word derives from the mistaken early belief that the disorder was caused by the bite of a tarantula spider.

Tarasoff decision Named after a famous California case, the decision that a psychotherapist must warn appropriate persons upon becoming aware that his or her client probably presents a risk to another person or persons. Therapist–client CONFIDENTIALITY is broken in such cases.

Tarchanoff phenomenon GALVANIC SKIN RESPONSE.

tardive Characterized by tardiness, lateness. Used of diseases and disorders in which the characteristic symptoms appear relatively late in the normal course of the disorder.

tardive dyskinesia Lit., a late-appearing abnormal movement, a disorder characterized by involuntary, stereotyped and rhythmic movements of the body and face, most commonly tongue protrusion, rolling movements, chewing, lip-smacking, abnormal finger movements, leg-jiggling and neck, trunk and pelvis movements. It is a side effect of long-term use of ANTIPSYCHOTIC DRUGS, and once it emerges it is extremely resistant to treatment. The neuropathology of tardive dyskinesia has not been established, although there are indications that compensatory increases in the functioning of DOPAMINE in the BASAL GANGLIA may be involved. The incidence of the disorder is lower with the newer group of ATYPICAL ANTIPSYCHOTIC DRUGS.

tardive dysmentia A late-emerging set of abnormal cognitive and emotional behaviours associated with long-term use of ANTIPSYCHOTIC DRUGS. Patients are emotionally volatile, socially inappropriate and may display many of the cognitive dysfunctions associated with schizophrenia. Like TARDIVE

DYSKINESIA, onset is insidious and once established exceedingly difficult to treat. The disorder is sometimes referred to as a type of IATROGENIC *SCHIZOPHRENIA. The incidence is lower with the use of the newer ATYPICAL ANTIPSYCHOTIC DRUGS.

target 1 In studies of memory and decision-making, the item that the subject searches for in an array or sequence of items. If more than one item is searched for, the several are collectively called the *target set*. **2** In perception, the specific stimulus the subject is to focus upon (the rest of the field is called the *background* or the *surround*). **3** In physiology, the cell or the type of cell that is affected by a particular chemical or nerve fibre; often called the *target cell*. **4** In research generally, the behaviour or event that an investigator searches for. Also called the *target response*.

target cell TARGET (3).

target response TARGET (4).

target set TARGET (1).

target stimulus TARGET (2).

Tartini's tone DIFFERENCE TONE. See the discussion under COMBINATION TONE. The term honours an 18th-century Italian violinist who first noted the existence of difference tones during double-stopping of a violin string; he used them as a cue to assist in the tuning of his instrument.

task Generally, something that needs to be done, an act that one must accomplish. The term enjoys enormous latitude in usage: it is used of simple physical movements as well as life-goals, and it covers personal tasks set by an individual as well as external demands established by others. It is, because of this generality of meaning, usually qualified to delimit the type of task under consideration.

task analysis Loosely and generally, breaking down any complex task into the component sub-tasks that need to be carried out and the skills, knowledge and operations needed to complete each. The term enjoys wide use in education, psychotherapy and industrial/organizational psychology.

task demands Those aspects of a particular task which, implicitly or explicitly, require of the individual the use of particular actions or particular patterns of thinking or feeling in order to accomplish the goal of the task. See also DEMAND CHARACTERISTICS and SET (2).

task-oriented A term descriptive of persons who tend to focus their attention and energy toward the fulfilment of a given task. The task-oriented individual is goal-directed and less concerned with the affective or aesthetic aspects of a task than with its completion.

taste 1 Originally the meaning of *taste* was *to sense*, taken broadly, and embraced any sense and any stimulus. Gradually the usage was narrowed, first to *touch* and the act of touching, with the connotation of appreciation of that which was touched (a meaning that still exists in many senses of the term), and finally to: **2** The *gustatory* sense, where information about the chemical composition of a solution is conveyed via TASTE BUDS on the tongue and to a lesser extent, the soft palate, pharynx and larynx. There are five known primary tastes, BITTER, SALTY, SOUR, SWEET and UMAMI, with some suggestions of a sixth for fatty acids. Each taste is conveyed by the absorption of particular proteins by specific receptor sites (see TASTE CELL) within individual taste buds. Taste, however, is only one part of gustatory experience; temperature, spiciness, astringency, odours, pressure and texture (see MOUTH FEEL) all play a role. See FLAVOUR. **3** The ability to make well-reasoned and valid aesthetic judgements concerning art, music, decoration, etc.

taste aversion A learned aversion to, and accompanying avoidance of, a particular food which has been associated with some painful outcome or toxic reaction. Also called by a variety of other names. See CONDITIONED *AVERSION and TOXICOSIS.

taste blindness The inability to taste particular substances at particular concentrations. The original work suggested that some people were totally 'blind' to the taste of certain chemical compounds. It now appears that they are not completely insensitive but simply have high thresholds for those compounds and can taste them if the concentration is increased sufficiently.

taste buds Individual sense organs clustered around small protuberances (*papillae*)

and containing the receptor cells for mediating the sense of taste. Taste buds are found over the surface and sides of the tongue, on the soft palate and on parts of the pharynx. Some taste buds contain only one kind of TASTE CELL and respond to only a restricted class of chemical compounds; others appear to contain several kinds of cells and hence respond to various compounds. The life of a taste bud is approximately 10 days.

taste cell The individual cell within each TASTE BUD which functions as a receptor for the sense of taste.

taste tetrahedron A four-sided solid figure presented originally by Henning as a schematic model for the representation of the relations between taste qualities. The presumed four tastes (bitter, salty, sour, sweet) sit on the corners and other tastes are seen as spatial locations assigned by combinations of these. The discovery that there are five primary kinds of TASTE has rendered the model moot.

TAT THEMATIC APPERCEPTION TEST.

tau (τ) coefficient of correlation A measure of correlation developed by the statistician M. G. Kendall (and often called *Kendall's tau*) based upon comparisons between the rank order of each item (or subject) on each of two variables or tests.

tau effect An illusion based on the interaction between time and physical space. In the classic case, three equally bright lights A, B and C are arranged to be equidistant from each other and then flashed in succession. If the time between A and B is less than between B and C, A and B will be perceived to be closer together than B and C. A similar illusion occurs in daily life. If you take two equally long trips, the journey that takes less time will be sensed as having been shorter. See also KAPPA EFFECT.

taurine An amino acid suspected of being a neurotransmitter.

tautology 1 Generally, an unnecessary repetitiveness in language, e.g. 'As a rookie in his first year of play.' **2** In logic, an expression wherein an argument is stated as equivalent to itself: $x = x$. **3** By extension, a circular argument which proves nothing.

taxis 1 A response of an animate organism

with respect to a particular stimulus. The response may be toward the stimulus (*positive taxis*) or away from it (*negative taxis*). Taxes are regarded as genetically controlled, species-specific reactions to particular stimulus events. adjs., *taxic, tactic*; pl., *taxes*. **2** A similar response in plants, a TROPISM. Properly, *taxis* should be used for animals and *tropism* for plants but this nicety is rarely observed.

-taxis A suffix used with words of Greek origin to denote specific taxes; e.g. *phototaxis* is a movement toward light, as displayed by moths.

taxometric procedures A broad class of data analytic procedures that allow one to determine if a TAXON exists. Used in biology, epidemiology and clinical research to identify natural categories, or clusters of symptoms that appear to constitute a disease or disorder. Generally, a number of analytic hurdles must be passed in order to determine whether a taxon exists; procedures include those based on FACTOR ANALYSIS and identification of a CUTOFF *SCORE.

taxon A natural class or category such as a species, a family or an identifiable disorder, whose members are qualitatively different from non-members. pl., *taxa*.

taxonicity The empirical clustering of features or symptoms into an organized and discrete class or category. Contrast with CONTINUITY.

taxonomic constraint The principle that, in learning new words and concepts, children assume that labels refer to objects at the same taxonomic level rather than to actions or objects that are thematically related (i.e. cross category level). For example, although children thematically relate doctors to offices and medical procedures, when asked to say what 'doctor' means or makes them think of, they generalize taxonomically and name specific doctors or say 'nurse'. They rarely mention pills, vaccines or offices.

taxonomy From the Greek, meaning *laws of arrangement*, any systematic set of principles for classification and arrangement. Most commonly, the term applies to hierarchical organization. adj., *taxonomic*, adv., *taxonomically*.

Tay–Sachs disease An inherited disease characterized by severe neurological deterioration and accompanying mental and physical retardation. The deterioration, which is always fatal (usually within the first 18 months of life), results from a lack of a single enzyme necessary for proper metabolism. Also known as *infantile amaurotic idiocy*, the disease occurs approximately 100 times more often in Jewish children, especially those of Ashkenazi ancestry, than among other racial and ethnic groups.

TBI TRAUMATIC BRAIN INJURY.

TCU See TURN-TAKING.

T data R. B. Cattell's shorthand term for any data based on the use of standardized testing procedures.

t distribution DISTRIBUTION, t.

teaching machine A general term for any device used in systematic programmed instruction. It was first introduced by operant conditioners when they extended their research from simple learning to issues of pedagogy. See also COMPUTER-ASSISTED INSTRUCTION, PROGRAMMED INSTRUCTION.

tears A mildly saline solution secreted by the lacrimal glands which functions as lubrication.

teat The nipple of a mammary gland.

technique A fairly specific, learned procedure or set of procedures for accomplishing some specific goal. Typically the term is used with the connotation that these procedures are skilled and mastering them reflects a certain level of expertise. Usage is very broad and typically a qualifier is appended, e.g. statistical technique, experimental technique. Compare with METHOD and PROCEDURE.

technology That aspect of a culture which applies the findings, procedures and principles of systematic investigation to the identification and solution of problems. *Technology* is used more broadly than *science* and more generally than *engineering*.

technopsychology PSYCHOTECHNOLOGY.

tectorial membrane A membrane that is part of the ORGAN OF CORTI in the inner ear. It is a rather rigid structure to which the cilia of the hair cells are attached.

tectospinal tract One of the VENTROMEDIAL PATHWAYS, this travels from the tectum to the spinal cord and coordinates movements of the head and trunk with those of the eyes.

tectum The dorsal portion of the midbrain, consisting of inferior and superior colliculi.

tegmentum The portion of the midbrain that contains the red nucleus, the substantia nigra and the nuclei and roots of the oculomotor nerve.

teknonymy The practice of referencing a parent through his or her offspring, e.g. 'She is Max's mother.'

telaesthesia A general term for those hypothesized paranormal abilities to perceive events, objects, thoughts, etc. without the use of normal sensory systems, e.g. *clairvoyance*, *telepathy*. See PARAPSYCHOLOGY for a general discussion.

telalgia Lit., distant pain. Used of any pain experienced away from the locus of the stimulus causing it, e.g. REFERRED *PAIN.

tel(e)- Combining form meaning: **1** *End* (from the Greek *telos*). **2** *Far* or *distant* (from the Greek *tele*).

teleceptor A DISTANCE RECEPTOR. vars., *teleoreceptor*, *telerecepter*.

telegnosis Lit., knowing at a distance; in PARAPSYCHOLOGY, knowledge of events supposedly acquired by extrasensory means.

telegraphic speech Roger Brown's term for a highly reduced form of speech in which the unessential words are dropped out. This selective omission is similar to what one would leave out of a message to be sent as a telegram. It is observed in the early stages of language learning in children and occasionally in some forms of aphasia. Also called *telegraphese*.

telekinesis PSYCHOKINESIS.

telencephalon A major subdivision of the forebrain. Its principal structures include the cerebral cortex, the basal ganglia and the limbic system. Also called the *end brain*.

teleo- Combining form meaning *perfect*, *complete*.

teleological Pertaining to TELEOLOGY, to purposes, ends or goals.

teleological regression PROGRESSIVE TELEOLOGICAL-REGRESSION HYPOTHESIS.

teleology Any of several theoretical and philosophical perspectives that share, in one form or another, a presumption that purpose and purposeful striving toward ends or goals is an essential component of all events. The term is most often associated with the doctrine that everything proceeds toward some divinely specified ultimate end, that all reality is infused with a *vitalist* spirit (see VITALISM) that directs this process. This point of view is usually branded as a fallacy, on the grounds that, taken to its logical extreme, it entails the notion that the future has a causal impact on the present. Within psychology proper, at least two major theoretical positions have had teleological aspects: McDougall's HORMIC PSYCHOLOGY and Tolman's PURPOSIVE PSYCHOLOGY. Neither ran foul of the teleological fallacy for both used the concept of purpose as a controlling or driving force behind behaviour rather than a leading or enticing force. However, both positions suffered from other shortcomings; see each for details. On occasion Piaget's theory of cognitive development has been called teleological. This is a mistake which comes from misreading his argument that the stage of formal operations is the end point of cognition toward which ontogeny strives. Actually, Piaget argued that his 'end point' was the result of modifications in cognition resulting from conflicts produced by more primitive cognitions of earlier stages. It was a natural outcome of unsatisfactory modes of thought, not a predetermined aim. See PIAGETIAN.

teleonomic Generally, characterizing behaviour that is purposeful. The nominal form, *teleonomy* is used by some as a euphemism for TELEOLOGY in an effort to mark the sense that evolution appears to be moving toward some goal without falling into fallacy. The lexicographic trick fails.

teleopsia A visual disorder in which objects are perceived as being further away than they are and the sense of depth generally is exaggerated.

teleoreceptor DISTANCE RECEPTOR. vars., *teleceptor*, *telereceptor*.

telepathy The hypothesized ability for direct mental contact between two or more persons. See PARAPSYCHOLOGY.

telephone scatalogia A PARAPHILIA marked by recurrent and intense sexual urges involving the making of erotic or obscene telephone calls to nonconsenting individuals.

telephone theory THEORIES OF *HEARING.

telereceptor DISTANCE RECEPTOR. vars., *teleoreceptor, teleceptor*.

telesis The use of social and natural processes in a conscious and rational manner to achieve specified societal aims. Also called *social telesis*.

telestereoscope A STEREOSCOPE that produces an exaggerated sense of depth.

telic Pertaining to that which has purpose or can be viewed as goal-directed. See TELEOLOGY.

telic change Change, particularly social change, that has occurred because of systematic planning aimed at achieving some purpose or goal.

temazepam A BENZODIAZEPAM used primarily for insomnia.

temper 1 Anger. 2 Mood or disposition, especially when conceived of as a personality trait, e.g. even-tempered.

temperament An aspect of an individual's general make-up characterized by dispositions toward particular patterns of emotional reactions, mood shifts and levels of sensitivity resulting from stimulation. The standard view is that temperament has a significant genetic disposition largely because fairly striking differences in reactivity to stimulation can be observed in neonates, especially to stimuli such as loud noises, bright lights, sudden movements, touching and physical contact. Similar differences have been observed in the young of many other species reinforcing the importance of evolutionary mechanisms.

temperature regulation THERMOREGULATION.

temperature sense The sensory system that responds to temperature and temperature changes. It includes the perception of stimuli below the adaptation level of the skin (see COLD) and those above it (see WARMTH). Also known as the *thermal sense* or

thermic sense. See also ADAPTATION LEVEL and THERMOREGULATION.

temperature spots COLD SPOT, WARM SPOT.

temper tantrum TANTRUM.

template (matching) model An early theory of PATTERN RECOGNITION which assumes that various internal representations (i.e. templates) of objects are stored in memory and new stimuli are processed by comparing them with the templates until a match is found. The theory fared poorly; it cannot account for the fact that we recognize that *A*, **A** and *a* are instances of the same letter.

temporal Pertaining to: 1 Time. 2 The temple area of the head. 3 The area of the cortex under the temples.

temporal avoidance conditioning An operant-conditioning procedure in which an aversive stimulus (typically an electric shock) is presented at regular intervals (e.g. every 10 sec.). When the organism (usually a laboratory rat) makes the proper response (e.g. a bar press), the shock is delayed by a fixed amount of time (e.g. 20 sec.). The procedure thus can be seen to have two independent variables: the *shock–shock (S–S) interval* and the *response–shock (R–S) interval*. Typically, good temporal avoidance conditioning develops and the animal learns to avoid the noxious events without the presence of any external stimulus. Since much of the original work with this procedure was carried out by M. Sidman, it is occasionally referred to in the literature as *Sidman avoidance conditioning* or *procedure*.

temporal lobe The lobe of the cerebrum located below the lateral fissure and in front of the occipital lobe. Auditory projection and association areas are found here as well as structures that process higher-order visual information. In addition, the MEDIAL TEMPORAL LOBE contains structures critical for memory, spatial representation and emotion.

temporal lobe amnesia AMNESIA, TEMPORAL LOBE.

temporal lobe epilepsy EPILEPSY, TEMPORAL LOBE.

temporal summation SUMMATION, TEMPORAL.

temporary threshold shift (TTS) Quite literally, the temporary (upward) shift in the threshold for a stimulus. For example, a TTS in hearing occurs following exposure to high-intensity sounds.

temptation 1 A desire or urge to behave in a manner contradictory to what is socially accepted. **2** The object or the circumstances which elicit this urge.

tendency 1 An internal state such that particular behaviours are likely to occur or can be learned relatively easily. This sense is intended when the object of discussion is an animate organism. See DISPOSITION and SET, both of which are used in similar ways. **2** A directionality or focusing of a large number of scores or events. This meaning is applied very generally, particularly in statistics, e.g. *central tendency*.

tender-minded William James's term for a category of persons characterized by idealism, optimism and intellectualism, and a tendency to be rational in thought, to be religious and to believe in free will. James contrasted such persons with the *tough-minded*, whom he characterized as materialistic, realistic and pessimistic, and with a tendency to be irreligious and fatalistic. Despite the intuitive sense that these groups of characteristics really do adhere in particular persons, factor-analytic studies have consistently failed to identify such personality types.

tendon Fibrous connective tissue by which muscles are attached to bones.

tendon reflex A reflexive muscular contraction elicited by a sudden stretching of a tendon. The KNEE-JERK REFLEX is the classic example.

tenet Any general principle, belief or dogma adhered to by a group or by a particular school of thought.

tense 1 adj. Generally, characterized by tautness, rigidity, stretched tight as in a muscle or fibre. **2** adj. Characterized by an emotional state of nervousness or strain, particularly a feeling of being pressured or stressed by events. **3** adj. In phonetics, a DISTINCTIVE FEATURE (2) descriptive of speech sounds produced by deformation of the vocal tract away from its resting position; the opposite of LAX. **4** n. In linguistics, a verb-inflection category marking the time of action as past, present or future. **5** vb. To make or become tense, to create a state of TENSION.

tension 1 Generally, the act of straining or stretching or the state of being so strained or stretched. **2** The sensation associated with contraction of a muscle, muscle group and/or the associated tendons, membranes and ligaments. **3** An emotional state characterized by restlessness, anxiety, excitement and a general, diffuse preparedness to act. Note that this last usage is quite loose and that there are a variety of connotations which may be implied by its use depending on the preference of the writer. **4** A state of strained mutual relations between members of a group, characterized by antagonism and a lack of cooperation; also called *social tension*.

tension reduction Lit., the lessening of tension. Occasionally used as a synonym of DRIVE REDUCTION.

tensor tympani A muscle in the tympanic membrane that controls the tension of the membrane and the amount of sound that is passed to the middle ear.

tentorial notch The opening in the dura mater through which the brainstem passes.

tentorium 1 Generally, any tent-like structure. **2** Specifically, the fold of dura mater that separates the cerebellum from the cerebrum.

teratogen Anything that produces abnormalities in the developing foetus. *Physical teratogens* include such drugs as thalidomide, which, when taken by the mother during early pregnancy, can produce a physically deformed infant. Those substances that do not produce gross physical abnormalities but may affect behavioural, emotional or cognitive processes are called *behavioural* or *psychological teratogens*.

teratology The study of birth defects, specifically the biochemical agents (see TERATOGENS) that cause them.

Terman giftedness study A long-term study begun in 1921 by L. M. Terman and colleagues designed to follow the lives of a large group of gifted children (IQs over 135). Although the lives led through the decades by the participants were highly variable, there was a tendency for the 'termites', as they came to be called, to live longer and be more satisfied with life than contemporaries. However, the study is generally regarded as flawed, not the least by Terman's initial aims, which were fuelled by an unhappy allegiance with the EUGENICS movement.

terminal behaviour In operant conditioning, the desired, final behaviour being shaped. See SHAPING.

terminal bulb TERMINAL BUTTON.

terminal button The enlarged, button-like structure at the end of the branches of an axon containing neurotransmitter substances. Also called by various other names including: *terminal bulb, terminal knob; synaptic bulb, button* and *knob*; and *end bulb, button* and *knob*. See also SYNAPSE and related entries.

terminal factor PRIMARY *FACTOR.

terminal insomnia INSOMNIA, TERMINAL.

terminal knob TERMINAL BUTTON.

terminal reinforcement In circumstances in which reinforcements are received for partial completion of an extended task, the final reinforcement received at the end. Grades and credits are reinforcements for a student, but the degree or the diploma awarded at graduation is the terminal reinforcement.

terminal stimulus The maximum stimulus along some specified dimension that an organism is capable of responding to.

termites TERMAN GIFTEDNESS STUDY.

territorial aggression AGGRESSION, TERRITORIAL.

territoriality The tendency to defend or protect one's space against invasion or incursion. The term is used broadly, so that the territory defended may be a real, physical one or a psychological or personal one; see PERSONAL SPACE. See also the following entries delineating the various kinds of territory that may be involved.

territory, primary A territory possessed and exclusively used by a particular organism or group. A home or a nest is such a territory, as is the area marked by an animal (usually by urinating round the perimeter). Encroach-

ment is a serious affront and the possessor will generally defend against it vigorously.

territory, public (or **free**) Any territory to which almost anyone has free access. Generally the access to and occupancy of such territories is limited and constrained by social or legal convention. Examples are beaches, restaurants, parks and trains.

territory, secondary A territory that is usually a blend of the private and the public. Such territories are not so clearly associated with the total control by one person of a PRIMARY *TERRITORY, but more control is exercised over access than in PUBLIC *TERRITORY. Private social clubs or fraternal organizations are examples.

terror management theory (TMT) A theory, derived from the writings of the anthropologist E. Becker, that argues that activation of the sense of mortality produces the potential for a sense of panic or terror. Such disruptive emotions are generally assuaged by learned and culturally transmitted beliefs that provide individuals with a sense that they are valuable members of an enduring and meaningful world. These beliefs promote self-esteem, which buffers the anxiety. The theory, developed and refined by J. Greenberg, T. Pyszczynski and S. Solomon, is supported by a wide range of evidence that making people momentarily aware of death (increasing 'mortality salience') tends to increase their liking for people and institutions that support their own world view and to engender hostility toward those associated with alternative perspectives. Intriguingly, mortality salience also functions implicitly. The classic TMT reactions emerge even when individuals are unaware of the manipulation.

tertiary circular reaction CIRCULAR REACTION.

test 1 n. Most generally, any procedure used to measure a factor or assess some ability. Included in this encompassing sense of the term are intelligence tests, which yield IQ measures, medical tests, which assess the presence or absence of disease, aptitude tests, which measure potential in some area, various personality tests, which assess aspects of personal style, belief systems and attitudes, statistical tests, which determine the significance of experimental results, etc. To prevent confusion amid this plethora of assessment devices, it is usual to append a qualifier to denote the type and form of test under consideration. Specialized tests are found elsewhere under the names by which they are commonly known. **2** n. In logic, a criterion or critical operation that can be used to assess the validity of a proposition, the truth of a statement, the correctness of an argument, the accuracy of a theory, etc. **3** vb. To undertake to administer any of the assessment devices or procedures covered by 1. **4** vb. To carry out the criterial operations outlined in 2.

testable Characterizing a hypothesis, proposition or theory that lends itself to some kind of systematic evaluation for assessing its validity or applicability. Testability is a hallmark of a good scientific theory. See also FALSIFICATIONISM.

test age AGE, TEST.

test anxiety Quite literally, anxiety about taking a test. When high, such anxiety can depress scores.

test battery A collection of tests the results of which can be combined to produce a single score or profile of scores. Test batteries are used on the assumption that the errors inherent in each separate test cancel each other out and that the single score obtained is, therefore, maximally valid.

test bias BIAS (5).

testee One who takes a test.

test-enhanced learning TESTING EFFECT (2).

testes pl. of TESTIS.

test, group Any test that has been designed so that it can be administered to more than one person at a time.

testicle TESTIS.

testicular Relating to a TESTIS or *testicle*.

testicular-feminizing syndrome ANDROGEN-INSENSITIVITY SYNDROME.

test, individual Any test designed to be administered to individuals one at a time.

testing effect 1 The effect that taking a test has upon the attitudes or opinions that the test is designed to evaluate. It is a source of

error in survey research, particularly when pretests are used which may alter attitudes independently of any experimental manipulation. **2** The phenomenon that studying and then being tested results in better recall than studying alone, even if no feedback is provided. Also called *test-enhanced learning*.

testis A male gonad or sex organ. One of two reproductive glands located in the scrotum which produce spermatozoa and the male hormone TESTOSTERONE. pl., *testes*. syn., *testicle*.

test item Any specific question or specific component of a larger test.

test, mastery Generally, any test designed to determine whether a student has mastered a particular subject-matter.

test–operate–test–exit TOTE.

testosterone The most potent of the naturally occurring ANDROGENS. It is the primary testicular hormone in men, although small quantities are produced by the adrenal cortex of both males and females and by the ovaries in females. Testosterone accelerates tissue growth, causes maturation of the male genitals and the production of sperm, and stimulates the development of the secondary sex characteristics, including growth of facial, axillary and genital hair, voice changes, shifts in hairline (resulting, in many cases, in baldness), muscle development and the redistribution of body fat. It also plays an important role in aggression and dominance.

test, power of POWER OF A TEST, STATISTICAL.

test–retest reliability RELIABILITY, TEST–RETEST.

tests and measurements A generic term for the broad subfield within psychology that focuses on the development, design, administration, evaluation and application of psychological tests of all kinds.

test scaling The process of setting up a scale for a given test. The usual procedure is to administer the test to a sample group of persons and assign values to each item based on the scores obtained from the sample individuals.

test sophistication The extent to which a person has had experience with (psychological) tests and hence is aware of the general nature and procedures in use. In general, such *test-wise* individuals have an advantage over those who are naïve about tests and testing.

test, standardized Any test that has been subjected to a sufficiently thorough development and empirical analysis for an adequate set of NORMS (1) to have been developed and a reasonable assessment of its *reliability* and *validity* to have been obtained.

test-wise TEST SOPHISTICATION.

tetanizing shock Electric shock strong enough to cause TETANUS (1).

tetanus 1 Sustained tonic muscular spasms.

tetany 1 The point at which neural signals to a muscle are rapid enough to cause continual contraction rather than spasmodic contractions. **2** A condition marked by intermittent tonic muscular spasms, usually in the extremities. It is usually caused by changes in extracellular calcium resulting from parathyroid dysfunction.

tetartanopia An extremely rare form of DICHROMATISM marked by diminished sensitivity to yellow and an inability to distinguish blues and yellows.

tetra- Combining form meaning *four*.

tetrachoric correlation CORRELATION, TETRACHORIC.

tetrachromatic theory OPPONENT-PROCESS THEORY OF COLOUR VISION. See THEORIES OF *COLOUR VISION.

tetrahydrocannabinol THC.

textual In Skinner's behaviourist analysis of language, a class of verbal operants controlled by visual verbal stimuli like words and symbols.

texture gradient GRADIENT OF TEXTURE.

T-group SENSITIVITY TRAINING.

thalamic Pertaining to the THALAMUS.

thalamic theory of emotion Also called the *Cannon–Bard theory*. See THEORIES OF *EMOTION.

thalamotomy A form of psychosurgery in which thalamic fibres are severed. It has been used in a few cases of extremely violent patients or extremely hyperactive children. See PSYCHOSURGERY for a discussion of the ethics of such procedures.

thalamus The largest subdivision of the diencephalon of the forebrain. It is a complex, two-lobed structure with one lobe on each side of the massa intermedia, which runs through the third ventricle. It functions as a kind of relay station for afferent information in that all sensory stimuli (except olfactory) are received by it and projected to the cerebral cortex. A number of specific nuclei are found in the thalamus: some receive specific afferent inputs and project them to specific cortical *areas* (e.g. the LATERAL GENICULATE BODIES and MEDIAL GENICULATE BODIES); others relay to the cortex but do not receive specific afferent inputs (e.g. the DORSOMEDIAL NUCLEUS); yet others project diffusely to other thalamic nuclei as well as to the cortex (e.g. the MIDLINE NUCLEUS and RETICULAR NUCLEUS).

thanato- Combining form meaning DEATH. See also NECRO- and related terms.

thanatology The study of the psychological and medical aspects surrounding death and dying.

thanatomania 1 A homicidal or suicidal mania. **2** Wasting away and ultimate death following awareness that one has transgressed seriously some societal taboo or in the belief that one has been bewitched. Also called *voodoo death*.

thanatomimesis DEATH FEIGNING.

thanatopsy An autopsy.

Thanatos The Greek god of death. In Freud's usage, *Thanatos* refers to the theoretical generalized instinct for death and destruction as expressed in such behaviours as denial, rejection and aggression. Compare with EROS.

that's-not-all technique A two-step device for obtaining compliance, common in sales, whereby a deal just offered is immediately sweetened, before the consumer can respond, by either lowering the cost or raising the gain to the consumer. Contrast with the REJECT-THEN-RETREAT TECHNIQUE, whereby the target must reject the initial request before the deal is sweetened. Compare with LOW-BALLING.

THC The abbreviation for *tetrahydrocannabi-nol*, which, for obvious reasons, tends to be used in place of the full scientific term. THC, the active ingredient in marijuana (see CAN-NABIS for details), is known to stimulate specific receptors in various locations in the brain, including the *cerebellum*, the *caudate nucleus*, the *hippocampus* and the *substantia nigra*. It has also been shown to have a variety of medical benefits, including the reduction of nausea caused by drugs used for cancer, lessening of the severity of asthma attacks, and decreasing the pressure on the eye caused by glaucoma. It also has side effects, such as altering mood, disrupting concentration, interfering with memory, modifying visual and auditory perception, and distorting the sense of time. These are the primary effects for those who use THC as a recreational drug.

thelarche (*thelar'kee*) The onset of breast development at puberty.

thema H. Murray's term for a unit of behaviour made up of a NEED and a PRESS. See e.g. THEMATIC APPERCEPTION TEST.

Thematic Apperception Test (TAT) A projective technique developed by Henry A. Murray and his co-workers. The person being tested is given a number of black-and-white pictures of various scenes which are capable of being interpreted in any number of ways and is asked to tell a story about each. The stories are often analysed in terms of the *thema* which the person introduces into each narrative. The thema are, according to Murray's theory of personality, assumed to reflect deep needs, desires, fears, conflicts, etc. See PROJECTIVE TECHNIQUE for further discussion.

theomania A delusionary condition in which an individual believes that he or she is God or has, more modestly, direct, divine inspiration for thoughts and actions.

theophylline A mild stimulant found in tea. It also relaxes the bronchial muscles. Grandma was right: drink hot tea for a cold.

theorem 1 A proposition that has been proved logically, or a corollary thereof. **2** A proposition that can be subjected to a logical proof (or disproof). Distinguish from HYPOTHESIS, POSTULATE and THEORY.

theoretical equation EMPIRICAL *EQUATION.

theory This term has three distinct uses, ranging from the highly formal and precise of the philosophy of science to the loose and informal of popular language. To wit: **1** A coherent set of formal expressions that provides a complete and consistent characterization of a well-articulated domain of investigation with explanations for all attendant facts and empirical data. Such a theory is ideally conceptualized as beginning with the induction of a set of primitive terms and AXIOMS. These axioms are then used to deduce THEOREMS, which are then tested for their truth value, their ability to encompass known facts and, one hopes, their ability to predict new phenomena the existence of which is not yet documented. Needless to say, such theories are rare indeed, even in the more developed natural sciences; in the social sciences there are few contenders and none of any generality. However, psychology abounds with theories of the following variety: **2** A general principle or a collection of interrelated general principles that is put forward as an explanation of a set of known facts and empirical findings. This is the pragmatic sense of the term and is applied widely to proposed explanations which fall well short of the formal criteria of meaning 1. For example, Freud's theory of personality development fails the test of unambiguous deduction of theorems, which is one reason why many have argued that it cannot be rigorously tested; it is, nevertheless, called a theory. To get some sense of how broad the coverage of this pragmatic meaning of the term is, consult the entries THEORIES OF *COLOUR VISION and STIMULUS-SAMPLING THEORY on one hand and the entry PERSONALITY on the other. It will be clear from these that the term is awarded to almost any honest attempt to provide an explanation of some body of fact or data. **3** In popular parlance *theory* takes on exceedingly loose meanings. It even loses some of its explanatory connotations and becomes a kind of catchword for any reasonable set of ideas or principles that are deemed dismissible or suspect. This meaning is often conflated with the above senses, particularly meaning (2). Sometimes this confusion is accidental and results from a failure to appreciate the role theories actually play in science. Other times it is a deliberate confounding of issues as, for example, the claim by defenders of CREATIONISM that evolution is 'only a theory'.

theory-begging The practice of giving a theoretical assumption the name of a well-established fact, thereby conferring apparent credence upon it.

theory-laden Of a term or concept the reference of which can only be understood in the light of a particular theory. The notion of 'unresolved Oedipus complex' only makes sense within the context of classical psychoanalysis.

theory of mind (TOM) A somewhat odd phrase used to refer to an individual's recognition of the concept of mental activity in others. The term, while in principle free of any connotation concerning developmental level, tends to be used with regard to children. That is, a child with a theory of mind is a child who: (a) recognizes that people have mental lives, beliefs, dreams and desires, and (b) has an explanatory framework to account for the actions of others. There is considerable argument in the field over just when a child first develops a theory of mind, with most guesses being in the 3–4-year-old range although different methodologies yield different estimates. See FALSE-BELIEF TASK for a common test used to determine whether a child has a TOM.

theory theory No, that's not a typo. This oddly named theory of cognitive development maintains that infants and children learn by forming and revising theories about the world around them. The view is based on an analogy between cognitive development and the crafting of scientific theories and assumes similar underlying mechanisms.

therapeutic From the Greek, meaning *treatment*. **1** Pertaining to the curative results of treatment. **2** Having some curative properties. **3** Characterizing any effective healing agent or procedure.

therapeutic alliance Loosely and generally, a cooperative working relationship between therapist and client. There are many who maintain that establishing such a rapport is essential for successful psychotherapy.

therapeutic community A social, cultural setting established for therapeutic reasons and within which persons needing therapy live. The term is not used of just any psychiatric facility but those established on the grounds that the whole social milieu, if properly controlled, can have a beneficial impact. See MILIEU THERAPY.

therapeutic crisis A turning point, a CRISIS (1, 2) in psychotherapy which, as per the meaning of the core term, can be either positive or negative.

therapeutics A generic label for any branch of science or medicine concerned with treatment and cure of disease or other abnormal conditions.

therapeutic window In psychopharmacology, the range of plasma concentration of a drug that has significant therapeutic value. The lower limit is the base below which only placebo effects occur, the upper limit is that beyond which the drug's side effects negate its therapeutic effects.

therapeutist THERAPIST (1).

therapist 1 A generic label for any individual trained in and practising the treatment of diseases or other abnormal conditions. **2** An abbreviation of PSYCHOTHERAPIST.

theraplay An occasional synonym of PLAY THERAPY.

therapy An inclusive label for all manners and forms of treatment of disease or disorder. Because the term is so broad, both connotatively and denotatively, qualifiers are typically used to designate the form of therapy referenced. Some combined phrases follow, others are listed under their qualifying term.

therapy, active A general term for any therapeutic approach in which the therapist takes an active, directing role, e.g. RATIONAL EMOTIVE (BEHAVIOUR) THERAPY. Also called *directive therapy*. Contrast with PASSIVE *THERAPY.

therapy, didactic A kind of DIRECTIVE THERAPY in which the therapist instructs the client, explains things in detail and attempts to teach the client various specific ways to overcome his or her problems.

therapy, passive Generally, any therapy in which the therapist maintains a low profile and makes little or no attempt either to control the direction of therapy or to direct changes in the client, e.g. CLIENT-CENTRED THERAPY.

therapy, physical Generally, the use of any physical agent in a therapeutic fashion, e.g. massage, exercise, heat.

therapy, preventive Any therapy that is designed to prevent a serious condition from developing.

therapy puppet A puppet used in PLAY THERAPY.

therapy, reality A cognitive therapy that emphasizes the need for individual change and personal responsibility. It focuses on helping people take control over their own lives and learn to make effective choices to fulfil their needs. It is a *directive therapy* in that the therapist makes concrete suggestions about ways to cope with stress and recommendations for adaptive thought and action.

theriomorphism The attribution to humans of nonhuman traits, characteristics and qualities. The term is typically used to refer to the invocation of explanatory mechanisms and principles derived from animal experimentation and observation for theoretical characterizations of human behaviour. Contrast with ANTHROPOMORPHISM. syn., *zoomorphism*.

thermal 1 From the Greek, meaning *pertaining to heat*. **2** By extension, pertaining to temperature in a broad sense.

thermalgesia A condition of hypersensitivity to temperature in which relatively mildly warm stimuli are experienced as painful. var., *thermoalgesia*.

thermalgia A form of neuralgia characterized by intense burning sensations, pain and reddening of the skin. Also called *causalgia*.

thermal sense TEMPERATURE SENSE.

thermanaesthesia Insensitivity to temperature changes; an inability to experience normal warmth and cold. vars., *thermoanaesthesia, thermanesthesia, thermoanesthesia*.

thermanalgesia A pathological condition in which the normal painful reaction to hot stimuli is not experienced. var., *thermoanalgesia*.

thermanesthesia THERMANAESTHESIA.

thermic sense TEMPERATURE SENSE.

therm(o)- A combining form meaning *warmth, heat* or *hot* that is also used with reference to the full temperature range, including the experiencing of cold. The point is that there is only one physical dimension here, that of kinetic energy, and the subjective classifications of cold, warm, hot, etc. are dependent upon *adaptation levels* and *temperature gradients*.

thermoalgesia THERMALGESIA.

thermoanaesthesia THERMANAESTHESIA.

thermoanalgesia THERMANALAGESIA.

thermoanesthesia THERMANAESTHESIA.

thermocouple A device for measuring temperature change.

thermoregulation The various adaptive processes in the body for regulating heat production and heat loss so that normal temperature is maintained. Centres in the hypothalamus have been identified as critical parts of the general temperature-regulation system. They are stimulated by afferent cutaneous neural impulses and by the temperature of the blood; in turn, they regulate adaptive behaviours such as vasoconstriction and -dilation, panting and sweating.

thermotaxis THERMOTROPISM.

thermotropism An orienting response (see TROPISM) to a stimulus of a particular temperature. The term applies to such responses made to either warm or cold stimuli. *Thermotaxis* is used more or less synonymously, although, strictly speaking, *-taxis* is applied to animals and *-tropism* to plants.

theta rhythm (or **wave**) A pattern of electrical activity in the brain characterized by a very slow rhythm of 4 to 8 Hz. It is observed in states of meditation or quiet focus, during some memory activities and phases of sleep. Also called *theta cycle* or *theta band*.

they-group OUT-GROUP.

thinking As G. C. Oden put it, 'Thinking, broadly defined, is nearly all of psychology; narrowly defined, it seems to be none of it.'

Given the subtle truth of this quip, we might be able to find a middle ground if we treat the term as denoting, most generally, any covert cognitive or mental manipulation of ideas, images, symbols, words, propositions, memories, concepts, percepts, beliefs or intentions; in short, as encompassing all of the mental activities associated with concept-formation, problem-solving, intellectual functioning, creativity, complex learning, memory, symbolic processing, imagery, etc. Few terms in psychology cast such a broad net and few encompass such a rich array of connotations and entailments.

Certain components none the less lie at the core of all usages: (a) *Thinking* is reserved for symbolic processes; the term is not used of behaviours explicable by more modest processes, such as that of rats learning a simple maze. (b) *Thinking* is treated as a covert or implicit process that is not directly observable. The existence of a thought process is inferred either from reports of the one doing the thinking or by observing behavioural acts that suggest thinking is going on, e.g. seeing a complex problem solved correctly. (c) *Thinking* is generally assumed to involve the manipulation of, in theory identifiable, elements. Exactly what these elements of thought are is anybody's (and sometimes, it seems, everybody's) guess. Various theorists have proposed muscular components (Watson), words or language components (Whorf), ideas (Locke), images (Titchener), propositions (Anderson), operations and concepts (Piaget), scripts (Schank) and so forth. Note that some of these hypothesized entities are quite elemental and others quite holistic. No matter: all are serious proposals and all have at least some evidence to support their use in the process of thinking.

Because of the breadth and looseness of the term, qualifiers are often used to delimit the form of thinking under discussion. Some combined phrases follow, others are listed under their qualifying term.

thinking, convergent Thinking which is characterized by a bringing together or synthesizing of information and knowledge focused on a solution to a problem. Such thinking is often associated with problem-solving, particularly with problems that have but a single correct solution. Compare with DIVERGENT *THINKING.

thinking, critical A cognitive strategy consisting largely of continual checking and testing of possible solutions to guide one's work. Critical thinking is often contrasted with *creative thinking* (see CREATIVITY) in that the latter leads to new insights and solutions while the former functions to test existing ideas and solutions for flaws or errors.

thinking, divergent Thinking that is characterized by a process of 'moving away' in various directions, a diverging of ideas to encompass a variety of relevant aspects. Such thinking is frequently associated with creativity since it often yields novel ideas and solutions. Compare with CONVERGENT *THINKING.

thinking type One of Jung's hypothesized personality types. See FUNCTION TYPES.

thinning In operant conditioning, gradually shifting the contingencies of reinforcement from a schedule in which most or all responses are reinforced to a widely spread, intermittent schedule. See SCHEDULES OF *REINFORCEMENT.

thiopental An ultra-short-acting BARBITURATE. Also known as *sodium pentothal* and *trapanal*.

thioridazine One of the PHENOTHIAZINES used as an ANTIPSYCHOTIC DRUG.

thioxanthines A group of ANTIPSYCHOTIC DRUGS, including *chloroprothixene* and *thiothixene* developed for use in schizophrenia. They have a number of side effects including cardiac arrhythmias and have been largely replaced by more effective treatments.

third ear Theodor Reik's metaphorical term for the intuitive perceptual 'processor' of the skilled clinician, which, he argued, can and should be used as the primary instrument in gathering data for clinical, psychiatric diagnosis.

third moment The SKEWNESS of a distribution. See also MOMENT (2).

thirst 1 An internal, physiological state that results from water deprivation. **2** A subjectively experienced internal state that results from water deprivation and is usually characterized by a dryness in the mouth, the throat and the mucous membranes of the pharynx. **3** A drive state resulting from water deprivation that produces a desire for fluids, specifically water, and motivates water-seeking behaviour. **4** By extension, a desire or drive for something, e.g. a thirst for power or knowledge.

thirst, osmometric Thirst produced by an increase in the relative osmotic pressure of extracellular fluids as a result of a loss of cellular fluids.

thirst, volumetric Thirst produced by a decrease in the amount of extracellular fluid in the body.

thoracic Pertaining to the THORAX.

thoracolumbar system A synonym of *sympathetic nervous system*; see AUTONOMIC NERVOUS SYSTEM for details.

thorax The part of the mammalian body between the neck and abdomen specifically demarcated by the diaphragm.

Thorndike–Lorge list A list of several tens of thousands of English words tabulated for frequency of usage as revealed in a variety of written materials, including children's books, novels and magazines. The full compilation, published in 1944, was the first thorough word count in English; several more comprehensive and up-to-date lists have appeared since.

Thorndike puzzle box One of the earliest (if not *the* earliest) pieces of laboratory apparatus specifically designed for studying learning. It was invented by E. L. Thorndike in the 1930s and consisted of a box built of wooden slats into which an animal was locked. Through the bars the animal could see a food reward but could not obtain it until some mechanism was manipulated (usually a lever that had to be pushed) to open the box. Once in common use Thorndike's invention has now been superseded by the SKINNER BOX as the apparatus of choice for the study of operant behaviour.

thought **1** A general term for the cognitive processes discussed under THINKING. **2** A single but complex idea, proposition, etc.

thought–action fusion The belief that

thinking something is the moral equivalent of actually doing it.

thought broadcasting Experiencing one's thoughts as being broadcast from one's head out loud so that they can be heard by others. It is a common symptom of some forms of schizophrenia.

thought disorder An umbrella term for any disturbance in speech, communication, thinking, etc., including delusions, flight of ideas, pathological perseveration and the like. When the disruption is in the form or structure of thinking rather than in the content, the term *formal thought disorder* is used.

thought disturbances A general term for any erratic, disoriented, bizarre thinking. It is found primarily in the clinical literature, where such disturbances are cited as symptomatic of some neurotic and psychotic conditions.

thought experiment MENTAL *EXPERIMENT.

thought impulses A psychoanalytic term for those aspects of dreams hypothesized to result from the ordinary stresses and experiences of everyday life. It is used to distinguish these mundane dream elements from those hypothesized to derive from deeper, unconscious conflicts. See also DAY RESIDUE.

thought insertion An experiencing of thoughts as though they were not one's own but rather were put (i.e. inserted) into one's mind. A common symptom of schizophrenia, it should be distinguished from auditory hallucinations, the apparent hearing of voices that do not exist (also a symptom of schizophrenia).

thought-stopping Quite literally, the stopping of a train of thought, whereby the therapist interrupts an undesirable thought process by the simple expedient of yelling 'Stop!' The client is then instructed on how to use the technique outside the laboratory in everyday life to interrupt counterproductive ways of thinking.

thought, supervalent A pattern of thinking which obsessively hovers around a particular topic. See OBSESSION.

thought withdrawal The experience that somehow one's thoughts have been taken away or removed from one's head. It is often accompanied by the sense that one has fewer thoughts left to use. It is a symptom of schizophrenia.

Thouless ratio The logarithmic transformation of the BRUNSWIK RATIO.

threat 1 Most generally, any action, gesture or response that indicates an intention to attack, harm or intimidate another. This meaning is found in various contexts: in lower animals threats are usually manifested by overt and relatively stereotyped actions; in humans they may be similarly direct, but more often are elaborated by verbal and symbolic forms shaped by our culture. **2** A symbol or sign that portends future unpleasantness. **3** An idea or image (and the accompanying emotional experiences) concerning anticipated events.

threat display Generally, any stereotyped pattern of behaviour that an organism uses to indicate that an aggressive act is imminent. Some use the term as though it does not apply to humans, noting that we have a propensity for the unannounced stealth attack upon our own kind. However, humans do have a number of ritualized bodily and facial displays that announce aggression and give others the opportunity to withdraw without harm coming to either party, which, of course, is the primary goal.

threat to self-esteem model A generalization about how HELPING BEHAVIOUR is viewed by the one being helped. If assistance is seen as supportive, it is appreciated, but if it is perceived as threatening, it tends to make the recipient feel inferior and dependent, and it and the helper are viewed negatively.

three-colour theory Another name for the *Young–Helmholtz theory*. See THEORIES OF *COLOUR VISION.

Three-Dimensional Block Construction Test As it says, a test of a patient's ability to construct three-dimensional block models. It is often used as supplementary to the BOSTON DIAGNOSTIC APHASIA EXAMINATION, as it is presumed to be sensitive to minor right-hemisphere damage.

three mountain task A task used to evaluate a child's PERSPECTIVE TAKING (1). A doll is placed in a variety of places in a display with three mountains and the child is asked to say what the doll can see.

threshold 1 The statistically determined point on a stimulus continuum at which the energy level is just sufficient for an observer to detect the presence of the stimulus. This is the so-called *absolute* (or *detection, objective* or *sensation*) *threshold*. **2** The statistically determined point on a stimulus continuum at which the energy level is just sufficient for one to be able to determine the identity of the stimulus. This is often referred to as the *subjective threshold*. **3** The point where the energy levels of two stimuli differ sufficiently for an observer to detect that the two are, in fact, different. This is the so-called *differential* (or *difference*) *threshold*. **4** The minimum stimulus energy sufficient to excite a neuron; see ALL-OR-NONE LAW (1).

These meanings derive from the vernacular meaning of the term (and its Latin form, LIMEN – see for details on usage) in which the clear connotation is of a point that separates one domain from another, just as the *threshold* of a house demarcates the interior from the exterior. In practice, however, psychological thresholds are only determinable through statistical procedures; they do not exist as unambiguous values. See here the discussions under MEASUREMENT OF *THRESHOLD, SIGNAL-DETECTION THEORY and SUBLIMINAL. syn., *limen*; adj., *liminal*.

threshold, dual This term refers to the fact that all stimulus dimensions basically have two thresholds, the objective and the subjective. See discussion under THRESHOLD (1, 2) for details.

threshold, measurement of Various psychophysical methods exist for determining the sensory THRESHOLDS (1, 2, 3) for any sensory modality. The following three are the most basic and derive from the original work of Gustav Theodor Fechner. They are used for establishing both absolute and differential thresholds, since the same procedural principles apply in each case: (a) *Method of limits* (also known as the *method of serial exploration* and the *method of minimal change*). For establishing a differential threshold a series of stimuli is presented in ascending and descending steps and the subject (or observer) reports whether each stimulus is more (in the sense of being bigger, brighter, louder, etc.), less, or the same as a comparison stimulus. For an absolute threshold there is no comparison stimulus and the subject simply reports whether the stimulus is detected or not; for a subjective threshold the subject attempts to identify each stimulus. The usual convention is to take the 50% point as determining the threshold – the point at which the subject detects the stimulus half the time (for absolute thresholds) or determines that it is detectably different from the comparison stimulus on half the trials (for differential thresholds). (b) *Method of constant stimuli* (also called the *method of right and wrong cases* and the *frequency method*). Similar to the method of limits except that rather than using a graded series of stimuli presented in ascending or descending fashion, a number of fixed stimuli are selected and each is presented many times in random order for subjects to detect, identify, or discriminate. (c) *Method of adjustment* (also called the *method of average error, method of reproduction* and *equation method*). Here the subject adjusts the stimulus directly. For the differential threshold it is adjusted relative to a comparison stimulus; for the absolute threshold the subject finds the weakest value detectable. These represent the classical methods, not surprisingly, a number of variants exist but most are too arcane even for this volume. See also SIGNAL-DETECTION THEORY for further discussion.

threshold shift 1 Generally, any permanent or temporary shift in the threshold for a particular stimulus. **2** In the study of audition, an *increase* in the threshold for a sound stimulus, a partial deafness.

Thurstone-type scales A number of scales, mostly constructed to measure attitudes, are collectively referred to by this label. All derive from the work of the American psychometrician L. L. Thurstone and are based on the general psychophysical technique known as the METHOD OF *EQUAL-APPEARING-INTERVALS. The general procedure for constructing such scales is to take a number of statements reflecting particular attitudes with respect to some topic (e.g. capital punishment, abortion, apartheid) and develop a set of NORMS (1) for them. The norms can then be used to assess individual attitudes of new groups of people.

-thymia, -thymic -THYMO-.

thymine One of the four nucleotide bases that make up DEOXYRIBONUCLEIC ACID. In RIBONUCLEIC ACID, thymine is replaced by *uracil*.

-thymo- (-thymia, -thymic) 1 From the Greek, meaning *emotion, temper* or *soul*. Combining forms are used freely to connote a connection with emotionality, affect, mood, etc. **2** Combining form for terms relating to the *thymus gland*.

thymus (gland) A gland located in the upper thorax anterior to and above the heart. Small at birth, it grows rapidly during the first 2 years of life, reaches its maximum size at puberty and undergoes involution after that. It produces the hormone *thymosin*, which plays a role in the development of immune responses. Removal during childhood is associated with increased susceptibility to infections and disease in later life.

thyroid (gland) An endocrine gland located at the base of the neck. It has two primary lobes lying on either side of the point where the larynx and trachea meet. The secretions of the thyroid control general metabolism and are important in the regulation of growth. See HYPOTHYROIDISM and HYPERTHYROIDISM.

thyroxin The primary thyroid hormone. Its main effect is an increase in metabolism. Excessive secretions lead to HYPERTHYROIDISM, deficiencies result in HYPOTHYROIDISM. Untreated hypothyroidism in infancy leads to CRETINISM.

tianeptine An antidepressant drug, similar in structure to the TRICYCLIC COMPOUNDS except that it functions as a SELECTIVE SEROTONIN REUPTAKE ENHANCER and decreases the serotonin available for neurotransmission. Preliminary studies suggest that it has both antidepressant and anxiolytic effects although there are insufficient data to assess long-term efficacy and potential side effects.

tic A stereotyped, involuntary, spasmodic, nonrhythmic movement or vocalization. Tics are experienced as virtually irresistible, although mild forms can be suppressed to some extent. Stress and anxiety typically exacerbate the condition; concentrated activity and sleep ameliorate it. See TIC DISORDERS.

tic disorders A class of disorders marked by movement or vocal TICS and usually first manifested during childhood or adolescence. They are classified as either *chronic* or *transient*, with a one-year duration being the distinguishing criterion. See e.g. TOURETTE'S SYNDROME.

tic douloureux TRIGEMINAL NEURALGIA.

tickle A rather peculiar sensation with accompanying reflex-like muscle movements produced most readily by light stroking of the skin. Tickle is a rather complex experience and dependent upon the location on the body stimulated, the amount of pressure applied, who is doing the tickling, whether or not it is anticipated and other factors. It is usually accompanied by emotional qualities, often strong, which are both slightly aversive in that there is often an attempt to avoid the stimulus and pleasurable in that it is sought out under the proper conditions. If one attempts to tickle oneself, it is possible to produce the reflex muscular reactions but the emotional tone is missing.

tidal air The air that is inhaled and exhaled during normal breathing while at rest.

tilde (~) **1** In logic, the symbol for negation, ~*A* means *not* A. **2** In linguistics, a diacritical placed over a letter in writing to mark a modified pronunciation.

timbre Tonal quality, tonal character. The subjective experience associated with complex acoustic stimuli that results from the patterns of overtones, combination tones, harmonics and resonances.

time 1 n. A slippery concept indeed. As St Augustine puzzled over it: when someone asked him 'What is time?' he knew what it was, but no sooner had the question been posed than the answer eluded him. The difficulty, he argued, lay in the problem of measurement and in the tendency to look for analogy between spatial and temporal measurements. These problems have received a certain, albeit not totally satisfactory, resolution in the modern relational conception of time as an aspect of a four-dimensional space–time manifold. In this conception, time is not a separate phenomenon and it becomes metaphysically meaningless to talk of the 'flow' of time or the 'passage' of time. Rather, the full spatiotemporal structure of things is given by the changing distribution of matter.

The reason for going into this problem here is that this relational perspective is precisely the one psychologists adopt, perhaps without knowing it, when they speak of time, and it is the only even marginally satisfactory way in which to conceptualize the psychological experiencing of time, duration, extension and the varied connotations of words like *past, present, future, now* and *then*. Put simply, from a psychological point of view time is always dealt with relativistically; time is marked and phenomenologically experienced as events occurring relative to other events. See, in this context, PSYCHOLOGICAL *TIME, SOCIAL *TIME and SPECIOUS PRESENT. **2** n. For those who find the above unrevealing it will do quite well to think of time as the interval between the beginning and the ending of a thing or event as measured by some arbitrarily selected marking device such as a stopwatch or calendar. **3** vb. To evaluate or measure the duration of an event.

time-and-motion analysis In industrial-organizational psychology, a study of the time that it takes for particular actions or operations to be carried out.

timed test Any test that has time constraints imposed on the person taking it. See also SPEED TEST.

time error ERROR, TIME.

time out A period of time during which the behaviours under consideration are prevented from occurring, or if they occur they go unreinforced. In experimental research of operant behaviour a time out can be brought about by any number of techniques, including removing the experimental subject, removing the manipulandum, introducing distracting stimuli or simply turning off all lights and plunging the experimental chamber into darkness. As a technique in behaviour therapy it is used to weaken undesirable behaviour; e.g. a child throwing a temper tantrum is deposited gently but firmly in a room away from everyone else. abbrev., *TO*.

time perception The perception of the passage of time; the awareness of duration.

Application of the term is generally restricted to subjective time, the sense of the passage of time or the awareness of when an event occurred relative to other events. See the extended discussion under TIME (esp. 1).

time, psychological Experienced time, subjective time. The sense of duration independent of external markers like clocks, calendars and day/night cycles. It seems clear that this sense of time must be dependent upon internal, endogenous events. Some of these may be biological (see BIOLOGICAL CLOCK, CIRCADIAN RHYTHM), others may be mental or cognitive (see COGNITIVE MARKER).

time sample SAMPLE, TIME.

time score Quite literally, a score based on how long it takes to carry out a particular operation, solve a problem, identify a stimulus, etc.

time sense TIME PERCEPTION.

time series The arranging or organizing of data along a time dimension, usually with constant temporal categories marked. For example, changes in some behaviour may be coded along a temporal dimension in which observations are taken every day at noon, once a week, etc. Time series are common modes of analysis for phenomena that show cyclical fluctuation, e.g. CIRCADIAN RHYTHM.

time, social Time as marked and coded in accordance with significant events within a particular society or culture. The notions of astronomical time or clock time are not always present in this form of subjective time; the frame of reference becomes societal phenomena and, hence, concepts like 'before' or 'after' are relativistically marked but concepts like 'how long before/after' may not be. Social time scales may be very different from culture to culture.

time study TIME-AND-MOTION ANALYSIS.

tinnitus A subjective sensation of ringing or tinkling in the ears experienced in the absence of any external acoustic stimulus. It has a number of causes, including diseases of the outer, middle or inner ear, nerve damage and some drugs, such as quinine and aspirin, to which it can develop as a reaction.

tip-of-the-tongue (TOT) state A term coined by R. Brown and D. McNeill, albeit the concept that it denotes goes back to William James, who gave, in 1890, a most poetic characterization of this mental state in which one cannot quite recall a name or a word. As James put it: 'The rhythm of a lost word may be there without a sound to clothe it; the evanescent sense of something which is the initial vowel or consonant may mock us fitfully without growing more distinct. Everyone must know the tantalizing effect of the blank rhythm of some forgotten verse, restlessly dancing in one's mind, striving to be filled out with words.' In other words, the missing name or word is 'on the tip of the tongue'.

tissue Generally, any organic structure made up of cells with similar structures and common functions which are organized or bound together in some manner.

tissue need NEED, TISSUE.

titillate 1 To excite or arouse sexually. **2** To tickle.

titration Determining the concentration of a substance in a solution. In psychopharmacology, the process is used to find optimal levels of therapeutic drugs. Dosage may be gradually increased until an effective level is found or decreased to establish levels where side effects are minimal.

T-lymphocytes IMMUNE REACTIONS, SPECIFIC.

TM TRANSCENDENTAL MEDITATION.

T-maze A maze shaped like a T, consisting of an approach alley and two arms, either one of which the subject may choose.

TMS TRANSCRANIAL MAGNETIC STIMULATION.

TO TIME OUT.

tobacco dependence NICOTINE DEPENDENCE.

tobacco withdrawal NICOTINE WITHDRAWAL.

toilet training Simply, training an infant to urinate and defecate in the socially accepted place and manner. Considerable fuss has been generated round this process, stimulated primarily by the notion derived from psychoanalytic theory that the manner in which toilet training is carried out may have a lasting impact on an individual's personality. Specifically, harsh or severe toilet training has been hypothesized to lead to a neurotic perfectionism, stinginess and a generally ungiving and unforgiving personality. There is little (no?) evidence to support this presumed tie between personality and toilet training other than the obvious – that harsh and severe parenting in any and all aspects of child-rearing may lead to a neurotic personal style in adulthood.

token 1 An object taken to represent something or event, a SIGN. **2** A mark characteristic or indicative of some thing, idea or principle, a SYMBOL. **3** An object such as a coin that can be used as a medium of exchange; see TOKEN ECONOMY. **4** A specific utterance or written form of a linguistic expression. In 'Happiness begets happiness' there are three word tokens but only two word types; see TYPE (4) and TYPE–TOKEN RATIO.

token economy A form of behaviour therapy in which a therapeutic environment is established based on the use of TOKENS (3) as secondary reinforcers. Derived from the premises of theories of conditioning and learning, such economies have been introduced into mental institutions, prisons, educational programmes with problem children and the like. They operate according to three basic principles: (^) the patient (prisoner, child) is rewarded with tokens for appropriate behaviour; (b) the number of tokens for a response is proportional to the requirements of the response (e.g. more work means more tokens); (c) the tokens may be cashed in for real, valued rewards.

token-identity theory IDENTITY THEORY.

token reward A TOKEN (3).

tolerance 1 An attitude of liberal acceptance of the behaviours, beliefs and values of others. The term is used by some with very positive connotations, in the sense that tolerance embodies vigorous defence of others' values and recognition of the worth of pluralism and that the truly tolerant person will resist any attempt to inhibit his or her free expression. Others, however, use it in a vaguely negative sense, implying that tolerance is a kind of strained forbearance, a sort of gritting of one's teeth while putting up with the behaviour, beliefs and values of others. This latter usage derives from: **2** The ability to endure stress, strain, pain, etc.

without serious harm. **3** Short for DRUG *TOLERANCE.

tolerance, acute DRUG *TOLERANCE which develops very rapidly; on occasion a single dose may be sufficient. syn., *tachyphylaxis*.

tolerance, chronic DRUG *TOLERANCE which develops gradually over time with repeated doses. Two kinds of chronic tolerance usually distinguished are DRUG-DISPOSITIONAL ·*TOLERANCE and PHARMACODYNAMIC *TOLERANCE.

tolerance, cross DRUG *TOLERANCE for one pharmacological compound produced by chronic doses of another from the same family of drugs. For example, chronic use of heroin produces increased tolerance for all other opiates, even though they may never have actually been sampled.

tolerance, drug A condition of diminished responsiveness to a particular drug resulting from repeated exposure to it. Once tolerance has developed, increased doses are required to produce the effects achieved earlier with smaller doses. Various types of drug tolerance are distinguished: ACUTE *TOLERANCE, CHRONIC *TOLERANCE, DRUG-DISPOSITIONAL *TOLERANCE, PHARMACODYNAMIC *TOLERANCE.

tolerance, drug-dispositional CHRONIC *TOLERANCE for a drug characterized by an increase in the speed and effectiveness with which the body can dispose of the substance. The manner in which over time the body comes to metabolize alcohol more and more rapidly illustrates this kind of tolerance. Compare with PHARMACODYNAMIC *TOLERANCE.

tolerance level In pharmacology, the level of a drug which, if exceeded, will likely cause unwanted side effects.

tolerance of ambiguity AMBIGUITY, TOLERANCE OF.

tolerance of anxiety ANXIETY, TOLERANCE OF.

tolerance of uncertainty UNCERTAINTY, TOLERANCE OF.

tolerance, pharmacodynamic CHRONIC *TOLERANCE for a drug characterized by a gradual decrease in the effectiveness of the substance to act upon the bodily tissues. The barbiturates show this form of tolerance. Compare with DRUG-DISPOSITIONAL *TOLERANCE.

tolerance, reverse An *increase* in sensitivity to a drug with repeated administrations. It is rare but occasionally seen in central-nervous-system stimulants such as *amphetamine*.

Tolmanian The point of view associated with the work of the American psychologist Edward Chace Tolman (1886–1959). Tolman is probably best categorized as a neobehaviourist. Because of his strong affiliation with building a scientific psychology he embraced the core notion of BEHAVIOURISM – that what an organism *does* is the source of legitimate data – but, because he eschewed the atomism of the Watsonian approach, he advocated the use of intervening variables and focused on a number of very nonbehaviourist processes, such as *purpose* (see PURPOSIVE PSYCHOLOGY), *expectation* (see SIGN GESTALT), *belief* (see BELIEF–VALUE MATRIX) and *spatial representation* (see COGNITIVE MAP).

TOM THEORY OF MIND.

Tomatis method (or **therapy**) A therapeutic method developed by Alfred Tomatis to retrain auditory attention and language processing in individuals who experience difficulties in listening and language comprehension. The method involves switching music, speech or other auditory stimuli on and off while the person listens.

tomato effect A failure to recognize the usefulness of a drug or therapeutic procedure because it fails to mesh with currently accepted views. The term comes from the refusal of North Americans to eat tomatoes until the 1820s. Having been identified as a member of the nightshade family, they were assumed to be toxic despite the fact that Europeans had been consuming them with gusto for decades.

-tome, -tomy Combining form meaning *cutting*, *slicing* or an *instrument for cutting*.

tomography From the Greek *tomos* meaning 'section' or 'cutting', the creating of a three-dimensional slice through an object that reveals its internal structure and features, e.g. POSITRON EMISSION TOMOGRAPHY.

tonal Pertaining to tones. Note that *tonal* and *auditory* are sometimes (but not, strictly speaking, correctly) used interchangeably, particularly in combined phrases. For entries

not found below see those following AUDITORY.

tonal attributes Generally, any of the characteristics of auditory sensations that can be independently assessed. The standard analysis is that there are four such attributes: PITCH, LOUDNESS, VOLUME and DENSITY; see each for details. Also called *tonal dimensions* or, more generally, *auditory attributes* or *dimensions*.

tonal brightness A dimension of sensation accompanying auditory stimuli which seems, subjectively, to relate to a sense of the 'brightness' or 'dullness' of the sounds. High-pitched tones are typically called bright or sharp and low-pitched ones dull or soft. syn., *tonal brilliance*.

tonal character TIMBRE.

tonal colour TIMBRE.

tonal density DENSITY (3).

tonal dimension TONAL ATTRIBUTES.

tonal gap Quite literally, a gap or hole in auditory perception, a region along the frequency dimension where, for any number of reasons, an individual shows reduced sensitivity. Compare with TONAL ISLAND.

tonal interaction(s) Collectively, those interactions that occur between two or more tones sounded simultaneously and the properties of the cochlea of the inner ear. See e.g. COMBINATION TONE.

tonal intermittence AUDITORY *FLICKER.

tonal island Quite literally, an island in auditory perception, a region along the frequency dimension where a person displays normal hearing but which is surrounded by regions of reduced sensitivity. Compare with TONAL GAP.

tonality 1 PITCH. **2** A perceptual characteristic that each particular pitch has with its octaves. For example, a tone of 440 Hz shares tonality with one of 880 Hz even though it is obvious to a listener that they have different pitches.

tonal range TONAL SCALE.

tonal scale The full range of frequencies perceivable in normal human hearing. In the young adult whose ears have not been assaulted by the outrages of factories, subways, tubes and high-intensity rock music, the range is roughly 20–20,000 Hz. Also called *tonal range*.

tonal volume VOLUME.

tone 1 Any sound produced by a regular or periodic vibrating source. Tones are *simple* or *pure* (see TONE, PURE) when the source vibrates with a single frequency, and *compound* or *complex* (see TONE, COMPOUND (or COMPLEX)) when more than one frequency is present. The term NOISE is reserved for auditory stimuli in which no regular periodic component exists. Several different kinds of tone can be identified: see the following entries or the appropriate listing elsewhere. **2** In music, a standard unit that forms the basis for dividing up an octave. Different musical forms use different units; in the music of the Western world a whole tone corresponds to one-sixth of an octave, which yields 12 semitones. **3** A general body state in which organs, muscles, glands, etc. are functioning normally. **4** A state of normal muscular tension characterized by a slight contraction of muscle. Muscle tone is maintained by proprioceptive reflex and serves to keep the body in a general state of preparedness. syn., *tonus*, *tonicity*. **5** Loosely, emotional quality, mood or feeling. **6** In some languages (e.g. Chinese) a type of phoneme based on pitch and pitch contour. **7** Nontechnically, a characteristic quality of voice, as in the common admonishment 'Don't you use that tone of voice with me.'

tone colour TIMBRE.

tone, compound (or **complex**) Any tone made up of two or more simple tones. Any complex tone can be analysed into a number of pure, sinusoidal components by means of a FOURIER ANALYSIS.

tone deafness Loosely, any poorer-than-normal ability to detect difference in pitch. The term does not carry the usual connotations of *deafness* in that thresholds for individual tones may be normal. Also known as *asonia*.

tone, intermittence INTERRUPTION TONE.

tone, pure A tone produced by a single periodic vibration occurring at a fixed rate. Pure tones are approximated by good tuning forks, but the really pure tone is only heard when generated by sophisticated electronic equipment. Also called *simple tone*.

tone, summation COMBINATION TONE.

tonic 1 adj. Pertaining to muscle TONE (4) or *tonus*. **2** adj. Descriptive of languages that use TONE (6) phonemes. **3** n. Any substance that increases bodily TONE (3, 4). **4** n. The keynote of a scale or a chord founded on the keynote.

tonic-clonic epilepsy See MAJOR *EPILEPSY.

tonic-clonic seizure A seizure that has tonic features where muscles are in spasm followed by a clonic state where muscle spasms alternate with relaxations. syn., *grand mal seizure*. See EPILEPSY et seq.

tonic immobility A condition of complete immobility resulting from contraction of muscle groups. It serves as a protective reaction against predators in many animals. Also called FREEZING and DEATH FEIGNING; see each for details on usage.

tonicity The state of possessing TONE (3 or 4).

tonic spasm SPASM.

tonoclonic Both *tonic* and *clonic*; used occasionally of severe muscle spasm.

tonometer 1 A device for measuring muscle tone. **2** A device for measuring the pitch of a tone.

tonotopic representation The point-by-point relationship between the basilar membrane and its representation along the auditory cortex.

tonotopy TONOTOPIC REPRESENTATION.

tonus A slight, continuous contraction or tension in a muscle. See TONE (4); compare with CLONUS.

tool use Obviously, the use of tools. But this deceptively simple definition masks issues of importance to philosophers, ethologists and psychologists. Contemporary definitions usually go something like: 'Use of an object external to the organism that is held, carried or otherwise controlled by the organism in order to accomplish a goal.' Note that some reserve the term for artefacts and manufactured objects, referring to the goal-directed use of naturally occurring, unmodified objects such as rocks and sticks seen in a variety of species (corvids, nonhuman primates) as *proto-tool use*. This restriction is a relic from earlier models that viewed the use of tools as a hallmark of our species.

topagnosis A loss of the ability to localize the site of a tactile stimulus.

top-down A spatial metaphor used to characterize cognitive and perceptual systems and operations that utilize abstract and symbolic representations to analyse simpler, raw inputs. See PHONEMIC RESTORATION EFFECT and PROOF-READER'S ILLUSION (2) for two common perceptual effects, EXPLICIT *LEARNING for an acquisition system based on top-down functions and DEDUCTION for its use in logical analysis and problem-solving. Compare with BOTTOM-UP.

top-down processing Generally, cognitive or perceptual processing in which complex and abstract representations are applied in a TOP-DOWN manner to the analysis of inputs and lower-level representations. Compared with BOTTOM-UP PROCESSING, top-down processing is relatively slow and deliberative, utilizes conscious control mechanisms and works with material that is abstract and symbolic. Note that when the term is used in cognitive psychology the implication is that the processes are characterized by deliberative, conscious control; in perception this connotation is missing.

topectomy A variation of the frontal lobotomy in which small cuts are made through the thalamo-frontal tracts. See LOBOTOMY.

topiramate An ANTIEPILEPTIC DRUG that is also used in treatment of BIPOLAR DISORDER. It slows neurotransmission generally by blocking sodium channels. Predictably, its side effects include drowsiness and a slowing of motor action.

top(o)-, -topic, -topy Combining forms meaning *place, location*.

topographagnosia A neurological disorder marked by a loss in the ability to represent the TOPOGRAPHY of one's environment. A form of LANDMARK *AGNOSIA, the cause is usually a parietal lobe lesion.

topographic memory SPATIAL *MEMORY.

topographic organization A systematic,

spatial arrangement. See SOMATOTOPIC REPRESENTATION, RETINOTOPIC REPRESENTATION and HOMUNCULUS (2) for examples within the nervous system.

topography 1 Generally, a schematic representation of a region of the environment marking physical features. **2** A similar representation of a body or bodily part showing structural features and relations between them. This meaning is occasionally extended in a metaphoric sense to abstract entities as in the *topography of the mind*, a phrase often used of Freud's vertical representation dividing the psyche into the *conscious, preconscious* and the *unconscious*. **3** RESPONSE TOPOGRAPHY.

topological psychology A descriptive term often used of Kurt Lewin's FIELD THEORY. See also TOPOLOGY.

topology A branch of mathematics that deals with those properties of space which remain unchanged when the space is distorted. In psychology the principles have emerged in several areas, notably Lewin's FIELD THEORY and Piaget's arguments concerning the infant's representation of space.

-topy TOP-.

Torrance Tests of Creative Thinking Two test batteries developed by E. P. Torrance to measure creativity objectively. The widely used tests are based on evaluating fluency, flexibility, originality and elaboration, the processes that many argue underlie creative functions. It should be noted that there is no broadly accepted model of creativity and only fleeting evidence that scores on these (or any other) tests predict future displays of this elusive mental property.

torsion 1 Generally, the condition of being twisted or the act of twisting. **2** The minor rotation of the eye through the horizontal axis from the pupil to the back of the eye that occurs during normal eye movement. Also called (*ocular*) *torsional movement*.

total determination, coefficient of The square of the MULTIPLE CORRELATION COEFFICIENT; hence, a number reflecting the proportion of total VARIANCE accounted for by all the independent variables in a multiple correlation. Denoted as R^2.

total institution INSTITUTION, TOTAL.

total recall Loosely, the ability to recall completely all information committed to memory. Such perfect storage and retrieval of memories is a myth. The closest thing to it is seen in some extremely accomplished mnemonists, who develop rich and elaborate schemes for remembering material (see MNEMONIC DEVICE) and in rare cases of people with EIDETIC IMAGERY.

totem 1 An object or class of objects (usually but not always a species of animal or plant) which is viewed by members of a society or group as having a special, mystical and symbolic role in their community. **2** Any symbolic representation of the venerated object(s) in the above sense. In Freud's more speculative theorizing, the totem was taken as symbolic of the primal father.

TOTE (unit) An acronym for *test–operate–test–exit*. A hypothesized unit of planned, sensorimotor activity which is easiest to explain with an example. A person fills a bathtub and puts a hand in to check the temperature (*test*); finding it too hot, the person adds cold water (*operate*); finding it now satisfactory (*test*) the person turns off the water (*exit*). The TOTE unit was put forward some years ago as a model of behaviours in which actions to be taken are based on plans modified by feedback concerning actions already taken, a basic conceptualization borrowed from CYBERNETICS.

TOT (state) TIP-OF-THE-TONGUE (TOT) STATE.

touch Loosely and generally, the contact of some object with the body or the sensory experience which accompanies such contact. Since Aristotle we have been saddled with the notion that we possess a 'sense of touch', and although the popular press (and even some technical literature) still refer to it as such, properly touch is not a unitary sensory system but an aspect of a complex group of CUTANEOUS SENSES, which includes pressure, pain (of at least two kinds), the temperature senses and tickle.

touch blends Sensations which are a mixture of other cutaneous experiences. The classic example is wetness, which is produced by a blending of pressure and cold and can be experienced without any moisture at all, as anyone who has ever put on a rubber surgical glove can testify.

touch spot Loosely, any small local area of the skin that is highly sensitive to light touching.

tough-minded TENDER-MINDED.

Tourette's syndrome (or disorder) A neurological TIC DISORDER characterized, in mild form, by involuntary tics and movements and, in advanced cases, by large involuntary bodily movements, noises like barks and whistles, and in many instances an uncontrollable urge to utter obscenities.

Tower of Hanoi A classic problem-solving task consisting of a board with three pegs and a stack of (usually but not necessarily) five disks of decreasing diameter placed on one of the pegs. The aim is to move the stack of disks to one of the two other pegs in the fewest number of moves – with two restrictions: the disks must be moved one at a time, and at no time may a larger disk be placed on top of a smaller one.

toxaemia Any abnormal condition produced by toxic substances carried throughout the body by the bloodstream. var., *toxemia*.

toxic Pertaining to poison, poisonous.

toxicosis 1 Generally, any condition caused by poisoning. **2** Specifically, a synonym for CONDITIONED *AVERSION.

toxic psychosis Any psychosis that results from organic damage produced by a toxic substance, e.g. *alcoholic psychosis*.

toxoplasmosis A disease caused by a protozoan carried by mammals and birds. When contracted, it is usually through the handling of cat faeces. Infected adults rarely have symptoms but those with compromised immune systems may have flu-like symptoms. A congenital form that occurs when the parasite is transmitted to the foetus can cause cranial deformities, retardation and blindness.

toy tests A general label for any psychological test utilizing toys. Not surprisingly such tests are used almost exclusively with children and frequently involve free play with common objects like puppets, dolls and blocks. They are usually considered to be projective tests in that children are assumed to reveal attitudes and feelings through their manner of play.

trace 1 The hypothesized modification of neural tissue resulting from any form of stimulation. A MEMORY TRACE. **2** A minute amount of a substance. **3** A mark or sign.

trace conditioning An experimental conditioning procedure in which the onset of the unconditioned stimulus (US) does not occur until some time after the termination of the conditioned stimulus (CS). Thus, any conditioning that occurs depends upon a hypothetical trace that is left after the CS terminates. Trace conditioning, when it occurs, reveals the operation of a rather basic memory process. Compare with DELAY CONDITIONING.

trace, perseverative Hull's term for neural firing that continues after the stimulus has been removed. The more modern characterization of this general principle is found under SENSORY INFORMATION STORE.

tracking 1 Following a target. **2** In education, the separating of each grade into levels and the assigning of each child to a particular level based on assessments of his or her (presumed) ability to master the material. Tracking may take place within a given school, or separate schools may be established for different levels. Also called *streaming*.

tract 1 Generally, a pathway. **2** A bundle of nerve fibres that constitutes a particular functional and/or anatomical unit. **3** A group of organs that constitutes a continuous functioning pathway, e.g. the digestive tract. **4** In sociology, a small division of a city or urban area.

tradition Any social custom or belief, or a coordinated set of such customs and beliefs, that is handed down through the generations.

traditional authority AUTHORITY, TRADITIONAL.

tradition-directed In the terminology of D. Riesman, a tendency to conform to and follow a society's traditions. Like Riesman's other terms, INNER-DIRECTED and OUTER-DIRECTED, this one is used in reference to both the society that fosters such behaviour patterns and the individual who displays them.

train Loosely, to direct activities and/or functions so as to produce some specified end state or condition. The term is used broadly: one can train plants, animals and people.

trainability The degree to which a particular individual can profit from training.

trainable mentally retarded (TMR) MODERATE *MENTAL RETARDATION.

training Generally, any specific instructional programme or set of procedures designed to yield as an end product an organism capable of making some specific response(s) or engaging in some complex skilled activity. This broad definition encompasses essentially all contemporary usages of the term, from the programme of an animal trainer in a circus (who uses operant-conditioning procedures) to the physical regimen of an athlete or to a parent toilet-training a child.

training trial LEARNING *TRIAL.

trait Generally, any enduring characteristic of a person that can serve an explanatory role in accounting for observed regularities and consistencies in behaviour. This is the proper use of the term; it is misleading to use it for the regularities themselves. The point is that a trait is a theoretical entity, a hypothesized, underlying component of an individual that is used to explain that person's behavioural consistencies and the differences between the behavioural consistencies of different persons. In this sense the term has wide applicability: (a) in biology it refers to a distinguishing anatomical feature; (b) in genetics it denotes an inherited characteristic; (c) in a larger sense it covers any aspect of an individual's personality. Note, also, that as one moves through these various domains of usage the referent of the term becomes more abstract and more difficult to assess. The problems become particularly serious in the study of PERSONALITY; see that entry (esp. 2) and PERSONALITY TRAIT for details.

trait, acquired A trait that is the result of experience, a learned trait. Contrast with INHERITED *TRAIT.

trait anxiety ANXIETY, TRAIT.

trait, compensatory Very loosely, any trait hypothesized to have become a significant part of an individual's make-up in compensatation for the lack or reduced ability of some other function. See COMPENSATION (1, 2) for the general theory here.

trait, inherited A trait due to genetic factors, one independent of learning or experience. While this is the literal meaning, the term is used with the understanding that what is inherited in most cases is not a trait, per se, but a *predisposition* to display that trait. This connotation reflects the generally accepted view that biological and genetic factors interact with the experiential. Contrast with ACQUIRED *TRAIT.

trait negativity bias A tendency to let negative information about an individual have a greater impact on impression formation than positive information. Put simply, one bad trait may destroy a person's reputation no matter how many good traits are present. Politicians and image makers are acutely aware of this bias. Also called *dirty halo effect*.

trait organization A loose term generally taken to refer to some hypothesized set of interrelationships between an individual's various personality traits.

trait profile PROFILE ANALYSIS.

trait, source A hypothetical 'deep' trait which is presumed to account for the fact that many SURFACE *TRAITS show relatively high mutual correlations.

trait, surface 1 An interrelated group of behaviours and manners observed to occur across various kinds of environment settings and constraints. 2 A hypothesized trait which is identified by factor analysis and presumed to be responsible for these correlated behaviours.

trait, unique 1 Interpersonally, a rare trait, one found in but a few. 2 Intrapersonally, a trait that shows essentially no correlation with others.

trait variability Quite literally, the dispersion or scatter of scores of an individual on several tests measuring traits.

trance 1 From the Latin for *passage*, trance originally referred to the state of passage from life into death. 2 A state in which consciousness is fragile or missing, voluntary action is poor or absent and normal bodily functions are reduced, perhaps to the degree that an individual in a trance appears to be in a deep sleep. Meaning 2 carries some of the vestiges of meaning 1.

trance and possession disorder A temporary alteration in consciousness accompanied by a loss of sense of identity, a selective focusing on specific aspects of the environment, and stereotyped behaviours that are experienced as beyond one's control. These symptoms are accompanied by a belief that one is possessed by a spirit, power or other person. The term is only used of conditions that result in distress and dysfunction, and not of such states when they occur as normal components of religious or other cultural ceremonies. Recent evidence suggests that this disorder is the most common DISSOCIATIVE DISORDER reported in non-Western cultures.

trance disorder, dissociative An involuntary state of TRANCE (2) that is not regarded as a normal aspect of an individual's religious or cultural traditions. It is the most common symptom of the various CULTURE-SPECIFIC SYNDROMES.

trance, hypnotic Generally, a TRANCE (2) induced by the use of hypnosis. Its most compelling feature is the high suggestibility of the subject, who tends to give up control over his or her actions to the hypnotist. See HYPNOSIS.

trance, religious A trance induced by intense religious devotion. Actually the term *trance* here is misleading, because the state referred to typically does not show the reduced bodily function generally associated with a trance, rather it is manifested by an energetic, vigorous, even frenzied quality. Hence the term *ecstatic state* is preferred by some, although, to be sure, this has its problems with the connotations of *ecstasy*.

tranquillizer chair RUSH CHAIR.

tranquillizers A generic label for any of several classes of drugs all of which have one or more of the following properties: anti-anxiety, sedative, muscle-relaxant, anticonvulsant, antiagitation. The term is rarely used in the contemporary technical literature although it may still be found in some texts and in the popular press. When it is used, a distinction is often made between the *minor* and the *major* tranquillizers. The former are now classified as ANTIANXIETY DRUGS, or *anxiolytics*, and the latter as ANTIPSYCHOTIC DRUGS, or simply *antipsychotics*.

tranquillizers, major A general label for those drugs which are used primarily to improve the mood and behaviour of patients with severe psychiatric disorders. The term is a connotative nightmare and is no longer used in the technical literature. Indeed, these drugs should really never have been called tranquillizers since they have rather different actions from merely tranquillizing, and affixing the adjective *major* suggests that they are on a continuum with the MINOR *TRANQUILLIZERS, which is pharmacologically incorrect. The preferred term is ANTIPSYCHOTIC DRUGS because their most significant function is the alleviation of many of the symptoms of various psychoses.

tranquillizers, minor A general term for any of several classes of drugs that are used primarily in the treatment of anxiety and psychiatric disorders that have an anxiety-related component. The term is a misleading one in that it suggests that these drugs are on a continuum with the MAJOR *TRANQUILLIZERS, which is pharmacologically incorrect. The preferred term is ANTIANXIETY DRUGS (see for details) or, simply, *anxiolytics*.

trans- Combining form meaning *across*, *beyond*, *over* or *through*.

transaction A behavioural event or aspect thereof the essential nature of which is captured by interactions between the actor, other individuals involved and the environment. This very general meaning is carried into various areas of psychology: see the following entries for examples.

transactional analysis (TA) A form of psychotherapy originally developed by Eric Berne. It is practised in a straightforward group setting in which the primary goal is to have the client achieve an adaptive, mature and realistic attitude toward life – to have, in Berne's words, 'the adult ego maintain hegemony over the impulsive child'.

transactional psychology An extension of the basic ideas of transactionalism from the study of perception (see TRANSACTIONAL THEORY) to other areas of human behaviour, notably social interaction.

transactional theory (of perception) A theory of perception based on the notion that what is perceived is dependent on knowledge gathered from interactive experiences with the environment. Perception, in this view, results from acquired but unconscious assumptions about the environment, represented as probabilities of transactions occurring within it. The real 'out-there' world and its perceptual properties are, it is argued, to be created in the transaction. The theory shares some of the principles of Egon Brunswik's theory, although the notion of ECOLOGICAL VALIDITY central to Brunswik's arguments is downplayed. The famous AMES ROOM was used in many experiments of the transactionalists to reveal how one's expectations would lead one to make false perceptual inferences.

transactive memory (system) A system of shared and unshared knowledge interrelated by METAKNOWLEDGE and held by individuals forming a couple, group or organization. What is known collectively by the group is distributed among a number of individuals who, in principle, are capable of retrieving others' knowledge based on the knowledge that they have about what others do and do not know. The concept was developed initially by Daniel Wegner as a contemporary and less mysterious account of the notion of a GROUP MIND. It has achieved considerable currency in organizational psychology since most large, structurally complex organizations have immense amounts of such knowledge which is often not shared easily or voluntarily. Also referred to as *transactive knowledge (system)* or *transactive memory process*.

transcendence In METAPHYSICS, a state of consciousness that goes 'beyond' normal waking experience, indeed, beyond material existence. Hence, a mental state assumed to be indefinable by ordinary means. Some claim to have achieved such. Some are sceptical. The empirical evidence supports the latter group.

transcendental meditation (TM) A form of MEDITATION. See also MYSTICOTRANSCENDENT THERAPY and MEDITATION.

transcortical Lit., across the cortex. Typically used of neural pathways leading from one part of the cortex to another.

transcortical aphasia APHASIA, TRANSCORTICAL.

transcortical motor aphasia APHASIA, TRANSCORTICAL MOTOR.

transcortical sensory aphasia APHASIA, TRANSCORTICAL SENSORY.

transcranial magnetic stimulation (TMS) The application of magnetic pulses to the skull, which temporarily disables the cortical areas underlying the magnets. The effects are short-acting and reversible with fewer side effects than other, intrusive methods. By comparing the lost or diminished functions with the region of the cortex stimulated, researchers can analyse the roles of specific cortical areas. It is currently used primarily as a research tool although there are suggestions that the procedure may have therapeutic effects, particularly with depression and obsessive disorders. When a series of short, recurring pulses is used it is called *repetitive TMS* (rTMS).

transcription 1 In general, an exact copy of something. **2** In studies of language and communication, a complete record of what was said. When unqualified, it is assumed that normal orthographic forms have been used, i.e. that the transcription is written in ordinary script; a *phonetic transcription*, on the other hand, is one which has been rendered in the INTERNATIONAL PHONETIC ALPHABET, while a *phonemic transcription* is one in which the text is presented in phonemic notation. **3** In studies of nonverbal communication, a coded record of movements and gestures. **4** In the synthesis of genes and proteins, the process of duplication of information from aspects of deoxyribonucleic acid (DNA). Messenger ribonucleic acid (mRNA) is synthesized by transcription, the information being carried to ribosomes containing RNA.

transcutaneous electrical stimulation The use of electrical stimulation in ACUPUNCTURE; see that term for details.

transducer Generally, any device that converts energy from one form to another. The term is used very broadly; see TRANSDUCTION et seq.

transduction 1 Generally, the process by which something is transformed. The thing is usually specified, either by appending a qualifying term or by the context, hence: **2** In the study of sensory processes, the sequence of operations by which physical energy (e.g. sound waves, light) is transformed into patterns of neural impulses that give rise to sensory experiences. Often called *sensory transduction*. **3** In cognitive psychology, the operation of recoding information from one form into another. **4** In genetics, the transfer of genetic material from one cell to another through a vector.

transductive logic TRANSDUCTIVE REASONING.

transductive reasoning Piaget's term for the type of reasoning exhibited by the preoperatory-stage child. Transductive reasoning tends to proceed from instance to instance, with the common thread that the child is centring on one particular aspect. Hence, it is neither deductive nor inductive. Occasionally it is called *transductive logic*, although its alogical quality makes this the nonpreferred term.

transection A cutting made across the long axis of tissue or a neural fibre; a CROSS-SECTION (2).

transfer Loosely and generally, the process whereby experience on one task has an effect (either *positive* or *negative*) on performance on a different task undertaken subsequently. The underlying notion is that the knowledge or skill acquired in the first task either facilitates or interferes with carrying out the subsequent task. Since the term is so general, qualifiers are often used to denote the specific type of transfer under consideration.

transfer appropriate processing Encoding of a stimulus or a set of stimuli in a manner that facilitates POSITIVE *TRANSFER to a novel situation.

transferase An enzyme that catalyzes the transfer of particles from one chemical compound to another.

transfer, bilateral Transfer of performance to one side of the body following training of the opposite side, e.g. improved left-handed performance following right-handed training.

transference 1 Most generally, the passing-on or displacing (i.e. transferring) of an emotion or affective attitude from one person to another person or object. **2** Within psychoanalysis, the displacement of feelings and attitudes applicable toward other persons (usually one's parents but also siblings, a spouse, etc.) onto the analyst. **3** The emotional state that results from the process in 2. Transference here is often termed either *positive* or *negative*, depending upon whether the person develops pleasant or hostile attitudes toward the analyst. Note that many authorities regard transference as a state that is ubiquitous in human interaction. Its conspicuousness in psychoanalysis, they argue, is attributable simply to the calculated neutrality of the analyst, which allows it to be more unambiguously observed.

transference neurosis 1 Generally, a neurosis in which satisfaction is achieved by transferring one's libidinal investment from appropriate to inappropriate persons or objects. **2** Specifically, such a situation as it occurs during an ongoing psychoanalysis in which the analyst becomes the inappropriate object.

transference resistance 1 Generally, the failure to recognize or acknowledge the process of transference (2) during psychoanalysis. **2** The use of transference during psychoanalysis as a defence against anxiety. Sense 1 is a resistance *to* transference; sense 2 is the use *of* transference to resist something anxiety-provoking, e.g. unearthing the past or the prospect of terminating analysis and being forced to do without the protection of the analyst. *Transference-resistance* is often hyphenated in sense 2 to distinguish it from sense 1.

transfer function MODULATION TRANSFER FUNCTION.

transfer, negative Transfer in which knowledge or skill acquired in one context or on one task results in lessened performance in some other context or on some other task.

transfer, nonspecific Transfer in which general principles or rules learned in one situation are used in another even though there are few or no specific common elements. *Nonspecific* here is used to mean *abstract* or *rule-defined*. Compare with SPECIFIC •TRANSFER, the term used in more concrete cases.

transfer of training Transfer of learned skills from one situation to another. Some authors have used this term as a synonym of TRANSFER. This is not recommended, however, as the notion of training tends to be associated with motor acts and overtly displayed skills, whereas the term *transfer* is much broader, encompassing aspects that are symbolic and abstract. Put simply, *transfer of training* is best used only in behaviouristic discourses.

transfer, positive Transfer in which knowledge or skill acquired in one context or on one task results in increased performance in another context or on another task.

transfer RNA RIBONUCLEIC ACID.

transfer, specific Transfer in which there is a significant overlap in the specifics of the two tasks such that the knowledge or skill acquired in the learning of the first relates directly to performance on the second. *Specific* is generally used in this context to mean *concrete*. Compare with NONSPECIFIC •TRANSFER, in which that which is transferred is more abstract.

transformation 1 Generally, modification or change in the form or structure of something. Clearly, a very rich conceptual notion, and, not surprisingly, the term finds wide application in various specific domains. Hence: **2** In mathematics and statistics, the modification of an equation or set of values that is made without altering the underlying 'meaning' or the set of quantitative relations entailed in the equation or set of values. See e.g. ARC SINE TRANSFORMATION. **3** In logic, the systematic replacement of one set of symbols by another set according to rules which leave the two logically equivalent. Also called the *transformation rule* or *rule of inference*. **4** In psychoanalysis, the altering of a repressed impulse or emotion so that in its disguised form it can be admitted to consciousness. **5** In linguistics, a rule that operates on a string of symbols (usually called a *phrase-marker* TREE (2)) to convert it into a different string of symbols. For example, the phrase-marker $NP_1 + V + NP_2$, which can be shown (with some technical refinements not needed here) to underlie a sentence like 'Max ate the soup', can be converted by applying (with some even more technical refinements) the *passive transformation* into NP_2 + 'was' + V + en + NP_1, which underlies the sentence 'The soup was eaten by Max.' See also TRANSFORMATIONAL *GRAMMAR for more details.

transformational (generative) grammar TRANSFORMATIONAL *GRAMMAR, GENERATIVE *GRAMMAR.

transformational leader A leader who does more than simply lead: he or she stimulates others to transcend their own needs and interests for a common goal. Such leaders can run the full range from the most horrific (e.g. Adolf Hitler) to the most progressive (e.g. Nelson Mandela). Also called *charismatic leader*, although some make subtle distinctions between these terms; see AUTHORITY, CHARISMATIC.

transformational rule TRANSFORMATION (5).

transformation rule TRANSFORMATION (3).

transformed score SCORE, TRANSFORMED.

transgendered 1 Generally, characterizing individuals (or their behaviours) that differ in notable ways from the gender role assigned at birth. **2** Relating to patterns of behaviour that combine or span traditional male and female gender-specific behaviours. The term is neutral with regard to sexual orientation or preference; its use is confined to issues of identity relative to a society's currently accepted social norms. The question of whether a transgendered individual should be deemed as displaying a GENDER IDENTITY DISORDER has more to do with any depression and distress that may be experienced than with the behaviours themselves.

transient Temporary, transitory. Used widely to characterize neurological, psychiatric and behavioural conditions that resolve within a relatively short time. Just how short 'short' is depends on the condition and the classification system in use. For example, TRANSIENT GLOBAL *AMNESIA usually lasts less than an hour, *transient* TIC DISORDERS up to a year.

transient global amnesia AMNESIA, TRANSIENT GLOBAL.

transient ischemic attack ISCHEMIC ATTACK, TRANSIENT.

transient situational disturbance ADJUSTMENT REACTION.

transient situational personality disorder See ADJUSTMENT REACTION.

transient tic disorder TIC DISORDERS.

transition Movement from one area to another or change from one state to another. The term is used generally and freely.

transitional cortex A term used occasionally to refer to those cortical cells that are intermediate in form and function between the phylogenetically older areas of the cortex and the newer areas.

transitional object OBJECT, TRANSITIONAL.

transitivity Lit., the capability of passing over or through. Hence, a characteristic of a relation between elements x, y and z such that if x is related in a particular fashion to y and y in like fashion to z, then x is necessarily so related to z. 'Taller than' is such a relation, and, in general, unidimensional relations like this are transitive. 'Like better than' is not necessarily transitive, and, in general, such multidimensional relations do not display transitivity. See INTRANSITIVITY.

translation 1 In genetics, the process through which information coded in messenger RNA (see RIBONUCLEIC ACID) is used to produce a new protein molecule. The term derives from the fact that the original code is 'read' (from DNA) and 'translated' by messenger and transfer RNA into a ribosome. **2** In linguistics, the rendering of a message from one language into another. **3** By extension, interpretation of a message.

translation research A domain of biological and social science that seeks to find efficient and effective ways to transform knowledge available to the scientific community into measures for everyday use in clinical settings and public health practices. The range of problems, socio-political, economic and epistemic (in addition to the scientific) is large and daunting.

translocation CHROMOSOMAL ALTERATIONS.

translocation Down syndrome A rare form of DOWN SYNDROME.

translocation, reciprocal CHROMOSOMAL ALTERATIONS.

transmission 1 Generally, transferring or moving something from one location to another or the result of such a process. **2** In genetics, the passing of particular genes (and, by extension, their phenotypic manifestations as physical or behavioural traits) from one or both parents to their offspring. **3** In information theory, the passing of a message from the transmitter through some medium to the receiver. **4** In anthropology and sociology, the passing of traditions and customs to succeeding generations. See CULTURAL TRANSMISSION. **5** In physiology, the excitation of a neuron by another neuron. See NEUROTRANSMITTER (2).

transmitter 1 Generally, the source of a message; that aspect or component of any transmission system from which the information emanates. **2** In physiology, the substance that initiates the action of neural transmission whereby one neuron excites a neighbouring neuron. Usually called a NEUROTRANSMITTER, occasionally a *transmitter substance*.

transmitter substance NEUROTRANSMITTER.

transmutation The act of transforming something with a particular nature, form or condition into another thing with a different nature, form or condition. Occasionally the term is used to characterize the evolutionary emergence of one species from another.

transmutation of measures A relatively rare term for the process of transforming RAW *SCORES into some set of STANDARD *SCORES.

transmuted score TRANSFORMED *SCORE.

transneuronal degeneration Degeneration of a presynaptic or postsynaptic neuron that follows damage to the neuron with which it synapses. Such degeneration helps to explain why a lesion at one site in the central nervous system can have effects on a distant site. Also called *transsynaptic degeneration*.

transorbital lobotomy LOBOTOMY, TRANSORBITAL.

transparency 1 The property of an object such that light passes through it without significant distortion or significant reduction in its luminance. **2** By extension, an openness and ingenuousness in social interactions. This meaning carries the connotation that the individual is secure in that setting and has nothing to hide. **3** A kind of social 'invisibility' whereby a person tries not to be noticed. Seen often when a request is made for a 'volunteer' to perform some task.

transpersonality An analytic feature of social behaviour that is observed to occur across a variety of social settings and is not dependent on any one specific kind of social circumstance for its emergence.

transport Collectively, the mechanisms and processes involved in the movement of substances across a membrane. In physiological research, in which the membranes are biological, the term *biotransport* is frequently used.

transposition 1 Generally, an exchange between some aspect(s) of two or more elements in a system. This sense of the term is used broadly and those things transposed may be temporal placements, logical relations, functional roles, spatial locations, etc. **2** In learning, a pattern of behaviour in which the subject selects a response to two or more stimuli based on relational factors, not on the absolute physical characteristics of the stimuli. For example, a subject is first trained to choose a circle with a 4 cm diameter over one with a 3 cm diameter. On a later test, the stimuli are two circles with a 4 cm and a 5 cm diameter. Typically, the subject selects the 5 cm circle, showing transposition of the relational concept 'larger than'. **3** In music, shifting a composition to a different key. **4** In reading and writing, a TRANSPOSITION ERROR.

transposition behaviour TRANSPOSITION (2).

transposition error 1 Generally, any error resulting from transposing two or more stimuli or elements of them. **2** Specifically, in reading and writing, an error resulting from interchanging two or more letters, syllables or words.

transposition of affect The transferring of feelings from one OBJECT to another. The term carries the connotation that the object onto which the affect is transposed is not a socially appropriate one. The term is used by some as a synonym of DISPLACEMENT.

transsexualism A condition characterized primarily by a belief that one is of the wrong sex. Several criteria have been proposed for identifying the true transsexual: (a) discomfort with one's sexual anatomy; (b) a persistent, deep desire to be a member of the other sex; (c) a wish to change one's genitalia; and (d) absence of other psychological disorders or genetic anatomical abnormalities such as hermaphroditism. Transsexualism is usually classified as a GENDER IDENTITY DISORDER and is to be contrasted with HOMOSEXUALITY and TRANSVESTISM. Also known as *sex-role inversion*.

transsituational Characterizing a pattern of social behaviour that occurs across a number of social situations and is not dependent on a particular social context.

transsynaptic degeneration TRANSNEURO-NAL DEGENERATION.

transverse At right angles to the longitudinal axis of a body or organ.

transverse section SECTION (2).

transvestic fetishism A PARAPHILIA marked by intense and recurrent sexual urges and fantasies involving cross-dressing. An individual with the condition typically keeps a collection of women's clothes (the condition has only been described in males) and uses them to cross-dress when alone, usually masturbating to various fantasies. In many cases the cross-dressing progresses to public places and can even become the individual's standard mode of dress. Discomfort with one's gender (see GENDER DYSPHORIA) may or may not be present. Male professional entertainers who work as *female impersonators* may or may not be *transvestic fetishists*: the terms are not synonymous.

transvestism Loosely, the practice of wearing the clothing of the opposite gender. It is not a clean synonym of TRANSVESTIC FETISHISM since it often occurs without the features of a PARAPHILIA and is also displayed by females. Nor should assumptions be made about sexual preferences since it is found in both heterosexuals and homosexuals.

tranylcypromine A MONOAMINE OXIDASE INHIBITOR used as an antidepressant drug. Unlike most other drugs of this type, its effects last but a few hours after one stops taking it.

trapezoid body In the brain, a transverse neural pathway in the pons that arises from axons of cells in the cochlear nucleus. It carries fibres that eventually end up in the superior olivary complex on both sides of the brainstem and hence is an important pathway in the transmission of auditory information.

trauma From the Greek for *wound*, a term used freely either of physical injury caused by some direct external force or of psychological injury caused by some extreme emotional assault. pl., *traumas* or *traumata*.

traumatic aphasia APHASIA, TRAUMATIC.

traumatic brain injury (TBI) Brain injury resulting from traumatic events such as a fall, accident or repeated blows (see POSTCONCUSSION DISORDER, *dementia pugilistica*). Diffuse and pervasive in its effects, symptoms of a TBI may include mood disorders and fatigue along with difficulties in memory, problem-solving and executive functions such as judgement, impulse control and attention.

traumatic neurosis Loosely, any neurosis that develops as a result of some dramatic event such as severe fright or sudden serious injury. See GROSS *STRESS REACTION.

traumatic psychosis A general term for any serious psychotic-like disorder that results from physical injury, usually a brain lesion.

traumatic shock TETANIZING SHOCK.

traumatophilia Unusual accident-proneness. Generally used of individuals who somehow seem to put themselves repeatedly into situations in which something goes seriously wrong, resulting in injury to themselves or to others. Also called *traumatophilic diathesis*.

travelling wave In the study of audition, a term that describes nicely the mode of action of the basilar membrane when stimulated by a sound source above roughly 150 Hz. Specifically, with stimuli above this frequency there is a pattern of deflection of the membrane that begins at the stiffer, narrow end near the oval window and travels down the membrane to the apex. The point of maximum deflection is given by the frequency of the stimulus, with low-pitched stimuli at the apex and high-pitched at the stapes. Note, if the stimulus is below roughly 150 Hz the whole membrane responds nearly in unison. See also THEORIES OF *HEARING.

Treacher Collins syndrome A genetic disorder characterized by facial abnormalities, including a misshapen jaw, a retracted chin, a large nose and malformed ears. Most cases have normal intelligence, although hearing and visual impairments may lead to an erroneous diagnosis of mental retardation. Also known as *Treacher Collins-Franseschetti syndrome* and *mandibulofacial dysostosis*.

treatment 1 Generally, and loosely, the subjecting of some person or some thing to some action, agent, substance or other influence. **2** Any specific procedure designed to cure or to lessen the severity of a disease or other abnormal condition. This meaning is also rather general and is used to cover medical, pharmacological, surgical or psychotherapeutic procedures. **3** In statistics, analysing and interpreting data. **4** In experimental design, a particular experimental manipulation or procedure under which subjects are run. This sense is roughly synonymous with INDEPENDENT *VARIABLE.

treatment variable INDEPENDENT *VARIABLE.

tree (structure or **diagram) 1** In anatomy and physiology, any structure with a tree-like branching pattern. Hence, dendrites are called tree structures, as are the bronchial tubes and their branches and terminal arborizations. **2** In linguistics, the schematic diagram of a sentence which reveals the underlying linguistic components of the sentence and the manner in which the words and morphemes are grouped together. A tree diagram of this kind is also called a *phrase-marker*, because the basic phrases that make up the sentence are clearly specified and their grammatical status marked.

tremograph Any instrument for recording and measuring tremors.

tremor Generally, any quivering or trembling of a part or parts of the body.

trend Generally, any directional tendency, a drift of events. Usage here is very broad and

encompasses discernible patterns in data (e.g. TREND ANALYSIS, TREND TEST) and tendencies for persons to behave in particular ways (e.g. NEUROTIC TREND).

trend analysis Quite as it says, an analysis of trends, specifically with an eye toward being able to EXTRAPOLATE so as to predict future events. The mathematical basis in all trend analyses is the same as that used in INTERPOLATION. See DELPHI METHOD and CROSS-IMPACT MATRIX METHOD for some examples of trend analyses.

trend test Any of several statistical tests that assess whether two or more trends seen in data can be said to be reliably different from each other.

trepan TREPHINE.

trephine 1 To bore a small hole in the skull. **2** An instrument resembling a carpenter's circular saw for perforating the skull. var., *trepan*. The process is known as *trephination*.

treppe The increase in the contraction of a muscle when it is either stimulated constantly over a short period of time or stimulated at a rapid and regular rate. Also called *staircase phenomenon* (*treppe* is German for *staircase*).

tri- Combining form meaning *three*.

triads, method of An experimental procedure in which the subject is presented with three stimuli and must select the one that satisfies some criterion, e.g. the odd one, the middle one.

triage The process of screening the sick, wounded or injured in times of crisis and classifying them into three groups: those who are likely to recover eventually without therapy, those who are expected to die no matter what is done to assist them and those whose recovery is deemed to depend on their receiving adequate care. The last group is the *priority group* and the recipient of any limited resources. The term is also used figuratively in less dramatic situations, as when allocating resources in educational settings, community units and the like.

trial 1 Loosely, a try-out, a test, a single effort designed to accomplish something. **2** In experimental research, a single 'unit' in which a stimulus is presented and some response is made. In this sense, each trial is generally assumed to be one component of an extended series of such units, all of which taken together represent an experiment. **3** A large-scale plan for testing and evaluating the effectiveness of some drug or therapeutic procedure; also called a *clinical trial* or a *clinical study*.

trial-and-error learning LEARNING, TRIAL-AND-ERROR.

trial, extinction In studies of conditioning, a TRIAL (2) on which the reinforcing event is not presented or the unconditioned stimulus is omitted. See EXTINCTION.

trial, learning In studies of conditioning, a TRIAL (2) on which the reinforcement is delivered or the unconditioned stimulus is presented. Also called *training trial* and *acquisition trial*. See LEARNING.

triarchic theory of intelligence A theory of intelligent behaviour due to Robert Sternberg. It assumes three partially distinct abilities based on an ANALYTIC, a CREATIVE and a PRACTICAL *INTELLIGENCE. Overall, intelligence is treated as the effective functioning of a cluster of information processing mechanisms that are applied to a person's experiences, particularly novel ones. The theory has three 'subtheories', dubbed *componential, experiential* and *contextual*. The componential subtheory assumes three components (it's worth noting that Dr Sternberg has a preternatural affection for the number '3'), one comprised of *metacomponents* that plan, monitor and evaluate decisions, one that assumes a set of *performance components* that make the decisions and take action, and a third group of *knowledge acquisition components* that guide learning. The experiential subtheory is assumed to function by specifying the experiences to which these components are applied and monitoring how novel environments are dealt with. The contextual subtheory outlines how the specific context within which actions take place impacts on the choices made. Intelligent behaviour takes place in contexts where individuals can select, shape and adapt to the setting. The theory, admittedly cumbersome and difficult to falsify, has been influential as the first to break away from the psychometric approach to assessing intelligence by using

standardized tests. See also MULTIPLE INTELLI-GENCES THEORY.

triazolam A short-acting BENZODIAZEPINE with hypnotic and anxiolytic properties. Once popular, it is now rarely used because of side effects including increased aggressiveness, agitation and short-term memory loss and is banned in some locales (the UK for one). Trade name Halcion.

tribadism Rubbing together of the genitals, specifically when both partners are female.

trichaesthesia The tactile sensation experienced in the skin when a hair is touched or moved. var., *trichesthesia*.

trichi-, tricho- Combining forms meaning *hair*.

trichotillomania Compulsive pulling of one's hair, often to the point of pulling it out.

trichotomy Division or classification into three, not necessarily equal, parts.

trichromacy Normal colour vision. In operational terms, a trichromat can use three appropriately selected hues to match any other visual stimulus; hence, there are three colour systems operating. Also occasionally called by a variety of similar terms, including *trichromatism, trichromatopsia, trichromopsia, trichromia* and *trichromasy*. Compare with DICHROMACY.

trichromacy, anomalous A colour-vision abnormality that allows the matching of any target colour with a mixture of the three primary hues even though the mixtures are anomalous and quite different from those normally given. Such conditions are assumed to result from minor deficiencies in one pigment or another.

trichromasy TRICHROMACY.

trichromat One with normal colour vision; one with TRICHROMACY. Contrast with MONO-CHROMAT and DICHROMAT.

trichromatic theory Also known as the *Young–Helmholtz theory*. See THEORIES OF *COLOUR VISION.

trichromatism TRICHROMACY.

trichromatopsia TRICHROMACY.

trichromia TRICHROMACY.

tricyclic compounds A group of ANTIDE-PRESSANT DRUGS which function by preventing the reuptake of amines in cholinergic synapses. The resulting increase in these stimulants is apparently the basis for the drugs' antidepressant effects. Of the many tricyclics developed, the most commonly prescribed was IMIPRAMINE. Tricyclics were developed in the 1950s and quickly became the primary drugs of choice for depression. While their side effects are fewer than the MONOAMINE OXIDASE INHIBITORS, they can cause dry mouth, constipation, weight gain and sleep disturbances and patients need to be monitored carefully because overdoses can be lethal. Although their antidepressant effects are significant, they have been largely replaced by the SELECTIVE SEROTONIN REUPTAKE INHIBITORS and similar compounds.

tridimensional theory of feeling Wundt's theory that all feelings could be represented as being composed of three dimensions: pleasure–displeasure, excitement–depression and tension–relaxation.

trifluoperazine One of the PHENOTHIAZINES used to treat both adult and childhood schizophrenia. It has antianxiety effects but it is not recommended as an ANXIOLYTIC because long-term treatment is associated with various side effects, including TARDIVE DYSKINESIA.

trigeminal lemniscus LEMNISCAL SYSTEM.

trigeminal nerve The Vth CRANIAL NERVE. A mixed nerve with three afferent, or sensory branches and one efferent, or motor, branch. The afferent branches are the major ones: the *ophthalmic* extends to the forehead and scalp, the mucosa of the nasal cavity and sinuses, and the cornea and conjunctiva; the *maxillary* runs to the dura mater, the gums and teeth of the upper jaw, and the upper lip; the *mandibular* extends to the tongue, the gums and teeth of the lower jaw, the cheeks, the lower jaw and the lower lip. The motor branch is much smaller and carries fibres to the muscles of mastication.

trigeminal neuralgia A neuralgia of the TRIGEMINAL NERVE. The primary symptom is a sudden stab of (often excruciating) pain typically beginning in the jaw and radiating along whichever branch of the nerve is affected. Also called *tic douloureux*.

trigger zone The area of a neuron, usually part of the axon, that has the lowest threshold for initiating an action potential.

triglycerides Complex molecules containing GLYCEROL combined with the FATTY ACIDS. The body's reservoir of adipose or fatty tissue is filled with triglycerides.

trigram A three-letter sequence. Nonsense trigrams (e.g. *xqz*) are often used in memory research when stimuli that are difficult to encode are needed.

trimmed mean MEAN, TRIMMED.

trip The period of time during which a person is under the influence of a psychedelic or hallucinogenic drug such as LSD. Often qualifiers such as *bad* or *good* are appended as needed.

triple-X syndrome A chromosomal anomaly in which three X chromosomes are present. Such individuals are phenotypically female, sexually normal and usually fertile, although menstrual problems and early menopause are common. Severe mental retardation is the single most striking feature.

triptans A class of drugs that function as direct SEROTONIN-RECEPTOR AGONISTS. Their primary action is vasoconstriction and their main use is for migraine headaches.

trireceptor theory The theory of colour vision based on the assumption that there are three types of receptors in the retina. See THEORIES OF *COLOUR VISION.

trisomy 18 A genetic disorder in which there is a third, anomalous, 18th chromosome. The syndrome is characterized by mental retardation and various physical anomalies, the most common being low-set, malformed ears, flexion of the fingers, a small jaw and heart defects.

trisomy 21 A genetic abnormality characterized by the presence of a third 21st chromosome. The vast majority of persons with DOWN SYNDROME display this anomalous chromosome.

tritanopia An extremely rare form of inherited DICHROMACY characterized by a lowered sensitivity to blue light. The prefix *tri-* comes from the Greek for *third* and is used because the presumption is that the tritanope has a deficiency in the blue-light-absorbing pigment and blue is regarded as the third primary colour. The condition also occurs more commonly, as a result of retinal disease.

triune brain A term used by the psychologist Paul MacLean which captures the notion that the human brain can be conceptualized as three (more or less) independent aspects, each of which is viewed as having emerged at a different evolutionary time. The earliest to emerge was what MacLean jokingly called the neural chassis, composed of the spinal cord, hindbrain and midbrain, followed by the limbic system and the neocortex.

tRNA Abbreviation for *transfer* RIBONUCLEIC ACID.

trochaic bias *Trochee* (var., *troachee, choree, choreus*) is a poetic metre in which a stressed syllable is followed by an unstressed one. The 'bias' refers to: (a) the tendency of native English speakers to favour such stressed-unstressed syllable sequences, especially when talking to children (e.g. referring to a horse as 'hór – sie'); and (b) the suspicion that infants tend to perceive a stressed-unstressed sequence as a word.

trocular nerve The IVth CRANIAL NERVE. A mixed nerve, it contains efferent, or motor, fibres to the superior oblique muscles of the eye, and afferent, or sensory, fibres which convey proprioceptive information from the same muscles.

troilism A deep desire to have sexual relations in the presence of a third person.

troland A measure of illuminance that approximates that on the retina itself. Named after the physiologist L. T. Troland, it is, by definition, the illuminance of the retina that results when a surface luminance of 1 candle/m² is incident through an apparent pupil of 1 mm². Once the term *photon* was used for this measure but its commandeering by physics necessitated a change.

trophic hormones Anterior pituitary hormones with indirect action; that is, they affect secretions of other endocrine glands. Also known as *tropic hormones*.

troph(o)- Combining form meaning *food* or *nourishment*.

trophotropic Descriptive of processes that conserve energy and promote recovery after stress. Contrast with ERGOTROPIC.

tropic hormones TROPHIC HORMONES.

(-)tropin Combining form used to indicate the stimulating effect of a substance (especially a hormone) on an organ or other site.

tropism A generic term for any unlearned orientation or movement of an organic unit as a whole toward a source of simulation. Typically used in compounds with the Greek word for the stimulus source, e.g. *phototropism* = turning toward light, *heliotropism* = movement toward the sun. Properly, *tropism* is used of such automatic movements when made by plants and TAXIS of similar movements by animate organisms, although this nicety is often ignored.

tropism, negative When unqualified, *tropism* connotes movement toward a stimulus; *negative* is appended when the movement is away from the source.

Troxler's effect A visual phenomenon. When an observer maintains fixation on a point directly in front while attempting to view a stationary line off to one side, this peripheral stimulus disappears. It is especially striking at low illumination levels but occurs at high levels as well, when a sort of visual fog seems to creep in from the periphery, obscuring objects. A slight movement in the periphery causes the peripheral stimuli to reappear.

true 1 In logic, characteristic of a proposition which follows logically from the axioms in use and previous propositions the truth of which is known. **2** Characteristic of a proposition, statement or belief which corresponds with reality as it is known. Note that what is true in sense 1 is not necessarily true in sense 2. **3** In statistics, characteristic of values which are based upon a full population of scores and not upon samples from a population, e.g. TRUE *MEAN.

true value TRUE *SCORE.

true zero ABSOLUTE *ZERO.

truncated distribution A distribution in which the extreme scores (at either or both ends) have been cut off. Such truncation may result from a decision to eliminate these scores from consideration or simply through a failure to collect data from the extreme(s). A classic example of a severely truncated distribution is the frequency distribution of IQ scores in universities, in which the lower part of the full population has been removed by entrance requirements.

trust game A procedure used in BEHAVIOURAL ECONOMICS to study the role of mutual trust in financial settings. In the classic setting, one individual (A) gives money to another (B) to invest. The amount both can make is dependent on how much money A is willing to give B which, over time, gets adjusted by how much trust A has in B's decisions and honesty when splitting the profits.

tryptophan An amino acid required for normal growth and development. It functions as a precursor in the production of the inhibitory neurotransmitter *serotonin*. There is some evidence that it may have mild antidepressant effects.

T-scope Abbreviation for TACHISTOSCOPE.

T score A type of score based on the transformation of normalized standard scores to a scale based on a mean of 50 and a standard deviation of 10. T scores may be either linear or uniform. In the former, scores are computed directly from the obtained raw or normalized standard scores. In the latter, an extra step is applied to yield T scores that more closely approximate a *normal distribution*, a useful procedure when comparing scores across different scales.

TSD Abbreviation for *theory of signal detection*. *See* SIGNAL-DETECTION THEORY.

***t* test** Any of a number of statistical tests of significance based upon the *t* statistic. See the discussion under t *DISTRIBUTION for the principles involved.

TTR TYPE–TOKEN RATIO.

TTS TEMPORARY THRESHOLD SHIFT.

tubectomy SALPINGECTOMY.

tubocurarine CURARE.

Tukey honestly significant difference test A POST HOC TEST used after an analysis of variance or other test has shown overall significance. It enables one to compare all possible pairs of means while not changing

one's criterion for a TYPE I *ERROR at a given level of significance. Also called *Tukey HSD test*.

tulipmania **1** A MASS HYSTERIA in Holland during the early 1600s in which tulips were so insanely overvalued that some rare bulbs were selling for the same price as houses. **2** By extension, any economic spasm in which a commodity becomes bizarrely overpriced. They occur with surprising frequency.

tumescence A swelling of tissue or the condition of being swollen.

tuning fork A two-tined metal instrument constructed of highly tempered steel to reduce its overtones so that when struck it yields a nearly pure tone. A well-made set of tuning forks was once the pride of every experimental psychology laboratory; today they are hardly ever used, having been replaced by electronic tone generators.

tunnel memory MEMORY, TUNNEL.

tunnel vision A condition in which peripheral vision is severely reduced or lacking altogether and a person can see only that which is projected onto the central area of the retina. The term is also used metaphorically to characterize the manner of thinking of the narrow-minded and the dogmatic.

Turing machine An abstract automaton (i.e. a computer or other finite, well-defined machine) characterized theoretically by the British mathematician Alan M. Turing in the 1930s. Basically, a Turing machine consists of a tape and reading head. The tape moves back and forth under the head, marking and changing the symbols on it one at a time based on information fed to it. In Turing's terminology, the machine is 'completely described' when every mark on the tape tells the machine: (a) the next symbol it should write; (b) the place on the tape it should go to; and (c) whether to move the tape forward or backward one step. Turing machines have fascinated computer scientists because, in the final analysis, when stripped of all of its sophisticated components a modern computer *is* a Turing machine. Workers in ARTIFICIAL INTELLIGENCE and the COGNITIVE SCIENCES have been intrigued by the possibility that the human brain itself may be represented as a Turing machine.

Turing's test A 'test' of the adequacy of an artificial intelligence device based on the question of whether or not it can be said to think. As Alan Turing conceptualized it, one human, A, is linked to another human, B, via a teletype through which the two can converse without face-to-face interaction. At some point in time unknown to A, B is replaced with a computer. The test is whether this artificial device can so effectively simulate human responses that no matter what questions A poses, A cannot discern whether it is the computer or person B that is answering. According to Turing, any device capable of passing this test would have to be considered capable of human thought. See also ARTIFICIAL INTELLIGENCE.

turn construction unit TURN-TAKING.

Turner's syndrome A chromosomal anomaly in phenotypic females. The basic genetic defect is a missing sex chromosome, so that the total count is 45, X. The syndrome is marked by short stature and absence of ovaries. With female sex hormones administered at the age of puberty normal secondary sex characteristics appear, although the sterility cannot be corrected. Most cases display normal intelligence although mild deficits in arithmetic skills and spatial organization are often seen.

turn-taking A pragmatic conversation principle usually (but, heaven knows, not always) respected whereby each participant in a dialogue takes turns at speaking. A turn is often called a *turn construction unit (TCU)* to acknowledge that many facets of a turn (e.g. initiation, length, termination) are actively constructed by the speaker with, of course, cooperation of conversational partners. The rules that govern turn-taking are rather complex and involve subtle factors such as intonation, contour and pausing as well as the more straightforward invitations from the other person(s) to speak, such as questions and partial lead-ins.

twilight vision SCOTOPIC VISION.

twin One of two offspring gestated in the same uterus and born at the same time.

twin control The use of twins in experimental studies as a way of controlling for genetic and environmental factors. When monozygotic twins are used the control over the genetic factors is complete; with dizygotic twins it is not, although the use of the latter has advantages over the use of regular siblings in that the environment within which they are raised is held roughly constant. See TWIN STUDIES.

twins, dizygotic Twins resulting from the (near) simultaneous fertilization of two ova by sperm cells. Since each twin develops from a separate zygote, they are no more alike genetically than any two siblings born at different times. Also called *fraternal twins*.

twins, monozygotic Twins resulting from the spontaneous fission of a single fertilized zygote. Such twins are genetically identical. Also called *identical, uniovular* or *monovular twins*. When such twins share a common placenta they are called *monochorionic*, when each has its own placenta, *dichorionic*.

twin studies This term refers collectively to a large number of studies carried out on monozygotic and dizygotic twins raised together or apart from each other. The focus of these studies is to sort out the relative contributions of heredity and environment to human behaviour.

twitch A simple, spasmodic muscular contraction.

2AFC TWO-ALTERNATIVE FORCED CHOICE.

two-alternative forced choice (2AFC) An experimental method used widely in studies of memory and learning in which the subject is presented with two alternative stimuli and must select one. For example, in studies of memory, one of the stimuli has been seen before and one is novel; the subject's task is to pick out the previously encountered stimulus. The procedure is preferred over simple choice techniques whereby, for example, the subject is shown a stimulus and asked whether it has been seen before. This latter procedure is subject to bias owing to large individual differences in the tendency to respond 'yes' or 'no'.

two-factor theories Psychologists seem to be irresistibly drawn by the allure of theories based on hypothesizing two, presumably distinct, factors. Such theories have appeared in explorations of learning, emotion, memory, decision-making, intelligence and a host of social functions. A few of the more frequently referenced are given below. It is hoped that future generations can resist this temptation and similarly for DUAL-PROCESS MODELS.

two-factor theory of emotion The proposal put forward by Schachter and Singer to the effect that the experience of EMOTION is a two-step attributional process in which one first experiences physiological arousal and then searches for the cause of that arousal.

two-factor theory of intelligence An early model of INTELLIGENCE proposed by Spearman that assumed that intelligence was comprised of a GENERAL *FACTOR and group of SPECIFIC *FACTORS.

two-factor theory of learning/conditioning The generalization that conditioning consists of two distinct forms, one based on principles of CLASSICAL CONDITIONING and the other on OPERANT CONDITIONING.

two-factor theory of memory A generalization that MEMORY can be divided into two broad types, a SHORT-TERM *MEMORY and a LONG-TERM *MEMORY.

two-point threshold The minimum distance apart of two point stimuli on the skin at which they are perceived as separate rather than as a single stimulus point. Although commonly cited as the standard technique for establishing perceptual maps of the skin surface, the technique is known to have serious problems as a measure of the spatial resolution capacities of the skin senses. Between- and within-subject variability is high, establishing a set criterion for saying 'two points' is difficult, and underlying neural mechanisms do not correspond in any straightforward way with obtained data.

two-tailed test In testing for the statistical significance of an observed difference (either between two samples or between a sample and a theoretical distribution) the question of the *direction* of the difference emerges. The standard statistical practice is as follows. If one anticipates the possibility that a particular manipulation will result in either extreme, a two-tailed test should be used, e.g. in testing a new drug when it is not clear whether it should increase performance or depress it. In such a situation significance will result from data in either critical region of the distribution (i.e. in either of the two

tails). When one is utterly convinced that only differences in one direction can manifest themselves (e.g. the effects of practice on learning), one can, in principle, run a *one-tailed test* that evaluates significance in one critical region (i.e. in only one tail). A one-tailed test has the advantage that the entire critical region for concluding significance at a given level is contained in one tail, hence it is twice as likely to produce a significant result as is a two-tailed test. There are, however, good reasons for not recommending this rather standard statistical practice. Consider, for example, an experimenter who is running a study in which he or she is convinced that only one directional outcome can occur and, hence, elects to use a one-tailed test. Suppose now that the experimental subjects are run with a large number of densely massed practice trials and consequently display dramatically poorer performance than control subjects who are run with fewer (but spaced) practice trials. In principle, since the experimenter decided in advance to use a one-tailed test, the observed result is not significant and should not be reported in the literature. This, of course, is nonsensical in the extreme – no surprises would ever be publicly revealed. What would happen, of course, is that our experimenter would quickly reverse course and run a two-tailed test. One-tailed tests are, therefore, ill-advised. They increase the probability of Type 1 errors to an unacceptable level and, of course, will always be jettisoned in favour of two-tailed tests as soon as the scientist anticipates an interesting reversal of expectations.

two-word stage A stage in infant language development where verbal productions follow a fairly simple set of rules known as a PIVOT GRAMMAR.

tympanic Pertaining to the eardrum, the TYMPANIC MEMBRANE.

tympanic canal COCHLEA.

tympanic membrane The eardrum, the flexible membrane stretched across the end of the external auditory meatus. It vibrates with the incoming stimulus and transmits the vibration pattern to the auditory ossicles. Also called *tympanum*.

type 1 Generally, a class or group distinguished by possessing or displaying some particular characteristic. **2** An individual or thing which embodies such typical characteristics; a representative of a type in sense 1. See PROTOTYPE. **3** A pattern of traits or other characteristics which can serve as criteria for classifying persons (or objects) into groups. See the discussion of *type theories* under PERSONALITY. **4** A class of utterances or words defined so as to represent a coherent group for the purpose of determining a TYPE–TOKEN RATIO. See also TOKEN (4). *Type* is usually qualified by some other term or phrase to specify the reference; a few combined forms follow, others are listed under the relevant qualifier.

type A personality A temperament characterized by excessive drive and competitiveness, hostility, an unrealistic sense of time urgency, inappropriate ambition, a reluctance to provide self-evaluation, a tendency to emphasize quantity of output over quality and a need for control. Type A behaviour is believed by many to be associated with increased incidence of coronary disease. Contrast with TYPE B PERSONALITY.

type, body SOMATOTYPE.

type B personality A temperament characterized by a relaxed, easygoing approach to life, a focus on quality over quantity, low competitiveness and a tendency for self-reflection. Contrast with TYPE A PERSONALITY.

type fallacy The tendency to encapsulate persons, concepts, categories, etc. and thus reify each type and treat it as distinct from others. Most psychological variables lie along dimensions and the dimensions often have identifiable poles. However, once these poles have been labelled types, it is easy to be seduced into treating them as if they were distinct from each other rather than as points on a continuum. Although most contemporary thinkers are aware of and sensitive to this problem as it pertains to dimensions like introversion and extraversion, they often fail to appreciate that it also pertains to dimensions like race (black–white) and even gender (male–female).

type-identity theory IDENTITY THEORY.

Type I error ERROR (TYPE I and TYPE II).

Type-R conditioning A term sometimes used to refer to OPERANT CONDITIONING and/or INSTRUMENTAL CONDITIONING.

Type-S conditioning A term occasionally used to refer to CLASSICAL CONDITIONING.

type–token ratio (TTR) In studies of language, the ratio of the number of TYPES (4) to the number of TOKENS (4) in a corpus of language. In the most frequently used sense the count of tokens is the total number of words in the corpus and the count of types is the total number of different words. The closer the ratio is to 1.0, the greater the verbal diversity the person under consideration can be said to display. Such ratios are often used in analysis of the verbal sophistication of children. Note, however, that what serves as a *type* is really quite arbitrary and various other forms of analysis are possible. For example, parts of speech could be used (noun, verb, etc.), and the ratio would then reflect flexibility of usage of grammatical forms.

Type II error ERROR (TYPE I and TYPE II).

typicality The degree to which a given example of a category can be said to be close to the abstract PROTOTYPE of that category.

typing The process or operation of categorizing persons or objects.

typography The setting of type for printing. Many different type fonts, or styles, exist and there are good reasons for suspecting that they play a role in the READING process.

typology 1 Generally, the study of types and of the processes of classification into types. **2** Any scheme of classification in which various instances are grouped together according to specifiable criteria.

tyrosine An amino acid that serves as a precursor for DOPAMINE, EPINEPHRINE, L-DOPA and NOREPINEPHRINE.

U

UCR UNCONDITIONED RESPONSE.

UCS UNCONDITIONED STIMULUS.

U curve U-SHAPED CURVE.

UG UNIVERSAL *GRAMMAR.

-ulous Suffix meaning *tending toward*.

ultimate explanation In evolutionary biology, an explanation of the behaviour of a species in terms of the larger evolutionary factors that gave rise to the adaptive value of the behaviour. An ultimate explanation of the mating behaviour of the elephant seal, for example, would focus on the role of the size of the polygynous male in enabling it to defend his territory and his females from encroaching males and how this pattern of behaviour promotes more offspring than other patterns. Compare with PROXIMATE EXPLANATION.

ultimatum game A procedure used in BEHAVIOURAL ECONOMICS. In the classic setting, two people (A and B) are given an amount of money (e.g. €10) to be split among them. Person A decides the distribution but B makes the ultimate decision to accept or reject. If B accepts A's offer, they both get those amounts. If B rejects it, no one gets anything. A common finding is that B will reject offers deemed unfair or unjust and opt for nothing over something. For example, if A offers to keep €8 and give B €2, most people in B's situation will forgo a €2 profit rather than accept what seems to be an unjust division. See the similar DICTATOR GAME.

ultra- Combining form meaning *going beyond*, *extreme* or *excessive*.

ultradian rhythms Any of the many biologic rhythms that are shorter than one day.

ultrasonic Pertaining to sound waves with a frequency beyond the range of normal human hearing, i.e. above roughly 20,000 Hz. syn., *supersonic*.

ultraviolet Pertaining to electromagnetic radiation with a wavelength shorter than that to which the normal human eye responds, i.e. below roughly 400 nm.

umami One of the five primary qualities of TASTE (2). The term is Japanese for 'delicious' and is associated with glutamate and related proteins found in cheeses, meats and some vegetables. Monosodium glutamate, the food additive, is particularly intense. It is suspected that the glutamate binds with specific receptors in the TASTE BUDS. Also called *savoury* or *savory*.

umbilical cord The cord that connects the foetus with the placenta.

Umweg DETOUR PROBLEM.

Umwelt *Eigenwelt.*

un- A multifunctional prefix meaning *back*, *reversed* or *reversal of*, *negation of*, *annulment of*, *not*.

unambivalent Not ambivalent. Used in psychoanalysis of any two motives that are in harmony.

unbalanced bilingualism BILINGUALISM, UNBALANCED.

unbiased A term used in a variety of contexts to characterize operations or processes which display no bias, e.g. decision-making that reveals no prejudices, choice behaviour that manifests no uneven or inappropriate tendency to select particular stimuli, sampling in which the samples selected are representative of the underlying population, tests that assess fairly the factors they have been designed to assess, etc. See BIAS and related terms for a sense of the range and pattern of usage.

unbiased error CHANCE *ERROR.

unbiased estimate Any estimate made on the basis of representative sampling, i.e. sampling that is unbiased.

unbiased estimator Any statistic which, in principle, gives a value for any sample that is an unbiased estimate of the true value in the full population. The mean is an unbiased estimator.

unbiased sample REPRESENTATIVE *SAMPLE.

uncertainty 1 Generally, the state of belief when one does not fully believe, when one is unsure, particularly when confronting an upcoming event about which one has insufficient information to know what is likely to happen. **2** In information theory, the degree to which there are no constraints upon the choices one has available or upon the possible outcomes of a situation. See ENTROPY.

uncertainty, tolerance of The degree to which individuals are able to tolerate a state of UNCERTAINTY (1). Low tolerance is often seen as a marker of cognitive vulnerability to development of anxiety disorders. Because the psychologically important pole is the *lack* of tolerance, many authors use the term *intolerance of uncertainty* as the key term.

uncomplicated A term used loosely in psychiatric diagnosis to denote disorders that are not accompanied by any significant pathological features other than those that signal the existence of the primary disorder.

uncomplicated alcohol withdrawal ALCOHOL WITHDRAWAL.

uncomplicated bereavement Normal reaction to the death of a loved one. It consists of various expressions of sadness, anger, guilt, depression and the like that are deemed appropriate to one's experiences and interactions with the deceased while alive. In order to qualify as uncomplicated, any pronounced distress must resolve within a culturally appropriate time period, typically 1 year in Western societies.

uncomplicated sedative, hypnotic, or

anxiolytic withdrawal SEDATIVE, HYPNOTIC, OR ANXIOLYTIC WITHDRAWAL.

unconditional positive regard POSITIVE REGARD.

unconditional reflex This is the proper translation of Pavlov's original term, which is now generally rendered as UNCONDITIONED RESPONSE. *Unconditional* was converted to *unconditioned* by a translator's error; *reflex* was changed to *response* by theorists who wished to generalize the principles of conditioning beyond the domain of the reflexes, which were the primary focus of Pavlov's research on CLASSICAL CONDITIONING.

unconditional response UNCONDITIONAL REFLEX.

unconditioned reflex UNCONDITIONED RESPONSE, UNCONDITIONAL REFLEX.

unconditioned response (UCR, UR or Ru) Any response that is reliably elicited from an organism by a particular unconditioned stimulus. Such a well-established link between an unconditioned stimulus and an unconditioned response may be the result either of previous learning or of the organism's innate behavioural repertoire, but in either case it is a prerequisite for the establishment of CLASSICAL CONDITIONING.

unconditioned stimulus (UCS, US or Su) Any stimulus that reliably elicits from an organism a particular unconditioned response. See CLASSICAL CONDITIONING.

unconscious Three distinguishable patterns of usage exist for this term, each with noun and adjective forms: the first is more or less nontechnical, the second is broad and atheoretical, and the third is closely tied in with a particular point of view with respect to theories of the human condition. All three, however, make contact in some way with the general notion of a level of mind lacking in awareness. To wit: **1a** n. A state characterized by a lack of awareness; unconsciousness. **1b** adj. Characterizing an individual in such a state. When they occur in technical writings these meanings are roughly equivalent to those in everyday language; that is, they refer to that pole of the dimension of mental arousal that is exemplified by coma, fainting, deep sleep or the result of general anaesthesia. **2a** n. A state characterized by a lack of awareness of ongoing internal processes. **2b** adj. Characterizing those internal processes that proceed in an implicit manner outside of consciousness. While, strictly speaking, these two usages cover all processes occurring outside of an individual's awareness, the referents are typically the cognitive, emotional and/or motivational processes. Physiological processes, to be sure, take place largely without one's awareness (no one knows what their liver is doing) but are rarely intended by users of the term.

Note that in both 1 and 2 *unconscious* is not actually defined. In 1a and 1b it represents *loss* of consciousness; in 2a and 2b it represents that which is *not* conscious. This kind of lexicographic trickery never really solves problems; see CONSCIOUS and CONSCIOUSNESS for more on this. See also TACIT, IMPLICIT and AWARENESS for further discussions of these semantic issues. **3a** n. In the depth psychologies, especially psychoanalysis, a domain of the psyche encompassing the repressed id functions, the primitive impulses and desires, the memories, images and wishes that are too anxiety-provoking to be accepted into consciousness. **3b** adj. Characterizing these primordial, repressed desires, memories and images. Note that the unconscious (3a) is assumed to be populated by two varieties of psychic entity: that which was once conscious but has been exiled from awareness, and that which has never been in consciousness. See REPRESSION (1). Distinguish from PRECONSCIOUS, which is the domain of mind the components of which are not at any moment a part of one's consciousness but which may be retrieved by a simple exercise of memory. Note that Freud referred to sense 3 as the *dynamic unconscious*, owing to the actions of repression, and often used the term *descriptive unconscious* for the *preconscious* – causing no end of confusion.

unconscious cognitive process Generally, any process involving thinking, reasoning, judging, problem-solving, etc. which takes place without consciousness, without awareness. See e.g. IMPLICIT *LEARNING, INCUBATION (3).

unconscious drive An id drive or need. See also UNCONSCIOUS (3a, 3b).

unconscious ideation COLLECTIVE GUILT.

unconscious inference **1** Generally and literally, a judgement made on the basis of a limited amount of evidence or data and made without awareness. **2** Specifically, a principle first articulated by the great German scientist Hermann von Helmholtz as an explanation for many perceptual phenomena. Helmholtz's principle is really only the specification of the general, literal meaning of the term with respect to the conditions under which such judgements are made. For example, things placed in front of other things block them from view, and everyone has had extended experience with such stimulus conditions. Hence, when two things, A and B, are arranged before us such that A is partially blocking B, we unconsciously infer that A must be closer to us than B.

unconscious knowledge Knowledge that a person is not aware of possessing, knowledge that is TACIT (3).

unconscious memory MEMORY, UNCONSCIOUS.

unconscious motivation MOTIVATION, UNCONSCIOUS.

unconsciousness The state of being UNCONSCIOUS (esp. 1a).

uncontrolled **1** Unregulated, not controlled. **2** Not measured, not assessed. The term is generally used of variables in an experiment that were neither systematically varied nor specifically held constant.

uncoupling protein A protein found in mitochondria that is related to the speed with which calories are burnt. Individuals with high levels tend to have higher metabolic rates and seem to be 'immunized' against weight gain. Not surprisingly, there are explorations into its possible use in a drug to treat obesity.

underachiever One whose actual performance on a task or in some situation (most typically in a school setting) is below what one would have predicted. Usually intelligence tests are the basis for such prediction, but the term is often used rather more loosely and assigned to persons on the basis of subjective feelings about their potential. See and contrast with OVERACHIEVER.

undercontrollers EGO-CONTROL.

underdetermined Of situations in which there is insufficient evidence, data or information to determine a value or the correct alternative in a set of choices, etc. See OVER-DETERMINED.

underextension UNDERGENERALIZATION.

undergeneralization The use of a word for a smaller and more specialized category of objects, events or circumstances than it is normally used for. Such *underextensions*, as they are also called, are common in young children, e.g. restricting the label 'kitty' to but one cat. Contrast with OVERGENERALIZA-TION.

understand To comprehend, to appreciate the deep meaning of a thing or a process.

understanding 1 The process of comprehending something, of appreciating the meaning of a word, sentence, event, proposition, etc. **2** An elusive intuitive process whereby one succeeds in apprehending the deep significant meaning of an event, a concept, an idea, etc. Note, some use COMPREHEN-SION as a synonym of both 1 and 2. **3** A sympathetic appreciation of another person, particularly of their point of view on some matter or their belief on some issue. Here SYMPATHY is a near-synonym. **4** In older writings, a hypothesized mental faculty the function of which was to yield comprehension of the meanings of things.

underweight By convention, a condition in which body weight is 10% or more below the norms for a person's body type and age. Like OBESITY, the term is used rather loosely, since it is impossible to provide a definition that pertains uniformly to all persons – the 10% criterion is, of course, arbitrary and flexible.

undifferentiated Not differentiated. Used of wholes or of aggregates the several components of which are not distinguished from each other. For example, in embryology, undifferentiated tissue is that which has not yet developed into its characteristic forms and structures; likewise, undifferentiated perceptions are those that are seen as unified wholes, mobs are undifferentiated groups of people, etc. See DIFFERENTIATION.

undifferentiated schizophrenia SCHIZO-PHRENIA, UNDIFFERENTIATED.

undifferentiated somatoform disorder SOMATOFORM DISORDER, UNDIFFERENTIATED.

undinism UROPHILIA.

undistributed middle, fallacy of An argument that leads to an invalid conclusion because of the use of a premise that is not distributed. For example, given that 'All Communists are atheists' and 'Max is an atheist', to conclude that 'Max is a Communist' would be to fall prey to the fallacy. To rescue the syllogism one would need to have an additional premise, such as 'All atheists are members of the Communist party.' The obviously fallacious aspects are shown if the syllogism takes a more blatant form, such as 'Max is a man', 'Sam is a man', therefore 'Max is Sam'. Psychologists' interest in the fallacy stems from two observations: (a) some schizophrenics willingly accept such arguments, and would indeed find nothing wrong with concluding that Max and Sam were the same person; and (b) normal people are surprisingly susceptible to such invalid arguments and are open game for advertisers who exploit this; e.g. 'Distinguished people smoke Zonko cigars', 'I smoke Zonko cigars', therefore 'I am distinguished.' In both cases here the tendency is toward what is called OVERGENERALIZATION.

undoing A defence mechanism, usually associated with children, in which a person attempts to annul (i.e. undo) the unpleasant outcome of some act by mentally replaying or in some cases ritualistically re-enacting the sequence of events but with a different, more acceptable ending.

unfalsifiable NONFALSIFIABLE.

unfilled pause SILENT *PAUSE.

unfolding A type of MULTIDIMENSIONAL SCAL-ING developed by Clyde Coombs. The technique is based on having a subject rank order a number of stimuli according to preference. The resulting preference ordering reflects an ideal point and the individual preferences are then 'unfolded' mathematically to display the locations of the scaled objects in any number of dimensions relative to the ideal point.

uni- Combining form meaning *one, singular*. Although not a true synonym of HEMI- the two are often used interchangeably to refer to conditions that affect one side of the body. *Unineglect* is a synonym of *hemineglect*, *unilateral* of *hemilateral*.

uniaural Pertaining to a single ear; MONAURAL (preferred).

unicellular Single-celled.

unidextrous Preferring one hand over the other for most actions. n., *handedness*.

unidimensional Descriptive of variables with a range of values that can be expressed along a single dimension. Compare with MULTIDIMENSIONAL.

uniform distribution DISTRIBUTION, UNIFORM.

uniformity 1 Generally, IDENTITY (3) in all important respects. **2** In social psychology, a condition of universal (i.e. uniform), or at least widespread, agreement concerning some belief, practice or fact. The term is used loosely and relatively since there are probably few things which are truly believed uniformly by all members of a society. Compare with CONFORMITY.

unilateral Lit., pertaining to but one side. Hence: **1** Descriptive of actions or decisions made by one person or one group. **2** Pertaining to anatomical structures or processes on only one side of the body.

unilateral neglect NEGLECT.

unimodal Having only one MODE. Used to characterize distributions with one peak.

unintended memory INVOLUNTARY *MEMORY.

uniocular Pertaining to a single eye; MONOCULAR (preferred).

uniocular dichromat DICHROMAT, UNIOCULAR.

uniovular twins MONOZYGOTIC *TWINS.

unipolar cell (or **neuron**) A neuron with a single stalk leading from the soma. This neural process branches with the dendrites at one end and the axonal terminals at the other. In unipolar neurons, unlike neurons with more than one pole, information is transmitted from dendrite to end button without passing through the somatic membrane. Compare with BIPOLAR and MULTIPOLAR CELL.

unipolar depression DEPRESSION, UNIPOLAR.

unipolar mania MANIA, UNIPOLAR.

unique factor SPECIFIC *FACTOR.

unique hues PRIMARY *COLOURS (esp. 2).

unique trait TRAIT, UNIQUE.

unisexual Characteristic of a species in which each individual organism is either male or female but not both.

unit **1** One of something taken as a whole, a datum. **2** A standard amount used as the basis of measurement. This meaning may convey: (a) something extremely precise and objectively well defined, such as physical magnitude, e.g. a *second* as a unit of time, a *metre* as a unit of length; (b) something subjective but reasonably well defined, e.g. a *sone* as a unit of loudness; or (c) something quite loosely defined, e.g. an *utterance* as a unit of speech. adjs., *unitary* (1), *unit* (2).

unit character A characteristic or trait that is assumed to be genetically determined as a whole or as a unit. The notion is that there is no genetic parcelling-out of components; it is a case of all-or-nothing genetic transmission. Albinism is a good example, as is Down syndrome.

univariate Consisting of but one variable. An experiment using only one variable may be called a *univariate study*, although the term *single-factor study* (or *experiment*) is more common.

universal **1** adj. Pertaining to UNIVERSE in any of that term's meanings. **2** adj. Pertaining to those underlying aspects or characteristics of human beings, their psychological make-up, their modes of thought, action and affect, that are presumed to be common to all despite the vast observed array of diverse manifestations of them. The term is rarely used in this sense to refer to the mundane or the obvious, such as simple anatomical features; it is generally reserved for the assertion of deeper, abstract components, such as Jung's *archetypes*, Chomsky's *universal grammar*, and Freud's *instincts*. **3** n. Any one of those aspects that are assumed to be universal in sense 2. **4** n. In logic, a proposition predicated of all members of a class.

universal complex In psychoanalytic theory, a complex hypothesized to have its roots in a fundamental instinct, i.e. an instinct assumed to be UNIVERSAL (2), e.g. the *Oedipus complex*. Compare with PARTICULAR COMPLEX.

universal grammar GRAMMAR, UNIVERSAL.

universalism An approach to social theory in which standards of conduct are determined according to sets of principles assumed to reflect universal ethical standards. In this approach the tendency is to disregard mitigating circumstances or individual contexts. Contrast with the more relativistic approach of PARTICULARISM.

universals, linguistic Those linguistic aspects that are common to all NATURAL *LANGUAGES. These hypothesized universals are usually viewed as being of two types: *substantive universals*, which are common aspects of description of natural languages, such as distinctive features, catalogues of word classes and sets of semantic features; and *formal universals*, which represent the nature of generative rules of grammar.

universal symbol SYMBOL, UNIVERSAL.

universe 1 Most generally, all things everywhere taken as a totality. **2** More specifically, a collection of things, taken together according to some defining feature(s) or characteristic(s). This meaning is close to that of SET (1). **3** UNIVERSE OF DISCOURSE. **4** STATISTICAL *UNIVERSE.

universe of discourse The full set of things under consideration in a given discussion, study or experiment.

universe, statistical The full population from which samples are drawn and about which inferences, based on the samples, are made. For more detail see POPULATION (2) and SAMPLE et seq.

unlearned A term used rather literally to refer to behaviours, acts, tendencies, dispositions and so forth that emerge in the life of an organism without any special training or instruction – in short, *without learning*. Unlearned behaviour may be a simple reflex or a complex sequence of actions like walking upright. Note that labelling a behaviour unlearned does not necessarily mean that experiential or maturational factors do not play a role; even the most basic 'preprogrammed' behaviours, like fixed-action patterns in lower organisms, will not manifest

themselves if an organism is deprived of the usual environmental experiences of its species.

unlearning A very general term for any process or operation which leads to the elimination of previously learned behaviour. Some use it as though it were equivalent to EXTINCTION; others argue that one can only eliminate the effects of previous learning by acquiring a new response that is incompatible with the old one and thus takes its place in the behavioural repertoire. For these latter theorists, unlearning is closer to COUNTER CONDITIONING.

unmarked adjective MARKED–UNMARKED ADJECTIVES.

unobtrusive procedure A general term for any research technique for gathering data without the individuals (persons or animals) being observed becoming aware of the procedures. It covers a large array of techniques, from the use of public and private records (e.g. census data, school reports), to the use of hidden cameras, tape recorders and one-way mirrors for surreptitious observation of subjects, to hiding in the reeds beside a pond to record the natural behaviour patterns of water fowl (see NATURALISTIC OBSERVATION).

unpack A term borrowed from the computer sciences, where it refers to the recovery of original data that have been stored (i.e. packed) with other data. It is used as a metaphor for the process of retrieval of specific memories from a large store of other memories and knowledge.

unpleasant 1 Characterizing an emotional experience that has negative, aversive or disagreeable qualities. In this sense the experience is usually conceptualized as the negative pole of a *pleasantness* dimension along which all emotional experiences can be located. **2** Characterizing any environmental state of affairs or stimulus conditions under which an organism learns to make responses that result in its termination and doesn't learn to make responses that result in its presentation. This is the behaviourist's use of the term, which attempts to avoid invoking the internal, subjective notions of meaning 1 and relies, instead, on changes in behaviour as criterial.

unpleasure The emotional experience that

results from the exposure to stimuli that are *unpleasant*. This experience is usually treated as basic and primitive and resistant to conscious, introspective analysis. There is, admittedly, something strangely awkward about the term, although it serves well as the antonym of PLEASURE. Psychoanalysts often use it for the affective state produced when instinctual needs go unmet.

unreadiness, law of LAW OF *READINESS.

unreality, sense (or **feeling**) **of** Technical usage here is quite similar to common usage: a feeling that things experienced are somehow not 'real' or not 'right'. When this feeling occurs occasionally in normal living it is usually interpreted as a failure to be able to integrate an experience with one's previous knowledge of things – and, indeed, it occurs most often in strange or novel situations. When it occurs frequently or continuously it is regarded as pathological. See also DEREALIZATION.

unreflective Impulsive. With respect to cognitive style, see REFLECTIVITY–IMPULSIVITY.

unreliability An antonym of RELIABILITY in any of the meanings of that term.

unresolved Generally, of conflicts or problems not yet worked out (i.e. not yet resolved). This meaning is found in cognitive psychology with respect to problems not solved or decisions not made, and in psychotherapeutic discourse in reference to psychological problems or conflicts with which the client has not yet come to grips.

unselected Characterizing a sample drawn from a population strictly at random. The connotation is that there were no pressures to select any particular elements and therefore the sample should display no bias. Note, however, that while unselected sampling yields an approximately REPRESENTATIVE *SAMPLE, in actual practice getting the most representative sample often requires selected sampling techniques such as AREA *SAMPLING or STRATIFIED *SAMPLING.

unsociable UNSOCIAL.

unsocial Characterizing an individual who is lacking in *sociability*. The term is used both of those whose lack of socially interactive behaviour is of their own choosing, i.e. those who are *unsociable*, and of those who

are excluded from social interaction because their behaviour violates social norms of acceptability, i.e. those who are *unsocialized*.

unsocialized UNSOCIAL.

unspaced practice MASSED *PRACTICE.

unspecified NOT OTHERWISE SPECIFIED.

unstable Generally, characterizing that which is prone to change, that which is not stable. Hence: **1** Of an individual who displays erratic and unpredictable behaviours and moods. **2** Of an individual who is likely to display behaviours that are neurotic, psychotic or just plain dangerous to others. *Unstable personality disorder* is an occasional synonym for BORDERLINE PERSONALITY DISORDER. **3** Of a statistic or a measure that has high variability; see the discussion under STATISTICAL STABILITY. **4** Of an aspect of language likely to undergo variation over time. Phonetic aspects of languages are relatively unstable compared with syntactic aspects. n., *instability*.

unstressed In linguistics, a syllable that receives minimal accentuation in a word, e.g. the *-er-* in *brotherhood*. See STRESS (2).

unstructured interview An interview in which the topics to be covered are left unspecified at the outset and things are left to the unfolding interaction between the persons involved in the interview.

unstructured stimulus STRUCTURED STIMULUS.

unvoiced VOICING.

unweighted Characterizing scores which have not been subjected to any adjustments in terms of WEIGHT (2). Actually, this term is slightly misleading since unweighted scores are not really unweighted; rather, each has a nominal weight of 1.

up-and-down method In psychophysics, a variation on the *method of limits* (see MEASUREMENT OF *THRESHOLD) in which the ascending stimulus sequence is shifted to descending as soon as the subject changes response category and vice versa. Also called the *staircase method*.

upper motor neuron dysarthria DYSARTHRIA, UPPER MOTOR NEURON.

uppers (or **ups**) Street slang for any drugs

that have stimulating, arousing effects. Most such drugs are AMPHETAMINES or amphetamine-derived.

upper threshold 1 The upper bound of sensitivity for a particular stimulus dimension. In some cases it can be empirically determined, e.g. the pitch of a tone, for which the limit for the average, undamaged human ear is roughly 20,000 Hz. **2** The upper stimulus in a *difference* THRESHOLD (3). **3** The most intense stimulus that one can experience without pain.

UR UNCONDITIONED RESPONSE.

ur- A prefix from the German, meaning *original* or *primitive*. Used roughly synonymously with PROTO-.

uracil One of the four nucleotide bases that make up RIBONUCLEIC ACID. Uracil replaces the *thymine* in the *deoxyribonucleic acid* molecule.

urban ecology ECOLOGY, URBAN.

urban legend A story, invariably apocryphal but presented as true, about some event. Typically the event is one with a traditional motif that mirrors a subculture. The story is usually attributed to some friend, or a friend of a friend who heard it from another friend. Also known as *urban myth*. The internet has become a prime medium for the distribution of such legends.

uresis Passing urine. See ENURESIS.

urethra The tube from the bladder through which urine is passed.

urethral eroticism Sexual feelings associated with the urethral area. See e.g. UROPHILIA.

urge Nontechnical term for any strong desire.

urolagnia UROPHILIA.

urophilia A PARAPHILIA characterized by the deriving of erotic stimulation from the smell or taste of urine or from the viewing of a person urinating. Also called *urolagnia* and *undinism*.

US UNCONDITIONED STIMULUS.

use, law (or **principle**) **of** The not surprising generalization, first formalized around the turn of the last century by E. L. Thorndike, that responses, functions, associations, etc. which are practised, exercised or

rehearsed (i.e. used) are strengthened relative to those which go unused.

user Lit., one who uses a thing. The most common reference is to one who takes a drug, with the connotation that he or she does so excessively.

user illusion The virtually universal impression that one's conscious perceptions, actions and thoughts are immediate, coherent and seamless. The illusory element comes from the finding that cortical markers for the perception of a stimulus occur before one is aware of the stimulus, and for action before the individual is aware of deciding to act. Computer scientists first noted the effect and used the term to refer to the sense that the words and symbols the user types in feel 'real' while the strings of 1s and 0s in the computer are the operative elements.

U-shaped curve Quite literally, any distribution which is shaped like the letter U, with high frequencies (or probabilities) for very low and very high values and low frequencies (or probabilities) for moderate values.

uterine Pertaining to the UTERUS.

uterine descent MATRILINEAL DESCENT.

uterine fantasy In psychoanalysis, any fantasy associated with the uterus, the most common being about returning to the womb, with its warmth and protection.

uterus The womb. In mammals, the female organ in which the embryo is contained and nourished during gestation. It is a muscular, pear-shaped structure consisting of an expanded upper part, a somewhat constricted central area and the cervix, which joins the uterus with the vagina.

U test MANN–WHITNEY U.

utility 1 In biology, the degree to which a particular structure has value in promoting survival. **2** In statistics, the value of a test or a statistic. This meaning is rather loose and involves any of a number of factors, including validity, reliability, robustness, etc. **3** As derived from economics, the value of a commodity or of money. This last meaning has been taken up in various psychological theories of choice behaviour, decision-making, scaling, games, etc. Here, utility is taken as the value to an individual of making a particular choice, arriving at a particular decision, playing a game according to a particular strategy, etc. **4** In psychometrics, CONCURRENT *VALIDITY. See also VALUE (esp. 1 and 3). Note that all these meanings share a common connotation. The *utility* of any issue, concept, theory or programme is essentially the degree to which it fulfils the functions it was designed for or developed to accomplish.

utilization 1 Generally, the use to which something is put or its useful value. **2** In studies of FEEDING BEHAVIOUR, the variety of physiological processes involved in the consumption of food, including digestion, absorption, metabolism and excretion.

utopia The ideal society. Taken from Thomas More's 1516 work of the same name, the term refers to any visionary system of social, political and personal perfection. Various persons since More have had their hand in utopian prescriptions, the American beha-

viourist B. F. Skinner being among them. See WALDEN TWO. ant., *dystopia*.

utricle The larger of the two vestibular sacs in the inner ear. Like the SACCULE, it is roughly round in shape and has a layer of receptors on the bottom, or floor, that respond to shifts in orientation of the head.

utterance Very generally, a unit of speech or of talk. An utterance may be anything from a single simple vocal sound ('uh-huh') to an extended, multisentence discourse. Determining exactly where a particular utterance begins and ends is no easy matter. In normal conversations the act of TURN-TAKING usually marks the beginnings and ends of utterances.

uvula The soft structure that hangs from the back of the soft palate in the midline of the mouth.

V

V **1** Variable stimulus (also *v*). **2** VARIANCE. **3** *Photopic* LUMINOSITY COEFFICIENT (var., *V* λ).

V1, V2 ...V5 The 'V' stands for 'vision' and the number denotes a neuroanatomically distinct area of the visual system. See following for details.

V1 The area of the occipital region also known as the PRIMARY VISUAL CORTEX. Information arrives here from the LATERAL GENICULATE NUCLEUS and is transmitted to other visual areas, primarily v2, v4 and v5, through different neural streams. The *dorsal stream*, often oversimplified as the 'where' pathway, goes through V2 to V5 and to the inferior parietal lobule and is linked with object location, motion and the processing of visual information for controlling movement. The *ventral stream*, somewhat simplistically called the 'what' pathway, also carries information to V2 then to V4 and the inferior temporal lobe and is associated with form and object recognition and long-term memory. V1 is the evolutionarily oldest visual area, the most extensively studied and the best understood. It is keyed to processing information about objects, both stationary and moving and carries out basic pattern recognition functions. In all animals with a V1, there is a clear correspondence between a specific spot in the visual field and a specific cortical location. Also known by a host of other names including *retinotectal projection area*, *retinal projection area* and (somewhat ambiguously) *visual projection area*.

V2 An area of the occipital region that lies adjacent and anterior to v1. It receives inputs directly from V1 and sends information on to v3, v4 and v5. It also has feedback loops to V1. Anatomically it is split into four quadrants which function visuotopically (see RETINO-TOPIC REPRESENTATION) to provide a full representation of the external, visual world.

V3 A part of the visual cortex. It is less well-defined anatomically than other areas and is the only visual area that v1 does not project to. It lies just in front of v2, from which it receives inputs. It appears to have colour sensitive neurons and may play a role in perception of global motion, a fact that suggests that it may have, like V2, a full representation of the visual world.

V4 An area of visual cortex that lies in the occipitotemporal cortex, anterior to v2. It receives inputs from v1 and V2 and processes information about colour, spatial orientation, spatial frequency and geometric shapes. Most of what is known about it comes from work with macaques.

V5 The part of the visual cortex located in the extrastiate cortex of the *medial temporal area*. Projections come from v1, v2 and, probably, from v3; it transmits information to a wide variety of brain regions though a complex array of pathways. Its functions appear complex although there is compelling evidence for a primary role in processing movement. Lesions here cause a MOTION *AGNOSIA.

V¹ *Scotopic* LUMINOSITY COEFFICIENT. var., $V^1λ$.

v **1** Variable stimulus (also *V*). **2** Volume. **3** Volt.

vaccinate To produce immunity to a disease by inoculation.

vacuum activity An ethological term referring to the occurrence of a FIXED ACTION PATTERN in the absence of its usual external stimulus (or *releaser*). The assumption is that *action-specific* energy builds up, breaks through the inhibitory function of the *innate* *releasing mechanism* and causes the fixed action pattern to occur spontaneously. Also called *vacuum response* and, in keeping with the hydraulic metaphor that lies behind this and related concepts, *overflow activity*.

vacuum response VACUUM ACTIVITY.

vagabond neurosis See DROMOMANIA.

vagina The muscular membranous canal from the uterus to the exterior.

vaginism VAGINISMUS.

vaginismus Involuntary, painful spasms of the peri- and circumvaginal muscles of the vagina which make coitus either extremely painful or impossible.

vagitus The first crying of a newborn.

vagotomy A sectioning of the vagus nerve.

vagotonia Condition of vasomotor instability caused by overaction of the vagus nerve.

vagus nerve The Xth CRANIAL NERVE. A mixed nerve with widely distributed afferent and efferent branches, it innervates the external ear, pharynx, larynx, lungs, heart, kidneys, spleen, liver, stomach and intestines.

valence In Kurt Lewin's *field theory*, the psychological value of an object, event, person, goal, region, etc. in the *life space*.

valence, substitute The valence associated with an object that has, for any number of possible reasons, come to serve as a substitute for an original but unreached object.

valid Denoting the circumstances in which, by the principles of logic, a statement is unambiguously implied by the premises. In this sense, the truth of the argument or the accuracy with which it characterizes the real world are not issues. The validity of a proposition, conclusion, syllogism, etc. is given by formal adherence to proper reasoning; a perfectly valid conclusion can have no descriptive accuracy at all. See also VALIDITY (esp. 2).

validation 1 The process of determining the formal, logical correctness of some proposition or conclusion. Determination of VALIDITY (2). See also VALID. 2 The process of assessing the degree to which a test or other instrument of measurement does

indeed measure what it purports to measure. Determination of VALIDITY (3). On occasion, *validation* takes the place of *validity* in the various combined forms in which that term is used in sense 3; however, in this volume, all such forms can be found under *validity*.

validity 1 Generally and loosely, the property of being true, correct, in conformity with reality. This meaning, common in ordinary parlance, is typically *not* intended in the technical literature. 2 In logic, of an argument or conclusion, the property of being deemed VALID because of conformation with proper, logical principles. The fundamental notion here is that the reasoning process itself must be correct; an argument may have validity in this sense and not correspond with reality, but the fault will lie with assumptions and not the reasoning process. See also LOGIC. 3 In testing, of any measuring instrument, device or test, the property of measuring that which it is purported to be measuring. Validity here is not a simple notion; it is not a simple either–or property as in sense 2 and to some extent in sense 1. In the field of tests and measurements a large number of procedures have been developed to assess the validity of testing instruments, the most widely used of which are given below.

validity, coefficient of An index of a test's VALIDITY (3); the coefficient of correlation between the scores on a test and a set of CRITERION SCORES which are taken as reflective of the variable(s) the test is purported to measure. For example, for a test designed to assess scholastic aptitude the correlation would be between the test scores and academic performance as assessed by grade-point average (the criterion scores), and it would provide a measure of the test's validity.

validity, concurrent A kind of CRITERION-RELATED *VALIDITY in which the relationship between the test scores and between the criterion scores is established at the same time. Although similar in spirit to PREDICTIVE *VALIDITY, the procedure really uses *post*diction rather than *pre*diction. For example, one way of evaluating the validity of, say, a test for clerical skills would be to see how scores on the test correlate with the known clerical skills of a group of clerks whose performance has been evaluated in actual working conditions. Also called *status validity* or *diagnostic utility*.

validity, congruent A method of establishing the validity of a new test by correlating scores from it with scores from another test of established validity. The most typical case here is in intelligence testing, where newly developed tests are compared with the well-known tests like the Stanford–Binet or the Wechsler.

validity, construct A set of procedures for evaluating the validity of a testing instrument based on the determination of the degree to which the test items capture the hypothetical quality or trait (i.e. the construct) it was designed to measure. Thus, for example, if a test is supposed to provide a measure of intelligence one should ask: (a) What traits or qualities (or constructs) actually characterize intelligence? (b) Do the test items actually tap such constructs? The initial stages of test construction are usually concerned with construct validity. The estimate of construct validity is always changing with the accumulation of further evidence about the traits and qualities that underlie the construct. See also CONTENT *VALIDITY, of which construct validity is but one form.

validity, content An estimate of the validity of a testing instrument based on a detailed examination of the contents of the test items. *Contents* here means the actual constituent materials of the test items; the evaluation of them is carried out by reviewing each item to determine whether it is appropriate to the test and by assessing the overall cohesiveness of the several test items. For example, in order to have a respectable level of content validity, a test of arithmetical abilities should not phrase the items in such a way that verbal abilities are critical for the person taking the test to understand what is being asked. Further, the contents should be balanced so that all tested aspects are represented appropriately; the test should not be overloaded with, say, multiplication items to the neglect of addition items.

Establishing content validity relies on the judgements of 'experts' concerning the relevance of the materials used. It is also situation-specific, and estimates made in one circumstance may not carry over to others.

validity, convergent and discriminant
The degree to which any particular testing instrument has validity will reflect the extent to which scores on the test (a) correlate highly with factors that they, in principle, should correlate highly with, and (b) correlate poorly with factors that they, in principle, should correlate poorly with. *Convergent validity* is manifested by the former, *discriminant validity* by the latter.

validity, criterion-related Validity of a testing instrument assessed by determining the relationship between scores on a test and some independent criterion; CONCURRENT *VALIDITY and PREDICTIVE *VALIDITY are examples. Also called *external validity* or *criterion validity*. See also EMPIRICAL *VALIDITY.

validity, cue The degree to which a CUE signals or is indicative of a particular meaning or intent. For example, where speakers look is only a partially valid cue for discerning what they are talking about; where they point has higher cue validity. Note that VALIDITY is used here in a relatively nontechnical sense. The cue validity of a setting or a stimulus does not logically imply meaning; it is a stochastic or probabilistic feature that allows an organism to judge the likelihood of meaning and/or intent.

validity, differential The ability of a test to predict performance that the test should predict and to specifically *not* predict what it was not designed to predict.

validity, empirical Validity determined by purely empirical means rather than by means that are theoretically driven, as in using EXPLORATORY *FACTOR ANALYSIS rather than CONFIRMATORY *FACTOR ANALYSIS. See each for details.

validity, face Validity assessed by having 'experts' or lay people review the contents of a test to see if they seem appropriate 'on their face'. It really is a rather fuzzy procedure for validating a test, and, because of inherent subjectivity, is typically used only during the initial phases of test construction. While face validity seems superficially similar to CONTENT *VALIDITY, the two are actually quite different, assessment of the latter being a systematic procedure.

validity, factorial A type of CONSTRUCT *VALIDITY whereby several tests, subtests or items purported to measure the same underlying traits or constructs are factor-analysed to determine whether they share common variance and thus can be said to be tapping the same underlying constructs.

validity, incremental With respect to various tests of personality, the amount of additional, valid information provided by a test beyond that obtained by other procedures.

validity, internal 1 The degree to which each item on a test is related to other items purported to measure the same construct. Some prefer the term ITEM RELIABILITY, since no external criterion is used to evaluate validity. 2 The degree to which the structure and content of a study really do allow one to study the phenomena under consideration. Usually assessed by a MANIPULATION CHECK, a DEBRIEFING, or careful consideration of the phenomenon under study.

validity, intrinsic Validity of a testing instrument based on the items in the test manifestly displaying the fact that they are indeed evaluating the designated trait. For example, an item that asks the testee to spell a word is an intrinsically valid item in a test of spelling ability.

validity, predictive CRITERION-RELATED VALIDITY based on determining the extent to which the scores on a test are predictive of actual performance. A test designed to measure, say, skills in sales will have high predictive validity if it predicts who will and will not succeed in jobs in selling. Compare with CONCURRENT *VALIDITY.

validity, procedural The ability of a test, tester or procedure to produce the same results as a procedure previously evaluated and assumed to be valid. For example, if a newly constructed clinical interview administered by paraprofessionals or a computer yields diagnoses similar or identical to those produced by experienced diagnosticians, the former procedure has procedural validity.

validity, sampling A variety of CONTENT *VALIDITY based on an assessment of the extent to which the various traits assumed to underlie what is being measured by a test are represented in the test. It is, in practice, more of a control procedure to guard against introducing a bias into a test than a real measure of a test's validity.

validity, synthetic 1 Validity of a complex testing instrument or of a full test battery based on the relationship between a composite score that is taken to represent the various factors that are represented on the test and actual performance. The term derives from the notion that many elements or factors have been synthesized into a single value. 2 Specifically, a system used to establish statistical linkages between job selection procedures and job components so that tests and combinations of scores can be used to predict performance in jobs with specific demands.

Valium DIAZEPAM.

valproic acid An ANTIEPILEPTIC DRUG also used as a mood stabilizer, particularly in modulating the manic episodes of BIPOLAR DISORDER. While effective, it has potentially serious side effects, specifically liver damage, and patients need to be monitored carefully.

value 1 n. The quality or property of a thing that makes it useful, desired or esteemed. Note the pragmatic aspect implied by this definition: the value of a thing is given by its role in a (social) transaction; the thing itself does not possess value. 2 n. An abstract and general principle concerning the patterns of behaviour within a particular culture or society which, through the process of socialization, the members of that culture or society hold in high regard. These *social values*, as they are often called, form central principles around which individual and societal goals can become integrated. Classic examples are freedom, justice and education. 3 n. In economics, the net worth of a thing as determined by what it will bring in exchange, either in other goods or in some medium of exchange – usually money. This meaning, combined with 1, is very close to the meaning of UTILITY (esp. 3). 4 n. In mathematics, a quantity or magnitude as represented by a number. 5 n. In the Munsell system for classifying colours, the position along the brightness dimension. 6 vb. To assess the worth of a thing. 7 vb. To hold something in esteem based upon one's evaluation of it.

value, absolute A number or VALUE (4) expressed without regard to its sign. The absolute value of -3 is the same as $+3$ and is denoted as $|3|$.

value affirmation task An experimental task in which participants are asked to identify their personal values and views and reflect on those that are most meaningful to them. Commonly used as a task that primes an individual to feel that their opinions and values are important.

value analysis A type of CONTENT ANALYSIS which focuses on the tabulation of the frequency with which particular values are expressed in a message.

value judgement A perspective toward a person, object, principle, etc. based on how one values the properties or characteristics thereof.

values clarification A variation on moral education which emphasizes awareness and clarification of moral judgements and ethical considerations. Compare with VALUES EDUCATION.

values education An aspect of education focusing on specific instruction in moral and ethical values in society. The term is usually associated with the work of L. Kohlberg on MORAL DEVELOPMENT, which is based on the assumption that some moral positions are inherently better than others. Hence, the educational curriculum here is oriented toward raising the child's level of morality. Compare with VALUES CLARIFICATION.

value system Loosely, any reasonably coherent set of values. The values may be treated as individual, societal or absolute.

val variant See COMT GENE.

Vandenbergh effect The acceleration of the onset of puberty in female mice caused by a *pheromone* in the urine of a mature male.

variability 1 In statistics, the degree to which the scores in a sample differ from each other or, as more commonly expressed, differ from the mean of the sample. See DISPERSION for more detail. **2** In evolutionary biology, the degree to which changes are manifested from generation to generation in a species.

variable 1 n. That which changes, that which is subject to increases and/or decreases over time – in short, that which varies. Although for the most part a variable is taken as some 'thing' that undergoes

changes, it is strictly speaking an abstraction, an amount, a quantity. If the variable is intensity of a tone, it is the *intensity* that is the operative variable; if difficulty of a test is the variable in a study, the real variable is the *difficulty*. The *tones* and the *tests* used are but ways in which to allow *intensity* and *difficulty* to manifest themselves. In mathematics and logic, this notion is captured more explicitly by treating a variable as a *symbol* that represents not any particular thing or value but the class of things or the domain of values that satisfies the specified constraints. Compare here with PARAMETER (esp. 4). Within the social sciences several kinds of variables are distinguished, as indicated in the following entries. **2** adj. Changing, varying, characterizing that which is subject to change or variation.

variable, autochthonous A variable that comes from within. See AUTOCHTHONOUS.

variable, control A variable which, in a particular experiment, is held constant or *controlled*. The term is semantically confusing and not recommended. Moreover, it is too easily confused with *controlled variable*, which is an occasional synonym of INDEPENDENT *VARIABLE, which is specifically *not* held constant.

variable, criterion The variable used to establish the criterion or standard against which other scores can be evaluated. See e.g. CRITERION-RELATED *VALIDITY.

variable, dependent 1 Any variable the values of which are, in principle, the result of changes in the values of one or more INDEPENDENT *VARIABLES. In mathematics this notion of dependence is readily represented by an expression of the kind $y = f(x)$, where the values of y are dependent on the values of x. In psychology, the operative principle is that the behaviour of the subject under consideration is (like y) dependent upon the manipulation of some other factors (the analogue of x). See EXPERIMENT. **2** The variable(s) estimated from other, given values. This sense is found in studies using regression and correlation, and the underlying sense of causality in meaning 1 is absent here. One may estimate x from values of y if they are given or y from values of x if they are given, without concluding that either x or y is the direct cause of the other.

variable, independent 1 Any variable the values of which are, in principle, independent of the changes in the values of other variables. In an experiment, any variable that is specifically manipulated so that its effects upon the DEPENDENT *VARIABLES may be observed. Also called the *experimental variable*, the *controlled variable* and the *treatment variable*. See also the discussion under EXPERIMENT for more on relevant terminology. 2 In correlational analyses, the CRITERION *VARIABLE.

variable interval reinforcement SCHEDULES OF *REINFORCEMENT.

variable, intervening An internal variable not directly assessable but the properties of which can be inferred and interpreted on the basis of systematic manipulations in an INDEPENDENT *VARIABLE and observations of the concomitant changes in a DEPENDENT *VARIABLE. See also ORGANIC VARIABLE.

variable, mediating A variable that explains the relationship between a predictor variable and a criterion or dependent variable, and thus mediates the relationship between the two. For example, suppose we were to discover that childhood trauma is related to high levels of anxiety later in life. Then, follow-up studies reveal that what first looked like a direct relationship either disappears (what is called *full mediation*) or is significantly reduced (*partial mediation*) when the factor of *hardiness* is controlled. In this case, *hardiness* can be said to be 'mediating' between the two variables. Also called *mediator variable*.

variable, moderator A variable that acts to change the relationship between an independent and dependent variable. For example, if childhood trauma is related to anxiety symptoms in adulthood, but only for individuals who have never been in therapy, then therapy serves as a moderator variable.

variable, predictor A variable that is used to predict the values on some other variable. Most commonly used in a REGRESSION ANALYSIS but also found in general discussions of statistical analyses of situations where a variety of factors are assessed in terms of how they relate to (i.e. 'predict') some outcome. For example, motivation might turn out to be

strongly predictive of success in higher education.

variable, proxy A variable used as an indirect measure of another variable when that second variable is difficult to measure or observe directly. For example, the frequency of abuse of street drugs is difficult to measure but it can be studied through the *proxy variable* of hospitalizations for drug overdose.

variable ratio reinforcement SCHEDULES OF *REINFORCEMENT.

variable stimulus In psychophysics, each of the set of stimuli which is compared with the STANDARD (2).

variable time (VT) SCHEDULES OF *REINFORCEMENT.

variance 1 n. The STANDARD *DEVIATION squared. A measure of DISPERSION (or *variability*) of a set of scores, its most common use is in the statistical procedures known collectively as ANALYSIS OF VARIANCE. 2 Differences across members of a group or population. 3 Deviant human behaviour.

variance, between-group The variance which results from the different groups or conditions in an experiment. In an analysis of variance the between-group variance is compared with the within-group variance.

variance, shared Literally, the extent to which two variables co-vary. For example, height and weight have considerable shared variance since increases in one are generally associated with increases in the other. Shared variance is most commonly calculated as the square of the CORRELATION COEFFICIENT, yielding an index that represents the proportion of total variance in one measure that is accounted for by variance in the other.

variance, true The variance in a population of scores. The variance observed in a sample is an estimate of this actual (i.e. true) population variance.

variance, within-group The variance within an experimental group or condition. In an analysis of variance, the within-group variance is compared with the between-group variance.

variant That which differs in significant ways from other things that are regarded as belonging to the same category or type. The term is applied to cases of diseases and syndromes that are uncharacteristic, to organisms that have features not typically found in their species, etc.

variate 1 n. A synonym of VARIABLE (1). **2** n. A particular value of any variable.

variation 1 Generally, change – especially change in the state or condition of something. **2** In statistics, DISPERSION. **3** In biology, differences between members of a species.

vary To change – with the connotation that such change is not so great that identity has been lost.

vas In anatomy generally, any vessel or duct through which liquids travel. pl., *vasa*.

vascular Pertaining to blood vessels or to tissue rich in blood vessels.

vascular dementia DEMENTIA, VASCULAR and MULTI-INFARCT *DEMENTIA.

vas deferens The narrow, muscular duct from the testis to the prostatic urethra.

vasectomy The surgical procedure of cutting or tying off the vas deferens. Bilateral vasectomy is a common method of sterilization of males since it only prevents movement of the sperm from the testes and does not affect hormonal balances or sexual experience. See SALPINGECTOMY, the analogous procedure in females. Distinguish from CASTRATION.

vaso- Combining form meaning *vessel* or, more commonly, *blood vessel*.

vasoconstriction The constriction of a blood vessel.

vasodepression Depression of the blood circulation.

vasodilation The expansion or dilation of a blood vessel. var., *vasodilatation*.

vasomotor 1 Pertaining to the nerves that have control over the muscular walls of the blood vessels. **2** Pertaining to the two forms of action of these nerves, namely *vasoconstriction* and *vasodilation*.

vasopressin A hormone secreted by the posterior lobe of the pituitary gland that functions as part of the system maintaining water balance. It causes the kidneys to excrete a more concentrated urine, thereby retaining water in the body. Also called *antidiuretic hormone (ADH)*.

vector 1 In mathematics and physics, a quantity with magnitude and direction. Schematically, a vector is represented as an arrow, a directed straight line in which magnitude is given by length and direction by location of the tip. A number of physical quantities are vectors, such as force, momentum and velocity. This rich and well-known mathematics has encouraged some psychologists to attempt to use vectors as a basis for modelling psychological performance. The most ambitious attempt was Kurt Lewin's theory of the LIFE SPACE, in which vectors represented forces producing directed movement. Other more modest applications have been made in *psychophysics*, *factor analysis* and *scaling*. **2** In statistics, a schematic representation of a particular score or value as a line of appropriate length and direction relative to other scores or values. **3** A disease carrier, an animal that transmits disease-producing organisms from the infected to the noninfected; e.g. the mosquito is the vector for malaria.

veg The unit for perceived weight.

vegetative Pertaining to: **1** Plants. **2** Autonomic nervous system functions. **3** A state lacking in responsiveness, a VEGETATIVE STATE.

vegetative state A state of consciousness resulting from brain injury in which there is no evidence of conscious cognitive activity or true wakeful alertness, yet spontaneous eye, limb or mouth movements and sometimes even short vocalizations are present. The presence and persistence of movement distinguish the state from COMA. Also called *persistent vegetative state* and, in older texts, *apallic state*.

velar 1 adj. Pertaining to the VELUM. **2** n. In linguistics, a consonant produced by stopping or disturbing the air flow with the back of the tongue against the soft palate (the *velum*), e.g. the *k* in *like*, the *g* in go.

velocity 1 Rate of motion with both speed and direction specified in either a straight line (*uniform velocity*) or a curve (*angular velocity*). **2** More loosely, speed, swiftness.

velum The soft PALATE of the roof of the mouth.

venereal 1 (archaic) With a capital V, pertaining to Venus; *Venusian* is a corruption necessitated by the ascendance of the other meanings of *venereal*. **2** Pertaining to sexual intercourse. **3** Pertaining to conditions that arise from or are caused by sexual intercourse with an infected person; see VENEREAL DISEASE.

venereal disease See SEXUALLY TRANSMITTED DISEASE.

venlafaxine An ANTIDEPRESSANT DRUG that inhibits the reuptake of both serotonin and norepinepherine (see SNRI's). It also has anxiolytic properties and is used widely for treatment of generalized anxiety disorders and social phobias.

ventilation 1 In physiology, an estimate of the volume of air inhaled per day. **2** Oxygenation of the blood. **3** Refreshment of the air by circulation and the drawing-off of foul air. **4** Metaphorically, particularly in therapeutic discourse, the airing of one's problems, emotions, fears, etc; compare with CATHARSIS.

ventral From the Latin, meaning *pertaining to the belly*. Thus, in bipeds, toward the anterior or frontal part of the body; in quadrapeds, toward the lower, underside of the body. Compare with DORSAL.

ventral amygdalofugal pathway A neural pathway between portions of the amygdala and the forebrain.

ventral angular bundle A neural pathway connecting the CA1 region of the hippocampal formation with the amygdala. Damage to this pathway disrupts the acquisition of conditioned emotional responses.

ventral anterior nucleus A thalamic nucleus that receives input from the globus pallidus and projects to the frontal cortex.

ventral corticospinal tract CORTICOSPINAL PATHWAY.

ventral lateral nucleus VENTROLATERAL NUCLEUS.

ventral noradrenergic bundle CENTRAL TEGMENTAL TRACT.

ventral posterior nucleus A thalamic nucleus that projects to the somatosensory cortex.

ventral root SPINAL ROOT.

ventral stream See VI.

ventral tegmental area An area in the ventral midbrain. Part of the limbic system, its dopaminergic neural projections go to the mesocortical and mesolimbic systems.

ventricle 1 Generally, any small cavity in an organ. **2** Either of the two lower chambers of the heart. **3** Any of the four cavities in the brain. The two large lateral ventricles are in the cerebral hemispheres; they connect with the third ventricle, which in turn communicates with the fourth. The ventricular system is filled with cerebrospinal fluid.

ventricular folds The false vocal cords, folds of mucous membrane located just above the true vocal cords.

ventricular zone The inside of the neural tube. During development the FOUNDER CELLS here give rise to the central nervous system.

ventro- Combining form meaning *anterior, abdominal*; see VENTRAL.

ventrolateral nucleus A thalamic nucleus that receives inputs from the cerebellum and sends information to the primary motor cortex.

ventrolateral preoptic area PREOPTIC AREA.

ventromedial hypothalamic syndrome A behaviour syndrome observed in experimental subjects (usually rats) following lesioning of the ventromedial hypothalamus (VMH). It typically exhibits two stages. In the initial *dynamic* stage the animal develops hyperphagia (overeating) and resulting obesity. As weight gradually stabilizes the animal enters the *static* stage, in which it shows little willingness to work for food, or to put up with any aversive conditions associated with food, and extreme finickiness, so that only easily obtainable, palatable food is eaten. At first these characteristics led to the hypothesis that the VMH was a satiety centre that operated in a counterbalancing fashion to the lateral hypothalamus (see LATERAL HYPOTHALAMIC SYNDROME). The current view, however, is that the VMH is not so much a *centre* controlling feeding as it is part of a complex system, and that the VMH syndrome itself results from the disruption of neural tracts that pass through the region (the ventral noradrenergic bundle).

ventromedial hypothalamus HYPOTHALA-MUS.

ventromedial pathways Collectively, the RETICULOSPINAL TRACTS, the TECTOSPINAL TRACTS and the VESTIBULOSPINAL TRACTS, all of which are involved in the control of movement.

ventroposterior nucleus A group of cells in the THALAMUS that transmit messages from the spinal cord to the PRIMARY SOMATOSENSORY CORTEX.

verbal From the Latin for *word*, pertaining to, characterizing, characteristic of, concerned with, consisting of or expressed in words. Although there is a certain looseness in the manner of usage of the terms *verbal* and *oral*, the latter is derived from the Latin for *mouth* and should not be treated as a synonym of the former. However, given that the human mouth's most notable products are its words, a certain synonymity in usage has proven hard to resist. See ORAL for another distinction.

verbal behaviour Lit., behaviour that involves verbal responses, including speaking, reacting to words and memorization of verbal materials. It is also the euphemism of choice for those with a behaviourist bent and who study the psychology of language but eschew the mentalistic cognitive assumptions of the discipline of PSYCHOLINGUISTICS.

verbal conditioning 1 Generally, any conditioning in which verbal components are used as either stimuli or responses. **2** The operant conditioning of verbal behaviour. Specifically, the shaping-up of specific aspects of verbal behaviour by reinforcement. See GREENSPOON EFFECT.

verbal factor A factor found in many analyses of performance on intelligence tests or other tests of ability that emerges as a cluster of skills seemingly representative of a facility with language and verbal materials.

verbal generalization GENERALIZATION, VERBAL.

verbal image 1 The recoding of a visual image in verbal form. **2** An echoic memory; see SENSORY INFORMATION STORE.

verbal intelligence 1 Ability with language. **2** Intelligence as assessed by tests that rely upon ability with verbal materials.

Meaning 2 is, of course, a theoretical induction from meaning 1, based on the premise that there is a deep relationship between intelligence and various linguistic skills. See INTELLIGENCE and PERFORMANCE TESTS for more discussion.

verbalism 1 An utterance with form but no substance, a formal phrase used with little or no meaning. **2** The predominance of (mere) words over ideas.

verbalization 1 Generally, any verbal statement, an UTTERANCE. **2** The act of expressing oneself verbally. **3** Occasionally, verbosity. **4** In clinical practice, the expression of ideas, fantasies, emotional states and the like during the therapeutic process. Compare with VOCALIZATION.

verbal learning Generally, the study of learning using verbal stimulus materials and verbal responses. *Verbal* here is rather inclusive, covering printed and written as well as spoken materials. The study of verbal learning has historically embraced a number of procedures, including paired-associate learning, serial learning and verbal problem-solving. In recent years the term itself has lost currency, primarily because the area of research so labelled was developed by those with a behaviourist orientation. Such theorists tended to view the study of language as the study of VERBAL BEHAVIOUR and assumed that the general learning principles derived from their experiments could be used as the basis for a theoretical analysis of all linguistic phenomena. Few would defend such a position any longer and, as a result, the terms PSYCHOLINGUISTICS and *psychology of language* are now preferred as labels for the general field. These terms carry distinct cognitive as opposed to behaviourist connotations.

verbal-linguistic intelligence MULTIPLE INTELLIGENCES THEORY.

verbal-loop hypothesis The theoretical principle that sensory/perceptual information is acquired and retained by translating what is perceived into words and remembering them.

verbal masochism A form of *sexual* MASOCHISM where arousal is derived from verbal insults and humiliation.

verbal overshadowing A phenomenon, first reported by Jonathan Schooler, that providing a verbal or written description of an individual seen or an event witnessed compromises later recall of that person or event. The act of providing the description adds information, not all of it relevant, and later attempts at recall become confused and error-prone. The effect is quite general and has been reported in memory for colour, spatial arrays, music, problem-solving, analogical thought and, of course, faces. The findings have major implications in FORENSIC PSYCHOLOGY and the use of EYEWITNESS TESTIMONY.

verbal repairs REPAIR MECHANISM.

verbal scale Frequently used synonymously with VERBAL TEST. However, the designation *scale* is reserved by some for a component of a larger test.

verbal test Generally, any test that is ultimately linked in some way with language knowledge, verbal skills, etc. Verbal tests may be *specifically* verbal, such as vocabulary tests, or they may be indirectly verbal, such as the early IQ tests, in which the verbal scale was only determined when the test battery was factor-analysed. Contrast with PERFORMANCE TEST.

verbatim recall 1 Memory for the exact words used in the original presentation of a message. 2 A procedure for studying memory in which the subject's task is to attempt a word-for-word recall.

verbatim trace FUZZY TRACE.

verbigeration Excessive, meaningless and repetitive speech.

verbomania LOGORRHOEA.

vergence A cover term for any turning of the eyes, specifically the turning of one eye relative to the other. See e.g. CONVERGENCE, DIVERGENCE.

veridical Lit., truth-telling. Used primarily of statements that are true in the sense that they are substantiated by facts.

veridical perception DIRECT PERCEPTION.

verification The process of determining the truth or correctness of a hypothesis. In scientific parlance the term refers to the controlled process of collecting objective data to assess the truth of a theory or hypothesis. By extension, it also refers to the everyday act of scanning the environment in an informal manner to gather information about the appropriateness of one's perceptions, thoughts, suspicions, etc. vb., *verify*.

verificationism FALSIFICATIONISM.

verification time The time that it takes to determine the truth or falseness of a proposition. This measure is particularly useful in gauging the complexity of many cognitive processes since it is assumed that longer verification times imply more complex thought processes. See also REACTION TIME, which is a more general measure.

vermis The part of the cerebellum located at the midline. Auditory and visual information arrive here from the *tectum*, and cutaneous and kinaesthetic information from the spinal cord. It projects fibres via the *fastigial nucleus* to, ultimately, the *vestibulospinal* and *reticulospinal tracts*.

vernacular The everyday, colloquial speech of a group of persons or in a circumscribed area.

vernier A small, finely graduated scale used as an auxiliary scale to give a measuring device greater adjustment accuracy.

vernier acuity ACUITY, VERNIER.

vertebra Any one of the 33 bony segments of the SPINAL COLUMN. pl., *vertebrae*; adj., *vertebral*.

vertex 1 Generally, the top or summit of something. 2 In anatomy, the uppermost peak of the head. 3 In geometry, the point furthest from the base. adj., *vertical*.

vertical 1 Pertaining to the vertex, specifically the uppermost point of a thing. 2 By extension, pertaining to the line or plane perpendicular to the ground or to the base of an object. 3 Upright.

vertical décalage DÉCALAGE.

vertical group GROUP, VERTICAL.

vertical mobility Mobility between social or occupational classes. The term covers movement up or down in a social system, but it is most commonly used with the connotation of upward movement. Also called *vertical social mobility*.

vertical sampling SAMPLING, VERTICAL.

vertigo 1 Loosely, dizziness. **2** Technically, an inappropriate sensation of bodily movement (*subjective vertigo*) or object movement (*objective vertigo*) caused by disturbances of the sensory mechanism for equilibrium. Mostly it is a result of middle-ear disease but it also occurs in toxic conditions (e.g. excessive alcohol intake).

vesanic Loosely, pertaining to insanity, particularly to clearly marked psychoses.

vessel Generally, any duct, tube or canal through which flows some bodily fluid.

vestibular apparatus The bony cavity in the labyrinth of the inner ear, including the two vestibular sacs (the UTRICLE and the SACCULE) and the three SEMICIRCULAR CANALS. See each for details on how the system functions as the sensory mechanism for the perception of head position, acceleration and deceleration. See also VESTIBULE (2), which is occasionally used as a synonym.

vestibular canal COCHLEA.

vestibular dysfunction Compromised function of the VESTIBULAR APPARATUS. It can be bilateral or unilateral and have any of several causes including physical damage to the inner ear, lesions and adverse reaction to an antibiotic. Symptoms are highly varied depending on the cause but typically include vertigo, a shifting and blurring of the visual image, disturbances in the sense of body position, abnormal nystagmus and hearing loss.

vestibular nerve VESTIBULOCOCHLEAR.

vestibular nucleus A nucleus in the cerebellum that receives inputs from various other parts of the cerebellum, including *fastigial nucleus* and the *flocculonodular lobe*, and projects its outputs to the spinal cord.

vestibular sacs Two small sacs in the inner ear that respond to gravity and provide information about the orientation of the head.

vestibule 1 Generally, any small cavity at the front of a canal. **2** Specifically, the middle part of the inner ear in front of the semicircular canals containing the utricle and saccule. Occasionally the term is used to include the whole of the VESTIBULAR APPARATUS (see which for details).

vestibulocerebellum ARCHICEREBELLUM.

vestibulocochlear nerve The VIIIth CRANIAL NERVE. It has two tracts, a *vestibular nerve* that carries afferent information about head position from the vestibule and the semicircular canals and an *auditory nerve* (also called the *cochlear* or *acoustic nerve*) that transmits information from the inner ear.

vestibulo-ocular reflex The reflex-like adjustments in eye movements that compensate for head movement and permit the maintenance of a steady retinal image while one is moving about.

vestibulospinal tract One of the VENTROMEDIAL PATHWAYS, this runs from the *vestibular nucleus* to the grey matter in the spinal cord and is involved in the control of posture in response to information that arises in the vestibular system.

vestige 1 Generally, a thing that in its present form is a degenerate or imperfect representation of a fully developed form which existed in the past. **2** Specifically, in biology, an organ or organ part showing such characteristics. adj., *vestigial*.

Vexierversuch The original German term for what is known as a CATCH TRIAL.

VI Abbreviation for *variable interval*. See SCHEDULES OF *REINFORCEMENT.

viable 1 Of an organism, likely to live. **2** Of a seed or spore, likely to germinate. **3** Metaphorically, characterizing a theory or a hypothesis likely to stand up under stringent experimental test.

vibration Generally, periodic motion of matter. A full vibration cycle is from a given point through the full cycle and back to the original point, as in a sine wave. See also VIBRATION RATE.

vibration, forced (or **induced** or **sympathetic**) RESONANCE (1).

vibration frequency VIBRATION RATE.

vibration rate The frequency of vibrations per unit of time (usually seconds). The years have witnessed several changes in the official notation used with respect to the rate of vibrating stimuli. Originally, a full vibration cycle was called a *double vibration* (or *d.v.*), and references to the frequency of vibrations (as, for example, in the measurement of tones) were noted as *d.v.s.* (double vibrations per second). Later this rather cumbersome notation was simplified: *d.v.* was replaced by *cycle* and *d.v.s.* by *cps* (cycles per second). Today the term of choice for vibrations per second is HERTZ, abbreviated *Hz*.

vibratory sense The capacity to sense the rapid shifting back and forth of a vibrating stimulus. The PACINIAN CORPUSCLE is thought to be the receptor. There is a suggestion that there are distinct subsystems, one that is maximally sensitive to vibrations up to roughly 100 Hz and another that responds to more rapid vibrations.

vicarious Pertaining to or functioning as a substitute.

vicarious brain process Following lesion to one part of the brain, the assumption of its function by another.

vicarious functioning Generally, the replacing of one psychological process, which, for any number of reasons, has been thwarted, blocked, inhibited or repressed, by another. The substitute process itself is often called a *vicarious function*.

vicarious learning Learning by observing. See MODELLING (2) and OBSERVATION(AL) *LEARNING.

vicarious pleasure 1 Loosely, pleasure derived from observing others enjoying themselves. 2 Specifically, the enjoyment of a voyeur.

vicarious satisfaction 1 Loosely, satisfaction experienced by watching the success of others. 2 Specifically, such satisfaction as experienced by a parent when an offspring succeeds where he or she did not.

vicarious trial and error (VTE) The covert or mental process of thinking through a sequence of tentative responses prior to (or instead of) making overt responses. In board games like checkers, chess or go most players engage in a good deal of VTE behaviour.

video deficit A deficit in the ability of toddlers to understand a task after watching a video of a person performing it even though they perform quite well if they watch a real person. The cause is unclear; the best guess is the lack of implied social interaction when viewing the video.

Vienna circle A collection of logicians and philosophers (notably Carnap, Reichenbach, Gödel and Feigl) who have had more than a passing influence on modern psychology. The essential focus of the circle was scientific philosophy, with an attendant empiricism and a deep trust in logical analysis. See LOGICAL POSITIVISM, which embodies the tenets of the circle.

Viennese school Those psychoanalytic thinkers and practitioners who followed the classical tenets and theories of Sigmund Freud.

Vierordt's law The generalization that the TWO-POINT THRESHOLD is directly related to (a) the mobility of the part of the body and (b) the distance of the body part from the central axis.

viewing angle The angle between the surface being fixated on and the eye. Distinguish from VISUAL ANGLE.

viewing conditions A general term encompassing any and all of the factors present when a stimulus is viewed. Most writers restrict application of the term to the physical factors involved (e.g. light level, stimulus size, nature of the display, viewing angle); others, however, include covert factors (e.g. attentional focus, stress, emotionality).

vigilance Alertness, watchfulness. The term is used broadly, with respect to processes that are intentional and conscious as well as those that are covert or unconscious. See e.g. PERCEPTUAL VIGILANCE.

Vigotsky test VYGOTSKY BLOCKS.

Vincent curve (or method) A procedure for analysing data from experiments in which not all subjects have taken the same number of trials or the same amount of time to achieve a set criterion. The data from each subject are divided into fractions of trials or time and each fraction is treated as equivalent to that from another subject. For example, using $\frac{1}{10}$ (0.1) as the fraction: for a subject who took 20 trials to learn the material, the first data point is based on the average performance on the first two trials, the second on the next two trials, and so forth; for a subject who took 100 trials to reach criterion, the first point is the average of the first 10 trials, and so on. The full *Vincent* or *Vincentized curve* for all subjects is then based on the averages of these averages.

Vineland Adaptive Behaviour Scales An instrument designed to assess adaptive personal and social functioning. An updating of the original Vineland Social Maturity Scale, it is designed to assess communicative, social, daily living and motoric skills. It uses a rating form and, when needed, additional data from a semi-structured interview with parents or caretakers. Designed to be used broadly, the scales have forms for ages from infancy to 90.

Vineland Social Maturity Scale VINELAND ADAPTIVE BEHAVIOUR SCALES.

violation-of-expectation paradigm An experimental design in which subjects are presented with two events, one consistent with physical belief and one not, and their reactions are noted. Typically, circumstances that violate beliefs are looked at longer. The procedure is often used with children and preverbal infants. See PREFERENTIAL LOOKING METHOD.

violet The hue experienced when the human eye is exposed to short-wavelength light in the 400–440 nm range.

viraginity 1 Generally, the feeling in a woman that aspects of her have a male-like quality. **2** Specifically, a condition in which a biological female feels that she should be male. See TRANSSEXUALISM.

virgin 1 Generally, fresh, untouched, unused. **2** Specifically, a person who has not had sexual intercourse. The term is generally used only of those who have passed puberty, and some authors restrict its application to full adults, so that, speaking strictly definitionally, there are no 6-year-old but a goodly number of 16-year-old virgins. Note also that there is a tendency to apply the term only to females; while there is etymological justification for this limitation (*virgo* is Latin for *maiden*), modern usage includes males who fit the criteria.

virile Masculine, having the physical and biological characteristics of a mature male.

virilism The presence or development of

male secondary sex characteristics in an anatomical female.

virtual environment VIRTUAL REALITY ENVIRONMENT.

virtual lesion A loss of cortical function produced by TRANSCRANIAL MAGNETIC STIMULATION (TMS). The term accurately describes the impact of TMS in that it produces a functional lesion with no lasting neurological damage.

virtual pitch Literally, a perceived pitch that is not physically present in the sound. It is heard most commonly when a complex wave form is presented. The experienced pitch will be the FUNDAMENTAL TONE, as computed using a Fourier analysis. Also called the *missing fundamental* and *residue pitch*.

virtual reality environment (VRE) A perceptual environment produced through the use of modern computer techniques and input devices. *Desktop VREs* are visual environments presented on a computer screen, often along with auditory input and/or motor control via a mouse or joystick. *Immersive VREs* are delivered to the perceiver through a head-mounted display that provides the sensation of being inside a new environment. Kinaesthetic sensations can be added through other input devices. VREs are used in learning and perception studies, in some therapeutic settings and have been used to produce out-of-body experiences. Sometimes shortened to *virtual environment* or *virtual reality*.

virtue A general tendency to behave in a manner that is in agreement with the moral code of a society. The term connotes that such behaviour is voluntary: one who is impressed into obeying the code against his or her will is not considered virtuous. Some writers emphasize sex and sexual codes but this restriction is not necessary.

virulent Poisonous or dangerous, in the sense that a virulent substance is one capable of overcoming the body's natural defences.

viscera Generally, the internal organs located in a body cavity; usually the reference is to the abdominal cavity and the abdominal organs. sing., *viscus*.

visceral 1 Pertaining to the VISCERA. **2** Emotional, nonmental, even nonthinking. This meaning is as common as it is misleading. It is reflected in the old distinction between the *viscerotonic* and the *cerebrotonic* components of temperament (see CONSTITUTIONAL THEORY) and is manifested today in both the technical and nontechnical literatures by expressions like *gut-level feeling* or *gut reaction* to characterize an unanalysed sense of rightness of action. In one sense such an extension of the term is not wholly wrong: emotional expression is often accompanied by visceral action; in another sense it confounds the semantics of the original term because the equating of emotionality with the viscera is a theoretical issue and not a lexicographic one.

visceral drive VISCEROGENIC DRIVE.

visceral learning BIOFEEDBACK.

visceral sensations Sensations derived from receptors in the viscera. Although the motor fibres to the viscera are many compared with the sensory fibres from it, a variety of *visceral* (or *organic* as they are also called) sensations occur, including responses to distension, contraction, temperature changes and various chemicals. Pain in the viscera is often poorly localized; see REFERRED *PAIN.

viscero- Combining form meaning *pertaining to the viscera.*

visceroceptor An interoceptor in the viscera.

viscerogenic Lit., originating in the viscera.

viscerogenic drive Loosely, any drive based on physiological needs. Occasionally called *visceral drive.*

viscerotonia One of the three primary components of temperament assumed by CONSTITUTIONAL THEORY.

viscus The rarely used singular form of *viscera.*

visibility 1 The property of a stimulus that makes it easy to see. **2** The property of a stimulus that means the physical characteristics of the energy radiating from it or reflected off it are adequate for exciting a sufficient number of visual receptors for the experiencing of a visual sensation. See LUMINOSITY.

visibility coefficient(s) LUMINOSITY COEFFICIENTS.

visibility curve(s) LUMINOSITY CURVES.

visible spectrum SPECTRUM, VISUAL.

visible speech An obsolescent term for the visual representation of an acoustic stimulus (specifically speech) as displayed by a sound SPECTROGRAPH.

visile An individual with a preference for representing things in visual images and a sensitivity to visually presented material. In an early model of reading 'visile' children were compared with *audiles* who presumably preferred auditory inputs.

vision 1 The sensory modality for seeing; the sense for which the stimulus is electromagnetic radiation (light) between approximately 380 and 740 nm in wavelength, and the receptor for which is the eye, or, more precisely, the photosensitive cells of the retina. **2** The process of seeing itself. **3** The perceptual experience of seeing. **4** A visual hallucination. **5** Clarity or foresight.

vision, achromatic Vision using the rods, black–white vision.

vision, alternating The alternate use of the two eyes.

vision, binocular Vision with both eyes, specifically with both fixated on the same point in the visual field. In normal binocular vision there is fusion of the images from the two eyes into a single percept.

vision, central Vision using the FOVEA and the PARAFOVEA of the retina.

vision, chromatic Vision using the cones, colour vision.

vision, distance Defined arbitrarily as vision for objects that are 20 ft (approximately 6.1 m) or more from the viewer.

vision, fovea Vision with the fovea. For details see FOVEA and PHOTOPIC VISION.

vision, monocular Vision with one eye.

vision, near Defined arbitrarily as vision for objects that are 2 ft (approximately 61 cm) or less from the viewer.

vision, paracentral Vision using the area

of the retina surrounding the fovea, the PAR-AFOVEA.

vision, perimacular Vision using the area of the retina surrounding the MACULA LUTEA.

vision, peripheral Vision using the PERIPHERY OF THE RETINA.

vision, persistence of ICONIC (2).

vision, stereoscopic Three-dimensional vision produced largely by the fusion of two slightly disparate views of a scene, one on each retina.

vision, theories of THEORIES OF *COLOUR VISION.

visual Pertaining to vision.

visual acuity ACUITY, VISUAL.

visual adaptation A general term covering several processes by which the visual system adapts itself to viewing conditions. See e.g. CHROMATIC ADAPTATION, DARK ADAPTATION, LIGHT ADAPTATION.

visual agnosia AGNOSIA, VISUAL.

visual allaesthesia An ALLAESTHESIA (1) that occurs in visual perception. var., *visual allesthesia*.

visual angle A measure of the size of the projection of an object on the retina. In the figure, *n* is the *nodal point*, *h* the *height* of the object in the environment, *d* the *distance* of the object from *n* and α the *visual angle*. Visual angle as measured in degrees, where one degree corresponds roughly with the size of your index fingernail when held out at arm's length.

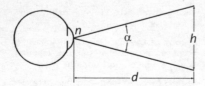

visual aphasia ALEXIA.

visual areas The cortical areas that play a role in vision and have been identified as neurologically and functionally distinct. The main ones are in the OCCIPITAL LOBES although up to 17 distinct areas found in the parietal, temporal and even the frontal lobes have been identified as playing roles in vision. Those most intimately linked to vision are V1, V2, V3, V4 and V5.

visual axis A straight line from the external fixation point through the nodal point of the eye to the fovea of the retina.

visual capture 1 The tendency for visual information to dominate when one's kinaesthetic information and visual information are discoordinate. For example, while wearing prisms which displace the visual world slightly to one side, one tends to 'feel' one's hand not as where it is physically but rather as where one sees it. **2** The tendency for sounds to be heard as coming from a plausible visual location, such as hearing a singer's voice as coming from the singer rather than the loud speakers on either side of the stage. Incidentally, visual capture is one reason why a good ventriloquist can be so convincing.

visual cliff An experimental apparatus designed to evaluate depth perception. It consists of a large box with a heavy glass top and a narrow board across the centre of the glass. On one side of the board there appears to be a sharp drop-off (the visual cliff); the other side appears shallow and safe. The subject (most commonly a newborn of a species) is placed on the board; consistent locomotion toward the safe side is taken to indicate an ability to perceive depth. Most species that can locomote at birth show an immediate avoidance of the 'cliff'. Human infants cannot be tested on the locomotor task for some months, but newborns placed face down directly over the cliff side usually show considerable distress, suggesting that depth perception may have an innate element.

visual cortex Loosely, any cortical area that mediates visual information. However, the reference is usually to PRIMARY VISUAL CORTEX (see also V1).

visual disparity RETINAL *DISPARITY.

visual dominance The perceptual dominance of an auditory or other stimulus by a visual one. If a visual stimulus and an auditory one are presented simultaneously, the visual is overwhelmingly likely to dominate awareness.

visual evoked potential EVOKED POTENTIAL.

visual extinction A form of visual NEGLECT in which a perceived stimulus in one visual field is no longer detected when another stimulus appears in the opposite visual field.

visual field 1 Objectively, all of the points in the physical environment that can be perceived by a stable eye at a given moment. **2** The subjective, phenomenological perception of the space being viewed at a moment in time.

visual field defect Generally, any limiting of the visual field. See, e.g. HEMIANOPIA.

visual fixation FIXATION, VISUAL.

visual flow OPTIC FLOW.

visual image IMAGE, VISUAL.

visual induction Generally, the induction of any visual perception of one stimulus resulting from another, adjacent, visual stimulus. A variety of phenomena have been reported, including induced-size effects (see EBBINGHAUS ILLUSION), induced-colour effects (see COLOUR CONTRAST) and induced-brightness effects (see MACH BAND).

visualize To form a visual image.

visually impaired Characterizing a person with a relatively serious vision loss but not to the point of being blind. The term is preferred by many over BLINDNESS and its various qualified forms.

visual-motor Referring to or characterizing motor responses which are coordinated with visual stimulation. A special case of *sensorimotor* in which the sensory modality is vision. var., *visuomotor*

visual-motor Gestalt test BENDER GESTALT TEST.

visual neglect NEGLECT.

visual noise NOISE.

visual organization A general term derived from the Gestalt psychologists and used to refer to the basic notion that visual perception is inherently dependent upon the manner of organization of the manifold aspects of the visual field. The basic issues here are discussed under PRINCIPLE OF *ORGANIZATION.

visual pigment(s) PHOTOPIGMENT.

visual projection PROJECTION, VISUAL.

visual projection area V1.

visual purple RHODOPSIN.

visual righting reflex A reflex-like shift in head position to the fixation of different visual points.

visual search Loosely, the process of searching through a visually presented display for a target stimulus. It is used as an experimental platform for studying attention, detection, and categorization and in clinical research to explore disorders such as visual NEGLECT and VISUAL *AGNOSIA.

visual space VISUAL FIELD (2).

visual span READING SPAN.

visual-spatial ability Loosely, pertaining to the capacity to comprehend and process information that requires coordination of the spatial elements of visual inputs. It is seen in functions such as navigating complex environments, reading maps and displaying flexibility in adjusting to changes in orientation. It is also a topic of controversy concerning possible gender differences and its role in intelligence (see MULTIPLE INTELLIGENCES THEORY).

visual-spatial intelligence See MULTIPLE INTELLIGENCES THEORY.

visual type VISILE.

visual yellow XANTHOPSIN.

visuomotor VISUAL-MOTOR.

visuomotor ataxia OPTIC *ATAXIA.

visuo-spatial Pertaining to visual perception of spatial relationships. vars., *visuospatial, visual-spatial*.

visuo-spatial agnosia AGNOSIA, VISUO-SPATIAL.

visuo-spatial sketchpad A form of WORKING *MEMORY in which a visual image is held in memory while input is interpreted or manipulated, e.g. remembering a string of numbers by forming a visual image of each number as it is presented. In Baddeley and Hitch's model of memory it functions alongside the PHONOLOGICAL LOOP, which processes auditory and language inputs. Also called *visuospatial scratchpad*, and written as *visuospatial* and *visual-spatial (sketchpad)*, with and without hyphens.

visuotopy RETINOTOPIC REPRESENTATION.

vital 1 Characteristic of or pertaining to life. **2** Making an essential contribution to life. **3** By extension, critical, important. **4** In studies of personality, vigorous, enthusiastic.

vital capacity The volume of air that can be expelled after full inspiration.

vitalism A philosophical point of view which holds that a 'vital force' not explicable by mechanical, chemical or physical principles is responsible for life. It is a form of PLURALISM (1), involving the vital force in addition to the mind and body of DUALISM.

vitality 1 Simply, that which differentiates the living from the nonliving. **2** By extension, the capacity to remain alive. **3** By further extension, movement, action or strength. **4** In the study of personality, a behaviour pattern marked by vigour, enthusiasm and endurance.

vital signs Generally, the indicators of life, e.g. respiration, pulse, normal body temperature.

vital statistics 1 Collectively, numerical data on information concerning births, deaths, marriages and the like in a given area. **2** Specific numerical data on a particular individual, such as height and weight.

vitamin Any of a large number of extremely complex organic substances essential, in small quantities, for normal metabolism, growth and development. Vitamins are distinct from other essential substances like proteins, carbohydrates, fats, minerals and salts. Moreover, they supply no energy of their own and do not add significantly to bodily substance. Their primary roles are as regulators of metabolic processes and aids in the transformation of other substances into energy.

vitreous humour The transparent jelly filling the eye between the lens and the retina. Also called *vitreous body*.

vivi- Combining form meaning *alive*.

vivisection Experimental surgery on a living animal for the purpose of anatomical, physiological or pharmacological investigation. In many countries governmental policies exist which regulate experimentation on live animals and in some, e.g. the UK, a licence is required to perform such research work.

VMH Abbreviation for the *ventromedial nucleus* of the HYPOTHALAMUS.

vocabulary 1 The full compendium of words that an individual knows. **2** The full list of words in use in a language. **3** Any specifically circumscribed list of words. When this last meaning is intended, a qualifier is typically used to denote the conditions.

vocabulary, active Generally, the VOCABULARY (1) used in speaking and writing (i.e. used actively). Compare with PASSIVE *VOCABULARY. Also called *productive vocabulary*.

vocabulary, passive Generally, the VOCABULARY (1) used in reading and listening (i.e. used passively). An individual's passive vocabulary is considerably larger than his or her ACTIVE *VOCABULARY. Also called *recognition* or *receptive vocabulary*.

vocabulary, sight In early readers, the words that can be read quickly (i.e. on sight) without the need to engage in any explicit phonetic decoding. Children taught to read using the whole-word approach typically have large sight vocabularies.

vocabulary test Generally, any test for assessing an individual's vocabulary. There are a truly remarkable number of variations here: one can simply count the words recognized, insist on the subject providing a definition for each word, require that the words be used properly in sentences, ask for words that match given definitions and so forth. Each method, of course, will yield a different approximation of an individual's vocabulary.

vocal 1 Pertaining to the voice. **2** Outspoken.

vocal cords The two muscular folds of tissue in the larynx which, by rapidly opening and closing, set up the vibration patterns for voicing. The name *cord* is slightly misleading, suggesting as it does a string-like affair; many authors prefer *vocal folds* or even *vocal flaps*, as these are anatomically more accurate.

vocal folds VOCAL CORDS.

vocality Generally, an aspect of an auditory sensation characterized as the extent to which it has vowel-like properties.

vocalization 1 Generally, the use of the vocal apparatus to produce sounds. This meaning is rather inclusive and encompasses all manner of sounds, language-like and non-language-like, made by humans (adult or infant) and other species. **2** Specifically, the production of sounds by *Homo sapiens* which are *not* part of true language, e.g. the babbling of infants. **3** The production of sounds by species other than *Homo sapiens*. *Vocalization* in sense 1 may be used as a synonym of VERBALIZATION, but in senses 2 and 3 it should not.

vocal tract The whole sequence of structures utilized in the production of vocal sounds, including the larynx, the pharynx, the mouth and the nose and all other associated structures.

vocation 1 Etymologically, the role in life to which one has been called. This meaning survives only in theological writings. **2** A job at which one works to earn a living.

vocational adjustment Quite literally, the degree to which one is suited, psychologically, to one's job.

vocational aptitude Potential for a particular vocation. The term is used with a predictive connotation; that is, it generally refers to an assessment of how likely it is that an individual will be successful and satisfied in a particular job given what is known about his or her interests, abilities, training, education, etc.

vocational counselling Lit., counselling a person concerning the selection of a vocation. The term is used broadly and encompasses specific testing of skills and abilities, and psychological assessment of personality, motivation, life goals, etc. Generally, counselling (or *guidance*) is aimed at helping an individual into an occupation for which he or she displays a high aptitude. Compare with VOCATIONAL SELECTION, the focus of which is on finding the individual for the position.

vocational guidance VOCATIONAL COUNSELLING.

vocational-interest blank See STRONG INTEREST INVENTORY.

vocational selection The process of attempting to select the person(s) with the highest likelihood of success in a particular position. The skills and aptitudes needed for the particular vocation are presumably already known; the selection process is focused on finding the optimal individual(s) to be hired. Compare with VOCATIONAL COUNSELLING, the focus of which is on finding the job for the person.

voice 1 Sound produced by the vocal apparatus. **2** The vibration of the vocal cords when uttering a sound. See VOICING.

voice box A nontechnical term for the LARYNX.

voice disorders Abnormalities in the voice, e.g. excessive hoarseness, high pitch, squeakiness.

voiced/voiceless VOICING.

voice key A switch activated by a voice. The older, crude models were not really *voice* keys since any sound would trigger them; more modern sophisticated models can be tuned to human voices.

voice onset time (VOT) The time between the beginning of the uttering of a sound and the vibration of the vocal cords. The easiest way to appreciate VOT is to say 'ba' and 'pa' with your fingers lightly touching your throat. The vocal cords vibrate at almost the same instant the lips are opened for 'ba' but there is a short lag (about 50–100 msec) in voicing for 'pa'. This lag time is the VOT.

voiceprint SPECTROGRAPH.

voicing In phonetics, a DISTINCTIVE FEATURE (2) marked by the presence or absence of vibration of the vocal cords. In English all vowels are voiced and several consonants can be distinguished from each other according purely to the presence or absence of this feature, e.g. the voiceless *t* in 'ta' compared with the voiced *d* in 'da'.

vol The unit of measurement of the psychological continuum of perceived volume of an auditory stimulus. A vol is defined as the apparent volume of a 1,000 Hz tone at 40 db. See VOLUME.

volar PALMAR.

volition 1 Generally and loosely, conscious, voluntary selection of particular action or choice from many potential actions or choices. **2** In the writings of the early introspectionists, a complex arrangement of kinaesthetic sensations and images that occurred along with a conceptualized goal or end of one's actions or thoughts.

volitional facial paresis FACIAL PARESIS.

volley The (near) simultaneous or synchronized firing of a number of neural impulses.

volley theory of hearing THEORIES OF *HEARING.

volume In psychophysics, the sense of how much space a stimulus appears to take up; the psychological equivalent of the physicist's definition. Volume is experienced most clearly with sounds, high-pitched tones being perceived as 'thin' and hence low in volume and low-pitched tones as 'larger' or 'fuller' and hence as more voluminous. The unit of volume is the VOL. The persistence of some radio and television manufacturers in mislabelling the *loudness* control *volume* (a practice arising from a mislabelling of the control for compensating for the human ear's deficiencies with low- and high-pitched tones as *loudness*) has produced more than its share of confusion. Many olfactory sensations also have a voluminous quality.

volume colour COLOUR, VOLUME.

volumetric thirst THIRST, VOLUMETRIC.

voluntarism The metaphysical doctrine that volition or free will is the prime force in reality. See FREE WILL and DETERMINISM for more on this issue.

voluntary 1 Characterizing that which is internally motivated, freely chosen, volitional. **2** Characterizing those psychological processes or behaviour patterns that are consciously modulated and deliberative.

voluntary admission Admission into a psychiatric institute or hospital undertaken voluntarily by an individual. The term is also used as a euphemism in the many borderline instances in which an individual is told by the appropriate authorities that either he or she request 'voluntary' admission or a court

order will be sought to impose admission. See COMMITMENT.

voluntary memory MEMORY, VOLUNTARY.

voluntary muscle Any muscle under voluntary control; for the most part, STRIATE *MUSCLES.

voluntary parenthood PLANNED PARENTHOOD.

volunteer bias A potential bias in any study in which the subjects are volunteers rather than persons who have been selected from the population using sampling procedures that protect against nonrepresentativeness. There is considerable evidence that volunteers are atypical: they are generally more highly motivated and tend to perform at a higher level on most tasks than control subjects who are selected at random.

vomeronasal organ A sensory organ that responds to various chemicals. In species that possess it (most, but not all, mammals) it mediates the effects of PHEROMONES. In nonhuman animals it plays a significant role in sexual behaviour; in humans it is sensitive to a variety of chemicals but a specific link to sexuality has yet to be discerned. Also called *vomeronasal system* and *Jacobson's organ*.

von Restorff effect If one in a series of stimuli to be learned (e.g. a list of words) is made physically distinctive in some way (e.g. printed in larger type or in a different colour from the others), it will be more easily learned and recalled. Also called the *isolation effect*.

voodoo A West African spiritual system of beliefs and rituals, some aspects of which are observable in the practices of populations descended from West African slaves in the Americas. Known by a host of other names including *voudou, vodoun, vudu,* and *djudju*.

voodoo death THANATOMANIA.

VOT VOICE ONSET TIME.

vowel A speech sound produced by vibrating the vocal cords without obstructing the passage of air through the vocal tract. Contrast with CONSONANT.

voxel Short for 'volume pixel', the smallest definable unit in a given three-dimensional space. Frequently used in neuroimaging where it defines a particular point in the brain.

voyeurism A PARAPHILIA characterized by a pattern of sexual behaviour in which the preferred means to sexual arousal is the clandestine observing of others when they are disrobing, nude or actually engaged in sexual activity. Interestingly, a voyeur does not usually derive pleasure from striptease shows, public nudity or pornography; arousal is dependent upon the observed person(s) not being aware of their being observed. See also SCOPOPHILIA.

VR Abbreviation for *variable ratio*. See SCHEDULES OF *REINFORCEMENT.

VRE VIRTUAL REALITY ENVIRONMENT.

VT Abbreviation for *variable time*. See SCHEDULES OF *REINFORCEMENT.

VTE VICARIOUS TRIAL AND ERROR.

vulnerability An individual's susceptibility to disease, to developing a disorder or otherwise failing to withstand adverse circumstances, stressful events or infectious agents. It is used in both biological and psychological contexts. See RESILIENCE and SUSCEPTIBILITY for more detail.

vulnerability marker MARKER, VULNERABILITY.

vulnerable Easily injured. Used with respect to physical, psychological or sociological circumstances.

vulva The external parts of the female genitals, consisting of the major and minor labia and the outer part of the vagina.

Vygotsky blocks A set of 32 wooden blocks differing in shape, height, width and colour. On the underside of each is written a nonsense word. In the standard design there are four nonsense words, one for all tall wide blocks, one for all low wide blocks, one for the tall thin ones and one for the low thin ones. Colour and shape are irrelevant. The blocks have been used in a variety of concept-formation studies and experiments on thinking, primarily with children as subjects. Interestingly, although they are called Vygotsky blocks after the Russian philologist, psychologist and philosopher, L. S. Vygotsky, who used them extensively in his work, Vygotsky himself credited a colleague, L. S. Sakharov, with developing them. The use of the full set of blocks is occasionally called a *Vygotsky test*. var., *Vigotsky*.

Vygotsky test VYGOTSKY BLOCKS.

W

W 1 *Weber fraction* (see WEBER'S LAW). **2** COEFFICIENT OF *CONCORDANCE. **3** *Weight* or *weighting factor* (also *w*).

Wada test A test of cerebral hemispheric function. Sodium amobarbital (or another similarly acting substance) is injected into one of the two carotid arteries, producing a period of hemispheric anaesthesia on the side of administration. Localization of language and spatial functions can be assessed since the side anaesthetized is nonfunctional.

WAIS WECHSLER ADULT INTELLIGENCE SCALE.

waist-to-hip ratio (WHR) The ratio of the circumference of the waist to the hips. A WHR of around 0.7 in women and 0.9 in men is associated with overall good health (it may be a better predictor of heart disease than the BODY MASS INDEX). These values are also associated with sexual attractiveness, although there are cultural differences.

waiting list effect The phenomenon that those on a waiting list for treatment or therapy show significant recovery or cure rates prior to receiving treatment. The effect is strong enough that many clinical trials include a *waiting-list control group*. See PLACEBO et seq.

waking centre A term once applied first to an area of the hypothalamus and later to a part of the reticular formation, each of which was implicated as the primary locus of cells that functioned to waken an organism. It is now generally agreed that there is no single such brain centre; both brainstem and forebrain structures are known to exert control over the extremely complex sleep–waking cycle. See SLEEP and related terms.

Walden Two The title of a novel by the American behaviourist B. F. Skinner, in which the principles of operant conditioning are applied to create a (or at least Skinner's characterization of a) utopia. See SKINNERIAN.

Wald–Wolfowitz runs test A nonparametric statistical test that evaluates whether two samples of data can be said to be drawn from the same population. The test analyses the pattern of RUNS (3) in the two samples and reflects differences between them. See RUNS TEST for a one-sample test.

Wallerian degeneration The *anterograde* DEGENERATION (1) of an axon when it has been separated from its cell body. The myelin sheath degenerates into a chain of small lipoid drops which can be stained, a procedure that permits the tracing of the course of the injured fibres. The neurilemma, if left intact, forms a hollow tube through which the axon can regenerate.

walleye 1 An eye with an abnormally light-coloured or white iris. **2** An eye with a dense, opaque cornea. **3** Divergent STRABISMUS.

ward A large room in a hospital for the use of many patients.

warming-up period WARM-UP PERIOD.

warm spot A point on the skin where a punctate stimulus that is below adaptation level evokes a sensation of warmth. It is not clear what specific sensory-receptor system is involved since examination of these warm spots reveals no special structures.

warmth 1 One of the skin senses. **2** The sensory experience resulting from a stimulus of a higher temperature than the normal temperature of the skin (32°C, 89°F). However, the experiencing of warmth is dependent upon the adaptation level of the skin and after immersing one's hand in water of 36°C (95°F) for a few minutes a stimulus of 34°C (92°F) is experienced as cool, not warm.

warm-up period In many complex learning situations, a period of time during which movements and responses are tentative and inexact. var., *warming-up period*.

Wason task A problem-solving task developed by Peter Wason based on four cards, each of which has one class of stimuli printed on one side and another on the other side, and a rule governing the relationship between them. In the classic condition letters are on one side and numbers on the other and the rule is 'vowels have even numbers'. Subjects get four cards with stimuli like H, A, 9, 4 showing and have to select two cards to turn over to make sure the rule has been followed. Subjects typically display a CONFIRMATION BIAS (picking 'A' and '4' or 'H' and '9'), failing to realize that the only sure test of the rule is to check for possible disconfirming cases (picking 'A' and '9' or 'H' and '4'). Also called the *four-card problem*.

Wassermann test A test for the presence of syphilis.

waterfall illusion A motion aftereffect most easily demonstrated by viewing a set of horizontal stripes moving downwards (like a waterfall) for a time. When the objective movement is stopped, the stripes appear to move upwards.

water-jar problem(s) A set of problems involving three jars of varying capacity. In a typical problem subjects are given jars with capacities of 115, 190 and 450 ml and asked how to obtain exactly 30 ml of water. The problems are usually presented as paper-and-pencil tests, although on occasion actual jars are used. They have been extensively used in the study of cognitive SET (2) in problem-solving. Also called *Luchins water-jar problem(s)* for Edith and Abraham Luchins who developed them.

water maze Not really a maze, it is a large vat of milky water with one or more small platforms just below the surface. A rat or other experimental animal is placed in the water and must find a platform to escape. The device is commonly used in studies of spatial learning and memory. Also called the

Morris water maze, after its developer, R. Morris.

Watsonian Referring to the psychological theory and philosophical point of view of the American behaviourist John Broadus Watson (1878–1958). The Watsonian approach was *pure* behaviourism; it was antimentalist to the extreme and regarded such cognitive experiences as thinking and feeling as mere epiphenomena that accompanied peripheral behaviours such as sublaryngeal movements or visceral and muscular responses. It also embodied a strict environmentalism in which genetic factors were assumed to be responsible for few (or none) of the observed differences between individuals. But as the term itself survives in contemporary writing, the strongest connotations are: (a) the advocacy of strictly objective methods in experimentation; and (b) the studied reliance upon only that which is publicly verifiable in attempts to theorize about, explain and predict behaviour. See BEHAVIOURISM.

wave 1 An orderly, periodic motion of particles manifested as a moving crest (as in water or any other liquid). **2** Any periodic vibration, e.g. as in a *sine wave*. **3** Any oscillation, particularly as observed on some recording device, such as an oscilloscope or a polygraph, that reflects some measured activity. See e.g. BRAINWAVES.

wave amplitude A measure of the energy in a wave given as the height of the wave measured from the trough to the crest.

wave frequency The number of complete waves occurring per unit of time. Usually measured in full cycles per second or HERTZ.

wavelength The distance between two equivalent points on adjacent waves. Usually measured as the distance between the crests, but any two points can be used. See COLOUR et seq. for details on the relationships between the wavelength of electromagnetic radiation (light) and vision.

wave of excitation 1 Generally, any neuronal impulse. **2** The propagation of an electrochemical charge along a neuron. **3** The excitatory impulses that travel through the conductile tissue of the ventricles of the heart resulting in the contraction of the chambers.

waxy flexibility CATATONIC WAXY FLEXIBILITY.

WB Scale WECHSLER–BELLEVUE SCALE.

WCST WISCONSIN CARD SORTING TEST.

weak law of effect LAW OF *EFFECT.

weaning The gradual process of accustoming a mammalian offspring to do without its mother's milk (or substitute thereof).

weaning aggression AGGRESSION, WEANING.

weaning, psychological 1 The process of gradually weakening and (one hopes) eventually breaking a child's psychological dependence upon his or her parents. **2** By extension, a client's gradual achievement of psychological independence from his or her psychotherapist; the process of dissolving TRANSFERENCE.

weapon-focus effect The tendency for individuals witnessing a crime like an armed robbery to focus on the weapon. This typically impairs their ability to identify the culprit. See also EYEWITNESS TESTIMONY.

weapons effect The tendency for aggressive behaviour to be increased simply because weapons are present. In a classic study, participants behaved more aggressively toward each other if there were guns and knives in the room than in control conditions in which sporting equipment was present.

Weber–Fechner law Since FECHNER'S LAW is derived from WEBER'S LAW, this combined term is occasionally used to encompass both generalizations. There is also some confusion in the older literature over whose law is called by which name, not a little of it stemming from Fechner himself in his generously referring to what we now call *Fechner's law* as *Weber's law* on the grounds that his general principle was a simple derivation from the law Weber had previously proposed.

Weber's law A psychophysical generalization due to the German physiologist Ernst Heinrich Weber. It states that the JUST-NOTICE-ABLE DIFFERENCES between stimuli are proportional to the magnitude of the original stimulus. Formally, $\Delta I/I = k$, where I is the intensity of the comparison stimulus, ΔI is the increment in intensity just detectable and k is a constant. The law holds reasonably well for the midrange of most stimulus dimensions but tends to break down when very low- or very high-intensity stimuli are used; e.g. for very low-intensity tones the Weber fraction is somewhat larger than it is for moderately loud tones. Note that the ratio is often rendered $\Delta R/R$, where R stands for *Reiz* (German for *stimulus*), as well as $\Delta S/S$, where S stands for *stimulus*. See also FECHNER'S LAW, which is derived from Weber's law.

Wechsler Adult Intelligence Scale (WAIS) One of the most frequently used tests of adult INTELLIGENCE, the WAIS was derived from the earlier WECHSLER–BELLEVUE SCALES and is based upon a series of subtests with two general categories of items: *verbal* and *performance*. Verbal items deal with general information, vocabulary, arithmetic tests, comprehension, similarities, etc.; performance items deal with picture arrangement and completion, block designs, spatial reasoning and the like. The most recent version of the test, published in 1997, is known as the WAIS-III, pronounced as 'wayss-three'.

Wechsler–Bellevue Scale(s) The first of the intelligence tests to separate systematically *verbal* and *performance* abilities. The Wechsler–Bellevue I was published in 1929 and the revised Wechsler–Bellevue II appeared in 1946. In 1955 further extensive revisions were made, and the test is now generally known as the WECHSLER ADULT INTELLIGENCE SCALE (WAIS).

Wechsler Individual Achievement Test (WIAT) An achievement test designed to assess oral expression, listening comprehension, reading, spelling, writing and arithmetic. Norms exist for ages 4 years through adulthood.

Wechsler Intelligence Scale for Children (WISC) An individually administered test of intelligence designed to be used with children ages 6 to 16. Like the WECHSLER ADULT INTELLIGENCE SCALE, from which it was developed, it has both *performance* and *verbal* components. The most recent version of the test, published in 2003, is the WISC-IV, pronounced 'wisk-four'.

Wechsler Memory Scale (WMS) A battery of tests designed to assess learning and memory functions. The scale has been revised several times, the current version is the WMS-III.

It consists of 11 subtests: six of these make up the basic test, the other five are supplemental. While the full battery is used to assess memory function, specific subtests are often used separately, particularly in cases of suspected neurological disorders of memory.

Wechsler Preschool and Primary Scale of Intelligence (WPPSI) An intelligence test designed for use with children aged 2.5 through 7.3 years. The most recent version of the test, published in 2002, is the WPPSI-III, pronounced 'whippsie-three'.

Wechsler scales A general label for the various Wechsler tests of intelligence, each of which is given above. Note that all the Wechsler scales are individually administered tests.

wedge lesion Any LESION that is shaped like a wedge or 'V'. Compare with FOCAL LESIONS, which are more point-like.

we-group IN-GROUP.

weight 1 Generally, the value of the impact of an observation, event or piece of data. The connotation here is of the degree to which a particular observation contributes to some overall conclusion or interpretation when measured against the impact or value of all other observed events or data. This meaning is paralleled in the standard legal language which one speaks of the 'weight of evidence' or of the 'weighing of testimony'. **2** In statistics, a multiplicative factor which adjusts the relative impact of one (or more) selected score(s) upon an overall statistic. For example, in calculating a grand mean from two separate means, each separate mean would be weighted to reflect the size of the sample from which it was calculated. Similarly, in psychological testing, the weight of subtests in a test battery is adjusted to improve overall predictive validity. The values by which each score is multiplied in such cases are called *weight coefficients*. **3** The proportional contribution of each variable in a complex multivariate system to the total variance. See FACTOR LOADING, which reflects essentially the same concept. Also called *nominal weight* (in sense 2) and *effective weight* (in sense 3).

weight coefficient WEIGHT (2).

weighting Determining the WEIGHT (1) of several scores under consideration so as to be able to assign the appropriate WEIGHT (2) to each.

Weigl–Goldstein–Scheerer Test A conceptual sorting task using a number of blocks of different colours and shapes. It has been used to study concept learning and, like the GOLDSTEIN-SCHEERER TESTS, to evaluate the disabilities that accompany various kinds of brain damage.

well-adjusted ADJUSTMENT.

Weltanschauung A German term best translated as *outlook on the world*; thus, one's overall philosophical perspective on all things.

Werner's disease A genetic disorder marked by diminished endocrine activity, stunted growth, premature aging and cognitive decline. Also called *progeria (adultorum)*.

Wernicke–Korsakoff syndrome Most cases of WERNICKE'S SYNDROME and KORSAKOFF'S SYNDROME (see each entry for details of symptoms) are associated with severe alcoholism and are often observed in the same individual, for whom this hybrid term is used. Note, however, that the two syndromes are really different diseases; the former responds well to thiamine, the latter has no known cure.

Wernicke's aphasia APHASIA, WERNICKE'S.

Wernicke's area A loosely circumscribed cortical area in the temporal region of the dominant hemisphere of the brain (i.e. the language hemisphere, which is the left for virtually all right-handed persons and the majority of left-handed persons). From a statistical point of view there is evidence that this general cortical region is involved in the reception and processing of *language*. However, it would be misleading to call it a *language-reception area* as some have done; there are extremely complex interrelationships between this area, the arcuate fasciculus that connects it with Broca's area, the neighbouring regions of auditory cortex and the many interconnections with the frontal lobes. For some sense of the kinds of functions that may be involved here, see APHASIA et seq., especially WERNICKE'S *APHASIA.

Wernicke's encephalopathy WERNICKE'S SYNDROME.

Wernicke's syndrome An acute brain disorder, with eye-movement dysfunctions, ataxia, orientation problems and general mental confusion being the primary symptoms. It is related to severe alcoholism and is, in the classic case, followed by *alcoholic amnestic disorder* (or KORSAKOFF'S SYNDROME), although this sequela can occasionally be prevented by large doses of thiamine. Also called *Wernicke's encephalopathy.*

Werther syndrome Named after the protagonist in Goethe's novel *The Sorrows of Young Werther*, the tendency for young people to attempt to take their own lives following a highly publicized suicide. The phenomenon, also called a CLUSTER SUICIDE, was identified when a rash of young male suicides followed the publication of Goethe's novel, in which the hero takes his own life.

Westermarck effect The tendency for sexually mature individuals to avoid persons with whom they were raised from infancy as sexual partners. First described in 1891 by E. A. Westermarck, it is a form of INBREEDING AVOIDANCE. The phenomenon has been documented in several studies, including one that found that Israelis raised on community farms known as *kibbutzim* often formed deep emotional relationships with those they were brought up with but rarely had sexual relationships with them. See INCEST.

wet dream A dream accompanied by seminal emission. Since such dreams usually occur at night they are also called nocturnal emissions, although this hardly seems an accurate term for the dream itself, more for the result.

wetware Lab slang for the brain and its associated neurological functions. If computers have software and hardware, the brain most surely must have its own internal mechanisms – in short, its wetware.

Wever–Bray effect COCHLEAR MICROPHONIC.

WGTA WISCONSIN GENERAL TEST APPARATUS.

white In vision, the visual sensation experienced when the eye is stimulated by a combination of wavelengths such that none dominates. White represents the extreme pole of the brightness dimension along the white–grey–black continuum. It may be produced by broad-spectrum light, as in normal daylight, or by careful balancing of complementary hues with high intensity. See also WHITE *NOISE for the auditory analogue.

white matter A general term for those parts of the spinal cord and the brain that contain a predominance of myelinated fibres. GREY MATTER reveals the predominance of cell bodies.

white noise NOISE, WHITE.

Whitney extension MANN–WHITNEY U.

Whitten effect LEE–BOOT EFFECT.

whole-learning method Simply, learning material (usually verbal) in its entirety as opposed to one small piece at a time (the so-called *part-learning method*).

whole object In psychoanalysis, an OBJECT that is responded to in a manner that makes it clear that the *whole* is the focus of the response and not any one aspect of it. Compare with PART *OBJECT.

whole-object assumption The assumption that a new word denotes an object and not some part of it. If, on a trip to the zoo, a parent says to a child 'Oh, there's a lemur', the child assumes the word refers to the animal and not to its long, ringed tail. See also MAPPING and OBJECT BIAS.

whole-word method A method of reading instruction in which the focus is on the relationships between particular configurations of letters (i.e. whole words) and their pronunciation. Often called the *look–say method.* Compare with PHONICS METHOD.

wholism HOLISM.

Whorfian hypothesis As put forward by the American linguist Benjamin Lee Whorf, the claim that language influences perception and thought. There are two forms of the hypothesis: a *weak form*, which argues that only perceptions are so influenced (e.g. Inuit, because of the many words in their language for snow, are hypothesized to distinguish variations in the quality of snow that would not be distinguished by a speakers of, say, English); and a *strong form*, which argues that abstract conceptual processes are so affected (e.g. the Hopi Indian language marks time in a relativistic fashion, compared with English's temporal breakdown into past, present and future, leading to the hypothesization that the very conceptualizations of time differ for the speakers of each language). There are some data, particularly from studies with children, that lend support but little that can be called definitive. It is likely that the complex interweaving of culture, social values, language and thought produces a rich representation of one's world knowledge which one's language can stretch or expand as necessary to encompass the perceptions and cognitions needed for effective verbal communication. Also known as the SAPIR–WHORF HYPOTHESIS (see which for reasons).

Wh-question In linguistics, any interrogative based on one of the *wh*- words: *what*, *which*, *where*, *when*, *why*, *who*, *whose* and *(w)how*. Wh-questions are always more information-seeking than YES–NO QUESTIONS.

WHR WAIST-TO-HIP RATIO.

WIAT WECHSLER INDIVIDUAL ACHIEVEMENT TEST.

wide-band procedures A term applied to the more subjective testing and evaluation procedures such as PROJECTIVE TECHNIQUES and INTERVIEWS. It was borrowed from information theory and implies that a broad spectrum of coverage is provided but at the price of relatively poor accuracy and dependability, just as a wide-band receiver gives access to a broad range of wavelengths but with poor selectivity of information.

Wilcoxon test An extension of the SIGN TEST, which evaluates the magnitude of differences as well as their direction in assessing the significance of differences between matched pairs of scores. Also called the *matched-pairs signed-ranks test*.

Wild Boy of Aveyron One of the more famous case studies in psychology. Victor, a *feral child*, was found in the early 1800s near the town of Aveyron, in France. Estimated to be about 7 years old at the time, he was trained and extensively studied by the French physician/educator Jean Marc Gaspard Itard. The growth and development of Victor intellectually, socially and, to a modest extent, verbally was described in loving detail by Itard over a period of many years and had a profound impact on educational theory and practice.

wilfulness A negative reactivity, a tendency

to resist the suggestions of, and/or attempts at manipulation by, others. The term generally carries a negative connotation, thus a wilful person is not viewed as mature and independent.

will 1 Generally, the internal, personal capacity for free determination of choice or action. Usually conceptualized as a conscious function whereby one decides to engage in some behaviours and refrain from others. See also FREE WILL (2). **2** The totality of a person. Sense 1 is somewhat archaic and rarely used in the technical literature these days, although the underlying notion lives on in any number of other terms, e.g. PURPOSE, VOLITION and FREEDOM (1); sense 2 is largely captured by the term SELF.

Williams syndrome A genetic syndrome caused by a missing gene and the surrounding DNA sequence on chromosome 7. Children with the disorder have abnormal calcium chemistry, various cardiac and circulatory defects, short stature, an 'elfinlike' face and mental retardation, which can run from quite mild to moderate. Despite the mental retardation the typical Williams syndrome child has good language ability and is highly social and friendly. Also known as (*infantile*) *hypercalcaemia* (syndrome), *Williams-Barratt syndrome* and *Williams-Beuren syndrome*.

will power A nontechnical term for self-control or the ability to resist temptation.

will to power Adler's term for the desire to dominate others or the striving for superiority over them

windigo A CULTURE-SPECIFIC SYNDROME observed in Algonquin Indians. A hunter imagines he is in the power of a flesh-eating supernatural monster.

win–shift lose–stay strategy The opposite of the WIN–STAY LOSE–SHIFT STRATEGY. The subject shifts to an alternative choice following each correct response but remains with the previous choice when wrong.

win–stay lose–shift strategy A commonly observed strategy in two-alternative choice experiments whereby the subject continues to make the same response when correct (win–stay) but abruptly switches to the other choice when wrong (lose–shift). Compare with WIN–SHIFT LOSE–STAY STRATEGY.

WISC WECHSLER INTELLIGENCE SCALE FOR CHILDREN.

Wisconsin Card Sorting Test (WCST)
Probably the most widely used of the card sorting tests, the WCST consists of a pack of 60 cards on which are printed from one to four circles, crosses, stars or triangles in either red, green, blue or yellow. The subject's task is to sort the cards according to one of three rules: sort by colour (all cards with red objects go together), by shape or by number. The key to the test is that after each run of ten correct responses the rule is changed. When the test was introduced, it was used primarily in detecting neurological lesions in the frontal lobes, since patients with frontal damage tend to perseverate after a rule change. However, performance is often disrupted by lesions in other cortical areas and the WCST is probably best thought of as a test of executive functioning that relies on the integration of function from several cortical regions.

Wisconsin General Test Apparatus (WGTA) A piece of laboratory apparatus designed at the primate research lab at the University of Wisconsin. It houses a single monkey in a cage and has a fairly flexible set of trays and platforms which hold various stimulus items for presentation.

wish 1 Generally, any longing or desire. Some authors use the term to mean either conscious or unconscious desires; others, however, prefer to limit it to one or the other. On some occasions it is used so that it is clear that the wisher makes no overt effort to gain the object(s) of his or her longing, in which case GOAL or AIM is used to refer to those things striven for. **2** The object of such desire.

wish fulfilment 1 In psychoanalysis, a complex process whereby id impulses are satisfied and, as a result, psychic tension is reduced. In the classical Freudian conception (which few adhere to today), dreams and parapraxes are vehicles for the action of wish fulfilment. In dreaming, for example, the primal id fails to distinguish between fantasies, images or hallucinations and reality, so the dreamer may represent as fulfilled in symbolic form wishes that would have otherwise disrupted sleep because of their unacceptability.

wishful thinking Thinking directed by, and along the lines of, one's wishes and desires rather than upon the objective constraints of reality. It is sometimes said that wishful thinking is not logical. This may be true in any given case but it is not a defining feature.

witchcraft The occult practice of sorcery. Beliefs concerning witchcraft and the role of its practitioners are found in many societies and with a wide range of variation. Witches themselves may be evil or *black* at one extreme or beneficent or *white* at the other. There is no doubt that in a culture with the proper deep belief patterns a witch is an extraordinary and powerful person who can cure or maim another: there is also no doubt that occult powers have nothing to do with these capabilities. See FAITH HEALING, PARAPSYCHOLOGY, PLACEBO EFFECT.

witch's milk An archaic term for the milklike secretion occasionally exuded from an infant's breast. It is stimulated by lactating hormone from the mother.

withdrawal 1 A pattern of behaviour characterized by a person removing him- or herself from normal day-to-day functioning and all of its attendant frustrations, tensions and disappointments. In this sense the term refers to a neurotic removal of self from normal social discourse, accompanied by uncooperativeness, irresponsibility and often a reliance on drugs and alcohol to facilitate this social remoteness. **2** A conscious removing of oneself from particular situations. Here the connotation is very different from that of sense l, withdrawal being the result of a calculated decision not to be involved for strategic, philosophical, political or other reasons. **3** In ethology, a pattern of behaviour exhibited by the loser of a battle, who gives a display of SUBMISSION and is allowed to leave the scene unmolested. **4** In psychopharmacology, the cessation of administration of a drug, especially one upon which a patient has developed a dependence. See WITHDRAWAL SYMPTOMS. **5** Eric Fromm's term for a neurotic lack of concern about the world to the point where a person's remoteness has self-destructive results. **6** Any sudden behavioural reaction to a painful or noxious stimulus. It may be mediated by reflex-like mechanisms in which case it will be rapid and stereotyped, such as pulling one's hand back from a hot stove or it may be a consciously modulated response reflecting deliberative features as in withdrawing from a deafeningly loud concert. **7** A method of birth control whereby the penis is removed from the vagina prior to ejaculation. Regular practitioners are known as *parents*.

withdrawal delirium Delirium caused by the WITHDRAWAL (4) of a drug upon which one has built up a severe dependence. See ALCOHOL WITHDRAWAL DELIRIUM and SEDATIVE, HYPNOTIC, OR ANXIOLYTIC WITHDRAWAL DELIRIUM for some specifics.

withdrawal symptoms A general term for any of the effects of the cessation of administration of a substance upon which one has built up a dependence; see DRUG *DEPENDENCE. In older writings this term tends to be used only with respect to drugs with well-known 'addictive' properties, such as the opiates. Contemporary usage reflects the recognition that an array of post-administration effects occurs with many substances and the particular withdrawal symptoms under consideration are classified and keyed to the substance or class of substances upon which the dependence has developed. See e.g. ALCOHOL WITHDRAWAL, SEDATIVE, HYPNOTIC OR ANXIOLYTIC WITHDRAWAL, NICOTINE WITHDRAWAL. See also TOLERANCE.

withdrawal syndrome, prolonged A syndrome in which the WITHDRAWAL SYMPTOMS associated with a drug continue for an extended period of time. See also TOLERANCE.

within-group variance VARIANCE, WITHIN-GROUP.

within-subjects design An experimental design in which each subject is used in all conditions. Compare with BETWEEN-SUBJECTS DESIGN.

Wittmaak-Ekbom syndrome RESTLESS LEG SYNDROME.

Witzelsucht From the German for 'uncontrolled joking', episodes of unrestrained and inappropriate punning, joking or telling of pointless stories, often accompanied by groundless levity, euphoria and laughter. It is thought to be due to frontal lobe lesions that disrupt inhibitory pathways. The term is used for pathological cases and not the alcohol-induced levity observed in pubs and bars.

WM WORKING *MEMORY.

WMS WECHSLER MEMORY SCALE.

wolf child FERAL CHILD.

Wolffian ducts The structures in the embryo that develop into the male internal sex organs.

wolf-man The sobriquet of one of Freud's more famous patients, a man whose dominant symptom was a recurring dream involving a marked fear of wolves. He was a Russian nobleman whom Freud analysed intensely and from whom he gathered much of his 'evidence' for childhood sexuality and the *Oedipus complex*.

womb envy An envy on the part of men for the reproductive capacity of women. Proposed by Karen Horney, some regard it as a serious psychoanalytic principle; others think that Horney (known for having a rich sense of humour) presented it as an unsubtle criticism of Freud's PENIS ENVY.

word The minimum free linguistic form. That is, the smallest (minimum) unit (form) in a language (linguistic) that can stand alone (free) in a written or spoken format. Oddly, while every literate person seems to understand implicitly what a word is, linguists have found it to be a rather slippery concept. The above definition, for example, is incomplete: Is 'um' a word? Is a cough? Are acronyms? What is a word in sign language? etc. Note also that MEANING is not part of this definition.

word association test An ASSOCIATION TEST using words. Francis Galton developed the first of such tests in the late 1800s to study individual differences in thinking. The procedure was adapted for clinical settings soon after by Emil Kräpelin and later picked up by psychoanalysts who used it as a PROJECTIVE TECHNIQUE. Its use survives in all three settings.

word blindness ALEXIA.

word-building test A variation on an ANAGRAM task in which the subject is asked to construct as many words as possible from a given letter set.

word-completion task STEM-COMPLETION TASK.

word configuration The overall shape of a word, its length, location of ascending and descending letters, placement of capital letters, etc. It is an important cue in the WHOLE-WORD METHOD of reading instruction.

word count A general term for any systematic assessment of the frequency of occurrence of words in written and/or spoken language. Often such counts are restricted to specific linguistic domains, e.g. first-year primers, parent–child interactions. However, several estimates of a full word count of a whole language have been made. Such counts are extremely useful research tools since they provide estimates of the familiarity which an average subject can be expected to have with the words used in a particular experiment. See e.g. THORNDIKE–LORGE LIST.

word deafness AUDITORY *APHASIA.

word-form dyslexia DYSLEXIA, WORD-FORM.

word–nonword task LEXICAL-DECISION TASK.

word salad An abnormal pattern of speaking in which the words seem as though they have been tossed randomly like a salad so that they come out in a discoordinated and uninterpretable jumble. It is seen occasionally in some forms of schizophrenia and JARGON *APHASIA.

word sentence HOLOPHRASE.

word stem-completion task STEM-COMPLETION TASK.

word-superiority effect (WSE) A phenomenon of letter recognition. A letter can be identified at a lower threshold and responded to more rapidly when it is part of a familiar word than if it is presented in isolation; e.g. the *d* in *dog* is recognized more readily than a *d* presented alone. First reported by J. McKeen Cattell in the 1880s, the effect is one of several CONFIGURATION SUPERIORITY EFFECTS.

working Assumed or used temporarily for the purpose of making further analyses, e.g. a *working mean* (see here ASSUMED *MEAN) or WORKING HYPOTHESIS.

working hypothesis An educated guess, a hypothesis about some issue that serves as the basis for further research until enough is learned about the phenomena to state a more formal hypothesis.

working mean ASSUMED *MEAN.

working memory MEMORY, WORKING.

working through A general term often used as characterizing the process of obtaining insight into one's problems during therapy.

work psychology A term preferred by many European psychologists to INDUSTRIAL/ORGANIZATIONAL PSYCHOLOGY.

work sample Quite literally, a sample of work taken as representative of the work of an individual.

work-up The process of obtaining as much data as possible for diagnosing a disease or a psychological disorder.

world hypothesis Steven Pepper's term for a global, philosophical point of view toward theory, science, methodology, etc. In some important respects a world hypothesis is similar to Kuhn's notion of a PARADIGM (4).

worry An unpleasant stream of negative cognitions that distract one from dealing with more painful tasks, images and emotions. It is hypothesized to be one of the two primary components of ANXIETY (1), the other component being *emotionality*.

wound 1 In medicine, any break or disruption in the integrity of tissue caused by physical trauma or violence. **2** By extension, in clinical psychology, a rent in the psychological fabric of a person caused by emotional trauma or violence.

WPPSI WECHSLER PRESCHOOL AND PRIMARY SCALE OF INTELLIGENCE.

write As part of the accelerating spillover of terms from the computer sciences this term is used as a synonym of *remember*. That is, *to remember* is often phrased *to write into memory*.

writer's cramp A spasm of the muscles used in writing.

writing disorder EXPRESSIVE WRITING DISORDER, DEVELOPMENTAL.

writing therapy Quite like it says, the use of writing in therapy. Benefits seem to result from desensitization to the anxiety-producing images and thoughts that are expressed.

WSE WORD-SUPERIORITY EFFECT.

Würzburg school A group of researchers at Würzburg University, led by Oswald Külpe, working around the turn of the last century. Although they were *introspectionists* they extended their scope of research beyond that of the Titchenerian form of STRUCTURALISM (1) and focused on the so-called higher mental processes of thinking, problem-solving, cognitive set and the like. See also IMAGELESS THOUGHT, SET (esp. 2) and related entries.

X

X 1 Any given raw score. **2** Any given value of an independent variable.

X̄ The arithmetic mean of a set of scores.

x A deviation from the mean of the *x*-variable.

Xanax Trade name for ALPRAZOLAM.

xantho- Combining form meaning *yellow.*

xanthocyanopia A form of colour blindness in which blues and yellows are distinguished but reds and greens are not. var., *xanthocyanopsia.*

xanthopsia Characterizing vision in which the sensitivity to yellow is heightened and everything has a yellowish tinge. It occurs as a visual defect in some individuals but can be artificially induced by adapting the eye with blue light. Also called *yellow-sighted.*

xanthopsin Visual yellow, a visual pigment produced when RHODOPSIN is bleached by light.

x-axis AXIS.

X chromosome CHROMOSOME.

x coordinate AXIS.

xeno- Combining form from the Greek for *strange* or *foreign.* var., *zeno-.*

xenogenous Pertaining to that which is caused by a foreign body.

xenoglossophilia A tendency to use unnecessary words which are strange, unusual or have foreign origins. The neologist who coined this term sublimely condemned him- or herself.

xenorexia A pathological condition characterized by the persistent swallowing of nonfood objects. See PICA.

xero- Combining form meaning dry.

XO syndrome TURNER'S SYNDROME.

x value The value of a score on the *x-axis*; see AXIS.

XX In genetics, the shorthand notation for the normal genotypic pattern for a human female in which two sex chromosomes are present; see CHROMOSOME.

XXX syndrome TRIPLE-X SYNDROME.

XXXY syndrome A variant of KLINEFELTER'S SYNDROME.

XXY syndrome KLINEFELTER'S SYNDROME.

XY In genetics, the shorthand notation for the normal genotypic pattern for a human male in which two sex chromosomes are present; see CHROMOSOME.

XYY syndrome A CHROMOSOMAL ANOMALY in which three sex chromosomes are present. Persons with the anomaly are phenotypically male and of above-average height and have normal genital development, but their fertility may be low owing to reduced sperm production. Some years back there was a flurry of studies carried out that seemed to implicate this chromosomal pattern in aggressive and criminally violent behaviour. Careful examination of large numbers of males, however, has failed to support any clear link between the XYY syndrome and aggression.

XYZ system A system of standard primaries taken as mathematical abstractions for a formal specification of colour. Unlike the RGB SYSTEM, in which the COLOUR EQUATION is based on 'real' colours, the XYZ primaries exist only as mathematical expressions.

Y

Y 1 Any given raw score of the *y*-distribution. **2** Any given value of a dependent variable.

y A deviation from the mean of the *y*-variable.

Yates correction A CORRECTION FOR CONTINU-ITY that improves the accuracy of CHI-SQUARE tests.

YAVIS syndrome YAVIS is an acronym for *y*oung, *a*ttractive, *v*erbal, *i*ntelligent, *s*uccess-ful – a half-joking description of the type of client that psychotherapists, in painfully simple terms, prefer to have in therapy. Persons displaying this syndrome make wonderful clients for a variety of reasons, not the least of which is that successful therapy is highly likely.

y-axis AXIS.

Y chromosome CHROMOSOME.

y coordinate AXIS.

yellow The PRIMARY *COLOUR experienced when the normal eye is exposed to light with wavelengths of approximately 575–585 nm, with a 'unique' yellow found, for most observers, at about 580 nm.

yellow-sighted XANTHOPSIA.

yellow spot MACULA LUTEA.

Yerkes–Dodson law The generalization that task difficulty and arousal interact such that on difficult tasks low levels of arousal improve performance relative to high levels, but on easy tasks the reverse is true, with high arousal levels facilitating performance relative to low levels.

Yerkish The artificial language developed by D. Rumbaugh and co-workers for communication with chimpanzees. It consists of a set of arbitrary symbols that stand for words or concepts and some simple grammatical rules for ordering symbols to express meaning. The name derives from the Yerkes laboratory in Georgia, USA, where the work was carried out.

yes–no question Any interrogative that takes either 'yes' or 'no' as the prescribed answer. There are three basic forms for such interrogatives: *auxiliary inversion* ('Did you do that?'), *tag questions* ('You did that, didn't you?') and a *rising-intonation contour* ('You did *that*?').

Y maze A MAZE shaped like a Y with a single approach alley and two arms, one of which the subject must choose.

yoga From the Sanskrit meaning *union*, a Hindu religious system of practices and beliefs the objective of which is the attainment of spiritual union with the Supreme Being. There are a number of distinct branches of yogic practice, some of which emphasize disciplined physical bodily control and others which are more cognitive or mental in orientation. See also MYSTICOTRAN-SCENDENT THERAPY.

yoked control An umbrella term for a number of research techniques all of which share the feature that the experimental and control subjects are linked (i.e. yoked) in some fashion, although only the experimental subjects receive a critical treatment or experience a particular procedure. For example, in a learning study experimental and control subjects both receive reinforcements at the same time but delivery is contingent only on the behaviour of the experimental subjects. Yoked subjects would therefore get the same number of reinforcements but independent of their behaviour. Resist the temptation to spell the term with an *l*.

Young–Helmholtz theory THEORIES OF *COLOUR VISION.

youth-bulge phenomenon The finding that when there is a large proportion of young people in a population (the 'bulge' on a frequency distribution), it is often accompanied by rapid social and political change, increases in the level of political upheaval and rebellion. The exact mechanisms for this link are not completely understood, but likely involve lack of civic knowledge, increased volunteerism, education, mistrust of government and economic factors.

y **value** The value of a score on the *y-axis*; see AXIS.

Z

Z Z-TRANSFORMATION.

z Z-SCORE.

zar A CULTURE-SPECIFIC SYNDROME found in north African and Middle Eastern societies marked by dissociative episodes that include odd behaviours like hitting one's head against a wall, singing, weeping and shouting. The afflicted believe they are possessed by a spirit with whom they feel they have an ongoing, close relationship.

Zeigarnik effect As first described by Bluma Zeigarnik in 1927: unfulfilled tasks are retained better than fulfilled tasks. The term is generally taken today to refer to the tendency of an individual to recall any task at which he or she is interrupted better than a task he or she is permitted to complete. Zeigarnik's original characterization, however, contained an important factor that often goes unmentioned in contemporary usage; specifically, that *fulfilment* is defined in terms of an individual's own sense of satisfaction: it does not equate simply with completion of a task but with satisfactory completion of it in terms of the goals of the person working on it.

Zeitgeber German for *time giver*. In the study of CIRCADIAN RHYTHMS the term is used to refer to whatever particular stimulus configuration provides the neural mechanisms of a particular species with information about temporal cycles. For most mammals, *light* is the *Zeitgeber*.

Zeitgeist German for *spirit of the times*. The term is used in a rather loose metaphysical manner to characterize the rich and varied matrix of ideas, trends, philosophies, economies, social structures, political climate, etc. that make up the tone of a culture during a given era. In historiographical work, the so-called *naturalistic approach* emphasizes the role of the *Zeitgeist* in directing and controlling events and is usually balanced against the so-called *personalistic approach*, which emphasizes the role of particular individuals. See GREAT-MAN THEORY.

Zen Buddhism A meditative school of Buddhism that focuses upon the 'stilling of the mind' with the aim of reaching the enlightened state (*satori*) in which one appreciates the true, mystical, unanalysed nature of things beyond the normal, rational, conscious manner of 'ordinary' knowing. See also MYSTICOTRANSCENDENT THERAPY.

Zener cards A deck of 25 cards used in research on extrasensory perception. Each card in the deck has one of five symbols on it (star, plus sign, wavy lines, circle, square) with each symbol appearing on five cards. Also called *ESP deck* (or *cards*), and *Rhine deck* (or *cards*), the latter after J. B. Rhine, who used the cards extensively in his work in PARAPSYCHOLOGY.

zeno- XENO-.

Zeno's paradoxes A set of four paradoxes of motion proposed by Zeno of Elea. One involves Achilles trying to catch a tortoise whose top speed is but one-tenth of his but who has an N metre head-start. By the time Achilles reaches the tortoise's start point the animal is N/10 metres ahead. When Achilles reaches that spot, the tortoise is now N/100 metres ahead, and so on. Hence, he can never catch the tortoise. Since mathematically we know that an infinite series can have a finite sum, the paradox is easily resolved and similar solutions exist for the others. However, they threw early Greek philosophy into a full intellectual crisis and have proved to be interesting platforms for examining human problem-solving.

zero, absolute The true zero point on any dimension; the point at which nothing of the variable under examination exists. The establishment of an absolute zero for a given variable is what permits measurement of that variable on a RATIO *SCALE rather than on an INTERVAL *SCALE. The classic example of this is the measurement of temperature. The establishment of an absolute zero at which all molecular action stops yielded the Kelvin scale, in contrast to the Fahrenheit and Celsius scales, on both of which the zero point is arbitrary.

zero-order Referring to ordinary correlation coefficients, i.e. coefficients calculated from the original data where none of the variables has been held constant, as is the case with PARTIAL *CORRELATIONS.

zero population growth (ZPG) The demographic condition in which the number of deaths in a population approximates the number of viable births, so that the total population remains stable over a period of time.

zero-sum-game GAME, ZERO-SUM.

zeta (ζ) A measure of the degree to which a given regression is linear.

Zipf curve ZIPF'S LAW.

Zipf's law A generalization due to George Kingsley Zipf, an early-20th-century scientist with a penchant for counting things. His law, in simplest terms, states that an equilibrium exists between uniformity and diversity. This notion is best expressed in the so-called *Zipf curve*, which displays the relation between the frequency with which a particular event occurs (e.g. a word in a language) and the number of events which occur with that frequency. When exploring the statistical nature of natural languages, Zipf curves occur with remarkable uniformity of shape; that is, in any language and in any circumscribed corpus of a language (e.g. novels, newspapers, comic books, etc.) there are a very large number of very short words which occur with high frequency and progressively fewer longer words which occur with progressively lower frequency. Zipf hypothesized (wrongly, it turns out)

that these uniformities were the result of a biological 'least effort' principle; they are now known to be merely the necessary result of particular stochastic processes. However, the basic principle codified in Zipf's name – the balance between uniformity and diversity – lives on.

ziprasidone An ATYPICAL ANTIPSYCHOTIC DRUG used to treat SCHIZOPHRENIA and BIPOLAR DISORDER, particularly instances with severe manic phases. It may produce changes in cardiac rhythm and should not be used with patients who have had heart attacks or have cardiac arrhythmias.

Zöllner illusion The vertical lines in the diagram, below, are all parallel.

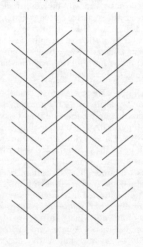

Zöllner illusion

zombie A kind of odd slang term used within the philosophy of mind for a hypothetical entity, a creature which is physically identical to a human being and acts exactly like one but lacks consciousness. Zombies jump and yell 'ouch' if they are shocked, complain about the heat, and act as if they are in love just like we do, but they do it all totally devoid of phenomenal experience. They know no pain, no exhaustion, no passion. The argument is that if such creatures are possible, consciousness cannot be explained in physical, material terms. While many philosophers of mind find this

MENTAL *EXPERIMENT intriguing, most psychologists think it rather silly.

zone of proximal development   An unfortunately cumbersome term introduced by Vygotsky to refer to the conceptual space or zone between what a child is capable of doing on his or her own and what he or she can achieve with assistance from an adult or more capable peer. As the term is used in his SOCIOCULTURAL THEORY, it carries some of the notions of READINESS (2), in that when a child is prepared to begin to undertake a task he or she can, through a process of SCAFFOLDING, be moved to a qualitatively different and functionally more sophisticated level of performance.

zo(o)-   Combining form meaning *animal*.

zooerasty   Sexual intercourse with an animal; see PARAPHILIA.

zoological psychology   See COMPARATIVE PSYCHOLOGY.

zoomorphism   THERIOMORPHISM.

zoophilia   A PARAPHILIA in which the preferred means of sexual arousal and gratification is with animals.

zoosemiotics   SEMIOTICS.

ZPD   ZONE OF PROXIMAL DEVELOPMENT.

z-score   A statistical score which has been standardized by being expressed in terms of its relative position in the full distribution of scores. A z-score is always expressed relative to the mean of the distribution and in standard deviation units, i.e. $z = (X - M)/SD$, where X = the individual score, M = the mean of the set of scores and SD = the standard deviation of the set of scores. Also known as the *standard score* and, in some older writings, the *sigma score*.

Z-transformation   A formula for transforming sample values of r (correlation coefficient) to make them correspond more closely to the normal distribution. Also called *Fisher's Z-transformation*.

Zürich school   A term used to refer collectively to the followers of C. G. Jung; see JUNGIAN for details.

Zwaardemaker olfactometer   A device for regulating the amount of gaseous materials delivered to the nose.

Zwaardemaker smell system   A system for classifying smells. It is based on nine fundamental odours: ethereal (fruits), aromatic (spices), fragrant (flowers), ambrosiac (musk), alliaceous (garlic), empyreumatic (coffee), hircine (rancid), foul (bedbugs) and nauseous (faeces). Compare with HENNING'S PRISM.

zygote   The fertilized cell produced by the union of two gametes; in higher animals the two gametes are a sperm and an ovum.

Appendix A: Simple Phobias

The term *phobia* comes originally from the Greek and to be etymologically correct the term for a specific phobia should use a Greek root; e.g. fear of being alone is properly *eremophobia* and not *autophobia* or *monophobia*, both of which use Latin roots. However, this nicety is not always followed and the following list of **simple phobias** contains many that use Latin, English and French roots. The first part of the list gives definitions of phobias; the second part provides the technical terms for particular fears.

One big problem faced by a lexicographer compiling such a list is what phobias to include. From an etymological perspective, the number of phobias is limited only by the number of nouns in the language, and with a little creativity all manner of phobias can be generated. However, from a clinical point of view the number of objects which are the focus of documented phobias is not all that large; the vast majority of phobic disorders involve relatively few phobic objects and/or situations (see PHOBIA et seq.). In what follows we have tried to include all those phobias to which we have been able to find some reference in the literature. Readers should feel free to generate their own at the slightest impulse; all you need is a Greek or Latin root and the suffix *-phobia*, e.g. *apiphobia* = bees, *aviophobia* = flying, *phasmophobia* = ghosts…

Part I

acarophobia 1 mites. 2 by extension, small insects or animals.

acrophobia heights.

agoraphobia being alone in a public place (see entry in main body of dictionary).

aichmophobia pointed instruments.

ailurophobia cats.

algophobia pain; that is, beyond the normal fear of pain.

amathophobia dust.

amaxophobia vehicles, riding in a vehicle.

androphobia 1 man (i.e. the species *Homo sapiens*). 2 the male sex. Distinguish from HOMOPHOBIA.

anemophobia 1 wind, drafts. 2 by extension, air.

anginophobia 1 generally, suffocation or being suffocated. 2 specifically, an attack of ANGINA (3).

anthrophobia 1 man (singly). 2 society (generally).

aphephobia being touched by another person.

aquaphobia 1 water. 2 by extension, swimming.

arachn(e)ophobia spiders.

astraphobia 1 lightning. 2 thunderstorms.

autophobia oneself, being alone.

bacillophobia bacilli (germs).

ballistophobia 1 missiles. 2 thrown objects.

basiphobia 1 generally, walking. 2 in extreme cases, standing erect and walking.

bathophobia 1 depth. **2** occasionally, looking down from a high place.

belonephobia sharp, pointed objects.

bibliophobia books; also used for an irrational *hatred* of books.

brontophobia thunder. Not used for the mild form commonly found in children.

cainotophobia 1 novelty. **2** new things. **3** new ideas. Also called *cenotophobia*.

cardiophobia heart problems.

catotrophobia 1 generally, mirrors. **2** specifically, breaking of a mirror.

cenotophobia 1 novelty. **2** new things. **3** new ideas. Also called *cainotophobia*.

cherophobia fun, gaiety.

claustrophobia closed spaces.

computerphobia computers, using computers. Also called *cyberphobia*.

coprophobia faeces; by extension, dirt, filth, contamination.

cyberphobia computers, using computers. Also called *computerphobia*.

cynophobia dogs.

cypridophobia 1 venereal disease. **2** sexual activity in general.

demophobia crowds.

dysmorphophobia imagined defects in appearance. However, see BODY DYSMORPHIC DISORDER.

enissophobia criticism.

epistemophobia knowledge.

eremophobia solitude, being alone.

ereuthrophobia blushing.

ergasiophobia 1 work. **2** by extension, responsibility. Also spelled *ergophobia*.

ergophobia 1 work. **2** by extension, responsibility. Also spelled *ergasiophobia*.

erotophobia sex.

erythrophobia 1 red objects. **2** by extension, blushing.

febriphobia 1 fever. **2** a generalized fear of body dysfunction produced by a rise in body temperature.

gamophobia marriage.

gatophobia cats.

geumaphobia tastes.

haematophobia 1 the sight of blood (preferred). **2** blood. Also called *haemophobia*.

haemophobia 1 the sight of blood (preferred). **2** blood. Also called *haematophobia*.

haphephobia being touched by another person.

heliophobia 1 the sun. **2** sunlight.

hierophobia 1 religion. **2** sacred objects associated with religion. **3** religious rites.

homophobia 1 when from the Latin root, man (i.e. the species *Homo sapiens*); a synonym of *androphobia*. **2** when from the Greek root, homosexuality.

hyalophobia glass.

hydrophobia 1 water. **2** Note, *hydrophobia* is also another name for rabies, the disease itself, not fear of it. See HYDROPHOBIAPHOBIA.

hydrophobiaphobia contracting the disease rabies. See HYDROPHOBIA.

hypertrichophobia growth of bodily hair, particularly excessive amounts.

hypnophobia falling asleep.

iophobia 1 being poisoned. **2** rusty objects.

kainophobia new things, new experiences, new situations.

kenophobia empty spaces.

keraunophobia 1 lightning. **2** by extension, thunder.

kopophobia becoming fatigued or exhausted.

lalophobia 1 generally, speaking. **2** specifically, stammering or committing errors while speaking.

levophobia things being on the left side of one's body.

macrophobia large objects.

microphobia small objects.

monophobia being left alone.

mysophobia 1 dirt. 2 contamination.

necrophobia 1 generally, death. 2 more specifically, dead things. 3 most specifically, human corpses.

neophobia 1 the new, the novel. 2 specifically, new foods. See DIETARY NEOPHOBIA.

nosophobia 1 illness. 2 acquiring some specific illness.

nyctophobia 1 night. 2 the dark, darkness. Not used for the common condition in children.

ochlophobia crowds, crowded places.

odontophobia 1 teeth. 2 having one's teeth worked on by a dentist.

ombrophobia rainstorms.

onomatophobia a particular word or name.

ophidiophobia snakes.

pan(t)ophobia everything! (A most unpleasant disorder.)

parturiphobia childbirth.

peccatophobia committing a sin.

phobophobia 1 fear. 2 acquiring a phobia.

phonophobia 1 generally, sound. 2 specifically, the sound of one's own voice.

ponophobia 1 pain. 2 work, being overworked.

pyrophobia fire.

rhypophobia 1 defecation – the process. 2 defecation – the product.

scopophobia being seen by others.

scotophobia the dark, darkness. Not used for the common condition in children.

stasibasiphobia standing erect and walking.

stasiphobia standing.

symbolophobia 1 symbols. 2 symbolic representations. It has been suggested, rather unkindly, that this disorder is caused mainly by long-term psychoanalysis.

taphophobia 1 graves. 2 being buried alive. var., *taphephobia*.

thalassophobia the sea.

thanatophobia 1 death. 2 dead things, especially human corpses.

theophobia 1 God. 2 retribution from God for one's sins (real or imagined).

toxophobia 1 poisons. 2 being poisoned.

tremophobia trembling.

trichopathophobia in women, facial hair. See TRICHOPHOBIA.

trichophobia generally, hair.

triskaidekaphobia The number that results from the operation of subtracting 1 from 14.

xenoglossophobia 1 foreign languages. 2 learning a foreign language.

xenophobia 1 generally, foreigners or strangers. 2 specifically, strange or foreign cultures or places.

zoophobia animals.

Part II

air anemophobia.

alone (being alone) autophobia, eremophobia or monophobia.

alone in a public place agoraphobia.

angina (or **an angina attack**) anginophobia.

animals zoophobia.

blood (or **sight of**) haematophobia or haemophobia.

blushing ereuthrophobia or erythrophobia (see also RED).

books bibliophobia.

bugs acarophobia.

buried alive taphophobia.

cats ailurophobia or gatophobia.

childbirth parturiphobia.

closed spaces claustrophobia.

computers computerphobia or cyberphobia.

contamination coprophobia or mysophobia.

corpses (especially human) necrophobia or thanatophobia.

criticism enissophobia.

crowds demophobia or ochlophobia.

darkness nyctophobia or scotophobia.

death (generally), dead things necrophobia or thanatophobia.

defecation (and its products) rhypophobia.

depth bathophobia.

dirt coprophobia or mysophobia.

dogs cynophobia.

drafts anemophobia.

dust amathophobia.

empty spaces kenophobia.

erotica (sexuality) erotophobia.

everything panophobia or pantophobia.

exhaustion (becoming exhausted) kopophobia.

faeces coprophobia.

fatigue (becoming fatigued) kopophobia.

fear phobophobia.

fever febriphobia.

filth coprophobia or mysophobia.

fire pyrophobia.

foreigners xenophobia.

foreign languages (or learning one) xenoglossophobia.

fun cherophobia.

germs bacillophobia.

glass hyalophobia.

God theophobia.

graves taphophobia.

hair (generally) trichophobia.

hair (excess amounts of bodily) hypertrichophobia.

hair (facial – in women) trichopathophobia.

heart problems cardiophobia (see also ANGINA).

heights acrophobia.

homosexuality (or homosexual persons) homophobia.

illness (or acquiring a specific illness) nosophobia.

knowledge epistemophobia.

large objects macrophobia.

left side (things being on the) levophobia.

lightning astraphobia or keraunophobia.

males, the male sex androphobia.

man (the species) androphobia, anthrophobia or homophobia.

marriage gamophobia.

mirrors, breaking a mirror catotrophobia.

missiles ballistophobia.

mites acarophobia.

name (a particular) onomatophobia.

night nyctophobia.

novel foods neophobia (SEE DIETARY NEOPHOBIA).

novelty, new things cainotophobia, cenotophobia, kainophobia or neophobia.

oneself autophobia.

pain algophobia or ponophobia.

phobia (acquiring one) phobophobia.

pointed instruments aichmophobia or belonephobia.

poison (being poisoned) iophobia or toxophobia.

public places agoraphobia.

rabies (catching the disease) hydrophobiaphobia.

rain, rainstorms ombrophobia.

red (objects) erythrophobia.

religion hierophobia.

responsibility ergasiophobia or ergophobia.

retribution from God theophobia.

riding in a vehicle amaxophobia.

rusty objects iophobia.

sacred (religious) objects hierophobia.

sea thalassophobia.

seen (by others) scopophobia.

sex erotophobia.

sexual activity in general cypridophobia.

sharp pointed instruments belonephobia.

sin (committing one) peccatophobia.

sleep (falling asleep) hypnophobia.

small objects microphobia.

snakes ophidiophobia.

spaces (empty) kenophobia.

speaking (committing errors while) lalophobia.

society (generally) anthrophobia.

solitude autophobia or eremophobia.

sound phonophobia.

sound of one's own voice phonophobia.

spiders arachn(e)ophobia.

standing stasiphobia.

standing erect and walking stasibasiphobia.

strangers (strange cultures or places) xenophobia.

sun, sunlight heliophobia.

swimming aquaphobia.

symbols symbolophobia.

tastes geumaphobia.

teeth (having one's teeth worked on) odontophobia.

thirteen (the number) triskaidekaphobia.

thrown objects ballistophobia.

thunder, thunderstorms astraphobia, brontophobia or keraunophobia.

touched by another person aphephobia or haphephobia.

trembling tremophobia.

vehicles amaxophobia.

venereal disease cypridophobia.

voice (one's own) phonophobia.

walking basiphobia.

water aquaphobia or hydrophobia.

wind anemophobia.

word (a particular) onomatophobia.

work (being overworked) ponophobia.

work (responsibility) ergasiophobia.

working ergophobia.

Appendix B: Authorities Cited

An asterisk (*) before a name indicates that there is a separate entry on that person under an adjectival-form entry, e.g. *Adler = Adlerian, *Watson = Watsonian.

Abney, William de Wiveleslie (1843–1920), English chemist and physiologist.
*Adler, Alfred (1870–1937), Austrian psychiatrist.
Ainsworth, Mary (1913–99), Canadian-born American developmental psychologist.
Allais, Maurice (b. 1911), French economist, physicist.
Allport, Floyd (1890–1978), American psychologist.
Allport, Gordon Willard (1897–1967), American psychologist.
Alzheimer, Alois (1864–1915), German physician and neurologist.
Ames, Adelbert Jr (1880–1955), American artist and educator.
Anderson, John Robert (b. 1947), Canadian-born American cognitive psychologist.
Anderson, Rose Gustava (1893–?), American psychologist.
Angell, James Rowland (1869–1949), American psychologist and educator.
Angelman, Harry (1915–96), English physician.
Anton, Gabriel (1858–1937), Austrian neurologist.
Apgar, Virginia (1909–74), American physician, anaesthesiologist.
Arago, Dominique (1786–1853), French physician.
Argyll-Robertson, Douglas M. C. L. (1837–1909), Scottish physician, ophthalmologist.
Arieti, Silvano (1914–82), Italian-born American psychiatrist.
*Aristotle (384–322 BC), Greek philosopher and educator.
Asch, Solomon E. (1907–96), Polish-born American psychologist.
Asperger, Hans (1906–80), Austrian psychiatrist.
Atkinson, John William (1923–2003), American social psychologist.
Aubert, Hermann (1826–92), German physician and psychologist.
Augustine, St (354–430), African-born philosopher and theologian.
Austin, John Langshaw (1911–60), English philosopher.
Babinski, Joseph F. F. (1857–1932), French neurologist.
Babkin, Boris Petrovich (1877–1950), Russian-Canadian neurologist.
Bach-y-Rita, Paul (1934–2006), American physician.
Baddeley, Alan D. (b. 1934), British cognitive psychologist.
Bales, Robert Freed (b. 1916), American social psychologist.
Balint, Rudolph (1874–1934), Hungarian neurologist.
Bandura, Albert (b. 1925), Canadian-born American psychologist.
Bárány, Robert (1876–1936), Austrian physician.
Bard, Philip (1898–1977), American psychologist.
Barnum, Phineas T. (1810–91), American showman, entrepreneur, charlatan.
Barr, Murray Llewellyn (1908–95), Canadian anatomist.
Barratt-Boyes, Brian G. (b. 1924), British cardiologist.
Barron, Francis X. (1922–2007), American psychologist.
Bartoshuk, Linda (b. 1938), American physiological psychologist.

Bates, Henry Walter (1825–92), British naturalist.
Bateson, Gregory (1904–80), British/American philosopher and anthropologist.
Bayes, Thomas (1702–61), English mathematician and clergyman.
Bayley, Nancy (1899–1994), American developmental psychologist.
Beck, Aaron Temkin (b. 1921), American psychiatrist.
Becker, Ernst (1925–74), American anthropologist.
Bekhterev, Vladimir M. (1857–1927), Russian physiologist and neurologist.
Bell, Charles (1774–1842), Scottish anatomist.
Bem, Sandra (b. 1944), American psychologist.
Bender, Lauretta (1897–1987), American neurologist and psychiatrist.
Benham, C. E. (*fl.* 1890s), English scientist.
Bennett, George Kettner (1904–75), American psychologist.
Berkeley, George, Bishop (1685–1753), Irish philosopher and theologian.
Berne, Eric (1910–70), Canadian-born American psychologist.
Bernheim, Hippolyte Marie (1837–1919), French physician and hypnotist.
Bernoulli, Daniel (1700–1782), Swiss mathematician and physician.
Bernreuter, Robert Gibbon (1901–95), American psychologist.
Bernstein, Basil (1924–2000), British sociologist, linguist.
Bessel, Friedrich W. (1784–1846), German astronomer.
Betz, Vladimir A. (1834–94), Russian anatomist.
Beuren, Alois J. (1919–84), German cardiologist.
Bezold, Johann Friedrich W. (1837–1907), German physicist.
Bidwell, Shelford (1848–1909), English physicist.
Biederman, Irving (b. 1939), American perceptual and cognitive psychologist.
Bierce, Ambrose Gwinnett (1842–1914(?)), American satirist.
Binet, Alfred (1857–1911), French psychologist.
Binswanger, Ludwig (1881–1966), Swiss psychiatrist, existentialist.
Binswanger, Otto (1852–1929), German physician.
Bleuler, Eugen (1857–1939), Swiss psychiatrist.
Bogardus, Emory (1882–1973), American sociologist.
Bonferroni, Carlo Emilio (1892–1960), Italian mathematician.
Boot, L. M. (*fl.* 1950s), Dutch biologist.
Boring, Edwin Garrigues (1886–1968), American psychologist and historian.
Boyer, Pascal (*fl.* 2000s), French-American anthropologist and psychologist.
Braid, James (1795–1860), British writer, coiner of the term *hypnotism.*
Braille, Louis (1809–52), French educator.
Brainerd, Charles (b. 1944), American psychologist.
Bray, Charles William (1904–?), American physician.
Brazelton, Thomas Berry (b. 1918), American physician, paediatrician.
Brentano, Franz (1838–1917), German philosopher, psychologist and theologian.
Breuer, Josef (1842–1925), Austrian physician.
Bridgman, Percy (1882–1961), American physicist and philosopher of science.
Briquet, Pierre (1796–1881), French physician.
Broca, Paul (1824–80), French physiologist and surgeon.
Brodmann, Korbinian (1868–1918), German neurologist.
Bronfenbrenner, Urie (1917–2005), Russian-born American developmental psychologist.
Brown, Roger (1925–97), American psychologist.
Bruce, Hilda Margaret (1903–74), Physiologist.
Brücke, Ernst Wilhelm (1819–92), German physiologist.
Bruner, Jerome Seymour (b. 1915), American developmental psychologist.
Brunswik, Egon (1903–55), Hungarian-born American psychologist.
Bucy, Paul Clancy (1904–92), American neurologist.

Bunsen, Robert Wilhelm (1811–99), German chemist.
Campbell, Donald Thomas (1916–96), American social psychologist.
Cannon, Walter B. (1871–1945), American physiologist.
Capgras, Jean Marie Joseph (1873–1950), French psychiatrist.
Carnap, Rudolph (1891–1970), German-born, Austrian/American philosopher.
Carr, Harvey A. (1873–1954), American psychologist.
Carroll, Lewis (Charles Lutwidge Dodgson, 1832–98), English mathematician, cleric and writer.
Cattell, James McKeen (1860–1944), American psychologist and publisher.
Cattell, Raymond B. (1905–98), British-born American psychologist.
Chalmers, David (b. 1966), Australian philosopher of mind.
Charcot, Jean Martin (1825–93), French physician, neurologist.
Charpentier, Pierre Marie Augustin (1852–1916), French physician.
Cherry, Colin (1914–79), English communications scientist and psychologist.
Chomsky, Avram Noam (b. 1928), American linguist, philosopher and psychologist.
Christie, Richard (1918–92), American social psychologist.
Clérambault, Gaëtan G. de (1872–1934), French physician.
Cohen, Jacob (1923–98), American psychologist and statistician.
Comte, Auguste (1798–1857), French philosopher and sociologist.
Condillac, Étienne Bonnot de (1715–80), French philosopher.
Cooley, Charles Horton (1864–1929), American sociologist.
Coombs, Clyde (1912–88), American psychologist.
Copernicus, Nicolaus (1473–1543), Polish astronomer.
Corti, Alfonso Giacomo Gaspare (1822–76), Italian anatomist.
Cotard, Jules (1840–89), French neurologist.
Coué, Émile (1857–1926), French pharmacist, therapist and phrase-maker.
Crespi, L. P. (*fl.* 1940s), American psychologist.
Creutzfeldt, H. G. (1885–1964), German neurologist.
Cronbach, Lee J. (1916–2001), American psychometrician.
Czikszentmihalyi, Mihalyi (b. 1934), Hungarian-American social cognitive psychologist.
Dalton, John (1766–1844), English chemist.
*Darwin, Charles (1809–82), English naturalist.
Dawkins, Richard (b. 1941), British evolutionary biologist.
Deese, James Earle (1921–99), American psychologist.
Deiters, Otto Friedrich Karl (1834–63), German anatomist.
Delboeuf, Joseph Remi Leopold (1831–96), French psychophysicist.
Dennett, Daniel Clement (b. 1942), American philosopher.
Derrida, Jacques (1930–2004), Algerian/French philosopher.
*Descartes, René (1596–1650), French philosopher and mathematician.
Dewey, John (1859–1952), American philosopher and educator.
Donders, Franciscus Cornelis (1818–89), Dutch physiologist and opthalmologist.
Doppler, Johann Christian (1803–53), Austrian physicist.
Down, John Langdon Haydon (1828–96), English physician.
Drever, James (1873–1951), British psychologist and lexicographer.
Duncan, David Beattie (1916–2006), Australian-born American statistician.
Durkheim, Émile (1858–1917), French sociologist.
Ebbinghaus, Hermann von (1850–1909), German psychologist.
Edwards, Allen L. (1914–94), American psychologist.
Ehrenfels, Christian von (1859–1932), Austrian philosopher and psychologist.
Eich, Eric (*fl.* 2000s), American-Canadian cognitive psychologist.
Ekbom, Karl-Axel (1907–77), Swedish physician
Ekman, Paul (b. 1934), American social and cognitive psychologist.

Ellis, Albert (1913–2007), American psychologist.

Emmert, Emil (1844–1911), Swiss ophthalmologist.

Engels, Friedrich (1820–95), German philosopher.

Erhard, Werner (b. 1935), American salesman.

Erikson, Erik Homburger (1902–94), German-born American psychoanalyst.

Estes, William Kaye (b. 1919), American psychologist.

Euclid (*fl. c.* 300 BC), Greek mathematician.

Ewald, Georg Heinrich August (1803–73), German semanticist.

Ewald, Julius Richard (1855–1921), German physiologist.

Eysenck, Hans Jürgen (1916–94), German-born English psychologist.

Fant, Louis Judson (1931–2001), American educator.

Fechner, Gustav Theodor (1801–87), German physician, physicist, philosopher, psychologist, psychometrician and essayist.

Feigenbaum, Edward A. (b. 1936), American computer scientist.

Feigl, Herbert (1902–88), Austrian-born American philosopher of science.

Féré, Charles S. (1852–1907), French neurologist.

Ferry, Edwin Sidney (1868–1956), American physicist.

Festinger, Leon (1919–89), American psychologist.

Fisher, Ronald Aylmer (1890–1962), English geneticist and statistician.

Fitts, Paul Morris (1912–65), American psychologist.

Flesch, Rudolph F. (1911–86), American philologist and psychologist.

Flynn, James R. (b. 1934), New Zealand moral philosopher.

Fodor, Jerry (b. 1935), American philosopher.

Fourier, Jean Baptiste Joseph (1768–1830), French mathematician.

Frank, Jerome David (1909–2005), American psychiatrist.

Frankl, Viktor (1905–97), Austrian-born American psychiatrist.

Fregoli, Leopold (1867–1936), Italian actor.

Freud, Anna (1895–1982), Austrian-born British psychoanalyst.

*Freud, Sigmund (1856–1939), Austrian neurologist and psychoanalyst.

Frisch, Karl von (1886–1982), Austrian zoologist, ethologist.

Fromm, Erich (1900–1980), German-born American psychoanalyst.

Fromm-Reichmann, Frieda (1889–1957), American psychoanalyst.

Frostig, Marianne B. (1906–85), Austrian-born American psychologist.

Fullerton, George Stuart (1859–1925), American psychologist.

Gabor, Dennis (1900–79), Hungarian-British physicist, born Gábor Dénes.

Galen (129–*c.* 199), Greek physician and philosopher.

Galileo Galilei (1564–1642), Italian astronomer and physicist.

Gall, Franz Joseph (1758–1828), German physician and phrenologist.

Galton, Francis (1822–1911), English natural scientist and psychologist.

Ganser, Sigbert (1853–1931), German psychiatrist.

Garcia, John (b. 1917), American psychologist.

Gardner, Howard (b. 1943), American psychologist.

Gauss, Carl Friedrich (1777–1855), German mathematician.

Geisser, Seymour (1929–2004), American statistician.

Gerstmann, Josef (1887–1961), Austrian neurologist.

Geschwind, Norman (1926–84), American neurologist.

Gesell, Arnold Lucius (1880–1961), American psychologist.

Gibson, James Jerome (1904–80), American psychologist.

Gilbert, Daniel (b. 1957), American social psychologist.

Goddard, Henry Herbert (1866–1957), American psychologist.

Gödel, Kurt (1906–78), Czech-born American mathematician and logician.

Goethe, Johann Wolfgang von (1719–1832). German writer.

Goffman, Erving (1922–82), Canadian-born American sociologist.

Goldenhar, Maurice (1924–2001), Belgian-American physician.

Goldstein, Kurt (1878–1965), German-born American psychologist.

Golgi, Camillo (1843–1926), Italian physiologist, histologist.

Goodenough, Florence Laura (1886–1959), American psychologist.

Goodman, Henry Nelson(1906–98), American philosopher.

Gosset, William Sealy (Student) (1867–1937), British statistician.

Gottschaldt, Kurt Bruno (1902–91), German psychologist.

Gould, Stephen Jay (1941–2002), American zoologist, palaeontologist and essayist.

Grassmann, H. (*fl.* 1850s), German scientist.

Greenberg Jeff (b. 1954). American social psychologist.

Greenhouse, Samuel W. (1918–2000), American statistician.

Greenwald, Anthony G. (b. 1939), American cognitive psychologist.

Greenspoon, Joel (b. 1921), American psychologist.

Gregory, Richard Langton (b. 1923), English psychologist.

Grice, H. Paul (1913–88), British/American philosopher.

Guilford, Joy Paul (1897–1987), American psychologist.

Guthrie, Edwin Ray (1886–1959), American psychologist.

Guttman, Louis (1916–87), American psychologist.

Haab, Otto (1850–1931), Swiss physician, ophthalmologist.

Hall, Granville Stanley (1844–1924), American psychologist.

Hall, Monty (b. 1921), Canadian-born American television game show host.

Halstead, Ward (1908–68), American neuropsychologist.

Harlow, Harry (1905–81), American psychologist.

Hartley, David (1705–57), English physician and philosopher.

Harvey, O. J. (b. 1927), American psychologist.

Head, Henry (1861–1940), English neurologist.

Hebb, Donald Olding (1904–85), Canadian psychologist.

Hegel, Georg Wilhelm Friedrich (1770–1831), German philosopher.

Heider, Fritz (1896–1988), Austrian-born American psychologist.

Helmholtz, Hermann Ludwig Ferdinand von (1821–94), German physiologist, psychologist.

Helson, Harry (1898–1977), American psychologist.

Henning, Hans (1885–1946), German psychologist.

Heraclitus (*c.* 540–*c.* 480 BC), Greek philosopher.

Herbart, Johann Friedrich (1776–1841), German philosopher and educator.

Hering, Heinrich Ewald (1866–1948), German physiologist.

Hering, Karl Ewald Constantin (1834–1918), German physiologist.

Hertz, Heinrich Rudolph (1857–94), German physicist.

Hess, Eckardt H. (1916–86), German-American psychologist.

Heschl, Richard L. (1824–81), Austrian anatomist.

Hick, William Edmund (1912–74), British psychologist.

Hilgard, Ernest R. (1904–2001), American experimental psychologist.

Hippocrates (*c.* 460–*c.* 377 BC), Greek physician.

Hiskey, Marshall S. (1908–98), American psychologist.

Hitch, Graham (*fl.* 1980s–2000s), British cognitive psychologist.

Hobbes, Thomas (1588–1679), English philosopher.

Hobson, Allan (b. 1933), American psychiatrist.

Höffding, Harald (1843–1931), German philosopher, psychologist.

Holland, John L. (b. 1920), American industrial psychologist.

Hollingshead, August B. (?–1975), American sociologist.

Holmgren, Alarik Frithiof (1831–97), Swedish physiologist.

Horn, John Leonard (1928–2006). American psychologist.

Horner, Matina Souretis (b. 1939), American psychologist.
Horney, Karen (1885–1952), German-born American psychiatrist.
Hovland, Carl (1912–61), American psychologist.
Hubel, David (b. 1926), American physiologist.
*Hull, Clark Leonard (1884–1952), American psychologist.
Hume, David (1711–76), Scottish philosopher and historian.
Hunt, Howard Francis (1918–2001), American psychologist.
Hunter, Walter S. (1889–1953), American psychologist.
Huntington, George (1850–1916), American neurologist.
Hurler, Gertrud (1889–1965), Austrian paediatrician.
Husserl, Edmund (1859–1938), German philosopher.
Hyman, Ray (b. 1928), American psychologist.
Ishihara, Shinobu (1879–1963), Japanese ophthalmologist.
Itard, Jean Marc Gaspard (1774–1838), French physician and educator.
Jackson, John Hughlings (1835–1911), English neurologist.
Jacobson, Edmund (1888–1983), American physician.
Jacobson, Ludvig Levin (1835–1911), Dutch physician.
Jacoby, Larry (b. 1944), American cognitive psychologist.
Jakob, A. M. (1884–1931), German neurologist.
*James, William (1842–1910), American psychologist and philosopher.
Janet, Pierre Marie Félix (1859–1947), French physician, psychiatrist.
Johansson, Gunnar (1911–98), Swedish psychologist.
Johnson, Marcia K. (b. 1943), American cognitive psychologist.
Jones, Alfred Ernest (1879–1958), British psychoanalyst, biographer.
Jost, Adolf (1874–1920), German psychologist.
*Jung, Carl Gustav (1875–1961), Swiss psychiatrist, psychoanalyst.
Julesz, Béla (1928–2003), Hungarian-American scientist.
Kahn, Eugen (1887–1973), German psychologist.
Kahneman, Daniel (b. 1934), Israeli–American cognitive psychologist.
Kanner, Leo (1894–1981), Austrian-born American psychiatrist.
Kant, Emanuel (1724–1804), German philosopher.
Kantor, Jacob Robert (1888–1984), American psychologist.
Katz, David (1884–1953), German-born Swedish psychologist.
Katz, Jerrold J. (1932–2002), American philosopher and linguist.
Keller, Frederick Simmons (1899–1996), American psychologist and educator.
Kelley, Harold (1921–2003), American social psychologist.
Kelly, George (1905–66), American psychologist.
Kendall, Maurice George (1907–1983), English statistician.
Kent, Grace Helen (1875–1973), American psychologist.
Kimble, Gregory Adams (1917–2006), American psychologist.
Kinsbourne, Marcel (b. 1931), Austrian-born, British-educated American neuroscientist.
Klein, Melanie (1882–1960), Austrian-British psychoanalyst.
Kleine, Willi (fl. 1920s), German psychiatrist.
Klinefelter, Harry Fitch (b. 1912), American physician, geneticist.
Kleffner, Frank R. (fl. 1950s–1980s), American audiologist and speech pathologist.
Klüver, Heinrich (1898–1979), German-born American neurologist.
Koffka, Kurt (1886–1941), German-born American psychologist.
Kohlberg, Lawrence (1927–87), American psychologist.
Köhler, Wolfgang (1887–1967), German-born American psychologist.
Kohs, Samuel Calmin (1890–1984), American psychologist.
Kolmogorov, Andrei Nikolaevich (1903–1987), Russian mathematician.
König, Karl Rudolph (1832–1901), German-born French physicist.

Korsakoff, Sergei Sergeievich (1854–1900), Russian neurologist.
Korte, A. (*fl.* 1910s), German psychologist.
Kräpelin, Emil (1856–1926), German psychiatrist.
Krause, Wilhelm (1833–1910), German anatomist.
Kretschmer, Ernst (1888–1964), German psychiatrist.
Kruskal, William Henry (1919–2005), American mathematician, statistician.
Kuder, George Frederic (1903–2000), American psychologist.
Kuhlman, Frederick (1876–1941), American psychologist.
Kuhn, Thomas S. (1922–96), American physicist, philosopher of science.
Külpe, Oswald (1862–1915), German psychologist.
Lacan, Jacques-Marie-Émile (1901–81), French psychoanalyst.
Ladd-Franklin, Christine (1847–1930), American mathematician and vision scientist.
Laing, Ronald David (1927–1989), Scottish-born psychiatrist.
Lamarck, Jean-Baptiste Pierre Antoine (1744–1829), French naturalist, evolutionist.
Lamaze, Fernand (1890–1957), French obstetrician.
Lambert, Johann Heinrich (1728–77), German mathematician, astronomer.
Land, Edwin Herbert (1909–91), American sensory psychologist and inventor.
Landau, William M. (b. 1924), American neurologist.
Landolt, Edmund (1846–1926), French ophthalmologist.
Lange, Carl Georg (1834–1900), Danish physiologist.
Lange, Cornelia de (1871–1950), Dutch physician.
Langer, Ellen (b. 1947), American social psychologist.
Lashley, Karl Spencer (1890–1958), American psychologist.
Leboyer, Frédéric (b. 1918), French obstetrician.
Lee, S. van der (*fl.* 1950s), Dutch biologist.
Leibniz, Gottfried Wilhelm von (1646–1716), German philosopher, mathematician.
Leiter, Russell Graydon (b. 1901), American psychologist.
Lesch, M. (b. 1939), American physician.
Levin, Max (b. 1901), Russian-born American neurologist.
Lévi-Strauss, Claude (b. 1908), French anthropologist.
Lewin, Kurt (1890–1947), German-born American psychologist.
Lewontin, Richard (b. 1929), American evolutionary biologist.
Liberman, Alvin Meyer (1917–2000), American psychologist and linguist.
Lifton, Robert Jay (b. 1926), American psychiatrist.
Likert, Rensis (1903–81), American social scientist.
Linehan, Marsha (b. 1943), American clinical and behavioural psychologist.
Lippitt, Ronald (1914–86), American psychologist.
Lissajou, Jules Antoine (1822–80), French physicist.
Lloyd Morgan, Conwy, *see* Morgan, Conwy Lloyd.
Locke, John (1632–1704), British philosopher.
Lombroso, Cesare (1836–1909), Italian criminologist.
Lorenz, Konrad Zacharias (1903–89), Austrian ethologist.
Lorge, Irving Daniel (1905–61), American psychologist.
Lotze, Rudolph Hermann (1817–81), German physiologist and psychologist.
Lovelock, James Ephraim (b. 1919). British physician, scientist and futurist.
Luchins, Abraham S. (1914–2005), American Gestalt psychologist.
Luchins, Edith H. (1922–2002), American mathematician and psychologist.
Luria, Alexander Romanovich (1902–77), Russian psychologist.
Luria, Salvatore Edward (1912–91), Italian-born American biologist.
Mach, Ernst (1838–1916), Austrian physicist and philosopher.
Machiavelli, Niccolò (1469–1527), Florentine statesman and political theorist.
Machover, Karen Alper (1902–96), American psychologist.

MacLean, Paul Donald (1913–2007), American physician.
Magendie, François (1783–1855), French physiologist.
Maharishi Mahesh Yogi (1917–2008), Indian mystic.
Maier, Norman R. F. (1900–1987), American psychologist.
Malthus, Thomas Robert (1766–1834), English economist and demographer.
Mandler, George (b. 1924), Austrian-born American cognitive psychologist.
Mann, Henry Berthold (1905–2000), Austrian-born American mathematician.
Marbe, Karl (1869–1953), German psychologist.
Marfan, Antoine Bernard Jean (1858–1942), French physician.
Markov, Andrei Andreievich (1856–1922), Russian mathematician.
Marx, Karl (1818–83), German social philosopher.
Maslow, Abraham Harold (1908–70), American psychologist.
Masoch, *see* Sacher-Masoch
Maxwell, James Clerk (1831–79), Scottish physicist.
May, Rollo (1909–94), American psychoanalyst, existentialist.
McCarthy, Dorothea (1906–74), American developmental psychologist.
McClelland, David (1917–98), American psychologist.
McClintock, Martha (*fl.* 1970s–2000s), American psychologist.
McCollough, Celeste (b. 1926), American psychologist.
McConnell, James Vernon (1925–90), American psychologist.
McDermott, Kathleen (b. 1968), American cognitive psychologist.
McDougall, William (1871–1938), British-born American psychologist.
McGurk, Harry (1936–98), British psychologist.
McNeill, David (b. 1933), American cognitive psychologist.
McNemar, Quinn (1900–1986), American psychologist and statistician.
Mead, George Herbert (1863–1931), American social philosopher.
Mead, Margaret (1901–78), American anthropologist.
Meehl, Paul Everett (1920–2003), American psychologist and philosopher.
Meissner, Georg (1829–1905), German physiologist and anatomist.
*Mendel, Gregor Johann (1822–84), Austrian monk and geneticist.
Ménière, Prosper (1799–1862), French physician.
Merkel, Friedrich Siegmund (1845–1919), German anatomist.
Merrill (James), Maud Amanda (1888–1978), American psychologist.
Merton, Robert King (Meyer R. Schkolnick) (1910–2003), American sociologist.
Mesmer, Franz Anton (1733–1815), German physician and hypnotist.
Meyer, Adolf (1866–1950), Swiss-born American psychiatrist.
Meyer, Max F. (1873–1967), American psychologist.
Mill, James (1773–1836), Scottish philosopher.
Mill, John Stuart (1806–73), English philosopher and economist.
Miller, George Armitage (b. 1920), American cognitive psychologist.
Miller, Wilfred Stanton (1883–?), American psychologist.
Mills, C. Wright (1916–62), American sociologist.
Minsky, Marvin Lee (b. 1927), American computer scientist and philosopher.
Mischel, Walter (b. 1930), American psychologist.
Molyneux, William (1656–98), Irish lawyer, politician and philosopher.
Moniz, Antonio Egas (1874–1955), Portuguese neurosurgeon.
Mooney, Craig M. (*fl.* 1950s), American cognitive psychologist.
More, Thomas (1477–1535), English lawyer, writer, saint.
Moreno, Jacob L. (1890–1974), Austrian-born American psychiatrist.
Morgan, Conwy Lloyd (1852–1936), English zoologist and psychologist.
Moro, Ernst (1874–1951), Austrian paediatrician.
Morris, Robert G. M. (*fl.* 1980s), British neuroscientist.

Morton, John (b. 1933), English cognitive psychologist.

Mowrer, Orval Hobart (1907–82), American psychologist.

Müller, Georg Elias (1850–1934), German psychologist.

Müller, Johannes Peter (1801–58), German physiologist.

Müller, Johann Friedrich Theodor (1822–97), German zoologist.

Müller-Lyer, Franz Karl (1857–1916), German psychiatrist and psychologist.

Munsell, Albert Henry (1858–1918), American artist.

Münchausen (or Münchhausen), Karl Friedrich Hieronymus von (1720–97), German soldier and fabulist.

Murphy, Gardner (1895–1979), American psychologist.

Murray, Henry Alexander (1893–1988), American psychologist.

Necker, Louis (1730–1804), Swiss mathematician and physicist.

Neill, Alexander Sutherland (1883–1973), British educator.

Neisser, Ulric Richard Gustav (b. 1928), American cognitive psychologist.

Newell, Allen (1927–92), American cognitive psychologist and computer scientist.

Newport, Elissa (b. 1947), American developmental psychologist.

Newton, Isaac (1642–1727), English physicist, mathematician, philosopher.

Nissl, Franz (1860–1919), German neurologist.

Nyhan, W. L. (b. 1926), American physician.

Ockham (Occam), William of (c. 1280–1349), English philosopher.

Oden, Gregg (b. 1948), American cognitive psychologist.

Ohm, Georg Simon (1787–1854), German physicist.

Olds, James (1922–79), American physiological psychologist.

Orbison, W. Dillard (1911–52), American psychologist.

Ornstein, Robert E. (b. 1942), American psychologist.

Osgood, Charles Egerton (1916–91), American psychologist.

Osten, Wilhelm von (fl. 1900s), German teacher and animal trainer.

Ostwald, Wilhelm (1853–1932), German physicist, chemist.

Pacini, Filippo (1812–83), Italian anatomist.

Paivio, Allan U. (b. 1925), Canadian cognitive psychologist.

Panum, Peter Ludwig (1820–85), Danish physiologist.

Pappenheim, Bertha (1859–1936), Austrian social worker.

Papez, James Wenceslas (1883–1958), American anatomist, physiologist.

Pareto, Vilfredo Frederico Domaso (1848–1923), Italian sociologist and economist.

Parkinson, James (1755–1824), English physician.

*Pavlov, Ivan Petrovich (1849–1936), Russian physiologist.

Peale, Norman Vincent (1898–1993), American preacher.

Pearson, Karl (1857–1936), English statistician.

Peckham, Elizabeth Maria Gifford (1854–1950), American naturalist.

Peckham, George William (1845–1914), American naturalist.

Peirce, Charles Sanders (1839–1914), American philosopher.

Pepper, Steven (1891–1972), American philosopher.

Perky, Cheves West (1874–1940), American psychologist.

Perls, Frederick (Fritz) S. (1893–1970), German-born American psychiatrist.

Peter, Lawrence J. (1919–90), Canadian-American educator.

Pfungst, Oskar (1874–1933), German psychologist.

*Piaget, Jean (1896–1980), Swiss psychologist.

Pick, Arnold (1851–1924), Prague psychiatrist.

Pinel, Philippe (1745–1826), French physician, psychiatrist.

Piper, Hans Edmund (1877–1915), German physiologist.

Pitres, Jean Albert (1848–1927), French neurologist.

Plateau, Joseph Antoine Ferdinand (1801–83), Belgian physicist.

Plato (*c.* 427–*c.* 347 BC), Greek philosopher.

Poetzl, Otto (1877–1962), Austrian psychiatrist.

Poggendorff, Johann Christian (1796–1877), German physicist.

Poisson, Siméon Denis (1781–1840), French mathematician.

Polanyi, Michael (1891–1976), Hungarian/British scientist and philosopher.

Popper, Karl Raimund (1902–94), Austrian-born English philosopher.

Porter, Eleanor Hodgman (1868–1920), American novelist.

Porter, Thomas Cunningham (1860–1933), English scientist.

Porteus, Stanley David (1883–1972), Australian-born American psychologist.

Prader, Andrea (b. 1919), Swiss paediatrician.

Premack, David (b. 1925), American psychologist.

Pribram, Karl Harry (b. 1919), Austrian-born American physician, psychologist.

Prince, Morton (1854–1929), American psychiatrist, psychologist.

Proust, Marcel (1871–1922), French novelist.

Pulfrich, Karl P. (1858–1927), German physicist.

Purkinje (Purkyně), Jan Evangelista (1787–1869), Czech physiologist.

Pylyshyn, Zenon (b. 1941), Canadian/American psychologist.

Pyszczynski, Thomas (b. 1954), American social psychologist.

Quételet, Adolphe (1796–1874), Belgian astronomer and mathematician.

Rank, Otto (1884–1939), Austrian psychoanalyst.

Ranvier, Louis Antoine (1835–1922), French physiologist.

Raven, John C. (1902–70), British psychologist.

Rayleigh, John William Stuart (1842–1919), English mathematician, physiologist.

Reber, Arthur Samuel (b. 1940), American cognitive psychologist and lexicographer.

Reich, Wilhelm (1897–1957), Austrian-born American psychoanalyst.

Reichenbach, Hans (1891–1953), German-born American philosopher.

Reid, Thomas (1710–96), Scottish philosopher.

Reik, Theodor (1888–1970), Austrian-born American psychoanalyst.

Reil, Johann Christian (1759–1813), German physician.

Reissner, Ernst (1824–78), German anatomist.

Renshaw, Birdsay (1911–48), American physiologist.

Rescorla, Robert (b. 1940), American experimental psychologist.

Restorff, Hedwig von (1906–62), German psychologist.

Rett, Andreas (1924–97), Austrian neurologist.

Rey, André (1906–65), Swiss psychologist.

Reyna, Valerie Frances (b. 1955), American psychologist.

Reynolds, George Stanley (b. 1936), American psychologist.

Rhine, Joseph Banks (1895–1980), American botanist and parapsychologist.

Ribot, Théodule A. (1839–1916), French psychologist.

Ricco, Annibale (1844–1919), Italian astronomer.

Richardson, Marion Webster (1896–1965), American psychologist.

Riesman, David (1909–2002), American sociologist.

Ringelmann, Max (1861–1931), French agricultural engineer.

Robin, Pierre (1867–1950), French dental surgeon.

Robinson, Edward Stevens (1893–1937), American psychologist.

Rock, Irvin (1922–95), American psychologist.

Roediger III, Henry L. (b. 1947), American cognitive psychologist.

Rogers, Carl (1902–87), American psychologist.

Rolando, Luigi (1773–1831), Italian anatomist.

Rolf, Ida Pauline (1896–1979), American biochemist.

Romberg, Moritz Heinrich von (1795–1873), German neurologist.

Rorschach, Hermann (1884–1922), Swiss psychiatrist.

Rosanoff, Aaron Joshua (1878–1943), American psychologist.
Roscoe, Henry Enfield (1833–1915), English chemist.
Rosenthal, Robert (b. 1933), American psychologist.
Rosenzweig, Saul (1907–2004), American psychologist.
Rotter, Julian Bernard (b. 1916), American psychologist.
Rozin, Paul (b. 1936), American cognitive and physiological psychologist.
Rubin, Edgar J. (1886–1951), Danish philosopher.
Rubin, Zick (1944–97), American social psychologist.
Ruffini, Angelo (1864–1929), Italian anatomist.
Rumbaugh, Duane (b. 1929), American psychologist.
Rush, Benjamin (1745–1813), American physician and diplomat.
Russell, Bertrand Arthur William (1872–1970), British philosopher, mathematician.
Rycroft, Charles (1914–1988), British psychoanalyst and lexicographer.
Ryle, Gilbert (1900–1976), British philosopher.
Sacher-Masoch, Leopold von (1836–95), Austrian lawyer and writer.
Sachs, Bernard Parney (1858–1944), American neurologist.
Sade, Donatien Alphonse François de (1740–1814), French essayist, novelist, revolutionary.
Sanson, Louis Joseph (1790–1841), French surgeon.
Sapir, Edward (1884–1939), American linguist.
Saussure, Ferdinand de (1857–1913), Swiss linguist.
Schachter, Stanley (1922–97), American psychologist.
Schacter, Daniel (b. 1952), American neurocognitive psychologist.
Schank, Roger (b. 1946), American linguist, cognitive scientist.
Scheerer, Martin (1900–1961), German-born American psychologist.
Scheffé, Henry (1907–77), American mathematician.
Schmeidler, Gertrude Ruffel (b. 1912), American parapsychologist.
Schooler, Jonathan (b. 1959), American cognitive social psychologist.
Schröder, Heinrich (1810–85), German biologist and educator.
Schwann, Theodor (1810–82), German anatomist.
Searle, John (b. 1932), American philosopher.
Seashore, Carl Emil (1866–1949), Swedish-born American psychologist.
Sebeok, Thomas Albert (1920–2001), Hungarian-born American linguist.
Sechenov, Ivan Mikhailovich (1829–1905), Russian physiologist.
Seligman, Martin E. P. (b. 1942), American psychologist.
Selye, Hans (1907–82), Austrian-born Canadian endocrinologist and psychologist.
Semon, Richard (1859–1918), German biologist.
Shannon, Claude Elwood (1916–2001), American applied mathematician.
Shaw, George Bernard (1856–1950), Irish playwright and critic.
Sheldon, William H. (1898–1970), American psychologist.
Shepard, Roger Newland (b. 1929), American psychologist.
Sherif, Muzafer (1906–68), Turkish-born American social psychologist.
Sherrington, Charles Scott (1861–1952), English physiologist.
Sidman, Murray (b. 1923), American psychologist.
Simenon, Georges, J. C. (1903–89), Belgian-French novelist.
Simon, Herbert Alexander (1916–2001), American economist, philosopher, psychologist.
Simon, J. Richard (b. 1929), American psychologist.
Simon, Théodore (1873–1961), French psychologist.
Singer, Jerome F. (b. 1924), American psychologist.
Skaggs, Ernest Burton (fl. 1920s–1940s), American psychologist.
*Skinner, Burrhus Frederic (1904–90), American psychologist.
Smirnov, Nikolai Vasilevich (1900–1966), Russian mathematician.
Snellen, Hermann (1834–1908), Dutch ophthalmologist.

Sobel, Michael E. (b. 1950), American social statistician.
Solomon, Richard L. (1918–95), American behavioural psychologist.
Solomon, Sheldon (b. 1953), American social psychologist.
Sotos, Juan F. (b. 1927), Spanish-American endocrinologist
Spearman, Charles Edward (1863–1945), English psychologist and psychometrician.
Spence, Janet Taylor (b. 1923), American psychologist.
Spencer, Herbert (1820–1903), English philosopher.
Spielberger, Charles D. (b. 1927), American psychologist.
Spitz, René A. (1887–1974), Austrian-born American psychologist.
Spooner, William A. (1844–1930), English cleric.
Steele, Richard (1672–1729), English essayist and playwright.
Stern, Wilhelm (1871–1938), German psychologist.
Sternberg, Robert J. (b. 1949), American psychologist.
Stevens, Stanley Smith (1906–73), American psychologist, psychophysicist.
Stilling, Jakob (1842–1915), German ophthalmologist.
Stratton, George Malcolm (1865–1957), American psychologist.
Strong, Edward Kellogg, Jr (1884–1963), American psychologist.
Stroop, John Ridley (1897–1973), American psychologist.
Student, *see* Gosset, William S.
Sullivan, Harry Stack (1892–1949), American psychiatrist.
Sutton, Willie (1901–80), American bank robber.
Sydenham, Thomas (1624–89), English physician.
Sylvius, Franciscus (1614–72), Dutch anatomist.
Szasz, Thomas Stephen (b. 1920), Hungarian-born American psychiatrist.
Talbot, William Henry Fox (1800–1877), English physicist and photographer.
Tannen, Deborah Frances (b. 1945), American linguist.
Tarasoff, Tatiana (*c.* 1950–69), American college student.
Tarchanoff, Ivan Romanovich (1846–1908), Russian physiologist.
Tartini, Giuseppe (1692–1770), Italian violinist.
Tay, Warren (1843–1927), American physician.
Terman, Lewis Madison (1877–1956), American psychologist and psychometrician.
Teuber, Hans L. (1916–77), German/American physiological psychologist.
Theodorson, Achilles G. (*fl.* 1950s–1960s), American sociologist and lexicographer.
Theodorson, George A. (*fl.* 1950s–1960s), American sociologist and lexicographer.
Thorndike, Edward Lee (1874–1949), American psychologist and lexicographer.
Thorpe, William Homan (1902–86), English ethologist.
Thurstone, Louis Leon (1887–1955), American psychologist and psychometrician.
Tinbergen, Nikolaas (1907–88), Dutch ethologist.
Titchener, Edward Bradford (1867–1927), English-born American psychologist.
Toffler, Alvin (b. 1928), American writer, social commentator.
Tomatis, Alfred (1920–2001), French physician.
*Tolman, Edward Chace (1886–1959), American psychologist.
Torrance, Ellis Paul (1915–2003), American psychologist.
Tourette, Georges Gilles de la (1857–1904), French psychiatrist.
Treacher Collins, Edward (1862–1932), British neurologist.
Trivers, Robert (b. 1943), American evolutionary biologist.
Troland, Leonard Thompson (1889–1932), American psychologist.
Troxler, Ignaz Paul Vital (1780–1866), Swiss physician and philosopher.
Tukey, John Wilder (1915–2000), American statistician.
Tulving, Endel (b. 1927), Estonian-Canadian cognitive psychologist.
Turing, Alan Mathison (1912–54), English mathematician, philosopher, computer scientist.
Turner, Henry Herbert (1892–1970), American endocrinologist.

Tversky, Amos (1937–96), Israeli-American cognitive psychologist.
Twitmeyer, Edwin B. (1873–1943), American psychologist.
Urban, Frank M. (*fl.* 1910s–1920s), American(?) psychologist.
Vandenbergh, John G. (b. 1935), American biologist.
Vierordt, Karl (1818–84), German physiologist.
Vygotsky, Lev Semionovich (1896–1934), Russian developmental psychologist.
Wada, Juhn Atsushi (b. 1924), Japanese-Canadian neurosurgeon.
Wade, Marjorie (*fl.* 1940s), American psychologist.
Wagner, Allan (b. 1934), American experimental psychologist.
Wald, Abraham (1902–50), Hungarian-born mathematician.
Wallach, Hans (1904–98), German-born American psychologist.
Waller, August Volney (1816–70), English physiologist.
Wallis, Wilson Allen (1912–88), American economist and statistician.
Walters, Richard (1918–68), Canadian/American psychologist.
Wason, Peter Cathcart (1924–2003), British cognitive psychologist.
*Watson, John Broadus (1878–1958), American behavioural psychologist. ˙
Weber, Ernst Heinrich (1795–1878), German physiologist and psychophysicist.
Wechsler, David (1896–1981), Romanian-born American psychologist.
Wegner, Daniel (b. 1948), American psychologist.
Weigl, Egon (1902–79), German engineer and neuropsychologist.
Weiskrantz, Lawrence (b. 1926), British neuropsychologist.
Werner, Carl Otto (1879–1936), German physician.
Wernicke, Karl (1848–1905), German neurologist.
Wertheimer, Max (1880–1943), Czech-born American psychologist.
Westermarck, Edvard (1862–1939), Finnish anthropologist.
Wever, Ernest Glen (1902–91), American psychologist.
Whitney, Donald Ransom (1915–2001), American mathematician and statistician.
Whitten, Wesley K. (b. 1918), Australian physiologist.
Whorf, Benjamin Lee (1897–1941), American linguist and chemical engineer.
Wiener, Norbert (1894–1964), American mathematician.
Wiesel, Torsten (b. 1924), Swedish-American physiologist.
Wilcoxon, Frank (1892–1965), Irish-born American chemist and statistician.
Willi, Heinrich (1900–1971), Swiss paediatrician.
Williams, J. C. P. (*fl.* 1960), New Zealand physician.
Wilson, Edward O. (b. 1929), American entomologist and sociobiologist.
Wilson, Timothy (b. 1951), American social psychologist.
Wittmaak, Theodor (*fl.* 1860s), German physician.
Wolff, Kaspar Friedrich (1733–94), German anatomist.
Wolfowitz, Jacob (1910–81), Polish-born American statistician.
Wolpe, Joseph (1915–97), South African-born American psychiatrist.
Woodworth, Robert Sessions (1869–1962), American psychologist.
Wulf, F. (*fl.* 1920s), German psychologist.
Wundt, Wilhelm Max (1832–1920), German physiologist, psychologist, philosopher.
Yates, Frank (1902–94), British statistician.
Yerkes, Robert Mearns (1876–1956), American psychologist.
Young, Thomas (1773–1829), English physician and physicist.
Zajonc, Robert (b. 1923), American social psychologist.
Zeigarnik, Bluma (1900–1988), Russian psychologist.
Zener, Karl E. (1903–64), American psychologist.
Zipf, George Kingsley (1903–50), American philologist.
Zöllner, Johann Karl Friedrich (1834–82), German physicist.
Zwaardemaker, Hendrik (1857–1930), Dutch physiologist.